Proceedings of the XIII International Congress of Nutrition

Proceedings of the XIII International Congress of Nutrition

Held under the auspices of the International Union of Nutritional Sciences, Brighton, UK, August 18–23 1985

Editors

T. G. Taylor *Southampton*

N. K. Jenkins *Liverpool*

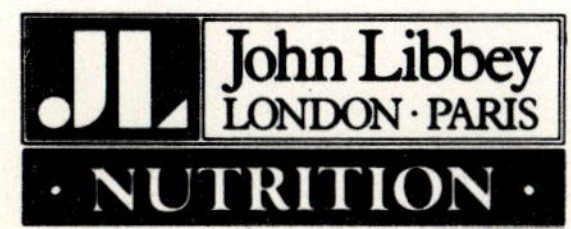

John Libbey
LONDON · PARIS

· NUTRITION ·

British Library Cataloguing in Publication Data
International Congress of Nutrition (*13th*)
   Proceedings of the XIII International
   Congress of Nutrition: under the auspices
   of the International Union of Nutritional
   Sciences
   1. Nutrition
   I. Title   II. Taylor, T. Geoffrey
   III. Jenkins, N. K.   IV. International
   Union of Nutritional Sciences
   613.2   TX353

ISBN 0-86196-066-1

Published by
John Libbey & Company Ltd
80/84 Bondway, London SW8 1SF, England (01) 582 5266
John Libbey Eurotext Ltd
6 rue Blanche, 92120 Montrouge, France (1) 47 35 85 52

Typeset by Activity Ltd, Salisbury, Wilts
Printed in Great Britain by Whitstable Litho Ltd, Whitstable, Kent

Preface

The scientific programme of the XIII International Congress of Nutrition was organized in five distinct categories: *Key-note lectures* on topics of major importance given by world authorities to plenary sessions of the Congress; *Symposia*, which consisted of a series of review papers on broad general subject areas; *Colloquia*, which comprised a number of shorter research papers in specific fields; *Workshops*; which took the form of discussions among small groups of specialists, often on topics not covered in the more formal sessions of the Congress (rather more than half of the workshop organizers submitted reports for publication in the Proceedings); and *Original communications*, all of which were published in the book of abstracts given to delegates at registration. This programme was organized by the Scientific Programmes Committee under the chairmanship of Professor Michael Gurr. The detailed planning of the symposia and colloquia was delegated to sub-committees and the administration of the workshops was undertaken by Dr Marie Coates.

The Congress sought to identify the most pressing problems that face nutritionists today and to give prominence to recent research directed to the solution of these problems. Particular emphasis was given to the problems of developing countries and the longest chapter of the book is devoted to this topic. A further aim was to integrate, where appropriate, research on fundamental aspects of nutrition carried out on farm animals, laboratory animals and on human subjects in the same symposium or colloquium. Other major topics highlighted in the Congress included nutrition education, nutrition and anthropology and the inter-relationships between diet and disease and between nutrition and food science.

Apart from the workshop reports, all of the papers in the book are by invited speakers, and our functions as editors were, therefore, somewhat limited: in conducting the scientific editing our main roles were to check with authors any points that appeared to us to be obscure or erroneous and to condense those papers that exceeded the space allocated. Our major regrets are that we were forced by economic considerations to abandon the Harvard system of references originally adopted and that a number of invited speakers failed to submit their manuscripts for publication.

After editing the typescripts, we grouped them into a logical series of chapters. The sequence of these chapters do not bear any relationship to the order in which the components were presented at the Congress and key-note lectures, symposia and colloquia papers and workshop reports are brought together in relation to their subject matter. However, the table on pages viii to x includes each category of the scientific programme in numerical order to help the reader locate any particular part of the original programme.

T. G. Taylor
N. K. Jenkins
July 1986

Contents

THE SCIENTIFIC PROGRAMME

Lectures and Key-note papers

Symposia

Colloquia

*Also VI (359) and X (532).

Workshops

Other numbers — no workshop report received

†Also VI (357)

I: Global issues

Food and people

Sir Kenneth BLAXTER
President, XIIIth International Congress of Nutrition, The Royal Society, 6 Carlton House Terrace, London SW1, UK.

We have gathered, some from close at hand, others from the far reaches of the earth, to discuss and advance the subject we all profess — Nutrition. Our programme in the ensuing days rightly emphasises the scientific dimensions of our subject for it is only through the application of advances in the physical and biological sciences, by the adoption of new approaches engendered through scientific discovery, that advances come. Yet, beyond the reductionism that such activities imply stretch the immensity and reality of the world, that is the immense and real problems of securing a nutritional adequacy for the world's peoples, now and in future.

It is on these wider issues that I wish to dwell. The problems are not new; they have plagued man for millennia. They have been subject to able comment and conjecture in times past and warnings and exhortations, not all of which have been heeded. My reasons for discussing the relation between people and their food supply are firstly that this has always been, and will for ever be, the greatest issue that has faced mankind, and secondly because it illustrates the integrative nature of nutritional studies. After all, nutrition is best defined as the relations between an organism and the substrate of food on which it depends, a definition which provides a unity of purpose between those concerned with physiological and biochemical detail and those whose endeavours embrace the generality of nutritional policy formulation.

The age-old problem. We can commence with what has been called 'the dismal theorem', namely the ideas promoted by Thomas Robert Malthus almost 200 years ago when he was a curate at Albury, a village about 25 miles from us here in Brighton. Malthus proclaimed 'I say that the power of population is indefinitely greater than the power in the earth to produce subsistence for man. Population, when unchecked, increases in a geometrical ratio. Subsistence increases only in an arithmetical ratio'. Malthus identified the checks to population as preventive and positive ones and their sum resulted in nothing other than 'misery and vice' for mankind. William Hazlitt, the essayist, took matters further by propounding 'the utterly dismal theorem' as a corollary to Malthus' proposition, namely that the sum total of vice and misery in the world would increase since population would expand to use all available resources for its subsistence.

World population 200 years ago when Malthus wrote was about 800 million and was growing at the rate of 0.25 per cent/annum, implying a doubling every 300 years. Now world population is in excess of 4400 million with a growth rate of 1.7 per cent, implying, were the underlying mortalities and fertilities to continue, that population would double in 41 years. In the 200 year period world population has increased five-fold; the supply of food must equally have increased five-fold, for the population has been sufficiently nourished to reproduce. Taking the world as a whole and neglecting the incidence of local and periodic famine, the dire consequences of Malthus' algebra are not in evidence. The question which arises is whether the production of food can continue to keep pace with population growth and whether we can continue to regard Malthus' inexorable logic as a tale to frighten the children of the world. This entails assessing likely future numbers of people, their demand for food and the potential food production that the world can achieve. Each of these entities is associated with uncertainty, yet to assess the magnitude of future problems we must make such estimates.

The numbers of people. Demography is not an exact science in the sense that it can make long-term predictions. Given sets of parameters of age-related fertility and age-related mortality, it can predict outcomes were these parameters constant over long periods of time. They have not been in the past and cannot be assumed to be so in future. Thus one can make predictions based on the assumption that the present crude rate of increase will continue. Then world population in 50 years time will be almost three times the present one. Alternatively one can assume that family planning results immediately and tomorrow in a net reproduction rate of 1.0. Then in 50 years time population will have increased by about 60 per cent. The latter increase arises from the enormous momentum that present surges in population have achieved in the less well developed countries of the world. Likely future population lies somewhere between these extremes.

Current thinking by the World Bank is that countries in the developing world which have populations growing at rates of over 3 per cent/annum and fertility rates of over five children per completed family, will achieve zero growth rates and net reproduction rates of 1.0 by the year 2030 or 2040. The major assumption is that these countries will follow the pattern of many Western ones, that demographic transition will occur and the fall in mortality which has led to increased life spans and to population growth, will inevitably be followed by falls in birth rate. A second assumption is that this transition will be completed in the next 50 years. Such assumptions are declarations of hope rather than precise predictions. Nevertheless they are probably reasonable bases for planning. They imply that the equilibrium population of the world will be about 11 000 million people achieved in about a century from now. More important, these estimates suggest that in the year 2000 world population will be 6100 millions, about a third more than its present one and only marginally less than that predicted from straightforward extrapolation of current rates of natural increase.

Nutritional needs. Were there to be no improvement in the diets of the world's peoples, then the demand placed on food provision would simply be that implied by projected population growth. I do not need to remind an audience of nutritionists of the inadequacies of food supplies in many areas of the world in terms of meeting basic requirements for energy and protein and of combatting known and preventable nutritional disease. In the African sub-continent as a whole, food supplies per capita have declined as population has augmented. Africa is not an isolated example; 58 of the world's 124 countries as listed by the World Bank are producing less food per head of their populations than they were 10 years ago. An increase in food production above that dictated by population growth is necessary in these countries simply to restore a former and inadequate nutritional status. What is a desirable level of food production per head of the population is a matter for debate. Lack of knowledge is in part responsible. Thus the low metabolic rate of peoples in the Indian subcontinent, their small stature and their low physical activity costs suggest that their energy requirements are much smaller than those of Europeans. It can be argued, however, that the low requirement represents homoeorhesis operating over generations. What is however evident from many surveys is that people demand better quality diets than those to which they have been habituated, better in the sense of more varied, nutritionally more adequate, more secure over time and more adequate in amount. It is usual to express this demand in economic terms, to make aspirations for food appear dependent on the purchasing power of the population. This may be the reality; it should not be the basis of planning. I see no reason why the food needs of everyone should not be assessed as those achieved in the affluent countries of the well developed world. If this is so, then the food needs of the average person in the world are a third higher than the amounts currently consumed.

If world population is to increase by a third in the next 15 years and a target is set to improve dietary intakes by a third, then food production must be increased by three-quarters before the turn of the century. Projecting even further ahead, if equilibrium population is indeed likely to be 11 000 million, then to support this number, food production must be increased by a factor of 3.3 in 75 years — in the life span of a man. Is this feasible?

Food production. The annual production of food depends on the area of land which can be cropped and the yield of human food obtained each year from unit area. In the past 200 years, population growth has been enabled firstly by increasing the land available and latterly by increasing yield per hectare. In the 30 year period from 1881 to 1910 Europe unloaded a fifth of her increase in population to fill the new lands of North America and Australasia and in the subsequent 30 years a further 15 per cent of Europe's increase was similarly disposed. Directly or indirectly these emigrants increased the area under cultivation.

The increase in food output in the last 50 years which has accompanied the massive increase in world population, has largely been due to an increase in crop yield. This has arisen from what can be called the industrialization of agriculture and the supplementation of farm resources by those derived from conventional industry. Such inputs include mechanical power, artificial fertilizers and agrochemicals for pest, disease and weed control, and the process has been taken far further in the highly developed economies of the world than in the developing countries. All these inputs involve the expenditure of fuel — to make tractors and to fuel them, to synthesise ammonia from the nitrogen of the air, to extract phosphatic and potassic ores for processing, to make herbicides and pesticides and to transport these industrial products long distances to the farm. The source of this energy has largely been the fossil fuel resources of the world. For example it takes 2 kg oil to manufacture 1 kg of nitrogen in a fertilizer. This massive change in the nature of food production, in which energy derived from past eras of photosynthesis has been used to augment current photosynthesis, continues and is increasingly being adopted to increase food production in the countries of the developing world. China, for example now uses more nitrogenous fertilizer than the whole of Western Europe.

Parallel to the industrialization of production of food commodities has been the industrialization of the whole food provision system, including secondary processing and distribution. As urbanization has proceeded — and in the developing countries population growth in urban areas far exceeds that in rural ones — so the energy dependence of the food provision system has grown. In the industrialized countries for every calorie of food consumed more than 10 calories of support energy are now expended to provide that food. This seems a profligate use of an essential resource.

The discernible limits to food production. Quite apart from the immediate problem of increasing food production by 75 per cent by the end of the century, there is the question of what are the limits to food production in the longer term. The determinants of the ultimate carrying capacity of the world are the area that can be cropped and the yield per unit area. During the last 10 years the area cropped in the developed countries has fallen but that in the developing ones has increased by 30 million hectares on a base of 680 million. The latter has been at the expense of grazing land and forests. The decline in the area of grassland and forest has been much greater than the increase in cropped land — almost 80 million hectares — and in addition a further 45 million hectares has been added to the land area which is no longer biologically productive. This land is now desert and urban or industrial land. The pattern of the last few decades is for farming to be carried out on poorer and poorer land, for most of the urbanization that is taking place occurs around old settlements where our forefathers wisely built to take advantage of the best quality of soil. Any new land brought into cultivation is poorer in terms of intrinsic fertility. Calculations made by Dutch soil scientists show that by the year 2000 the world area of highly productive land will have fallen by 22 per cent and the area used for non-agricultural purposes will have risen by 50 per cent. Clearly there is no massive reserve of land for agricultural use. In the long term the area at present cropped might be doubled but this would entail cropping inferior land and eroding forests and natural grasslands to a massive, and, in view of demands for timber and fuel wood, unacceptable extent.

Seventy per cent of the output from cropping consists of cereals and well over 50 per cent of man's diet consists of these grains consumed directly. The average yields obtained in the world as a whole amount to about 2 tonnes per hectare. There is much variation from area to area in yield; in the instance of wheat, the Netherlands obtained an average yield of 7 tonnes per hectare while in many areas marginal for the crop, average yields are less than 0.5 tonnes per hectare. There would seem to be clear scope for increasing mean output of wheat per unit area and this is true of other crops. There are, however, considerable problems in doing so. First, and as already indicated, soils vary and only about 15 per cent of the world's land is of the high quality of the Netherlands. Secondly much of present cropped land is limited in its productivity by lack of water. In the world as a whole, the water requirement of all crops amounts to 5.6 kg for every gram of dry matter produced. Under optimal conditions of water supply, and even under semi-arid conditions, this amount could be reduced by an order of magnitude. However, the efficiency of irrigated systems of farming, on which two thirds of the world population depends for its food, is incredibly low and over-use of water is rife. Over-use of water leads to salination and loss of productive land. The irrigated area of the world could be increased and crop yields augmented, but unless improved methods of water control, as exemplified by those in use in Israel and in central Chile, are adopted, greater irrigation could lead to little increase in average yield through losses by salination. Thirdly high yields imply high inputs of fertilizers. The production of every tonne of wheat, for example, entails the provision of 25 kg of nitrogen and the high yields obtained in temperate agriculture only come about by providing this nitrogen artificially. Other crop nutrients have also to be provided and the overall requirement for fertilizers to increase yield are immense. We have already noted that the provision of fertilizer is at present mainly dependent on the use of oil and natural gas as an energy source. Thus to increase yield implies a further erosion of world stocks of these fossil energy sources — unless some alternative and safe source of energy can be developed. Lastly, to increase yield in many areas implies a departure from traditional methods — an increase in scale of operation, a replacement of man and animal power by that of machines and the provision of an infrastructure for disposal of the crop commodities to provide food.

These problems and difficulties can be overcome, despite their magnitude, and the production of food increased. The necessary technologies could be developed and applied given the will and purpose. The process is not one without limits which can go on for ever, for the physics and chemistry of the photosynthetic process sets bounds and limits the extent to which yield can be increased in any given environment. It is pertinent to enquire what these limits might be.

For any given location one can compute from knowledge of the incoming solar radiation and of the steps in photosynthesis and the biogenesis of the organic molecules on which we depend, the yield of human food which could be achieved in the absence of constraints due to lack of water, lack of soil nutrients and presence of pests and diseases. This has been done for many crops and areas and the remarkable point arises that the world record yields are about 90 per cent of these maxima. Thus for wheat in the UK maximal theoretical yield is 16.5 tonnes per hectare; the world record yield held by a Mr Rennie in Scotland is 14 tonnes per hectare. As far as whole countries are concerned, the mean yields obtained at present by the most successful ones are about 40–50 per cent of those obtained by world record holders. In 1983, for example, the People's Republic of Korea had average yields of rice per hectare of 6.3 tonnes, about 45 per cent of the world record, while Israel produced a country-wide average yield of 44 tonnes of potatoes per hectare, 46 per cent of the world record yield. In other words several countries have already achieved average yields over the whole of their farmed areas which are close to half those which are physically possible. One can immediately ask whether these limits set by theory or by record holders are immutable. There is every reason to believe that they are not likely to be overtaken in the foreseeable future since they are set by the thermodynamics of energy transduction within the green leaf. Any advances in the limit to yield will have to come through changes in the biochemical processes of energy capture — an incredibly difficult task to accomplish if indeed it can be accomplished at all.

The carrying capacity of the world. These considerations all show that there are real and somewhat immediate limits to the ability of the earth to produce food. Taking realistic estimates of the land area that could be cropped and the yields likely to be obtained, the carrying capacity of the world in terms of people is probably about 7–8 thousand millions, that is not quite double our present population. This assumes, as I have already done, that diets for everyone are varied and adequate. Seven to eight thousand million people supported at a nutritional level similar to that realised in the more affluent countries is admittedly more than the six thousand million we will have to support in the year 2000 — 15 years ahead. It is however less than the numbers who will need to be supported a lifetime from now, on the assumption that all countries reach net reproductive rates of 1.0 within a few decades.

These considerations show that there are real, and immediate, limits to the capacity of the world to provide food for man and this limit is not too distant when the current rate of population increase and the effects of its momentum are considered. There can be no equivocation about this conclusion. Given the premises which I have outlined, taking into account the uncertainties and without exaggerating the limitations placed on food production, there is little doubt that we are approaching the limit of the earth's bounty in producing sustenance for man. The problem of people and the limits placed on them by their food supply is a future problem it is true, just as much as it was when Malthus propounded the dismal theorem two centuries ago. Then Malthus did not foresee the increase in land available through colonization of the Americas, Australasia and Africa or the scientific and technological advances that would lead to yield increases. Now we may not be able to see the future possibilities which would again make Malthus' argument apparently untenable.

The nutritional problems of the world. What an appalling set of dilemmas face mankind! If we all wish to live to a ripe old age then we must curtail our reproduction. If we wish to increase food production — even in the short term — then either we have to make inroads into reserves of forest and natural grasslands or embark on techniques of farming which are highly dependent on fossil sources of energy. If we wish to increase nutritional standards in developing countries then the methods available to us to increase output from slender land resources entails an erosion of traditional cultures. If we all wish to live in cities, then the provision of our food becomes more expensive in terms of finite resources, while in the enlargement of our urban settlements we will further reduce the amount of highly fertile land available to us.

These dilemmas are moral and social ones with which to tax the collective wisdom of mankind. They do however have a scientific dimension. It was Engels in 1844, in the year before he met Marx in Paris, who put the matter most succinctly when he too commented on Malthus' dreadful theorem. He wrote 'has it been proved that the productivity of land increases in an arithmetical progression? The extent of land is limited — that is perfectly true. But the labour power to be employed on this area increases along with population; and even if we assume that the increase in yield does not always rise in proportion to the labour, there remains a third element — namely science, the progress of which is just as unceasing and at least as rapid as that of populations. But science increases at least as fast as population. Science advances in proportion to the knowledge bequeathed to it by previous generations, and thus under the most ordinary conditions it also grows in geometrical progression — and what is impossible for science?'

The deliberations in this Congress about needs for nutrients, about the provision, availability and nutritional adequacy of food, about the metabolic consequences of nutrient deficiency and excess, about the environmental stresses that modify man's requirements, about the interaction of nutritional status with infective and non-infective disease and about the roles of different cultures on food habits and beliefs, are all part of this vast scientific progression. Many of the new findings will pose newer problems in their turn and our knowledge and understanding will grow, slowly perhaps, but inevitably and inexorably. Such is the breadth of nutritional study that we who are concerned with it are always aware of the wider problems of the world about which I have talked to you and the part that our own investigations play in contributing to the whole. It is from this vast accumulation of knowledge, in which we all play a part, and from its integration, that new hope for the world will arise to refute once more the proposition with which Malthus has troubled the conscience of the world.

The politics of food

The Rt. Hon. Edward HEATH
House of Commons, London SW1, UK.

Individualists have a major part to play in our society but they are not always welcomed with open arms by those responsible for organizations, by those responsible for bureaucracies and particularly by politicans. Politicians regard them as a complete nuisance, who should be got rid of if possible, but if not they should be put somewhere where most people cannot hear them and you just listen to whàt they have to say privately.

Lord Boyd-Orr was not prepared to accept that, and so he put his views as an individualist very forcibly and they were the views of an internationalist who believed that our problems world-wide could only be coped with by appropriate international organizations. It was characteristic of him that he accepted gladly the position of first Director of the Food and Agriculture Organization in 1945 and then, when he found the bureaucracy to his distaste, he resigned from it a year later. But the impact had been made and he made it clear throughout his life, in this country and throughout the world, that we could only solve our problems internationally.

We in the Brandt Commission would like to think that perhaps, 30 years later, we had also set in action a train of thought which would achieve results, most of which he wanted, but which had not followed from his own efforts. And this we did at a very important time in history. The Brandt Commission began to meet in 1977; we issued our first report in 1980: and our second report in January 1983. Both of those reports were very comprehensive about the problems of the relations between the developed countries and the developing world. We did not pretend to be omniscient and tell everybody what they knew in their own specialist field. We recognised our own limitations, but we did try to set out the main objectives for the rest of this century. In this decade all the international organizations created after the Second World War have been under direct challenge by those who do not share Lord Boyd-Orr's belief in international action.

We saw in the middle of the 70s the breakdown of the IMF, we have seen the World Bank limited in its activities during these past few years: we have seen the General Agreement on Tariffs and Trade under very great pressure from the protectionists on both sides of the Atlantic. Now why is this? The reason is that in the middle of the 70s the pressures that had grown up were too great for these international institutions to sustain. This was particularly the case in the world of international finance. Our predecessors after the Second World War wanted to create stability throughout the world financial system to enable business to flourish and prosper and the standard of living to be improved. And so they established the system and the machinery with which to deal with it. Similarly with the World Bank they wanted to see the difference between rich and poor diminished and for that purpose they created the Bank and gave it the resources that were required. And the General Agreement on Tariffs and Trade was to prevent the growth of protectionism which would impede the increase in world trade which was necessary to provide the improved standard of living. But then, in the middle of the 70s, the international financial system was subject, first of all, to the shock of the gold dollar standard being abandoned because of the burden on the USA of the Vietnam War, which meant that the world was covered with Eurodollars and other forms of dollars which prevented the system from working.

Then we were affected in 1973/4 and again in 1979/80 by the two enormous increases in world oil prices, which drained off a large part of the resources of the developed world. The developing countries at that time had no plans as to how to use them; it had all occurred so suddenly, and, as a result, unemployment spread rapidly in the developed countries. That unemployment made it more difficult psychologically for countries to carry out their international obligations.

Thirdly, as a result of these two things, at the beginning of the 80s we had an enormous increase in interest rates and that too, apart from creating additional unemployment in the developed world, put an enormous burden on the developing countries themselves. As a result of all these events we had not only a recession but also a depression, massive world unemployment and the developing world particularly effected by very high interest rates and the fall in demand for their commodities.

And so we reach our present position in which the International organizations have broken down. But more than that there is a change of psychology on both sides of the Atlantic which far from ignoring we must endeavour to change. The psychology can best be summed up in the phrase 'in difficult times we must first put our own house in order'. And when we have done that we can look out of the window and see if anything else needs doing outside.

That is a fatal approach from both points of view, internal and external. No country today in this modern world is capable of putting its own house in order, not even the USA itself and certainly not the other super power, the Soviet Union. And therefore it is entirely fallacious to say we must put our own house in order and then go to the rest of the world. We can only put our own house in order if we do it jointly with the rest of the world and that is the fundamental lesson which many generations have to learn and which we now have to bring home to them because they have forgotten the lessons of the aftermath of the Second World War. That is the first thing. And the second thing is to recognize that there are those who are opposed to any international effort of any kind. And these are the ones who have set out to destroy international organizations. You, the IUNS, are an international organization of great strength and you can resist all that. But the formalized international organizations have already been attacked. The first was the International Labour Office, by President Carter in the United States at the end of the 70s because they did not do everything that he wanted. But after two years the USA had to return; it could not afford to be outside the International Labour Office.

Now we see the attack on UNESCO by those who do not believe in an international culture or in each other helping to preserve other cultures which we believe to be of importance. It is always possible to find fault with an International Organization. We hear it constantly about the EEC in Brussels. When I point out to my constituents that the size of the bureaucracy in Brussels, running a community consisting of 320 million people, is smaller than the size of the bureaucracy in Edinburgh responsible for running Scotland with 5½ million people they show some surprise. UNESCO has its faults: some of its administration may be bad, some of its objectives may be intolerant. But that is all the more reason for those of us who believe in its primary aims to continue as members, and to ensure that as far as we can that UNESCO and other International Organizations follow the path appropriate to their activity.

Now let me turn to the Brandt Report, the Brandt Commission and what we ourselves consider to be the approach for the rest of this century. I first became interested in these matters when I led the British delegation to the first United Nations Conference on Trade, Aid and Development which then became known as UNTAD and exists today with its conferences every four years. It is well known that we British played a major part in creating UNTAD and I am glad to say that in the developing world we have received credit for it.

As a result of stratification, the developing countries saw that they could only achieve something by always taking up exactly the same position. Looking at it as impartially as I can, I believe that that was a mistake because it played into the hands of the enemies who did not want to help. And for this reason. They can say perfectly well 'Look at the difference now between the various developing countries as well as between the developed ones. You have the difference between the living standards of the United States and those of southern Italy. But in the developing countries you have the difference between the giants of Mexico, Brazil, Argentina, Nigeria and the smaller ones like Malaysia and Yugoslavia and you have the city-island states of Singapore, Hong Kong and Taiwan. Why should we apply exactly the same criteria to all those states which have such different conditions?'

We have to find a basis for our actions. There are those who say it should be Christianity and its obligations to our families, schools, universities, trade unions, employers, regiments. Others think it should be idealism, because it is such a strong factor among the young. The third basis is mutual interest. What we have to do is to show that there is a mutual interest in every proposal we put forward between the developed and developing countries. If we can do that we have a chance of mustering public opinion in order to achieve the results we want.

We recognise then the breadth of the problems, and in particular the basic one. We have sometimes been accused of ignoring these basic problems but that is not the case. The basic problem is one of food, health and housing; it is the problem of education and we only have to look at the figures to recognise how acute these problems are. And of course, water: and it is sometimes overlooked that this is the water decade of the United Nations which has promised that by 1990 every village in the world will have clean water. We are half-way through the decade but we are nowhere near half-way towards providing clean water. These basic needs all contribute towards the basic needs of the populace and another aspect is that we are seeing throughout the developing world a growth in the great cities, whether it is in Africa, India, or in Latin America. They are growing to disproportionate sizes because the basic things of life are not provided outside the cities. If people are not to be attracted into Bombay, Rio, Mexico City or any of the other great and fast growing cities that exist in the world the basic amenities of life must be provided for the rural communities.

Having then looked at the basic questions we come to the question of what are the major structural problems in this relationship between the developed and the developing countries. Immediately we come to a whole series of questions.

First there is the question of protectionism: you sold us the machinery, now you keep out our goods. Comparing it with the 30s, the extent to which protectionism has been resisted is remarkable. But at a time of mass unemployment in the developed countries, nearly 14 per cent in this country, it is very difficult to persuade people that they should lose their jobs in order that we can import materials from other countries, be they developed or developing.

And then there is the problem of maintaining a stable price for commodities. We have seen the burden of doing this in the EEC, first the cost of storage and secondly the expenditure on buying the goods from the farmers. To do this on a world-wide scale seems to most of us not a practical reality. The only way it can be dealt with is by an expansion of the world economy as a whole. When we create that through the changes in the world monetary system then we shall find the demand for all the commodities and the restoration of a better standard of living to the developing countries themselves. This means dealing with the problem of indebtedness and interest payments which afflicts the developing world to such a large extent. The developing countries were not responsible for the increase in oil prices; they were not responsible for the very high interest rates: they did not know there was going to be a world depression in which their income from commodities would fall to the lowest level since 1931. There is nothing to be gained by trying to blame the developing world.

Our primary aim must be to enable the developing world to have the resources with which to improve its situation. These resources include both technical and financial ones and they particularly affect agriculture. But again there is the problem of technology and how we are able to help with that.

The final factor is one of timing. Boyd-Orr became exasperated by the time it takes to get things done. We likewise. We have put forward specific proposals for dealing with the debt and interest rates. This was in 1980 and only now, 5 years later, have the developed countries seriously tackled the scale of the problems. A 1 per cent rise in interest rates means $3.5 billion more to be paid by the developing world. The only answer is a long-term reconstruction of the whole of this debt, and by long term I mean 15–20 years.

Let me remind you now how the Marshall Plan came into existence. General Marshall had an opportunity when he was awarded an Honorary Degree at Harvard and the Press Officer said to his secretary 'what's he going to say?'. The secretary replied 'I don't know: he is up in his bedroom writing it with his pencil'. When he made that speech, which was quite short, it contained one simple sentence — 'We Americans will pay for the re-creation of the European economy'. Afterwards it was learned that he had not told President Truman or anybody in the State Department or anybody in Congress, but he was backed by President Truman and the whole administration. Six weeks later they created the Organization for European Co-Operation which exists today as a major International Organization. Directly after that Congress voted $4 billion ($20 billion today) and at the end of the year another $15 billion ($120 billion today). That was the speed with which they worked in order to deal with an international problem and it was Governments who did it.

Those are the qualities which we need today to deal with the problems between the developed and the developing countries. The vision to see what is required: the imagination to create the means of dealing with it: the determination to see it through; in other words the political will to bring about the ends which we can all recognise as necessary.

The effect of development programmes on the nutrition of populations

C. GOPALAN
President, The Nutrition Foundation of India, B-37, Gulmohar Park, New Delhi-110049, India

Most developing countries of the world today face major problems of undernutrition among their people. One would normally expect that the several developmental programmes being now undertaken in these countries will overcome these problems and bring about rapid improvement in the nutritional status of their populations. But this expectation is not often borne out by actual experience. Nutritional improvement induced by 'development' in many of these countries, far from being rapid, is in fact proving to be painfully slow and difficult. Three major reasons for this can be identified.

First, the earliest and most tangible result of development in these countries has been a steep decline in death rates resulting in rapid growth of their populations. This had occurred long before 'development' had made any significant dent on their massive problem of poverty and undernutrition. The tremendous population growth thus unleashed by 'development' has been progressively magnifying the total quantum of their nutrition problem and increasingly straining their fragile economies, public services and institutions to the point when solution of that problem is becoming more difficult and further development itself is being slowed down. Secondly, these countries generally lack the material and manpower resources necessary to address *all* dimensions of their underdevelopment adequately and simultaneously. As a result, their total developmental effort has suffered from many inadequacies and imbalances. Nutritional improvement is hardly ever addressed as the direct objective of the planning process in these countries. It is overall economic growth that is perceived as the national goal, and nutritional improvement is expected to follow as a spin-off effect. This, however, does not always happen. Thirdly, some of the powerful modern technologies being currently used in these countries themselves generate side-effects which tend to aggravate the nutrition problem and developing countries often do not have the means to contain and control these side-effects.

Each of these aspects will now be considered in some detail.

Impact of demographic changes induced by development. For historical and other reasons, developing countries today are in no position to follow the same orderly developmental paths which the fortunate developed countries had earlier pursued so successfully (Fig. 1). Declines in death rates in Europe were achieved through better standards of living brought about by socio-economic development and progressive elimination of poverty and undernutrition and not so much as a result of health technology which had not then reached its present level of efficacy and sophistication. These declines were never as steep and precipitous as those now being witnessed in developing countries. At no time in all its developmental phase did the annual rate of population growth in Europe exceed 1.5 per cent. Socio-economic development did bring about a nearly three-fold increase in Europe's population; but this was spread

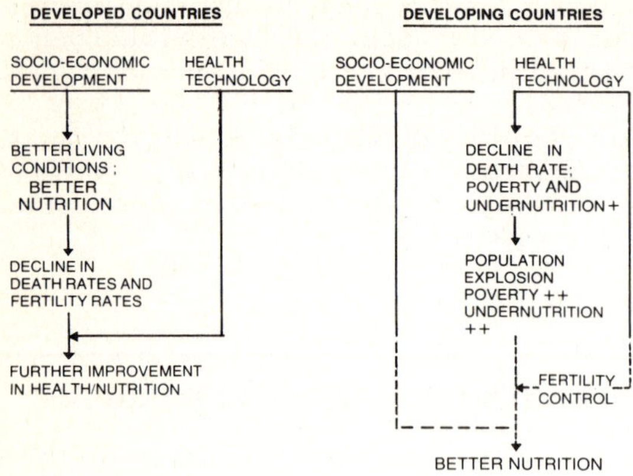

Fig. 1. *Contrasting developmental patterns.* See previous page.

over nearly 150 years, during which there was more than a four-fold increase in economic production. Emigration to colonies and empires outside Europe took care of nearly 20 per cent of the annual population growth. Demographic transition induced by development in Europe, therefore, far from hindering further development actually helped to stimulate it. The story, as far as developing countries today are concerned, is totally different.

Developing countries today have achieved their decline in death rates, and more recently are trying to achieve declines in fertility rates largely through vigorous application of health technology even in the face of continuing underdevelopment and poverty. This is a difference of crucial importance.

Population explosion. With the use of health technology, declines in death rates in developing countries have set in much earlier and faster than declines in birth rates. Since, unlike in developed countries, such declines have *preceded* socio-economic development, the resulting tremendous population explosion has not been associated with concurrent improvement in nutritional status. The absolute numbers of poverty-stricken and undernourished people in developing countries has, therefore, increased enormously during the last three decades. Of the 80 million people added to the world's population in 1984, 73 million belonged to the developing countries where 75 per cent of the world's population live.

As a result, a considerable part of the scarce resources of developing countries is now being used up to meet the needs of the *annual additions* to their populations and in expensive fertility control measures to limit population growth. Many countries have thus to struggle hard even to remain where they are in the developmental scale, and have, therefore, been unable to achieve substantial improvements in the nutritional status of their populations. It is a cruel irony that a good part of the scarce resources of developing countries is being used, not so much for development, which they sorely need, as for grappling with an intermediate by-product of the developmental process itself.

Thus is has been computed that just to take care of the annual addition to her population and to maintain status quo in the developmental scale, India has to produce *additionally* every year nearly 1.5 million tonnes of foodgrains, 220 million metres of cloth, 3 million houses, 15 000 new schools and 500 000 teachers and generate 5 million jobs over and above the previous year.

Better child-survival without better child nutrition. Steep declines in death rates without a concurrent dent in poverty are also responsible for the aberration being increasingly witnessed in some developing countries, namely better child survival without better child nutrition. Till very recently, declines in death rates in developing countries were largely accounted for by a reduction in adult death. Child mortality was still very high. Death-control strategies of health technology are now being specifically targeted to the under-fives in many developing countries. Better child-survival, though not better child-nutrition, can be achieved by strategies which are currently within the competence and resources of many developing countries. Through 'crisis-management' techniques like oral rehydration, timely treatment of major illnesses and nutritional intervention measures targeted to children in extremis — the so-called grade-three malnutrition — child mortality is now being substantially reduced in many developing countries even in the presence of dire poverty and undernutrition.

On the other hand, child nutrition calls for sustained inputs of a more exacting kind which developing countries are, as yet, often unable to provide. For this reason, vigorous death-control measures have not always gone hand in hand with equally vigorous measures aimed at eradication of poverty and under-nutrition. The result is that many developing countries are moving into the stage wherein child mortality is being substantially reduced with no corresponding dent in the problem of child nutrition. In short, better child-survival is being achieved without better child nutrition[4,10,14]. In India, the clear superiority of the State of Kerala with respect to 'child survival' in comparison to other States has not been matched with similar superiority with respect to child nutrition (Table 1).

Table 1. *Child survival and child nutrition.*

State	Death rate* (0–4 years)	'Moderate' and severe undernutrition in underfives**	
Kerala	12.6	38.3%	*SRS Registrar General of India, 1980
Karnataka	30.4	47.1%	**NNMB data (1975–79)
Uttar Pradesh	64.5	32.9%	
Madhya Pradesh	61.0	51.7%	

The object of development is not just to ensure that children *exist* but that they live full and healthy lives. This transitional phase of development which helps to increase the pool of substandard survivors will certainly not contribute to the improvement of the quality of human resources of any country and must therefore be traversed most expeditiously. This is not an argument against child survival measures; it is an argument against stopping short with such measures.

Distortions in development arising from inadequate resources. Development has two major dimensions, economic and social. Economic development which results in eradication of poverty and in raising income levels helps to provide individuals and families with better access to those services and facilities which are essential requisites for improved nutrition, namely food, health, a good environment including a safe water supply and family planning. Social development, of which the level of education (especially female education) is the hallmark, helps them to optimally utilise, and derive maximal benefit from, such essential services, to the extent that they may be available to them (Fig. 2). It should be the objective of the developmental process to provide the inputs needed for both economic and social development of the people. Unfortunately, however, in view of acute scarcity of resources, most developing countries are unable to provide all these inputs adequately and simultaneously, leading to inevitable distortions and imbalances in the transitional stages of development.

Several examples of situations which developing countries face as a result of these inadequacies and imbalances in their developmental process can be cited.

Inadequacies with respect to all dimensions of development, eg countries of the Sub-Sahara, ie the least developed countries. There are some unfortunate countries of the world which suffer from resource constraints of an order that prevents them from addressing *any* dimension of their underdevelopment adequately. These countries suffer from all-round underdevelopment — agricultural, industrial, social and economic. These countries face the persistent threat of acute food shortage, mass starvation and famine.

They have suffered over the years irreversible devastation of their agricultural system — large-scale loss of livestock and extensive denudation of forests (4 per cent of the national terrain in Ethiopia is now forest land as against 44 per cent at the beginning of the century). It has been estimated in a recent FAO study ('Land, food and people') that even with the best farming methods these countries cannot produce the food they need; also in view of their poor economic and industrial development they cannot import the food they require. From the nutritional point of view, these countries must be considered as most vulnerable.

Adequate food production at the national level with inequitable distribution at the household levels, eg India and China. Fortunately, most developing countries of Asia and Latin America now generally do not suffer from acute food shortage, and are no longer plagued with recurrent bouts of large-scale famines which used to afflict them earlier. However, many of these countries are still

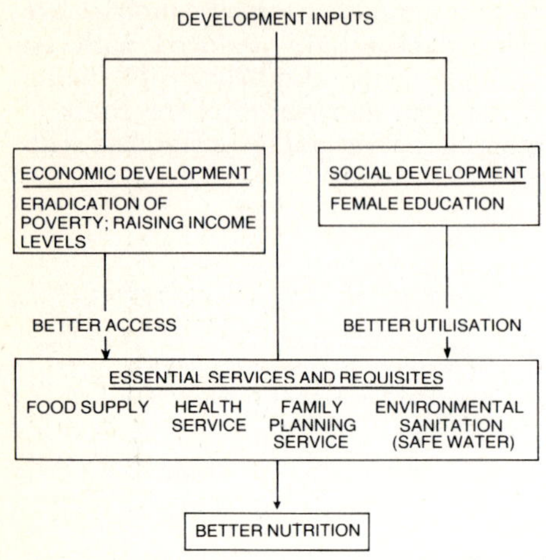

Fig. 2. *Impact of development on nutrition.*

encountering problems with regard to achieving equitable distribution of food among their population despite overall adequacy of food at the national level.

The experience of China and India, the two biggest countries of the world which, between themselves, today account for over 1700 million people (about 38 per cent of mankind) will illustrate this point.

Food production. It will be seen from Tables 2 and 3 that both countries have managed to keep their food production ahead of their population growth — not a small achievement, considering the tremendous increase in their populations.

With respect to achieving equitable distribution, the strategies adopted by the two countries have been necessarily largely conditioned by their political systems.

The Indian experience: India's remarkable success with respect to food production at the overall national level has unfortunately not been matched by similar success in the eradication of poverty among large sections of her people, and we witness today the cruel paradox of mounting food surpluses posing storage problems on the one hand and pockets of undernutrition on the other. India's buffer stocks are expected to reach an all-time high of 28 million tonnes this year. And yet some of the most florid forms of undernutrition are being seen among the poorest sections of her population.

India's developmental strategy has been based on the expectation that heavy investment in capital-intensive industries would generate sufficient jobs in industries which would help to siphon off the surplus rural agricultural work force. Unfortunately, the jobs generated in industry despite heavy investments, which have now made India the tenth largest industrial power in the world, have proved far too inadequate in relation to the tremendous ever-expanding rural work force. The result has been that the basic problem of poverty which lies at the root of the nutrition problem has not yet been adequately contained.

In recent years, other direct strategies for eradication of poverty have been initiated. Employment generation programmes and several other 'anti-poverty' programmes have been initiated but their impact has yet to be felt.

Table 2. *Overall nett availability (in million metric tons) and per caput availability of food grains in China* (World Bank Report No. 3391, June 1981)

	1957	1977	1979
Cereals	92.08	149.44	187.83
Pulses and soyabean	15.19	12.60	9.97
Total	107.27	162.04	198.4
Per caput availability (g/d):			
Cereals	399.3	436.0	533.3
Pulses	65.7	36.7	30.1
Total	465.0	472.7	563.4

Table 3. *Overall nett availability (in million metric tons) and per caput availability of food grains in India* (Economic Survey 1984–85, Ministry of Finance, Government of India)

	1956	1970	1982
Cereals	52.42	79.29	106.8
Pulses	10.23	10.20	10.07
Total	62.65	89.49	116.87
Per caput net availability, g/d:			
Cereals	360.5	403.1	414.5
Pulses	70.4	51.9	39.2
Total	430.9	455.5	453.7

The Chinese experience: It might be expected that, given its political system, China would have been able to achieve equitable distribution of its available food supplies. The indications, however, are that this has not been the case either. A World Bank Report[8] speaks of uneven

Table 4. *The Chilean model*

Health inputs	*Welfare inputs*
Hospital beds (350 000); clinics (1500)	Maternity leave (4½ months); breast-feeding allowance.
Chain of: health posts; nutrition rehabilitation centres special clinics for low-birth weight babies; hostels for rural mothers.	Allowance for families with children under 21 years, with pregnant women and with nursing women (up to 1 year after delivery)
Day care centres for 150 000 under-fives	Creches for children up to 6 years of age for working
One health worker per 200 of population.	mothers.
	Free education.
	Free milk distribution for infants, nursing women and under-fives.

Table 5. *Health care and environmental sanitation in South East Asia* (Bull. Regional Health Information WHO-SEARO, 1983)

Total population	— 1124.8 million	Percentage of population	— 38
Number of countries	— 11	with access to safe	
Percentage of children	— 26.1 (BCG)	drinking water	
under one year	29.3 (DPT3)	Percentage of population	— 16
immunised:	14.8 (OPV3)	with excreta disposal	
	0.5 (Measles)	facilities	

distribution of food supplies within the country leading to the persistence of substandard consumption levels in at least some areas.

A Chinese Communist Party Central Committee statement adopted in 1978 reported that more than 100 million people in rural areas suffered from a lack of grain. The World Bank Report states that 'despite secular improvements in the nutritional status of children in China, and despite the sufficiency of overall nutrient availability, significant numbers of children remain malnourished'. Other available reports speak of wide-spread prevalence of anaemia, iodine-deficiency and rickets, but extreme forms of PEM — kwashiorkor and marasmus — are apparently rare.

It is also widely recognised that children of the 'rice-eating' South of China are shorter and lighter for age than those of the north of the country; indeed the difference has been reported to be of such order that separate growth standards for assessment of growth retardation of children of the north and south had been suggested.

It will thus be seen that the *primary* focus in the transitional stages of development, in both countries, has been (understandably) on rapid achievement of overall national self-sufficiency in food supplies. For this purpose, inputs have been provided preferentially to those areas and sectors that promised quick results in this regard.

Heavy reliance on welfare and 'free services' to mitigate undernutrition, in the face of persistent economic underdevelopment and poverty, eg Chile. Compelled by their inability to solve the basic problem of poverty, the root cause of undernutrition, several Third World countries are now resorting to 'welfare' and 'nutrition intervention' programmes to mitigate under-nutrition in the presence of poverty. It has been claimed that despite widespread poverty, economic stagnation and rising unemployment, Chile has been able to achieve substantial reduction in infant mortality (108 to 21 per thousand) and improvement in child nutrition over the last two decades through massive health inputs and wide-ranging welfare and relief measures[11]. Chile, in some ways, is rather unique with more than 80 per cent of its relatively small population of 11 million concentrated in urban areas. The health-welfare-nutrition intervention inputs in that country are truly massive (Table 4) and of a scale which few developing countries today can afford. Table 5 sets out data provided by WHO with respect to the current status of health facilities and services in the South-East Asia region. This will show how far removed the present situation with respect to health infrastructure in these countries is from the picture presented by the Chilean model. The percentage figures in the table do not fully reflect the enormity of inadequacies of the health infrastructure in the countries among the poor because even these low percentages are mostly accounted for by facilities enjoyed by the relatively rich in these countries. The replicability of the Chilean model in most other developing countries, where even minimal health care facilities are lacking, appears doubtful. All the same, the Chilean experience serves to underscore the important contribution which basic health services can make to nutrition.

Cuba is also reported to have achieved notable reduction in child mortality through state-sponsored welfare measures. Sri Lanka has adopted for some years massive food transfer schemes which has resulted in significant reductions in child mortality; but the economic viability of this strategy has been questioned. Provinces within India are also attempting huge feeding operations targeted to children, and foodgrain subsidy schemes. Such measures do, no doubt, help relieve acute distress and undernutrition among the poor, to whose level the benefits of overall national economic development have not as yet percolated, but the important question is: Can poor developing countries with limited resources and a long way to go *permanently* rely on such massive give-away operations for sustaining health and nutrition of their populations. Unfortunately, food-for-work programmes which would seem to make more economic sense, are being operated more as mobile short-term relief operations rather than as part of a well-thought out strategy for promoting self-generating socio-economic development; and for this reason they have not had sustained impact on the nutritional status of populations.

In transitional stages of development such heavy reliance on welfare and 'give-away' programmes may be unavoidable and indeed may be even necessary, but this situation must not be considered as the final goal, since these programmes could inhibit, and restrict resources for sound non-populist programmes which alone in the long-term will help eradicate poverty.

The real challenge that many developing countries currently face is the need to evolve (and find resources for) a judicious mix of (a) welfare programmes which will address the hard realities of the immediate present and (b) less dramatic anti-poverty programmes (eg employment/income generation, land tenure reforms etc) which alone will lay the durable foundation for national development and are, therefore, more important from the long-term point of view.

Many Third World countries are in fact moving away from isolated welfare' charity operations and so-called 'nutrition intervention' programmes and are increasingly opting for 'integrated rural development programmes' in which nutrition intervention constitutes only one component, the major emphasis being on employment/income generation and promotion of female literacy and health care. Unfortunately, as yet, there have been far too few truly objective evaluations of such large-scale rural developmental programmes (as opposed to small scale projects under dedicated missionary leadership) and of their impact on nutritional status.

Prosperity associated with poor social development, inadequate service infrastructure, and undernutrition, eg the Gulf countries. While the association of undernutrition with poverty is the general rule, there are some notable exceptions. Within the last three decades, following on the unprecedented oil boom, the Gulf countries have become richer than the richest of developed countries, but this sudden prosperity has not been matched by parallel equally spectacular social development, using the term in a broad sense to include promotion of literacy, efficient health and social services, indigenous scientific and technical manpower, and entrepreneurship and managerial skills.

A recent study[12] of the nutritional status of the populations of five of these countries — Kuwait, Qatar, United Arab Emirates (UAE), Bahrain, and Oman — has revealed a high prevalance of marasmus in infants and children, and anaemia in both children and women. The use of commercial baby foods in infants is extremely high, and the practice of breast-feeding has been severely eroded. Thus, for example, in Kuwait only around 50 per cent of infants of even mothers of low social classes were receiving any breast milk at all at six months, while in UAE, less than 15 per cent of infants below three months were exclusively breast-fed. Indeed, these countries today provide the richest pasture for commercial baby food manufacturers. In the absence of adequate standards of personal hygiene and environmental sanitation, gastrointestinal diseases in infants and children take a heavy toll.

At the other end of the nutritional spectrum in the same populations, adults have been reported to exhibit the manifestations of overnutrition, high prevalence of obesity, degenerative heart diseases and diabetes. Sudden affluence and luxury had completely changed life-styles in the last two to three decades. With sedentary lives and a per capita energy intake of well over 3500 kcal (14.5 MJ) in many cases even among the lowest social classes, obesity has become a major problem especially among women.

The experience of Gulf countries underscores the fact that development has two dimensions, social and economic, and that socio-cultural advancement is an essential requisite for a society to successfully absorb and derive maximal benefit from economic prosperity.

Nutritional repercussions of developmental technologies.

Distortion of the pattern of food availability. Modern intensive agricultural technology has contributed greatly to the augmentation of foodgrain production in many developing countries during the last two decades. However, practically all the increase in foodgrains production achieved through modern intensive agricultural technology is attributable to increase in production of cereals, especially wheat and rice. Pulse production has been more or less static throughout all the agricultural boom generated by the green revolution. The trends regarding cereal and pulse production in China and India (Tables 2, 3) will show the profound distortion in the ratio of the overall availability of cereals on the one hand and pulses on the other. In India, this has resulted in an increase in the price of pulses relative to that of cereals of more than two-fold between 1950 and 1983. It is to be expected that this will be reflected in diminished intake of pulses by poor families. Since pulses are the major sources of lysine in poor vegetarian dietaries, this would mean deterioration of the protein quality of the dietaries of the poor. Fortunately, there is wide recognition of the need to correct this serious imbalance.

Hazards of pesticides. Yet another major hazard of modern intensive agricultural technology arises from the indiscriminate use of pesticides. With the propagation of high-yielding varieties of foodgrains, the use of a wide range of potentially toxic pesticides has become necessary. These are now being extensively used not only in agricultural operations but also for control of arthropod vectors of malaria and filariasis in many developing countries.

Unfortunately, however, these countries are in no position to strictly enforce the regulatory measures essential in the use of pesticides. In fact, several pesticides not permitted to be used in developed countries are being freely used in developing countries. The laboratory infrastructure and the analytical expertise needed to monitor levels of pesticide-residues in foods (of the type available in Japan, for example) just do not exist in most cases.

High levels of pesticide residues have been reported in developing countries not only in food-stuffs but also in human tissues[6]. Pesticide residues in human milk in China, India and Mexico are much higher than those reported from developed countries[13]. High levels of pesticide residues have also been reported in stored foodgrains, vegetables, milk, meat, eggs and cattle-feed in developing countries.

A syndrome of arthritis attributable to consumption of crabs with high levels of pesticide residues in their tissues has been identified in some parts of India[2].

Resurgence of malaria. The more disturbing claim, however, is that the development of resistance to insecticides on the part of *Anopheles* and *Aedes* mosquitoes may be attributable to the selection pressure resulting from the wide use of pesticides in agriculture[15].

The near-eradication of malaria in the sixties did far more to improve the health and nutritional status of millions of poor in India and other countries than any other single health operation or nutrition intervention. If the use of pesticides does contribute to a resurgence of malaria, the benefits derived from the use of pesticides with respect to foodgrain production would have been nullified to a considerable extent.

However, the problem of pesticide toxicity has to be seen in the total context of development. It may not be necessary to see the issue of pesticide use as a trade-off between high foodgrain yields and environmental protection and extreme positions in this regard are not of much help. Developing countries will continue to need pesticides in their agricultural and health operations; but there is considerable scope for avoidance of their indiscriminate use by (a) adopting such strategies as crop-rotation, intercropping etc., which will minimise the need for pesticides in agriculture; (b) minimising sole reliance on pesticides for control of vectors of communicable diseases by parallel use of other measures; (c) strict adherence to precautions in the handling and use of pesticides; and (d) improving laboratory analytical facilities for monitoring pesticide residues in foods.

Dams and irrigation projects. Modern agricultural technology also relies heavily on extension of irrigation. In their efforts to meet their developmental needs for irrigation and electricity, developing countries have resorted to the construction of huge dams and irrigation projects. The contribution that these have made to overall development in these countries cannot be disputed; but like most other developmental tools which are double-edged, dams and irrigation projects have also exerted some deleterious repercussions.

Effect on soil fertility. It has been claimed that the degradation of the soil in the command areas of irrigation projects due to the increase in soil salinity and water logging has brought about a reduction in fertility of soil downstream. Thus before the buiding of the Aswan Dam, it is reported that the Nile deposited 100 tonnes of silt per hectare annually over one million hectares of land in the Nile valley. The annual cost of fertilisers now required by Egypt to replace this loss is reported to be of the order of 100 million dollars a year[3].

Effect on fisheries. The impact of large-scale water projects on fisheries has also been quite considerable. The immediate effect of the construction of a reservoir is a dramatic rise in the population of some fish species but this short-lived increase is followed by eventual near-extinction of fish populations not only in the reservoir but in the entire river basin, the classic examples being Lake Volta and Lake Kariba.

Aggravation of malaria and schistosomiasis. The introduction of perennial irrigation following on construction of dams is also reported to have favoured the resurgence of malaria in many countries by providing for the vector vastly extended and highly favourable habitats. The incidence of schistosomiasis, which according to some estimates, accounts for 200 million victims all over the world today, is also aggravated. Large-scale water projects provide ideal habitats for both fresh water snails and the parasite and have created ideal conditions for the multiplication of the disease.

Aggravation of endemic fluorosis. In India, following on the construction of the huge Nagarjunasagar Dam, in an area earlier known to be endemic for fluorosis, there has been a marked aggravation and qualitative change in the fluorosis problem[9]. Marked bony deformities, genuvalgum, affecting children and young adults, which were earlier unknown in these areas, have now become so common as to involve the majority of adults in entire villages in the area, resulting in serious disabilities (Fig. 3).

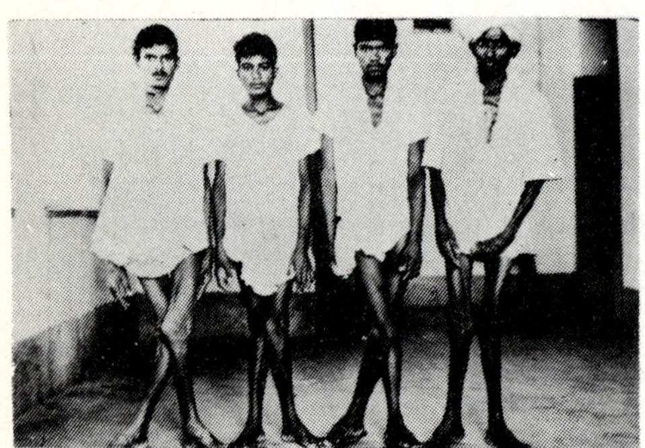

Fig. 3. *Sufferers from genuvalgum.* A consequence of the Nagarjunasagar dam.

All this implies that in the construction of dams and irrigation projects, the possible ecological repercussions should receive full consideration. It is now proposed that alternatives to gigantic water projects such as, for example, more efficient exploitation of ground water resources, should be considered wherever possible. Instead of a small number of huge hydroelectric plants, a relatively large number of small hydro works requiring relatively shorter water drops and resulting in much smaller water reservoirs causing negligible impact on the environment are now considered preferable. This is the strategy which China seems to have largely opted for.

Urbanisation. An equally important repercussion of modern development is *unplanned* urbanisation. The migration of rural labour to urban areas is an inevitable by-product of the developmental process and indeed the developmental strategy of many countries is based on a policy of siphoning off surplus agricultural labour from rural areas. It was estimated nearly ten years ago that around 200 million people live in urban areas under conditions of absolute poverty, characterised by lack of access to potable water, sewerage and adequate nutrition. About 56 per cent of these were estimated to live in Asia, 24 per cent in Latin America and 20 per cent in Africa. The World Bank has estimated that by the year 2000 AD, nearly 40 per cent of the world's population will be urbanised the fastest growing being the biggest cities, and within these cities the slums and squatter areas. According to a recent estimate, of the 10 million population in Calcutta, three million live in slums and one million are pavement dwellers.

Official urban health statistics hide the appalling health and nutritional conditions of urban slum dwellers and squatters, most of whom are not 'official' residents of the cities and therefore hardly get included in urban statistics. Nutrition surveys in Colombia and Morocco revealed that the nutritional status of the poorest urban socio-economic groups was worse than that of corresponding poor rural groups in those countries and a recent study by the Nutrition Foundation of India also reveals a similar picture. Because of overcrowding, less time which mothers find to look after their children, and heavy environmental pollution, the chances of gastro-intestinal infection in children in urban slums are far greater than in rural areas[1].

Increasing use of commercial milk foods in infant feeding. An undesirable result of urbanisation and industrialisation has been the increasing use of commercial milk foods in infant feeding by the poor who have neither the means to buy these foods in adequate amounts nor the facilities to use them hygienically. This practice is fortunately now largely restricted to the urban areas and the immediate rural environs of cities. A recent study by the Nutrition Foundation of India[5] in Bombay, Calcutta and Madras and the surrounding areas showed that commercial milk foods and commercial cereal foods were being used by a substantial number of the poor in urban and peri-urban areas (Table 6). Because of the highly inadequate amounts of these foods which the poor infants were getting, they were apparently conferring only marginal nutrition benefit to them. On the other hand, the unhygienic manner in which they were used contributed to a higher prevalence of gastrointestinal disorders, with the result that infants of the poor receiving commercial infant foods in urban slums were generally nutritionally worse off than those who were not.

Table 6. *Percentage of mothers using commercial infant foods in three cities of India by different income groups* (Gopujkar P.V. *et al*. Scientific Report-4, Nutrition Foundation of India, 1984)

Per caput income per month (rupees*)	Bombay	Calcutta	Madras
50 or less	8.9	24.5	37.4
51–100	21.1	48.2	60.8
101–150	24.1	66.4	65.9
150–200	25.7	77.2	80.0
201 +	30.5	92.9	75.0
Mothers' education			
Nil	19.4	26.1	33.6
Low	19.5	46.7	51.3
High	27.2	77.5	70.9

*10 Rupees = $US1

Problems of overnutrition in the developed countries. So far, I have considered the impact of development on problems of undernutrition in developing countries. This presentation will be incomplete without a brief reference to the problems of overnutrition which afflict the 'developed' countries of the world.

In the case of considerable proportions of populations of the countries of Europe and North Ameria, and of the highly affluent minority in developing countries, the developmental process has served to promote ill-health arising from overnutrition. Obesity, degenerative vascular diseases and diabetes now take a heavy toll among these population. Affluence, the hall-mark of development, permits, on the one hand, free access to foods of all kinds; and, on the other, has reduced the need for hard physical labour. Energy intakes, far in excess of energy needs, high level of intake of animal foods, fats, sugar, refined foods, elaborately processed foods (possibly with as yet unknown carcinogens), fast food and junk foods have all contributed to this scenario. Stresses and tensions, which are an inevitable part of the highly competitive industrial culture have compounded these effects of overnutrition.

It is sad to think that in the world of today in spite of all its spectacular technological advances, much less than one fourth of its people are properly nourished; good health and nutrition seem to have eluded considerable sections of populations even of developed countries that do not suffer from dietary and economic constraints.

Unfortunately, the response to this situation has been as yet inadequate. The problem of overnutrition is sought to be overcome through slimming exercises and work-outs, and multi-million dollar slimming industries and a whole array of gadgetry has sprung up. Obviusly sensible movements to discourage excessive consumption of food (food as a whole and not just fats) are relatively muted. Market forces are apparently at play to ensure that both food establishments and slimming industries flourish with mutual support.

The emphasis in the developmental process everywhere has been on the achievement of affluence and prosperity, and not so much on promoting life-styles and value-systems which will enable people to 'absorb' and derive the true benefits of such affluence and prosperity from the point of view of their physical and prosperity from the point of view of their physical and mental well-being. The culture of unbridled consumption which the developmental process tends to promote must be considered as its major weakness.

These problems are by no means confined to the countries of Europe and North America alone; there is as much, if not more, obesity and degenerative vascular disease among the affluent sections of populations of developing countries as well, and with economic improvement they will increase in the years ahead. As such the subject is of concern to all nutrition scientists of the world.

1 Basta, S.S. (1977): Nutrition and health in low income urban areas of the Third World. *Ecol. Fd Nutr.* **6**, 113–124.
2 Bhat, R.V. & Krishnamachari, K.A.V.R. (1977): Endemic familial arthritis of Malnad — an epidemiological study. *Ind. J. Med. Res.* **66**, 777–86.
3 Goldsmith, E. & Hildyard, N. (1984): *The Social and environmental effects of large dams*, pp. 58–59. The Ecological Centre.
4 Gopalan, C. (1984): Child survival and child nutrition. *Bull. Nutr. Found. India* **5**, 1–3.
5 Gopujkar, P.V., Chaudhuri, S.N., Ramaswamy, M.A., Gore, M.S. & Gopalan, C. (1984): Infant feeding practices with special reference to the use of commercial infant foods. *Sci. Rep. 4, Nutr. Found. India*.
6 Indian Council of Agricultural Research (1967): *Report of the special committee on harmful effects of pesticides*.
7 Institute of Paediatrics, Chinese Academy of Medical Sciences, Peoples' Republic of China (1975): *Studies on the Physical development of children and adolescents in New China*.
8 Jamison, D.T., Ho, T.J. & Townbridge, F.L. (1981): Food availability and the nutritional status of children in China. Suppl. Paper III, Annex B, Wld Bank Rep. No. 3391.
9 Krishnamachari, K.A.V.R. & Krishnaswamy, K. (1973): *Genu valgum* and osteoporosis in an area of endemic fluorosis *Lancet* **2**, 877–879.
10 Malcolm, L.A. (1974): Ecological factors relating to child growth and nutritional status. In *Nutrition and malnutrition — identification and measurement*, ed A.F. Roche & F. Falkner, pp 329–353. New York: Plenum Press.
11 Monckeberg, F. (1983): Socio-economic development and nutritional status: efficiency of intervention programmes. In *Nutrition intervention strategies in national development*, pp 31–39. New York: Academic Press.
12 Musaiger, A.O. (1984): Nutritional status in the Arabian Gulf countries. In Proceedings of the Fourth Asian Congress of Nutrition, pp. 549–553. Thailand: Aksomsmai Press.
13 Slorach, S.A. & Vaz, R. (1983): Assessment of human exposure to selected organochlorine compounds through biological monitoring. Paper prepared for UNEP and WHO by the Swedish National Food Administration, Uppsala.
14 Teller, C., Sibrian, R., Talavera, C., Bent, V., Del Canto, J. & Saenz, L. (1979): Population and nutrition: implications of socio-demographic trends and differentials for food and nutrition policy in Central America and Panama. *Ecol. Fd. Nutr.* **8**, 95–109.
15 WHO (1976): Tech. Rep. Ser. No. 585. Resistance of vectors and reservoirs of disease to pesticides.

Feeding, feedback and sustenance of primary health care

J.E. ROHDE
Management Sciences for Health, Box 2560, Port au Prince, 01622 Haiti.

Malnutrition is the major health problem in the world today. More than half of the next generation is growing up undernourished, deprived of the food needed for normal healthy growth. Of 850 million children under the age of 5 years, 350 million are undernourished and 100 million moderately or severely malnourished. Prospective studies in Bangladesh and India have shown the dramatic increased risk of death amongst these children. Those severely malnourished have a 20 times greater chance of dying than their normal peers. The large Pan American Health Organization study in Latin America showed malnutrition as an underlying cause in more than 50 per cent of child deaths. Many of these died from minor illnesses, eg diarrhoea or measles, which become fatal in the pernicious environment of malnutrition. Indeed, for the malnourished children of the world every infection is a potentially fatal illness.

Given the clarity of this situation, how ironic it is that nutrition remains the most neglected aspect of health care and most notably, of primary health care. One need only consult the budget of a health ministry to see that less is spent on nutrition activities than on even the simplest of drugs for symptomatic treatment. Health workers customarily spend little time in activities promoting good nutrition. Even the staffing of bureaucracies such as WHO or ministries of health reflects the neglected state of nutrition.

Why is nutrition so assiduously neglected? First, nutrition is an invisible attribute — only its absence is readily noticed and then, only in extreme cases. Second, while malnutrition can be measured or detected at a given point in time, normal nutrition in a child implies regular continuous growth. But growth, and growth faltering take place too slowly and too imperceptibly to attract the attention of mothers or health workers in the same way as do more acute, dramatic problems like fever, diarrhoea, or measles. To counter this difficulty, growth must be made perceptible. We must make growth faltering, the earliest sign of inadequate nutrition, as visible to the mother and the health workers as fever or a baby crying. By emphasizing visible *feedback* from growth monitoring as well as *feeding*, we can make nutrition efforts as attractive and satisfying as other health interventions. By creating a demand for this feedback, we involve each mother more actively and regularly in the assessment of her child's individual health. Frequent contact for regular assessment of growth will result in a rise in demand for primary health care activities, thereby increasing coverage of essential preventive and promotive services. Feeding and feedback through regular growth monitoring can become the driving force leading to universal primary health care.

Let me start by looking at the usual approaches to improving nutritional status. Why are they so neglected? To begin with, nutrition interventions are not discreet and well-defined as immunizations. By projecting nutrition as a continuous daily need, we relegate it to the category of natural behaviour, like breathing or excretion. Nutrition, and particularly feeding, is not considered a health intervention — it is just part of normal life.

Second, nutrition interventions require soliciting the participation of mothers. Clinical health workers are taught to respond to client demands for service. They are usually neither interested, nor skilful in selling ideas to a disinterested client. They are also frustrated by the fact that there is no single approach, no single message, no definitive answer to give a mother, and often no thanks in return.

Next, nutrition activities do not respond to an acutely-felt need as does oral rehydration for diarrhoea. In most cases, there is no demand on the part of consumers for nutrition, at least not until it is too late. Even fever or a runny nose in a fussy child attracts far more attention than poor nutrition from mother and health worker alike.

Nutrition is, frankly, a bore. It requires continuous action on a daily basis. It implies changing the approach over time and in response to a child's changing health conditions. But then, even correct behaviour which takes place despite these inhibitors results in a subtle outcome difficult to perceive and certainly long in coming.

Nutrition is further neglected because to date, actions aimed at the therapy of malnutrition or even its prevention do not seem to work. The extensive review of food supplement programmes by Beaton and Ghassemi convinced even the enthusiasts that nutritional status is not often affected by feeding programmes. Years of experience with nutrition education have resulted in little measurable effect in behaviour or resulting nutritional health of target children. Nutrition is neglected because from all experience, it does not work. Is it any wonder that health workers lose heart and shift their efforts to interventions that pay off?

Why is it that our efforts do not work? I believe that a major reason that nutrition interventions are so ineffective is because they all too often address only the final stages of malnutrition. Focus on the moderately or severely malnourished child, completely misses the opportunity to intervene at an early age when the most severe deficit in growth is occurring and opportunities for effective action are both pragmatic and affordable. Major *deviation* in growth occurs, in almost all malnourished populations, between 6 and 24 months of age. But, major *prevalence* of established malnutrition in these same populations is seen among children of 3 or 4 years of age. Our interventions are aimed too late at the victims suffering the late effects of early growth deprivation. No wonder nutritional rehabilitation is so unsuccessful.

Of equal concern even if we keep such children alive, is the clear loss of genetic growth potential in children who have suffered early malnutrition. When malnutrition has persisted long enough to become severe, stunting has almost always occurred, and catch-up growth even with aggressive feeding appears to be limited by attained height.

The answer is to intervene earlier, before the malnutrition becomes too severe to overcome and before permanent stunting occurs. To be effective, interventions must begin within the first year of life, and their major nutritional impact will be seen *before* the child reaches 30 months of age.

Why do most health systems miss this early opportunity for timely intervention? Because there is no trigger, no perceived problem, no effective stimulus for action. At the earliest age, hunger in a child so obvious in crying, is pacified by the breast and as long as milk production is adequate, growth is entitely normal. In almost all traditional societies, normal growth along Western standard curves is seen until 4 to 6 months of age. Beyond that age, however, growth often falters markedly, but that faltering is invisible. Hunger is still pacified by the breast or by provision of bulky foods which fill the child's stomach and stop its crying. Meanwhile, the child's growth begins to fall behind without the mother realizing it: she, in fact, has been responding to all the signals available to her. The situation may progress to the oft-described condition of breast addiction leading to the paradoxical suggestion to wean the child from his only source of high quality food in order to force him to eat more and overcome his malnutrition. At this stage, basal metabolic requirements may be fulfilled, and energy needs reduced through inactivity, but growth, the only real measure of nutritional adequacy, is silently ignored.

All living systems operate through a response cycle consisting of efferent action (something going out from the organism) and an afferent return message, sensing what has happened as a result of the efferent action. After judging the desirability of the afferent feedback, the organism then adjusts the efferent activity. Through a continuous series of efferent-afferent cycles the optimal status is achieved and maintained. Clinical care and health are monitored by both the patient and the health care provider by sensing measurable changes in such parameters as temperature, blood pressure, serum biochemical levels or even a subjective sense of well-being. The patient or physician then takes appropriate action in response to those changes. Recently, we have even seen external mechanisms — so-called biofeedback machines — used to control high blood pressure or to change brain waves. Indeed, it is not unreasonable to say that all effectively working systems are controlled in this fashion, by monitoring the results of action and feeding the results of that monitoring back to the action source.

We, in nutrition, have not created a viable, physiologically sound closed-loop feedback system. While, our efferent limb, our output, is highly developed, even hypertrophied, there are no clear, objective, measurable and visible effects to feedback into the response mechanism. We send out nutritional messages but we rarely learn whether they are internalized or acted upon. The mother who follows our nutrition messages, in turn, has no means to detect the results of her action. Yet, she is still expected to follow these directions, which all too often seem irrational or culturally alien to her, over a long period of time. How much blind faith can we reasonably expect? In short, in nutrition we lack the feedback or afferent component of the system that would serve to stimulate or modify continuing action on the part of the mother or indeed even the health worker who is guiding her.

Growth monitoring can provide that critical feedback, the afferent component. Growth monitoring measures growth by objective means and then records it in a manner which is visible and comprehensible by all persons involved, particularly the mother. By making perceptible the result of proper feeding, both when the child is well and particularly during and following acute infections, growth monitoring can stimulate further action on the part of the mother. By tying the provision of appropriate and practical nutritional messages and imparting pragmatic skills in response to a rise or fall of weight of the child on a growth chart, nutrition can become, for the mother, the most critical element of her child's health. Growth monitoring is, in a very real sense, the nervous system of individual health care. Successful feedings, as demonstrated by the visual record of adequate growth, assure the dynamic health of the child, while the demonstration of deficient growth, like crying, can now stimulate an appropriate corrective feeding response.

Growth monitoring, most frequently through regular weighing of the child and recording of the weight on a growth chart, allows the mother to see growth. The chart must be designed for her use and comprehension. She herself must perceive and internalize what she is measuring. This is why the mother herself should determine whether growth of her child has met her expectations over the interval since the last weighing. Mothers can't weigh accurately, can't understand graphs, can't mark the cards, can't read… say the critics. Ridiculous! … mothers can't because we won't teach them. We don't take the time, and we respect neither their capacity nor their motivation. We treat mothers like irresponsible, immature children, and wonder why they don't take our advice on how to rear their children. Whenever we have approached mothers in a culturally sensitive and intellectually respectful way, we have found responsive women able to weigh their children accurately and to interpret growth with the insight and subtlety of a trained nutritionist.

In market places throughout the world women weigh their wares with accuracy to satisfy the shrewdest gem dealer. Even illiterate women are often numerate, and most take pride in mastering the skill needed to place a mark properly on a growth card. Where designed with the help of mothers, cards with narrow growth channels make recognition of normal continuous growth easy, confused only by the obfuscation of nutritional status categories long cited by health workers as judgement on a child's attained size. Mothers know children come in all shapes and sizes. They know growth is a continuous process and they need help only to measure that growth in order to recognize health in their child. When their children have been shown not to grow, not to get bigger or heavier with time, mothers become quite susceptible to appropriate practical nutrition messages. For growth monitoring must be more than just the measurement of growth. It requires an effective response by the mother, aimed at sustaining normal growth or improving sub-optimal growth as revealed by the monitoring. An effective response to any stimulus requires four successive elements:

First, *Perception*: awareness of a problem or situation — the mother must first see, feel or perceive growth or lack of it in order to be able to respond.

Second, *Motivation* — She must then have, or develop, a desire to respond, to do something to promote growth. She must have a *felt need* to achieve growth in her child.

Third, *Knowledge and skills* — she must then know how to feed, what to feed, when to feed. In fact, the preparation and administration of appropriate food has been the major focus of traditional nutritional education.

Finally, *The means to act* — she must, in the last analysis, have food available to give the child. Classical nutrition programmes providing supplementary foods have tended to focus almost exclusively on this element.

Many elements have criticized growth monitoring programmes as being ineffective, and indeed many are. The reason is that they stop with the first of these elements, perception, or, in fact, they may even fail to provide that to the mother. How many of you have visited child weighing programmes in which the mothers line up with their children, the local health worker then takes the child from the mother and weighs it, marks the card, *closes it*, and then hands it and the child back to the mother, not even commenting on whether the weight has gone up or down? This sort of programme fails even to provide perception or awareness of growth or its faltering, never mind the required motivation and knowledge.

Perception of growth, desire by the mother for growth, knowledge of appropriate feeding, and the availability of food — these are the necessary elements for effective growth monitoring. The lack of any one results in an interruption in the cycle and failure of the system. Weighing a child and plotting his weight on a growth chart does not necessarily lead to comprehension on the part of the mother. But even if her perception is raised, weighing is surely not enough. She must be motivated, there must be a demand created where she wishes to take action and achieve growth in her child. She becomes responsive to the inputs of nutritional education and willingly assimilates the knowledge and skills imparted with appropriate nutritional message. Armed with these, the mother can find the means within her own home in most cases. After all, particularly in the youngest age child, the difference between adequate growth and growth faltering is a few hundred calories. A small redistribution within the family itself will often be enough. In those unusual cases, where even a motivated and informed mother cannot find the resources, food supplements clearly play a role. To be effective, growth monitoring must be linked with the motivational and knowledge transfer aspects of good nutrition education.

Nutrition education must be more, however, than simply instructing a mother in the basic principles of good nutrition or of child feeding and care. Nutrition messages all too often lack relevance to mothers, are impractical and are too general, too vague and unfocussed. Once mothers have seen a clear indicator or trigger to initiate their response, have gained the necessary feedback from growth monitoring, they must receive *precise, prescriptive* and *practical* directions which they can carry out in their home. Such messages can provide motivation, knowledge and the means to feed, all in one. The patient who has learned to control his hypertension with a biofeedback machine may eventually be able to give up that external mechanical feedback channel and use only the internal mechanisms developed with the help of the machine. So the mother may eventually, after much effective nutritional education, need only the feedback of a falling growth curve to trigger an appropriate feeding response. But in the meantime, for most mothers, weighing must be accompanied by additional motivational and educational inputs in order to bring about appropriate behavioural responses.

Recent experiments in behavioural modification applied to nutrition provide important insights into motivation on the part of mothers, called by our colleagues in the marketing business demand creation. We in health and nutrition have long focussed on the supply side, the food, the knowledge, the skills, the weight cards, the scales, the health workers all supplying products to the mother. But marketing experts look at 'demand' as the missing function and have turned to the consumers themselves to learn how to create that demand. This early consumer consultation, is called *feed-forward* by Manoff. It attempts to define in what the consumer is interested: what does she think and what are her reactions to various presentations of a product or idea. Applying this approach to nutrition, by starting with the mother and addressing *her* concerns and perceptions of nutrition and growth in her child, we may have a better chance of adjusting our nutrition messages so that they will be credible, appropriate, and will be acted upon.

A remarkable proof of this approach was demonstrated in a study in Indonesia by Manoff and associates. Using 'feed forward' techniques such as focus groups, interviews, and surveys, they determined the major concern of mothers about feeding their children at different ages and under different circumstances, all focussing on the first 24 months of life. They then developed recommended practices specific to each locality, by observing actual food preparation methods used in village homes, investigators cooking along with the mothers. In an effort to make more interactive educational materials, they developed 'action posters' which stimulated the mother to record on the poster each time she carried out a recommended feeding activity. The central forum for continuing motivation and transfer of these recommendations was a monthly weighing post held in each village. Viewed not as a medical encounter or a data collection visit, but as the ideal educational opportunity, growth over the previous months became the trigger for specific educational messages unique to each child and his growth pattern, his age, his health situation, and his developmental status. It was, in Manoff's words, 'the precise delivery of the precise message to the precise mother at the precise time of her precise need. This is social marketing's primary tactic, a focus on priority need, when, where and for whom it is essential, and a minimization of all extraneous factors.' How little does traditional nutritional education conform to this definition.

The results achieved in the Indonesian trial are nothing less than dramatic. Dietary surveys documented increased food consumption and nutrient intakes by comparison with control children in similar villages. The mean weight of project children was almost 1 kg higher than controls after 23 months. Almost one half a standard deviation separated the mean Z score in weight for age of the intervention and control groups.

Notably, the sizeable effect of maternal formal education on nutritional status of the child was virtually absent. In Indonesia, as elsewhere in the developing world, maternal educational level has been shown to be a prime determinant of nutritional status of the child. Yet, this differential, seen among control children, was eliminated in the experimental group, as all mothers, schooled or not, changed their feeding behaviours and brought improved growth to their children. This improved growth correlated well with the mother's nutritional knowledge score. The usual effect of mother's education on nutrition is, as we might expect, related to maternal appreciation for adequate feeding and feeding behaviours in the face of a variety of situations affecting the growing child. Effective nutrition education resulting in measurable behavioural change can overcome the great social deficits noted by Mosley and Caldwell to underlie all of child health and mortality in developing societies for which maternal education has been, hitherto, an appropriate proxy measure.

The implications of this observation are profound, for it means that we do not have to wait for universal female education before we can hope to improve child survival. Such critical areas as nutrition and other child rearing practices can be transferred effectively to mothers with resulting dramatic changes in nutritional status and by implication, survival. Growth promotion through monitoring and active learning processes involving mothers offer a cost-effective strategy for short-cutting the lengthy process of inter-generational progress through female education and alleviation of economic deprivation. Properly done, growth monitoring offers health to each child, today. Nutrition interventions have classically occurred too late. Initially, school feeding programmes were attempted, but after evaluation were found to have little nutritional effect. In recent decades preschool feeding has taken over but once again, its effect on the overall nutritional status of populations has been shown to be minimal. Effective intervention must occur during the weaning period. It is weanling growth monitoring programmes that must command our major attention if we are to effectively address the problem of malnutrition. An analysis of the weight deficits of children in low class communities in New Delhi compared to high class communities showed that, of a 2.46 kg difference which had occurred by age 5 years, 84 per cent of this difference had occurred prior to 30 months of age, while only 16 per cent of the deficit, 0.4 kg, had occurred in the second 30 months of life. It is this period before age two, when the major impact of nutritional education can be realized, and fortunately, it is precisely during this time that modest behavioural change and redistribution of family food resources is most possible for the mother.

Interestingly, it is this same age period when maximal mortality and morbidity are seen in developing country population. Infancy is the peak age of diarrhoeal and pneuomonia deaths. The second year of life sees the major deaths from immunizable diseases and vitamin A deficiency. This is the time when the need for health care as well as nutritional intervention is greatest, when health care can hope to have its largest impact on mortality and morbidity in entire populations, yet children and adults are by far the major beneficiaries of Primary Health Care resources.

What primary health care needs is a mechanism for getting mothers to pay more attention to the health of their children and for getting medical providers out of the clinics and into contact with mothers at a more accessible location. We in the nutrition community have constantly wrestled with the question of how to integrate nutrition into primary health care. In fact, it seems quite obvious that the more appropriate approach is that of integrating primary health care into growth monitoring. By making measured growth the criterion of good health observable by both mother and health workers alike we provide an important missing link in the entire cycle of primary health care for young children which has heretofore been lacking.

Primary health care remains unfortunately, in most instances, passive, confined to clinics or health posts, and responsive only to periodic illness brought to the facility or occasional orchestrated attempts at preventive health care such as mass immunization campaigns. Regular monitoring of growth can draw primary health care workers into interaction with the community on a continuing, regular basis, with a clear overall goal which can be measured — growth for all, now. The monthly weighing activity is the appropriate forum for the health worker to provide instruction on the use of oral rehydration therapy, to distribute chloroquine for malaria or to provide periodic high doses of vitamin A. The whole spectrum of primary health care activity, not only those aimed at the child but also the mother, with contraceptive services, iron-folate tablets for anaemia, and screening for high risk pregnancies, can be carried out during growth monitoring sessions. And like curative activities (and unlike many preventive activities) growth monitoring has a measurable result, healthy growth, which can provide feedback and positive reinforcement to the health worker too, keeping her coming back month after month to the community.

Growth monitoring provides a handle for all health education. Illness is a major cause of malnutrition. Yet exhortations to eat during and after acute illness are clearly beyond the realm of cultural acceptability in almost every society. Recovery of pre-illness weight, however, can be understood as a definition of full recovery from illness and can be accepted by mothers everywhere. Extra feeding, then, can become a very clever, time-limited and goal-oriented response to illness rather than a general and somewhat vague exhortation from health workers. Illness of any kind can then be interpreted as a clear demand for action with expected results. Illness and lack of appetite is the trigger, feeding is the response, the result is growth and recovery of pre-illness weight. As a very specific action, with clear goals and time-limited nature of the expected response, this approach is far more acceptable and more likely to be followed.

Many primary health care interventions are likely to be ineffective in the absence of effective nutrition interventions. While oral rehydration effectively avoids death from acute diarrhoea, there is considerable evidence to suggest that most diarrhoeal deaths occur among malnourished children in whom diarrhoea has become chronic. A recent study in India found more than three quarters of all diarrhoeal deaths to be in children who were malnourished and with chronic illness. In an urban slum of Haiti, with 3 per cent of all children suffering third degree malnutrition, some 10 per cent of children coming to rehydration centres were severely malnourished, 35 per cent of those admitted to the hospital with diarrhoea were severely malnourished and 65 per cent of all those who died were from the same severely malnourished group. Clearly, malnutrition was a major determinant of mortality and thereby an important limiting factor on the overall impact of oral rehydration on diarrhoea-related mortality in that city. Black and colleagues have shown in Bangladesh increased severity and duration of diarrhoeal illness in malnourished children. Rehydration therapy without effective convales-cent feeding and growth recovery, at best, simply delays death. Primary care without growth can hardly be considered health care — it is palliative only.

Growth monitoring has, in many countries, been handed over to the communities themselves. In Haiti, rural community health agents recruited from their villages, were previously expected to pay household visits on each of more than 500 families a month, a task they almost never accomplished. Now mothers gather in convenient nearby locations, often under a shady tree or at the house of a well-known friendly village woman for monthly weighing, advice and the provision of other essential primary health care services. Some community health agents have taught the mothers to do most of the work themselves but often attend to provide curative services for children who may be sick, vaccines for those who are not yet fully immunized and advice to all participating mothers on the newest acitivities in health care.

On the opposite side of the world, in Indonesia, more than 25 000 villages with 40 000 mothers' groups, originally organized as family planning acceptor groups, have taken up growth monitoring as a means to ensure the health of their children (in now, substantially smaller families, thanks to their wide acceptance of family planning provided at the village level). In thousands of these villages, monthly weighing carried out by mothers has become the driving force for all health activities. When properly organized, near home, by a small group of mothers, with appropriate guidance and occasional professional support from the health system, growth monitoring forms the basic recurring activity of Indonesian village level primary health care. The monthly health and social occasion is looked forward to by the village women as a chance to see their friends, pick-up practical tips on improving their home environment and assuring that their child is healthy or that appropriate interventions are taken even before he may appear to be sick or undernourished. Convenient, enjoyable, affordable and relevant, growth monitoring in the village, with accent on dialogue, and timely health intervention, is a practical means to high coverage community involvement in promotive child health.

Furthermore, village-based growth monitoring activities pull primary health care out of the health facilities and into the community itself. Villages have begun to demand services at the monthly rallies, asking for immunization, ORT, deworming, contraceptive resupply, vitamin A and simple curative care in the village. There, it becomes relevant, demand responsive and achieves high coverage of the most needy population.

The feedback cycle, so important to the individual child and mother pair, works also to stimulate primary health care. Health workers themselves find growth monitoring a rewarding means of measuring the impact of their own interaction with mothers and of other programmes designed to improve the health of the communities. In Indonesia, villagers record the level of participation in their weighing programme and the percentage of children gaining weight, recognizing that weight gain in the village as a whole is a reflection of the general health of the entire community. Low levels of weight gain have been the first indicator to detect epidemic illness, food shortage and impending large scale hunger, recognizing that the youngest members of the community are the most susceptible to even modest changes in food availability. Feedback as a measure of nutritional health becomes the motivating tool for health workers and their supervisors can immediately see which communities are prospering and which need more attention.

For too long, the nutrition community has abdicated its natural place in the hierarchy of public health programmes. Let us speak out with far greater clarity and purpose to carry our message beyond even the realms of health care providers to those in positions of political power and responsibility. Let us clearly state that there cannot be health without proper nutrition, that regular growth in the first 2 years is the critical foundation of health throughout a lifetime, and that only through monitoring that growth can mothers be expected to perceive, appreciate and act to assure normal growth. Let us offer regular growth monitoring, with all appropriate concern for culturally sensitive, practical involvement of mothers in the understanding and implementation of healthy child rearing, as a strategy uniquely tailored to the needs of each and every child, whatever his circumstances of birth. This same strategy, offered to health planners will assure that primary health care will reach the largest number of needy people in the most timely and cost effective manner possible. Feeding and feedback — the way to a healthy child, and to a universal system of primary health care.

Nutrition and fertility

F.T. SAI
World Bank, Washington, D.C., USA.

The common observation that people in the less developed countries (LDCs) tend to produce more children than those in the industrialized countries has misled some observers into believing that mild/moderate malnutrition and the existence of poverty are themselves stimulants to higher reproduction in the human. This is probably a false interpretation of the observed facts. The higher reproduction in LDCs is probably a function of poverty and the conditions of living which make people feel they want to have more children rather than actual biological factors which influence their fertility.

Human reproduction can be broken into two components. One is fecundity which may be described as the latent capacity for reproduction. The other is fertility, the ability to get pregnant, to carry a pregnancy to term and produce a live offspring. The influence of nutritional status on both of these has been analysed extensively in many animals. However, findings with animals cannot be completely translated to the humans. In studying these interactions in the human there have been many serious problems. The effects of extreme malnutrition such as severe famines are clear enough but those of marginal malnutrition which are the most widespread types of malnutrition have proved difficult of study and interpretation. The problems are due to: (1) inadequacies in the methodologies available for measuring relative states of moderate malnutrition; (2) the complexity of confounding factors which interact with nutrients and influence several components of the reproductive cycle and their measurement; and (3) incomplete understanding of adaptive and physiological mechanisms that are mobilized during pregnancy when dietary inadequacies occur.

Much of the evidence that marginal malnutrition, particularly with respect to micronutrients, has functional reproductive consequences comes from demographic statistics and epidemiological studies; and their interpretation is not easy, since such studies only provide data on associations and definitive linkages cannot be affixed to them. There have been all too few studies on nutritional status methodology designed to come up with measurements which mean something in terms of survival, health and reproductive performance. There may also be a lack of a formalized system to digest and act upon data even when these are available. Efforts to tackle these problems are urgently needed.

Fecundity and nutrition. The capacity to reproduce, or fecundity, can be determined by different biological factors. These include: (a) age at menarche; (b) age at menopause; (c) regularity of ovulation among menstruating women; (d) the quality and quantity of sperm; (e) prevalance of primary sterility; and (f) ovulation inhibiting effect of breast-feeding. From studies based on blockaded European cities during World War I, on the Spanish Civil War and from others based on concentration camps in World War II, from the Leningrad Siege and from the classic analyses of the Hongerwinter of the Dutch cities during October 1944 to May 1945, many important findings relating to severe malnutrition and fecundity have been reported[33,34]. Women in these famine situations reported amenorrhoea and it was believed that they also had anovular cycles from gonadal atrophy. The conclusion that such amenorrhoea was entirely due to malnutrition is not clear cut since it is known that psychological stresses such as fear of death and anxiety may precipitate amenorrhoea[4]. In fact, people who have been observing young women changing roles and positions in life have sometimes come across inexplicable periods of amenorrhoea.

People displaced or incarcerated during World War II reported that amenorrhoea tended to occur after 2 or 3 months' internment. However, after about 18 to 20 months of internment without too many changes in the living and food conditions the amenorrhoea disappeared and regular cycles were re-established[25]. This would tend to support the belief that the amenorrhoea is not only caused by the nutritional changes to which they were being subjected. American doctors who were interned in Japanese camps during the war[39] tended to believe that psychological factors had a very important role to play. It was not so much the low level of the daily ration in absolute figures which was the cause of the amenorrhoea as the sudden deterioration of the diet, both in quality and quantity[35]. It is thus likely that the amenorrhoea, although related to nutrition in the beginning, had other causes and in the end adaptive forces came into play which re-established regularity of menstruation.

Anorexia nervosa, a severe form of self-inflicted, chronic malnutrition, is accompanied by amenorrhoea or irregularity of ovulation. Here again, it is difficult to separate the purely nutritional reasons for the amenorrhoea from the psychological state which precipitated the self-induced starvation in the first case. In the classic experiment of Keys *et al.*[20] male voluteers who were subjected to a 50 per cent reduction in energy intake for 23 weeks demonstrated a loss of libido, decrease in sperm motility and longevity. Starvation appeared to depress the functions of the sex organs. Women also appeared to lose libido in periods of starvation. When feeding was re-established the effects of severe starvation or famine on fecundity seemed to disappear completely. These must, therefore, be considered as temporary.

The menarche. Human fertility in a woman is, to a certain extent, dependent on the duration of time between the menarche and the menopause. In Western societies with relatively reliable historical data, a decline in the age of menarche of about 3 years has taken place since the end of the last century[41]. In the 1800s in Scandinavia, for example, 16 years was the average age of menarche. It is now about 13 years[10]. Averages in developing countries are typically higher and vary very substantially both between countries and, in many cases, within countries. For example, Cuba with relatively good nutrition and health status has an average age at menarche of 12.4[16]. It is 15.7 in Bangladesh[6] and 18.8 among the Bundi in New Guinea[16].

A direct link between the age at menarche and nutritional status has been established in studies in the United States and Europe. Well-nourished girls in United States have been found to start menstruating some two years earlier than under-nourished girls[11]. Similarly, an Indian study concluded that girls whose diets were higher in energy and protein had earlier menarche[2]. In an effort to explain the link between nutrition and menarche, many have tried to point out that there is a critical weight at which menarche typically occurs. Frisch & McArthur[13] postulated that the maintenance of regular ovulatory cycles in women is dependent on the maintenance of a minimum weight for height; and went on to state that there is a critical weight at which menarche typically occurs. Frisch & McArthur[13] postulated that the maintenance of regular ovulatory cycles in women is dependent on the maintenance of a minimum weight for height; and went on to state that there was a critical fat storage requirement for the establishment of regular cycles. This has been questioned by others. However, in favour of the theory of critical weight and fat stores may be put the fact that ballet dancers and athletes tend to have delayed age at menarche and high incidence of irregular cycles and amenorrhoea. When intense activities are decreased the regular menstrual cycles return.

The available evidence regarding the determinants of age at menopause is conflicting and inconclusive. The confusing results are probably due in part to enormous methodological problems in obtaining accurate age information and research is complicated by the fact that menopause is a gradual phenomenon and not so well defined as menarche. No conclusive evidence regarding nutritional influence on age at menopause is provided by the studies Bongaarts analysed[4]. On the other hand, Frisch[12] concluded that there was a time trend discernible for Western populations; that the average age at menopause in 1850 was between 45 and 50 years and the average age for present day women is about 50 years or more. The chances, however, are that in modern society the age of menopause is unlikely to influence fertility to any great extent because by the time women approach menopause, the majority of those in developed countries would have long since stopped childbearing. LDC programme efforts are emphasizing this too.

Regularity of ovulation, another component of fecundity, has been very difficult to measure directly. It is measured as the number of months between the occurrence of the first postpartum menses, an indicator of the resumption of ovulation, and the next conception[4]. Two prospective studies of poorly nourished women in Bangladesh[36] and Guatemala[3] were specifically designed to test the effect of nutritional status on mean waiting time to conception. In both populations contraceptions and induced abortions are little used. The mean waiting time for groups of women with different weights were not statistically significant in the Bangladesh study after controlling for the confounding effect of age and absences of husband. There was no correlation between other anthropometric measures and mean waiting time. In the Guatemala study nutritional status was differentiated into low, medium and high categories based on a composite nutrition index, and according to Bongaarts & Delgado[3], there was no relationship between nutritional status and mean waiting time.

The evidence would suggest that behavioural factors such as breast-feeding, frequency of sexual activity are far more significant determinants of these intervals as discussed later than the nutritional status of the population.

Fertility and nutrition. Nutritional deprivation of considerable severity as has occurred in famines or mass starvation is associated with large, but temporary, reduction in fertility[4]. Some evidence from 17th and 18th century Europe indicate that the malnutrition that followed food crises with rises in food prices led to declines in birth rates. Few of these studies have reported the systematic effects of famines on the determinants of fertility. Notable exceptions are the account of Valaoras[38] on the effect of the famine in Greece 1941–1942 on births, deaths and child growth and on the effects of the siege of Leningrad in 1943 on fertility and perinatal morbidity and mortality[1]. The best documented is the Dutch famine which took place from October 1944 to May 1945 in an otherwise well-nourished population[33]. The birthrate did not change during the actual period of famine, but some 9 months later fertility was reduced by more than 50 per cent. A fertility decline of nearly the same magnitude was observed after the 1974–75 famine in Bangladesh where the birthrate declined from about 45 per thousand population before the famine to 27.5 for the period of April 1975 to March 1976[26]. In all cases there was a marked increase in miscarriages.

This finding has been supported by Ifekunigwe[17], who says of the Biafran experience: when pregnancy took place the incidence of miscarriage was also markedly raised. Whether some micronutrients are implicated or whether this is due to general intrauterine deprivation is not clear.

In the Dutch population a steep rise in conceptions immediately after the liberation marked the restoration of susceptibility to fertilization. The immediate recovery of fertility in the population suggests that there was immediate physiological recovery of sexual activity, normal ovulation and fecundity in general. The excessive fetal loss also ceased.

Perhaps the most important lesson to be learned from famines is the great resilience of human populations exposed to the harshest nutritional psychological and environmental forces, especially as regards the maintenance of reproductive capacity.

Moderate undernutrition and pregnancy outcome. The evidence of a link between moderate maternal malnutrition and fetal mortality is still being researched. A study of this subject is limited by methodogical problems in measuring the prevalence of interuterine mortality, especially during the early months of gestation[23]. Estimates of total fetal mortality rates do not differ substantially between well-nourished and relatively undernourished populations, although still-birth ratios are somewhat higher among poorly nourished women[1,39]. The absence of a statistically significant difference in the fetal mortality rates of the developed and the developing countries would tend to suggest that nutrition does not have a very large effect.

Independent studies in the United States and Sweden have yielded estimates for fetal mortality ranging from 12.5 to 33.9 fetal deaths per 100 conceptions[23]. Similar investigations in underdeveloped countries report figures within the range of 14.9 per cent in Matlab Thana, Bangladesh[5] and 16 to 19 per cent and 30 per cent in two surveys in India. Low birth weight and prematurity are the commonest causes of death in the neonatal period, not counting neonatal tetanus in some settings. These are both correlated to maternal prepregnancy weight and pregnancy weight gain. Studies on maternal nutrition and the birth weight of infants have not yielded uniform results. A review of the literature and data from the INCAP longitudinal study in Guatemala[22] confirmed that maternal nutrition both before and during pregnancy has an effect on birth weight. They suggested that there appeared to be a minimum level of nutrients which must be made available in order to obtain adequate birth weight. However, above this minimum level pregnant women may adapt themselves to a wide variety of food intake — both in quantity and quality — without affecting birth weight of the child. There is no comment on what happens below the minimum level. The authors also concluded that nutritional supplementation programmes for malnourished mothers have been successful in increasing birth weight in spite of the usual range of barriers to successful implementation.

Other factors, such as physical activity, prevalence of disease and magnitude of the maternal nutritional stores before pregnancy, are also important determinants of the relative contribution of energy, protein and other nutrients to increments in birth weight.

Many other studies have not supported these findings. On the whole the evidence would seem to indicate that manipulation of supplements to the mother, particularly during the final trimester, manages to increase the birth weight of the child an average of 300 g only. Studies in Gambia of pregnant women during various seasons would tend to support the findings that when food is short during pregnancy, supplementation made a great deal more difference to the final weight of the child than during seasons when food is plentiful according to the local situation, although in both seasons the women were consuming a lot less than the recommended dietary allowance.

The fetus is not a completely efficient parasite so it is affected to some extent by shortages in the mother. Cretinism of infants of goitrous mothers, vitamin A deficiency of infants and infantile beriberi are examples. On the other hand, pregnancy may denude a mother of nutrients. Iron and folic acid anaemias, deficiencies of some vitamins of the B group in the mother are all aggravated by pregnancy.

Breast-feeding and postpartum amenorrhoea. Recent research has looked into the relationship between breast-feeding and resumption of menstruation, resumption of ovulation, birth intervals or subsequent pregnancy. The conclusion is that breast-feeding delays resumption of menstruation, inhibits ovulation and reduces the likelihood of conception, thus making a substantial contribution to birth spacing and fertility control in many parts of the world[32]. However, breast-feeding cannot be depended on as a predictably safe birth spacing method for an individual woman.

In many parts of the world a positive correlation has been demonstrated between the duration of breast-feeding and the length of postpartum amenorrhoea, and this relationship is least consistent among groups in whom breast-feeding is relatively short — 12 months or less —or relatively long — over 20 months. In the intermediate range, however, each additional month of breast-feeding means an average of almost one additional month of amenorrhoea[18,19,28]. Again, owing to difficulties of detecting ovulation, studies in resumption of ovulation are few and small with widely varying results. In some eight studies, the percentage of breast-feeding women identified as ovulating before the first menses ranged from 12 to 78 per cent[30] and the longer the time since delivery the more likely ovulation is to precede menstruation. A Chilean study[29] concluded that ovulation before first menses was most likely in non-breast-feeding women, intermediate in partially breast-feeding and least likely in fully breast-feeding women. Because duration of breast-feeding and the length of postpartum infecundity are linked, any substantial shortening of the average duration of breast-feeding is likely to lead to higher fertility unless contraceptive use increases fast enough to counteract this effect. In some populations, especially in urban areas where women are exposed to modernizing influences, fertility may already be increasing largely because of declines in breast-feeding without compensating increase in the use of contraception[27].

Suckling and fecundity. The ovulation and menstruation-inhibiting effect of breast-feeding and also the differential effect of breast-feeding patterns are believed to be due to a neurally mediated[8] hormonal reflex system initiated by the suckling stimulation of the breast nipple. The hormone prolactin secreted by the anterior pituitary gland as a result of an infant suckling stimulates the production of breast-milk. The same hormone is believed to inhibit the ovary and the corpus luteum. A woman's level of prolactin is highest and the duration of amenorrhoea and anovulation longest when the infant continues suckling at the breast. The more frequent the suckling, the higher the levels of prolactin and the longer the duration of amenorrhoea. As suckling frequency decreases, prolactin levels fall and ovulation resumes[30]. Studies of the direct link between suckling intensity and frequency and duration of infecundity are few. In cultures where maternal infant contact is continual and where there is easy unrestricted access to the breast, as is typical for rural Bangladesh, among the nomadic Kung-Hunter gatherers[21] and some areas of Africa[14], lactational amenorrhoea may last 12 to 18 months or longer and birth intervals are as long as 24 to 36 months or more — four years, among the Kung. Animal studies have also shown that the anovulatory period lasts longer with stronger and more frequent suckling.

Effect of supplementary food on suckling and ovulation. By 6 months, virtually all infants need some complementary food to add to the breast-milk. Although there are conflicting and non-conclusive reports from the pre-industrial world, most studies would indicate that the lactational amenorrhoea period ends shortly after complementary food is introduced[7,37]. The question is how do poor mothers who want to regulate their fertility adequately meet the nutritional needs of the nursling for complementary food while maintaining the full contraceptive effects of breast-feeding? Among well-nourished lactating women in Scotland[24], infant food supplementation was associated with a rapid decrease in the total duration of suckling, a decline in the maternal serum prolactin levels and the resumption of ovarian activity. The return of fertility among these well-nourished women was attributed to a decrease in suckling duration, presumably a consequence of the reduction of the infant's dependence on breast-milk for meeting his full nutritional needs. In contrast to this, among very marginally nourished rural African tribes[14] where there was no dietary substitute for mother's milk, introduction of semi-solid local food as a breast-milk complement, which occurs as early as 15 to 21 days post partum while maintaining natural on demand access to the breast, did not influence maternal prolactin levels. The volume of milk produced by these women was uniformly small and the child suckled constantly. Mean serum prolactin levels among these women remained above the threshold where ovulation recurs in this population up to approximately 15 months[9].

Maternal nutrition and lactational amenorrhoea. The extent to which chronic malnutrition itself lengthens the period of amenorrhoea and infecundity in breast-feeding women is not known. The question which arises is whether improvement in maternal nutrition would shorten amenorrhoea and thereby increase fertility. The bulk of evidence would appear to indicate that maternal nutrition *per se* does not play a major role in determining the length of postpartum amenorrhoea. The strongest evidence for an association between dietary intake and postpartum amenorrhoea is indicated in studies in the Gambia in which lactating women were provided with a biscuit-based supplement resulting in a mean net increase in energy intake of over 700 kcal (2.9 MJ) per day. The supplement produced a slight initial improvement in maternal body weight and subcutaneous fat stores but did not increase milk output or fat content[8,31]. However, this substantial supplementation of the mothers' diets lowered prolactin levels. Lactational amenorrhoea as evidenced by oestrogen levels lasted about 10 months in the women who received food supplements compared to about 16 months in women who received no supplements. The researchers speculate that prolonged high prolactin concentrations found in under-nourished mothers may enhance milk synthesis when food intake is limited by preferentially channelling nutrients towards the breast. Alternatively, the lower hormonal levels associated with improved maternal nutrition may shorten the period of postpartum infertility, despite prolonged breast-feeding. A major finding in this study is the relationship between prolactin levels, diet and season. During the wet season, a time of food shortages and low energy intakes and high energy expenditure caused by agricultural demands, the prolactin levels remained highest. Prolactin levels were intermediate during the dry season but when diets were supplemented during the dry season, prolactin levels were lowest.

Fertility regulation. Many of the fertility-regulation methods that are used today have at least a potential for interacting with nutritional levels and nutrients or with the metabolism of the woman. Oral contraceptive agents have been known to cause metabolic changes in women which, in theory at least, may influence requirements for certain vitamins and minerals. In a review of the literature[36] cited studies found increased requirements for zinc, pyridoxine, folic acid, riboflavin and ascorbic acid along with lower requirements for iron, calcium, copper, niacin and vitamin A. Since then, several investigations have been done but no convincing evidence has been found. It must be stressed that the formulations which were being studied then are not the ones in use today and the changes with the current formulations are likely to be of much smaller orders of magnitude. No real need for supplements has therefore been demonstrated.

The old formulations of the pill appeared to have quite marked effect on breast-milk production. The oestrogen component has generally been blamed for reduced milk yield and/or reduction in the duration of breast-feeding. By contrast, nearly all studies of progestin only contraceptives, whether pills or injectables, have found either a beneficial effect, an increase in milk volume or no measurable effect. The newer formulations of the contraceptive pill would appear to have little or no effect on maintenance of lactation once it has been properly established. Some later studies have refuted this and appear to prove that on even newer combined pills breast-milk production is lessened in quantity and duration. However, since it is recognized that in malnourished populations, the return to fertility is unlikely to be under 12 months, starting to give combined pill contraceptives before this period is not advisable. Small amounts of contraceptives are transmitted to the infant in breast-milk and although no serious immediate effect has been noticed, long-term effects need to be studied. The reason for concern about infants receiving hormones is that naturally produced hormones are known to influence normal physical development at various points. For example, early fetal exposure to hormones can lead to birth defects[40] or in the well known instance of the oestrogen diethylstilbestrol (DES) induces vaginal cancer when a daughter exposed *in utero* reaches adolescence[15].

Voluntary sterilization is an appropriate postpartum fertility control method for breast-feeding women who deliver in hospitals or health centres and want permanent protection against another pregnancy. It has been reported that postpartum sterilization has no adverse effects on breast-feeding. However, one study has found that women sterilized 4 to 6 days after delivery produced less milk for as long as 2 weeks postpartum. This suggests that an adverse effect may occur; however the determination of whether this is from the type of anaesthesia has not been done and more studies would be useful.

Conclusions. What is known so far would suggest the need for much more research on the effect of marginal malnutrition on reproductive efficiency, much more work on complementary feeding of mothers and the outcome of pregnancy, and more multi-centre studies on the interaction of breast-feeding and contraception. A better identification of when to initiate hormonal contraception in LDCs is very necessary. There should be a search for a safe contraceptive that will enhance lactation without being secreted in the breast-milk. Programmes to improve maternal health an nutrition should include family planning, so that such improvement does not lead to a shortening of the interval between births.

1 Antonov, A.N. (1947): Children born during the siege of Leningrad in 1942. *J. Pediatr.* **30**, 250–259.
2 Bhalla, M. & Shrivastava, J.R. (1974): Indian adolescent females on diets with greater protein and calories reach menarche sooner. *Indian Pediatr.* **11**, 487–493.
3 Bongaarts, J. & Delgado, H. (1977): Effects of nutritional status on fertility. Intl. Popn. Conference, Mexico, 1977, p. 17.
4 Bongaarts, J. (1980): Does malnutrition affect fecundity? A summary of evidence. *Science* **208**, 564–569.
5 Chen, L.C., Ahmed, S., Gesche, M. & Mosley, W.H. (1974): A prospective study of birth interval dynamics in rural Bangladesh. *Popn. Stud.* **28**, 277–297.
6 Chowdhury, A.K.M., Huffman, S.L. & Curlin, G.T. (1977): Malnutrition, menarche, and marriage in rural Bangladesh. *Soc. Biol.* **24**, 316–325.
7 Delgado, H., Brineman, E., Lechtig, A., Bongaarts, J., Martorell, R. & Klein, R.E. (1979). Effect of maternal nutritional status and infant supplementation during lactation on postpartum amenorrhoea. *Am. J. Obstet. Gynec.* **135**, 303–307.
8 Delvoye, P., Delogne-Desnock, J. & Robyn, C. (1976): Serum-prolactin in long lasting lactational amenorrhoea. *Lancet* **2**, 288–89.
9 Delvoye, P., Desmaegd, M., Uwayitu-Nyampeta & Robyn, C. (1978): Serum prolactin, gonadotropins, and estradiol in menstruating and amenorrheic mothers during two years' lactation. *Am. J. Obstet. Gynec.* **130**, 635–639.
10 Eveleth, P.B. & Tanner, J.M. eds (1976): *Worldwide variation in human growth.* London: Cambridge University Press.
11 Frisch, R.E. (1972): Weight at menarche: similarity for well-nourished and under-nourished girls at differing ages, and evidence for historical constancy. *Pediatrics* **50**, 445–450.
12 Frisch, R.E. (1978): Population, food intake and fertility. *Science* **199**, 22–30.
13 Frisch, R.E. & McArthur, J. (1974): Menstrual cycles: fatness as a determinant of minimum weight for height necessary for their maintenance or onset. *Science* **185**, 949–951.
14 Hennart, P. & Vis, H.L. (1980): Breast-feeding and postpartum amenorrhea in Central Africa. 1. Milk production in rural areas. *J. Trop. Pediatr.* **26**, 177–183.
15 Herbst, A.L., Scully, R.E., Robboy, S.J. & Welch, W.R. (1978): Complications of prenatal therapy with diethylstibestrol. *Pediatrics* **62**, 1151–1159.
16 Hiernaux, J. (1968): Ethnic differences in growth and development. *Eugen. Q.* **15**, 12–21.
17 Ifekunigwe, A. (1971): In *Famine*, ed G. Blix, Y. Hofvander & B. Vahlqvist, pp. 144–154. Uppsala: Almqvist Wiksell.

18　Jain, A.K., Hsu, T.C., Freedman, R. & Chang, M.C. (1970): Demographic aspects of lactation and post partum amenorrhea. *Demography* **7**, 255–271.

19　Jain, A.K. & Sun, T.H. (1972): Inter-relationships between socio-demographic factors, lactation and postpartum amenorrhea. *Demography India* **1**, 3–15.

20　Keys, A.B., Brozek, J., Henschel, A., Michelson, O. & Taylor, H.L. (1950) *The biology of human starvation*, pp. 745–763. Minneapolis: University of Minneapolis Press.

21　Konner, M. & Worthman, C. (1980): Nursing frequency, gonadal function, and birth spacing among !Kung Hunter Gatherers. *Science* **107**, 788–791.

22　Lechtig, A., Delgado, H., Martorell, R., Yarbrough, C. & Klein, R.E. (1979): Materno-fetal nutrition. In *Human nutrition, Vol. 2*, ed D.B. Jelliffe. New York: Academic Press.

23　Leridon, H. ed (1977): *Human fertility: the basic components*. Chicago. University of Chicago Press.

24　McNeilly, A.S., Howie, P.W. & Houston, M.J. (1980): Relationship of feeding patterns, prolactin, and resumption of ovulation post-partum. In *Research frontiers in fertility regulation*, ed G.I. Zutuchi, M.J. Labbok & J.J. Sciarra, pp. 102–116. New York: Harper and Row.

25　Mondot-Bernard, J.M. (1977): Relationships between fertility, child mortality and nutrition in Africa. Technical paper for Organization for Economic Cooperation and Development, Paris.

26　Mosley, W.H. (1979): In *Patterns and determinants of natural fertility*, ed J.A. Menken & H. Levidon. Liege: Ordina.

27　Nag, M. (1979): How modernization can also increase fertility. *Center for Policy Studies Working Paper No. 49.*, p. 49. New York: Population Council.

28　Perez, A., Vela, P., Mesnick, G.S. & Potter, R.G. (1972): First ovulation after childbirth: the effect of breast-feeding. *Am. J. Obstet. Gynecol.* **114**, 1041–1047.

29　Perez, A., Vela, P., Potter, R. & Masnick, G.S. (1971): Timing and sequence of resuming ovulation and menstruation after childbirth. *Popn. Stud.* **25** (3): 491–503.

30　Population Reports Series J.24 (1981): *Breastfeeding, fertility and family planning*. Population information program. Baltimore, Maryland: The Johns Hopkins University.

31　Prentice, A.M., Roberts, S.B., Watkinson, M., Whitehead, R.G., Paul, A.A., Prentice, A. & Watkinson, A.A. (1980): Dietary supplementation of Gambian nursing mothers and lactational performance. *Lancet* **2**, 866–888.

32　Rosa, F. (1974): Breast-feeding and family planning (Editorial). *J. Trop. Pediatr. Envir. Child Hlth* **20**, 273–274.

33　Stein, Z. & Susser, M. (1978): Famine and fertility. In *Nutrition and human reproduction* ed W.H. Mosley. pp. 123–145. New York: Plenum Press.

34　Stein, Z., Susser, M., Saenger, G. & Marolla, F. (1975): *Famine and human development: the Dutch hunger winter of 1944–45*. New York: Oxford University Press.

35　Sydenham, A. (1947): Amenorrhea at Stanley Camp, Hong Kong, during internment. *J. Clin. Endocr. Metab.* **7**, 659.

36　Theuer, R.C. (1972): Effect of oral contraceptive agents on vitamin and mineral needs: a review. *J. Reprod. Med.* **8**, 13–19.

37　Underwood, B.A. & Hovrander, Y. (1982): Appropriate timing for complementary feeding of the breastfed infant. *Acta Paediatr. Scand. (Suppl.)*, 1–32.

38　Valaoras, V.G. (1946): Some effects of famine on the population of Greece. *Milbank Mem. Fund Q.* **24**, 215–234.

39　Whitacre, F. & Barrera, B.(1944): War amenorrhea: a clinical and laboratory study. *Am. Med. Ass. J.* **124**, 399–403.

40　Wilson, J.G. (1973): *Environment and birth defects*, p. 305. New York: Academic Press.

41　Zacharias, L. & Wurtman, R.J. (1969): Age at menarche. Genetic and environmental infuences. *New Eng. J. Med.* **280**, 868–875.

★　★　★

THE CONTRIBUTIONS OF THE UN AGENCIES TO NUTRITION

The contribution of the World Health Organization to nutrition

A. PRADILLA
Nutrition Unit, WHO, 1211 Geneva 27, Switzerland.

Most members of the international nutrition community know of the World Health Organization (WHO), even if not all may understand precisely the role it plays in nutrition. Many people I have met during the 7 years I have been part of WHO have frankly questioned whether health plays any role in the preventive aspects of malnutrition and it is useful to elaborate on the nature of the WHO, the kind of support it provides its members, and how these factors combine to influence its basic orientation towards nutrition.

The structure of WHO. WHO, which was established in 1948, is a specialized agency of the United Nationals system. Its objective is the attainment by all peoples of the highest level of health, which its constitution describes as a state of complete physical, mental and social well-being and not merely the absence of disease or infirmity.

The organization consists of member states associated for the purpose of cooperating among themselves and with others, for example nongovernmental and voluntary organizations, to protect and promote the health of all peoples. In 1948 WHO had fewer than 60 Member States; today it has 166. It functions through three main organs. The World Health Assembly, which meets once a year, is the Organization's supreme decision-making body. The Executive board, which meets twice a year, is composed of 31 health professionals designated by as many member states on a rotating basis. The main function of the board is to give effect to the decisions and policies of the Assembly. In addition, it is responsible for submitting to the Health Assembly, for its consideration and approval, a general programme of work covering a specific period. The Board acts on behalf of the whole membership of the organization and not only those countries that have been elected to represent its members. The WHO Secretariat is the organization's staff as a whole, throughout the world, comprising the Director-General as its chief technical and administrative officer and such other staff as may be required.

The main role of the Secretariat is to support member states in their national and international action for health, to facilitate technical cooperation among them, and to ensure technical cooperation between WHO and the individual members on the basis of internationally agreed policies.

The headquarters of WHO are in Geneva. However, a characteristic feature of the organization is its high degree of decentralization. It has six regional organizations: one for Africa, with the regional office in Brazzaville; one for the Americas, with the regional office in Washington; one for South-East Asia, with the regional office in New Delhi; one for Europe, with the regional office in Copenhagen; one for the Eastern Mediterranean, with the regional office in Alexandria; and one for the Western Pacific, with the regional office in Manila. Membership in the regional organizations is mainly, but not necessarily, geographically determined, since member states are free to select the region to which they wish to belong.

According to the constitution, each regional organization is an integral part of the organization and consists of a regional committee and a regional office. The head of each regional office is the Regional Director, who is appointed by the Executive Board after nomination by the regional committee.

Finally, the organization also includes the International Agency for Research on Cancer (IARC), which was established by the World Health Assembly in 1965 as an autonomous body within WHO, having its own statutes, membership and budget. IARC has its headquarters in Lyon, France and its main objectives are to generate and disseminate information useful for the primary prevention of cancer, through both intra- and extra-mural activities.

WHO's general programme of work. The constitution of the WHO requires its Executive Board to submit a general programme of work covering a specific period. The Assembly has thus far adopted seven general programmes of work, the latest covering the period 1984–1989. These programmes were formulated by the Executive Board, approved by the World Health Assembly, and subsequently adapted to regional needs by the regional committees. The current programme of work provides the framework for all the organization's actions. It is made up of a number of specific programmes, each consisting of activities directed towards the attainment of specific objectives. The totality of the programmes organized as just described is called a classified list of programmes, which is used not only for the general programme of work but also for all the components of the WHO managerial process.

The foundations of WHO's nutrition policy. Let us now focus more directly on nutrition, not by leaving WHO's structure and programme of work, but by linking these two all-important elements with the organization's view of the role of nutrition in health, the role of the health sector in nutrition, and the role of WHO in supporting the health sector.

The nutrition policy of the WHO should be viewed in the light of the two overriding concepts that govern all of the organization's work:

Health for all by the year 2000, which is the main social target of governments and WHO calling for the attainment by all people of the world by the year 2000 of a level of health that will permit them to lead a socially and economically productive life; and

Primary health care, the key to attaining the goal of health for all, which is essential care made accessible at a cost the country and community can afford, with methods that are practical, scientifically sound and socially acceptable, and which involves related sectors in addition to the health sector.

In accordance with the 1978 Declaration of Alma-Ata, the *promotion of food supply and proper nutrition* is one of the eight essential elements of primary health care.

Defining malnutrition: the perspective of the WHO. As measured by growth performance in children and body size and composition in adults, malnutrition is a major public health problem the world over, and not just in developing countries where wasting and stunting are but its most conspicuous signs. In industrialized countries, too, malnutrition is rampant, with obesity ranking first together with its allied conditions: hypertension, cardiovascular disorders and, probably, a number of cancers.

Nutritional status is the result of a complex interaction of a multitude of individual, household, community, national and international factors. Food must first be produced and procured, whether directly by the individual or through cash payment, in exchange for labour, or by some other means. Food must be prepared, cooked and consumed. Dependent persons — the very young, the very old and the infirm — must be fed. Ingested food must be digested, absorbed and utilized by the body.

In ideal circumstances nutritional status is largely the result of individual choice, tempered by knowledge and perceived needs. Malnutrition in most industrialized countries, where choice is genuine, and among a growing number of elite sub-populations in the developing world, is thus characterized by an excess of nutrients or a nutrient imbalance. By the same token, the most common forms of malnutrition in developing countries are also present in what have been referred to as pockets of poverty in otherwise well-off societies. The number, variety and complexity of factors associated with malnutrition, and their effects on populations both within and between countries, are such that it would be foolhardy to prescribe standarized solutions. It is no different when trying to assign a precise mix of sectoral roles and responsibilities for ensuring balanced nutrition. Nevertheless, I believe that it is useful to explore briefly the role of the sector I know best — the health sector — in the prevention, detection and management of malnutrition.

The role of the health sector in dealing with malnutrition. It is obvious that one sector, acting alone, cannot expect to cope with all, or even most, of malnutrition's causes and contributing factors. Although there is agreement that this is the case of the health sector, as with any other, there is considerably less certainty within the international nutrition community as to the exact role health has to play in this regard. What does the WHO consider the role of the health sector to be and what is the Organization's nutrition programme in support of this view?

WHO considers that the health sector has both a *direct* and an *indirect* role to play in dealing with malnutrition:

Direct: in terms of identifying the major causes of malnutrition in specific epidemiological circumstances; promoting appropriate dietary and health habits; preventing detecting and managing transmissible diseases through improvements in environmental health and at the level of service delivery; promoting and facilitating convenient and desired reproductive behaviour; and detecting and managing disease and malnutrition to prevent further deterioration and death, while striving to reverse the process through appropriate rehabilitative care.

Indirect: in terms of monitoring the overall nutritional situation and calling planners' and decision-makers' attention to problems and their consequences; acting together with other sectors so as to ensure that the numerous non-health factors contributing to malnutrition are addressed; serving as an advocate for an intersectoral approach to malnutrition prevention and management; and advising other sectors of the probable consequences of action proposed or taken by them.

The nutrition programme of the WHO. This programme is geared to implementing *health interventions that have an impact on the nutritional status* of individuals, families and communities; to including *specific nutrition concepts and activities* at all levels of the health system; and to undertaking *joint action* with other sectors, agencies, organizations and so forth for improving nutritional status.

The first and most critical programme component is the development of an appropriate infrastructure for the delivery of nutrition-related services. At the same time ways must be found to stimulate the use of these services and increase awareness by people and communities of their responsibility for self-care and for family and community care. The precise technical content of health services, whether nutrition-specific or not, will vary depending on local circumstances. What will not vary, however, is the need for an appropriate delivery system. The nutrition programme has a dual orientation, first and most obviously towards the health sector and all of the health-related means for promoting proper nutrition and combatting malnutrition; and second, given the multiple non-health causes and contributing factors of malnutrition, towards close collaboration with others.

In the final analysis, improvement in nutritional status can only occur through national efforts. WHO's support of the development of national infrastructure, including the strengthening of national capabilities in nutrition, is the central focus of all its nutrition activities. This approach, which may appear to have little or no result in the short term, often yields maximum sustainable results in the longer term. This challenge is implicit in every aspect of the nutrition programme.

Although targets and outcomes will vary according to the specific needs of countries, there are three broad means at the organization's disposal for implementing its nutrition programme:

(1) Promoting awareness of the prevalence of the major nutritional deficiencies, their causes, and their effects on the health of vulnerable groups.

(2) Supporting the development and promoting the application of improved methods of malnutrition prevention, detection and control.

(3) Providing technical and other support to countries for strengthening their capabilities for preventing and managing malnutrition, including problem definition; programme formulation, implementation, monitoring and evaluation; and the development of suitable training activities, in collaboration with bodies and organizations of the United Nations system, and with the support of bilateral development agencies.

Summary and conclusion. The scale and seriousness of the health problems caused by inappropriate dietary intake are enormous. The prevalence of malnutrition in both the developing and developed world is also staggering. The tragedy of these problems is based on the gap between already available knowledge, technologies and resources and the present commitment, feasibility and impact of policy in countries.

Many of the fundamental causes of malnutrition can be controlled by the health system, and even though wider action by other sectors is indispensable for its complete control, the health sector is capable of preventing the major consequences of less-than-optimal dietary intake. What is more, the technology to fulfil this promise is in large part available now. The role of the WHO as the United Nations specialized agency responsible for matters of health, is to stimulate the development of appropriate national and international commitment at policy and operational levels, provide the necessary technical support for the development of effective national health systems, and facilitate the introduction of health objectives in the development objectives of other sectors. This role is played, where nutrition is concerned, as part of a coherent blend of action within the health sector and beyond.

Some WHO publications relating to nutrition.
A36/7 — Infant and young child nutrition, including the nutritional value and safety of products specifically intended for infant and young child feeding and the status of compliance with and implementation of the international code of marketing of breast-milk substitutes (1983).

A37/6 — Infant and young child nutrition (Progress and evaluation report; status of implementation of the international code of marketing of breast-milk substitutes). (1984)

'Health for All' Series:
1 'Alma-Ata 1978: primary health care' (1978)
2 'Formulating strategies for health for all by the year 2000' (1979)
3 'Global strategy for health for all by the year 2000' (1981)
4 'Development of indicators for monitoring progress towards health for all by the year 2000' (1981)
5 'Managerial process for national health development: guiding principles' (1981)
6 'Health programme evaluation: guiding principles' (1981)
7 'Plan of action for implementing the global strategy for health for all and index to the 'Health for all' series, No 1–7' (1982)
8 'Seventh general programme of work, covering the period 1984–1989' (1982)

NUT/83.3 — Report of the Meeting of Regional Advisers in Nutrition, WHO/HQ, 8–13 December 1982
Draft Report of the Meeting of Regional Advisers in Nutrition, WHO/HQ, 24, 27 and 28 May 1985
World Health Forum, Vol 4, No. 1 — 'Nutrition — a health sector responsibility' by J.-P. Habicht 1983
Draft Report of the Programme Advisory Committee in Nutrition Meeting, WHO/HQ, 20–23 May 1985.

The contribution of FAO to nutrition

Francesca RONCHI-PROJA
Food Policy and Nutrition Division, Food and Agriculture Organization of the United Nations, Via delle Terme di Caracalla, Rome 00100, Italy.

The Food and Agriculture Organization of the United Nations (FAO) is the leading international organization for the development of agriculture, fisheries and forestry. Founded in 1945 it now has a membership of 156 nations. The FAO member nations have pledged themselves to raise the levels of nutrition and standards of living of their peoples; to improve production and distribution of food and agricultural products, and to better the conditions of their rural populations, especially the poorest.

The work of FAO can be classified into four main categories:

Collection, analysis and dissemination of information.

Advice to governments on policy and planning

Promotion of consultation and cooperation among member nations.

Provision of technical advice and assistance.

The main priorities guiding FAO programmes in the current and forthcoming biennia (1984–5 and 1986–7) are the promotion of food production, increase in food security, consolidation of information systems, emphasis on training, cooperation among developing countries, ensuring impact at the field level. Among the regions, Africa has been given priority due to the critical food and economic situation being faced by many of its countries. Many of FAO's activities in the field of nutrition are carried out in cooperation with other agencies and programmes such as WHO, UNESCO and World Food Programme (WFP), as well as through the Administrative Committee on Coordination/Subcommittee on Nutrition (ACC/SCN) with other UN and bilateral bodies.

Nutrition in agricultural and rural development. A methodology for introducing nutrition objectives and nutrition interventions into agricultural and rural development programmes has been developed by FAO in response to a recommendation by member nations at the FAO conference in 1977. The question was raised at that conference because doubts had been expressed concerning the expected nutrition advantages of major agricultural programmes. Some delegations asked whether the nutritional programmes had been sufficiently taken into account. Had any consideration been given by planners to ensure that no deterioriation of the nutritional conditions of the poorest would derive from major changes caused by these programmes?

The methodology developed by FAO was first tested through case studies and is now often introduced in current programme planning. It includes a preliminary analysis at the planning stage of such programmes of the potential effect (direct or indirect) on nutritional status and food consumption. Subsequently it requires the collection of nutritional indicators as baseline data to be utilized for a continuous evaluation of the nutritional effects of programmes, so that guidance can be provided to prevent negative results at any stage of programme development. Where indications exist that nutrition may be affected negatively, advice is provided to introduce, if necessary, nutrition interventions focussed on the most vulnerable groups of the populations covered.

We are at present assisting some countries in Africa (Burkina Faso and Niger) to introduce the methodology into their agricultural and rural development projects. On the other hand, workshops have been carried out in Africa and Asia to acquaint planners with the subject, as well as with food and nutrition planning strategies. Action has been started to introduce the methodology into fisheries and forestry projects assisted by FAO.

Nutrition interventions. The distribution of supplementary foods to selected vulnerable groups (mainly pre-school and primary school children, pregnant and nursing women) is a classic intervention in which FAO has been active for many years, assisting governments not only on nutritional aspects (selection of the right types of food, introduction of associated nutrition education activities), but also on the management side, to improve the utilization and preparation of the foods distributed.

Food aid has had an important role to play in these programmes, but we consider it to be a temporary measure alongside others aimed at helping countries and beneficiaries to achieve self-sufficiency in food. We are nutrition advisers (together with the WHO) to the WFP, which handles the multilateral food aid assistance. Our role includes both policy and technical advice as well as support to those governments which receive WFP food aid in a variety of projects. Considerable problems are faced in the implementation of these projects in several countries, due on the one hand to logistic difficulties and on the other to the lack of properly trained national staff able to handle, prepare safely and distribute the food. It is on the latter aspects that we have concentrated our assistance to governments, training their personnel through regional and national seminars and courses, developing and distributing manuals, guidelines and other training material for their use.

Another problem which has been under discussion in recent years is the effectiveness of food aid programmes in terms of their nutritional impact. The subject of the evaluation of nutritional impact, as well as the most suitable, yet simple, methodology, applicable under the conditions in developing countries, has been debated in the forum of the ACC/SCN, where a Working Group including several UN agencies is still studying it together with many other important issues. In the meantime, efforts are continuing to introduce (at least in a few projects) elements for an evaluation of impact, mainly by the collection of data on specific indicators such as heights and weights of children.

Nutrition education and training are the bases on which nutrition programmes are built. Without a group, albeit small, of well trained nutritionists, it is impossible to count on well planned and well implemented programmes. The importance and priority of manpower development in all fields of concern to FAO have been emphasized by the FAO Regional Conferences in recent years. In the field of nutrition we have concentrated our attention on *ad hoc* training in food policy and planning, on introducing human nutrition elements into the curricula of agricultural schools and colleges, on the in-service training of medium-level extension workers, on training in food control methods and on group feeding management. Guidelines and training materials on some of these subjects have been developed, tested, and translated into several national languages. These are now being used, often with FAO's assistance, in Africa, Asia and Latin America. Similar activities are starting in the Near East Region.

One important tool has proved to be the Field Programme Management Training Pack Food and Nutrition which emphasizes the management elements required for planning, implementation and evaluation of projects. Improvement in the staff capacities of management has been stressed as a felt need in several countries as well as at recent international meetings. One important intervention is nutrition education, especially at primary school level where it can be directed to children who will become the future parents, and will be the builders of their country's society and development. In the past, FAO has given attention to this subject, as can be seen by the several documents, publications, and seminar reports. Applied nutrition programmes, a classic intervention of the 1960s and '70s had major elements of nutrition education. In consultation with UNESCO, efforts are now being resumed to introduce nutrition education into the basic training of primary school teachers.

Food quality control. In recent years in both developed and developing countries, increased emphasis has been given to formulating or strengthening strategies for food quality control, by establishing national food control systems. This is due to the recognition of the existing problems of contamination and adulteration of foodstuffs, and of the need to ensure protection of the consumer against health hazards and commercial frauds. Adequate food laws and food control infrastructure are necessary to face these problems successfully.

FAO's assistance in this field is provided through several instruments, one of which is the FAO/WHO Codex Alimentarius Commission (where 122 countries are presently represented), and its technical committees. In addition, countries are assisted in training national staff in laboratory methods of food control, in the setting up of such laboratories and in planning and establishing national policies and legislation for food control, as well as in improving food handling practices at the village and household levels.

Nutrition and food security. The World community today is able to respond more rapidly and effectively to famine situations, but the problem remains of the chronically hungry and malnourished amongst the poorest groups of the population. The concept of food security (which was interpreted and applied in the past at the international level in terms of national security to ensure stocks of foods for a nation's needs) is now extended to cover household food security, thereby aiming at supporting projects which assist the poorest groups to produce or procure sufficient food for their nutritional needs. Within this enlarged scope of food security, FAO has implemented a programme which aims at promoting the production and consumption of so-called minor crops, or under-exploited food plants — two perhaps inappropriate terms which indicate a number of often traditional food plants which are now showing a tendency to disappear in developing countries, supplanted as they often are by imported cereal (in particular wheat and rice) which although more easily utilized, are not as easily produced in those countries.

This programme, which has so far been limited to the arid and semi-arid zones of Africa (our priority region) includes the preparation and distribution of two basic documents, one of which contains a list and description (with nutritional details) of selected food plants: *Food plants in arid and semi-arid lands: their composition and importance for human consumption with reference to Eastern Africa*, intended for use by planners and extension supervisors; and a second document, for policy makers: *Broadening the food base with traditional food plants*. Case studies on the subject are being undertaken with FAO's support in five African countries (Ethiopia, Kenya, Tanzania, Zambia and Zimbabwe) with technical advice from the London School of Hygiene and Tropical Medicine. A Workshop will be held later this year in Zimbabwe to examine the results of the studies and finalize the first document mentioned above.

At the same time promotion acitivities have been started by giving financial and technical support to a Workshop organized by the Zambian Alliance of Women/International Alliance of Women, which took place in Zambia in May this year. Participants, who were representatives of the International Alliance of Women from 13 African countries, contributed with considerable enthusiasm to the discussion concerning problems related to the use of a number of traditional food crops. With FAO's assistance they are now preparing proposals for promoting projects within their own countries, to be implemented in the near future. These concerted efforts will hopefully lead to the orientation of planners at national levels when making decisions on food and nutrition policies.

United Nations strategy against nutritional blindness. One major programme in which FAO is participating is the UN 10-Year Strategy Against Vitamin A Deficiency and Nutritional

Blindness, launched by the ACC/SCN in 1985. Within this strategy, FAO plans to deal with the long-term prevention programme — namely the production and consumption of foods rich in vitamin A. Obviously, this requires the mobilization not only of FAO's Food Policy and Nutrition Division, but also of other Divisions of FAO concerned with production: those dealing with animal production, fisheries, forestry and plant production and protection. The Plan will be ready later this year and will be discussed within the forum of the ACC/SCN together with other agencies concerned: WHO, which is the leading agency in this Plan; UNESCO and UNICEF.

The role of women in food security. The role of rural women in food production and food security has been the theme of FAO's studies and activities during the Decade of Women in Development. FAO's international and regional meetings have provided opportunities for joint discussion of problems and for planning interventions in support of rural women, which are implemented in several countries.

The nutritional implications of women's hard work in rural areas, especially in Africa, influence the family's nutrition and food consumption, child feeding practices and child care. The actual energy requirements as related to intakes are subjects of great interest which FAO is helping to clarify through studies and surveys in selected countries. As regards women in food security, FAO has produced a film which is being distributed this year to all member nations.

FAO as a source of information on nutrition subjects. Another important role of FAO is the collection, review and dissemination of information of wide interest to the international world. In the field of nutrition, this role is accomplished on specific subjects, some examples of which are: nutritional requirements, food composition and food consumption. The subject of nutritional requirements is constantly reviewed, in cooperation with the WHO, the nutrients under consideration at the present time being energy and protein and vitamin A and iron. The latest report on energy and protein will be issued later this year, while vitamin A and iron requirements will be discussed at a technical meeting to be held later this year. Less emphasis is presently being given by FAO to food composition, after the very intensive activities which led in the past to the publication of numerous food composition tables (for international use as well as for each region of the world). This subject is now being pursued through participation in the INFOODS network at the international level.

Updating data on food production, supply and consumption both at the world and at national levels is important for food and nutrition surveillance, and even more so for policy and planning. The Fifth World Food Survey is presently being finalized in FAO. This basic document will give an overall picture of food supply and food production versus estimated requirements. At the national level assistance is concentrated on the training of national staff in the techniques of data collection, analysis and interpretation, using the available modern methods of computerization. Occasionally, this training is carried out at FAO Headquarters on an individual basis.

Finally, our biannual review *Food and nutrition* highlights the world developments in food policy and nutrition through articles written by outstanding scientists as well as by FAO nutritionists. The review also gives worldwide news on meetings, training courses and publications.

The contribution of the World Food Programme to nutrition

D.J. SHAW
World Food Programme, Rome, Italy.

The World Food Programme (WFP) has given high priority to the improvement of nutrition in Third World countries since its inception over two decades ago. WFP, the food aid arm of the United Nations system, is the principal international organization concerned with providing that form of assistance. The Programme is essentially a funding agency, which works like the international financing institutions, providing grant food aid instead of money.

WFP began operations in 1963. In the past 22 years, it has provided about $6.8 billion of assistance to 1300 development projects in 120 countries and $1.6 billion of aid in 800 emergency operations in 96 countries. WFP's resources have grown significantly in recent years. It is now the largest single source of development assistance in the United Nations system apart from the World Bank group. In 1984, the Programme committed $925 million of assistance for development projects. In addition, $234 million of emergency aid was approved[13]. All WFP assistance is provided on a project basis within which the people to benefit and the development objectives are explicitly defined. WFP gives priority to assisting poor people in low-income countries. About 86 per cent of its development assistance went to low-income, food-deficit countries in 1984.

Nutrition improvement projects. By its very nature, WFP's food aid reaches very poor people and helps to improve their food intake and standard of nutrition. From its inception, WFP has given particular consideration to supplementary feeding programmes for this nutritionally vulnerable group and to the provision of meals in primary schools. About 30 per cent of its assistance, involving about $2 billion of aid, has been provided for some 250 projects of this type. At present, there are over 60 projects in operation in this field, involving about 10 million beneficiaries (1.3 million mothers, 4.1 million pre-school children and 4.6 million primary school children) and over $700 million of aid. These numbers are small in relation to global requirements. In certain countries, however, a large number of beneficiaries in these groups are reached.

The provision of emergency food aid to the victims of natural and man-made disasters[9], including refugees and displaced persons, has played a vital, often life-saving, role in sustaining people at basic nutritional levels both for their survival and to enable them to engage in self-help activities during the immediate period leading to reconstruction, rehabilitation and development. About 17.6 million people received WFP emergency food aid in 1984.

Pregnant women, lactating mothers and pre-school children. Pregnant and lactating women and pre-school children are particularly vulnerable to nutritional deficiencies in the developing world. Food supplements for pregnant and lactating women and the weanling child have proved to be highly cost-effective in certain cases in protecing the lives and health of young children[12]. Food supplements for at-risk pregnant women have been shown to be effective in helping to prevent low birth-weight. As low birth-weight is associated with perhaps one third of all infant death in the developing world, food supplements in pregnancy can be a powerful lever for raising levels of child health and survival. Supplementing diets with specific micronutrients can also be a highly cost-effective way of protecting children's lives and promoting growth[4,10].

Food aid has played a synergistic role in helping to establish closer co-operation among different government ministries and departments so that the interrelationships of nutrition, health and education have been brought together in a seamless robe of concerns in a relationship of cumulative causation[15]. The provision of food aid has acted as a stimulus to encourage governments to invest more in human resource development and to extend health and nutrition services for the poor. It has also supported and fostered the involvement of local communities, including women and voluntary organizations in supplementary feeding programmes for vulnerable groups.

Such programmes have also contributed to institution-building. Organizational, managerial and logistical systems have been set up, often for the first time, to reach out to the poor to provide them with food and basic health and nutrition services. Day-care centres have been established for children, thereby easing the burden of mothers working outside the home, facilitating the employment of women in income-earning activities and providing a facility for controlling the health and nutrition of their children.

While improvements in health and nutrition have been observed, in many cases these have not been scientifically measured. Assessment methodologies, based on appropriate indicators, are required to monitor and evalute the full nutritional and non-nutritional benefits of such programmes. Important, sometimes unintended, benefits may not be recorded because evaluation is focused narrowly on quantitative nutritional outcomes[1]. In-depth evaluations are costly and difficult to implement. WFP is designing low-cost monitoring and evaluation systems to be built into the design of projects which have explicit objectives.

The outreach of supplementary feeding programmes is limited to the distribution centres and logistical facilities available. Reaching those in greatest need is often difficult and food supplies may be irregular or disrupted. Targeting on the most needy individuals has proved particularly difficult; take-home rations designed for them may be shared among the household, thereby diluting their effect. WFP has focused on this problem, in concert with other agencies, by giving consideration to criteria for beneficiaries selection and by addressing the needs of the poor household as a whole through, for example, providing food for all household members by combining supplementary feeding and food-for-work programmes (see below).

Supplementary feeding programmes may create a disincentive to local food production and adverse effects on dietary patterns and food habits, leading to dependence on imported foods and a decrease in breast feeding. There are, of course, many factors which create these disincentives and adverse effects and to extricate the effect of food aid is difficult. A recently completed desk study[3], representing a first effort to start a deeper study on the effects of food aid on food habits, concluded that there are insufficient data available to make an assessment and there has been comparatively little research in the developing world on why and how food habits change.

Nutrition education, health services and training raise other issues. If supplementary feeding programmes are not associated with well designed nutrition education and health services then, at best, they may only help, as a temporary measure, to prevent a decline in the nutritional status of the beneficiaries. Shortage of adequately trained staff can result in inadequate supervision, defective recording and reporting or lack of compilation and analysis of data. In such situations, food aid may become a handout and stimulate a curative rather than a preventative approach. WFP has provided advice on the organization and management of food distribution at centres and has encouraged the training of staff.

The total costs, and components of cost, of supplementary feeding programmes need to be more carefully assessed. This would enable comparisons to be made with benefits, design of the most cost effective delivery systems for food aid, examination of how costs might be reduced and decisions to be made on whether programmes could be enlarged or replicated, with or without modifications.

Primary school children. WFP assistance for providing meals or snacks in primary schools has the dual and interrelated objectives of improved nutrition and education. Health and nutrition both affect whether children can attend school regularly and whether they have the mental and physical energy to learn. The provision of meals at school can also help to reduce the dropout rate and increase the range of school enrollment, including girls. Food is provided at school to complement that received at home in order to make up for deficiencies in proteins, fat and certain minerals and vitamins, the absence of which could lead to greater exposure to disease and to undermining the general health of children.

Experience has shown that primary school feeding programmes are relatively easier to implement than supplementary feeding programmes for mothers and pre-school children. It is important to ensure, however, that the necessary logistical conditions exist, including the provision of kitchen facilities for the preparation of meals, sufficient eating utensils and adequate funds to use the food aid provided effectively.

Teachers and officials have reported improvement in the health, alertness and proficiency of the pupils receiving school meals. Attempts have been made in some projects to measure the impact of improved nutrition on a scientific basis. For the majority of school feeding programmes, however, no proper study of nutritional impact has been undertaken owing to a shortage of qualified personnel and the absence of appropriate base-line information.

Apart from their intrinsic nutritional and health value, primary school feeding programmes can be used as a vehicle to train children in improved food habits and the hygienic handling of food. To bring this about, teachers will need to be given instruction as to how to use such programmes for putting the theories of nutrition education into practice rather than seeing them only as a means of feeding children.

The importance of opportunity cost as a factor affecting school attendance is often overlooked in designing school feeding programmes[8]. The income of earnings which would have to be foregone in attending school often present a barrier to actual attendance by children of low-income households. Those children make a significant contribution to total household subsistence or income. To provide adequate incentive for them to attend school, therefore, food aid would have to offset the opportunity cost involved. Rather than providing only a meal at school for the individual child concerned, therefore, it may be necessary to give additional food for the household as a whole. This approach would augment the stock of human capital by improving the nutrition and health of the household, increasing schooling and providing income transfers to the poor and disadvantaged in such a way as to enable them, perhaps for the first time, to make longer-term investments that would raise their productivity and increase their income-generating potential. Seen, in this way, as a transfer of income, the food aid provided would be demand-enhancing rather than merely supply-augmenting.

In common with other aid organizations[11], experience has shown that recipient governments cannot be expected to take over the costs involved in running feeding programmes for vulnerable groups within a short period of time. Extensions of WFP assistance have, therefore, been frequent. In agreement with governments in recipient countries, however, WFP makes provision for them gradually to assume greater responsibility for programme financing as its assistance is phased out. Ideally, each country should develop an overall plan, with short and long-term objectives, which makes provision for the phasing-over of responsibility for funding gradually from the aid organizations concerned.

Other approaches. As hunger and malnutrition is an outcome of poverty, WFP aims to link supplementary feeding programmes designed to reduce the current incidence of malnutrition with longer-term activities devised to increase local food production, employment, income and self-reliance generally at the community level. Seen in that context, food aid can have a number of functions in addition to providing a nutrition transfer through supplementary feeding programmes. Some examples of those other functions are summarized below.

WFP has provided food aid to help communities settle on new agricultural lands over the initial period in their new locations until an adequate level of production is reached. Family rations have been provided which have acted as an income transfer, sustained productivity and expedited the process towards self-sufficiency.

The provision of food through food-for-work schemes to households either as part-payment of wages or as an incentive for community self-help acitivites has also been an important nutritional support during periods of the year when food is in short supply, or when access of the poor to food is limited by seasonal unemployment and reduced purchasing power. Food aid could be used more deliberately to reduce or remove some of the more accute effects of the seasonal dimensions of poverty among poor, rural communities when food is short, food prices are high and the workload in agricultural activities, such as land preparation and harvesting, at their peak[2].

A more integrated approach to nutrition projects has also been adopted[14]. There is growing awareness that sustained nutrition improvement depends on improvements in women's educational levels and access to independent incomes as well as social infrastructural support (especially potable water and fuel), health and health-related services and training. WFP has, therefore, encouraged and stimulated the design of programmes which encompass both supplementary feeding for vulnerable groups and income-generating activities for the household, including women, so that the beneficiaries are better able to take over responsibility for their own nutritional and general wellbeing on the termination of external assistance.

The Programme is also looking at the various functional roles that food aid could play in enhancing nutritional improvement. For example, WFP is carefully considering the concept of the income-transfer effect of food aid on nutrition[7]. As all payments in kind transfer income, this concept argues that people will consume more food when they receive a food aid commodity which conveys more income rather than more energy (calories) per unit of cost.

Food aid, as well as other forms of aid, will work best in a policy environment within which governments in developing countries give a strong commitment to achieving self-reliance, reducing poverty and improving nutritional status of the poor. WFP, therefore, seeks to give its support to effective development policies and programmes and to assist in the process of 'adjustment with a human face'[5]. UNICEF has drawn attention to the serious adverse effects of the world recession on children[6]. Food aid has a special role to play in rescuing and preserving some essential parts of national support programmes for children, and for the poor and disadvantaged generally, which are threatened by financial stringency. In this connection, food aid can act as a cushion during the process of short-run, balance-of-payments adjustment. The importance of supplementary food supplies in a food-deficit situation if a sharp rise in food prices are to be avoided is one example.

Government pricing policy for producers and consumers can have a powerful effect on nutrition levels. There is need to resolve the dilemma of providing incentive prices to producers without pricing poor consumers out of the market. Food aid, and its counterpart funds, could be used during an interim period of price policy adjustment which would take account of both producer and consumer prices. In Mali, for example, a number of donors, including WFP, are co-operating with the government in a programme involving the reform of grain pricing and marketing arrangements, thereby increasing food production and food security. The food aid is sold and the proceeds deposited in a common counterpart fund and dispersed in support of this programme. In Senegal, a similar approach is being adopted whereby the common counterpart fund will be used to support the government's initiative to shift consumption away from imported wheat and rice toward locally produced sorghum, millet and maize.

It is especially important to give more attention to the links between emergency and development assistance. Enhancement of national food security systems and the promotion of disaster prevention and preparedness measures, which address the root causes of recurrent emergencies, require priority attention. This approach is required particularly in sub-Saharan Africa: otherwise what is already a chronic and perennial state of emergency, with adverse nutritional and other effects, will become a quite intractable problem. This is one of the biggest challenges facing governments in the afflicted countries and the international community over the next decade.

Co-ordinated action. WFP has emphasized that while an important, often vital, ingredient, food aid alone is not enough to address the nutrition-related issues confronting Third World countries. The causes of malnutrition and undernourishment are multidimensional. Their irradication calls principally for specifically focused development policies and investment programmes by governments in the developing countries themselves. Those policies and programmes should be supported cohesively and consistently with different types of assistance from donor countries and organizations through aid co-ordination arrangements such as the World Bank consultative groups and UNDP round tables.

WFP seeks to co-operate with other aid organizations, both within and outside the United Nations system, in the knowledge that food aid will work best when associated with other forms of aid. In most of the projects it supports, WFP aid is linked to that of other multilateral, bilateral or non-governmental organizations. The underlying rational for this collaborative co-operation is the harmonizing of the various inputs of the United Nations system to meet the development needs of countries in the most effective and expeditious manner. In this fundamental sense, the question to be asked should not only be what WFP's contribution is to nutrition but what are the concerned organizations of the United Nationals system doing in concert to improve nutrition in the Third World.

1 Beaton, G.H. & Ghassemi, H. (1979): *Supplementary feeding programmes for young children in developing countries*. New York: UNICEF.
2 Chambers R. & Longhurst, R. eds (1981): *Seasonal dimensions to rural poverty*. London: Frances Pinter.
3 Coles, A.M.S. (1984): *The effects of food aid on dietary patterns and food habits*. Rome: FAO.
4 Figa-Talamanca, I. (1985): *Nutritional implications of food aid: an annotated bibliography*. Food and Nutrition Paper 33. Rome: FAO.
5 Jolly, R. (1985): *Adjustment with a human face*. The Barbara Ward Lecture 1985, Society for International Development. 18th World Conference, Rome.

6 Jolly, R. & Cornia, G.A. eds (1984): *The impact of world recession on children*. Oxford: Pergamon Press.
7 Reutlinger, S. (1983): Project food aid and equitable growth: income-transfer efficiency first! In *Report of the World Food Programme/Government of the Netherlands Seminar on Food Aid*, pp. 167–177. Rome: WFP.
8 Schuh, G.E. (1983): Increasing the effectiveness of food aid: offsetting the opportunity costs of schooling. In *Report of the World Food Programme/Government of the Netherlands Seminar on Food Aid*, pp. 101–105. Rome: WFP.
9 Sen, A.K. (1981): *Poverty and famines: an essay on entitlement and deprivation*. Oxford: Oxford University Press.
10 Singer, H.W. (1978): *A survey of studies of food aid.* (Document WFP/CFA:5/5–C). Rome: WFP.
11 Taylor, E.B. (1985): *Survey report: Seminar on improving the development impact of the PL-480 Title II schoolfeeding programme.* Newton, Maryland, USA: International Nutrition Communication Service.
12 UNICEF (1985): *The state of the world's children 1985*, pp. 103–107. Oxford: Oxford University Press.
13 WFP (1985): *Annual report of the Executive Director on the development of the Programme: 1984.* (Document WFP/CFA: 19/4). Rome: WFP.
14 WFP (1985): *Breadwinners at home and at work.* WFP information paper for 1985 World Conference on the United Nations Decade for Women. Nairobi, July 1985.
15 World Bank (1980): *World development report, 1980.* Part II. Poverty and human development, pp. 68–70. New York: Oxford University Press.

The work of UNICEF in relation to nutrition

R. JOLLY
UNICEF, New York, USA.

The urgency and opportunity for action. Rising malnutrition has become a worldwide problem of the 1980s. The world has been made dramatically aware of the emergency situation in Africa. But economic problems are having disastrous consequences on child nutrition in other parts of the world too. In Latin America, where levels of development and child welfare are basically much higher than in Africa, there is evidence from a number of countries of rising levels of malnutrition, in some cases of rising infant mortality, particularly among the poor and vulnerable.

The *causes* of rising malnutrition are a tragic interaction of both national and international factors. The cut-backs and adjustments that many countries are making reflect in part the severe constraints imposed by the international economic system and in part the way countries have re-formulated their policies in response to those pressures. The *challenge* is to work urgently towards a solution in the short as well as the long run.

It is a challenge to be taken up by Governments, donor agencies, voluntary and international agencies; research institutions; scientists; communicators .... UNICEF's response has been to advocate for the need for adjustment with a human face, to argue that for reasons of sound economics as well as social justice the needs of children, especially children under five, must not be deferred, and to stress that though the costs of urgent and necessary action will not be trivial neither will they be so enormous that they cannot be met.

Early beginnings. The International Union of Nutritional Sciences and UNICEF both came into being shortly after the end of World War II. It is sobering to recall that much of the scientific and technological basis for action to control malnutrition was available at that time. In 1947, a joint committee of specialists in nutrition and paediatrics was appointed by FAO and the WHO Interim Commission at the request of what was then called the International Children's Emergency Fund of the United Nations, and prepared an advisory report on Child Nutrition which provided basic information on such matters as the energy and protein requirements of various age groups, the importance of breastfeeding, the deleterious effects of infections on nutritional status and the effects of deficiencies of micro-nutrients such as iodine, iron and vitamin A.

At that time relief and rehabilitation requirements were taking priority. Much of the promise of the 1930s for more enlightened approaches to food and nutrition problems had faded. In

1937, having studied the situation in which widespread hunger and malnutrition existed in a time of high level production but poor distribution of foodstuffs, the Mixed Committee of the League of Nations issued a report emphasizing the need for multisectoral approaches to these problems, including the involvement of economists, and for the marriage of health and agriculture. Sir John Boyd Orr had documented the association between poverty and malnutrition in Great Britain. But after the success of the World War II food policy the world to a large extent was allowed to forget many of the lessons of the past, though Boyd Orr and others tried to keep the vision alive in an international context: the account of FAO's first 10 years of international cooperation toward freedom from want was entitled 'So bold an aim', recalling phrases used by Lester Pearson at its birth. Thus UNICEF and others were destined to a long journey on two tracks — *one*, to promote and deliver as much programming as possible to give immediate and near-term relief, especially to those in greatest need, and, *two*, to promote better global understanding of nutritional needs and problems and to work towards long-term solutions. In these efforts UNICEF was often helped by leaders in the IUNS and at times there were more specific joint efforts, as in the holding of special conferences on the nutrition of the pre-school child.

Evolving UNICEF perspectives. UNICEF's experience since that time endorses the relevance of both direct and indirect approaches to good nutrition. In very broad terms one can detect in the course of UNICEF's history four main eras, or areas of emphasis, although there is of course much overlapping. Durings its first decade UNICEF concentrated on direct child feeding and food conservation programmes: these were the days when milk reigned supreme (partly perhaps because of positive experience in Britain before and during World War II), and the dairy industries in many third world countries owe their initial development to UNICEF support.

The second era dates from the later 1950s, when a longer-term approach was introduced. What became known as applied nutrition programmes (ANP) had an essentially educational purpose, with a strong training component, emphasising increased local production and consumption of nutritious foods. During the 1960s the interactions of nutrition and infection became increasingly appreciated, and by the late 60s and early 70s ANP with the technical support of FAO, WHO and UNESCO was giving strong attention to the triangle of education, health care, and local food production and utilisation.

The third era, characterised by introducing nutrition strategies into regional and national development planning, had its beginnings in the 1960s but received major impetus from the World Food Conference in 1974 which called on UNICEF, together with other UN agencies, to cooperate with governments in the development of food and nutrition plans and policies, and asked governments to consider specific measures designed to improve nutritional conditions of mothers and childen in low-income families. Those measures included recognition of the major role to be played by women in the development process. To a considerable extent this represented a restitution of the philosophical position that the world was gaining at the time of the great upheaval of World War II. But now there was a greater understanding of the development process, which led to the formulation of concepts that have had a profound effect on the operational approach to nutrition, especially the *basic needs and services* concept, and the *primary health care* (PHC) approach.

From UNICEF's perspective a fourth era may be identified as starting around the beginning of the 1980s, with an enhanced focus on the young child and with a special emphasis on low-cost actions which families can take themselves to reduce infant and child mortality. Activities that have been identified as central to what UNICEF has termed the Child Survival and Development Revolution (CSDR), and suitable for national application, all reflect the synergism between nutrition and infection: the promotion of exclusive breast-feeding for the first few months of life, and better weaning practices; immunisation against the six EPI diseases; oral rehydration therapy for the control of diarrhoea; and regular growth monitoring of the child primarily in order to help the mother to play her role in promoting growth. These activities are relatively low-cost, do-able, politically neutral, and effective. It should be stressed that they represent only a first core: other activities suitable for widespread application and responding to the specific needs of the situation can and must be identified, for instance, iodised oil/salt for eradicating cretinism, prophylaxis for malaria, etc. More problematic for national application but highly relevant are food supplementation (necessary in some cases, perhaps most importantly for the pregnant woman), female literacy, and family (or birth) spacing: it has been argued that the demonstration of increased survival is a necessary condition for the voluntary acceptance by parents of a small family.

The most important aspect of this strategy is not the techniques as such but the emphasis on putting the family at the centre, with the goal of empowering families with the knowledge and confidence to take more effective action themselves. This has lead to a strong emphasis on mass communications and social mobilisation which in a number of countries has led to dramatic nation-wide action justifying the term revolution. It has been possible to arouse to an unforeseen extent the social perceptions of society and mobilise a whole range of non-government groups such as the churches, the Red Crescent and Red Cross, boy scouts and girl guides, as well as professional and government groups, many of them not normally involved in health. The phenomenal progress of the CSDR is chronicled in UNICEF's annual State of the World's Children Reports, but it is important to realise that UNICEF is now but one of many actors, and in no sense claims the Revolution as its own.

UNICEF's current support to nutrition. In consequence of UNICEF's traditional decentralised style of country programming with governments, based on an analysis of the situation of children in a given country in relation to perceived opportunities for action, our programmes of cooperation in the approximately 130 developing countries where we presently work will collectively include direct or indirect support to virtually all of the activities referred to earlier, and many others barely touched upon. (These latter will include programmes to combat specific nutrient deficiencies, assistance in the establishment of surveillance systems, support to country-related research studies, introduction of nutrition into school curricula...). Rarely however will food itself be provided, for if an external source is necessary this would, within the UN system, normally be the WFP.

Recently of course the shadow of Africa has overlain UNICEF concerns for nutrition. We have felt that the crisis has emphasized the relevance of the CSDR strategy, and support for training, provision of vaccines and essential drugs, strengthening of the immunisation cold chain, and so forth, have been accelerated and sometimes re-directed to areas of critical need. But a priority concern has been food. Although UNICEF occasionally has purchased food grains locally for distribution as a temporary measure until a major bilateral or WFP programme can be established, or more often provided special high-energy foods for rehabilitation of malnourished children, most support has been for logistics or surveys to establish needs. A pioneering approach has been built on the recognition that starvation often arises even when foods are available through a lack of entitlement or purchasing power. UNICEF has supported some cash-for-food projects in Ethiopia and elsewhere, which have prevented displacement of a population in search of relief, encouraged community development, and promoted self-sufficiency.

Health measures are central to a new initiative that was taken in 1982, when UNICEF and WHO together established the joint nutrition support programme (JNSP) with special funding. The programme's impact objectives are the reduction of infant and young child mortality and maternal nutrition. It aims to improve the nutritional status of children and mothers, and thus is able to support a broad range of activities, including immunisation, oral rehydration therapy, improved sanitation, income generating activities for women... as well as what would commonly be thought of as more conventional nutrition activities. The exact mix depends on country programming, supported by the combined and complementary traditions of WHO and UNICEF. JNSP uses the PHC approach, and provides support at community, intermediate and central levels in order to strengthen national capacities to plan, manage, and evaluate. Projects are in various stages of development in 18 countries, and will contribute to understanding means of involving communities, and of how best to manage and coordinate multisectoral programmes.

Special attention is being given to extending and improving the practice of growth monitoring, both to provide basic information needed to develop a national food security and nutrition strategy, as done in Botswana where the country's policy makers intend that this should link short-term drought relief efforts to long-term planning strategies, but also as the focus for relevant child care education. Improved income, or family food sufficiency, are not in themselves sufficient conditions for the alleviation of malnutrition in young children. Environmental factors are of course important, but often the understanding of mothers about the desirable nature and frequency of supplementary feeding is a critical issue. So while continued support will be given for breastfeeding, which studies show is being eroded even in rural strongholds, emphasis will be shifted towards the weaning process.

Increased attention is being given to women's concerns, the UNICEF Board noting at its 1985 session the many circumstances in which an improvement in the general conditions of women is essential to the implementation of strategies for child survival and development, and also that women-centred activities should be development-oriented rather than welfare-based. In most countries women have a key role in family food production, which should be promoted with due weight given to environmental as well as to social and economic aspects. Consensus seems to be growing that success will largely depend on the extent to which communities are genuinely involved, *small* farmers and especially women able to benefit, and ecological principles respected: old truths re-learned.

Amongst the micro-nutrients enhanced attention is being given to the prevention of vitamin A deficiency, as evidence increases of the significance of its non-ocular effects. The extent of iodine deficiency disorders seems to have been underestimated in the past, and increased efforts are now being made towards their prevention and eradication.

The use of nutritional indicators to illuminate socio-economic change and influence policy has an important and exciting potential.

A new challenge. This potential has special relevance to the introduction of nutritional concerns into the adjustment process, which would link immediate humanitarian concerns with the dominant contemporary international economic issue. Specifically, adjustment of this sort would involve three considerations:

First, a clear acknowledgement in the goals of adjustment policy of concern for human welfare and a commitment to protect the minimum living standards of children and other vulnerable groups.

Second, a broader approach to the conventional adjustment process, embracing three new components: (a) actions to maintain a minimum floor of nutrition and other basic human needs, related to what the country can in the long term sustain; (b) restructuring within health, education and other social sectors, to ensure maximum benefits from constrained resources; (c) restructuring the economy to put more emphasis on small scale enterprises and the informal sector, with special support for women. Such an approach would endorse the PHC and basic services strategies, and make maximum use of the CSDR opportunities.

Third, a system for monitoring the human situation during the adjustment process. We need to be concerned not only with the growth of GNP, balance of payments and inflation but with the growth of children, food balances and the proportion of children falling below the basic poverty line.

In this 40th anniversary year of the United Nations it would be fitting indeed for its various agencies, and national and professional bodies, to enter into a new partnership with governments for tackling nutrition problems worldwide, and in so doing to recapture the vision and idealism that characterised the period that led to its birth, the optimism that was sustained by the concept of bold action based on sound science. The challenge is clear. Do we have the vision and the determination to respond?

UNICEF (1984): *The impact of world recession on children*, ed R. Jolly & G.A. Cornia. Oxford: Pergamon Press.
UNICEF (1984): *The state of the world's children 1985*. London: Oxford University Press.
UNICEF (1984): Going to scale for child survival and development. *Assignment Children* (65/68). UNICEF, Geneva.
UNICEF (1985): Within human reach — a future for Africa's children. UNICEF, New York.

Nutrition and the World Bank

A. BERG
World Bank, Washington DC USA.

Over the past decade, the World Bank has undertaken or financed 55 pieces of nutrition-related research, much of it of an economic nature, and in 16 countries what we call sector studies of malnutrition problems and their determinants. Bank research, aside from health-related effects of malnutrition, examined the economic value of improved nutrition, the effects of food supplements on productivity, and the effects of malnutrition on the future earning capacity of children. Also, a major part of the Bank's experience has derived from its participation in nutrition projects of member countries.

The main findings of Bank research and sector work are simply that increasing incomes and agricultural production are not expected to resolve malnutrition problems within a generation in most developing countries. Most governments are not reaching the very poor, especially the rural poor, with nutrition benefits, and few central ministries have the resources or organizations to mount a substantial national effort to combat malnutrition.

More than half of the malnourished in the countries we studied were families of landless agricultural labourers, farmers with land holdings that were too small to be within the scope of most rural development programmes, small-scale fishermen, and the urban unemployed. Nutrition problems were evident in all ages and both sexes. Apart from whether or not sufficient food was available, malnourished people often did not have the economic and sometimes the physical access to food, and in some cases were not always using limited resources in nutritionally efficient ways.

Parallel to this research and sector work and in an effort to learn more about how a UN agency like ours might respond with projects to the problem, the Bank initiated four large nutrition projects between 1976 and 1980 in Brazil, Colombia, India, and Indonesia and 53 nutrition components in other Bank-assisted projects. Concentration here will be on the four nutrition projects.

While addressing the special needs of target populations, the four projects shared some common features. All included one or more institution-building components and several operational components, usually including the delivery of nutrition services through primary health care systems, and a nutrition education component. The projects in Brazil, Indonesia and Colombia were multisectoral, comprising nutrition-related elements affecting agriculture, water supply and sanitation, and food marketing, in addition to direct nutrition actions. The project in Tamil Nadu (India) concentrated on fewer activities.

The four, largely experimental, projects were designed, in part, to draw lessons for future nutrition-related activities of these countries and secondarily of the Bank. What were these operational lessons?

Targeting food supplies. The consumer food subsidy experiments and the institutional feeding programmes used a variety of approaches to identify the specific populations that needed nutritional help and to direct appropriate nutrition services to those groups. The main lesson was that some form of targeting are feasible and can indeed lower costs.

The consumer food subsidy programmes in Brazil and Colombia promoted the idea of selective participation. In Colombia targeting was by geography, with the poorest areas selected and groups within these areas. In Brazil, selection was based on income. The pilot project in Recife distributed food through several government-run supermarkets to coupon holders selected on income criteria. It demonstrated the difficulty of targeting by income in a setting where income reporting can be very arbitrary. The programme showed that food coupon programmes are more effective at reducing levels of child malnutrition if the subsidies are high enough to sustain participation — several levels were tried. However, it also showed that heavy bookkeeping and related administrative costs are required to conduct an effective food coupon programme, that down payments for coupons pose a barrier to the lowest income group, and that the system must adapt to the frequent small purchases that low-income families are forced to make.

Building on lessons from the evaluations conducted during project implementation, the Brazilian consumer subsidy component was modified, with apparent success, by confining it to small shops in very low income neighbourhoods, making everyone eligible without requiring coupons or down payments. Even though there may have been modest leakage of benefits to non-target groups, the cost of this to the programme was less than the costs of administering the food coupon system. The new administration in Brazil is currently expanding this effort throughout the northeast.

One of the most important findings from the Bank's experience in Brazil was that it was possible to reduce food prices for low-income families solely by reducing the costs of delivering food, through a more efficient food marketing system.

Targeting in direct institutional feeding programmes was tried several ways but best achieved through the weight-monitoring programme set up in Tamil Nadu, designed to screen children for admission to a feeding programme when their growth faltered and release them once weight increased satisfactorily. A recent evaluation published by the Tamil Nadu government reported that:

'The net decline in severe malnutrition is 40 per cent among children 12–36 months of age. It declined by 23 per cent
(from 20.4 to 15.7) in the pilot block while in the control it rose by 19 per cent (from 15.0 to 17.8)....
'The average weight of children in the pilot project increased while decreasing in the control. The advantage in weight gain increases and continues even after 36 months of age. The difference in weight gain was 1.75 kg in children 49–60 months of age. It supports the assumption that interventions during the critical period in a child's life viz. 6–36 months give a "head start" that benefits the child in later stages of growth'.

The relationship of nutrition to family planning and primary health care. From the Bank's experience, it seems that the delivery of family planning and nutrition services can be organized to complement each other. In Indonesia, for instance, the family planning agency credited growth-monitoring and related nutrition activities with having provided an important inducement for villagers to get together to discuss and become involved in family planning work. In the design of a second Indonesian nutrition project, going to our Board for approval next month, nutrition at the village level is closely linked to family planning services.

Community nutrition workers from the 9000 villages in the project in Tamil Nadu have been cited by family planning staff there as the best sources for successfully identifying couples who would participate in family planning programmes. This is largely because of their village base and close contact with mothers. Further, the full-time community nutrition worker in Tamil Nadu provides simple health services (eg deworming, diarrhoea control, provision of vitamin A, and iron and folic acid), and at the weighing sessions and through regular home visits promotes use of health centres.

A study of the Indonesian programme demonstrated that village-level services were likely to offer a more efficient and more equitable use of resources than comparable services offered higher up in the health system, at a subdistrict health centre, for example. The Colombian experience showed that a nutrition project, in this case a consumer food subsidy, could be designed in a way to lead to an improved primary health care system. In Colombia a main element was that potential food coupon holders needed to visit local health centres to qualify and receive coupons for their rations, redeemable in a commercial market.

Nutrition education. Efforts appear to be most effective when designed to modify highly specific behaviour, rather than when designed to convey the kinds of general nutrition messages commonly used in the past. Rohde refers elsewhere (this book: pp. 24, 25) to the new concepts employed in Indonesia as part of the Bank-assisted project. These involved working with target audiences, learning their perceptions, and allowing them to try different approaches to improve their specific nutrition problems and to help formulate new approaches before designing messages for use in the project. (One of the keys to success was the work of a nutrition anthropologist who lived in Javanese villages during most of the 14-month period of programme formulation.) The objectives of the programme were based on what people could and would do. They addressed a few priorities, and they were transmitted in simple ways and effectively by village workers in home visits and growth monitoring sessions. These efforts were reinforced by radio. The project was successful because it was built on the use of resources that already existed in the community. These concepts will be part of a second project with Indonesia, scheduled for negotiations in October.

The Brazilian experience indicated that nutrition education for mothers, along with providing nutrition and intellectual stimulation in a school setting for preschool children, had a marked effect in reducing subsequent school drop-out and repeater rates.

Community participation. All of the projects tried to mobilize both resources and volunteers in the community — leading to construction of nutrition and health facilities in Brazil; construction of water and sanitation systems in Colombia; mothers' working groups in Tamil Nadu; and nutrition education through village nutrition workers in Indonesia.

Generally, participation by members of the community generated enthusiasm in the project, raised nutritional awareness, and improved the chances that project activities would continue after the project ended. On the other hand, part-time volunteers with limited skills took more time than regular workers to get a job done, there were more of them to be trained, tasks had to be fewer and simpler, and quality control and supervision was more difficult. And in areas where not enough volunteers were available, services suffered. There are cost savings in a volunteer programme but there are also costs to both the project and the participants that should be weighed when a volunteer system is being considered. The same applies to the desirable goal of community involvement in determining the content of a project. Extended delays thus caused in preparation of a nutrition project requested by the Senegalese government contributed to the project eventually being dropped.

Opportunities for what commonly is called community participation are culture-specific. The concept assumes that autonomous, rural communities exist in some democratic form and that they can be mobilized to manage their own collective welfare in an egalitarian manner. These assumptions are not valid for many societies, and striving to incorporate community participation where it is alien to the culture may be an elusive goal. Where extensive community participation is deemed feasible, experience from the Bank's nutrition projects suggests that the main ingredients for success are appropriate training and adequate supervision.

Project design. The Bank experience with nutrition projects indicates that the initial three as originally planned were too complex, trying to test numerous approaches and optimistically assuming a high degree of management and organizational skills. These were administratively cumbersome, cutting across organization lines in governments and in the Bank. Communications and coordination among agencies were sometimes poor, particularly at the headquarters level; less so at the field level.

Part of the complexity was created by the desire to add productive components. In stressing the need for directly productive components (such as food gardens in Colombia and Indonesia, and food industry activities in Brazil), a key point about the value of investment in nutrition was missed, that is, better nutrition makes all the other sectors more productive.

A less ambitious, more narrowly focussed project consisting of no more than three or four well-integrated nutrition interventions, and carefully designed to limit needs for managerial skills, is more likely to be successfully implemented. Although nutrition projects should be more limited in scope than were the first three projects, successful experience in Tamil Nadu demonstrates that they need not be confined to one sector. Also, the early projects, planned to last 4 or 5 years, were also unrealistically short to demonstrate the expected changes in nutritional status.

Costs. The annual cost of Bank project components on which aggregated data are available ranged widely. Many obvious factors contributed to the differences — the size and nature of the project; the size of the food transfer, if any; the extent of targeting; and so on. Costs also varied by country, because of differences in wages, food prices, and food consumption patterns. Annual costs per beneficiary ranged from $2 in Indonesia's nutrition education programme to $35 and $21 in the Colombian and Brazilian consumer food subsidy programmes respectively.

To what extent can governments afford nationwide interventions? This depends on a number of factors, not the least being the importance a government assigns to the malnutrition problem and its willingness to commit resources in this area.

Many low-income countries are now spending 6 per cent of their budgets or less on health and nutrition together. However, a number of countries have devoted substantial portions of their budgets to consumer food subsidies, generally not perceiving or budgeting them as nutrition programmes. In 1975, such subsidies accounted for 21 per cent of Egypt's total government expenditures, 19 per cent of Korea's, 16 per cent of Sri Lanka's, and 12 per cent of Morocco's. In 1981, the urban food subsidy in China accounted for 13 per cent of government expenditures. Although for many countries these levels have proved too high to sustain in the long run, the examples suggest substantial resources are made available, albeit sometimes with objectives other than just improved nutrition in mind. Costs for the nutrition actions taken under the Bank-assisted projects would, if carried out on a national scale, range from 0.1 to 2.6 per cent of national budgets.

Cost-effectiveness. To more fully assess the appropriateness of nutrition interventions, it is of course necessary to attempt to quantify their effects or benefits and then relate such measures to costs. Much attention has been given to attempting to measure effect in these projects.

In Indonesia, the nutrition status of children up to 24 months of age in five areas where nutrition education under the project was offered can be compared with that in five areas that received more standard nutrition assistance, including more conventional nutrition education. One year after the full implementation of the communications strategy, there were significantly smaller proportions of malnourished children in the project villages, as measured by weight for age — half a standard deviation difference. Forty per cent of children in the programme improved nutrition status over what would have been expected. There were no significant differences between the villages before the nutrition education project and no other factors were found to explain the improvements. One of the standard government programmes with which it was compared cost nearly three times as much to cover a population of 100 000 and had lesser nutrition impact.

The cost per child in Tamil Nadu of ending malnourishment ranges from $33 to $126 per year, depending on the severity of the condition. These costs are stikingly lower than those of well-documented, more traditional nutrition rehabilitation programmes in some countries, where improvement was estimated to cost $600 per child and the cost to eliminate a case of third-degree malnutrition compared with control groups was $3600.

In short, compared with many of the earlier interventions (which often had either indiscriminate coverage or, if targeted, often involved one-on-one treatment and oversight from highly trained professions), the large-scale concepts tried under the projects by these four governments appear to have shown the feasibility of pushing per capita beneficiary costs down to relatively low levels. Even at the high end of the cost spectrum, a consumer food subsidy programme, *if targeted properly*, is affordable in certain contexts. The low-cost nutrition education as practised in Indonesia looks particularly attractive. Evaluations have shown that it was — at each step — increasing knowledge, bringing about behavioural change, increasing food consumption, and growth. That it was cheaper than programmes requiring distribution of food comes as no surprise; the question is whether it was effective. The evidence has shown that nutrition education alone *can* make a difference in improving nutritional status. Nutritionists have long held out the promise of this possibility; the Indonesian experience is the first time it has been demonstrated in a operational setting.

The numbers of nutrition projects and the contributions by the World Bank in this area are modest compared to other development assistance agencies. A good deal of energy has been spent in determining whether or not nutrition is a legitimate World Bank activity. A review by top Bank management last year concluded that it was.

The Bank's management has recognized malnutrition as an important development problem, and one the institution should address. Because of the obvious relationships between nutrition, population, and health, much of the Bank's work in the future will be in the context of integrated programmes. However, free-standing nutrition projects in some situations may be appropriate. These may follow one or more of the following approaches: (1) reduce infant and child morbidity and mortality and promote child growth (a Tamil Nadu-style 'food as medicine' approach); (2) improve formation of human capital and labour productivity by enlarging the family food basket and contributing to physical and intellectual development rather than concentrating on a curative activity; and (3) control the major micronutrient deficiency diseases — iron-deficiency anaemia, iodine-deficiency goitre, and of vitamin A deficiency. Experience has shown that free-standing nutrition projects focus attention on malnutrition problems in say, finance and planning ministries, and attack them in ways that, at least for now, other Bank projects have not been able to.

Experience with the nutrition projects has shown that several nutrition actions with demonstrated benefits are technically feasible, cost-effective, and affordable. Whether these can be mounted and effectively administered on a national scale depends, of course, on available resources, but most importantly, on the existing infrastructure. The limitations in absorbing external assistance for such efforts in some countries, particularly in sub-Saharan Africa, pose special problems. In general, however, the type of analysis employed and some of the underlying principles of these actions may merit consideration for being transferable.

Animals in the service of human nutrition

Elsie M. WIDDOWSON
Department of Medicine, Level 5, Addenbrooke's Hospital, Hills Road, Cambridge CB2 2QQ.

I feel extremely honoured to have been invited to give the McCollum Lecture at this Congress, especially as Professor McCollum has been one of my heroes for the past 50 years. I only saw him once, in 1936, when, as a young and inexperienced research worker, I went to the United States for the first time. I knew of his work and I very much wanted to meet him so I wrote to him and told him so. He invited me to visit him in his laboratory at Johns Hopkins, which I did. He was a great man and I was a nobody, yet he treated me with courtesy and kindness, shared his sandwich lunch with me and made me feel as though I was someone who mattered. I have never forgotten his lesson and example.

When I was given the title of my lecture by the organisers of the Congress I realised that it could be interpreted in more than one way, so I want to make it clear at the outset that I am not going to talk about the nutritional value of meat or milk. What I propose to do is first to say something about the history of the use of animals in research on human nutrition, second to refer to the application of the results of studies on animals to man, and third, to say a few words about the use of animals in research on nutrition in relation to the difficulties many are experiencing in doing such research at the present time.

Some highlights of history. Nutrition is a subject that lends itself to experimental work with animals, and thousands of experiments have been made on numerous species in which the diet has been unusual in one respect or another, and the effect on the animals has been followed in various ways. Many of the early studies, however, were made on animals fed on supposedly adequate diets, and measurements were made of their metabolism of energy and protein. England and France led the way in nutritional work with animals and the era of energy metabolism may be said to have opened with Priestley, Crawford and Lavoisier in the latter part of the 18th century. These men were not employed to do this work. Priestley, for example, was a clergyman and Lavoisier was supposed to be concerned with agriculture. Crawford wrote a book in 1778 entitled 'Experiments and observations on animal heat', five years before the publication of the classical paper of Lavoisier and Laplace. Crawford and Lavoisier both used guinea-pigs. Lavoisier and Laplace put a guinea-pig inside a bell jar surrounded by ice and left it there for 10 hours. They commented that they chose this animal because it is docile and will go for a long time without food and drink. The ice gradually melted and they measured the water from it and calculated the amount of heat given out by the guinea-pig which melted the ice. The carbon dioxide in the expired air was also measured.

Lavoisier also studied his own respiratory exchanges and those of his friends. Among other things he showed that oxygen uptake and carbon dioxide output were raised by a fall in environmental temperature, by exercise and by the processes of digestion after a meal. Sadly these were among Lavoisier's last experiments, for in May 1794, at the age of 51, Lavoisier was guillotined. The results were never published in full but they are described in a letter written in November 1790 to Joseph Black, discoverer of carbon dioxide. This letter is reproduced in the earlier editions of Davidson and Passmore's book *Human nutrition and dietetics*. For some reason it has been omitted in later editions.

The principle Lavoisier initiated of making parallel studies on man and animals was handed down to his French pupils, who passed it on to those who came to France from Germany over the next 50 years. Liebig studied in Paris around 1822, and when he returned to Germany he trained Voit who trained Rubner, Pettenkoffer, Bischoff and others, and throughout their work we can see the influence of Lavoisier. These German investigators used experimental animals, particularly dogs, side by side with man, in their studies of energy and protein metabolism. Rubner built an animal calorimeter, and Voit and Rubner made a great many studies on the basal metabolism of man and animals. Rubner formulated his surface area law, which stated that the basal metabolism is proportional to the surface area of the animal, provided that the measurements of different species are made at the same environmental temperature. Some of the German work was undoubtedly inspired by the famines that had devasted Europe from time to time through the centuries, and the effects of starvation on the metabolism of protein, fat and carbohydrate were carefully worked out on dogs. Professional fasters provided the human comparison, and the physiological effects of starvation on man were compared and contrasted with the effect on animals.

While the dog was the experimental animal of the German investigators at the end of the 19th century, the rat was undoubtedly the animal that contributed most to the discovery and disentangling of the vitamins during the first two decades of the present one, but other species played their part, chickens, pigeons, guinea-pigs, mice and dogs. Eijkman, a prison medical officer in the Dutch East Indies, noticed that chickens developed a paralysis when they were fed on polished rice which was similar to that characteristic of the prisoners suffering from beri-beri so he made some experiments. When he gave the birds unmilled rice or a water extract of rice polishings they did not develop the paralysis. Eijkman's paper was published in 1897.

In the days of sailing ships the voyages were long, and there were often outbreaks of disease among the sailors, who lived on dry foods. Japanese sailors, like prisoners, lived on polished rice, and they also got beri-beri, but it was found that this could be prevented with fresh food. The Norwegian navy was also in trouble and Hölst, working in the University of Christiania, now Oslo, became involved early in the 1900s. He supposed the Norwegian sailors had beri-beri too and he repeated Eijkman's studies on chickens, but he used pigeons because these animals are cheaper than chickens and do not take up so much room. He got a similar result. Then, for some reason which is not revealed, Hölst and his colleague Frölich gave a cereal diet to guinea-pigs, expecting them to develop the paralysis of beri-beri, but they became ill in a different way which is described in marvellous detail in their paper published in 1907 in the *Journal of hygiene*. This was of course, scurvy, which was what was affecting sailors in the Norwegian navy, as it was the British sailors in Captain Cook's day. Captain Cook had successfully treated it by giving his crew fresh food, and when the Norwegian guinea-pigs were given fresh cabbage or potatoes along with their cereal the disease did not occur. Hölst and Frölich made the further observation that the 'nutriment' they postulated the cabbage contained was partially lost by boiling it in water for half an hour.

Hopkins knew nothing of all this when he embarked on his famous studies on rats. As a matter of fact his work on vitamins was rather a sideline to him, and among biochemists he is far more famous for his isolation of tryptophan and glutathione than vitamins. It was his studies on tryptophan when he used mice as experimental animals that seem to have given him the idea which he propounded in an address to the Society of Public Analysts in 1906 'No animal can live upon a mixture of pure protein, fat and carbohydrate, and even when the necessary inorganic material is carefully supplied the animal still cannot flourish. The animal body is adjusted to live either upon plant tissues or the tissues of other animals, and these contain countless substances other than proteins, carbohydrates and fat.' Hopkins made some preliminary experiments around this time, but the paper describing his main experiment was not published till 1912. When he later discovered that he was not the first to suggest that unknown nutrients were essential or to make animal experiments to investigate it he was anxious to make amends, which he did in his Nobel lecture in 1929. He shared the Nobel prize with Eijkman.

Hopkins had groups of four to six animals weighing 30–50 g, housed two to a cage for, as he said, rats progress more normally when they have a companion than when kept singly. He fed them all on a diet consisting of casein, raw potato starch, cane sugar, lard, and mineral salts produced by incinerating equal parts of oatmeal and dog biscuits. He stated specifically that he provided no roughage. To one group of animals in each experiment he gave fresh milk, 1, 2 or 3 ml per rat per day. Those having milk grew, while those not having milk ate less food and failed to grow and soon began to lose weight, so that after about 20 d the experiment had to be terminated. If after 18 d the treatment was reversed, those now given milk started to grow, while those deprived of milk lost weight. Hopkins postulated that the milk contained something that was essential for growth and health of the animals. So far so good. But nobody could repeat these experiments and the reason was the usual one; nobody did exactly what Hopkins had done, and the main trouble was that he did not describe in his original paper every experimental detail of his procedure. Raw potato starch, which was used as the principal source of carbohydrate, is not as well digested as other forms of raw starch, or cooked starch, or sugar. Undigested potato starch reaches the caecum where it ferments, causes the caecum to enlarge and the caecal contents to have an acid pH, and it also results in the synthesis of B vitamins, which are then absorbed. This process is known as refection.

Anyone following what Hopkins said he did in his original experiments could not have got the results he got for they would have found that the rats grew splendidly whether they had milk or not. In fact Hopkins found this out when he repeated his original experiments 30 years later. One thing was done in the original experiments which was not mentioned in the paper, except to say that it was not done, and this was to give the animals roughage in the forms of strips of filter paper dipped in a weak sugar solution before they were fed. The filter paper must have prevented refection, prevented synthesis of B vitamins in the caecum, so the animals became deficient in B vitamins, and the milk given them must have provided just enough of the B vitamins for their needs, although it is difficult to see how such very small amounts of milk could have done so. Hopkins' paper inspired a large amount of work, and even though his Nobel prize seems to have been awarded for the publication of one rather doubtful paper and a big idea, the honour done to him met with general approbation because it was recognised that he was responsible for opening up a new and rapidly developing field of discovery; discovery which largely depended on the use of the young rapidly growing rat.

In 1906, when Hopkins' thoughts were turning to those 'countless substances other than proteins, fats and carbohydrates', McCollum obtained his PhD degree at Yale and in 1907 he obtained a post in the Department of Agricultural Chemistry at the University of Wisconsin. Unlike Hopkins, McCollum was a great reader of the literature, and he soon found that a number of investigations had been made between 1873 and 1906 in which small animals, usually mice, had been fed on restricted diets of isolated proteins, fats and carbohydrates. In every instance he wrote 'they promptly failed in health, rapidly deteriorated physically and lived only a few weeks'. He concluded that the most important problem in nutrition was to discover what was lacking in such diets. He reasoned that he must use small experimental animals with a short life span, and like Hopkins, he decided to use rats. Rats did not seem to be available at the University of Wisconsin, and McCollum did not get much enouragement from the Dean of the College of Agriculture, who refused to provide any money, so he had to get the rats himself. He describes how he did this in a letter he wrote to Dr Salmon of the Alabama Polytechnic Institute in 1948. Dr Prebluda kindly sent me a copy of this letter. Even in 1907 McCollum was evidently aware of Hopkins' early experiments and ideas for he wrote 'In the autumn of 1907 I decided to try to take up studies of the effects of purified food mixtures where

Professor F.G. Hopkins had left off the preceding year. Because of total lack of comprehension of what such studies meant in the way of experimental management of animals I decided upon using wild grey rats. Accordingly I caught 17 one afternoon in the horse barn at the Wisconsin Experiment Station Farm and set out to feed them experimental rations. They were so terrified and ferocious when I tried to do anything to them that I soon gave it up and chloroformed them. I then bought a dozen "albino" rats from an animal dealer in Chicago. He was a pet stock man. I do not remember his name. I began with this stock, and soon had sufficient experimental young animals for my small resources'.

He subsequently acquired other rats which he interbred with his own, and so set up his hybrid colony. What McCollum does not say in this letter is that he had to buy his first 12 rats from the pet stock man himself, and then pay for their cages. Later, Professor Hart, head of the Department of Agricultural Chemistry, allowed him to spend 50 dollars for two animal units. The carpenter, who was sorry for him, made him three units for the price of two. So in January 1908 he was ready to start. He had the notion that the reason rats did not do well on purified diets was because these diets were unpalatable. This led him nowhere, but it was not until 1911 that he gave up the idea. He devoted much of his time to his rat colony during those early years, caring for them himself, but he badly needed help, and this came providentially in the shape of Miss Marguerite Davis. She was a graduate who wanted to study biochemistry with McCollum. When she learned about his rat colony and how he was doing everything himself she volunteered to look after the animals for him. This she did for 5 years without pay, and it was only in the 6th year that Dr McCollum managed to get a small salary for her. Her practical help led to a fruitful collaboration and the publication of 11 joint papers. I cannot go into all the work in detail, for there was so much of it. Among their important discoveries were that the substance present in whole cereals that prevents polyneuritis in chickens and pigeons was also necessary for rats. Further, even when the diet contained whole cereals young rats needed something else which was contained in butter fat but not in lard or olive oil. Thus McCollum and Davis have the credit for discovering that two factors, fat-soluble A and water-soluble B, were necessary for the growth of rats. One outcome of this work was that the colony of rats, which had been barely tolerated in the Wisconsin College of Agriculture, now became important because they had been used to prove that butter was superior to olive oil and lard, and this was great news for the dairy farmers of Wisconsin.

When Miss Davis left in 1916 she was replaced by Miss Nina Simmonds, and it was during the collaboration of McCollum and Simmonds that it was discovered that green leaves had activity similar to that of fat-soluble A, and that the fat-soluble factor A had functions other than promoting growth. Deficiency of it produced eye lesions, and McCollum and Simmonds introduced the word xerophthalmia to describe the condition.

Now we come back to England to Mellanby. Mellanby studied in Cambridge and in 1906 he spent a year working under Hopkins in the crowded old physiological laboratories. He then went to London to qualify in medicine and in 1913 was appointed Professor of Physiology at King's College for Women in Kensington, London. In 1914 the Medical Research Committee, which later became the Medical Research Council, held a meeting, at which Hopkins was present. Rickets was still a great scourge in Britain, and Hopkins suggested that the nature and cause of rickets would be a suitable subject for investigation. Hopkins recommended that Mellanby should be invited to undertake the work. Mellanby knew that puppies got rickets so he chose them as his experimental animals. There was nowhere at the college in Kensington to keep the puppies, so they were housed in Cambridge. At that time rickets was believed to be due to lack of exercise, or to an infection, but after a long series of experiments Mellanby was able to prove that a dietary deficiency was the cause, and the essential nutrient was present in animal fat, especially in cod liver oil, but was lacking in vegetable oil. It therefore seemed to correspond with McCollum's fat-soluble A factor. However, in 1920 Mellanby published a paper showing that two unknown factors must exist, because some fats cured the lesion of the eyes which McCollum had named xerophthalmia and others cured rickets. Cod liver oil would cure both. Mellanby made some preliminary communications, and his full publication 'Experimental rickets' appeared in 1921.

In 1917 McCollum moved to Johns Hopkins, taking some of his rats with him. The others remained in Wisconsin with Hart and Steenbock. In 1918 he noticed that rats developed a rachitic condition if they were fed on cereals and an abnormal calcium to phosphorus ratio. This could be prevented by giving small amounts of cod liver oil. McCollum devised the line test — a line of calcification in the bone of a deficient rat when it was given a source of vitamin D. So McCollum and Mellanby between them separated the two fat-soluble vitamins A and D, and thanks to their studies on animals, and those of Dame Harriette Chick and her colleagues on children in Vienna after the first World War, widespread rickets in Europe and America virtually disappeared. Not so xerophthalmia and blindness due to a deficiency of vitamin A. In spite of all the work of McCollum 70 years ago vitamin A deficiency is still with us, and it is a sad reflection on the world today that 5 million children every year suffer from xerophthalmia, of whom 250 000 become blind.

The story of how the B vitamins were sorted out is a long one and I do not propose to go into it except to say that it was Elvehjem's observations in 1937 that black tongue in dogs, which is similar to human pellagra in many ways, was cured by nicotinic acid that gave the clue to the cause of pellagra, and Sebrell's studies, also with dogs, helped to solve the problem of riboflavin deficiency.

The work of Hopkins, McCollum, Mellanby and other pioneers was followed by many studies on rats, some very good, some less so. In the 1930s about 3000 papers a year were published on some aspect of vitamin research, generally involving the use of rats as experimental animals. New and important work was opening up at this time on trace elements. Those with the longest history are iodine and iron, and in both instances the original observations were made on man.

By 1928 Hart, in Wisconsin, was himself using rats, presumably from McCollum's colony, and with colleagues mastered the technique of feeding them on purified diets containing all the essential mineral elements apart from the trace element they were studying. They discovered that copper as well as iron was necessary for blood formation, and in 1931 showed that manganese was essential for normal ovarian function. In 1934 they demonstrated that zinc was essential for growth and development.

McCollum had been interested in inorganic nutrients since 1909. His early studies concerned the phosphorus requirement of laying hens, part of his agricultural commitments. Then in the 1930s with his student Elsa Orent, he began investigating the effects of magnesium deficiency on young rats and puppies. In 1931 they showed that a deficiency of manganese caused degeneration of the testes and sterility in male rats. Manganese-deficient females produced their young normally but did not suckle or care for them. The newspapers got hold of this and reported that manganese was necessary for the maternal instinct.

So much for the use of animals in the discoveries of vitamins and trace elements. In 1939 came the Second World War, and the war years and those following them saw the revival of interest in deficiencies of energy and protein. The description by Cicely Williams working in the Gold Coast in the 1930s of a protein deficiency disease which she called kwashiorkor sparked off a large amount of work after the war both on children and on experimental animals. The Medical Research Council set up research units in Uganda and Jamaica for studies on children, and centres were set up by the United States, Sweden and other countries in various parts of the world. India too played an important part in research on human malnutrition. Investigations were also made in many countries in the 50s and 60s on the effects of deficiencies of energy and protein on rats, pigs, dogs, primates and other species. We made some ourselves, but I think the important fundamental obervations were made, and are still being made, on children and their mothers in Africa, Jamaica, Central America and elsewhere.

In the developed countries obesity, cardiovascular disease and the importance of dietary fibre are the aspects of human nutrition of most concern. Are animals helping us over these problems? So far as cardiovascular disease and dietary fibre are concerned the important observations are being made and will probably continue to be made on man. The problem of obesity and the regulation of energy balance is being studied on man and experimental animals with calorimeters and by other means, just as the German investigators were doing 100 years ago. I think the heyday of animals in the service of human nutrition was in the first two decades of this century and that is why I have devoted much of my lecture to this period. New techniques have now made it possible to make studies on man that would hitherto have been out of the question. Much of this Congress has concerned observations made directly on man.

The applicability of results on animals to human nutrition. I want now to discuss briefly the applicability of results obtained on animals to human nutrition. There are of course important differences between man and animals, and for those of us who are interested in comparative nutrition these provide the fun. However, if our concern is primarily with human nutrition there are certain things we must bear in mind. There are a few real species differences in metabolism, for example the ability of animals except man and the guinea-pig to synthesise vitamin C, and the peculiarities of the cat as regards its metabolism of fatty acids and amino acids. But most of the species differences are quantitative, due to differences in size, rate of metabolism, growth, maturation and reproduction and hence nutrient requirements. These can be an advantage or a disadvantage as the case may be. The rapid growth of small animals like the rat, with their correspondingly high requirement for nutrients, was vital in the identification of the various accessory food factors. In using animals as models for man, whether at birth, during childhood, as adults or in old age it is important to know the characteristics of the species of animal you have chosen. Claude Bernard was so right when he wrote in his *Introduction to the study of experimental medicine* in 1865 'The solution of a physiological or pathological problem often depends solely on the appropriate choice of the animal for the experiment'.

Problems of today. I know that investigators in many countries are very troubled at the present time about how long their experimental work with animals will be allowed to continue. Do not despair. They were having the same problems in Britain in 1890 when Thomas Henry Huxley wrote about them, and in France in 1865 when Claude Bernard was doing the same thing. Animal experiments must go on, for who knows what discoveries lie ahead? I have used many species including the human one in my investigations, and in fact I have to confess that for the first 20 years of my research life I never touched an experimental animal at all. Professor McCance and I worked entirely with human beings, ourselves included, studying the response to salt deficiency, the absorption and excretion of calcium, magnesium, iron, and other elements under various conditions, the voluntary intake of food, the expenditure of energy, the response to undernutrition and the nutritive value of different kinds of bread for undernourished children. It was only after we returned to Cambridge from Germany, in the early 50s, that we started to work with animals, and since then pigs, cats, dogs, rats, mice, guinea-pigs, rabbits, and even seals, eels and trout, not to speak of blackbirds and thrushes, have been used by us to investigate some aspect of nutrition and growth. It always seemed strange when I was busy with studies on human beings in the 1930s and 1940s that, while all animal experiments in UK were strictly controlled, there were no regulations about experiments on man. Now human experiments are under the supervision of ethical committees, but this is a recent development and I think Professor McCance's paper on 'The practice of experimental medicine' in 1951 was one of the first to draw attention to this matter. As long ago as 1876, however, in the UK the Cruelty to Animals Act was passed. I always think this is rather an unfortunate title. The Home Office not only licences every institution in which experiments are made and supervises them by inspection, but issues licences and certificates to individual investigators, all of whom have to be approved beforehand as competent and responsible persons. The types of experiments they are permitted to perform, and the conditions they must fulfil, are all clearly laid down and all experiments have to be reported to the Home Office. No experiment which is likely to cause pain is permitted unless the animal is anaesthetized. Legislation is soon to be introduced to make the control over the use of experimental animals even tighter. Not only the scientists but each of their projects will have to be approved beforehand. I have never resented the Home Office regulations concerning animal experiments — in fact I have welcomed them as providing a form of protection and help. I do not know the situation in other countries so I must leave you to compare our way of dealing with the supervision of animal experiments with your own.

Animals have served human nutrition well over the past century, they are still doing so, and will do so in the future. However, I think man is becoming more important as a subject of study, and it seems as though we are rediscovering the philosophy of Alexander Pope early in the 18th century that 'The proper study of mankind is man'.

The suitability of animal models for research in human nutrition: a workshop report

C. BEYNEN and C. E. WEST (Organizers)
*Department of Laboratory Animal Science, State University, P.O. Box 80.166, 3508 TD Utrecht;
Department of Human Nutrition, Agricultural University, De Dreijen 12, 6703 BC Wageningen, The
Netherlands.*

The workshop discussion was introduced by the presentation of data on the use of animals in biomedical research. The total number of animals used in the United Kingdom in 1982 was 4.2 million[1]. For the United States in 1980 and the Netherlands in 1983 these figures were 20 to 70 and 1.3 million, respectively[2,3]. As a rough guide, this is equivalent to one animal per ten residents per year in each of these countries. Put in another way, seven animals are used for each of us during our lifetime. Mice (56 per cent) and rats (28 per cent) represent about 80 per cent of the total animals used[3].

There are no data available on the number of animals used in human nutrition research. In volumes 35 – 38 of the *American Journal of Clinical Nutrition*, which is a journal that particularly focuses on human nutrition research, 76 (17 per cent) of the original research papers involved animal studies. In 51 (67 per cent) of these papers rats were the experimental animals used. About half of these rat papers dealt with aspects of lipid or mineral metabolism.

After the introduction, the workshop took the form of a general discussion on two major topics concerning the use of animals in human nutrition research, followed by a presentation of four specific examples. The general discussion commenced with summaries of statements submitted prior to the meeting by 21 participants, which were prepared by the organizers. These statements could be divided into two types: those with which there was unanimous agreement, and those which were controversial to a greater or lesser degree. Immediately after presentation of the statements, and prior to a discussion of them, consensus was reached on the issue of whether animals should be used *per se*. *It was concluded that it is legitimate to use animals in the service of man for human nutrition research.* However, there are certain limitations which were discussed.

The first question addressed was: 'Why use animal models in human nutrition research?' All participants agreed on the following points: greater control over the variables (including diet) being studied; reduction of the variability between subjects; more ability to carry out demanding and invasive studies; ability to carry out lifespan (endpoint) and multigeneration studies; use of the specific sensitivity of animals at the species, strain or individual level, and reduction of cost.

Although cost is an important factor, the workshop agreed that in fact this was not and should not be the primary reason for using animals in human nutrition research. The general advantages of the use of animals were thus highlighted. The major disadvantage lies in the fact that animals are not humans, and therefore extrapolation of animal data to man has to be done with great caution. The participants agreed upon a number of *guide-lines for animal experimentation*: only those experiments to be carried out which have potential to contribute useful knowledge — as seen by outside observers possibly comprising a committee capable of providing peer review; use of the minimum number of animals consistent with statistical analysis of the results anticipated (journal editors should help here!), and reduction of discomfort to animals as far as possible. It should not be implied that experimental animals always suffer discomfort. Any intervention should be within acceptable limits established by investigators and society as a whole; a peer-review system would represent the interests of both these groups.

The choice of the proper animal model was scrutinized. The question addressed was: *'What are the criteria for the choice of animal models in human nutrition research?'* All participants agreed on the following points. The animal must exhibit, as closely as possible, the biological phenomenon to be examined or it must be possible to induce such a phenomenon. The animal husbandry used must not impose unreasonable constraints on the animal, on the experimental design or on the investigator. The experience (in both meanings of the word) of research workers plays a role in the choice of animal model to be used. The availability and price of animals also plays a role.

The workshop was seen by all present as a very useful exercise. It performed a valuable function in defining the role, advantages and problems of using animals in human nutrition research. The participants were of the opinion that the deliberations and conclusions of the workshop should reach as wide an audience as possible. They also proposed that the topic of the workshop should be included in the programme of future international nutrition congresses.

We thank the following persons for their written contributions submitted prior to the workshop: C.A. Barth, J.E. Bauer, W. Becker, R. Bressani, K.K. Carroll, M.I. Gurr, J.E. Halver, B.S. Hetzel, K. Imaizumi, A.G. Low, Y.-F. Lu, R. van der Meer, R. Noack, B. Ratcliffe, E. Renner, A.A. Rerat, D.C.K. Roberts, E.J. Sinkeldam, A.M. Snoswell, M. Sugano, and B. Tucker. The following persons are thanked for expressing prior to the workshop their willingness to contribute to the discussions at the workshop from the floor: G.B. Brubacher, M.E. Coates, N. DiMarco, D. Frape, A.R. Johnson, D. Kritchevsky, G.U. Liepa, G.T. Steel and A. Wise.

1 Home Office (1982): *Statistics of experiments on living animals (Cmnd 8986)*, London: HMSO.
2 Institute for Laboratory Animal Resources (1980): *International survey on the supply, quality and use of laboratory animals (NIH Public. No. 80–2091)*. Washington DC: US Department of Health and Human Services.
3 Sectie Dierproeven van de Veterinaire Hoofdinspectie van de Volksgezondheid (1984): *Zo Doende 1983*. Leidschendam: Ministerie van Welzijn, Volksgezondheid en Cultuur.

II: Problems in the developing world

Undernutrition and the quality of life

M. GABR
Department of Paediatrics, Faculty of Medicine, Cairo University, Egypt

Food deprivation is unquestionably the most pervasive problem of mankind. Improved nutrition is part and parcel of a better quality of life. The case for national support for nutrition essentially rests on two bases, a welfare or quality of life rationale and an economic rationale. The pay-off of the first is qualitative and must be appraised in the light of the values in a society[1]. I will elaborate here on those human factors related to dietary intake which might affect the quality of life, viz disease response, reproductive competence, cognitive functions, work output, productivity, social and behavioural functions. Functional failure in any of these domains can have profound consequences affecting the pattern of human activity and may even have broader consequences for society through alteration in individual behaviour and psychosocial well-being[6].

Nutrition and child-bearing women. Several studies have demonstrated the low energy and nutrient intake of pregnant women in developing countries. The average daily intake of non-privileged Ethiopian pregnant women for different nutrients varied between 40–70 per cent of FAO/WHO recommendations[19]. The same is true for lactating women (Table).

Table. *Daily energy intakes of child-bearing women in some developing countries.[19]*

		kcal	MJ			kcal	MJ
Pregnancy:	Gambia (wet season)	1350–1450	5.6–6.1	Lactation:	Gambia (wet season)	1200–1300	5.0–5.4
	(dry season)	1600–1700	6.7–7.1		(dry season)	1600–1750	6.7–7.3
	New Guinea	1360	5.7		India	1300–1620	5.4–6.8
	India	1400–1920	5.7–8.0		Guatemala	1600	6.7
	Ethiopia	1540	6.4				
	Tanzania	1850	7.7				
	Guatemala	1500–2060	6.3–8.6				

Protein-energy malnutrition of the pregnant mother is an important cause of low birth-weight which may be as high as 25 per cent compared to 4 per cent in Western countries[16]. It was reported that a 10 per cent increase in a mother's weight for age resulted in a 2.4 per cent increase in a child's weight for age[3]. Furthermore, the incidence of abortions, miscarriages, still births and congenital malformations is highest in malnourished mothers.

Studies in Guatemala have demonstrated that maternal energy supplementation is causally related to birth-weight and the length of pregnancy. The proportion of low-birth-weight (below 2.5 kg) and short gestational age babies (less than 36 weeks) in the group of low-supplemented mothers was 19 and 18 per cent as opposed to 9 and 4 per cent in highly-supplemented mothers respectively[12].

Low-birth-weight babies are more liable to infections because of their poor immunological capabilities. This results in much higher perinatal and neonatal infant mortality and morbidity rates. There is evidence that the immunological defect might persist till late childhood even after catch-up in physical growth is achieved. The harmful effect of nutrient deficiencies on the brain is severest when it affects the fetus. The resulting mental, psychological and educational handicaps are not completely reversible, with a marked effect on social and economic productivity of the nation.

Except in extreme maternal undernutrition, the concentration of energy and protein in breast milk is usually maintained. In Gambia, the energy content dropped by about 10 per cent when intake was 1100 kcal (4.6 MJ)/d. The vitamin content, particularly of water-soluble vitamins, is very sensitive to dietary intake. It is the volume of milk which suffers greatly from maternal undernutrition. Studies in Zaire, Gambia and Kenya have shown that the fall in milk volume becomes critical as early as the 4th month. In a recent study in Egypt, it was shown that certain anti-infective factors in human milk are also affected by maternal undernutrion which might affect neonatal gastrointestinal defence of the newborn[10].

Furthermore, the decreased physical performance secondary to undernutrition of the pregnant and lactating mother in many developing countries greatly affects her work productivity at home and in the fields, contributing to further undernutrition in family and community.

Nutrition and infection. The interaction between nutrition and infection has been established for decades both in animal and human field studies. Infections contribute to undernutrition through several factors: increased tissue catabolism, nitrogen loss in urine, reduced appetite, vomiting, decreased absorption, protein loss in gastrointestinal tract, rapid sequestration of nutrients and their utilisation in the production of acute-phase reactant proteins, antibodies, complement and other host-protective factors[7]. Diarrhoeal disease in particular is an important cause of undernutrition. Absorption of protein has been reported to be decreased by 20–30 per cent, that of carbohydrates by 73–77 per cent while fat excretion is reported to be increased by 6–14 per cent. The mechanism of malabsorption in diarrhoea is related to pancreatic malfunction, bacterial overgrowth with fermentation, abnormal conjugation of bile salts, morphological changes in the villi as well as increased intestinal transit time. Furthermore, intestinal parasites compete with host requirements. The common cultural practice of withholding food during diarrhoea exaggerates the resultant malnutrition.

The synergistic effect of malnutrition and infection contributes to the social and health misery of the poor; death from measles is 200–400 times greater in malnourished children than in Western nations. While mortality of measles is 0.01 per cent in Sweden, it varies between 5–25 per cent in Africa. Complications of measles have been reported in over 60 per cent of malnourished children in Nairobi. Measles is known to precipitate acute malnutrition in the marginally-nourished child and there is evidence that improving the nutritional status is an effective measure in reducing the fatality from diarrhoeal disease and measles[20].

It is encouraging however to note that with better socioeconomic development and better nutrition the rate of childhood mortality is declining in many African countries.

Nutrition and the immune response. Undernutrition interferes with immunocompetence in several ways. The skin of the malnourished infant is thin and breaks easily while the epithelium of the eye is defective. Gastric acidity is impaired. The bacterial killing capacity of the polymorphs is reduced. Many of the natural, cellular and humoral factors responsible for immunocompetence are impaired in malnourished individuals.

Protein-energy malnutrition (PEM) results in decrease of the total haemolytic complement as well as reduced levels of many complement components, particularly C_3. Transferrin levels are low in PEM. Humoral immunity in malnutrition is only impaired for those antigens needing the help of T lymphocytes or macrophages. There is a diminished number of IgA-secreting cells in the jejunal mucosa of children with PEM.

Cell-mediated immunity is greatly impaired in malnourished children who are more susceptible to infections by organisms such as tuberculosis, measles, herpes simplex, hepatitis, pneumocystis carinii and Gram-negative septicaemia. There is marked reduction in the population of T lymphocytes together with increase in the number of nul cells. The proportion of rosette-forming T lymphocytes and of T-helper cells is reduced while suppressor cells are increased. Delayed cutaneous hypersensitivity is demonstrated in PEM being more marked in kwashiorkor than marasmus. These changes are also observed in a lesser degree in the much more prevalent marginal or moderate malnutrition both in children and adults[7]. Nutritional rehabilitation restores the defective immunological capabilities except in fetal malnutrition where impaired malnutrition may persist for several years. Nutritional deficiencies may also impair immune functions. Reduced cell-mediated immunity and impairment of bacterial killing by leucocytes has been reported in iron-deficiency anaemia[10].

Nutrition, infant and child mortality. Malnutrition is the single most important associated factor responsible for the high mortality rate in developing countries. A recent World Bank review related energy deficits to life expectancy, child and infant mortality and child growth[12]. Cases of PEM have a high fatality rate[5].

It is estimated that 24 000 children die in Ghana annually due to kwashiorkor[15]. Nutritional deficiency was found to be the underlying associated cause of death in 55 per cent of child deaths in Latin America. Infant mortality rates are 20 times higher in certain developing countries than developed countries. The 1–4 year child mortality which is 1 per cent in most Western countries was as high as 36 per cent in Ethiopia.

Nutrition and fertility. Better nutrition affects women's fertility by influencing the ages of menarche, menopause, the success of each pregnancy, the duration of post-partum sterility and fecundity during the menstrual cycle. Females from better-nourished populations have earlier menarche and later menopause than females from malnourished populations.

On the other hand, reduction in infant and childhood mortality associated with better nutrition has been shown in several field studies to be a prerequisite for accepting family planning services which should be made available together with nutritional rehabilitation programmes. Family planning is maximal when parents are assured that their offspring will survive.

Furthermore, better maternal nutrition extends the period of lactation and does so to such a degree that the duration of post-partum infecundity of the lactating mother may in fact be extended rather than shortened by improving maternal nutrition.

Nutrition, intellectual development and cognitive functions. There is a concensus of opinion that severe malnutrition affects intellectual development specially if it occurs during the first 6 months of life and possibly the first 2 years. In these cases, the detrimental effects seem irreversible whereas the effects of malnutrition occurring later in life seem less persistent.

Nutrition, behaviour and socio-emotional functions. Most studies deal with the effect of malnutrition on cognitive functions, while only a few studies deal with the effect of undernutrition and child behaviour. Such studies are important for several reasons. (1) Cognitive performance is dependent on motivational factors including attention, persistence and self-confidence. (2) Animal studies proved the great impact of undernutrition on such behavioural characteristics as activity levels, emotional control, attention to novel stimuli and social responsiveness. (3) There is evidence that social and emotional capacities are more vulnerable to chronic environmental insult than are cognitive functions. Under certain conditions, eg iron-deficiency, changes in nutrient intake will influence behaviour prior to measured physical parameters. There is evidence that lasting behavioural problems may result from social deprivation. Malnutrition in infancy is a particular type of environmental deprivation, since infant-feeding occurs with an interactive contact, thus constituting in itself a type of social stimulation; therefore interference with it results in decreased interaction with physical and social environment. (4) There is a shift on part of educators and psychologists from cognitive to social competence as the major criterion for evaluating the physiological functioning of children[2].

Socio-emotional competence of the undernourished child is affected in two ways: (1) general social interaction characteristics including interaction with peers, behaviour towards adults, response to physical environment, affection and activity level; (2) characteristic response to specific types of situations particularly to stressful or pressured situations including response to competition, frustrating problems, physical stress or discomfort, another person in distress, an unfamiliar environment or demand to control impulses etc[2].

The inadequately-nourished child shows characteristics of apathy, non-responsiveness, non-goal-directed behaviour, impulsivity, failure to respond normally in social interactions and difficulty to cope with stress or frequent daily demands.

There is evidence that deficits in family function, and in social behaviour of those caring for children, and their interaction with infants affect their nutritional state. Recent studies demonstrated identifiable differences in child care and social behaviour between families whose children develop PEM and those who do not[9]. Those caring for children usually respond to the undernourished child less often, and with less enthusiasm, than to the well-nourished, probably due to the former's less demanding attitude. This sets up a vicious circle with the malnourished child withdrawing from social interaction, having lowered self-esteem and ultimately having a lowered physical activity.

Studies on adult human volunteers have shown that adults develop similar behavioural changes following food deprivation. They become apathetic, have difficulty in concentration and become less physically active.

Malnutrition and physical performance. Poor working efficiency amongst undernourished populations has been a frequent observation for decades. Experiments on human volunteers revealed a reduction of muscle strength by nearly 30 per cent and of precision movements by 15–20 per cent at the end of a semi-starvation period. Adaptation to malnutrition seems to be achieved in part through reduction in voluntary activity.

Malnutrition in early childhood affects the working capacity in adult life mainly through its effect on body weight and there is a direct relationship between body size and the capacity to perform work. In certain agricultural occupations, better nutrition leads to a body composition with a high proportion of fat-free mass which represents an investment in human capital. Similarly, improved levels of energy and protein during the preproductive phase of life cycle, when these lead to taller adults, represent an investment in human capital resulting in significantly increased life-time earnings[18].

Recent studies using modern ergometric psychomotor tests, suggest that marginal degrees of malnutrition affect the ability to perform more complex work functions such as precision control, multilimb coordination, rate control, arm/hand steadiness, finger dexterity, reaction time and aiming.

On the national level, the decreased working capacity of the malnourished labourer adversely affects productivity. A vicious circle is established when the diminished physical capacity of the malnourished farmer affects food production. The beneficial effects of dietary improvement on production not only increases productivity, but also improves employees' morale, labour management relation and health with significant reduction in illness, absenteeism and number of accidents[8].

Nutrition and educational capabilities. The impaired cognitive functions interact with the socio-emotional incompetence, decreased activity and physical capabilities and the higher risk of infection of the undernourished child to interfere with the learning process. Malnutrition interferes with education later in life, not only because the malnourished child's ability to concentrate and learn are impaired, but because of frequent absenteeism secondary to nutritionally-related illnesses. Malnutrition contributes to poor performance, low aspiration towards higher levels of education and to substantial rate of scholastic failure or drop-out often found among the poorly fed. The child's chances of advancement are greatly restricted if he is malnourished no matter what else he may be offered by education or other means.

Breast-feeding and quality of life. Malnutrition, diarrhoeal disease and infant mortality rates are much higher among artificially-fed infants compared to breast-fed infants. Out of 924 cases of kwashiorkor in India, none were breast-fed and only five out of 29 cases of marasmus were breast-fed. In a study in three Arab villages, 28.6 per cent of bottle fed-infants, 6 months' old were below the 3rd percentile against 1.6 per cent of breast-fed infants of the same age group. Infant mortality rates in artificially-fed infants are 5–10 times higher than breast-fed infants. In Egypt, diarrhoeal disease was four times more prevalent in bottle-fed than breast-fed infants. The protective value of breast-feeding in this crucial period is a blessing in underprivileged communities which cannot provide a safe and adequate replacement.

Post-partum plasma prolactin levels of lactating mothers are much higher than those of non-lactating mothers, affording a long protective period of amenorrhoea. It was estimated that the 'couple-years protection' provided by breast-feeding in developing countries may be as high as 35 million annually[11].

Specific deficiencies. Certain specific deficiencies might have sustained life-long sequelae on the health productivity and welfare of the community. Vitamin-A-deficiency is one of the main causes of blindness in developing countries. The efficacy, simplicity and cheapness by which this can be overcome should encourage all governments to take the most suitable intervention action. The mental retardation and occasional deafmutism of endemic cretins born to iodine-deficient goitrous mothers can also be prevented. Iron-deficiency anaemia is known to affect the immune response, physical activity, cognitive and socio-emotional functions. Because of its prevalence among schoolchildren, its effect on learning ability is greater than is commonly recognized. Recent studies indicate that the same defects are also observed in subclinical cases of iron-deficiency. Iron-fortification and iron-therapy should be part of all nutritional intervention programmes.

Cost of malnutrition. Malnutrition constitutes a costly drain on a national economy so that policies and plans to improve human nutrition will spare funds and make them available for other development programmes. An attempt to quantify the cost of malnutrition is required in order to justify allocating a reasonable share of available resources for its combat. The economic losses of undernutrition include: (1) direct costs related to prevention, treatment and rehabilitation of nutritional disorders as well as treatment of nutritionally-related infections, and child wastage through miscarriage abortion, stillbirth and increased mortality, as well as the costs of infant formula, if breast-feeding is declining; (2) indirect costs due to loss of productivity secondary to impaired cognitive functions, physical performance, learning abilities, behavioural changes, the negative effect on family planning and the lack of an individual's ability to enjoy life. A great part of these indirect costs of malnutrition are not easy to quantify.

An attempt to estimate economic benefits of better nutrition in the United States concluded[14] that these — measured in US dollars — can accrue in five areas: physical performance 6.4–25.5 billion; morbidity 201–502 million; mortality 68–157 million; education 6.4–19.2 billion and intergenerative effects 1.3–4.5 billion.

The social and economic costs of reproductive losses and the associated fetal and infant wastage—inefficient reproduction— is effectively a loss of investment in human capital. Reproductive inefficiency results in heavy nutrient wastage.

Cost of infant and child waste through increased mortality related to malnutrition has been estimated in Jamaica in 1968–69 to be 110 US $ for an infant and 188 US $ for a child 1–4 years old giving a total value of 317 250 US $ for 148 deaths secondary to nutritionally-related disease in a population of 2.7 million inhabitants[8]. It is difficult to estimate the cost of prevention, treatment and rehabilitation of malnutrition. A critical review of intervention programmes revealed that the cost of a successful intervention programme providing a supplement of 300–400 kcal (1.25–1.67 MJ)/d was 15–25 US $ per person per year. In 1972 it was estimated that 250 000 US $ were spent yearly in Ghana to treat malnourished children[16]. In Jamacia (1968–69) the estimated total annual cost of inpatient treatment of childhood PEM was 1.3 million US $.

Food loss that can occur with decline in breast-feeding is tremendous. It was estimated that in Tanzania, the annual production of human milk was approximately 40 million gallons. Its value if substituted for powdered milk would have been US $ 22 million/year (1963 estimate), a sum which considerably exceeds the whole Ministry of Health budget. Although breast-feeding is the norm in Ivory Coast, if it were to increase so that every infant was breast-fed for 2 years the savings would amount to 16–28 million US $ annually. Each family would save 600 to 730 US $ on cost of goods and time plus any savings that might result from avoidance of disease or malnutrition caused by bottle-feeding as well as the loss of the beneficial contraceptive effect of lactation. It was reported from Trinidad that it costs twice as much to import infant formula to bottle-feed babies than to import commodities required for supplementary feeding of lactating mothers. This does not take into account the other unquantifiable losses if breast-feeding is abandoned.

The loss of productivity of adult workers due to childhood malnutrition and the cost to the educational budget because of lowered efficiency of learning are not easily quantifiable. It has been postulated that if all of the 25 000 malnourished children in Chile in 1973 were given a food supplement in the first 2 years, the total gain in earning would represent 100 million escudos, or more than 1 per cent of the gross domestic production, a very large absolute return from a single programme[17].

Conclusion. In the third world where economic resources are limited, policies to improve human nutrition must have strong justification, in order to receive the necessary priority so that sufficient funds may be allocated for that purpose. The adverse effects of malnutrition on the quality of life and its implications on national productivity and socioeconomic development is the strongest argument that would convince policy makers. Unless the vicious circle is broken human beings will continue to be undernourished because they were born poor and will continue to be poor because they are undernourished.

Thanks to the establishment of new techniques there has been a tremendous advance in our knowledge of the relationship between nutrition and the various parameters affecting the quality of life, viz fetal wastage, mortality, morbidity, fertility, immunity, cognitive functions, behaviour, socio-emotional competence, educational capability, physical performance, productivity and last but not least the drain on national economy. Scientists, however, should always seek to fill in gaps in our knowledge. More research is needed, to standarize new techniques and methodologies, to settle areas of conflict, to determine economic sequences of undernutrition and find out innovative intervention approaches.

Establishment of valid and reliable instruments, techniques, methodologies and their standardisation on an international basis is required for better assessment and evaluation. This is specially needed for studies related to social, emotional, cognitive and physical capabilities. Recent advances in computers, electronics and applied mathematics have given rise to development of quantifiable techniques. Attempts to simplify these methods and render them less costly to be adapted for application in developing countries is needed.

Because of the interaction between early nutritional history and the ongoing nutritional experience as well as the possible intrusion of environmental and cultural factors into the nutritional situation, interdisciplinary research is needed to distinguish irreversible functional residues of early malnutrition from the effects of past or present adverse biological and social conditions including recent nutritional conditions. This might explain the discrepancies in the long-term effects of undernutrition, reported from different countries.

Recent studies suggest that nutritional intervention can reduce cognitive insult following early undernutrition if carried out as late as 36–48 months of age[13]. More research is needed to increase our understanding of the potential reversibility of the functional sequelae of undernutrition.

More studies are also required to clarify the role of socioeconomic and cultural characteristics of the mother and the family in determining the functional sequelae of undernutrition in their children. The compatibility of the mother's job with care of her children, and the welfare of children of working mothers, need more studies in different sociocultural and economic settings.

Although the functional consequences of marginal malnutrition seem to be well-established, more research is needed to clarify the magnitude and specific functional handicap of the marginally undernourished as well as its economic consequences. The possibility of adaptation in the chronically-malnourished, if it exists, has to be studied in depth. More research on the effect of malnutrition on human capital is needed in order to quantify the cost effectiveness of its combat within the existing socioeconomic and cultural constraints. Innovative feasible, cheap and effective intervention programmes, utilizing optimally the most recent scientific knowledge, are needed to break the vicious circle of malnutrition, and underdevelopment. The precise quantitative and qualitative relationship between nutrition, infection and immunological capabilities remains to be defined. The relationship between deficiency of a specific nutrient and functional or immunological incompetence needs further research. Replacement of this nutrient might permit a desirable response.

Research on the various physiological and biochemical derangements following undernutrition might aid in preventing, minimizing or treating certain sequelae of malnutrition. If animal experiments demonstrating depletion of biogenic amine neurotransmitters, particularly nor-adrenaline and dopamine in malnourished animals, are shown to have their counterparts in the human, it may be possible to use sympathomimetic drugs to correct behavioural disturbances in the undernourished child.

These and other areas of research, should stimulate nutritionists to investigate more in depth the relationship between nutrition and quality of life and its effects on socioeconomic development. The International Union of Nutritional Sciences should take the lead in this respect. Being an international, non-political, non-governmental organization, it is in a unique position to carry out multinational standarized studies in many of the forementioned areas.

Through cooperation between scientists in developed and developing countries, new methods and techniques can be established, tested, standardized and made use of in understanding the causes and effects of malnutrition. These would also help in the development of better intervention programmes focusing more on specific causes and vulnerable targets. Studies can be carried out in different settings and different countries helping in advancement of our knowledge to attain better nutrition for all. These studies will ultimately convince policy makers that investments to improve nutritional standards are justifiable not only on welfare and humanitarian grounds but also as stimulants to economic growth.

1 Barg, B. (1973): Nutrition and national development. In *Nutrition, national development and planning*, ed A. Berg, N. Scrimshaw & D.L. Call, p. 66. Cambridge, Mass.: MIT Press.
2 Barrett, D.E. (1984): Conceptualization, assessment and an empirical study of social emotional function in malnutrition and behavior. In *Malnutrition and child behavior*, p. 280 ed J. Brojek, & B. Schurch, Lausanne, Switzerland: Nestlé Foundation.
3 Battad, J.E. (1978): Nutritional status of preschoolers. *Philipp. Econ. J.* **17**, 154–167.
4 Beaton, G.H. & Ghassemi, H. (1982): Supplementary feeding programs for young children in developing countries. *Am. J. Clin. Nutr.* **35**, 864–916.
5 Berg, A., ed (1981): Malnourished people, a policy view. Poverty and Basic Needs Series. Washington DC: The World Bank.
6 Calloway, D.H. (1982): Functional consequence of malnutrition. *Rev. Infect. Dis.* **4**, 736–745.
7 Chandra, R.K. (1982): Malnutrition and infection. In *Nutrition policy implementation*, ed N. Scrimshaw & M.B. Wallerstein, p. 3. New York: Plenum Press.
8 Cooke, R. (1971): The cost of malnutrition in Jamaica. *Ecol. Food Nutr.* **1**, 61–66.
9 Frank, D.A. (1984): A view from the bedside in malnutrition and behavior, *Malnutrition and child behavior*. p 307, J. Brojek & B. Schurch, (Editors), Nestlé Foundation Publication Series, Lausanne, Switzerland.
10 Gabr, M.K. (1983): Malnutrition and immune response. In *Proc. XVII Int. Congr. Pediat.* (Manila, Philippines).
11 Jelliffe, D. & Jelliffe, E.P. (1978): *Human milk in the modern world*, London: Oxford University Press.
12 Neumann, C.G., Jelliffe, D.B. & Jelliffe, E.P.F. (1980): Interaction of nutrition and infection, *Clin. Pediat.* **17**, 807–812.
13 Pollitt, E. (1982): Comment on the impact of malnutrition on behavior. In *Nutrition policy implementation*, p. 37, ed N. Scrimshaw, & M.B. Wallerstein, Plenum Press, New York.
14 Popkin, B.M. (1972): Economic benefits from the elimination of hunger in America. *Public Policy* **20**, 133–153.
15 Reutlinger, S. & Alderman, H. (1980): The prevalance of caloric deficit diets in developing countries. *Wld Devel.* **8**, 399–411.
16 Sai, F.T. (1972): Nutrition as a priority in national development. In *Nutrition, a priority in African development*, ed. B. Vahlqvist, pp. 137–148. Stockholm: Almqvist and Wiksell.
17 Selowsky, M. & Taylor, L. (1973): The economics of malnourished children: an example of disinvestment in human capital, *Econ. Develop. Cultural Changes*, **22**, 17–30.
18 Viteri, F.E. (1982): Nutrition and work performance. In *Nutrition policy implementation*, ed. N. Scrimshaw & M.B. Wallerstein, p. 3. New York: Plenum Press.
19 Whitehead, R.G., ed (1983): *Maternal diet, breast-feeding capacity, lactation and infertility*. Tokyo: The United Nations University.
20 Wray, J.D. (1978): Direct nutrition intervention and the control of diarrheal disease in preschool children, *Am. J. Clin. Nutr.* **31**, 2073–2082.

★   ★   ★

UNDERNUTRITION AND MENTAL AND PHYSICAL FUNCTION

The effect of childhood malnutrition on mental development

Sally GRANTHAM-McGREGOR
Tropical metabolism research unit, University of the West Indies, Mona, St. Andrew, Jamaica.

The association between poor mental development and both severe and chronic undernutrition is well-established; however, we remain uncertain as to the precise relationship. There are three main problems. First, the confounding effects of poor social background on mental development are difficult to separate from those of malnutrition. Secondly, the outcome variable itself, mental development, is difficult to measure, particularly in communities where there are no standardised indigenous tests[33].

Thirdly, the diagnosis of malnutrition itself is far from adequate. PEM is not a specific disease but embraces many different clinical conditions, ranging from an acute attack of oedema (kwashiorkor) to less severe undernutrition which may extend for most of childhood and even begin in the intrauterine period.

Mechanism. PEM is caused by an inadequate supply of different nutrients, complicated to a greater or lesser degree by repeated infections. Which nutrient deficiencies are responsible for particular syndromes is still not clear. It may be that a deficiency of a single nutrient or any one of several nutrients are responsible for different syndromes such as oedema or stunting. The effects on mental development will depend on how these deficiencies together with repeated illness effect functioning.

Hypotheses. Excluding the possibility of a purely indirect association with unstimulating environments, there are several different hypotheses concerning the mechanism of the relationship between poor mental development and PEM. Anatomical and/or metabolic alterations of the nervous system may cause impaired functioning either during the period of malnutrition or permanently. Decreased activity and exploration due to energy deficit or other deficiency or imbalance may lead to failure to acquire skills and develop at a normal rate. Decreased responsiveness of people, especially the mother, towards the child may occur as a consequence of the child's apathetic behaviour. The quality of the environment may modify the outcome from any of the above mechanisms.

Anatomical and metabolic alterations. Permanent changes have been demonsrated in the brains of undernourished animals and children and the main question is, do these alterations affect functioning? (Dr. Smart addresses this question in this volume, pp. 74–78.

Lack of activity. It has been shown[40] that activity is reduced as energy uptake is restricted. In addition, several studies of undernourished children have shown they have decreased activity and exploration — see[15] for review.

It has been demonstrated that poor Guatemalan children had reduced energy intakes when they were ill[27]. This may explain the association, described by Pollitt[32], between morbidity in the first 6 months of life and developmental levels at 8 months in Taiwan children.

Responsiveness of environment. It has been shown that when children were given nutritional supplementation, not only did their own behaviour change, but their parents became more stimulating towards them[6]. This suggests that the unstimulating behaviour of parents of malnourished children is in response to the children's apathetic behaviour. Conversely, it has been found that unresponsive maternal behaviour preceded the onset of PEM[8].

Severity and duration. The outcome from any of the above mechanisms would probably depend on both the severity and duration of the insult, as well as the stage of development when the child is exposed. Wasting (per cent expected weight for height) is thought to reflect recent nutritional experiences[42]. It gives some indication of severity and probably of energy deficit in particular. Oedema reflects severity in terms of mortality risk. Stunting (per cent expected height for age) is thought to reflect duration of PEM[42]. However, the relationship between stunting and duration is not straightforward.

It has been shown that, in communities where PEM is endemic, poor environmental conditions explain more of the variance in height than genetic predisposition[26]. However, stunting can be remedied given an appropriate supportive environment, at least if this is begun early enough[43], so that several years of malnutrition in early life may not be apparent if catch-up has subsequently occurred. It has also been shown[40] that given adequate protein, as energy intake is restricted, activity is reduced before growth is stopped, suggesting that at certain levels of energy intake, activity may be reduced in the presence of normal growth in height. In communities where PEM is endemic, stunting is usually more closely related to children's development than wasting[24,34,35].

We have shown, in Jamaica, that within one month of children leaving hospital, having recovered from severe PEM, their developmental quotients (DQs) were related to their degree of stunting on admission to hospital, but not their degree of wasting or presence of oedema[14] (Table). This suggests that, when considering mental development, duration of PEM as reflected by stunting, the commonest form of childhood malnutrition, may be more important than severity. Most studies have not used any measure of duration, instead they have used the Wellcome[1] or Gomez classification[13], both of which depend on the degree of weight deficit and the presence of oedema. Lack of a measure of duration may be responsible for some of the inconsistencies in findings.

Table. *The relative effect of independent variables on developmental quotients of 39 children one month after recovery from PEM.*

Independent variables	Standardised regression coefficient
Intervention	0.37**
Age	0.17
% Expected height for age	0.49**
% Expected weight for height	0.16
Presence of oedema	0.05

**$P<0.01$.

Severe PEM. Recent studies of survivors of severe PEM have found that several years after recovery, they have lower scores at tests of IQ[11,12] and specific cognitive functions[31]. These studies used retrospective case-control designs, comparing survivors with either siblings or carefully matched peers for controls. In an attempt to further control for social background inequalities, some investigators have measured social and economic variables and allowed for these in the analyses.

None of the study designs were completely satisfactory; siblings were usually undernourished themselves in early childhood, and it is impossible to control for all social background factors which may affect mental development. Techniques for measuring children's environment are still crude and often lack reliability and validity, so that controlling for these variables statistically may be misleading.

It would appear at this stage that little is to be gained by repeating studies using these same designs. Only truly experimental designs can demonstrate cause and these are not possible in humans when considering severe PEM, for obvious ethical reasons. Consequently, I suggest we use epidemiological guide-lines to determine when we can reasonably attribute cause to association. In this respect, biological plausibility, temporality, strength, specificity, the presence of a biological gradient and experimental evidence have to be looked for[19].

Any of the possible mechanisms discussed above are biologically plausible. Only one study has considered temporality and it[8] showed that children had normal development preceding the onset of severe PEM.

The association between marasmus or mixed PEM and poor mental development has been demonstrated to be not only consistent but strong, in many different populations by different investigators: Lebanon[29], Uganda[20], South Africa[39] and Chile[30]. Findings from survivors of kwashiorkor have not been quite so consistent, and at least two have failed to find a disadvantage[3,9]. However, children with kwashiorkor tend to be less stunted than those with marasmus, implying PEM of a shorter duration. If duration is the important criterion for mental development, then little difference would be expected between a chronically-undernourished sibling and a child who suffered an acute attack of oedema superimposed on the same degree of chronic undernutrition.

A biological gradient was demonstrated in the longitudinal study in Guatemala whereby the amount of nutritional supplementation consumed was related to children's scores in tests of cognitive functioning[23]. The only reservation is that the children were not randomly assigned to different supplementation levels but were self-selected.

Specificity cannot be established because poor mental development is caused by many factors including poor social background. However, there is considerable experimental evidence from animals, that PEM effects some types of learning.

Interaction with environment. Children from developed countries who become malnourished secondary to other illnesses show only slight or no difference in mental development several years later[22]. It is possible that stimulation at the time of malnutrition protects the child from poor mental development.

It is also possible that the children improved after an initial deficit[25]. Malnourished Korean children who were adopted by North American families showed normal levels of IQ and school achievement several years later, although their IQs remained associated with their initial degree of malnutrition[43]. This study, however, had no measures of development in the early stages.

In Jamaica, we studied a boy who survived severe PEM and was adopted by a middle class family two years later[16]. He was one of a group of 17 severely malnourished children on whom we carried out regular development assessments from the time of leaving hospital. The adopted boy made remarkable improvement gaining 30 IQ points, and scoring over 2 s.d.s above the mean for the group (Fig. 1).

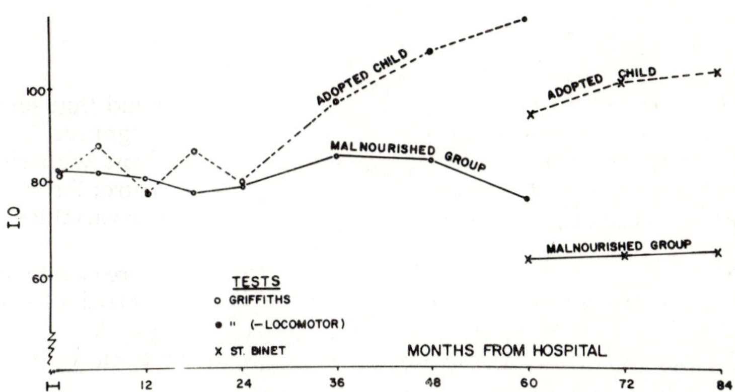

Fig. 1. *Developmental levels on the Griffiths test and intelligence quotients (IQ) on the Stanford Binet, of an adopted boy who survived severe malnutrition, compared with 16 similar children who remained in their own homes*

Rehabilitation following severe PEM. The above studies suggest that an enormous amount of improvement can take place if children are exposed to vast improvements in their environment. It is important to determine how much improvement can occur in the children's own homes.

Programmes of short term psychosocial stimulation while the children were treated in hospital have produced only transient improvements in children's development[7,29]. The only reported programme of long-term psychosocial stimulation with severely malnourished children is one we have just completed in Jamaica[17]. It was designed to be integrated into the existing primary health care services and comprised an hour's play a day while the children were in hospital, followed by home visiting for 1 hour a week for 2 years, then every 2 weeks for a further year. At the visits community health aides demonstrated the use of home-made toys to the mothers, who were encouraged to play with their children between the visits. The intervened malnourished group's development was compared with that of two other groups which received standard medical care only; one severely malnourished and one adequately nourished. The children in all three groups were patients in the same hospital at the beginning of the study.

On admission to hospital both malnourished groups were seriously behind the adequately nourished group on developmental testing. The non-intervened malnourished group remained behind the adequately nourished children for the following 4 years, showing little sign of catching up. The intervened malnourished children improved in DQs and were significantly ahead of the non-intervened malnourished group by the time they left hospital. They continued to improve and 12 months later their DQs were similar to those of the adequately-nourished group. They maintained this position until intervention stopped (Fig. 2). It is important to know how long the benefits gained will last.

Locomotor development was the only area of development which did not catch up to the adequately nourished children at any stage. In addition both malnourished groups remained stunted with smaller head circumferences than the adequately nourished group. The intervention did not include nutritional supplementation after leaving hospital, and greater improvements may have occurred if it had. We need to examine the effects of giving supplements to these children after recovery from the acute stage with and without stimulation.

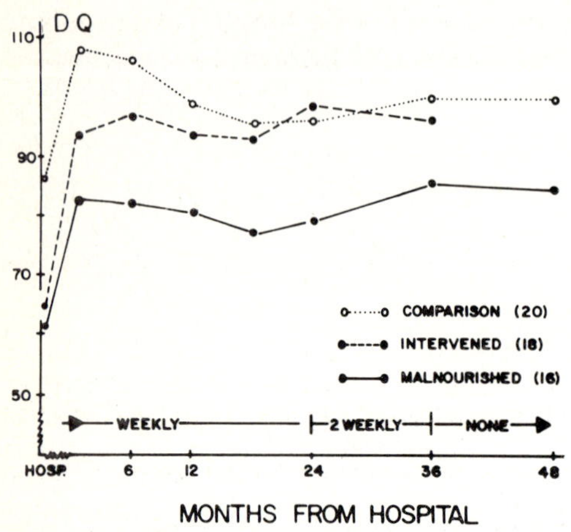

Fig. 2. *Mean developmental quotients (DQs) on the Griffiths test, from admission to hospital to 3 years later, of three groups: Intervened (by psychosocial stimulation) and non-intervened malnourished, and adequately nourished comparisons.* Frequency of home visits is indicated above the horizontal axis.

Behaviour. Recently investigators have focused attention on the behaviour problems of malnourished children, which may be more important than deficits in intelligence quotients. Survivors of severe PEM have been found to have attention disorders, to be lacking in energy, to make poor social relationships and be emotionally immature[20,36,37]. These studies however, depended on mothers or teachers' reports which are of doubtful validity, especially when teachers are aware of the children's school grades.

Observations of chronically-undernourished children have shown that they have low levels of activity and exploration[15]. An innovative approach also showed[2] that highly-supplemented children were more sociable, happy, or angry, and less anxious, and coped better with stressful situations than poorly-supplemented children. There is a need for more observations of children's behaviour in real life situations.

Nutritional supplementation in nutritionally-deprived pregnancy and early childhood.
In New York, nutritional supplementation given to high-risk women during pregnancy, had no benefit on the children's development at one year of age,[38] but in a well-designed study in Taiwan[21] supplementation to mothers in pregnancy and lactation was found to have a significant benefit on children's scores on the motor scale of the Bayley Test at 8 months of age, but not on the mental scale.

Three major studies of the effects of supplementation during pregnancy and early childhood have been concluded in Latin America. In one it was found that supplemented children attained higher scores on the Gesel schedules in all areas of development, between 6 and 60 months of age[5]. However, it appears that these children received extra attention which may have accounted for at least some of the improvement, also groups were not randomly assigned.

In Bogota[41] pregnant mothers were randomly assigned to groups, one received food supplementation, one received increased stimulation alone, a third group received both supplementation and stimulation. By 36 months of age, the children receiving supplementation whether or not stimulation was included, had the highest scores on all subscales of Griffiths Test, with the greatest effect on locomotor development. The benefits gained were, however, very small.

In both these studies some benefits persisted in school performance at primary school[4,18]; these were larger in the Mexican study but it is not clear whether supplementation was still continuing, whereas in the Bogota study it stopped at three years of age.

A third study in Guatemala[10] compared highly-supplemented children with poorly-supplemented ones and found a significant association between the amount of supplement taken and cognitive functioning. However, the amount of variance explained by supplementation was small, and the long-term benefits are not yet clear. The problem in this study is that the supplemented children were self-selected, so that the highly-supplemented children may have been different from the poorly-supplemented ones at the outset.

Supplementation failed to produce benefits in chronically undernourished 3-year-olds in Cali, Colombia. When supplementation was added to stimulation, large benefits ensured, but it is not clear whether they were entirely due to the stimulation alone, or whether supplementation played a part[28].

Acknowledgements. The Jamaican studies referred to were funded by the Ford Foundation, USA, the Overseas Development Administration, UK and the Medical Research Council, UK.

I thank W. Schofield, C. Powell, L. Harris, E. Burke, I. Halstead and M. Lewis for assistance, and Professor J.C. Waterlow for encouragement.

1 Anon (1970): Leader—Classification of infantile malnutrition. *Lancet* **2**, 30.

2 Barrett, D.E. (1984): Malnutrition and child behaviour: conceptualization, assessment and empirical study of social-emotional functioning. In *Malnutrition and behaviour: critical assessment of key issues*, ed J. Brozek & B. Schurch, pp. 280–306. Lausanne, Switzerland: Nestlé Foundation.

3 Bartel, P.R., Griesel, R.D., Burnett, L.S., Freiman, I., Rosen, E.V. & Geefhuysen, J. (1978): Long term effects of kwashiorkor on psychomotor development *S Afr. Med J.* **53**, 360–362.

4 Chavez, A. & Martinez, C. (1981): School performance of supplemented and unsupplemented children from a poor rural area. In *Nutrition health and disease and international development. Symposia from the XII International Congress of Nutrition*, eds A.E. Harper & G.K. Davis, pp 393–402. New York: A.R. Liss.

5 Chavez, A. & Martinez, C. (1982): Neurological maturation and performance on mental test. In *Growing up in a developing community* (INCAP).

6 Chavez, A., Martinez, C. & Yaschine, T. (1975): Nutrition, behavioural development and mother-child interaction in young rural children. *Fed. Proc.* **34**, 1574–1582.

7 Cravioto, J. & Arrieta, R. (1980): Stimulation and mental development of malnourished infants. *Lancet* **2**, 899.

8 Cravioto, J. & Delicardie, E. (1972): Environmental correlates of severe clinical malnutrition and language development in survivors from kwashiorkor or marasmus. In *Nutrition, the nervous system and behaviour*, pp. 73–94. PAHO Sci. Pub. No. 251.

9 Evans, D.E., Moodie, A.D. & Hansen, J.D.L. (1971): Kwashiorkor and intellectual development. *SA Med. J.* **25**, 1413–1426.

10 Freeman, H.E., Klein, R.E., Townsend, J.W.L. & Leghtig, A. (1980): Nutrition and cognitive development among rural Guatemalan children. *Am. J. Publ. Hlth.* **70**, 1277–1285.

11 Galler, J., Ramsey, F., Solimano, G. & Lowell, W.E. (1983): The influence of early malnutrition on subsequent behavioural development, II Classroom behaviour. *J. Am. Acad. Child. Psychiat.* **22**, 16–22.

12 Galler, J., Ramsey, F., Solimano, G., Lowell, W. & Mason, E. (1983): The influence of early malnutrition on subsequent behavioural development 1. Degree of impairment in intellectual performance. *J. Am. Acad. Child Psychol.* **22**, 8–15.

13 Gomez, F., Ramos-Galvan, R., Frenk, S., Cravioto, J.M., Chavez, R. & Vasquez, J. (1956): Mortality in second and third degree malnutrition. *J. Trop. Pediat.* **2**, 77–83.

14 Grantham-McGregor, S.M. (1982): The relationship between developmental level and different types of malnutrition in children. *Hum. Nutr: Clin. Nutr.* **36C**, 319–320.

15 Grantham-McGregor, S.M. (1984): The Social background of malnourished children. In *Malnutrition and behaviour: critical assessment of key issues* ed J. Brozek & B. Schurch. Lausanne, Switzerland: Nestlé Foundation.

16 Grantham-McGregor, S.M. & Buchanan, E. (1982): The development of an adopted child recovering from severe malnutrition. Case report. *Hum. Nutr.: Clin. Nutr.* **36C**, 251–256.

17 Grantham-McGregor, S.M., Schofield, W. & Harris, L. (1983): Effect of psychosocial stimulation on mental development of severely malnourished children: an interim report. *Pediat.* **72**, 239–243.

18 Herrara, G. & Super, C. (1983): *School performance and physical growth of underprivileged children: results of the Bogota project at seven years.* Report to World Bank. Cambridge: Harvard School of Public Health.

19 Hill, A.B. (1965): The environment and disease: association or causation. *Proc. R. Soc. Med* **58**, 295–300.

20 Hoorweg, J. (1976): *Protein-energy malnutrition and intellectual abilities.* The Hague: Mouton.

21 Joos, S.K., Pollitt, E., Mueller, W.H. & Albright, D.L. (1983): The Bacon Chow study: maternal nutritional supplementation and infant behavioral development. *Child Devel* **54**, 669–676.

22 Klein, P.S., Forbes, G.B. & Nader, P.R. (1975): Effects of starvation in infancy (pyloric stenosis) on subsequent learning abilities. *J. Pediat.* **87**, 8–15.

23 Klein, R.E., Irwin, M.H., Engle, P.L. & Yarbrough, C. (1977): Malnutrition and mental development in rural Guatemala. In *Advances in cross-cultural psychology*, ed. N. Warren. New York: Academic Press.

24 Lasky, R.E., Klein, R.E., Yarbrough, C., Engle, P.L., Lechtig, A. & Martorell, R. (1981): The relationship between physical growth and infant behavioural development in rural Guatemala. *Child Devel.* **52**, 220–226.

25 Lloyd-Still, J.D., Hurwitz, I., Wolff, P.H. & Shwachman, H. (1974): Intellectual development after severe malnutrition in infancy *Pediat.* **54**, 306–311.

26 Martorell, R. (1984): Genetics, environment and growth: issues in the assessment of nutritional status. In *Genetic factors in nutrition*, eds Velasquez & Bourges. New York: Academic Press.

27 Martorell, R. & Yarbrough, C. (1983): The energy cost of diarrhoeal diseases and other common illnesses in children. In *Diarrhea and Malnutrition*, ed L.C. Chen & N.S. Scrimshaw. New York: Plenum.

28 McKay, H., Sinesterra, L., McKay, A. & Gomez, H. & Lloreda, P. (1978): Improving cognitive ability in chronically deprived children. *Science* **200**, 270–278.

29 McLaren, D.S., Yatkin, U.S., Kanawati, A.A., Sabbagh, S. & Kadi, Z. (1973): The subsequent mental and physical development of rehabilitated marasmic infants. *J. Ment. Def. Res.* **17**, 173–181.

30 Monckeberg, F. (1968): Effect of early marasmic malnutrition on subsequent physical and psychological development. In *Malnutrition, learning and behavior*, ed N. Scrimshaw & J.E. Gordon, pp 267–269. Cambridge MA: MIT Press.

31 Nwuga, U.C.B. (1977): Effect of severe kwashiorkor on intellectual development among Nigerian children. *Am. J. Clin. Nutr.* **30**, 1423–1430.

32 Pollitt, E. (1983): Morbidity and infant development: A hypothesis *Int. J. Behav. Devel* **6**, 461–475.

33 Pollitt, E. & Thomson, C. (1977): Protein-calorie malnutrition and behaviour. A view from psychology. In *Nutrition and the brain*, ed R.J. Wurtman & J.J. Wurtman, Vol. 2, pp 261–306. New York: Raven Press.

34 Powell, C.A. & Grantham-McGregor, S. (1985): The ecology of nutritional status and development in young children in Kingston, Jamaica. *Am. J. Clin. Nutr.* **41**, 1322–1331.

35 Richardson, S.A. (1979): Severity of malnutrition in infancy and its relation to later intelligence. In *Behavioural effects of energy and protein deficits*, ed E. Brozek, pp. 172–184. U.S. Department of Health, Education, and Welfare. NIH Pub. No. 79–1906.

36 Richardson, S.A., Birch, H.G. Grabie, E. & Yoder, K. (1972): The behaviour of children in school who were severely malnourished in the first two years of life. *J. Hlth Soc. Behav.* **13**, 276–283.

37 Richardson, S.A., Birch, H.G. & Ragbeer, C. (1975): The behaviour of children at home who were severely malnourished in the first two years of life. *J. Biosoc. Sci.* **7**, 255–267.

38 Rush, D. (1984): The behavioural consequences of protein-energy deprivation and supplementation in early life. An epidemiological perspective. In *Human nutrition. A comprehensive treatise*, ed J. Galler, pp 119–154. New York: Plenum Press.

39 Stoch, M.B., Smythe, P.M., Moodie, A.D. & Bradshaw, D. (1982): Psychological outcome and CT findings after gross undernourishment during infancy: a 20-year developmental study. *Develop. Med. Child Neurol.* **24**, 419–436.

40 Torún, B. & Viteri, F.E. (1981): Energy requirements of pre-school children and effects of varying energy intakes on protein metabolism. In *Protein-energy requirements of developing Countries: evaluation of new data*, ed B. Torún, V.R. Young & W.M. Rand. *UNU Fd Nutr. Bull.* Suppl. 5, 229–241.

41 Waber, D.P., Vuori-Christiansen, L., Ortiz, N., Clement, J.R., Christiansen, N.E., Mora, J.O., Reed, R.B. & Herrara, M.G. (1981): Nutritional supplementation, maternal education, and cognitive development of infants at risk of malnutrition. *Am. J. Clin. Nutr.* **34**, 807–813

42 Waterlow, J.C. & Rutishauser, H.E. (1974): Malnutrition in Man. In *Early malnutrition and mental development* ed J. Cravioto, L. Hambreus & B. Valhqvist, pp 13–25. Uppsala: Almqvist and Wiksell.

43 Winick, M., Meyer, K.K. & Harris, R.C. (1975): Malnutrition and environmental enrichment by early adoption. *Science* **190**, 1174–1175.

Undernutrition, learning and memory: review of experimental studies

J. L. SMART
Department of Child Health, University of Manchester, The Medical School, Oxford Road, Manchester M13 9PT, UK.

There is no doubt that undernutrition early in life can have permanent effects on brain growth: that is, effects which are irrecoverable even after prolonged refeeding[1,3]. What is less certain, in spite of much investigation, is whether this matters for the proper intellectual functioning of the animal, human or otherwise.

I have attempted to make an exhaustive review of all published studies which meet the criteria laid down below. Many reviews represent the verification of an opinion: they are undertaken from a particular standpoint and the evidence is assessed accordingly. The understandable tendency is to emphasise the confirmatory evidence and to play down or ignore the contradictory. I have tried to avoid this trap by accepting all the published evidence at its face value and, as far as possible, adopting only numerical or statistical reservations. In a further attempt at objectivity the evidence has been translated into an algebraic sum of experiments for or against the hypothesis that early undernutrition impairs learning ability, with each experiment contributing one unit to the sum.

It is, of course, a problem with this sort of numerical analysis that poor studies carry as much weight as good ones. One of the most obvious indications of poor experimental design is the use of too few animals drawn from even fewer litters, and in one of the analyses (Table 1, Analysis B) criteria are employed to exclude such studies. Perhaps an even more intractable problem is the possibility of bias with respect to which kind of result is published and which is not. Positive results with respect to the hypothesis that early undernutrition impairs learning ability might possibly find more favour with reviewers and editors than negative results. In my opinion, it ought not to be so, and there is some degree of reassurance that this has not occurred to any marked extent in the large number of negative findings in the literature (Table 1). Happily, this kind of consideration has little bearing on the analyses which compare the effects of different periods of undernutrition (Table 2) or which compare performance on different learning tests (Table 3).

Table 1. *Numbers of experiments indicating superior performance by C (well-nourished control) or PU (previously undernourished) animals or no significant difference (n.s.).*

			Analysis A†			Analysis B†		
Species	*No. of papers*	*No. of expts.*	*C*	*PU*	*n.s.*	*C*	*PU*	*n.s.*
Rat	68	137	59	10***	68	39	6***	38
Mouse	7	19	14	2**	3	12	0**	3
Pig	2	6	5	0	1	0	0	0
Cat	1	1	1	0	0	1	0	0
Monkey (2 species)	2	2	1	0	1	0	0	1
TOTAL	80	165	80	12***	73	52	6***	42

†Criteria for Analyses A and B: A, significant differences; B, significant differences and adequate numbers of animals (see text for further details).
*$P < 0.05$, **$P < 0.01$, ***$P < 0.001$ (Sign test, two-tailed, comparing observed frequencies with null hypothesis, equal frequencies of C and PU superiority.) A list of source references may be obtained from the author.

Table 2. *Numbers of experiments indicating superior performance by C (well-nourished control) or PU (previously undernourished) rats or no significant difference (n.s.) in relation to the timing of the undernutrition.*

		Analysis A†		
Period of undernutrition	*No. of expts.*	*C*	*PU*	*n.s.*
Gestation	16	9	0**	7
Gestation and suckling	38	22	1**	15
Suckling	60	19	8	33
Suckling and early post-weaning	17	9	1*	7
Early post-weaning	6	0	0	6

†As for Table 1.

Table 3. *Numbers of experiments indicating superior performance by C (well-nourished control) or PU (previously undernourished) rats or no significant difference (n.s.) on different tests of learning ability.*

	No. of expts.	Analysis A†		
Test		C	PU	n.s.
Hebb-Williams maze	21	11	1**	9
Multiple-T and Lashley III mazes	12	5	1	6
Radial maze	13	6	0*	7
Visual discrimination	32	14	0**	18
Extinction	10	7	0*	3
Latent learning	6	2	0	4
Long-term memory	9	4	1	4
Active avoidance	31	8	6	17
T-maze (left vs right)	12	3	2	7
Reversal learning	17	3	2	12

†See Table 1. Certain experiments are represented twice above, in which initial learning was followed by reversal learning or extinction.

Characteristics of the review. The characteristics of the review are described in detail elsewhere[6] and will be outlined only briefly here. It is confined to studies of non-human mammals in which a period of protein-energy malnutrition was imposed early in life (some time between conception and the early post-weaning period) and was followed by a period of refeeding *ad libitum* on a good quality diet for a period of at least 1 month before the testing of behaviour. Almost always the period of refeeding exceeded the earlier period of undernutrition and usually it was much longer than 1 month. Well-nourished control animals are designated C and previously undernourished animals PU.

The analysis is in terms of experiments for and against the hypothesis that early nutritional privation impairs later capacity to learn and hence it is necessary to clarify what is meant here by an experiment. Two quite different tests on the same animals (eg Lashley III maze and pole jump avoidance) are counted as two experiments. However, two-part tests (eg initial learning followed by reversal learning or by extinction) are counted as one experiment, unless stated otherwise. Slow extinction is taken to be maladaptive. Where there are more than two treatment groups simultaneously under study, the number of experiments is deemed to be the number of appropriate comparisons of well-nourished control with previously undernourished groups. Where results are presented separately for males and females from the same investigation, these findings are counted as two experiments. Not all possible comparisons have been included: for example, one between brain-lesioned C and PU rats was not thought to be appropriate in the present context and was omitted.

Experiments were categorised as indicating superior performance by the C or by the PU group ($P < 0.05$) or no significant difference, on the basis of the authors' own statistical analysis. In recent years there has been increasing use of more complex experimental designs, through which researchers have sought to investigate the interaction of under-nutrition with some other factor such as the complexity of the rearing environment. The correct statistical treatment in these instances is analysis of variance followed, where appropriate, by pair-wise comparison between groups. Problems arise for the categorisation exercise with cases in which pair-wise comparisons are not reported, even when they ought to have been carried out. One is left, where possible, to perform t-tests using means and standard errors derived from tables and even graphs, and to exclude cases in which this cannot be done. Instances in which there was no statistical analysis are omitted, as are findings from tests of passive avoidance.

Presentation and discussion of the findings of the review. The rat has been by far the most popular species, having been the subject of 85 per cent of all papers published (Table 1). The observed frequencies of experiments demonstrating superior performance by C animals or by PU animals are compared with the theoretical expectation of equal frequency of occurrence using the Sign test (Table 1). The instances of C superiority were highly significantly predominant for the rat and the mouse and over all. Nevertheless, it should be pointed out that 'no difference' cases, ignored in the analysis by Sign test, constitute a major category. Analysis B in Table 1 shows the results of the same form of analysis but excluding studies with inadequate numbers of animals. Experiments with fewer than eight animals per group or with less than four litters represented per group are omitted. This has the effect of removing 39 per cent of all experiments, but it does not influence the results of the analysis by Sign test. Well-nourished control superiority still predominates strongly.

The succeeding, more detailed analyses are of the rat data only, because of the paucity of papers on other species, and include all relevant experiments irrespective of numbers of animals or litters. One of the questions that can be posed of this kind of analysis is whether there is a vulnerable period for the effects of undernutrition on later learning ability? This is best done by comparing individual periods of approximately equal duration (gestation, suckling, or early post-weaning) and, in the first instance, ignoring combined periods which are obviously longer and hence complicate the analysis by introducing duration as a factor in addition to timing. On this basis, gestation is found to be the most vulnerable period, in that it is the only one which results in a significant majority of experiments in which C rats perform better than PU (Table 2). Taking account of the combined periods does not affect this conclusion.

The suggestion that gestation is the most vulnerable period is of particular interest since it would appear to conflict with the evidence for brain development which strongly implicates the suckling period as the most vulnerable stage in the rat, at least in terms of most gross parameters of brain growth[3]. The key to the puzzle may be the fact that in the forebrain most neuronal proliferation, including all division of large neurons, occurs prenatally in mice and rats[5]. Hence, gestational undernutrition may possibly result in deficits in cerebral neuron number or other disturbances of neuronal development, with deleterious consequences for later intellectual functioning.

A further question which ought to be amenable to the present form of analysis is whether some abilities are more affected than others by early undernutrition? This would certainly appear to be the case (Table 3). The ability to run complex mazes would appear to be fairly reliably impaired, whereas performance in a simple T-maze is not. Visual discrimination too is often found to be deficient, and the extinction of learned responses is often slow in PU rats. There are too few studies of long-term memory and latent learning (usually unrewarded learning about aspects of the environment) to discern a pattern of results with any confidence, but there are indications that they too may be vulnerable. Active avoidance, left/right discrimination in a T-maze and its reversal (learning to turn left, having originally learned to turn right etc) are not consistently impaired. It may be noteworthy that the last three are all simple tasks.

Latent learning and memory are probably the aspects of learning which are most deserving of further investigation in PU animals. Whether it is proper to call memory an aspect of learning is debatable, but it most certainly contributes to observed performance of any learned task and might account in part or even wholly for differences between groups in performance. Memory has too seldom been a subject for investigation in its own right in this field and merits study in relation, for instance, to the postulated 'working' and 'reference' memory processes and to retention over long periods of time.

Female rats have been much less studied in the context of early undernutrition than males, probably because the permanent stunting of body growth consistently reported for males is less marked in females[8]. Indeed, there had been so few investigations of female PU animals in the period up to 1977 that that analysis had virtually to be confined to results from male animals. Female rats have since been tested in several experiments. Instances of C superiority comprise 50 per cent of all experiments on male rats but only 26 per cent of all experiments on female rats (Table 4). The tendency for C superiority is, therefore, rather more marked in males. The effect of early undernutrition on learning may be less severe in females, or perhaps it is merely more difficult to demonstrate significant effects in females because their oestrous cycle increases variance.

Table 4. *Numbers of experiments indicating superior performance by C (well-nourished control) or PU (previously undernourished) rats or no significant difference (n.s.) in relation to gender.*

	No. of	Analysis A†		
Gender	expts.	C	PU	n.s.
Male	94	47	6	41
Female	19	5	0	14

†See Table 1. Experiments in which the sex of the animals was not stated or in which the results for males and females were combined are excluded.

Comparing the frequencies of C, PU and n.s. results for males and females: $\chi^2 = 6.075$ (2 d.f.), $P < 0.05$.

Probably the main change over all since 1977 is that the percentage of non-significant findings has decreased markedly. For experiments on male rats, the proportion of non-significant results fell from 53 per cent in papers published before 1977 to 30 per cent in papers appearing more recently. A likely reason for this is that researchers have been employing better experimental designs and larger numbers of animals in recent years, thus increasing the likelihood of revealing significant effects. In support of this, the proportion of experiments excluded on grounds of inadequate numbers of animals or litters (Table 1) is much diminished now compared with 1977. The majority of recently-added results are instances of C superiority, giving more substance to the general conclusion that C superiority is the predominant result where the groups are found to differ at all.

The present paper glosses over many of the problems which beset this field. For instance, it is impossible to measure 'learning ability' because it is a quality intrinsic to the animal. All that can be done is to record 'performance', which reflects ability to a greater or lesser extent, on a particular test or series of tests[2,6]. Also there has been no mention of the mechanism(s) through which the effects of undernutrition may be mediated, whether directly through effects on brain growth or indirectly through environmental changes like altered maternal care which may be concomitants of undernutrition procedures[4,7]. However mediated, there would certainly appear to be a tendency for PU animals to perform less efficiently in tests of learning than their well-nourished controls.

Acknowledgements. I am grateful to the Medical Research Council and to the National Fund for Research into Crippling Diseases for financial support.

1 Bedi, K.S. (1984): Effects of undernutrition on brain morphology: a critical review of methods and results. In *Current topics in research on synapses*, Vol. 2, ed D.G. Jones, pp. 93–163. New York: Liss.

2 Crnic, L.S. (1976): Effects of infantile undernutrition on adult learning in rats: methodological and design problems. *Psychol. Bull.* **83**, 715–728.

3 Dobbing, J. (1981): Nutritional growth restriction and the nervous system. In *The Molecular basis of neuropathology*, ed R.H.S. Thompson & A.N. Davison, pp. 221–233. London: Arnold.

4 Levine, S. & Wiener, S. (1976): A critical analysis of data on malnutrition and behavioral deficits. *Adv. Pediat.* **22**, 113–136.

5 Rodier, P.M. (1980): Chronology of neuron development: animal studies and their clinical implications. *Devl Med. Child Neurol.* **22**, 525–545.

6 Smart, J.L. (1977): Early life malnutrition and later learning ability: a critical analysis. In *Genetics, environment and intelligence* ed A. Oliverio, pp. 215–235. Amsterdam: Elsevier/North-Holland.

7 Smart, J.L. (1984): Animal models of early malnutrition: advantages and limitations. In *Malnutrition and behavior: critical assessment of key issues*, ed J. Brožek & B. Schürch, pp. 444–459. Lausanne: Nestlé Foundation.

8 Williams, J.P.G., Tanner, J.M. & Hughes, P.C.R. (1974): Catch-up growth in female rats after growth retardation during the suckling period: comparison with males. *Pediat. Res.* **8**, 157–162.

Nutrition and work performance: physiological aspects

G.B. SPURR and J.C. REINA
Departments of Physiological Sciences and Pediatrics, Universidad del Valle, Cali, Colombia; Department of Physiology, Medical College of Wisconsin, and Research Service, VA Medical Center, Milwaukee, Wisconsin, USA.

This paper will be limited to the effects of chronic, naturally occurring malnutrition on physiological work performance in adult males and school-aged boys. A more detailed review of the subject has been presented elsewhere[17].

Adults. *Malnutrition and physical work capacity ($\dot{V}o_2$ max).* When the physical work capacity (PWC) of several groups of young Guatemalan adults was compared it was found that all of those who had existing, or evidence of past, chronic malnutrition had lower maximum oxygen consumptions ($\dot{V}O_2$ max) than those subjects who had never been exposed to nutritional deprivation[24]. It was concluded that the differences in $\dot{V}O_2$ max were due to body composition, not to differences in muscle cell function.

We have studied three groups of chronically undernourished adult males who were classified as having mild (M), intermediate (I) and severe (S) malnutrition based on a combination of weight/height ratios, serum albumins and daily creatinine excretion[6]. The most severely-malnourished of these subjects were also studied in a hospital metabolic ward during a 45-d period of adequate energy intake and the same level of protein they were ingesting prior to entry into the study (27 g/d). This was followed by increasing protein intake to 100g/d for 79 d while continuing the same energy intake[7]. Measurements of $\dot{V}O_2$ max were made on all subjects before, during and at the end of the dietary repletion regime and compared with determinations

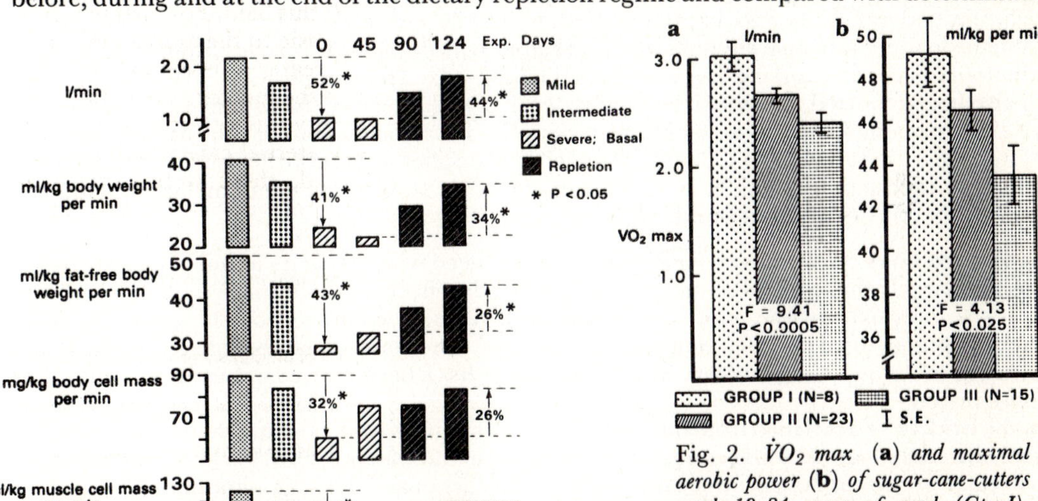

Fig. 2. $\dot{V}O_2$ max (**a**) *and maximal aerobic power* (**b**) *of sugar-cane-cutters aged 18–34 years of good (Gp I), average (Gp II) and poor (Gp III) productivity. F ratio values are from a one-way analysis of variance. Correlation coefficients (r) between productivity and maximum oxygen consumption were 0.55 (P < 0.0002) and 0.34 (P < 0.02) when calculated as l/min and ml/kg body weight per min, respectively*[20].

Fig. 1. $\dot{V}O_2$ *max expressed in terms of various body compartments for the undernourished subjects and during dietary repletion for up to 124d of the most severely malnourished*[17].

made in nutritionally normal agricultural workers. All groups had the same maximum heart rates, but exhibited a marked and statistically significant progressive depression in $\dot{V}O_2$ max which was related to the severity of their nutritional deprivation. We were unable to do body composition studies in the nutritionally normal subjects so that the results presented in Fig. 1 are discussed in terms of the differences in $\dot{V}O_2$ max between the mild and severely malnourished subjects and in the latter during the dietary repletion regime. All differences between M and S subjects were significantly different despite the expression of the results in terms of various body compartments, but over 80 per cent of the difference was accounted for by the differences in the muscle mass of the two groups (Fig. 1). The remaining difference may be accounted for by lower oxygen carrying capacity of the blood since the severely malnourished subjects had average blood haemoglobin values $< 10\,g/100\,ml$. Even 124 d of dietary repletion was not sufficient to restore $\dot{V}O_2$ max to the level observed in group M. Evidently, the recovery process is a long one, particularly when carried out under the sedentary conditions of the metabolic ward. It would be interesting to study the effects of a physical training regime on the time course and progress of this recovery process.

Productivity and physical work capacity. Having established a direct relationship between nutritional status and PWC, attention can now be directed to the association between $\dot{V}O_2$ max and productivity. Productivity in the present context is limited to the quantity of the end-product of moderate to heavy physical work and is measured in those tasks where piece-work is the basis for payment of the worker. A positive correlation has been found between $\dot{V}O_2$ max (estimated from submaximal measurements) and productivity in the logging industry[12] and in sugar-cane cutting[10,11]. We have also studied nutritionally-normal sugar-cane workers in Colombia, where the tasks of cutting and loading cane are performed by separate gangs of men. The cutters were divided into good (Gp I), average (Gp II) and poor (Gp III) producers according to daily tonnage cut. They worked at about 35 per cent of their $\dot{V}O_2$ max during the 8-h work day[18], which is close to the maximum that can be sustained for this period of time[4,14]. The relation of productivity in sugar cane cutting to $\dot{V}O_2$ max is shown in Fig. 2. There was a statistically significant positive correlation between $\dot{V}O_2$ max expressed both as 1/min and ml/kg min[20]. Productivity in the sugar cane loaders was also significantly correlated with $\dot{V}O_2$ max[19]. In addition to $\dot{V}O_2$ max, productivity in sugar-cane-cutting was related to body size and composition[19]. Similar findings have also been reported for industrial factory work of less intensity than sugar-cane-cutting[15].

The description of the relationships between $\dot{V}O_2$ max and nutritional status, and between $\dot{V}O_2$ max and productivity in Colombian men[6,18,19] implies a relationship between nutritional status and productivity which is in agreement with studies in Guatemalan agricultural workers[13,25] and African road builders[8,26].

School-aged boys. With the recognition that the reduced work capacity found in malnourished adults was largely the result of reduced muscle mass, the effect of chronic marginal malnutrition, which is so prevalent in the poorer segments of developing countries, on the growth of work capacity in school-aged children was then investigated. There are few studies of exercise and work capacity in malnourished children, and most of these have been carried out using sub-maximal exercise testing[1,9,16].

In the work to be described from our laboratory, all subjects were boys and had to present their official birth certificate as a first condition of inclusion in the study ($n = 1013$). They were grouped into five age groups at 2-year intervals from 6 to 16 years of age. Using Colombian standards of normal growth, children were selected who had weight for age and weight for height > 95 per cent (but < 110 per cent) of predicted as being nutritionally normal (N) and without a history of undernutrition. Those with a weight for age < 95 per cent but weight for height > 95 per cent of the standard were called the low weight for age (W-A) group and were considered to have a history of nutritional deprivation but to be nutritionally normal at the time of the study. A 3rd nutritional group was formed from those children with both weight for age and height < 95 per cent of the standard. These children were considered to be undernourished at the time of study and are referred to as the low weight for height (W-H) group.

The children were also recruited according to socioeconomic status: an upper socioeconomic group (UU) recruited from three of Cali's private schools with high tuition costs, a 2nd lower

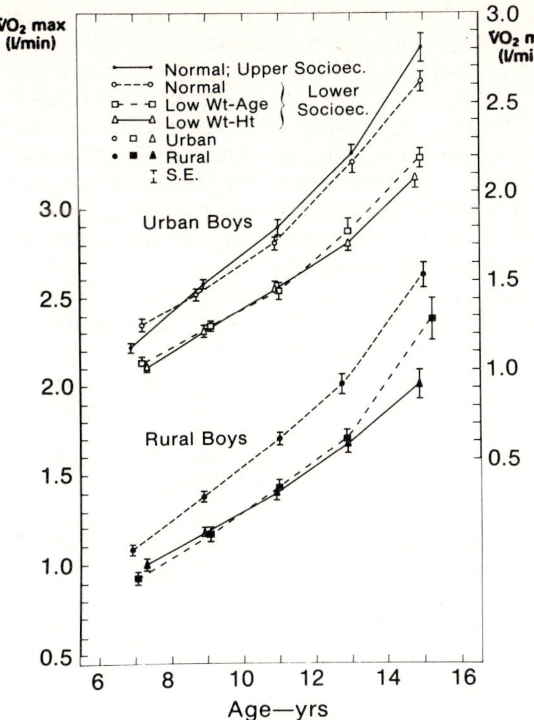

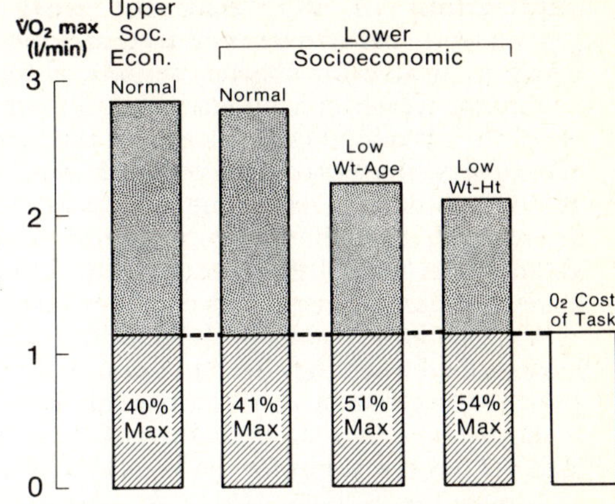

Fig. 4(above). *Average $\dot{V}O_2$ max of the four groups of 14 to 16-year-old urban boys showing the relative work load in the lower socioeconomic groups of a work task selected to be 40 per cent of the $\dot{V}O_2$ max of the upper socioeconomic group[21].*

Fig. 3(left). *$\dot{V}O_2$ max of nutritionally normal, low weight for age and low weight for height boys, plotted as a function of average group ages[21]: urban boys, right hand scale; rural boys, left hand scale.*

socioeconomic group from public schools located in several of the poorest city barrios (LU), and a 3rd lower socioeconomic group from three rural villages located outside of Cali (LR). Consequently, each of the two lower socioeconomic groups (LU, LR) had three nutritional groups each (N, W-A, W-H) while the upper urban socioeconomic boys had only N subjects. The details of the selection process and the methodology employed in the anthropometric, maturation[22], and direct $\dot{V}O_2$ max[21], measurements have been described previously.

Anthropometry and maturation. The three groups of nutritionally normal boys followed growth curves which varied between the 50th–25th percentiles of the US National Center for Health Statistics (NCHS) standards for both height and weight for age. The two nutritionally deprived groups followed a growth pattern which was on or considerably below the 5th percentiles of the NCHS data for both height and weight for age[19]. It was possible to remeasure height and weight 6–12 months after the first measurements in 53 per cent of the boys and so to calculate height and weight growth velocity curves which demonstrated a statistically significant delay in the adolescent growth spurt. Furthermore, the boys in the 12 to 13.9 and 14 to 16-year-old age groups displayed a significant retardation in sexual maturation based on Tanner Scores[23]. All of these observations are cardinal features of malnutrition in growing children and demonstrate that the selection process identified boys who were at least marginally malnourished.

Growth of work capacity ($\dot{V}O_2$ max). The growth of $\dot{V}O_2$ max (l/min) in the children described above is shown in Fig. 3. There were no significant differences between the N-UU and N-LU boys, nor between the urban, W-A, and W-H children, but the $\dot{V}O_2$ max of the nutritionally deprived boys was significantly lower ($\sim$ 85 per cent) than the N children throughout the age range studied. A similar pattern is seen in the LR subjects (lower panel, Fig. 3). Consequently, the $\dot{V}O_2$ max (l/min) of these boys follows a pattern similar to the growth of their height and weight and the reduced PWC would appear to be principally the result of smaller body size.

Implications of $\dot{V}O_2$ max for work and productivity. The relative intensity of a given work task can be expressed as per cent $\dot{V}O_2$ max, with higher intensities (% $\dot{V}O_2$ max) being endurable for shorter periods of time[4]. Approximately 40 per cent VO_2 max is the maximum which can be sustained for an 8-h working day when working at a continuing pace[3,14,18]. Work tasks which exceed this intensity can therefore be sustained for shorter periods of time or, when $\dot{V}O_2$ max is reduced for whatever reason (body size, malnutrition), carried out at lower absolute levels of energy expenditure. In either case, the result may be lower levels of productivity in moderate to heavy physical work[5,17]. In Latin America, for example, where about 55 per cent of the economically active adult male population is engaged in moderate to heavy physical labour[17], this can have serious economic implications[13].

What do these results portend for the work capacity, and productivity, of the young boys we have studied when they become adults? Figure 4 presents the $\dot{V}O_2$ max of the four groups of 14 to 16-year-old urban boys in comparison to the O_2 cost of a work task artificially set at 40 per cent of the N-UU children. In the case of the N-LU children, this amounts to about the same work load (41 per cent), but for the W-A and W-H boys, it amounts to 51 per cent and 54 per cent of $\dot{V}O_2$ max, respectively, which are well in excess of the maximum relative loads which can be sustained for an 8-h working day. Even at 40 per cent of their $\dot{V}O_2$ max, these nutritionally disadvantaged and smaller boys will probably produce, on the average, at a lower level than the N boys when they achieve adulthood. The economic implications of allowing a considerable segment of the world's population to grow up as second-rate producers is evident. Results have been reported[13] which support the hypothesis that nutritional improvements during childhood are forms of human capital investment which result in higher lifetime earnings in certain occupations and may be associated with upward social and occupational mobility during adulthood. Again, it must be underlined that these considerations apply to a large segment of the population[2] which will become involved in heavy physical work.

1 Areskog, N-H, Selinus, R. & Vahlquist, B. (1969): Physical work capacity and nutritional status in Ethiopian male children and young adults. *Am. J. Clin. Nutr.* **22**, 471–479.

2 Arteaga, L.A. (1976): The nutritional status of Latin American adults. *Basic Life Sci.* **7**, 67–76.

3 Åstrand, I. (1967): Degree of strain during building work as related to individual aerobic capacity. *Ergonomics* **10**, 293–303.

4 Åstrand, P-O. & Rodahl, K. (1977): *Textbook of work physiology.* New York: McGraw-Hill.

5 Barac-Nieto, M. (1984): Body composition and physical work capacity in undernutrition. In *Malnutrition: determinants and consequences,* ed P.L. White & N. Selvey, pp. 165–178. New York: A.R. Liss.

6 Barac-Nieto, M., Spurr, G.B., Maksud, M.G. & Lotero, H. (1978): Aerobic work capacity in chronically undernourished adult males. *J. Appl. Physiol.: Respirat. Environ. Exercise Physiol.* **44**, 209–215.

7 Barac-Nieto, M., Spurr, G.B., Dahners, H.W. & Maksud, M.G. (1980): Aerobic work capacity and endurance during nutritional repletion of severely undernourished men. *Am. J. Clin. Nutr.* **33**, 2268–2275.

8 Brooks, R.M., Latham, M.C. & Crompton, D.W.T. (1979): The relationship of nutrition and health to worker productivity in Kenya. *E. Afr. Med. J.* **56**, 413–421.

9 Davis, C.T.M. (1973): Physiological responses to exercise in East African children II. The effects of shistosomiasis, anaemia and malnutrition. *J. Trop. Ped. Environ. Child Hlth.* **19**, 115–119.

10 Davis, C.T.M. (1973): Relationship of maximum aerobic power output to productivity and absenteeism of East African sugar cane workers. *Br. J. Indust. Med.* **30**, 146–154.

11 Davies, C.T.M., Brotherhood, J.R., Collins, K.J., Dore, C., Imms, F., Musgrove, J., Weiner, J.S., Amin, M.A., Ismail, H.M., El Karim, M., Omer, A.H.S. & Sukkar, M.Y. (1976): Energy expenditure and physiological performance of Sudanese cane cutters. *Br. J. Industr. Med.* **33**, 181–186.

12 Hansson, J.E. (1965): The relationship between individual characteristics of the worker and output of logging operations. *Studia Forestalia Suecia No. 29,* pp. 68–77. Stockholm: Skogshogskolan.

13 Immink, M.D.C., Viteri, F.E., Flores, R. & Torun, B. (1984): Microeconomic consequences of energy deficiency in rural populations in developing countries. In *Energy intake and activity,* ed E. Pollit & P. Amante, pp. 355–376. New York: A.R. Liss.

14 Michael, E.D., Hutton, K.E. & Horvath, S.M. (1961): Cardiorespiratory responses during prolonged exercise. *J. Appl. Physiol.* **16**, 997–1000.

15 Satyanarayana, K., Nadamuni Naidu, A., Chatterjee, B. & Narasinga Rao, B.S. (1977): Body size and work output. *Am. J. Clin. Nutr.* **30**, 322–325.

16 Satayanarayana, K., Nadamuni Naidu, A. & Narasinga Rao, B.S. (1979): Nutritional deprivation in childhood and the body size, activity and physical work capacity of young boys. *Am. J. Clin. Nutr.* **32**, 1769–1775

17 Spurr, G.B. (1983): Nutritional status and physical work capacity. *Yearbook Phys. Anthrop.* **26**, 1–35.
18 Spurr, G.B., Barac-Nieto, M. & Maksud, M.G. (1975): Energy expenditure cutting sugar cane. *J. Appl. Physiol.* **39**, 990–996.
19 Spurr, G.B., Maksud, M.G. & Barac-Nieto, M. (1977): Energy expenditure productivity, and physical work capacity of sugar cane loaders. *Am. J. Clin. Nutr.* **30**, 1740–1746.
20 Spurr, G.B., Barac-Nieto, M. & Maksud, M.G. (1977): Productivity and maximal oxygen consumption in sugar cane cutters. *Am. J. Clin. Nutr.* **30**, 316–321.
21 Spurr, G.B., Reina, J.C., Dahners, H.W. & Barac-Nieto, M. (1983): Marginal malnutrition in school-aged Colombian boys: functional consequences in maximum exercise. *Am. J. Clin. Nutr.* **37**, 834–847.
22 Spurr, G.B., Reina, J.C. & Barac-Nieto, M. (1983): Marginal malnutrition in school-aged Colombian boys: anthropometry and maturation. *Am. J. Clin. Nutr.* **37**, 119–132.
23 Tanner, J.M. (1962): *Growth and adolescence.* Oxford: Blackwell.
24 Viteri, F.E. (1971): Considerations on the effect of nutrition on the body composition and physical working capacity of young Guatemalan adults. In *Amino acid fortification of protein foods*, ed N.S. Scrimshaw & A.M. Altshull. pp. 350–375. Cambridge, Mass: MIT Press.
25 Viteri, F.E. & Torún, B. (1975): Ingestión calorica y trabajo fisico de obreros agrícolas en Guatemala. Efecto de la suplementación alimetária y su lugar en los programs de salúd. *Bol. Of. Sanit. Panamer.* **78**, 58–74.
26 Wolgemuth, J.C., Latham, M.C., Hall, A., Chester, A. & Crompton, D.W.T. (1982): Worker productivity and the nutritional status of Kenyan road construction laborers. *Am. J. Clin. Nutr.* **36**, 68–78.

Nutrition and performance: the social dimension

K. SATYANARAYANA

National Institute of Nutrition (Indian Council of Medical Research), Hyderabad — 500 007 (A.P.), India.

A careful nutritional anthropometric survey of 9000 Indian school children belonging to well-to-do and low-income groups (1971) concluded that well-to-do Indian boys were comparable to their American counterparts in both height and weight between 5–14 years and the Indian girls were comparable to American girls up to 12 years of age[22]. It was also pointed out that among Indian children only the upper 5 per cent from the low-income group were as tall as an average well-to-do child, but the weight of none of the low-income group children equalled that of an average well-to-do child. Data from Guatemala also support the contention that children from affluent sections of the population attain a body size comparable to European and American children[10]. An examination of about 3000 preschool children from rural Hyderabad showed heights of between 50 per cent and 100 per cent of American reference values. Wider deficits were observed in weights[12].

A hypothesis has been put forward that half to three-fourths of children from developing countries possess normal anthropometric measurments and claiming that most of the malnutrition (80–90 per cent) seen was of an odd kind; children were short for their age, but of an appropriate weight for height[19,20]; accordingly it did not matter if children had a large deficit of weight for age. Extensive available data on children from India was avoided in these views[19,20]. Stating that 'smallness' is a product of poverty, the author (Seckler[19,20]) proceeded to separate smallness due to poor socio-economic environment from smallness due to undernutrition. Apparently the first category, constituting 80 to 90 per cent of all under-nourished children, were small but healthy as they had no evidence of functional impairment. This argument is untenable in the absence of convincing data to prove their normal functional performance, either in childhood or in later life.

Gopalan[5] challenged these misguided concepts and reiterated that all growth retardation (apart from that genetically determined or due to hormonal defects) is a reflection of undernutrition and of nothing else. Seckler's data base[19,20] is inadequate both in the sphere of growth and development of children as well as on normal functional capacities or absence of functional impairment of small but healthy children and/or adults.

Growth and development of small individuals. Our observations on rural Hyderabad

Table 1. *Classification of rural Hyderabad boys in longitudinal study by height for age at 5 years of age.*

Groups	s.d. Class	Height range (cm)	Nutritional category	Subjects in main study No.	%	Subjects* completing study No.	%
	Deviation of height for age from Boston standards (110.3±4.5 at age 5)						
I	Mean to mean −2 s.d.	110.3–101.3	Normal	186	(20.8)	107	(26.3)
II	Mean −2 s.d. to Mean −4 s.d.	101.2–92.3	Mild and moderate undernutrition	534	(59.7)	247	(60.5)
III	Less than mean −4 s.d.	<92.2	Severe under nutrition	174	(19.5)	54	(13.2)
			Total	894	(100.0)	408	(100.0)

*These subjects attained adult height (linear growth was less than 1 cm/year, after adolescence).

Table 2. *Influence of early nutritional plane on adult height and weight in male subjects.* Values are: mean ± s.d. L = longitudinal; CS = cross-sectional.

Growth study place	N	Initial values Age (yr)	Height (cm)	Weight (kg)	Final values Age (yr)	Height (cm)	Weight (kg)
Rural Hyderabad study(L)							
Group I	107	5.03±0.24 [a]	104.7±2.90 [a]	15.3±1.40 [a]	20.4±1.29 [a]	167.8±6.26 [a]	51.5±6.60 [a]
Group II	247	5.07±0.23 [a]	97.4±3.03 [b]	13.4±1.18 [b]	20.5±1.22 [a]	163.8±5.43 [b]	48.7±5.17 [b]
Group III	54	5.04±0.29 [a]	89.2±4.02 [c]	11.5±1.08 [c]	20.7±0.96 [a]	157.8±6.09 [c]	44.0±3.91 [c]
London[4] (CS)		5.0±	108.3	18.5	18.0±	174.7	63.0
Well-to-do Indian[8] (CS)		5.0	108.0	18.3	20.0	171.8	59.6

Between Gps I, II and III mean value with different superscrips[a,b,c] are significantly different, $P < 0.05$ or more.

children indicate that only about a fifth of them could be considered normal, with height-for-age values between the mean and mean −2 s.d. of Boston reference values (Table 1)[13]. Shortness seen in the mild and moderately malnourished boys (Gp II) was of the order of 11 cm deficit and about 5 kg weight deficit compared to well-to-do Indian children at the 5th year of life (Table 2). Thus, they had deficits in both height and weight for age. These deficits were not due to any regulatory process but were brought about by stormy and tumultuous processes in which the very survival of the child is often in doubt[5]. The shortest group had a deficit of 21 cm compared to Boston children (Table 2) and about 19 cm deficit compared to well-to-do urban Hyderabad children[7] and 7 kg weight deficit at 5th year of life. Data from a longitudinal study revealed that short children even of Gp II had significant height and weight deficits in their 20th year. Seckler's hypothesis, described above[19,20], conveniently left out data on Indian well-to-do children and adults[8] and Guatemalan well-to-do children and adults.

Unlike well-to-do families in urban areas, the majority of socially deprived rural households consist of families with no land of their own, an illiterate mother and father eking out a living based on seasonal agricultural wage-labour. We have evidence from our longitudinal study that only about one-sixth of children from such poor families can be considered as normal. On the other hand more than half the children from landlord families with more than 5 acres of wet land were found to be normal ie height for age within the mean −2 s.d. of reference value in their 5th year of life. It is unfair to science and against social justice to brand a substantial segment of undernourished young men who are mostly illiterate, paid lower wages for manual work in agriculture and without much prospect for a change in life-styles, as 'small but healthy' and adjusted to their environment.

Economic hypotheses on nutrition and productivity. David & Richard[3] put forward two hypotheses, rejecting the first one — 'malnutrition is in and of itself a major deterrent to economic development' as basically not amenable for testing. Their second hypothesis was that 'malnutrition in a society results in a degradation of the human being which in and of itself is a social problem that cries for solution'. A closer look at the available evidence indicates that there is sufficient proof for the first hypothesis itself. An economist has recently reviewed studies regarding the influence of better health on greater wealth[6].

Results of macro-studies. Health and nutrition together could account for 5 per cent of economic progress of nine Latin American countries[2]. Better health status, as indicated by low infant-mortality rate[11] and longer life expectancy[9], was associated with higher economic growth rate. Most of the variation in output change could be accounted for by two health indicators, ie infant mortality rate and the population:physician ratio.

A most sophisticated 'simultaneous model' approach to the relationship between health and economic output[24] led to the view that 'in simultaneous estimates for the 1960s, changes in life expectancy appeared to contribute significantly to change in output'. Up to this point, this analysis agreed with all other earlier studies. Macro studies in general support the conclusion that quality of human resource in terms of health and nutrition and other social indicators play an important role in the economic development of societies.

Most of the research carried out at field level was related to one of two aspects, ie (1) changes in current energy intake and (2) the role of body size and lean body mass (nutritional anthropometry) as an indication of previous nutritional history. Two Indian studies failed to show any improvement in the productivity of workers who received supplements[1,14] despite the fact that the workers had put on weight and felt better. In both instances methodological and organizational constraints, other than health improvement, were in operation. Since then scientists have attempted to avoid such methodological problems by looking at the nutritional status of the workers as indicated by body size, body composition and biochemical parameters rather than by alteration in current energy intakes as a determinant of work output in real life and/or physical work capacity as a proxy for work output. Rapid progress was achieved as refinement after refinement was incorporated in these studies. More than a dozen studies are available involving one or other of the two major aspects of nutritional status outlined above and in most cases where current nutritional anthropometry was taken as a parameter, there was some kind of positive relationship between nutritional compromise and work output or work capacity. Productivity among sugar-cane cutters was positively influenced by some indicators of nutritional status and functional capacity[21]. Work output has been shown to be related directly to body weight (r = 0.72) or lean body weight (r = 0.74) in the absence of obesity in men[15,16]. In women workers output increased with body weight until a point of obesity was reached, after which it fell off sharply. Better-nourished Guatemalan peasants were able to complete their assignment in about half the time as compared to poorly nourished peasants who were receiving no supplements[23].

The final proof of a connection between childhood nutrition background, adolescent growth, work capacity and wages earned by adolescents came from a longitudinal study from India[17,18]. Chronically-undernourished adolescents had significantly low physical work capacity, 60 per cent that of normal adolescents. They had to strain themselves to handle a standard work load (300 kpm/min), while their normal counterparts could do the job with relative ease, as it was not a major load relative to their total capacity.

Wages earned by the 151 adolescent boys employed by the farmers were significantly related to age (r = 0.42), body weight (r = 0.61) and height (r = 0.52) at the time of the study[18]. Better-paid boys weighed more at corresponding ages; and a greater proportion of them had a better nutritional background at age 5 years than those who were paid less. Better-nourished boys were sought after by the farmers and were assigned to the more demanding agricultural jobs and were paid the higher wages that went with these jobs. These observations illustrate the important influence of nutritional anthropometry on agricultural wages in real-life situations.

As far as physical work capacity or work output is concerned, our data indicated a linear relationship up to a point, which plateaued and fell sharply as obesity became very clear cut. It is the total lean body mass of the individual that is important in explaining variations in performance and there was no group that could be designated 'small but healthy', as the handicap was proportional to lean body weight or body weight in these communities where frank obesity is not a public health problem. Poorly nourished young men could never compete with normally-nourished matched counterparts either for work capacity or wages earned.

Since adult nutritional anthropometry was markedly influenced by adverse nutritional background during early childhood and adolescence, it would appear that nutritional status, through its effect on body size, influences both working and earning capacities. Nutritional and health situations (governed by social, economic and political factors) which lead to lower adult nutritional anthropometry may therefore be expected to be associated with reduced work output in real-life situations, even when maximum work capacity is not involved. Labour (social) productivity and social contribution to the humanity at large, have been shown to be limited in undernourished groups in several studies due to a limitation of growth and development, physiological capabilities and acquisition of skills.

1 Belavady, B. (1966): Nutrition and efficiency in agricultural labourers. *Indian J. Med. Res.* **54**, 971–976.
2 Correa, H. & Cummins, G. (1970): Contribution of nutrition to economic growth. *Am. J. Clin. Nutr.* **23**, 560–565.
3 David, L.C. & Richard, L. (1972): Evaluation of the economic consequences of malnutrition. *In Western Hemisphere Nutrition Congress*, ed P.L. White & S. Selvey, pp. 312–317. New York: Future Publishing Co.
4 Eveleth, P.B. & Tanner, J.M. (1976): Europeans in Europe and European descendents in Australia, Africa and the America. *In World wide variation in human growth*, I.B.P. Vol. No. 8, pp. 15 and 51. London: Cambridge University Press.
5 Gopalan, C. (1983): 'Small is healthy'? for the poor, not for the rich! *Nutr. Foun. India Bull.* October, 1–5.
6 Gwatkin, D.R. (1983): *Does better health produce greater wealth?* pp. 1–37. Washington: Overseas Development Council.
7 Hanumantha Rao, D., Satyanarayana, K. & Sastry, J.G. (1976): Growth pattern of well-to-do Hyderabad pre-school children. *Indian J. Med. Res.* **64**, 629–638.
8 Hanumantha Rao, D. & Sastry, J.G. (1977): Growth pattern of well-to-do Indian adolescents and young adults. *Indian J. Med. Res.* **66**, 950–956.
9 Hicks, N. (1980): cited by Gwatkin[6]
10 Johnston, F.E., Wainer, H., Thissen, D. & Macvean, R.B. (1976): Hereditory and environmental determinants of growth in height in a longitudinal sample of children and youth of Guatemalan and European ancestry. *Am. J. Phys. Anthop.* **44**, 469–475.
11 Malenbaum, W. (1970): cited by Gwatkin[6].
12 Pralhad Rao, N., Darshan Singh & Swaminathan, M.C. (1969): Nutritional status of pre-school children of rural communities near Hyderabad city. *Indian J. Med. Res.* **57**, 2132–2246.
13 Reed, R.B. & Stuart, H.C. (1959): Patterns of growth in height and weight from birth to eighteen years of age. *Pediatrics* **24**, 904–921.
14 Satyanarayana, K., Hanumantha Rao, D., Vasudeva Rao, D. & Swaminathan, M.C. (1972): Nutrition and working efficiency in coal-miners. *Indian J. Med. Res.* **60**, 1800–1806.
15 Satyanarayana, K., Nadamuni Naidu, A., Chatterjee, B. & Narasinga Rao, B.S. (1977): Body size and work output. *Am. J. Clin. Nutr.* **30**, 322–325.
16 Satyanarayana, K., Narasinga Rao, B.S. & Srikantia, S.G. (1979): Nutrition and work output. *Indian J. Nutr. Diet.* **16**, 170–174.
17 Satyanarayana, K., Nadamuni Naidu, A. & Narasinga Rao, B.S. (1979): Nutritional deprivation in childhood and the body size, activity and physical work capacity of young boys. *Am. J. Clin. Nutr.* **32**, 1769–1775.
18 Satyanarayana, K., Nadamuni Naidu, A. & Narasinga Rao, B.S. (1980): Agricultural employment, wage earnings and nutritional status of teenage rural Hyderabad boys. *Indian J. Nutr. Diet.* **17**, 281–286.
19 Seckler, D. (1982): 'Small but healthy': a basic hypothesis in the theory, measurement and policy of malnutrition. In *Newer concepts in nutrition and their implications for policy.* ed P.V. Sukhatme, pp. 127–137. Pune, India: Maharashtra Association for the cultivation of Science Research Institute.
20 Seckler, D. (1982): Malnutrition: an intellectual odyssey. (ibid pp. 139–148).
21 Spurr, G.B., Barac-Nieto, M. & Maksud, M.G. (1977): Productivity and maximal oxygen consumption in sugar cane cutters. *Am. J. Clin. Nutr.* **30**. 316–321.
22 Vijayaraghavan, K., Darshan Singh & Swaminathan, M.C. (1971): Heights and weights of well-nourished Indian school children. *Indian J. Med. Res.* **59**, 648–654.
23 Viteri, F.E. (1971): Considerations on the effect of nutrition on the body composition and physical work capacity of young Guatemalan adults. In *Amino acid fortification of foods* ed N.S. Scrimshaw and A.M. Altschul, pp. 350–375. Boston, Massachusetts: MIT Press.
24 Wheeler, D. (1980): cited by Gwatkin[6].

Effects of drought in Africa: a workshop report

A. OMOLOLU (Organizer)
Department of Nutrition, University of Ibadan, Nigeria.

Introduction (by the organizer). The drought in Africa started in the Sahel area of West Africa in the early 70s. Since then, it had spread to Central and East Africa affecting Chad, Sudan, Ethiopia and Somalia. In the past 2 years, the Southern parts of Africa too have been affected by drought — Mozambique, Angola, Malawi, Zambia and Zimbabwe. Thus, countries of Africa along both tropics — Cancer and Capricorn — seem to bear the brunt of the drought, though the effects on nearby countries over the past 15 years are also enormous. The international communities have suddenly, over the past year, been brought face to face with the calamity through the mass media, and have generously responded with food aid. The problems, however, are more basic. The economics of most of these countries have been seriously affected over the past 10 years; rural and urban development have been at a standstill, desertification has increased, migration of populations have occurred. How can we face and solve these problems — apart from stopping deaths from famine, improving the infrastructure and ensuring agricultural production?

Mahgoub described the present problem in Sudan. He noted that the drought was compounded by continuing desertification which resulted from overgrazing, bad cultivation of marginal areas, woodcutting and deforestation for fuel and building, bush fires and the lowering of the water-table due to increased use and over use of bore holes. He noted that both drought and desertification started some 15 years ago. The sudden influx of refugees from Ethiopia, Chad, Uganda and Zaire (about 1.2 million of them) as well as the inernal movement of people from the drought affected parts of Sudan to the towns and areas of better rainfall (about 1.8 million people) have made the problem worse. He noted that the development of the affected areas and of the country as a whole had been adversely affected. Health, education, services and production experienced some setback and the effect on the nutritional status of the whole population had affected their working and production abilities.

The response of both national and international organisations had been marvellous. Aid had come in forms of money, food, drugs, shelter, clothes and other items. It was estimated that 300 million dollars worth of aid had been spent in Sudan by 1985. The nutrition relief has had success with intensive feeding and medical care, distribution of free food and concèssionary sales of cereals. The poor infrastructure in the country — bad roads, poor bridges, disorganisation of transportation and lack of lorries — has slowed down the work. On rehabilitation, FAO/WHO had proposed 37 rehabilitation projects that would combat and prevent future drought and desertification in the Sudan. The paper from the Economic Commission for Africa was prepared by the Secretary, *A. Adedeji* and presented by Dr. *Sarr* of the commission.

Socio-economic effect of drought in Africa. The first part dealt with the background to the current economic crisis in Africa. Most African economies still had the following characteristics, the effects of colonial domination which lasted for decades: (1) overspecialization in raw material production; (2) overdependence on foreign factor inputs including foreign capital, technology and even raw materials, as well as on foreign markets for raw materials exports in spite of the highly inelastic supply of these products and the price instability on international markets; (3) development of economic units that constitute real enclaves as they have little or no link with other sectors or with human resources base; (4) insufficient attention paid to the development of human resources in terms of education, training and skill development, health and other basic services; (5) persistence of undesirable scars on the psychology of the African people resulting in a loss of self-confidence which is essential in the battle for economic and social development.

An aggravating factor had been an unfavourable and deteriorating international economic environment with (1) a continuous long-term decrease in commodity prices, (2) a stagnation and decline in Official Development Assistance in real terms, (3) rising interest rates on loans and debts, (4) sharp currency fluctuations and (5) increased protectionism. These factors have interacted to exacerbate the escalating social and economic crisis. It was against this background and because of it, that the Lagos Plan of Action and the Final Act of Lagos were formulated at the second extraordinary session of the Assembly of Heads of State and Governments of the Organisation of African Unity held in Lagos from 28 to 29 April 1980. The plan was later presented to the general assembly of the United Nations and became an integral part of the International Development Strategy for the Third United Nations Development Decade.

The Lagos Plan of Action is based on six main pillars, namely (a) Africa's huge resources must be applied principally to meet the needs, and purposes of its people; (b) Africa's almost total reliance on the export of raw materials must change; (c) Africa must cultivate the virtue of self-reliance without cutting itself off from outside contributions which should only supplement Africa's national and collective efforts; (d) as a means to achieve increased self-reliance, Africa must mobilize its entire human and material resources for its development; (e) in pursuing all embracing economic, social and cultural activities, African countries must ensure that both the efforts put into and the benefits derived from development are equitably shared; (f) efforts towards African economic integration must be pursued with renewed determination in order to create a continent-wide framework for the much needed economic co-operation for development based on collective self reliance.

In spite of the adoption of the Lagos Plan of Action by the African heads of state and government, the structural weaknesses of African economics have prevailed. The African social and economic conditions rather than improving have become progressively worse culminating in the present widespread drought.

In the 4 years since the adoption of the Lagos Plan of Action in 1981, the performance in the African region was far below the objectives and targets envisaged. Africa's gross domestic product fell, in real terms, by 1.3 per cent in 1981; increased by only 1.3 per cent in 1982 and stagnated in 1983 and 1984.

In per caput terms, the loss in output was around 10 per cent relative to 1980. Agricultural output recorded a growth rate of only 0.1 per cent per annum during the period 1981–84, whilst the overall current account deficit was US \$31.8 billion in 1981, \$24.5 billion in 1982, \$17.3 billion in 1983 and \$10 billion in 1984. It is to be noted that the reduction in the deficit over the period 1981–1984 was achieved through a drastic reduction of essential imports and consequently at a heavy cost in terms of growth.

It was against this background that drought struck. Although Africa had been confronted with drought in the past — especially in the early 70s, the situation since 1983/84 was markedly different and more ominous. At the beginning of 1984 and as a result of poor harvest especially in West, and Southern Africa, 24 countries were declared abnormally dependent on food aid. By October 1984, the number had increased to 27. It should be noted that the food aid requirements of the affected African countries had increased sharply from 3.3 million tons in 1983/84 to over 7 million tons in 1984/85. Put in another way, by the end of this year, one in five Africans will be living solely on imported food aid.

The drought had brought in its train other crises namely: (a) water supply; (b) transportation, storage and distribution of food and other emergency supplies; (c) massive population displacements; (d) deteriorating health conditions; (e) worsening nutritional status of vulnerable groups; (f) loss of livestock; (g) increased need for income-generating relief projects; (h) increased energy shortage. The provision of food aid, though important, is simply not enough.

In the very lively discussions that followed comments were made about lack of planning and inadequacies of some African Governments in wasting their resources; the lack of political will and follow through of plans and strategies. Questions were asked about the use and monitoring of the large sums of money now being donated. Was there any way of monitoring these monies so that they would be used not only for relief but also for the much needed rehabilitation and strengthening of infrastructures? The need to involve African nutritionists, economists and workers in the ongoing programmes so that they could follow through with the work when the international organisations and foreign voluntary organizations left.

It was noted that the Organisation of African Unity at the 21st summit in July 1985 adopted a Special Programme of Action which included short, medium and long-term measures. Among the short-term measures were the establishment and strengthening of national early warning systems that would monitor crop conditions, meteorological as well as other data on seasonal variations that affect food production, quantity of crops and food security; packages of incentives for increasing production and productivity in the agricultural sector. In the long-term measures, emphasis was laid on research and development of drought resistant and quick-maturing crop varieties, harnessing of waters of rains, rivers and lakes for irrigation and the restoration of ecological balance through the introduction of suitable farming systems.

After the discussions, the Workshop resolved to: (1) record thanks to countries and international organisations that have responded so gallantly, quickly and generously to the present situation in Africa. The response had saved millions of lives and brought hope to many. There was however, need to remind individuals, voluntary organisations, national and international bodies that there was a greater need for greater and more sustained support to African Governments in their plans for rehabilitation and long-term programmes so that drought, desertification and poor agriculture will not recur; (2) express fears about the lack of evaluation and proper coordination of the activities of the many and various relief organisations and bodies, and the large sums of money collected and being expended. There was the need for cost-effective systems and better utilization of monies as well as progress reports on attainments, costs of personnel, transport, logistics etc. Voluntary, national and international agencies that collect money for relief should be accountable; (3) ask all agencies involved in drought relief in Africa to ensure that more and more Africans be coopted into the planning and execution of their programmes. At the end of the acute phase, the rehabilitation and long-term problems will need to be solved by Africans. There is therefore an urgent need to include African nutritionists, managers, dietitians, economists and planners in all the ongoing programmes.

Ethics and ideology in the battle against malnutrition: a workshop report

C. SCHUFTAN (Organizer)
Dept of Pediatrics, Louisiana State University Medical School, 1542 Tulane Avenue, New Orelans LA 70112 2822, USA.

Discussants: Wenche Barth Eide (University of Oslo, Norway); M. Latham (Cornell University, USA); J. Rivers, London School of Hygiene and Tropical Medicine, UK. Chairman: R. Sharp, World Food Assembly, London UK.

Introduction (by the organizer). 'What have we been achieving all these years? Have we been using the appropriate armamentarium and strategies in the battle against hunger and malnutrition? We cannot afford to say "This is what science has taught me to do and anything beyond it is none of my business". Who are we cheating? Ourselves? The people we pretend to work for? Both?' These are some of the questions for the workshop to consider.

There was a broad measure of agreement on the proposition that the nutrition profession needed to take much more account of the underlying and basic causes of malnutrition — economic, political or ideological — which at present it chose largely to ignore. Most nutrition interventions were at the micro-level of symptoms and immediate causes. But people in this field should not delude themselves with the idea that they could steer clear of politics: to decline to take a stance on fundamental policy issues was in itself a vote for the status quo. Ignoring the macro causes, nutritionists still dreamt that their goals could be reached if only they did their technical work better.

In fact, nutrition workers were in many cases contributing to the perpetuation of maldevelopment. To rectify this, they needed to engage in a serious debate on the strategies and tactics they should adopt vis-à-vis governments, international agencies and transnational corporations. Various lines of action were possible. In the speaker's view, the first thing requiring clarification was the role of nutritionists as advocates and change agents.

A minority of institutions was recognised to be working seriously for a more equity-oriented development. Two or three of these were United Nations agencies but the majority were non-governmental groups and grassroots organisations, many of whom were not allied under the umbrella of the World Food Assembly. A new alternative was emerging and all concerned with issues of food policy were urged to take note and consider joining the movement. Nutritionists could exercise a considerable influence on policy, and science was on their side. The prime question was how they could best use these resources to bring about meaningful change.

W. Barth Eide, while agreeing with much of Dr Schuftan's thesis, did not believe that science today was on the nutritionist's side. A lot of it had been very unscientific. Nevertheless, the answer was not to reject science but to strive for a more scientific approach. Science might also be a better ally if people in the profession were clearer about the answers they were looking for.

Efforts should be made to achieve a common value basis for all nutritional work, whether by people's movements or by official agencies, so that all interventions would lead in the same direction and thus help to reinforce each other. In seeking an effective link between practical action and advocacy, the human rights approach to food offered considerable promise. More work was needed before nutritionists could be sure of precisely what they should advocate, but this was a tremendous challenge since a new nutritional ethic could contribute importantly to the conceptual and practical basis of human rights.

Latham quoted from one of his articles in which he asserted that the solution of the world's nutrition problems depended on political decisions and regretting that nutritionists were not willing to discuss more openly the politics that profoundly affected the problems they sought to solve. It was 16 years since he had written those words and things had still not changed much. Many people at the Congress would regard this workshop as irrelevent, but in fact it was essential for nutritionists to be advocates and though this could be difficult for expatriates working in the third world there were still many things they could do. They should (1) make sure that their actions did not exploit the poor, (2) ally themselves with the people in the country trying to tackle these problems, (3) ensure that their own activities mainly benefitted the poor, and (4) look at the health and nutrition impact of a whole range of the government's policies.

Rivers said that the first problems needing to be resolved were those concerning the ideas, structures and influence of the nutrition profession itself. Nutritionists were part of the 20th century priesthood of scientists involved with problems of humanity: they had great power to influence policy, which was important for one thing because resources allocated on their advice were unavailable for other purposes. This meant that millions of dollars could be channelled into research on brain development when in many places even the basic conditions of life were lacking.

Once the younger generation of nutritionists reached a consensus on the kind of professional change they wanted, there was a real danger that the structures they developed would embody as many vicissitudes as those they now saw in existing institutions. Before marching into action they needed to be clearer in their minds about *how* to act. Before trying to do good it was important that they put their own house in order.

General discussion. Interventions from the floor illustrated practical ways in which people have sought to take account of this broad range of issues in their work. There were examples from South Africa of work that had achieved a dramatic reduction in malnutrition and of collaboration among health workers to resist the oppressive controls of apartheid. 'Success stories' from other countries were also reported.

In conclusion, it was proposed that everyone personally concerned with these issues of nutritional ethics should aim to direct their energies into two channels — firstly, to seek ways to enable people to define and solve their own nutrition-related problems, and secondly, to widen this debate within the profession in order to raise awareness of the nutritionist's role as an agent for change.

The workshop was attended by more than 50 participants from about 20 countries and it stimulated a lively and thoughtful discussion on the politics of hunger and the nutritionists' role.

★ ★ ★

NUTRITION AND RISK FACTORS FOR MORBIDITY AND MORTALITY IN THE UNDER FIVES

Vitamin A and mortality

A. SOMMER, I. TARWOTJO, K.P. WEST, R. TILDEN, B. HAWKINS, L. MELE and E. DJUNAEDI
The International Center for Epidemiologic and Preventive Ophthalmology Dana Center for Preventative Ophthalmology, Wilmer Institute, Room 120, Johns Hopkins Hospital, Baltimore, Maryland, 21205, USA; the Department of Health, Government of Indonesia; and Helen Keller International, New York.

It has long been known that vitamin A is important for more bodily functions than simply dark adaptation and normal functioning and appearance of the eye. While children with severe vitamin A deficiency and malnutrition were known to experience extremely high mortality[4] it was only recently discovered that mild vitamin A deficiency was associated, in a population setting, with reduced survival[6]. In a longitudinal prospective study of 4000 preschool Indonesian children who were re-examined every 3 months over an 18-month period of time, those with mild pre-existing xerophthalmia (night-blindness and/or Bitot's spots) experienced four to 12 times the mortality of their non-xerophthalmic peers. This relationship was dose-dependent: mortality rose with progression from night-blindness to Bitot's spots to the two conditions together, which parallels the degree of mild vitamin A deficiency[5]. In addition to being dose-dependent, increased mortality was present after adjustment for age and anthropometric status.

The mild vitamin A deficiency was also associated with an increased risk of diarrhoea and respiratory disease, the two conditions responsible for most deaths in preschool children[7]. In fact, the risk of respiratory disease and diarrhoea was more closely correlated with xerophthalmic status than it was with general anthropometric status.

As the result of early animal work and autopsy studies[1,8] it has been known that vitamin A is necessary for the production of normal mucus-secreting epithelia in a wide variety of organs. In the absence of vitamin A, mucous epithelium becomes transformed by keratinizing metaplasia into skin-like stratified squamous epithelium. This may well account for observations of increased rates of urinary tract colonization, if not frank infection[2,3].

Despite these observations, it was necessary to establish that the correlation between xerophthalmia and mortality was not due to an unrecognized third factor, and to demonstrate that vitamin-A-supplementation could have a measurable impact. For these reasons, a population-based, randomized community trial was carried out in Aceh province, Sumatra, Indonesia. The Government of Indonesia was rapidly expanding vitamin A capsule distribution programmes throughout the country, especially to those areas shown in a nation-wide study to have a high rate of disease. It was impossible, however, to begin distribution in all villages at the same time. In Aceh province, distribution was to be phased in over a 5-year period. By randomly allocating villages that would receive distribution during the 1st and 3rd year, the following study could be carried out.

Methods. Approximately 450 villages containing 30 000 preschool children were randomly assigned to one of three distribution mechanisms: the standard, community-based volunteer programme in which a local villager was instructed to distribute a vitamin A capsule to all children aged 1 to 6 years every six months; the UGKP villages, in which vitamin A distribution was included in a package of maternal and child health activities, and control villages. It was soon discovered that there were insufficient UGKP villages for comparison and these were dropped from the allocation scheme. An advance team visited each of the villages in turn, mapping and censusing the village, and identifying all houses containing children less than 6 years of age. Because of local taboos, and the fact that children below 1 year of age are not provided with capsules under the Indonesian distribution scheme, these are not included in the analyses that follow.

After census and mapping, a village was visited by one of two standardized field teams, composed of an ophthalmologist, a nurse-assistant, a nutritionist, and five field workers. Historical and socio-demographic data were collected on all children at their homes; the eyes of all available children were examined by the ophthalmologist, and anthropometric and dietary data were obtained for all children with xerophthalmia, matched controls, and a random subsample of the entire study population. The same team returned approximately 12 months later to up-date information and re-examine all children initially enrolled in the study. Children born or entering into households since the baseline examination are not included in the analysis.

Following initial baseline examination, the regular government health structure carried out routine training for vitamin A capsule distribution volunteers. They were provided with basic information about the importance of vitamin A and the need for administering vitamin A capsules to every child between 1 and 6 years of age immediately, and again 6 months later. In theory every child in the supplementation villages received two capsules, one within a month of the baseline examination, the 2nd 6 months later, approximately 4 to 6 months before the final examination. The capsules contained 200 000 IU vitamin A and 40 IU vitamin E as provided by UNICEF. Specially-trained supervisors visited supplementation villages following the scheduled capsule distribution and subsampled households to ensure distribution had indeed been carried out. Where coverage was below 80 per cent the volunteer distributors were encouraged to find unsupplemented children and provide them with a capsule.

Any child found to have evidence of xerophthalmia at the baseline survey was treated regardless of his village allocation. In addition, all local clinics and health centres were sensitized to the potential seriousness of vitamin-A-deficiency, provided with vitamin A capsules, and encouraged to treat all children who presented with vitamin-A-deficiency as well as their neighbours (because of the previously documented clustering effect[5]). For these reasons the control villages were not entirely uncontaminated: approximately 1 per cent of all children in these villages in fact received the vitamin A capsule during the period between the surveys.

Results. Preliminary results show that the levels of distribution in supplemented villages were high, with 85 per cent of children receiving at least one capsule and 75 per cent of children two capsules according to the mother's history. In contrast, only 1 per cent of children in non-supplemented villages were said to have received a capsule during the inter-survey period. Supplemented villages contained a total of 12 761 children aged 1 to 5 years at the baseline examination and non-supplemented villages 11 572 children. Overall mortality rate in the non-supplemented villages was 50 per cent higher than in the supplemented villages. The relative risk was only 1.1 for children in the 2nd year of life, but reached a peak of 2.9 for children during the 3rd year of life. Thus, vitamin-A-supplementation reduced childhood mortality in children from 1 to 6 years of age (at original baseline) by 35 per cent.

Discussion. The tremendous impact that vitamin-A-deficiency had on this population is consistent with the early clinical studies and the recent results of the longitudinal observational study in Java[6]. They are probably typical of those that could be achieved in other areas of vitamin-A-deficiency. The baseline survey demonstrated a Bitot's spot rate of approximately 1–2 per cent, which is common in many areas of Asia. The area was therefore not one in which vitamin-A-deficiency was particularly prevalent; nor were the children particularly malnourished.

The results probably underestimate the impact of vitamin-A-supplementation. Preliminary data indicate that children who needed the vitamin A most were least likely to have received it; vitamin A distribution was only carried out for a single year, precluding any benefit from long-term accumulation of vitamin A stores in young children, and perhaps more importantly, in women of child bearing age. The control villages were not entirely uncontaminated, precautions having been taken to sensitize the health workers and ensure adquate treatment of all affected children and at least some of their neighbours. The most vulnerable group, children with frank xerophthalmia at baseline examination, were all treated and therefore excluded from the analyses.

Acknowledgements. This project was carried out under the Cooperative Agreement AID/DSAN-CA/0267 between the Office of Nutrition, USAID, and ICEPO; and with partial financial support from the Government of Indonesia, Helen Keller International, USAID, IBM International, Hoffman-LaRoche, and the Ford Foundation.

1 Blackfan, K.D. & Wolbach, S.B. (1933): Vitamin A deficiency in infants. A clinical and pathological study. *J. Pediatr.* **3**, 679–706.
2 Bloch, C.E. (1924): Blindness and other diseases in children arising from deficient nutrition (lack of fat-soluble A factor). *Am. J. Dis. Child.* **27**, 139–148.
3 Brown, K.H., Graffar, A. & Alamgir, S.M. (1979): Xerophthalmia, protein-calorie malnutrition, and infections in children. *J. Pediatr.* **95**, 651–656.
4 Sommer A. (1982): *Nutritional blindness: xerophthalmia and keratomalacia.* New York: Oxford University Press.
5 Sommer, A., Hussaini, G., Muhilal, Tarwotjo, I., Susanto, D. & Saroso, J.S. (1980): History of nightblindness: a simple tool for xerophthalmia screening. *Am. J. Clin. Nutr.* **33**, 887–891.
6 Sommer, A., Hussaini, G., Tarwotjo, I. & Susanto, D. (1983): Increased mortality in children with mild vitamin A deficiency. *Lancet* **1**, 585–588.
7 Sommer, A., Katz, J. & Tarwotjo, I. (1984): Increased risk of respiratory disease and diarrhea in children with preexisting mild vitamin A deficiency. *Am. J. Clin. Nutr.* **40**, 1090–1095.
8 Wolbach, S.B. & Howe, P.R. (1925): Tissue changes following deprivation of fat-soluble A vitamin. *J. Exp. Med.* **42**, 753–777.

Wasting and stunting as risk factors for morbidity and mortality

F.L. TROWBRIDGE
Division of Nutrition, Centers for Disease Control, 1600 Clifton Road NE, Atlanta, Georgia 30333, USA.

Since their introduction by Waterlow[15], the terms 'wasting' and 'stunting', defined as low weight-for-height and low height-for-age, respectively, have been increasingly used to characterize the nutritional status of children. The cross-classification of weight-for-height and height-for-age permits children with more acute malnutrition to be distinguished from those with more chronic nutritional deficiency, an extremely valuable distinction that allows intervention activities to be targeted to those most in need.

It has been proposed that the highest priority for intervention should be children who are both wasted and stunted, followed by children who are wasted but not stunted, with third priority to children who are stunted only[16]. A central purpose of this paper is to review the extent to which subsequent investigation has supported these priority rankings, and to consider how well wasting and stunting perform in identifying risk compared with other anthropometric classifications. These issues will be addressed in the context of considering several key, specific questions about wasting and stunting as nutritional classifications.

How well do wasting and stunting represent nutritional status? The use of weight-for-height to describe and compare current nutritional status assumes that normal weight-for-height is relatively constant across different age, sex and race groups. However, all these assumptions are open to question. Some have argued that age differences in weight-for-height should be taken into account in classifying children[9], but it has been generally assumed that these differences are quantitatively of minor significance. Sex differences in weight-for-height also occur, but sex-specific reference standards are available so that variations can be taken into account. Genetically based differences in body proportions may also affect weight-for-height[3], but the quantitative significance of these effects has not been widely assessed.

Differences in body composition stemming from genetic and/or dietary factors are other factors potentially affecting weight-for-height. Peruvian children with very low height-for-age were found to have high weight-for-height values that averaged above the 60th percentile[14]. However, these children had low body fat as indicated both by low skinfold thicknesses and by a relatively high percentage of body weight as water, measured by stable isotope dilution techniques. Moreover, the increased weight-for-height was not explained by body proportions: their sitting height to total height ratio was only 2 per cent greater than that of North American reference children. Thus, children with high weight-for-height may have relatively poor current nutritional status as reflected in depleted body fat. Moreover, high or low weight-for-height may have different nutritional implications in children from different genetic, environmental, and dietary backgrounds.

The presumption that stunting can be taken to represent chronic undernutrition seems somewhat less controversial than the relationship of weight-for-height to acute malnutrition. Genetically based differences in linear growth potential exist, but are quantitatively small compared with the impact of environmental factors such as inadequate diet and infection[4,5]. Thus, for public health purposes the prevalence of stunting, calculated in relation to the international growth reference[18], appears to be a reasonable indicator of chronic under-nutrition[17].

Are wasting and stunting causally related to morbidity and mortality outcomes? Many studies have examined the association of wasting and stunting with morbidity and mortality. Cross-sectional studies have shown higher rates of recent diarrhoea among children who are wasted, and particularly among those who are wasted and stunted (Table 1)[10]. These results conform with the priorities suggested by Waterlow for intervention[16]. Longitudinal studies suggest that wasting is significantly related to the duration, but not the incidence, of diarrhoea episodes[1]. Moreover, wasting and especially stunting are related to overall mortality risk[2], although measles mortality was not related to preexisting nutritional status in other longitudinal studies[7].

Table 1. *Percentage reporting diarrhoea in each nutritional category in El Salvador 1978 Studies[10]*

	January–March survey (Dry season)	July–September survey (Rainy season)
Normal	21.4	28.1
Stunting only	21.3	26.3
Wasting only	28.9*	38.7**
Wasting and stunting	34.2**	48.7**

*Significantly greater than control ($P<0.05$);
**Significanly greater than control ($P<0.01$).

Table 2. *Sensitivity and specificity of indicators in identifying children with diarrhoea[10]*

Indicator	Prevalence (%)	Sensitivity (%)	Specificity (%)
Wasting (<90% of median)	8.6	12.0	92.4
Low arm circum-ference (<13.5 cm)	10.1	18.2	92.2
Low weight-for-age (<75% of median)	10.5	14.6	90.6

Other data indicate the important effects of morbidity, such as diarrhoea, on nutritional status. Wasting can occur rapidly in children with acute infection, and stunting is clearly related to the extent of previous diarrhoea[8]. Diminished height growth related to diarrhoea has been observed even in relatively short-term, 3-month observations of Brazilian children[5]. It appears from these observations that wasting and stunting are often as much a reflection of previous morbidity as they are a predictor of future illness[14]. The relationships of wasting and stunting to morbidity and mortality do not necessarily reflect causal links but rather the common association of malnutrition and child morbidity/mortality with poverty.

Are wasting and stunting the most efficient anthropometric indicators for identifying risks? Assessment of the relative performance of wasting and stunting in comparison with other anthropometric indicators may best be conceptualized in terms of sensitivity and specificity.

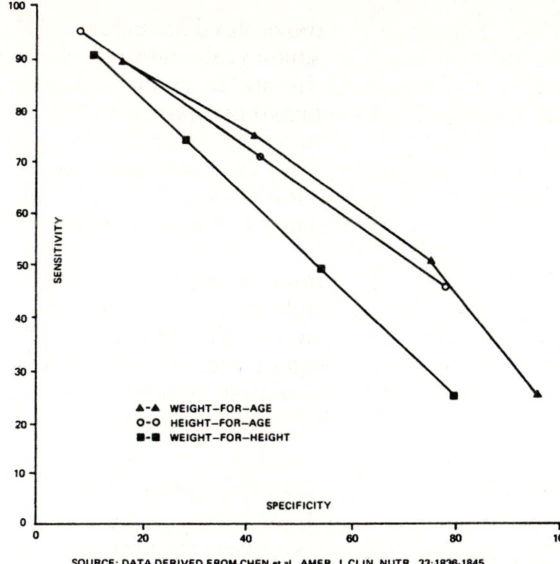

Figure. *Sensitivity and specificity of weight-for-age, height-for-age and weight-for-height in identifying children dying within 2 years[2].*

Sensitivity relates to the ability of the indicator to identify positive cases while specificity describes the ability to properly exclude negatives ones. A study in El Salvador using this approach found that low weight-for-height displayed similar sensitivity and specificity compared with low arm circumference and low arm-circumference-for-age in identifying children below 75 per cent of median weight-for-age, but was less sensitive than arm circumference indicators in identifying children below 60 per cent of median weight-for-age[13].

Taking diarrhoea morbidity as the reference point, data from El Salvador[10] may be used to calculate that, at a similar prevalence and specificity, the indicator of wasting gave a lower level of sensitivity than did arm circumference; weight-for-age gave a slightly higher sensitivity but at a lower specificity (Table 2). Thus, wasting offered no particular advantage for identifying children with recent diarrhoea.

In regard to mortality risk, weight-for-age and height-for-age provided greater sensitivity than weight-for-height at all levels of specificity tested (Figure)[2]. Even shorter-term (0–5 months) mortality risk was not as well identified by weight-for-height as by other anthropometric indicators. It may be that weight-for-height is more sensitive than other indicators to short-term weight fluctuations, introducing an added level of variability which weakens its ability to discriminate long-term mortality risk.

Overall, weight-for-age and arm circumference-for-age had the greatest ability to discriminate mortality risk over a 24-month period; height-for-age and arm circumference-for-height were intermediate while weight-for-height showed the lowest ability to discriminate mortality risk[2]. Another study in Bangladesh[12] found the sensitivity and specificity performance of simple arm circumference in identifying mortality risk to be better than arm circumference-for-height, a conclusion which is consistent with the findings in the Chen study. Low weight-for-age was also shown to be significantly related to mortality risk in Indian children[6] but sensitivity and specificity estimates were not made.

Discussion and conclusions. The definition of wasting and stunting as indicators capable of distinguishing acute from chronic malnutrition has been a significant advance in classifying protein energy malnutrition in children. The proposal that the highest risk for morbidity and mortality would be found in children who are both wasted and stunted, has been generally supported by subsequent investigations. Wasting without stunting has been related to diarrhoea morbidity but wasting has not performed well as an indicator of long-term mortality risk. Moreover, body composition studies suggest that normal or even increased weight-for-height can occur in children with poor nutritional status as reflected in reduced body fat. Thus, the interpretation of weight-for-height appears to be rather complex, and the morbidity, mortality implications of low weight-for-height may vary from one population to another.

These findings should not be interpreted as indicating that wasting and stunting lack value and validity as a means of nutritional assessment and classification. Weight-for-height is a useful index of acute malnutrition and has the significant advantage of not requiring age determination. Height-for-age remains the most logical and useful index available to assess chronic malnutrition. Although it is becoming clear that comparisons among populations in regard to weight-for-height status need to be made with caution, comparisons within the same population over time can be highly useful for defining changes in the prevalence of malnutrition or monitoring the effects of interventions. At the same time, the excellent performance of other anthropometric indicators in identifying morbidity and mortality risks suggests that other measures may also be useful in assessing risks and monitoring trends in malnutrition.

1 Black, R.E. & Brown, K.H. (1984): Malnutrition is a determining factor in diarrheal duration, but not incidence, among young children in a longitudinal study in rural Bangladesh. *Am. J. Clin. Nutr.* **37**, 87–84.
2 Chen, L.C., Chowdhury, A.K.M.A. & Huffman, S.L. (1980): Anthropometric assessment of energy-protein malnutrition and subsequent risk of mortality among preschool-aged children. *Am. J. Clin. Nutr.* **33**, 1836–1845.
3 Garn, S.M. (1976): The anthropometric assessment of malnutrition. In *Proc. 3rd Nat. Nutr. Workshop for Nutritionists on University Affiliated Facilities*, ed M.A. Harvey-Smith, pp. 3–16. Child Development Center, University of Tennessee, Memphis.
4 Graitcer, P.L. & Gentry, E.M. (1981): Measuring children: one reference for all. *Lancet* **2**, 297–299.
5 Guerrant, R.L., Kirchoff, L.V., Shields, D.S., Nations, M.K., Leslie, J., de Sousa, M.A., Araujo, J.G., Correia, L.L., Sauer, K.T., McClelland, K.E., Trowbridge, F.L. & Hughes, J.M. (1983): Prospective study of diarrheal illnesses in Northeastern Brazil: patterns of disease, nutritional impact, etiologies, and risk factors. *J. Infect. Dis.* **148**, 986–997.
6 Kielmann, A.A. & McCord, C. (1978): Weight for age as an index of risk of death in children. *Lancet* **1**, 1247–1250.
7 Koster, F.T., Curlin, G.C., Aziz, K.M.A. & Haque, A. (1981): Synergistic impact of measles and diarrhea on nutrition and mortality in Bangladesh. *Bull. WHO* **59**, 901–908.
8 Martorell, R., Habicht, J-P., Yarbrough, C., Lechtig, A., Klein, R.E. & Western, K.A. (1975): Acute morbidity and physical growth in rural Guatemalan children. *Am. J. Dis. Child.* **129**, 1296–1301.
9 McLaren, D.S. & Read, W.W.C. (1972): Classification of nutritional status in early childhood. *Lancet* **2**, 146–148.
10 Stetler, H.C., Trowbridge, F.L. & Huong, A.Y. (1981): Anthropometric nutritional status and diarrhea prevalence in children in El Salvador. *Am. J. Trop. Med. Hyg.* **30**, 888–893.
11 Trowbridge, F.L., Newton, L.H. & Campbell, C.C. (1981): Diarrhea reporting in relation to nutritional status (letter). *Lancet* **1**, 1375.
12 Trowbridge, F.L. & Sommer, A. (1981): Nutritional anthropometry and mortality risk, (letter). *Am. J. Clin. Nutr.* **34**, 2591.
13 Trowbridge, F.L. & Staehling, N. (1980): Sensitivity and specificity of arm circumference indicators in identifying malnourished children. *Am. J. Clin. Nutr.* **33**, 687–696.
14 Trowbridge, F.L., Lopez de Romana, G., Marks, J.S., Boutton, T.W. & Klein, P.D. (1985): Body composition of growth stunted Peruvian children with increased weight-for-height. *XIII International Congress of Nutrition* (Brighton, UK), Abstract.
15 Waterlow, J.C. (1972): Classification and definition of protein-calorie malnutrition. *Br. Med. J.* **3**, 566–569.
16 Waterlow, J.C. (1974): Some aspects of childhood malnutrition as a public health problem. *Br. Med. J.* **4**, 88–90.
17 Waterlow, J.C., Buzina, R., Keller, W., Lane, J.M., Nichaman, M.Z. & Tanner, J.M. (1977): The presentation and use of height and weight data for comparing the nutritional status of groups of children under the age of 10 years. *Bull. WHO* **55**, 489–498.
18 World Health Organization (1978): A growth chart for international use in maternal and child health care. Geneva: WHO.

Mortality, morbidity and malnutrition in relation to birth-weight. A longitudinal study of 5914 Brazilian children

C.G. VICTORA, F.C. BARROS and J.P. VAUGHAN
Department of Social Medicine, Universidade Federal de Pelotas, C.P. 464, 96100 Pelotas, RS, Brazil; Department of Maternal and Child Health, Universidade Católica de Pelotas, Av. Dom Joaquim, 982, 96100 Pelotas, RS, Brazil; Evaluation and Planning Centre, London School of Hygiene and Tropical Medicine, Keppel Street, London WC1E 7HT, UK.

Birth-weight is a very important determinant of child survival, both in rich and in poor countries[5,8,10]. However, there are very few studies from developing countries in which a substantial number of children were followed up from birth to assess the long-term health effects of low-birth-weight and other perinatal factors. The present cohort study provides information

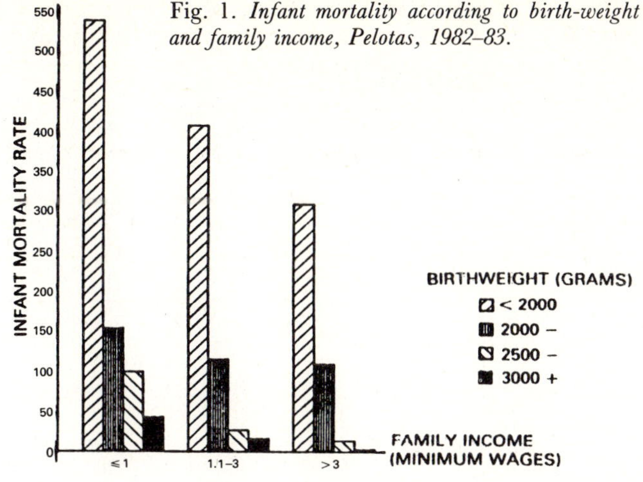

Fig. 1. *Infant mortality according to birth-weight and family income, Pelotas, 1982–83.*

on the influence of birth-weight on infant mortality, on hospital morbidity and on subsequent nutritional status.

Methods. All children born in hospital in Pelotas (Southern Brazil, population 210 000 in 1982 were studied. Of this original cohort of 5914 live-borns, representing over 99 per cent of all births in that year, 233 are known to have died, 4931 were examined in 1984, and the remaining 750 (12.7 per cent) could not be located[13]. Mothers were interviewed soon after delivery, and their babies were weighed. The first follow-up visit took place in January–March 1983, and children born in the first 4 months of 1982 were visited when aged 9–15 months (average 12 months). The second visit was carried out a year later and covered children born in the whole year of 1982, when they were aged 12–27 months (average 20 months). All 69 000 urban households in the city were visited and 87.3 per cent of the original cohort were located. In both visits, children were weighed and measured according to standardized methods[6], and information was collected on hospital admissions and on a number of other variables. The accuracy of the information on hospital admissions was validated by a review of 120 hospital records chosen randomly. Mortality data were obtained through the monitoring of deaths reported at hospitals, registries and health authorities. In addition, interviewers asked about recent child deaths when all urban households were visited in 1984.

Results. The incidence of low-birth-weight (below 2500 g) was 8.1 per cent among live-born singletons, with a mean birth-weight of 3202 g and a standard deviation of 577 g. The infant mortality rate was 42 per thousand.

The Table shows a very strong association between birth-weight and neonatal death rates. Post-neonatal mortality was also much higher among low-birth-weight babies, there being an 11-fold differential between those weighing less than 2000 g and those with 3500 g or more. A similar relative risk was observed for the 87 deaths due to infectious diseases occurring in the first 2 years of life. There were also important variations in diarrhoea and respiratory deaths, although the numbers are small.

Family income is an important determinant of the risk of infant death and it is also strongly associated with birth-weight[2]. It could therefore act as a confounding factor in the relationship between birth-weight and mortality. This possibility was investigated first by stratifying for income and examining mortality risks by birth-weight groups (Fig. 1), and also by estimating income-adjusted risks through logistic regression. Both approaches showed that the effect of birth-weight is largely independent from that of income.

By the age of 20 months, 46.1 per cent of all children born with less than 2000 g had been admitted to hospital, against 23 per cent for those with 3500 g or more. Similar ratios were observed for admissions for diarrhoea and respiratory infection (see Table).

The Table also shows the prevalences of malnutrition — defined as 2 s.d. or more below the North American NCHS standards[11] — at the first and second follow-ups, according to birth-weight. At around 12 months of age, there was virtually no malnutrition among children born with 3000 g or more, while about half of those born with less than 2000 g were malnourished according to weight and length for age.

At around 20 months, the effect of birth-weight on nutritional status was still very strong. It appeared to be most marked on low length for age, but this is due to the higher prevalance of stunting in that age group. Children born with a low birth-weight were 4.9 times more likely to

Table 1. *Mortality, hospital admission and malnutrition rates according to birth-weight, Pelotas, 1982–84.*

| | Birth-weight groups (g) | | | | | |
Outcome	<2000	2000–2500	2500–3000	3000–3500	3500+	All groups
Mortality rates (per 1000)						
Early neonatal	304	64	8	6	3	18
Late neonatal	43	22	5	1	1	4
Post-neonatal	87	41	27	10	8	18
Infant	435	127	41	16	12	41
Infectious diseases mortality						
Diarrhoea	12	10	7	2	5	5
Respiratory infections	37	38	11	5	2	9
All infections	81	54	23	9	8	17
Hospital admissions (%)						
All causes	46.1	38.7	31.6	25.4	23.3	27.3
Diarrhoea	16.9	16.7	10.1	8.1	7.2	8.9
Respiratory infections	13.5	16.4	12.2	9.6	8.4	10.3
Malnutrition (%)[a]						
At ≃12 months[b]						
Low weight for age	60.9	21.8	9.0	1.1	2.5	5.4
Low length for age	43.5	21.8	8.2	3.2	1.1	5.3
Low weight for length	13.0	7.7	1.5	0.2	0.9	1.3
At ≃20 months						
Low weight for age	23.9	19.9	8.9	3.9	1.4	5.5
Low length for age	45.7	31.4	18.6	10.6	4.3	12.2
Low weight for length	3.3	3.7	1.7	0.8	0.5	1.2
Number of births[c]	161	314	1201	1943	1541	5160

[a]Percentage of children 2 s.d. or more below the median of the NCHS reference; [b]Based on a 30% sample of births; [c]Excluding children lost to follow-up (750) and those with unknown birth-weight (4) but including known deaths (233).

have a low weight for age than those born with 2500 g or more. The relative risks for low length for age and low weight for length were 3.4 and 3.7, respectively.

To study the relationship between birth-weight and weight at around 12 months in different socio-economic groups, separate regressions were calculated for the five income categories. In Fig. 2, both birth-weight and weight for age at 9–15 months are expressed as z-scores. The slopes of the lines were quite similar, meaning that, within all five income groups, a given difference in birth-weight was associated with a similar absolute difference in weight at 12 months. In other words, there was no interaction between birth-weight and income. The correlation coefficients were also similar in the five income groups.

On the other hand, the intercepts of the lines in Fig. 2 increased with income. For example, a boy born with 3.3 kg (z-score at birth = 0) would weigh on average 10.7 kg (z-score = 0.5) at 12 months if he belonged to a family in the highest income bracket. If a boy with the same birth-weight was born to a family in the lowest income group, he would weigh on average 9.65 kg (z-score = −0.55) at one year of age. A similar picture was observed for length at age, but the findings for weight for length were not as clear cut, which might be expected since this indicator reflects only current nutritional status.

The positive effect of birthweight on the duration of breast-feeding is shown in Fig. 3. This effect was apparent throughout the range of birth-weights, although it was more marked for babies at the lower end of the scale.

Discussion. The above results emphasize the overwhelming importance of an adequate birth-weight in ensuring child health. In relation to most other studies from developing

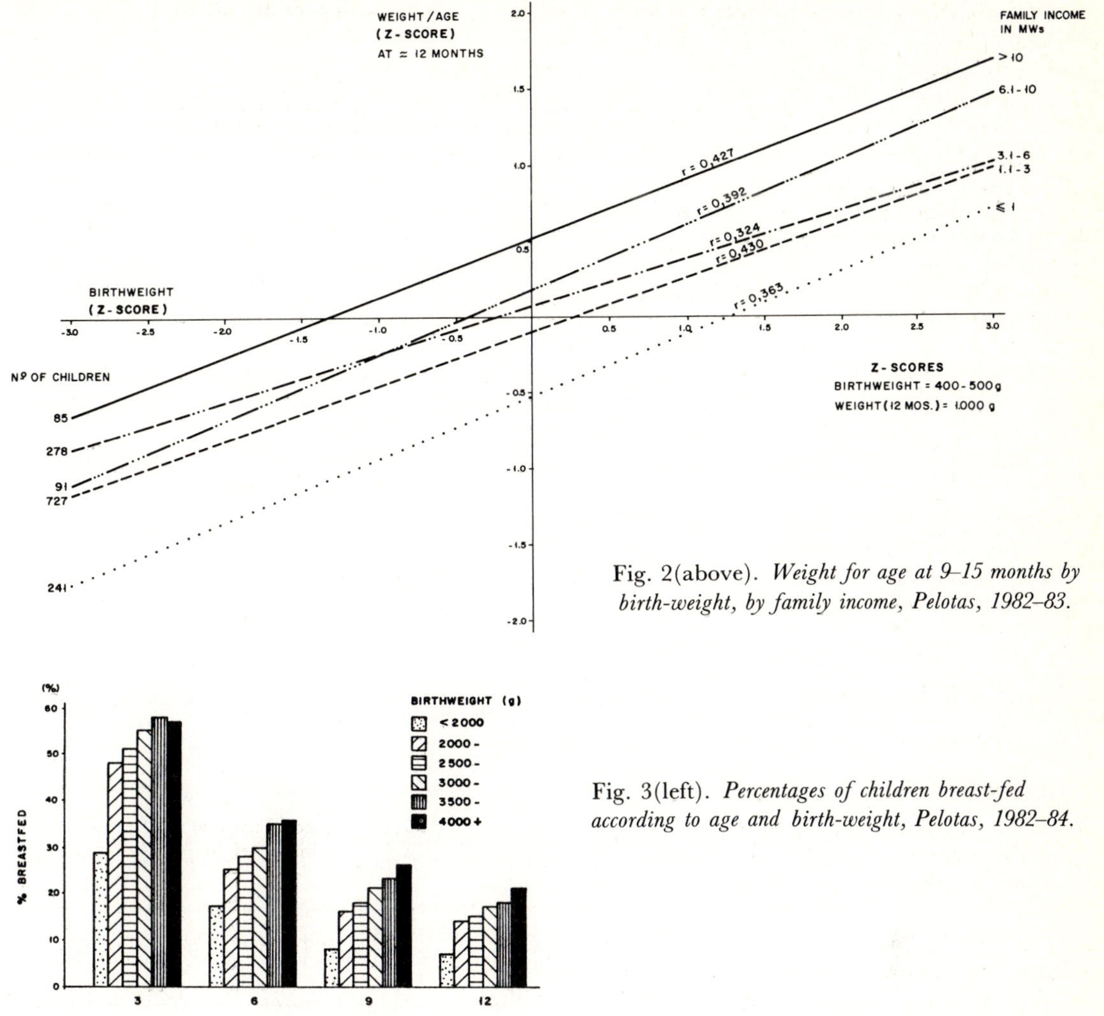

Fig. 2(above). *Weight for age at 9–15 months by birth-weight, by family income, Pelotas, 1982–83.*

Fig. 3(left). *Percentages of children breast-fed according to age and birth-weight, Pelotas, 1982–84.*

countries, our results have the advantages of (a) being population-based; (b) having been collected prospectively; (c) having covered a very large number of births; (d) having obtained the birth-weight of nearly all (99 per cent) of them, and (e) in following-up a high proportion of the children.

The findings on mortality confirm many of the results of earlier studies, such as the Inter American Investigation of Mortality in Childhood[12]. However, information on cause-specific infant mortality by groups of birth-weight does not seem to have been previously available for developing countries[1]. The above findings, although limited by the relatively small numbers of deaths, suggest that children born with a low-birth-weight are 5.2 times more likely to die of infectious diseases, 2.6 times for diarrhoea and 6.8 times for respiratory infections.

Information on hospital admissions by birth-weight is available from developed countries[9] but we were not able to find any such studies for less developed countries. There was a two-fold differential in hospital admissions between the lightest and the heaviest babies, confirming that LBW babies exert a heavy demand on scarce hospital services. This may be partly due to a higher disease incidence among LBW babies but also, given the same disease situation, paediatricians may be more likely to admit low-weight babies than heavier ones.

The association between birth-weight and subsequent nutritional status emphasises the lasting effects of low-birth-weight. Virtually no children weighing 3000 g or more at birth were found to be malnourished at around one year of age. At around 20 months of age, very few of those with a birth-weight of 3500 g or more were malnourished. The study of weight and length at 12 months relative to birth-weight, within the five socio-economic groups, shows the very strong and independent effects of both birth-weight and income. Within each income group, children who were lighter at birth were likely to remain lighter and shorter one year later. However, depending on its social class, a child of average birth-weight would be well above or well below the standard at age one.

A final finding was that the duration of breast-feeding was also strongly influenced by birth-weight. Although it is well-known that very small babies are less likely to be breast-fed, the present finding of an effect throughout the range of birth-weights is relatively new. We were able to find three other studies with similar findings[3,4,7], but the potential impact of this association was apparently not realised. Since children who are heavier at birth are both healthier and likely to be breast-fed for longer periods, birth-weight is a confounding variable which should be taken into account in all studies of the effects of breast-feeding on health.

A low-birth-weight child, therefore, is not only directly at increased risk, but is also less likely to receive the protective effects of breast-milk. Ensuring that as many children as possible are born with an adequate weight is essential in lowering infant mortality and in improving child health in developing countries.

Acknowledgements. Study financed by the Overseas Development Administration (United Kingdom) and by the International Development Research Centre (Canada).

1 Ashworth, A. & Feachem, R.G. (1985): Interventions for the control of diarrhoeal diseases among young children: prevention of low birthweight. *Bull. WHO* **63**, 165–184.

2 Barros, F.C., Victora, C.G., Granzoto, J.A., Vaughan, J.P. & Lemos, Jr. A.V. (1984): Saude perinatal in Pelotas, RS, Brasil: fatores soiais e biologicos. *Rev. Saude Publ. S. Paulo* **18**, 301–312.

3 Biering-Sorensen F., Hilden, J. & Biering-Sorensen, K. (1980): Breast-feeding in Copenhagen, 1938–1977. Data on more than 365,000 infants. *Danish Med. Bull.* **27**, 42–48.

4 Butz, W.P. & DaVanzo, J. (1981): *Determinants of breastfeeding and weaning patterns in Malaysia.* Santa Monica: Rand Corporation.

5 Chamberlain, R.N. & Simpson, R.N. (1979): *The prevalence of illness in childhood.* Tunbridge Wells: Pitman.

6 Jelliffe, D.B. (1966): *The assessment of the nutritional status of the community.* Geneva: World Health Organization (WHO Monograph Series no. 53).

7 Lopez Bravo, I., Cabiol, C., Arcuch, S., Rivera, E. & Vargas, S. (1984): Breast-feeding, weight gains, diarrhea and malnutrition in the first year of life. *Bull. Pan Am. Health Organ.* **18**, 151–163.

8 McCormick, M.C. (1985): The contribution of low birthweight to infant mortality and childhood morbidity. *New Engl. J. Med.* **312**, 82–90.

9 McCormick, M.C., Shapiro, S. & Starfield, B.H. (1980): Rehospitalization in the first year of life for high-risk survivors. *Pediatrics* **66**, 991–999.

10 Mata, L. (1978): *The children of Santa Maria Cauque. A prospective field study of health and growth.* Cambridge, Mass.: MIT Press.

11 National Center for Health Statistics (1976): *NCH growth charts.* Rockville, MD: National Center for Health Statistics (DHEW Publication no. (HRA)76–1120; Monthly Vital Statistics Report Vol. 25 no. 3).

12 Puffer, R.R. & Serrano, C.V. (1973): *Patterns of mortality in childhood.* Washington, DC: Pan American Health Organization (Scientific Publication No. 262).

13 Victora, C.G., Barros, F.C., Martines, J.C., Beria, J.U. & Vaughan, J.P. (1985): Estudo longitudinal das crianças nascidas em 1982 em Pelotas, RS: metodologia e resultados preliminares. *Rev. Saude Publ. S. Paulo* **19** 58–68.

Maternal nutritional risk assessment in Bangladesh

Sandra L. HUFFMAN and Katherine KRASOVEC
The Johns Hopkins University School of Hygiene and Public Health, Baltimore, Maryland, USA.

Maternal malnutrition plays a major role in the problem of low-birth-weight perinatal, neonatal and infant mortality in developing countries. In areas where the prevalence of maternal malnutrition is high, health services are usually limited and often are incapable of providing necessary care for the majority of pregnant women. The use of risk indicators that will select out those women with particularly high risk can enhance the effectiveness of a maternal and child health programme, by enabling the programme to focus efforts on those at greatest risk. The determination of risk indicators that are the easiest to use by community health workers with low literacy levels and that are easily transportable, and inexpensive will lead to a more widespread and effective usage, therefore enhancing the efficacy of the programme.

We will assess here the role of nutritional risk indicators in predicting women at risk to poor pregnancy outcomes in Bangladesh. We will assess the relationship of the following maternal risk factors and the risk of perinatal and neonatal deaths: maternal pre-pregnant weight, arm circumference, maternal height, weight gain during pregnancy and change in arm circumference.

Assessing the value of a risk indicator is best done by the use of sensitivity, specificity, and positive predictive value. The adaptation of the case-control method for use with data collected in demographic surveys, with characteristics of survey children (controls) compared to those of children who have died (cases) has recently been suggested[3]. If exposure is greater in the cases (for example, exposure defined as low maternal height), it suggests an increased risk associated with the exposure factor.

The sensitivity of an indicator used to predict the risk of low-birth-weight or infant mortality is defined as the per centage of cases (perinatal or neonatal deaths) who are identified by the risk indicator (such as low maternal height). The specificity is the per centage of those not at risk (survivors) who are identified as such by the indicator (normal height). The positive predictive value is the per centage of those identified as being at-risk mothers (eg, due to low heights) who were in fact at risk (with a perinatal or neonatal death). The Figure illustrates the characteristics of risk indicators and the calculations used to determine them.

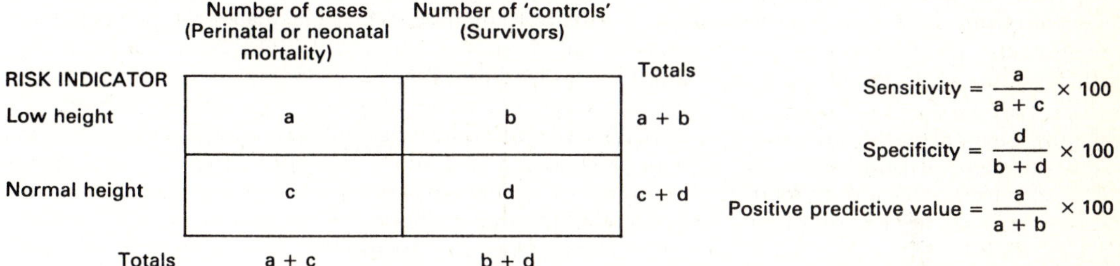

$$\text{Sensitivity} = \frac{a}{a + c} \times 100$$

$$\text{Specificity} = \frac{d}{b + d} \times 100$$

$$\text{Positive predictive value} = \frac{a}{a + b} \times 100$$

Figure. *Characteristics of risk indicators*

Methodology. Our data were collected in a longitudinal study of nearly 2500 women followed between 1975 and 1978 in Bangladesh. Anthropometric measures, information on fertility status (pregnancy, lactational amenorrhoea), outcome of pregnancy, and child survival were collected at monthly intervals in 14 villages in Matlab, a rural area 40 km south of Dhaka. Information on birth-weight was not available.

The sample used in this study consisted of a total of about 1000 pregnancies. Included were women with live births and still births for whom information on date of last menstrual period was available with an accuracy to within one week. Not included in these analyses were women who conceived during post-partum amenorrhoea ($n = 175$) and women for whom a date of last menstrual period was not known to within 1 week. The numbers included in the analyses differ because of missing values at different months of interview at different times during the pregnancy.

The Table summarizes the sensitivity and specificity analyses conducted for pregnant women followed through the first post-partum month. Still-birth and neonatal deaths have been combined to form the case group and all others are considered controls (survivors). As indicated, pre-pregnant weight and arm circumference give the highest positive predictive values at similar levels of sensitivity and specificity. However, none is particularly high. These

Table. *Maternal nutritional status and perinatal and neonatal mortality, Matlab, Bangladesh.*

Pre-pregnant weight	Cases		Controls		Total		
	n	%	*n*	%	*n*	%	
<43kg	83	(82)	348	(64)	431	(67)	Sensitivity = 82%
≥43 Kg	18	(18)	194	(36)	212	(33)	Specificity = 36%
	101		542		643		Positive predictive value = 19%
Height							
<152 cm	101	(83)	563	(79	664	(80)	Sensitivity = 83%
≥152 cm	20	(17)	149	(21)	169	(20)	Specificity = 21%
	121		712		833		Positive predictive value = 15%
Pre-pregnant arm circumference							
<23 cm	84	(81)	406	(69)	490	(71)	Sensitivity = 81%
≥23 cm	20	(19)	182	(31)	202	(29)	Specificity = 31%
	104		588		692		Positive predictive value = 17%
Weight gain in first 2 trimesters							
<4kg	37	(71)	321	(67)	358	(68)	Sensitivity = 71%
≥4kg	15	(29)	157	(33)	172	(32)	Specificity = 33%
	52		478		530		Positive predictive value = 10%
Arm circumference change							
<0.5 cm	47	(87)	407	(78)	454	(79)	Sensitivity = 87%
≥0.5 cm	7	(13)	114	(22)	121	(21)	Specificity = 22%
	54		521		575		Positive predictive value = 10%

indicators also perform the best when the combination of sensitivity and specificity are examined.

Conclusion. Numerous studies have illustrated the positive relationship of pre-pregnant weight and weight gain during pregnancy on pregnancy outcome[1,4,7–11]. None has reported their results in terms of sensitivity analyses as we have done.

In contrast to this study, researchers in Tanzania noted a strong relationship of maternal height with perinatal and neonatal deaths. The close relationship between arm circumference and outcome of pregnancy has also been reported in Chile[2] and Guatemala[12]. The use of arm-circumference change during pregnancy to predict early mortality has not been previously reported. Our results point to a possible role for this indicator in predicting women at risk, especially in populations where health outreach into the community is limited. The ease and lesser cost of obtaining arm-circumference measures in contrast to weight is relevant when resources are limited.

The efficiency of an indicator is tied to the intervention[5]. Indicators that are responsive to dietary supplementation with energy (such as weight gain) may be more suitable if feeding is the intervention to be employed, while interventions of referral for hospital delivery for at risk cases, height may be the appropriate indicator. In reality, however, often services may be unable to separate out the various classifications of risk. The decision on which cutoffs to use will be based on the country's resources and the severity of malnutrition and the relationship of maternal nutritional status to perinatal, neonatal and infant mortality. The consequences of missing cases, costs of treatment and screening need to be assessed in choosing the correct cutoff for a given situation[6].

A review of the literature on risk indicators to predict women at risk to poor pregnancy outcome illustrates that few investigators compare the effectiveness of different indicators within the populations studied, although often several have been included in the research. There is a need for sensitivity-specificity analyses, as conducted in this paper, to do this in order to compare the degree that individual indicators can predict women at risk. These results then can be combined with information on resource availability and costs of training and logistics associated with the use of the selected indicators.

1. Arteaga, A. (1983): Nutrition intervention programs in Chile for pregnant and nursing mothers: the issues. In

Nutrition intervention strategies in national development, ed B. Underwood. New York: Academic Press.
2 Atalah, E. (1983): Sensitivity and specificity of arm and calf circumferences in identifying undernourished pregnant women. Department of Nutrition, Faculty of Medicine, Santiago, Chile. (Unpublished paper).
3 Gray, R.H. (1985): Demography and the biomedical sciences: the integration of demographic and epidemiologic approaches to studies of health in developing countries. Paper prepared for IUSSP General Conference, Florence Italy, June 5–12.
4 Gueri, M., Jutsum, P. & Sorhaindo, B. (1982): Anthropometric assessment of nutritional status in pregnant women: a reference table of weight-for-height by week of pregnancy. *Am. J. Clin. Nutr.* **35** 609–616.
5 Habicht, J-P. and Yarbrough, C. (1981): Efficiency in selecting pregnant women for food supplementation during pregnancy. In *Maternal nutrition during pregnancy and lactation*, ed H. Aebi & R.G. Whitehead. Bern: Hans Huber.
6 Habicht, J.P., Yarbrough, C. & Martorell, R. (1978): Anthropometric field methods: criteria for selection. In *Human growth*, ed D.B. & E.F.P. Jelliffe. New York: Plenum Press.
7 Naeye R.L. (1981): Maternal blood pressure and fetal growth. *Am. J. Obstet. Gynecol.* **140**, 780–787.
8 Naeye, R.L. (1983): Effects of maternal nutrition on fetal and neonatal survival. *Birth* **10**, 109.
9 Rosso, P. (1985): A new chart to monitor weight gain during pregnancy. *Am. J. Clin. Nutr.* **41**, 644–652.
10 Shah, K.P. (1978): Surveillance card for married women for better obstetric performance. *J. Obstet. Gynecol. India* **28**, 1005–1020.
11 Shah K.P. & Shah P.M. (1981): 'The mother's card' — a simplified aid for primary health workers. Appropriate technology for health. *WHO Chronicle* **35**(2), 51–53.
12 Vaquera, M.V., Townsend, J.W., Arroyo, J.J. & Lechtig, A. (1983): The relationship between arm circumference at birth and early mortality. *J. Trop. Ped.* **29**, 167–174.

Nutritional status as a risk factor for mortality in children in the highlands of Papua New Guinea

P.F. HEYWOOD
Papua New Guinea Institute of Medical Research, P.O. Box 378, Madang, Papua New Guinea.

Numerous studies of the growth of young children in the highlands of Papua New Guinea (PNG), have revealed marked retardation in growth as compared to international standards[2,5–8,10]. However, the implications of this apparent growth retardation are unclear for several reasons. First, it is argued by some that international growth standards may not be appropriate for this population and that their implicit use as growth goals may result in incorrect estimates of the extent of malnutrition. In the same vein, some have advanced the general argument that reduced body size may represent an adaptation to environmental stress rather than a pathological response[9], the implication being that low growth rates may not represent malnutrition at all.

A second problem in the interpretation of many of the earlier growth studies in PNG is their reliance on weight measurements. Height was not always measured and, as a result, weight was seldom related to height. As Waterlow[11], and many others, have pointed out a child can be low weight-for-age (W/A) because he or she is low length-for-age (L/A) or low weight-for-length (W/L), or both and for this reason reservations have been voiced about the use of W/A as the sole index of nutritional status in community studies.

A third reason for uncertainty in interpretation of growth data derives from failure to separate use of information about growth as a general index of health status, which is essentially retrospective in nature, from its use as an index of nutritional status, for which the implications are prospective. In the latter case nutritional status is seen as possibly having an effect on the future risk of morbidity and mortality.

It is in this latter sense that nutrition is viewed as a risk factor for mortality. The child is exposed to a risk factor (varying degrees of growth retardation) which may affect the specific outcome under consideration (in this case, mortality). However, it is also known that the pattern of growth retardation is related to age and that mortality often varies with age. In that age is related to both the risk factor and the outcome of interest, age is likely to be a confounding factor[1].

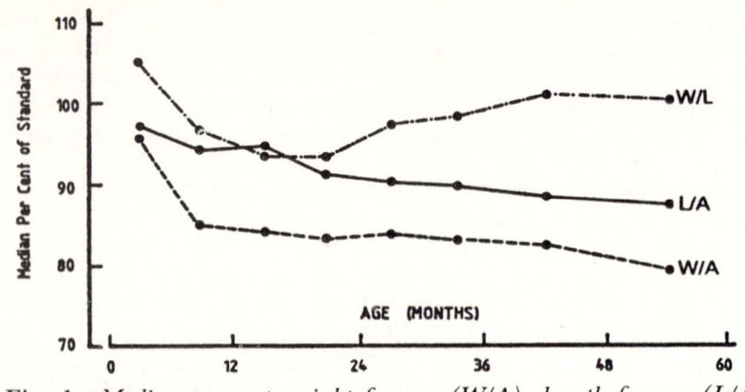

Fig. 1. *Median per cent weight-for-age (W/A), length-for-age (L/A) and weight-for-length (W/L) by age.*

Growth and mortality in highland children. *(a) Pattern of growth.* The typical growth pattern of highland children in PNG is illustrated by the results of a cross-sectional study carried out in the Tari basin of Southern Highlands Province in 1978–79, a summary of which is shown in Fig. 1 (Heywood & Smith, unpublished). W/A, L/A and W/L are all calculated using the Harvard standard. The mean W/A falls rapidly during the first year and then much more gradually to approximately 80 per cent in the 5th year of life. Mean L/A falls gradually to under 90 per cent during the 5th year. Mean W/L falls from approximately 105 per cent of the standard in the first 6 months to a low of approximately 95 per cent at 18 months, then rises gradually to approximately 100 per cent during the 4th year of life.

(b) Nutritional status and mortality. Within the Nutrition Research Programme of the PNG Institute of Medical Research we have been attempting to determine the significance of this growth pattern for health. Our first approach has been to carry out a prospective study of the relationship between nutritional status, as assessed by length and weight, and mortality. This has been done through the Tari Research Unit, established in the Tari basin of the Southern Highlands Province by Dr Ian Riley in the early 1970s. In recent years this unit has been operated by the Institute of Medical Research in conjunction with the Southern Highlands Province under the supervision of Dr Deborah Lehmann. The majority of the population in this area live at an altitude of approximately 1500 metres above sea level. Demographic surveillance of a population of approximately 25 000 people has now been carried out for more than a decade. Ages, particularly in those people born in the last 10 years, are known to at least the month and, in most cases, the day, and mortality is closely monitored.

In this paper, the final results for the relationship between nutritional status and mortality in children 6–29 months of age at the beginning of the study are summarized. Preliminary results have been presented previously[4].

Weight and length were measured in a total of 1232 children who were between 6 and 30 months of age at the beginning of the study and for whom definite information was available as to whether they were dead or alive 2 years later. Each child was assigned to three cohorts — one according to W/A, one using L/A and another using W/L. A total of 71 children died within 2 years of initial measurement.

Because age, which may be related to overall mortality and to the pattern of growth, is a possible confounding factor the data relating each index of nutritional status to mortality were initially analysed by log-linear analysis[1] using four 6-month age categories. For each index of nutritional status the data were adequately described by a model which included the three main effects (survival, nutritional status and age) together with the two-way interactions of (survival × nutritional status index) and (nutritional status index × age). The three-way interaction (survival × nutritional status × age) was not significant for any of the three indices of nutritional status (W/A, L/A, and W/L). (In the case of W/L the three-way interaction was found to be not significant only after declaring empty two cells which yielded results clearly contrary to the overall trend of the data.) The two-way interaction of (survival × age) was also found to be not significant. Thus, further analysis of survival by nutritional status was carried

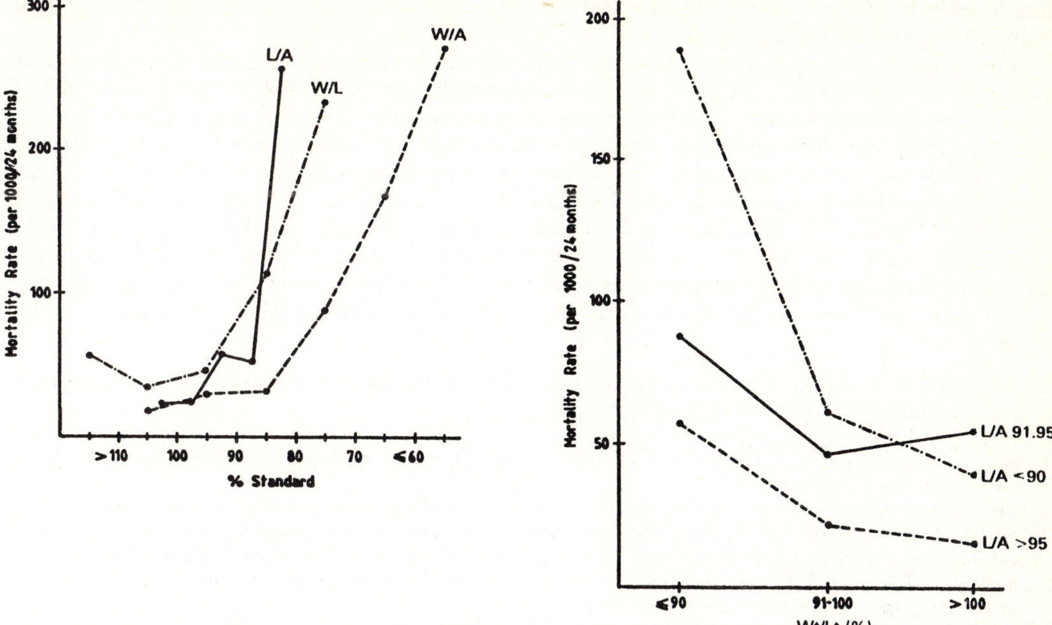

Fig. 2. *Prospective mortality rate by nutritional status.*

Fig. 3. *Prospective mortality rate by length-for-age (L/A) and weight-for-length (W/L).*

out with the data summed across age categories. The results for W/A, L/A and W/L are presented in Fig. 2. In each case the test for trend in proportions is highly significant (P < 0.0005).

For W/A there is a gradual increase in mortality rate from 18/1000 per 24 months to 32/1000 per 24 months as the level falls from above 100 to 81–90. Below 80 per cent W/A the mortality rises steeply to reach 273/1000 per 24 months for children less than 60 per cent.

For L/A mortality rises from 24/1000 per 24 months for those above 95 per cent to approximately 55 for those whose L/A is between 86 and 95. There is then a sharp rise in mortality to 258/1000 per 24 months for those less than 85 per cent L/A.

For W/L there is a smooth rise in mortality rate as the level falls below 90 per cent. The rate rises to 235/1000 per 24 months for children below 80 per cent W/L.

The joint effect of L/A and W/L is shown in Fig. 3. As there was no four-way interaction of (L/A × W/L × survival × age) the data have been aggregated across age categories. As with the previous analysis there were independent effects of W/L and L/A on survival. The interaction between W/L, L/A and survival was not significant. At a given L/A survival decreases with a decrease in W/L. This effect is most marked in children whose L/A is less than 90 per cent. Similarly, at a given W/L survival decreases with decrease in L/A. The effect is most marked with children whose W/L is less than 90 per cent.

Discussion. For each of the three indices of nutritional status used in this study (W/A, L/A, W/L) there is a clear and significant increase in mortality rate as the value of the index decreases. In the case of W/A and W/L there is a graded rise in mortality with departure from the standards. The relationship between L/A and mortality showed a more threshold-like relationship with a sharp increase in mortality for those children below 85 per cent of the standard.

In the only other similar study in the literature a threshold-like relationship was shown for each of the indices of nutritional status[3]. This appears to be true for only L/A in the present study. The level of L/A at which mortality rate rises is also very similar in the two studies.

In addition to the difference in shape of the relationship between W/A and W/L and mortality between the two studies, the mortality rate rises at a higher level of those two indices in PNG than in Bangladesh. A mortality rate of 100 is reached at a W/A of 70 per cent in PNG and 55 per cent in

Bangladesh. For W/L a mortality rate of 100 is reached at approximately 85 per cent in PNG and at 70 per cent in Bangladesh.

Thus all three indices of nutritional status are potent indicators of prospective risk of death in both studies. However, the level at which risk increases is much higher for W/A and W/L in PNG than in Bangladesh. The reasons for this are unclear. The leading causes of death in the two studies are different, diarrhoea in Bangladesh and pneumonia in the highlands of PNG. There are many important environmental and human differences between the two areas. Nevertheless it seems clear that highland children in PNG are compromised at higher levels of W/A and W/L than those in Bangladesh, raising the question of whether the level of an index at which the risk of mortality rises is the same across populations. This issue is of particular relevance to PNG where lowland children at any given age are in general taller and thinner than those in the highlands[5]. Studies addressing this question are currently being carried out.

Acknowledgments. Dr David Smith participated in the initial data collection for this study which was funded, in part, by the Southern Highlands Rural Development Project.

1 Anderson, S., Auquier, A., Hauck, W., Oakes, D., Vandaele, W. & Weisberg, H. (1980): *Statistical methods for comparative studies.* New York: John Wiley.
2 Bailey, K.V. (1964): Growth of Chimbu infants in the New Guinea highlands. *J. Trop. Pediat.* **10**, 3–16.
3 Chen, L.C., Chowdhury, A.K. & Huffman, S.L. (1980): Anthropometric assessment of energy-protein malnutrition and subsequent risk of mortality among preschool aged children. *Am. J. Clin. Nutr.* **33**, 1836–1845.
4 Heywood, P.F. (1982): The functional significance of malnutrition — growth and prospective risks of death in the highlands of Papua New Guinea. *J. Fd Nutr.* **39**, 13–19.
5 Heywood, P.F. (1983): Growth and nutrition in Papua New Guinea. *J. Hum. Evol.* **12**, 133–143.
6 McKay, S.R. (1960): Growth and nutrition of infants in the Western Highlands of New Guinea. *Med. J. Aust.* **1**, 452–459.
7 Malcolm, L.A. (1966): *Growth and development in New Guinea — a study of the Bundi people of the Madang District.* Institute of Human Biology Monograph Series No. 1 Madang, Papua New Guinea.
8 Ooman, H.A.P.C. & Malcolm, S.H. (1965): *Nutrition and the Papuan child.* South Pacific Commission Tech. Paper No. 118.
9 Segraves, A.B. (1977): The Malthusian proposition and nutritional stress: differing implications for man and for society. In *Malnutrition, behavior and social organisation,* ed L.S. Greene, pp. 173–218. New York: Academic Press.
10 Venkatachalam, P.S. (1962): *A study of the diet, nutrition and health of the people of the Chimbu area (New Guinea).* Papua New Guinea Department of Public Health Monograph 4.
11 Waterlow, J.C. (1976): Classification and definition of protein-energy malnutrition. In *Nutrition in preventive medicine,* eds G.H. Beaton & J.M. Bengoa, pp. 530–555. Geneva: WHO.

Role of health services in improving nutrition and health

L. MATA
Instituto de Investigaciones en Salud (INISA), University of Costa Rica, Ciudad Universitaria Rodrigo Facio, Costa Rica.

A quick glance at the present world disribution of malnutrition and famine reveals its concentration in the tropics and subtropics. Undoubtedly, negative environmental factors in such regions make it more difficult to attain an adequate level of nutrition and development than in temperate regions. Deficiencies in food availability and in sanitation are considered the primary determinants of malnutrition[16]. In recent times, however, infection is receiving increasing emphasis in many less developed countries since a close examination of food balance sheets, family dietary histories, and individual records of food intake by small malnourished children do not consistently reveal a limitation in food availability or consumption[8,9]. On the other hand, it is clear that infection itself can induce acute and chronic malnutrition and growth retardation and can diminish survival[9,10].

Infection alters host nutrition in many ways[1,8,16]. Reduction of food intake and nutrient wastage are important effects in rural children. Furthermore, lack of knowledge and resources to care for children with diarrhoea or respiratory infection results in failure of mothers to provide an adequate diet during convalescence. On the other hand, malnutrition, whether induced by recurrent infections or by food restriction as in famine or both, may alter the immune system[18] but infection itself suppresses some manifestations of the immune response[4].

If the previous statements are correct, the effective control and prevention of infectious diseases, at least the bulk of them, should result in a demonstrable improvement in nutrition and health, particularly in children. A recent analysis of longitudinal data from two field studies, 'Cauqué and Puriscal', seemed to indicate that the remarkable differences between the two populations are accountable primarily by dramatic differences in the burden of infection, but not by differences in food consumption levels[10,11].

Interventions affecting nutrition and survival. During the 1960s the prevailing idea was that an improved diet was *sine qua non* to increase nutrition and survival of children. This paradigm was challenged by the demonstration, through long term prospective observation, that infection itself is a main inducer of malnutrition, important precipitating factor of the severe forms, and a main determinant of death[8,9]. It follows, therefore, that infection has to be controlled in order to improve nutrition[1]. Today, it is widely recognized that education of mothers, prenatal care and child spacing, along with improved water, oral rehydration, breast-feeding, immunization, and control of devastating diseases like malaria and tuberculosis are fundamental steps to attain an adequate level of health[2,3,7,9,13,19,20]. The former emphasis on food has diminished as communities like Costa Rica[11,12], Chile[14] and Kerala[15] improved their health indicators without a demonstrable marked change in food consumption levels. On the other hand, village diets previously considered insufficient were not really so, while most health workers recognized that adequate performance can be attained with energy levels of about 80 per cent of the international recommendation[8,9].

The case of Kerala deserves special mention because its population has the lowest *per caput* food intake while exhibiting the lowest infant mortality and best health status of the whole of India[6,15]. Similarly, societies in which there is an adequate food supply in most homes still exhibit high infant mortality due to infections derived from an inadequate environment and traditional life-styles[7,18]. If the infection paradigm is correct, one would expect to see whole nations improve their health condition by controlling infection without modifying food consumption in a significant way. On the other hand, an improved diet would not lead to better nutrition and survival if infection remains unchecked, as was the case of the population of Cauqué.

National control and prevention of infection. In Costa Rica, public health emphasis has been, over the past four decades, on control and prevention of infectious diseases. The approach included strengthening of education, building roads, improving the infrastructure of villages and towns and extending primary health care to cover more than 70 per cent of the rural population (Table 1). The first accomplishment was the control of malaria in the 1950s and 1960s which made the Caribbean and Pacific coastal areas suitable for development. In the 1960s, improved education had resulted in a drastic reduction in fertility (Table 2). The rural health programme which began in 1971 emphasized immunizations, prenatal care, health education, family planning, control of intestinal parasites and vector-transmitted diseases and community organization[8,12]. Significant changes in health indicators were readily noted (Table 2). Diarrhoeal diseases and acute respiratory diseases were sharply reduced as a result of improved living conditions[11,12]. Poliomyelitis and diphtheria were last recorded in 1973. Measles, tetanus and pertussis are practically controlled. Otitis media, scarlet fever and rheumatic fever have decreased drastically.

Interestingly, no significant changes were detected in mean consumption levels of protein and energy while a marked improvement in the nutritional status of infants and preschool children was recorded at the national level; the proportion of overweight and obese children has increased significantly. Severe malnutrition has declined dramatically and the few cases still observed are associated with chronic disease, child battering, massive parasitosis, cerebral palsy and congenital defects[5].

Table 1. *Development of the health sector in Costa Rica, 1940–1980.*

	1940	1950	1960	1970	1980
Per caput health expenditure, $*	15	8	14	37	65
Expenditure as % gross domestic product	..	2.2	3.0	5.6	7.4
Hospital beds, per 1000	5.6	5.1	4.6	4.1	3.3
Hospital discharges, per 1000	..	9.5	10.1	11.1	11.7
Medically certified deaths, %	55	60	65	71	84
Physicians, per 10 000	2.7	3.1	2.8	5.6	7.8
Population covered by illness & pregnancy insurance, %	0	8	15	39	78
Population with piped water, %	..	53	65	75	84
Population with sewage disposal, %	..	48	69	86	93
Population covered by primary health care, %	..	..	..	10	60

*Data deflated with the internal price index (US $ 1 = 5.09 Costa Rican colones, 1970).

Table 2. *Changes in host and environment in Costa Rica, 1966–1980.*

	1966	1978–1980	% change
Education			
% literate	84.4[d]	90.1	+7
% in school, 18–23yr olds	4.0[d]	21.0	+425
Sanitation			
% water connection, rural	34.0	62.0	+82
% water connection, urban	90.0	98.0	+9
% with *Ascaris*[a]	21.7	3.5	−84
% with *Trichuris*[a]	56.7	4.6	−92
% with hookworm[a]	10.2	2.9	−72
Nutrition			
Energy,[b] kcal	1894.0	2020.0	+7
Protein,[b] g	53.6	54.0	+1
Iron,[b] rural, mg	15.4	14.4	−6.5
Iron,[b] urban, mg	16.3	12.7	−22.1
Retinol,[b] rural, µg	206.0	326.0	+58.3
Retinol,[b] urban, µg	586.0	672.0	+14.7
% low-birth-weight	12.5	7.0	−44
% stunted[c]	16.9	7.6	−55
% wasted[c]	14.2	7.8	−45
% II degree malnutrition[c]	12.0	3.9	−68
% III degree malnutrition[c]	1.5	0.2	−87
% overweight[c]	3.8	9.9	+161
Health services			
% rural population covered	10.0[d]	60.0	+500
% deliveries in clinics	50.0[d]	90.7	+81
Birth rate per 1000	48.3[d]	31.2	−35
Global fertility, children	7.3[d]	3.7	−49
Mortality			
Diarrhoea per 100 000	104.4	11.8	−89
Acute respiratory infections per 100 000	144.7	76.1	−47
Infant per 1000 live-births	69.8	17.7	−75
1–4 yr olds per 1000	5.5	0.7	−87
Maternal per 1000	1.4[d]	0.3	−79

[a]In 1966, 2–4yr olds; in 1982, all ages; [b]Daily consumption, average per person; [c]Preschool children, Gomez classification; [d]Data for 1960.

The only explanation for an improved nutrition is reduced nutrition wastage as a consequence of fewer and milder (smaller doses) infections in the Costa Rican community. The dramatic increase in vitamin A consumption during the 70s resulted from fortification of sugar and might have favoured a lower infectious morbidity, which in turn might have favoured nutrition. Vitamin A deficiency has been found related to increased infectious morbidity[17]. A better nutrition *in utero*, an improved infant nutrition promoted by breast-feeding, and a lesser risk of infection coupled with better health services to prevent and treat serious diseases, seem to explain the dramatic improvement in survival observed in Costa Rica[11]. Infant mortality in 1983 was 18.2 per 1000 live-born.

Infection has negative effects on the pregnant woman, fetus, infant, and young child. The outcomes are malnutrition, stunting, and increased risk of death, evident at any stage of fetal and child development. The nutritional damage and risk of death associated with infection is enhanced by inappropriate child care, lack of prompt and proper treatment and inadequate feeding during convalescence. The risk of death is greater for preterm and small-for-gestational-age infants, particularly if they are wasted and/or stunted; well-nourished children also are at risk of death in very hostile environments. Stunted women in turn may give birth to preterm or retarded neonates, thus perpetuating the problem. Then, interventions should focus on mother's education and child-spacing, improved environmental sanitation and personal hygiene and better child-rearing and child care practices.

Populations suffering from acute food shortage constitute an exception and in such cases food distribution should be given the first priority. A practical way of knowing whether control of infection should be the target of public health action in a given ecosystem, is to assess the prevalence of undernutrition and mortality across age groups. An excess frequency of malnutrition and deaths in all ages and social classes indicates that food is the main limiting factor (best illustrated in famine). The constraint in most developing countries, however, is not an inadequate food intake, since most children frequently consume more than 90 per cent of recommended energy. It is expected that improvement of water supplies, environmental sanitation, expanded primary health services, and health education (emphasizing women's education), will influence nutrition worldwide, without necessarily demanding a drastic increase in food consumption.

 1 Beisel, W.R. (1977): Magnitude of the host nutritional responses to infection. *Am. J. Clin. Nutr.* **30**, 1236–1247.
 2 Faechem, R.G. (1983): Interventions for the control of diarrhoeal diseases among young children. Supplementary feeding programmes. *Bull. Wld Hlth Org.* **61**, 967–979.
 3 Henry, F.J. (1981): Environmental sanitation, infection and nutritional status of infants in rural St. Lucia, West Indies. *Trans Roy. Soc. Trop. Med. hyg.* **75**, 507–513.
 4 Isliker, H. & Schürch, B. (1980): *The impact of malnutrition on immune defense in parasitic infestation.* Bern: Hans Huber.
 5 Jiménez, P. *et al.* (1985): Desnutrición severa en Costa Rica: una reinterpreación de su causalidad. *Acta Med. Cost.*, in press.
 6 Krishnan, T.N. (1984): Infant mortality in Kerala State, India. A preliminary analysis. *Assignment Children* **65/68**, 293–308.
 7 Longhurst, R.W. (1979): Malnutrition and the community — the social origins of deprivation. *Proc. Nutr. Soc.* **38**, 11–16.
 8 Mata, L.J. (1978): *The Children of Santa María Cauqué. A prospective field study of health and growth.* Cambridge, Mass: MIT Press.
 9 Mata, L. (1978): The nature of the nutrition problem. In *Nutrition planning. The state of the art,* ed L. Joy, pp. 91–99. Surrey, England: IPC Science and Technology Press.
10 Mata, L. (1982): Malnutrition and concurrent infections. Comparison of two populations with different infection rates. In *Viral diseases in South-East Asia and the Western Pacific,* ed J. S. Mackenzie, pp. 56–76. Sydney: Academic Press.
11 Mata, L. (1983): Evolution of diarrhoeal diseases and malnutrition in Costa Rica. The role of interventions. *Assignment Children* **61/62**, 195–224.
12 Mohs, E. (1982): Infectious diseases and health in Costa Rica: the development of a new paradigm. *Ped. Infect. Dis.* **1**, 212–216.
13 McDermott, W., Deuschle, K.W. & Barnett, C.R. (1972): Health care experiment at Many Farms. *Science* **175**, 23–31.
14 Medina, E. & Kaempffer, A.M. (1983): An analysis of health progress in Chile. *PAHO Bull.* **17**, 221–232.
15 Panikar, G.K. & Soman, C.R. (1982): *Inter-sectoral action for health: Kerala study.* Trivandrum: Centre for Development Studies.
16 Scrimshaw, N.S., Taylor, C.E. & Gordon, J.E. (1968): *Interactions of nutriton and infection.* Geneva: World Health Organization, Monograph Ser. 57.
17 Sommer, A., Katz, J. & Jarwotjo, I. (1984): Increased risk of respiratory disease and diarrhea in children with preexisting mild vitamin A deficiency. *Am. J. Clin. Nutr.* **40**, 1090–1095.
18 Suskind, R.M. (1977): *Malnutrition and the immune response.* Kroc Found. Ser., Vol 7. New York: Raven Press.
19 Walsh, J.A. & Warren, K.S. (1979): Selective primary health care. An interim strategy for disease control in developing countries. *New Engl. J. Med.* **301**, 967–974.
20 Weller, T.H. (1983): Too few and too little: barricade to the pursuit of health. *Rev. Inf. Dis.* **5**, 994–1002.

NUTRITIONAL IMPLICATIONS OF DIARRHOEA IN YOUNG CHILDREN

Nutrient intake during diarrhoea in young children

A.M. TOMKINS
*Department of Human Nutrition, London School of Hygiene and Tropical Medicine, Keppel Street, London,
WC1E 7HT, UK.*

It is well-recognised that nutrient intake is reduced during diarrhoeal syndromes which are severe enough to require hospitalisation but it is not clear whether milder episodes which affect young children in developing communities so frequently[12] also result in decreased food intake. There are still methodological problems in assessing the relationship between diarrhoea and nutrient intake.

Methodology. *(1) Breast-milk intake.* A high proportion of nutrients comes from breast-milk, especially in the younger child. Measurments of milk intake, particularly in relation to the requirements for growth, are beset with difficulties. Unfortunately the recent innovative approach, using deuterium to measure breast-milk consumption, is only suitable for steady-state conditions so some form of test weighing is still necessary to detect the rapid changes which could occur during diarrhoea. Twenty-four hour consumption has been estimated from a 12-h daytime measurement with a correction factor (24 h intake = 12 h intake/0.52)[4]. The study showed a seasonal change in breast milk consumption among Bangladeshi village children[5]. When seasonality was allowed for in the analysis there was evidently no significant affect of diarrhoea on breast-milk consumption. Others also demonstrated that breast-milk consumption did not decrease in children with diarrhoea which was severe enough to require hospitalization[7].

(2) Food intake. Accurate measurements of food intake in children are also difficult. Studies using direct weighing of portions consumed by children demonstrate the importance in considering differentials in food distribution within the family[1]. Such methods have shown a decrease in nutrient intake in protracted diarrhoea among children in an urban community in the Gambia[13]. Brown[5] showed that febrile illness, but not diarrhoea, was associated with decreases in food intake in his community study whereas Hoyle *et al*[7] showed marked reduction in food intake in children from the same area but who had more severe disease. Alternative methods, regularly performed 24-h or 7-d recall, were used in Guatemalan villages and showed significant reduction in food intake when the data were analysed for association with diarrhoea[9,10].

(3) Clinical features. There are considerable variations in severity, type of illness and enteropathogen responsible for diarrhoea and the differences in the impact of acute watery diarrhoea, dysentery and protracted diarrhoea and nutritional impact in the community require better methods of evaluation of clinical features in community-based studies.

(4) Socio-cultural aspects. Nutrient intake during diarrhoea is not only dependent on availability of food and the child's appetite but on attitudes of parents/guardians/medical advisers on the types of preferred foods and the time to offer these. Different feeding practices may well explain the differences in the severity of malnutrition and mortality accompanying diarrhoea which occur in different continents and communities. Practices involving excessive dilution of feeds, witholding breast-milk, avoidance of certain nutritionally adequate foods are all likely to be detrimental to child growth.

Nutrient intakes in different diarrhoeal syndromes. Low energy intakes have been found (of about 70 kcal (290 kJ)/kg body weight per d) in children with severe diarrhoea due to Rotavirus, *Vibrio cholerae*, enterotoxin producing *E. coli* and *Shigella*[11]. This was despite being offered a variety of tempting alternative food dishes. Consumption gradually increased over the days after admission till intakes reached about 100 kcal (420 kJ)/kg B.W. per d by day 4. Intakes were even higher (130 kcal (545 kJ)/kg B.W. per d) during the remainder of that week and repeat measurements after clinical improvement showed intakes of around 100 kcal (420 kJ)/kg B.W. per day. Intakes were lowest among children with Rotavirus. This may reflect a greater anorectic effect of this infection but this group was significantly younger. A previous study[7] of a group of children with a variety of enteropathogens showed that mothers provided with a variety of cooked foods and nutrition education could not improve on the voluntary intake of children who were less intensively managed. A study of slightly older children with protracted diarrhoea in the Gambia showed that food intake at home was about 70 kcal (290 kJ)/kg B.W. per d despite the presence of adequate food and mothers with adequate time to encourage their children to eat. After successful treatment of the diarrhoea intakes increased to over 120 kcal (500 kJ)/kg B.W. per d[13].

Most studies therefore show a decrease in food intake but breast-milk intakes are maintained during severe diarrhoea whereas milder episodes, though frequent and potentially important cumulatively, have minimal effect on food intake.

Mechanisms of reduced nutrient intake. Anorexia has been recognised for many years in adults with malabsorption syndromes such as coeliac disease and tropical sprue where the degree of weight loss relates more closely to impaired food intake than malabsorption of nutrients.

Abdominal pain, vomiting and distension will all decrease appetite as will fever[3] and the metabolic problems associated with infection[14]. It may be that biochemical and neuro-endocrine mechanisms are important in the control of appetite. The subject is complex and reviewed by James[8] but among the hormones which are released from the gastro-intestinal tract during gut infection it is possible that cholecystokinin, pancreatic glucagon and enteroglucagon are important by their effect on hypothalamic appetite centres. The profiles of these hormones are markedly affected by the type of feeding[2] and are deranged in infective diarrhoea.

Zinc deficiency, a known experimental cause of anorexia, occurs in some children with protracted diarrhoea, especially those who are malnourished. The mechanisms involved to produce anorexia may include a direct effect on the buccal epithelium affecting peripheral taste receptors, increased blood ammonia levels and toxic levels of plasma amino acids because of the marked disturbances in nitrogen metabolism that occur during Zn deficiency. Folic acid therapy in tropical sprue is associated with a significant increase in food intake, long before the malabsorption state has improved. Oral rehydration regimes particularly those containing bicarbonate may improve appetite via the reversal of metabolic acidosis as well as by improving the ability to chew and swallow.

Despite the best intentions to maintain nutrient intake during diarrhoea, there are problems associated with certain foods whereby intestinal losses are increased thereby discouraging further eating. These include osmotic diarrhoea due to carbohydrate malabsorption (both disaccharide and less commonly monosaccharide), gastro-colic reflex, and dietary allergy to cow's milk protein, gluten and possibly other antigens. These feeding-associated diarrhoeas have resulted in a number of 'bowel-rest' strategies by parents and physicians alike which may include the witholding of breast-milk and food and delayed re-introduction of the latter. There is no evidence that withdrawal of breast-feeding is ever beneficial. On the contrary a recent study in Burma shows that breast-feeding reduces the number of stools during diarrhoea, possibly by the beneficial effects of milk which is hydrolysed to substrates which promote sodium and water transport across the enterocytes.

The stage at which the re-introduction of food, or formula feeds if bottle-fed, and the concentrations at which they should be given is still debated. A slow 'regrading' with gradually increasing quantities has the benefits of limiting the problems of increased intestinal losses or vomiting but has an obvious nutritional cost. This may be unimportant in a well-nourished child but could contribute to the problems of children who are already malnourished. Studies on more rapid 'regrading' are needed as there are few data on how this affects dietary intake, nutrient balance and growth. The use of low lactose feeds or formulae made from proteins other than cow's milk may be highly beneficial in certain children. It has to be emphasised that even in clinical situations with investigations and a variety of diets available, it is difficult to establish a single feeding regime that will eliminate refeeding problems in all children.

The social and economic constraints on child-care during infection cannot be overemphasised and are geographically and culturally varied. A greater understanding of these is essential if nutrition education approaches are to be more effective within diarrhoeal disease control projects in primary health care.

A policy implication from this review is that the nutritional status of young children in poor communities is unlikely to improve by increasing food availability alone. The wretched child who is undernourished is often the same child who lives in a deprived environment where diarrhoeal disease is more a way of life than an illness.

An interactive analysis. We may propose a rather over-simplified schematic model (Figure) in which the interactions of various factors affecting nutrient intake during diarrhoea in children are displayed. The value of an integrated approach towards development has been stated repeatedly[6] but unfortunately this is rarely utilized. Nevertheless, within these constraints, it is possible to implement programmes which optimise the intake of whatever appropriate nutrients are available. Breast-milk is probably the most important.

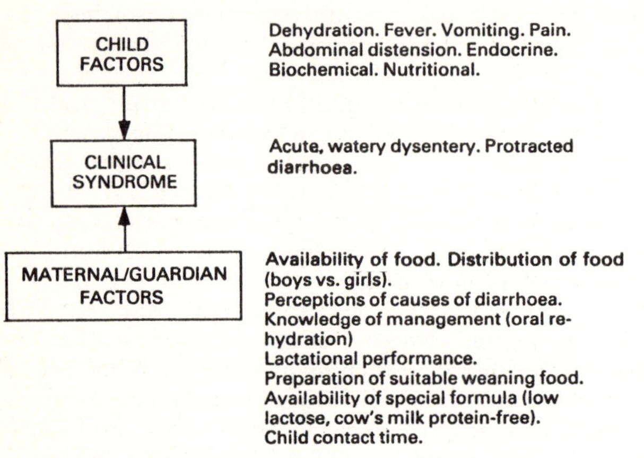

Figure. *Factors affecting nutrient intake in childhood diarrhoea.*

The success of such interventions in the future requires concentration on improved, basic methods of disease management especially those which improve appetite. This should be accompanied by innovation in establishing the best means of re-feeding during the early recovery phase of diarrhoea.

1 Abdullah, M. & Wheeler, E.F. (1985): Seasonal variations and the intra-household distribution of food in a Bangladeshi village. *Am. J. Clin. Nutr.* **41**, 1305–1313.
2 Aynsley-Green, A. (1985): Metabolic and endocrine interrelations in the human fetus and neonate. *Am. J. Clin. Nutr.* **41**, 399–417.
3 Beisel, W.R., Sawyer, W.D., Ryll, E. & Crozier, D. (1967): Metabolic effects of intracellular infections in man. *Ann. Intern. Med.* **67**, 744–749.
4 Brown, K.H., Black, R.E. & Robertson, A.D. (1982): Clinical and field studies of human lactation: methodological considerations. *Am. J. Clin. Nutr.* **35**, 745–756.
5 Brown, K.H., Black, R.E., Robertson, A.D. & Becker, S. (1985): Effects of season and illness on the dietary intake of weanlings during longitudinal studies in rural Bangladesh. *Am. J. Clin. Nutr.* **41**, 343–355.
6 Chen, L.C., Chowdhury, Akma & Huffman, S.L. (1979): Seasonal dimension of energy protein malnutrition in rural Bangladesh; the role of agriculture, dietary practices and infection. *Ecol. Fd. Nutr.* **8**, 175–187.
7 Hoyle, B., Yunus, M. & Chen, L.C. (1980): Breast feeding and food intake among children with acute diarrhoeal disease. *Am. J. Clin. Nutr.* **33**, 2365–2371.
8 James, W.P.T. (1985): Appetite control and other mechanisms of weight homeostasis. In *Nutritional adaptation in man*, ed K. Blaxter & J.C. Waterlow, p. 141–153. London and Paris: John Libbey.
9 Martorell, R., Yarborough, C., Yarborough, S. & Klein, R.E. (1980): The impact of ordinary illnesses on the dietary intakes of malnourished children. *Am. J. Clin. Nutr.* **33**, 345–350.
10 Mata, L.J., Cromal, R.A., Vrrutia, J.J. & Garcia, B. (1977): Effect of infection on food intake and the nutritional state: perspectives as viewed from the village. *Am. J. Clin. Nutr.* **30**, 1215–1227.
11 Molla, A.M., Molla, A., Sarker, S.A. & Rahaman, M. (1983): Food intake during and after recovery from diarrhoea in children. In *Diarrhoea and Malnutrition*, ed L.C. Chen & N.S. Scrimshaw, New York and London: Plenum Press.

12 Rowland, M.G.M., Cole, T.J. & Whitehead, R.G. (1977): A quantitative study into the role of infection in determining nutritional status in Gambian village children. *Br. J. Nutr.* **37**, 441–450.

13 Tomkins, A.M. (1983): Nutritional cost of protracted diarrhoea in young Gambian children. *Gut* **24**, A459.

14 Tomkins, A.M., Garlick, P.J., Schofield, W.N. & Waterlow, J.C. (1983): The combined effect of infection and malnutrition on protein metabolism in children. *Clin. Sci.* **65**, 313–324.

Absorption of macronutrients in children during acute diarrhoea and after recovery

A.M. MOLLA, Ayesha MOLLA and Naseha KHATUN
International Centre for Diarrhoeal Disease Research, GPO Box 128, Dhaka-2, Bangladesh.

Acute diarrhoea is one of the most common causes of morbidity and mortality particularly in children below 5 years of age in the developing countries. The median mortality rate from diarrhoea amounts to about 20 per 1000 children[12]. It has been estimated that at least 20 per cent of the physical growth retardation in the disadvantaged children can be attributed to diarrhoeal disease[1,2].

Nutritional impact of diarrhoea is due to several factors, including (1) decreased intake due to anorexia or withholding of food, (2) direct loss or malabsorption of nutrients, and (3) increased catabolism. The effect of these factors becomes prolonged in recurrent or chronic diarrhoea[2]. In 1948 it was clearly shown[5] that nitrogen absorption was directly related to the feeding of high, medium and low-energy diets. The study further showed that a substantial absorption of nitrogen and fat occurred if food was given during acute diarrhoea, while no positive absorption occurred during the period of starvation. A recent study in Peru has shown that in acute diarrhoea nitrogen and fat absorption was clearly related to the amount of energy[3]. Malabsorption of glucose, xylose, and lactose, and fats has been demonstrated earlier[4,6,7,10]. There is scanty information available on the absorption status of macro and micro-nutrients in acute diarrhoea in children, especially in diarrhoea due to specific aetiology. Such information is essential to arrive at a decision to justify continued feeding during acute diarrhoea.

The present study at the International Centre for Diarrhoeal Disease Research, Bangladesh was undertaken to quantitatively estimate the absorption of macronutrients like carbohydrate, energy nitrogen and fat in children with acute diarrhoea due to different aetiologies.

Patients and methods. Sixty-eight children of age 1–5 years suffering from acute diarrhoea due to cholera (29), rotavirus (17), *E. coli* (ETEC) (13) and shigella (nine) with moderate dehydration were admitted into the metabolic ward of the International Centre for Diarrhoeal Disease Research, Bangladesh during July 1982 to June 1984. After initial rehydration was done by using intravenous fluid, patients were fed a nonabsorbable charcoal marker followed by a familiar Bangladeshi meal of known composition[8], fed *ad libitum* but accurately measured. The first appearance of the marker in the stool was taken as 'zero' hour. The length of time between feeding and the appearance of the marker in the stool was defined as 'transit time' and was recorded during acute stage and after recovery from diarrhoea. Accurate record of the quantity of food consumed was maintained for 72 h after feeding the first marker. Collection of stool, urine and vomit was started at 'zero hour' until the appearance of the second marker fed at the end of 72 h. Food of all kinds and stool, urine or vomit were stored at −40°C. Samples from aliquots of food, stool, urine or vomit were analysed for energy, carbohydrate, nitrogen and fat. Calculations were done to estimate the coefficient of absorption of nutrients by using the formula[9]: Intake-output/Intake × 100. Weight and height of each patient was measured on admission and on discharge. The relation of nutrients absorption to the nutritional status of the children was determined. One-hour blood xylose test was done by feeding 5 g xylose solution (100 g/l) on an empty stomach a day after the admission. Patients were followed up 2 and 8 weeks after recovery from diarrhoea and the balance study was repeated.

Table 1. *Clinical characteristics of the study patients on admission (adm).* Values are means ± i s.d.

Variable	Cholera(29)	Rotavirus(17)	E. Coli(13)	Shigella(9)
Age (months)	42.4±12.9	24.8±13.5	33.0±11.4	30.0±18.5
Body Wt (kg)	9.5±1.8	9.0±2.2	9.8±1.9	9.6±2.1
Diarrhoea at adm (h)	20.0±18.5	22.7±16.7	22.5±23.4	11.5±9.0
Purging rate (ml/kg.d)	162.9±119.9	51.5±31.5	34.5±25.2	79.8±57.6
Serum sp. gr.	1.027±0.003	1.026±0.002	1.026±0.001	1.025±0.003

Table 2. *Absorption of xylose in diarrhoea due to known aetiologies.*

	Serum xylose (mg/100ml ± s.d.)	
Aetiologies	Acute	Recovery
Cholera	19.8±8.2	30.4±8.4
ETEC	16.8±6.5	26.0±8.5
Shigella	24.3±13.4	30.0±6.7
Rotavirus	14.5±8.6	27.8±6.4

Results. Table 1 shows the clinical characteristics of the patients. Cholera and shigella patients were older and comparatively malnourished. Rotavirus patients were younger and relatively better nourished. One hour serum xylose levels are presented in Table 2. Xylose absorption was normal ($\geqslant$ 20 mg%) except for patients with rotavirus and ETEC in whom absorption became normal within the first week after recovery from diarrhoea. Table 3 presents the relation between the xylose absorption and nutritional status. The mean values of the coefficient of absorption of carbohydrate during acute diarrhoea and after recovery are presented in Table 4. The mean absorption of carbohydrate was between 76 to 91 per cent of the intake in the acute stage of diarrhoea. Nitrogen absorption in relation to nutritional status is presented in Table 5. Nitrogen absorption was lower than carbohydrate absorption but malnourished children showed an equal ability to absorb nitrogen. Table 6 shows the loss of different nutrients in diarrhoea due to different aetiologies. Rotavirus patients showed more loss of all nutrients. In the recovery stage this loss decreased but ETEC patient continued nitrogen loss for a longer period.

Table 3. *Relation between nutritional status and xylose-absorption in children with acute diarrhoea and after recovery.*

	Serum xylose (mg/100 ml ± s.d.)			
	Acute		Recovery	
Aetiology	GR A	GR B	GR A	GR B
Cholera	20.3±8.9	20.8±8.2	27.3±9.5	31.4±6.8
Rotavirus	13.2±5.4	17.3±14.4	29.5±6.7	23.9±3.6
ETEC	17.5±6.9	13.0±2.8	25.6±8.6	28.7±10.2
Shigella	24.3±13.4	'–'	30.1±6.7	'–'

GR A = Wt/Ht 90% NCHS; GR B = Wt/Ht 71–89% NCHS;
'–' Shigella patients with severe malnutrition were not studied.

Table 4. *Coefficient of absorption of carbohydrate during acute diarrhoea and after recovery in healthy children.*

	Coefficient of absorption (mean ± s.d.)	
Aetiology	Acute	Recovery
Cholera	87.8±19.5	92.8±6.9
Rotavirus	78.0±22.5	90.0±5.4
ETEC	91.0±5.6	88.7±9.2
Shigella	76.5±27.0	83.3±18.0

Table 5. *Relation between nutritional status and absorption of nitrogen in acute diarrhoea and after recovery.*

	Coefficient of absorption (mean ± s.d.)			
	Acute		Recovery	
Aetiology	GR A	GR B	GR A	GR B
Cholera	53.3±32.3	50.6±30.7	70.9±8.9	79.1±13.9
Rotavirus	57.2±12.9	51.6±8.3	72.3±12.8	66.6±16.9
ETEC	58.2±18.6	65.4±6.5	46.7±34.2	67.2±27.9
Shigella	25.0±54.9	'–'	65.1±15.9	'–'

GR A = Wt/Ht 90% NCHS; GR B = Wt/Ht 71–89% NCHS;
'–' Shigella patients with severe malnutrition were not studied.

Table 6. *Loss of nutrients (g/kg per d) in acute diarrhoea and after recovery.*

	Acute				Recovery			
Aetiology	Fat	N_2	CHO	kcal	Fat	N_2	CHO	kcal
Cholera	0.54	0.16	1.2	12.2	0.27	0.12	1.4	9.9
Rotavirus	1.0	0.13	2.0	20.7	0.36	0.09	1.3	10.5
ETEC	0.41	0.11	1.3	10.8	0.43	0.16	1.7	14.5
Shigella	0.80	0.15	2.2	17.7	0.30	0.12	2.9	17.4

Discussion. The present study showed very clearly that even in acute diarrhoea due to most aetiologies, nutrient absorption, particularly of carbohydrate, remains almost unaffected. In rotavirus and *E. coli* diarrhoea absorption of all nutrients is comparatively decreased in the acute stage and protein malabsorption continues for a longer time. This study however, did not distinguish between exogenous and endogenous losses of nitrogen. Several other studies have also indicated some special aspects of *E. coli* diarrhoea: loss of α_1 antitrypsin is high[10] and children who suffered from this diarrhoea remain more stunted[1]. Study in this centre showed lack of correlation between the transit time and absorption in acute diarrhoea. Thus further research is necessary to explain the malabsorption of different nutrients in acute diarrhoea of specific aetiology. Further work is necessary to correlate the actual absorptive functions with the digestive enzymatic status, possibly mucosal integrity, in children of the tropical countries in diarrhoea due to infective aetiology.

Recommendation. Since absorption of nutrients is satisfactory in acute diarrhoea in children, continued feeding should be encouraged during the acute episode and following recovery.

1 Black, R.E., Brown, K.H. & Becker, S. (1984): Effects of diarrhoea associated with specific enteropathogens on the growth of children in rural Bangladesh. *Pediatrics* **73**, 799–805.
2 Black, R.E., Brown, K.H., Becker, S., Alim, A.R. & Hug, I. (1982): Longitudinal studies of infection and physical growth of children in rural Bangladesh. II. Incidence of diarrhoea and association with known enteropathogens. *Am. J. Epidemiol.* **115**, 315–324.
3 Brown, K.H., Gilman, R.H., Khatun, M. & Ahmed, Md. G. (1980): Absorption of macronutrients from rice vegetable diet before and after treatment of ascariasis in children. *Am. J. Clin. Nutr.* **33**, 1975–1982.
4 Brown, K.H., & MacLean, W.C. (1984): Nutritional management of acute diarrhoea: an appraisal of the alternatives. *Pediatrics* **73**, 119–125.
5 Chung, A.W. (1948): Effect of oral feeding at different levels on the absorption of foodstuffs in infantile diarrhea. *J. Pediatr.* **33**, 1–13.
6 Einstein, L.P., Mackay, D.M. & Rosenberg, I.H. (1972): Paediatric xylose malabsorption in East Pakistan: correlation with age, growth retardation and weanling diarrhoea. *Am. J. Clin. Nutr.* **25**, 1230–1233.
7 Lindenbaum, J. (1965): Malabsorption during and after recovery from acute intestinal infection. *Br. Med. J.* **2**, 326–329.
8 Molla, A., Molla, A.M., Sarker, S.A. & Khatun, M. (1983): Whole-gut transit time and its relationship to absorption of macronutrients during and after recovery. *Scand. J. Gastroenterol.* **8**, 537–543.
9 Molla, A. *et al.* (1983): Effects of acute diarrhoea on absorption of macronutrients during disease and after recovery. In *Diarrhoea and malnutrition: interactions, mechanisms, and interventions* ed L.C. Chen & N.S. Scrimshaw, p. 143–154. New York and London: Plenum.
10 Rahaman, M.M. & Wahed, M.A. (1983): Direct nutrient loss and diarrhoea. In *Diarrhoea and malnutrition: interactions, mechanisms, and interventions,* ed L.C. Chen & N.S. Scrimshaw, pp. 155–160. New York and London: Plenum.
11 Rosenberg, I.H. & Scrimshaw, N.S. (1972): Workshop on malabsorption and nutrition: I and II. *Am. J. Clin. Nutr.* **25**, 1046–1226.
12 Snyder, J.D. & Merson, M.H. (1982): The magnitude of the global problem of acute diarrhoeal disease: a review of active surveillance data. *Bull. WHO* **60**, 605–619.

Growth faltering in diarrhoea

M.G.M. ROWLAND and S.G.J. Goh ROWLAND
International Centre for Diarrhoeal Disease Research, Bangladesh. P.O. Box 128, Dhaka-2, Bangladesh.

The importance of the relationship between nutrition and infection has long been recognised[26] and there is now a wealth of evidence that diarrhoea is the most important non-dietary cause of growth faltering in young children in developing countries. Diarrhoea is a symptom with many causes and varying pathology and there may be wide variation in the amount of diarrhoea experienced by individuals, even of the same age and within the same community[12].

In The Gambia[25], there could also be a tremendous variation in its effect on the growth of children at different seasons of the year; sometimes growth was highly dependent upon the amount of diarrhoea experienced by individuals and at other times was almost unaffected by it. This supported other work showing that not all children who have an attack of diarrhoea suffer growth impairment as a result[13]. Here we explore some of the possible reasons for these variations and attempt to identify some of the more specific characteristics of subjects and disease episodes involved in the impact of diarrhoea on growth.

Who suffers growth faltering in association with diarrhoea? *Age.* Diarrhoea and malnutrition in their endemic or seasonally recurrent form are both essentially diseases of early childhood. Peak rates of diarrhoeal incidence and prevalence in the community tend to occur within the second half of infancy or the second year of life[4,16,24]. The largest deviations from normal growth in terms of weight-for-age tend also to occur around this time. By three years of age the situation is often improving with respect to both factors; diarrhoea rates are much lower[1,27] and growth velocities tend to approach normal[19] though attained weight does not reach normal levels for many years. It would be natural therefore to expect that the main strength of the interaction between diarrhoeal illness and growth might occur before 3 years of age. In practice, most longitudinal community studies designed to systematically investigate this relationshhip have not encompassed wide age ranges. In Guatemala a relationship between diarrhoea and growth in children up to the age of 7 years has been shown[25]. Though age did not appear to affect this relationship the authors did not systematically quantify the impact on growth through this age range. The same limitation is true of the Gambian analysis, where it was calculated that between age 0.6 and 3 years, the mean impact of diarrhoea on growth was of the order of 100 g month and that growth rates were being more or less halved by the level of diarrhoeal illness experienced there[5,25].

Sex. Both diarrhoeal morbidity and rates of malnutrition in childhood may vary according to sex. In general boys tend to suffer higher attack rates of diarrhoea than girls, for reasons largely unknown. Girls may be disadvantaged with respect to malnutrition and, in some communities at least, there is evidence that discriminatory practices with respect to food intake and other aspects of child care may play a part in this. Surprisingly few of the analyses relating growth and infection have taken sex into account. In one example where it was, the Bacon Chow study[1], no sex difference in the relationship between diarrhoeal disease and linear growth of infants was found.

Feeding practices. The pattern of infant-feeding has a marked effect on diarrhoeal morbidity. Wherever studied, and particularly in the youngest children in underprivileged societies, the frequency and lethality of diarrhoeal illness is higher in bottle-fed, mixed-fed, or weaned children than in exclusively breast-fed children[6]. The hazards of supplementary infant-feeding in conditions of bad environmental hygiene have been clearly demonstrated, and a causal relationship with diarrhoea has been suggested by at least one study[3]. This has led people to realise the importance of avoiding unnecessarily early supplementation. Unfortunately this is not easily translated into practice and carries with it the risk of producing or aggravating undernutrition if carried out over zealously[7]. This in itself may predispose to diarrhoeal illness of increased duration[23] and possibly of severity also[10,14]. It is this balance of risks that led to the term 'weanling dilemma' being coined.

The growth-infection relationship has been best documented when children in traditionally breast-feeding communities are entering this transitional phase of feeding when other foods are being introduced in addition to continued breast-feeding, the so called weaning period[9]. Waning immunity, increasing mobility and exposure to environmental contaminants all predispose to this overall problem. Nevertheless remarkably little attention has been given to the quantitatively assessment of the impact of diarrhoea on growth in exclusively breast-fed as against mixed-fed or weaned children.

There has been, however, some suggestive evidence from Keneba, The Gambia, on this score[29]. It was found that infants with above average intakes of breast-milk were given supplementary feeds later than others. In these children pre-weaning diarrhoeal attacks appeared to be mild and only 12 per cent suffered diarrhoea-induced weight loss. The first attack of diarrhoea which produced growth-faltering also tended to occur later and these children were significantly heavier at the end of one year than those receiving lower than average breast milk intakes and starting weaning earlier.

Perhaps surprisingly in view of this, it has been reported that, in breast-fed neonates in particular, infection with pathogenic bacteria such as *Shigella* may not be accompanied by diarrhoea, but weight faltering may still occur[18].

Nutritional status. One might equally well wonder to what extent baseline nutritional status influences the impact of diarrhoea on growth. Again there has been remarkably little attention to this aspect. It has been observed[16] that infants with evidence of fetal growth retardation suffered greater nutritional sequelae (stunting) than did others in the Guatemalan cohort. In a systematic re-working of Morley's Nigerian data[22], it was found that weight-faltering associated with diarrhoea tended to be more severe in smaller (lighter) subjects than in the heavier ones, but this relationship could be demonstrated only in late infancy[8]. In our own unpublished data derived from a recent study of young urban Gambian children, the impact of diarrhoea on growth appeared to be most marked in the second half of infancy but this has not yet been related either to the individual's feeding (weaning) pattern or to the nutritional status of the subject. Other authors have claimed to have found a negative relationship between nutritional status and the impact of diarrhoea on growth but this appears to be largely based on individual case histories rather than on systematic analysis[17]. Thus the evidence is far from conclusive and this relationship deserves more attention.

Apparently at variance with these observations is the finding by one group of investigators that malnourished children in the post-diarrhoeal recovery phase actually appear to have enhanced nutrient absorption compared with their better nourished counterparts[20].

Which diarrhoeal episodes are associated with growth faltering? *Frequency, prevalence, duration, severity.* Relatively little attempt has been made to systematically investigate the relationship between diarrhoeal attacks of varying description and growth. Of course there appears to be much variation in the impact of individual attacks but its nature is not well understood. In an earlier study of Gambian children up to the age of 18 months[13], it was found that 63 per cent of diarrhoeal episodes were associated with weight faltering but the variation could have been associated with different patterns of feeding[29].

In the Bacon Chow study[1] the authors concluded that the number of episodes, rather than duration or severity, was important in determining the effect of growth during infancy. In our own Gambian study referred to earlier, some of the variation in impact on growth was presumably due to prevailing dietary factors. In general when dietary intakes appeared satisfactory there was a strong negative linear correlation between prevalence and growth during 2-month periods. No attempt was made to differentiate between the effect of frequent attacks of short duration and of fewer more prolonged attacks. In studies in rural Bangladesh[2] it was noted that it was the prolonged attacks lasting more than 10 days which appeared to have the greatest effect on growth.

Pathogen specific diarrhoea. Most of the knowledge in this area has been derived from field and hospital studies by the International Centre for Diarrhoeal Disease Research, Bangladesh. In the former situation a significant negative relationship was shown between growth in weight over a 2-month period and enterotoxigenic *Escherichia coli* diarrhoea and between growth in length and *Shigella*-associated diarrhoea[2]. In the latter case this relationship could be demonstrated over a 1-year period. In approximately half of the attacks of diarrhoea suffered by these children, aged 2–60 months, no pathogen could be identified. In these cases no significant relationship between diarrhoea and growth could be demonstrated over a 2-month period.

It is worth noting here, however, that all of those subjects irrespective of aetiology showed some acute weight faltering (some of it presumably due to dehydration). In subjects unaffected in the long term, initial pre-attack weight was regained within 2 weeks; weight predicted by their premorbid growth trajectory was achieved after a further 4 weeks. It is important therefore that any studies on the diarrhoea-growth relationship take into account the distinction between early transient weight loss and the less common deficit that may be detectable months later. In fact growth, even in normal children, is not a smoothly progressive phenomenon[29] and most community studies have been more concerned with deficits measured over a period of one month[13,17], 2 months[2,24], 6 months or even 1 year[2,15]. That an effect can be discerned in some children so long after the original illness could presumably be due, in very simple terms, to chronic dietary constraints (often permitting maintenance but not catch-up growth), persisting pathology impairing gut function, such as in the post-enteritis syndrome[28] or some combination of both.

It is important to note also that most hospital-based studies of intake, absorption and the effect of various therapeutic regimes on unspecified or pathogen-specific diarrhoea are, for very obvious reasons, carried out over a relatively short period of time. One attempt to get over this problem has been to admit children for reassessment several weeks after recovery. In these circumstances prolonged anorexia following acute rotavirus gastroenteritis was demonstrated[21], a finding which is perhaps surprising since rotavirus was not found by others[2] to be significantly associated with prolonged growth faltering. This raises another issue. Community studies are in general based on fairly frequent questionnaire surveys and tend to document diarrhoeal morbidity fairly comprehensively. Most hospital studies are carried out on children selected for admission on the basis of more or less severe dehydration (as in the case of most of the Bangladesh studies) or severe concomitant malnutrition (as would tend to occur in The Gambia). This aspect must be considered when trying to relate the various findings and particularly when trying to determine the basis for interventions or strategies aimed at reducing malnutrition during diarrhoea.

1 Baumgartner, R.N. & Pollitt, E. (1983): The Bacon Chow Study: analyses of the effect of infectious illness on growth of infants. *Nutr. Res.* **3**, 9–21.

2 Black, R.E., Brown, K.H. & Becker, S. (1983): Influence of acute diarrhea on the growth parameters of children. In *Acute diarrhea: its nutritional consequences in children*, ed J.A. Bellanti, pp. 75–84. Nestlé Nutrition Workshop, Volume 2. New York: Raven Press.

3 Black, R.E., Brown, K.H., Becker, S., Alim, A.R.M.A. & Merson, M.H. (1982): Contamination of weaning foods and transmission of enterotoxigenic *Escherichia coli* diarrhoea in children in rural Bangladesh. *Trans. Roy. Soc. Trop. Med. Hyg.* **76**, 259–264.

4 Black, R.E., Brown, K.H., Becker, S. & Yunus, M. (1982): Longitudinal studies of infectious diseases and physical growth of children in rural Bangladesh. 1. Patterns of morbidity. *Am. J. Epidemiol.* **115**, 305–314.

5 Cole, T.J. & Parkin, J.M. (1977): Infection and its effect on the growth of young children: A comparison of The Gambia and Uganda. *Trans. Roy. Soc. Trop. Med. Hyg.* **71**, 196–198.

6 Cunningham, A.S. (1981): Breastfeeding and morbidity in industrialized countries: an update. In *Advances in international maternal and child health*, Vol. 1. ed D.B. Jelliffe, & E.F.P. Jelliffe, pp. 126–168. Oxford: Oxford Medical Publications.

7 Editorial (1977): A Swedish code of ethics for marketing of infant food. *Acta Paed. Scand.* **66**, 129–132.

8 Fullerton, P. (1978): Malnutrition and infection: an examination of the effects of diarrhoeal disease and other infections on the growth of children up to three years of age. pp. 58. University of London: D.T.P.H. Thesis.

9 Gordon, J.E., Chitkara, I.D. & Wyon, J.B. (1963): Weanling diarrhea. *Am. J. Med. Sci.* **245**, 345–377.

10 Gordon, J.E., Ascoli, W., Mata, L.J., Guzmán, M.A. & Scrimshaw, N.S. (1968): Nutrition and infection field study in Guatemalan villages 1959–1964. VI Acute diarrheal disease and nutritional disorders in general disease incidence. *Arch. Environ. Hlth.* **16**, 424–437.

11 Leeuwenberg, J., Gemert, W., Müller, A.S. & Patel, S.C. (1978): Agents affecting health of mother and child in a rural area of Kenya. VII The incidence of diarrhoeal disease in the under-five population. *Trop. geogr. Med.* **30**, 383–391.

12 Lloyd-Evans, N., Pickering, H.A., Goh, S.G.J. & Rowland, M.G.M. (1984): Food and water hygiene and diarrhoea in young Gambian children: a limited case control study. *Trans. Roy. Soc. Trop. Med. Hyg.* **78**, 209–211.

13 Marsden, P.D. & Marsden, S.A. (1965): A pattern of weight gain in Gambian babies during the first 18 months of life. *J. Trop. Pediatr.* **10**, 89–99.

14 Martínez, C. & Chávez, A. (1979): Nutrition and development of children from poor rural areas. VII The effect of nutritional status on the frequency and severity of infections. *Nutr. Rep. Internat.* **19**, 307–314.

15 Martorell, R., Habicht, J-P., Yarbrough, C., Lechtig, A., Klein, R.E. & Western, K.A. (1975): Acute morbidity and physical growth in rural Guatemalan children. *Am. J. Dis. Child.* **129**, 1296–1301.

16 Mata, L.J. (1983): Epidemiology of acute diarrhea in childhood. In *Acute diarrhea: its nutritional consequences in children*, ed J.A. Bellanti, pp. 3–22. Nestlé Nutrition Workshop Series, Vol. 2. New York: Raven Press.

17 Mata, L.J., Kronmal, R.A., Urrutia, J.J. & García, B. (1977): Effect of infection on food intake and the nutritional state: perspectives as viewed from the village. *Am. J. Clin. Nut.* **30**, 1215–1227.

18 Mata, L.J., Urrutia, J.J., Abertazzi, C., Pellecer, O. & Arellano, E. (1972): Influence of recurrent infections on nutrition and growth of children in Guatemala. *Am. J. Clin. Nut.* **25**, 1267–1275.

19 Mata, L.J., Urrutia, J.J. & Beteta, C.E. (1978): Growth and development in infancy and early childhood. In *The Children of Santa Maria Cauqué* ed L.J. Mata, pp. 167–201. Cambridge MA: MIT Press.

20 Molla, A., Molla, A.M. & Khatun, M. (1985): Effect of nutritional status of children on intake and absorption of nutrients. In *Child Health in the Tropics*, ed R. Eeckels & O. Ransome-Kuti. The Hague: Martinus Nijhoff Publishers.

21 Molla, A.M., Molla, A., Sarker, S.A. & Rahaman, M.M. (1982): Food intake during and after recovery from diarrhoea in children. In *Diarrhea and Malnutrition*. ed L.C. Chen & N.S. Scrimshaw, pp. 113–123. New York: Plenum Publishing Corporation.

22 Morley, D., Bicknell, J. & Woodland, M. (1968): Factors influencing the growth and nutritional status of infants and young children in a Nigerian village. *Trans. R. Soc. Trop. Med. Hyg.* **62**, 164–199.

23 Palmer, D.L., Koster, F.T., Alam, A.K.M.J. & Islam, M.R. (1976): Nutritional status: A determinant of severity of diarrhoea in patients with cholera. *J. Inf. Dis.* **134**, 8–14.

24 Rowland, M.G.M., Barrell, R.A.E. & Whitehead, R.G. (1978): Bacterial contamination in traditional Gambian weaning foods. *Lancet* **1**, 136–138.

25 Rowland, M.G.M., Cole, T.J. & Whitehead, R.G. (1977): A quantitative study into the role of infection in determining nutritional status in Gambian village children. *Br. J. Nut.* **37**, 441–450.

26 Scrimshaw, N.S., Taylor, C.E. & Gordon, J.E. (1968): Interactions of nutrition and infection. *W.H.O. Monogr. Ser.* No 57, pp. 329.

27 Snyder, J.D. & Merson, M.H. (1982): The magnitude of the global problem of acute diarrhoeal disease: a review of active surveillance data. *Bull. W.H.O.* **60**, 605–613.

28 Walker-Smith, J.A. (1979): Delayed recovery after gastroenteritis. In *Diseases of the small intestine in childhood*, 2nd edn. pp. 234–236. Tunbridge Wells, Kent: Pitman Medical.

29 Watkinson, M. (1981): Delayed onset of weanling diarrhoea associated with high breast-milk intake. *Trans. R. Soc. Trop. Med. Hyg.* **75**, 432–435.

30 Whitehead, R.G. (1979): Dietary allowances of energy and nutrients. In *International Reviews of Biochemistry: Biochemistry of Nutrition*, ed A. Neuberger & T.H. Jukes, pp. 281–325. Baltimore: University Park Press.

Health education as a strategy for improving the management of diarrhoea

R. MARTORELL, D. FOOTE and C. KENDALL
Food Research Institute, Stanford University, Stanford, California 94305; Applied Communication Technology, 1010 Doyle Street, Suite 17, Menlo Park, California 94025; Agency for International Development, Room 702D, SA 18, Washington DC 20523, USA.

The Diarrhoeal Disease Control Programme of the World Health Organization (WHO) has advocated a four-point strategy for decreasing the mortality and morbidity associated with diarrhoeal diseases through mutually reinforcing and complementary measures[2]. First, the plan calls for better management of episodes of diarrhoea and emphasizes the use of oral rehydration therapy and the appropriate feeding of children during diarrhoeal illness and convalescence[4].

The second strategy seeks to increase host resistance to infection through a variety of measures such as improved maternal and child nutritional status, appropriate infant-feeding practices including breast-feeding, and adequate coverage of immunization, particularly against measles. Improved child nutrition is viewed, therefore, as a key mechanism for enhancing immunocompetence. The third and fourth strategies are to reduce the transmission of the pathogenic agents of diarrhoeal disease and to control and/or prevent diarrhoea epidemics. Improvements in the standard of living, particularly in water supplies and waste disposal and better hygiene practices, are essential for interrupting the transmission of diarrhoeal disease pathogens. Unfortunately, the intractable problem of poverty and the staggering cost of even very simple water supply and sewage systems makes effective environmental sanitation a long-term prospect for most people in all but a few countries. Prospects for health education seem more hopeful and it has been proposed that in spite of the poverty of developing countries, the level of health could be significantly improved through the adoption of more appropriate health practices[1].

Until recently, the history of health and nutrition education was disappointing[3]. Little was achieved by programmes which focused on knowledge acquisition and on such irrelevant concepts as the four food groups. Recent attempts to apply 'social marketing', which uses the techniques of commercial advertising and product design strategies, have been more successful. The objectives of this paper are to describe one such project which took place in Honduras and to present some key findings.

The Honduras mass media and health practices project. The project was an undertaking of the Honduran Ministry of Public Health and was implemented by the Academy for Educational Development based in Washington DC. Our group at Stanford University was in charge of the evaluation. The programme used a combination of radio, printed material, and interpersonal communication through health workers to teach mothers to prevent and treat acute diarrhoea. The programme focused on the promotion of a prepackaged oral rehydration solution (ORS) that mothers could mix and administer at home when their children were ill. Supplementing messages about ORS administration were messages on prevention behaviours such as continued breastfeeding, feeding during diarrhoea, basic hygiene, and appropriate food preparation for children. The prepackaged salts for the mixture were produced in Honduras using the WHO formula. The package of salts was mixed with a litre of water, and hence received the name 'Litrosol'.

The intervention was distinguished by several features. The steps that must be taken and the resources that are required before an action in health behaviour is carried in the local setting were identified and taken into account in the design of the campaign. Local vocabulary and beliefs were incorporated into campaign messages and these focused on a carefully specified set of feasible objectives and stressed a few key behaviours rather than general knowledge acquisition. Other aspects were pretesting of as many messages, materials, and procedures as possible and careful monitoring and modification of the campaign as it progressed. Over the course of two years, the programme took advantage of an extensive network of private and public radio stations to transmit thousands of radio spot announcements and dozens of weekly health programmes which repeated Litrosol mixing instructions and reminded mothers when to seek care at health centres. A variety of posters, instructional pamphlets, and photonovelas were developed for both health workers and rural mothers. Hundreds of health workers were trained by the project on how to teach mothers to use Litrosol properly.

Evaluation design. The programme was targeted to a region containing approximately half a million people. To measure the effects of the intervention, a panel of 750 families with young children were studied for 2 years. Families were recruited into the study from 20 communities under a stratified sampling plan with random selection within communities.

A model was developed to help guide the evaluation. In order for any changes in behaviour or in health status to take place, a complex sequence of events had to occur (Fig. 1). For a successful campaign, the target audience needs to be exposed to the campaign effort. Next, it is required that the audience learn from that exposure and that messages be remembered and accepted in order for behavioural change to occur and for this change to result in improved health status.

Evaluation findings. In general, the population had good access to radio, interpersonal contact through the health care system, and printed materials, as well as high exposure to the campaign components. For example, 80 per cent of the families owned at least one radio. After asking them to turn the radios on to demonstrate that they worked, 67 per cent of the families had working radios. Radio had a very high penetration in rural areas and was listened to very frequently. An average of 60 per cent of mothers reported listening to the radio on the previous day.

Exposure to campaign message through the different channels is the second step of the evaluation model. Radio coverage with campaign messages was extremely high and 73 per cent of women listeners remembered hearing at least one radio spot the previous day. Listeners reported hearing an average of 3.3 spots.

A great deal of learning of the specific content of the campaign messages took place as exemplified by knowledge about Litrosol and breast-feeding (Fig. 2). In assessing these changes, three types of samples were studied. There was concern that repeated visits to households might

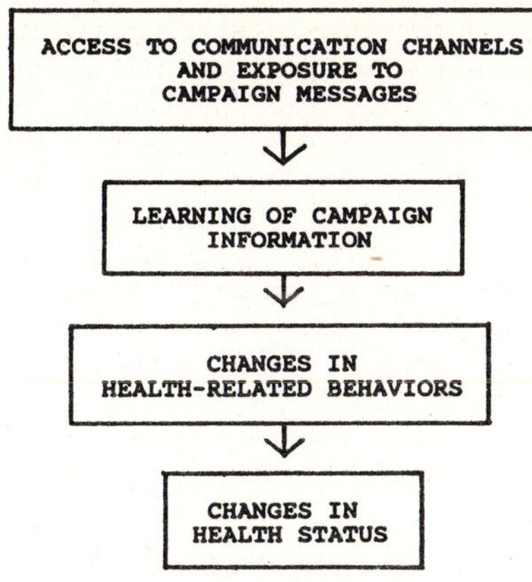

Fig. 1. *Simplified version of process model used in Honduras evaluation.*

cause mothers to become more aware of the campaign. For this reason, in the case of measures of learning and exposure, the experimental sample was randomly divided into two equal groups. The first group was visited four times and is called the 'High-frequency interview' group. The second group was not questioned about media aspects until the end of the intervention and is referred to as the 'Low-frequency interview' group. Also, a sample outside the study area was included as a further check. This last group came from villages that received all the elements of the campaign but which were not visited by the field team till the end of the campaign. This group is called the 'sample outside study area'.

The name 'Litrosol', was introduced with the campaign and within 6 months after broadcasts began, half of the mothers could name Litrosol as the medicine being promoted, a figure which rose to nearly 80 per cent almost two years later. Values for the two other samples, the low-frequency interview group and the outside study area group, are around 10 percentage points lower suggesting a small effect of repeated visits.

The campaign also emphasized the benefits of breast-feeding. Figure 2 shows the percentage of correct responses about the benefits of breast-milk as a percentage of all possible responses. Examples of correct answers are its lack of contamination and its anti-infective properties. There was a clear rise in knowledge in the high-frequency interview group. Between the third and fourth surveys the breast-feeding messages were intense and a clear rise occurs. Knowledge in the two control samples was only slightly lower suggesting a true campaign effect. These data are misleading in that they suggest mothers knew very little about the benefits of breast-milk. This is unlikely. Rather, the campaign may have taught mothers how to express the benefits of breast-feeding in concrete terms and more importantly it may have generated more positive attitudes towards breast-feeding among rural women.

Through a morbidity questionnaire, the percentage of episodes which were treated with Litrosol in the 2 weeks previous to the interview were monitored. These data were collected through five surveys. A few months into the campaign, 10 per cent of cases were being treated with Litrosol, a figure which rose to 37 per cent in the final survey. Younger children were more likely to be treated than older ones and boys were just as likely to be treated as girls. The probability of Litrosol use rose with the seriousness of the episode, either as perceived by the mother or as defined by signs of severity and dehydration.

Feeding behaviours, particularly breast-feeding and feeding during episodes of diarrhoea, were also targets of the campaign. Breast-feeding appears to have been increased by the campaign: early in the intervention, 65 per cent of children under 18 months were breastfeeding; by the end of the campaign, the number had risen to 81 per cent of children under 18 months ($P < 0.005$). Similarly, bottle-feeding dropped from 64 per cent to 50 per cent over the same time period ($P = < 0.005$). Continuation of breast-feeding and bottle-feeding during episodes of diarrhoea was at about the same level. That is, virtually all mothers who were breast-feeding or bottle-feeding reported that they continued to do so during episodes of diarrhoea. There was a slight rise in the giving of other liquids during episodes.

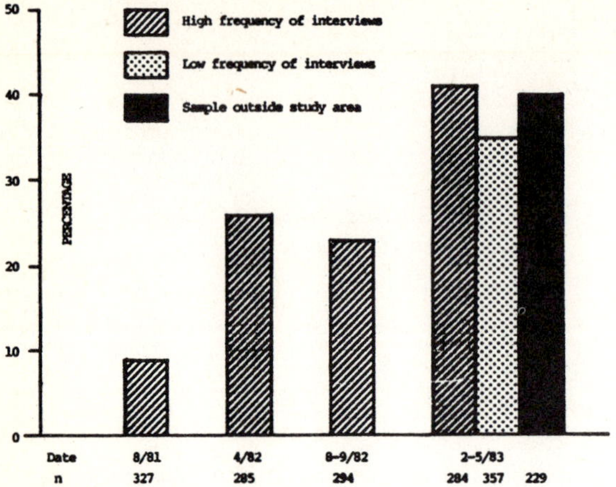

Fig. 2. *Correct responses about the benefits of breast-milk as a percentage of all possible responses.*

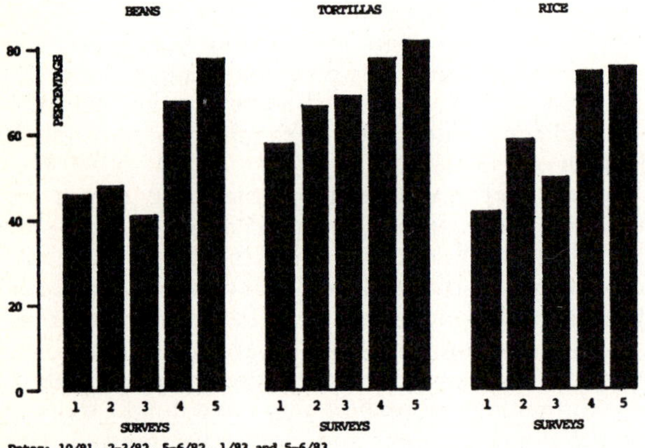

Fig. 3. *Percentage of children consuming staple foods during episodes of diarrhoea within the last 2 weeks.*

There appears to have been an increase in food consumption during episodes of diarrhoea as shown in Fig. 3. This is suggested by three simple indicators of food consumption; namely, the percentage of children who consumed beans, tortillas, and rice. These foods are the three principal staples and together usually account for most of the food intake. There is a clear overall tendency towards greater food consumption during diarrhoea over the course of the study period and this tendency is evident for all three staples.

Data from the official death registry was used to assess mortality changes. Data for all deaths in children less than 5 years in the three county seats where the study villages are located were transcribed for a period from late 1978 through March of 1983 by a Honduran physician who was experienced in rural health care. The cases were then classified into two groups: cases involving diarrhoea as a primary or secondary cause of death and cases not involving diarrhoea. The total cases of death in children less than 5 years of age available for analyses was 378, with 206 occurring before the intervention and 172 after the intervention.

Registry data are unreliable for estimating true rates because many deaths go unreported.

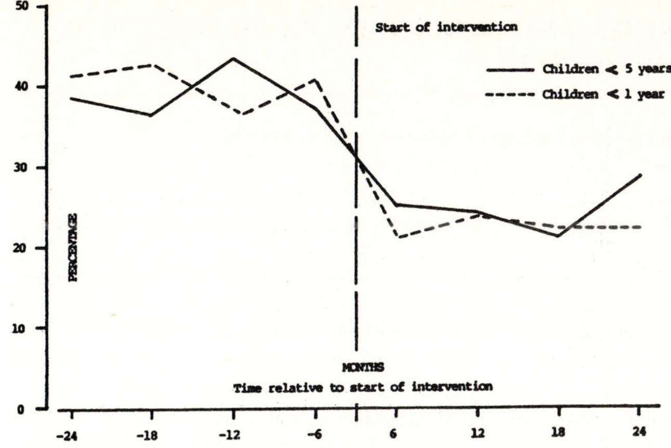

Fig. 4. *Percentage of deaths that involve diarrhoea in any way, for 2 years before and after the start of the intervention.*

For these reasons, changes in the proportion of deaths associated with diarrhoea are emphasized. In Fig. 4, data are presented for 2 years before and 2 years after the intervention. In children less than 5 years of age, the proportion of deaths involving diarrhoea declined from 39.8 per cent before to 24.4 per cent after the intervention, similar to the decline observed in children less than 1 year old. These declines were statistically significant ($P < 0.01$).

Two clear-cut findings emerge from this analysis. One is that reported diarrhoeal mortality was sharply lower after the campaign than before, and that this drop occurred precisely and suddenly at the introduction of the ORT campaign. The second is that this effect was stable over time and across age groups, so it is unlikely to be the result of random fluctuations.

Caution must be exercised in interpreting these data. The mortality data are of unknown validity and it may not be true that diarrhoeal mortality decreased. For example, it is entirely possible that with the saturation of messages about diarrhoea and ORT that mothers somehow became less likely to report diarrhoea as a cause of death. Some mothers may have been ashamed to admit that their child died of diarrhoea at a time when a highly publicized care was available at no charge.

Conclusion. Compared to commercial campaigns, the Honduras project was enormously successful. It is clear that there was good access to all the communications channels used by the campaign and that the target audience was heavily exposed to campaign messages through those channels. The exposure resulted in learning gains across virtually all the topics covered by the campaign messages and the audience adopted the promoted behaviours at high rates. Finally, there is the possibility that mortality due to diarrhoea was reduced by half.

Acknowledgement. The research reported here has been supported by the Offices of Education and Health of the Bureau for Science and Technology, United States Agency for International Development under Contract AID/DSPE-C-0028.

1 Feachem, R.G. (1984): Interventions for the control of diarrhoeal diseases among young children: promotion of personal and domestic hygiene. *Bull. Wld Hlth Org.* **62**, 467–476.
2 Feachem, R.G., Hogan, R.C. & Merson, M.H. (1983): Diarrhoeal disease control: reviews of potential interventions. *Bull. Wld Hlth Org.* **61**, 637–640.
3 Hornik, R.C. (1985): *Nutrition education: a state-of-the-art review.* Nutrition Policy Discussion Paper No. 1. Rome: FAO.
4 NRC (National Research Council) (1985): *Nutritional management of acute diarrhea in infants and children.* Washington, DC: National Academy Press.

MICRONUTRIENT DEFICIENCIES AND DISEASE IN THE DEVELOPING WORLD

Selenium-deficiency and endemic Keshan disease in China

G.Q. YANG
Institute of Health, China National Center for Preventive Medicine, 29 Nan Wei Road, Beijing, China

Keshan disease (KD), an endemic cardiomyopathy of extremely poor selenium (Se) status, and of unknown origin was first reported by Yang and Wang in the first National Symposium on the Etiology of KD in Shenyang, China in 1973 (Yang & Wang, unpublished,[20]). Since the selenite-supplementation trial was effective in preventing against KD in 1974[9] and that was later confirmed in 1975[15], it was finally concluded that KD is a Se-deficiency-related endemic disease[2,8,9]. Several aspects of KD have been recently reviewed elsewhere[6].

Epidemiologic surveys before the 1950s indicated that the prevalence of KD was a very severe problem not only due to its high fatality, usually higher than 80 per cent, but also its high incidence. Since young women are more susceptible, it was not uncommon that in sites where 'foreign' immigrants, ie Chinese migrants from distant places, gathered, most men remained single or families were forced to leave their homes and wandered about elsewhere in early days during heavy prevalence. However, at present its epidemiologic characteristics have changed somewhat. On the one hand, the prevalence of this disease became far milder, ie the average morbidity of acute and subacute cases steadily decreased to only 3.6 per hundred thousand in 1981 in North China even though in some of the affected areas the poor Se status remained. On the other hand affected areas have expanded but in the new affected area only children became sick[22]. Such a noticeable change in epidemiologic characteristics has not yet been satisfactorily explained. On the basis of the early accumulated data in this field in connection with recent work on Se, the author proposed that it is likely that people may be able to adapt to low Se intakes after long residence in a low Se area[18].

Selenium-deficiency and Keshan disease. Although Se-deficiency was found a necessary factor for the pathogenesis of KD, other factors must be involved. Among factors suspected such as vitamin E, protein, methionine, Pb, Cd, Hg and As, only methionine was found to promote the bioavailability of dietary Se. Consistent differences in plasma vitamin E levels have not been found between affected and nonaffected areas, but occasionally they were at levels of marginal deficiency[17]. It was found that Se-supplementation protected Se-deficient mice against the heart lesions induced by Coxsackie B4 virus isolated from the blood of a KD patient[1]. It is likely that some detrimental factor(s) eg unknown factor in the food[14] has not yet been clearly defined.

Possible mechanisms of the effects of selenium. It is expected that in patients with low glutathione peroxidase activity in their heart tissues, biomembrane of cells may be damaged. Histochemical study of patients' heart tissues showed that acid phosphatase activities increased in the area surrounding the necrotic foci[5]. It was also found that the phospholipid content of patients' erythrocytes was lower than normal[11], and that ATPase activity and cytoskeletal component of the membranes were abnormal in KD patients[16]. Also morphological changes in the myocardium resembled the changes caused by ischaemia and hypoxia[13]. Recent studies *in vitro* indicated that the haemoglobin of KD patients seemed more sensitive to the pro-oxidant effect of the autoxidation of dihydroxyfumaric acid (Ju, D. 1985 personal communication).

Epidemiology of KD. Low Se areas have been described in New Zealand (NZ)[12], Finland (Koivistoinen, 1985 personal communication) and other countries. Why has KD so far appeared only in the low Se areas of China? The Se contents of the main foods and the Se intakes by the residents in both low Se areas of China and New Zealand are comparable (Table 1). New Zealanders obtained 82 per cent of their Se intake from animal sources which have a rather high

Table 1. *Comparison of Se contents of foods and dietary Se intakes in low Se areas in China and NZ.*

Country (Reference)	Food (µg/g)				Dietary Se intake (µg/d)	Sources (%)		
	Cereals	Cabbage	Egg	Pork muscle		Cereals	Animal foods	Drinking water
Nz[12]	0.011	0.0008	0.24	0.057	6 – 70	14 – 18	82	negligible
China[19,20]	0.006	0.0007	0.06 0.18	0.030	4 – 11	75	6.9	negligible

Table 2. *Se status of residents in low Se areas in China and NZ.*

Country	Se content						Ref
	Blood (ng/ml)	Plasma (ng/ml)	Erythrocyte (ng/ml)	Toe-nails (µg/g)	Milk (ng/ml)	Urine (µg/day)	
NZ	59	48	74	0.26	7.6	12.7 13.1	Robinson 1984 (pers. commun.) [19,21]
China	18	22**	31**	0.17	2.6	4.8	

**Xi, GZ. (1985) personal communication

amount of Se in comparison with plant sources, while Chinese derived 75 per cent of their Se from cereals, and animal sources accounted for only 6.9 per cent. Table 2 shows that the Se status of Chinese residents is only 1/2 to 1/3 of New Zelanders. The blood Se level of 59 ng/ml in NZ residents is similar to the average level of 52 ng/ml in residents in KD area after receiving selenite-supplementation for 6 months. This treatment was shown to be effective in protecting against KD in the previous trial in 1974 in Mianning county[8]. KD appeared only under extremely poor Se status. Furthermore, KD is not a pure Se-deficiency disease, other unknown factor(s) are involved.

Evidence of possible human adaptation to low Se intake. Results from early epidemiologic surveys (Ju, D. 1956 personal communication) indicated that foreign residents were much more sensitive to KD in the endemic area of Heilongjiang province, 1955–1956. The ratio of local to foreign is 1.0 : 2.0 for total residents while it was 1.0 : 6.0 for KD deaths.

Study of the population of 60 villages in Beian county revealed that the larger the proportion of foreign immigrants in the villages, the more severe the incidence of KD (Table 3). Incidence of KD is greater in areas with both poor Se status and a larger proportion of foreign immigrants.

KD has become milder but the affected area has expanded in recent years. The successful Se intervention and the general improvement of nutritional status in rural populations is important, but the rural population has remained relatively stable. Since 1949, grain production has tripled. Logically the Se concentration of staple cereals would drop in low Se areas. In the newly affected areas the adaptation of children to low Se intake may not yet have been well developed. D.V. Frost (1985 personal communication) pointed out that Se deficiency is a growing problem world-wide. The adaptation of microorganisms and animals to high Se has already been reviewed[10]. Evidence obtained here in China seems to indicate that adaptability of humans, to low Se may also be important.

Minimum selenium requirement of humans. Three methods were used for estimation. Principally they are based on measuring minimum amounts either to protect the residents from KD by actual dietary survey or to maintain plasma GSHPx activity at plateau by supplementing subjects with graded amounts of seleno-DL-methionine[19]. Another method for estimating the minimum Se requirement was to calculate the intake from the Se content in staple cereals. This marginal level is around 0.02 ppm[21]. In the rural population around 70 per cent of the dietary Se is derived from cereals. This permitted us to calculate the daily minimum Se intake. If a 20 per cent loss from milling and cooking was taken into account[3,7], the average intake was 18 µg/day (Table 4).

Table 3. *Population origin in relation to varying prevalence of KD in 60 villages in Beian county from 1953 to 1956.*

| | Mild | | | Medium | | | Heavy | | |
Population	Total population	Died of KD	Mortality (per 1000)	Total population	Died of KD	Mortality (per 1000)	Total population	Died of KD	Mortality (per 1000)
Local residents and local immigrants	8283	22	2.6	2491	32	12.8	1051	19	18.1
Foreign immigrants	2416	16	6.6	1403	48	34.2	844	85	100.7
Total	10 699	38	3.6	3894	80	20.5	1895	104	54.9
Mortality ratio (local/ foreign)		0.39			0.37			0.18	

Table 4. *Minimum daily selenium requirements of adults estimated by different methods.*

Method	Male (μg)	Female (μg)	Average (μg)	Proposed minimum daily safe allowance (μg)
Dietary survey	19.1	13.3	16	
Calculation	19.2	16.0	18	40
Plasma GSHPx activity at plateau	40.9	–	–	

It can be seen that minimum Se requirements obtained either by calculation or by survey are doubled to take into account other variables and the amount obtained is fairly comparable with the value obtained by the GSHPx activity plateau method. It also agrees well with the minimum daily safe intake 50 µg/day suggested by the US National Research Council[4]. In China normal Se intakes excluding seleniferous area, fell into the range of 20–160 µg/day (Yang & Zhou 1985 unpublished).

1 Bai, J., Ge, K.Y., Den, X.J., Wu, S.Q., Wang, S.Q., Xue, A.N. & Sue, C.Q. (1982): The effect of selenium intake on myocardial necrosis induced by viral infection in mice. *Acta Nutrimenta Sinica* **4**, 235–241.
2 Chen, X.S., Yang, G.Q., Chen, J.S., Chen, X.C., Wen, Z.H. & Ge, K.Y. (1980): Studies on the relations of selenium and Keshan Disease. *Biol. Trac. Elem. Res.* **2**, 91–107.
3 Ferretti, R.J. & Levander, O.A. (1974): Effect of milling and processing on the selenium content of grains and cereal products. *Agr. Fd Chem.* **22**, 1049–1051.
4 FNB/NRC (Food & Nutrition Board/National Research Council, USA) (1980): *Recommended Dietary Allowances,* Washington DC: National Academy of Sciences.
5 Ge, K.Y., Chen, C.S., Xue, A.N., Bai, J., Wang, S.Q. & Menh, G.S. (1982): Morphological and histochemical observation of myocardium of Keshan Disease. *Acta Nutrimenta Sinica* **4**, 91–97.
6 Ge, K.Y., Xue, A.N., Bai, J. & Wang, S.Q. (1983): Keshan Disease — an endemic cardiomyopathy in China. *Virchows Arch. (Pathol. Anat.)* **401**, 1–15.
7 Higgs, D.J., Morris, V.C. & Levander, O.A. (1972): Effect of cooking on selenium content of foods. *Agr. Fd Chem.* **20**, 678–680.
8 KCAM (Keshan Disease Research Group of the Chinese Academy of Medical Sciences) (1979): Epidemiologic studies on the etiologic relationship of selenium and Keshan Disease. *Chin. Med. J.* **92**, 477–482.
9 KCAM (1979): Observations on effect of sodium selenite in prevention of Keshan Disease. *Chin. Med. J.* **92**, 471–476.
10 Levanded, O.A. (1972): Metabolic interrelationships and adaptations in selenium toxicity. *Ann. N.Y. Acad. Sci.* **192**, 181–192.

11 Li, F.S., Guan, J.Y., Li, L., Zhao, Y.H. & Bai, Q.F. (1982): Changes of Selenium content and composition of lipids in erythrocytes and plasma of children suffered from Keshan Disease, and their pathogenic significance. *Acta Nutrimenta Sinica* **4**, 221–226.

12 Thomson, C.D. & Robinson, M.F. (1980): Selenium in human health and disease with emphasis on those aspects peculiar to New Zealand. *Am. J. Clin. Nutr.* **33**, 303–323.

13 Wang, F. (1962): Discussion of the etiology of Keshan Disease based on the pathological findings. *Chin. Med. J.* **48**, 17–21.

14 Wang, G., Li, G.S. & An, R.Q. (1982): Studies on the etiologic relationship of molybdenum deficiency to Keshan Disease. *Acta Nutrimenta Sinica* **4**, 271–276.

15 XMC (Xian Medical College) (1979): Observations on the effects of sodium selenite for preventing acute Keshan Disease. *Chin. Med. J.* **59**, 457–460.

16 Yang, F.Y., Huang, F., Ling, Q.H., Zhang, K. & Shi, B.P. (1984): Alteration in biomembrane of patients suffered from Kaschin-Beck Disease in Yungshou county in *Investigation on Kaschin-Beck Disease in Yungshou*, pp. 366–371, ed Central Office on Prevention of Endemic Disease, Shenyang.

17 Yang, G.Q. (1983): On the relationship between selenium and the etiology of Keshan Disease. *Shenli Kuoxie Jinzhan* **14**, 313–317.

18 Yang, G.Q. (1985): Comment on the recent epidemiologic characteristics in relation to the possible existence of adaptation to low selenium intake in residents residing long in Keshan Disease areas. *Wesheng Yanjiu*, In the press.

19 Yang, G.Q., Zhu, L.Z., Liu, S.J. & Gu, L.Z. (1984): Studies of human selenium requirement in China. *Proceedings of the 3rd International Symposium on Selenium in Biology and Medicine, in Beijing.* In the press.

20 Yang, G.Q., Wang, G.Y., Yin, T.A., Sun, S.Z., Zhou, R.H. & Zhai, F.Y. (1982): Relationship between the distribution of Keshan Disease and selenium status. *Acta Nutrimenta Sinica* **4**, 191–200.

21 Yang, G.Q., Chen, J.S., Wen, Z.H., Ge, K.Y., Zhu, X.Z., Chen, X.C. & Chen, X.S. (1984): The role of selenium in Keshan Disease. In *Advances in nutrition research* ed H.H. Draper, pp. 203–231. New York: Plenum.

22 Yuan, C.H. (1983): A discussion on the etiology of Keshan Disease based upon the epidemiologic point of view. *Difang bing Tongxun* **47**, 35–38.

Nutritional status and cancer mortality in China

J. CHEN, R. PETO, J. LI and T.C. CAMPBELL
Institute of Health, China National Center for Preventive Medicine, 29 Nan Wei Road, Beijing, China; Clinical Trial Service Unit, Radcliffe Infirmary, University of Oxford, Oxford, UK; Cancer Institute, Chinese Academy of Medical Sciences Longtan Lake, Beijing, China; Division of Nutritional Sciences, Cornell University, Ithaca, NY 14853, USA.

During the past 20 years, there has been a renewed emphasis on the role of food in the development of cancer. More recently, an awareness has emerged that nutrients can also contribute to cancer risk[1]. Many published epidemiological studies have shown that total food intake, fat, selenium, ascorbic acid, vitamin A and carotene, are related to human cancer incidence or mortality[2]. However, most of these studies were only focused on single nutrients or based on questionnaire and survey. The present study was based on the assumption that cancer is a complex disease and can be affected by a considerable variety of food and nutrients. Therefore, multiple risk factors in China were studied and correlated with the available cancer mortality data for 14 cancer sites collected in 1973–75.

Survey protocol. Sixty-five rural counties with a population over 100 000 were systematically selected from a total of approximately 2000 counties. These counties represent the range of county, sex and organ-specific cancer mortality of rural population in 1973–75 in which seven main organ-specific cancers in China (nasopharynx, oesophagus, stomach, liver, lung, colon/rectum and breast) were included. A three-stage random cluster sampling procedure was used to select the survey commune and production teams. The household and individual subjects under investigation were also randomly selected.

The following information was collected: (a) intakes of foods, nutrients and other constituents of 30 households per county; (b) blood and urine assays for various nutrient and non-nutrient risk indicators of 100 subjects per county; (c) life-style/medical history by questionnaire obtained from 100 subjects per county.

Assays on blood, urine and food. Plasma: total/HDL cholesterol, triglyceride, selenium/glutathione peroxidase, retinol, retinol binding protein/RBP, carotene, tocopherols, ascorbic acid, pre-albumin, ferritin, transferrin, uric acid, trace elements, HBV antigen and antibody. Red blood cell: Fatty acid profile, folate, glutathione reductase. Urine: Ascorbic acid, riboflavin, creatinine, sulphate, N-nitroso compounds. Food: Trace elements, dietary fibre (neutral detergent fibre, cellulose, hemicellulose, lignins).

Statistical analysis. Ecological studies are being conducted on the county base between the sex specific cancer death rate (each cancer site) of the truncated age group of 35–64 years and the diet and nutrition data obtained in each county. Univariate correlation and multiple regression analysis of different methods are being used.

In order to maximize the collection of meaningful data at a minimal cost and carry out as many pertinent assays as possible, individual blood and urine samples were pooled sex specifically within each of the two survey sites in one county. Thus, there were four pools for each county. Validation tests have been carried out to compare the mathematical means of individual results with the results of pools. In all the assays, the analytical results of pool and the mean of individuals are very close to each other.

Preliminary results. The survey was completed in 1983 and most of the assays have been completed. Statistical analysis has just started.

A wide range of mortality data was observed in all of the main forms of cancer in the 65 counties (Table 1). There were few differences between the two survey sites within one county, but significant differences between the 65 counties in the biochemical and nutritional survey data.

Single correlation analysis (Pearson method) was carried out by using the transformed (log or square root) mortality data and some of the results obtained are listed in Table 2.

Table 1. *Range of annual cancer mortality rates (per 100 000) for males, 35–64 years- old, in 65 counties.*

Cancer sites	Range of mortality rates	Cancer sites	Range of mortality rates
Nasophaynx	0.9 – 75	Colon/rectum	1.3 – 68
Oesophagus	1.4 – 480	Lung	3.5 – 98
Stomach	6.0 – 386	Leukaemia	0.7 – 9.1
Liver	6.0 – 354	Total	35.0 – 782

Table 2. *Examples of univariate correlations showing the statistically significant (P <0.05) positive (+) or negative (−) correlations between the measured parameters and the organ or sites of recorded cancer in mortality records for male (m) or female (f) subjects in the survey.*

Measured parameter and trend (+ or −) of correlation	Organ or site of cancer
Plasma total cholesterol (+)	Liver (m,f), colon/rectum (m), lung (m), leukaemia (m,f), total (m)
Plasma β-carotene (−)	Stomach (m)
Plasma selenium (−)	Oesophagus (m,f), stomach (m,f)
Plasma ascorbic acid (−)	Oesophagus (m), stomach (m), total (f)
Plasma RBP (−)	Nasopharynx (f)
Protein intake (+)	Oesophagus (m,f), stomach (m,f), colon/rectum (f), lung (f), leukaemia (m,f), total (f)

Very preliminary multiple regression analysis showed that total plasma cholesterol, plasma ascorbic acid, plasma selenium, lignin intake and urinary N-nitroso compound excretion are synergistically significantly correlated with oesophagus and stomach cancer mortality.

1 Doll, R. & Peto, R. (1981): The causes of cancer: quantitative estimate of avoidable risks of cancer in the United States Today. *J. Natl. Cancer Inst.* **66**, 1191.
2 Committee on Diet, Nutrition and Cancer, National Research Council (1982): *Diet, Nutrition and Cancer.* Washington DC: National Academy Press.

Nutrient deficiencies and malaria: a curse or a blessing?

D.I. THURNHAM
The Wolfson Research Laboratories, Queen Elizabeth Medical Centre, Birmingham, and Clinical Investigation Unit, Dudley Road Hospital, Birmingham B18 7QH, United Kingdom.

There have been several suggestions in the literature that malnutrition may give man some protection against malaria and refeeding has been associated with recrudescence of latent infections. This paper will examine some of the experimental work on the effects of specific nutrient-deficiencies on host-parasite relationships and discuss its relevance in man.

Experimental studies. *Vitamin A and protein energy malnutrition.* The influence of a nutrient deficiency on the *in vitro* development of malaria parasites does not necessarily predict the effect of that deficiency on the parasite within the host. Only biotin deficiency was reported to have a direct and appreciable effect on the development of *Plasmodium knowlesi* in culture[20].

In contrast, within experimental host-parasite systems, most nutritional deficiencies depress parasite growth although some have the opposite effect. For example the multiplication of *P. berghei* was stimulated in vitamin-A-deficient rats[12]. In the well-nourished, control rats, the host's immunity was able to overcome the infection, parasiteaemias remained low and no animal died over the 5-week experiment. In vitamin-A-deficient rats, however, the parasitaemias increased rapidly and all animals died by 7 days. There was a leukopenia and the immune response to antigen was impaired.

The pair-fed controls in these experiments however were protein and energy malnourished since they received restricted amounts of food and their weight gain was gradually reduced to negligible amounts around 7 to 10 weeks to match the vitamin-A-deficient rats. Immune response was impaired in these animals also, since mortality was 100 per cent although parasitaemias were only slightly increased.

Folate and 4-aminobenzoic acid (PABA) deficiencies. Malaria species require folate for their growth but can synthesise their requirements from PABA. Thus folate deficiency is probably more damaging to the host than the parasite and it has been suggested that it may enhance maternal immunosuppression in pregnancy and derange the fetal immune system[2].

By contrast, deficiencies of PABA in rats[14] and monkeys[3] caused by feeding milk diets, suppress parasite development directly, allowing the host to overcome the infection.

Protein-deficiency. The effects of protein-deficiency on rodent malaria were recently described[7]. They used an actively growing form of *P. berghei* in young, non-immune rats and obtained an 80 per cent mortality. They showed that by restricting the quantity of protein, in otherwise iso-caloric diets, the parasitaemia was reduced and all rats survived. As the response to the reduced protein intake was so rapid, the authors suggested it was unlikely that the protection was due to developing immunity, but more likely that the supply of essential amino acids was directly limiting parasite growth. Support for this idea was obtained by supplementing the 4.2 per cent casein diet with the essential amino acids threonine, isoleucine and valine which produced a considerable increase in the level of infection[7].

Tocopherol, ascorbic-acid and riboflavin (B_2) deficiencies. Deficiencies of tocopherol, ascorbic acid and riboflavin also depress parasite growth, but, in contrast to essential amino acids or PABA, most animals deficient in E and B_2 succumbed to the infection. Vitamins E and C, and also riboflavin via its coenzyme role in the regeneration of reduced glutathione (GSH), have antioxidant properties. The mechanisms by which deficiencies of these latter nutrients depress parasite growth but fail in the case of vitamins E and B_2 to prevent the hosts' mortality are only partially resolved but recent research suggests some intriguing possibilities.

We recently undertook some experiments involving riboflavin-deficient rats infected with *P. berghei*[11]. We anticipated that the riboflavin-deficiency would interact with the parasite in a similar manner to the effects of glucose-6-phosphate dehydrogenase (G6PD) deficiency. In G6PD deficiency, the red cell becomes more susceptible to oxidant damage since the supply of NADPH for the synthesis of GSH is impaired. When the system is under oxidative stress, riboflavin availability may control the regeneration of GSH from GSSG in the red cell. Hence if the red cell is unable to meet the oxidative stress imposed by the presence of the parasite, it ruptures prematurely liberating the parasite before it can multiply.

Riboflavin-deficiency could indeed inhibit development of parasites, sometimes totally, in inverse proportion to the riboflavin status. In spite of this, however, all animals died after only a slightly longer duration of infection than in the control groups. Deaths would not have been expected from riboflavin-deficiency alone and the cause of death in the face of such low parasite counts is difficult to explain, but we suspect that an associated factor may have been anaemia. There was more evidence of haematuria in the cages of the infected, riboflavin-deficient animals than in those of infected controls. In addition, anaemia has also been indicated as a complicating factor in the deaths of vitamin-C-deficient monkeys[16] and in vitamin-E-deficient rats[6] infected with malaria.

The reduced parasitaemias in all three systems may therefore be explained by the cell-rupture hypothesis, but why does this not terminate the infection? The malaria parasite generates peroxide[8] and haemoglobin can react with peroxide to produce superoxide[9]. Superoxide can pass through plasma membranes[13] but is not particularly damaging itself[10]. Drugs which generate superoxide produce hydroxyl radicals in malaria-infected rats[5], free iron or porphyrin[4] will catalyse the formation of hydroxyl free-radicals which are much more potent oxidising agents of unsaturated lipid in plasma membranes than superoxide. Antioxidants stabilize the unsaturated lipid in membrane structures thus, the reduced antioxidant concentration occasioned by the vitamin deficiencies will increase red cell vulnerability to haemolysis. More haemolysis will increase the amount of porphyrin iron in the plasma to catalyse the formation of more hydroxyl radical. Thus a vicious cycle may be established where the increasing haemolysis increases the production of the hydroxyl radical, causing damage not just to red cells but also to the vascular endothelial lining, and contributing to cerebral damage and pulmonary and renal insufficiency, particularly when blood vessels become congested with adhering parasitized red cells.

Vitamin-C-deficiency in the monkeys differed from deficiencies of tocopherol and riboflavin in rats in that the infection appeared to be contained by the deficiency long enough in most cases for the immune system to act. In the riboflavin experiments, the rats were too immature to mount an immune response but if older rats had been used or a different host, where the immune system was more developed, these animals may also have contained the infection. If this is the case, then such deficiencies with the support of the immune system should protect against malaria, but in the non-immune person such deficiencies could well augment the disease process. In this context it is interesting that while the two acute and serious forms of malaria — viz blackwater fever and cerebral malaria — occur frequently in association with G6PD deficiency, they also commonly occur in non-immune immigrants in malaria-endemic areas[15,19].

Malaria in man. Extensive haemolysis is a well-known feature of malaria for which there is still no satisfactory explanation. Could it be connected with deficiencies of vitamins E, C or B_2? It has been suggested that vitamin E deficiencies limit the severity of malaria in herding peoples in Eastern Niger where the diet consists of defatted and rancid milk derivatives[6] and following the provision of grain there was a recrudescence of latent malaria[17]. Such diets are uncommon, but riboflavin deficiency is likely to be far more common in many malaria-endemic areas, due to the lack of milk products in the diet. Riboflavin deficiency however has not been associated with any protective effects against malaria in man apart from the one study in Papua New Guinea where five cases of malaria occurred in 87 infants under 12 months[21]. Not only was the riboflavin status of the malaria-infected infants significantly better than that of the non-infected infants but also the density of parasites in the blood was inversely proportional to the riboflavin status. That is the heaviest infection was present in the activation coefficient and *vice versa*. The numbers involved in this study were too small to be very convincing but workers in the Gambia have recently showed that a significantly greater parasite density was found in 86 children who were supplemented for 3 months with riboflavin, thiamin, vitamin C and iron than in 76 who received the placebo[1]. The effect was small in spite of the fact that the status of vitamins C and B_2 and of iron was poor in the placebo group. However clinics were on hand for treatment so the chance of a large difference developing between the two groups was unlikely.

Lastly, prevalence of malaria in infants in Papua New Guinea following i.m. iron or placebo has been reported[18]. The relative risk of malaria at both 6 and 12 months was doubled in the iron-supplemented group. An excess of iron may stimulate the formation of hydroxyl radicals, exacerbate membrane damage and increase the severity of the disease.

Acknowledgements. the author is supported by the Department of Health & Social Security, UK.

1 Bates, C.J., Powers, H.J., Lamb, W.H., Gelman, W. & Webb, E. (1985): Effect of supplementary vitamins and iron on malaria indices in rural Gambian children. *Trans R. Soc. Trop. Med. Hyg.* In press.
2 Brabin, B.J. (1982): Hypothesis: the importance of folacin in influencing susceptibility to malaria infection in infants. *Am. J. Clin. Nutr.* **35**, 146–151.
3 Bray, R.S. & Garnham, P.C.C. (1953): Effect of milk diet on *P. cynomolgi* infections in monkeys. *Br. Med. J.* **7**, 1200–1201.
4 Chance, B., Sies, H. & Boveris, A. (1979): Hydroperoxide metabolism in mammalian organs. *Physiol. Rev.* **59**, 527–605.
5 Clarke, I.A. & Hunt, N.H. (1983): Evidence for reactive oxygen intermediates causing haemolysis and parasite death in malaria. *Inf. Imm.* **39**, 1–6.
6 Eckman, J.R., Eaton, J.W., Berger, E. & Jacob, H.S. (1976): Role of vitamin E in regulating malaria expression. *Trans Ass. Am. Physiol.* **89**, 105–113.
7 Edirisinghe, J.S., Fern, E.B. & Target, G.A.T. (1981): Dietary suppression of rodent malaria. *Trans R. Soc. Trop. Med. Hyg.* **75**, 591–593.
8 Etkin, N.L. & Eaton, J.W. (1975): Malaria-induced erythrocyte oxidant sensitivity. In *Erythrocyte structure and function*, ed G.J. Brewer, pp. 219–232. New York: Liss.
9 Friedman, M.J. (1982): The biochemical ecology of intracellular parasites. *Trends Biochem. Sci.* **7**, 332–334.
10 Halliwell, B. & Gutteridge, J.M.C. (1985): In: *Free radicals in biology and medicine*. Oxford: Clarendon Press.
11 Kaikai, P. & Thurnham, D.I. (1983): The influence of riboflavin deficiency on *Plasmodium berghei* infection in rats. *Trans R. Soc. Trop. Med. Hyg.* **77**, 680–686.
12 Krishnan, S., Krishnan, A.D., Mustafa, A.S., Talwar, G.P. & Ramalingaswami, V. (1975): Effects of vitamin A and undernutrition on the susceptibility of rodents to a malaria parasite *Plasmodium berghei*. *J. Nutr.* **106**, 784–791.
13 Lynch, R.E. & Fridovich, I. (1978): Permeation of the erythrocyte stroma by superoxide radical. *J. biol. Chem.* **253**, 4697–4699.
14 Maegraith, B.G., Deegan, T. & Sherwood Jones, E. (1952): Supression of malaria (*P. berghei*) by milk. *Br. Med. J.* **2**, 1382–1384.
15 Manson-Bahr, P.E.C. & Apted, F.I.C. (1982): Malaria and babesiosis, In *Manson's tropical diseases*, ed P.E.C. Manson-Bahr & F.I.C. Apted, 18th edn, pp. 38–71. London: Ballière Tindall.
16 McKee, R.W. & Geiman, Q.M. (1946): Studies on malaria parasites. V. Effects of ascorbic acid on malaria. (*Plasmodium knowlesi*) in monkeys. *Proc. Soc. Exptl Biol. Med.* **63**, 313–315.
17 Murray, M.J., Murray, A.B., Murray, M.B. & Murray, C.J. (1976): Somali food shelters in the Ogaden famine and their impact on health. *Lancet* **1**, 1283–1285.
18 Oppenheimer, S.J., Gibson, F.D., Macfarland, S.B., Moody, J.B. & Hendrickse, R.G. (1984): Iron supplementation and malaria. *Lancet* **1**, 389–390.
19 Phillips, R.E., Looareesuwan, S., Warrell, D.A., Lee, S.H., Merry, A. & Weatherall, D.J. (1985): Anaemia and P. falciparum malaria. *Quart. J. Med.* In the press.
20 Trager, W. (1977): Cofactors and vitamins in the metabolism of malaria parasites. Factors other than folates. *Bull. WHO* **55**, 286–289.
21 Thurnham, D.I., Oppenheimer, S.J. & Bull, R. (1983): Riboflavin status and malaria in infants in Papua New Guinea. *Trans R. Soc. Trop. Med. Hyg.* **77**, 423–424.

Immune response and infection in relation to vitamin A and iron deficiency in children

P. BHASKARAM
National Institute of Nutrition, Indian Council of Medical Research, Jamai Osmania PO, Hyderabad 500007, India.

Single-nutrient deficiencies are uncommon in humans. They often co-exist with protein-energy malnutrition (PEM) and there are interactions between micronutrient-deficiency, infection and immunity in the case of vitamin A, iron and B-complex-deficiencies in children of apparently normal nutritional status.

The role of vitamin A in offering resistance against infection was recognized by Larsen 56 years ago[19]. Epidemiological and clinical investigations indicate consistent synergism between vitamin-A-deprivation and infection.

Hypovitaminosis A. *Vitamin A and infection.* Chronic laryngitis was reported in adults with hypovitaminosis A[30]. McLaren observed higher mortality attributable to vitamin A deficiency among malnourished children[22]. Higher mortality rates and increased risk due to infections in children with mild vitamin-A-deficiency have been recently reported[27,28]. Though the exact mechanism of precipitation of infections by vitamin-A-deficiency is not clear, alterations in mucosal surfaces and altered immune status have been proposed.

Several workers demonstrated disturbances in circulating vitamin A levels during acute and chronic infections[13,25]. Recent studies reported from National Institute of Nutrition emphasize these observations in children with measles[7] and in those with bronchopneumonia[6]. The extent to which measles causes disturbances in vitamin A levels was investigated in an urban slum. This longitudinal study in children aged below 5 years was carried out as a part of the Indo-US collaborative project on comprehensive studies in the prevention of nutritional blindness. Serum retinol and retinol-binding protein (RBP) levels were estimated before, during, and 8 weeks after the development of measles. A significant decrease in serum vitamin A levels was observed during measles from the premeasles level, the latter being determined about 2 to 7 days prior to the onset of measles. However, the vitamin A levels returned to premeasles levels within 8 weeks without any nutritional intervention. Serum RBP levels closely followed retinol levels (Fig. 1,[24]). The pathophysiological consequences of these short-term disturbances of serum vitamin A levels in common childhood infections are not clear. However, in developing countries where PEM and infectious diseases are often co-existent, disturbances in vitamin A level though of short duration might be significant.

Vitamin-A-deficiency and immune response. Immunological studies were carried out in children aged below 6 years and suffering from signs of vitamin-A-deficiency manifesting as Bitot's spots or nightblindness. Children with severe PEM or associated infection were excluded from the study. Children matched for age, sex and nutritional status served as controls. Humoral immune response as assessed by the percentage of B cells in circulation and the antibody response to a challenge with tetanus toxoid were not affected[18]. However, lysozyme levels in serum as well as in leukocytes in vitamin-A-deficient children were found to be decreased compared with the controls[23]. Cell-mediated immune response (CMI) was assessed by determining the percentage of lymphocytes in peripheral circulation and lymphocyte proliferative response was determined by measuring the incorporation of ^{3}H thymidine into DNA by *in vitro* lymphocyte cultures on stimulation with PHA. The T-lymphocyte counts showed a slight but significant decrease while the proliferative response remained unchanged in the deficient children compared with the controls[5]. Treatment with vitamin A improved the total circulating T cell number[6] (Fig. 2).

These observations indicate that the effect of vitamin-A-deficiency on cell-mediated immune system is marginal and reversible. Though the mechanism of the reduction of total circulating T cell number is not clear, the adjuvant role of vitamin A in lymphocyte proliferation is proposed[1].

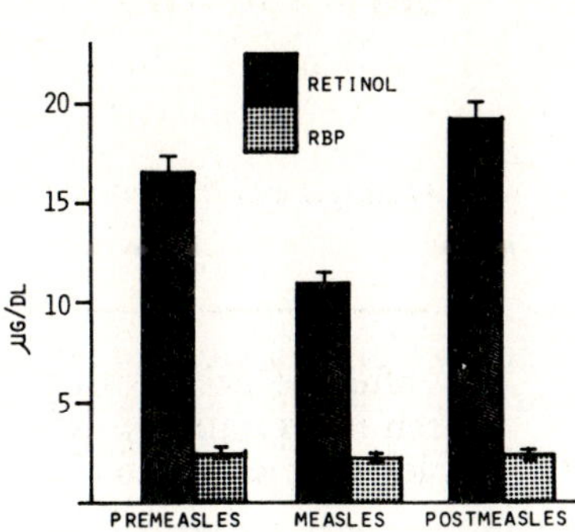

Fig. 1. *Serum retinol levels in measles.*

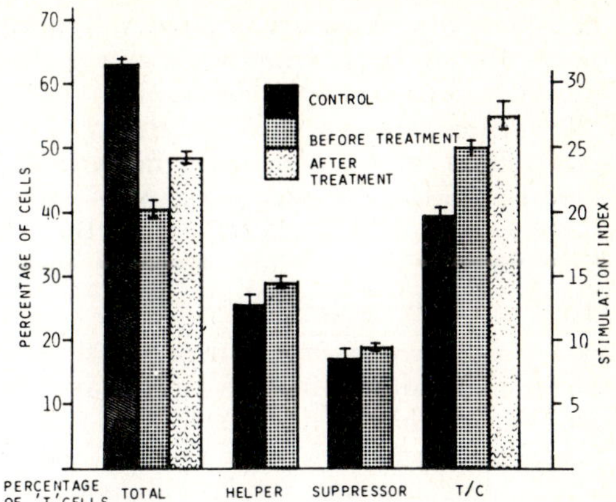

Fig. 2. *Cell-mediated immune response in vitamin A deficiency.*

Iron-deficiency. Nutritional anaemia is one of the public health problems of the developing countries affecting people of all ages and causing significant disturbances. Iron deficiency has been found to be by far the commonest cause of nutritional anaemias. Anaemia is, however, a late stage of manifestation of iron-deficiency and is preceeded by a period of tissue iron deprivation described as latent iron-deficiency. Amongst its other roles iron is a cofactor for the function of many enzymes that govern proliferation of cells including those of immune system.

Anaemia and infection. Epidemiological observations have demonstrated the association of iron-deficiency anaemia and increased risk of infections[2]. The association between lesions of herpes viral infection and iron-deficiency anaemia has been described[8]. Decrease in the frequency of infections in iron-deficient children following supplementation with iron has been reported[3].

However, some clinical and community studies suggested the protective role of iron-deficiency anaemia against infections[21] and the lack of significant effect of iron supplementation in decreasing the morbidity due to infections[10,14]. These reported interactions between iron-deficiency and infection need careful scrutiny.

Immune response in severe iron deficiency anaemia. Bactericidal activity (BCA) of neutrophils was low in severely anaemic children[29]. The impaired function was due to decrease in the levels of myeloperoxidase, an important iron-dependent bactericidal system in the neutrophils[26].

Normal B lymphocyte counts and immunoglobulin levels were reported in a study of humoral response[4]. Antibody response to tetanus toxoid was also satisfactory. However, serum complement levels were low in severely anaemic children[15].

CMI response was significantly impaired in severely anaemic children. The T cell percentage, as well as lymphocyte proliferative response, were grossly impaired. Delayed cutaneous hypersensitivity reaction tested with phytohaemagglutinin (PHA) was negative in five out of nine children. Reinvestigation of these children 4 weeks after adequate therapy with iron showed an increase in T lymphocyte count, but the proliferative response of lymphocytes remained unchanged. Nor did the skin test show much improvement over the original observation[5]. These observations on severe iron-deficiency anaemia on various immune functions are in agreement with a number of other reports[9,16,20].

However, no alterations in CMI status of children with iron-deficiency anaemia were observed by one group[17]. These differences in observations could be due to the differences in patient population and/or the tests employed, to assess the immune functions.

One could conclude that iron-deficiency anaemia would lead in general to alterations in immune response contributing to increased risk of infections. Reversal of the defects with iron therapy further supports this contention.

Milder grades of anaemia and host-resistance. Though severe iron deficiency anaemia is not an uncommon observation in the community, children suffering from milder grades of anaemia outnumber those with severe anaemia. It is important to investigate the immuno-competence of these children to understand the degree of interactions between anaemia and morbidity which might affect the vaccination programmes in communities where anaemia is prevalent and to draw priorities for programmes planned for prevention and control of anaemia.

Bactericidal activity of neutrophils and CMI status were assessed in children having various Hb levels. Both these functions were significantly impaired in children having Hb levels <10 g/dl compared with those having Hb >10 g/dl. Children with Hb levels <8 g/dl however, had the lowest values. Both the functions were restored to normal levels 12 weeks after administration of adequate dose of iron[29].

Latent iron-deficiency and immune response. Fifteen per cent of the children in the study had Hb levels more than 10 g/dl but had low iron status suggesting the presence of latent iron-deficiency. These children showed decreased BCA of neutrophils and also had low CMI response[30].

These observations highlight the public health importance of the functional deficits caused by iron-deficiency anaemia and latent iron-deficiency and explain the perpetuation of infections among iron-deficient children in the community.

B-complex deficiency. Experimental studies have clearly demonstrated impaired immune response in B-complex deficiency. However, information available in humans is meagre. Our studies in children suffering from angular stomatitis and glossitis showed no effect on cell-mediated immune status[5].

However,[11] and[12] demonstrated impaired CMI response in folate deficient children and women respectively.

1 Allison, A.C. & Davis, A.J.S. (1971): Requirement of thymus dependent lymphocytes for potentiation by adjuvants of antibody formation. *Nature Lond.* **233**, 330–332.

2 Andelman, M.B. & Sered, B.R. (1966): Utilization of dietary iron by term infants. A study of 1,048 infants from a low socio-economic population. *Am. J. Dis. Child.* **111**, 45–55.

3 Arberter, A., Echevens, C., Franco, D., Munson, D., Velez, H. & Velez, J.J. (1971): Nutrition and infection *Fed. Proc.* **30**, 1421–1428.

4 Bagchi, K., Mohan Ram, M. & Reddy, V. (1980): Humoral immune response in iron deficiency anemia. *Br. Med. J.* **280**, 1240–51.

5 Bhaskaram, C. & Reddy, V. (1975): Cell mediated immunity in iron and vitamin deficient children. *Br. Med. J.* **3**, 522.

6 Bhaskaram, P., Mathur, R., Rao, V., Madhusudan, J., Radhakrishna, K.V., Raghuramulu, N. & Reddy, V. (1985): Pathogenesis of corneal lesions in measles (In press).

7 Bhaskaram, P., Reddy, V., Raj, S. & Bhatnagar, R.C. (1984): Effect of measles on the nutritional status of preschool children. *J. Trop. Med. Hyg.* **87**, 21–25.

8 Chandra, R.K. (1985): Trace element regulation of immunity and infection. *J. Am. Coll. Nutr.* **4**, 5–16.

9 Chandra, R.K. & Saraya, A.K. (1975): Impaired immunocompetence associated with iron deficiency. *J. Pediatr.* **86**, 899–902.

10 Damodaran, M., Naidu, A.N. & Sharma, R.K.V. (1979): Anemia and morbidity in rural preschool children. *Ind. J. Med. Res.* **69**, 448–456.

11 Das, K.C. & Hoffbrand, A.V. (1970): Lymphocyte transformation in myeloblastic anemia morphology and DNA synthesis. *Br. J. Haematol.* **19**, 459–468.

12 Gross, R.L., Reid, J.V., Newberne, D., Burgers, B., Marson, R. & Huff, W. (1975): Depressed cell mediated immunity due to folic acid deficiency. *Am. J. Clin. Nutr.* **28**, 225–232.

13 Harris, A.D. & Moore, T. (1978): Vitamin A in infective hepatitis. *Br. Med. J.* **1**, 553–558.

14 Howell, D. (1971): Consequences of milk iron deficiency in children. In *Proceedings of workshop on extent and meaning of iron deficiency in the US*, ed G. Goldsmith, p. 65 Washington DC: National Research Council.

15 Jagadeesan, V. & Reddy, V. (1979): Serum complement levels in malnourished children. *Ind. J. Med. Res.* **70**, 745–749.

16 Joynson, D.H.M., Murray Walker, D., Jacobs, A. & Dolby, A.E. (1972): Defect on cell mediated immunity in patients with iron deficiency anemia. *Lancet* **2**, 1058–1059.

17 Kulapongs P., Vithayasai, V., Suskind, R. & Olson, R.E. (1974): Cell mediated immunity and phagocytosis and killing function in children with severe iron deficiency anemia. *Lancet* **2**, 689–691.

18 Kutty, P.M., Moharam, M. & Reddy, V. (1981): Humoral immune response in vitamin A deficient children. *Acta. vitaminol. Enzymol.* **3**, 231.

19 Larsen, H.C.A (1930): Vitamin A deficiency and resistance to specific infection. *J. Hyg.* **30**, 300.

20 MacDougall, L.G. & Jacobs, M.R. (1978): The immune response in iron deficient children. *S. Afr. Med. J.* **53**, 405–407.

21 Masawe, A.E.J., Muindi, J.M. & Swai, G.B.R. (1974): Infections in iron deficiency and other types of anemia in the tropics. *Lancet* **2**, 314–317.
22 Mclaren, D.A. (1964): Xerophthalmia: a neglected problem. *Nutr. Rev.* **22**, 289.
23 Mohanram, M., Reddy, V. & Misra, S. (1974): Lysozyme activity in plasma and leukocytes in malnourished children. *Br. J. Nutr.* **32**, 313–316.
24 National Institute of Nutrition, (1983): Annual Report, pp. 54–62.
25 Oomen, H.A.P.C. (1958): Clinical experience on Hypovitaminosis A. *Fed. Proc.* **17**, Suppl 2, 103–143.
26 Sivaprasad, J. (1979): Leukocyte function in iron deficiency anemia. *Am. J. Clin. Nutr.* **32**, 550–552.
27 Sommer, A., Tarwotjo, I., Hussaini, G. & Susanto, D. (1983): Increased mortality in children with mild vitamin A deficiency. *Lancet* **2**, 585–588.
28 Sommer, A., Katz, J. & Tarwotjo, I. (1984): Increased risk of respiratory disease and diarrhoea in children with pre-existing mild vitamin A deficiency. *Am. J. Clin. Nutr.* **40**, 1090–1095.
29 Srikantia, S.G., Bhaskaram, C., Sivaprasad, J. & Krishnamachari, K.A.V.R. (1976): Anemia and immune response. *Lancet* **1**, 1307.
30 Stell, P.M. & Mclonghlin, M.P. (1972): Vitamin A and chronic laryngitis. *Lancet* **1**, 147–158.

Micronutrient deficiencies in the aetiology of anaemia

Hilary J. POWERS
University of Cambridge and Medical Research Council, Dunn Nutrition Unit, Milton Road, Cambridge CB4 1XJ, UK.

West Kiang is a subsistence farming region of The Gambia. Reports of an iron-responsive anaemia, in association with the seasonal incidence of hookworm and malaria, were published as early as the 1960s[5,12]. Our investigations into the functional significance of marginal vitamin-deficiencies, and of riboflavin in particular, have included controlled supplementation trials in West Kiang during a time when food is scarce, and malaria and hookworm have peak incidence[6,8]. These studies have enabled us to clarify the current situation regarding the aetiology of anaemia among men and lactating women in this region.

Observations. Among the men (80) prior to receiving iron (200 mg $FeSO_4$) or riboflavin (5 mg) daily, there were a few cases of frank anaemia, and the high proportion of cases with low mean cell haemoglobin concentrations (62 per cent) and low plasma iron (79 per cent) suggested that iron-deficiency was the most important determinant of anaemia (Table 1). Subclinical

Table 1. *Haematology and biochemical status of 80 men and 63 women prior to supplementation.* (Numbers in parentheses denote references).

Variable*	Mean		Range		Lower limits of normality		% Falling outside normal range	
	Men	Women	Men	Women	Men	Women	Men	Women
Hb (g/dl)	11.86	12.00	4.90–14.5	9.1–14.1	13.0[3]	12.0[13]	71.8	41
PCV (%)	35.6	33.8	19.0–43.0	23.9–39.8	40.0[3]	36[13]	88.7	75
MCV (fl)	77.2	81.7	51.0–96.0	65–100	77.0[3]	77[3]	46.5	15
RBC (10^{12}/l)	4.63	4.80	3.44–6.33	3.21–5.17	4.5[3]	3.8[3]	46.5	21
Plasma:								
iron (μmol/l)	9.14	9.52	0–24.43	3.70–17.61	13.0[3]	8.9[13]	78.9	44
ferritin (ng/ml)	25.1	24.9	0–87.6	4.6–83.2	10[4]	10[9]	29.4	8
ascorbic acid (ng/ml)	0.44	0.15	0.02–1.32	0.02–0.56	0.10[10]	0.1[10]	10.9	31.9
folic acid (ng/ml)	2.6	1.96	0.3–10	0–5.0	2.0[2,10]	2.0[2,10]	46.2	53.1
RBC folic acid (ng/ml cells)	254	159	42–535	0–425	100[2,10]	100[2,10]	9.7	16.9
EGRAC	2.42	2.30	1.59–3.58	1.31–3.06	1.3	1.30	100	100

*Abbreviations: Hb — haemoglobin. PCV — packed cell volume. MCV — mean cell volume. RBC — red blood cell. EGRAC — erythrocyte glutathione reductase activation coefficient (>1.30, with the exception of subjects deficient in glucose-6-phosphate dehydrogenase).

riboflavin-deficiency was evident in all subjects, with the exception of those with glucose-6-phosphate dehydrogenase (G6PD) deficiency[11] and folic acid and ascorbic acid status was also low in some of the men. The haematological status of the lactating women (63) prior to receiving daily supplements of riboflavin (5 mg), iron (30 mg $FeSO_4$) or riboflavin in addition to iron was generally not as poor as that observed among the men (Table 1). Strong correlations between Hb and plasma iron ($P < 0.001$) and plasma ferritin ($P < 0.001$) indicated that iron lack was the major cause of the poor haematology. Subclinical riboflavin-deficiency was evident in all women with normal G6PD activity, and ascorbic acid and folate status were generally poor.

Table 2. *Relationship between poor folate status and macrocytosis, prior to supplementation.* (For abbreviations see Table 1).

	Men		Lactating women	
	MCV <90 fl ($n = 64$)	*MCV >90 fl* ($n = 8$)	*MCV <90 fl* ($n = 52$)	*MCV >90 f* ($n = 11$)
RBC folate (ng/ml cells)[a]	264 ± 17	160 ± 14*	158 ± 9	144 ± 26
Percentage of subjects with RBC folate levels below 100 ng/ml cells	9.4	12.5	15.4	36.4***

Comparison between groups differentiated on the basis of MCV: *$P<0.05$ (t-test), ***$P<0.001$ (X^2 test)
[a]mean ± s.e.m.

There was some evidence for a macrocytic response to low folate status in some of the men and lactating women (Table 2). A subgroup of men with initial mean cell volume (MCV) >90 fl had significantly lower levels of RBC folate than the rest of the sample. In addition, whereas circulating Hb in this subgroup fell during the 6-week study the remaining subjects showed an improvement, and the difference in the response of the two groups was significant ($P < 0.05$). Similarly, a chi-squared analysis of the percentage of women with RBC folate <100 ng ml, compared with that in a subgroup having MCV >90 fl, was significant at $\chi^2 = 11.6$ and $P < 0.001$.

After 6 weeks, supplemental iron had elicited a response in a number of haematological variables in the men, but the presence of riboflavin in addition to iron enhanced the haematological improvement. In a subgroup of men with initially low Hb (<11.5 g/dl) the benefit of riboflavin in addition to iron was especially clear-cut (Table 3). Whereas the effect of 30 mg $FeSO_4$ given to the women was evidently sufficient merely to prevent a deterioration in haematological status; the presence of riboflavin, in addition to the iron, had the effect of increasing both circulating plasma iron and plasma ferritin, which reflects hepatic iron stores (Table 4). Neither folic acid nor ascorbic acid status in men or women was influenced by iron or riboflavin-supplements. Riboflavin status, however, showed a dramatic improvement in both men and women in response to riboflavin in the supplement. All subjects received malaria prophylaxis during the studies and hookworm severity and incidence were very low[6,8].

Conclusions. It is clear that subclinical deficiencies of riboflavin, ascorbic acid, iron and folic acid occur in West Kiang in the rainy season, all of which have some role to play in normal erythrokinetics, and that there are equally clear seasonal fluctuations in the incidence of malaria and hookworm. The major dietary determinant of anaemia in this community is iron deficiency, but the enhanced recovery observed when riboflavin is given in addition to iron-supplements is consistent with a role for riboflavin in promoting iron-utilization. A number of animal studies have indicated that iron release from ferritin may be flavin-dependent and that in consequence riboflavin-deficiency may impair the mobilisation of iron stores and possibly iron absorption as well[1,7,8,14]. Riboflavin deficiency in this community may compromise iron-utilization. Very poor folate status appears to contribute to the anaemia observed in some men and women and may have limited the response to iron-supplements. The extent to which poor ascorbic acid

Table 3. *Mean haematological changes ($\pm$ s.e.m.) in men with initial haemoglobin of 11.5 g/dl or less to 6 weeks of supplementation with iron or iron plus riboflavin.*

| | | Supplement | |
Variable	Placebo	Iron	Iron plus riboflavin
Hb (g/dl)[1]	0.46 ± 0.31	1.90 ± 0.64†	2.27 ± 0.76††
PCV (%)	-1.71 ± 1.49	2.17 ± 1.47	5.83 ± 2.91**
MCV (fl)	6.29 ± 1.67	8.54 ± 1.04	10.17 ± 1.90**
MCH[a] (pg)	1.76 ± 0.56	5.17 ± 0.70†	4.20 ± 0.34*
RBC $\times$ $(10^{12}/l)$	-0.14 ± 0.15	-0.11 ± 0.15	0.39 ± 0.39*
Plasma iron (μmol/l)	-2.39 ± 1.86	5.36 ± 2.04	6.92 ± 2.39*
Transferrin saturation (%)	-6.33 ± 4.40	9.99 ± 4.10	9.82 ± 3.69†
Plasma ferritin (ng/ml)	-7.14 ± 6.56	19.99 ± 8.27	33.50 ± 13.22**

Change significantly different from placebo: *$P<0.05$, **$P<0.02$, †$P<0.01$, ††$P<0.001$

[a]MCH — mean cell haemoglobin. For other abbreviations see Table 1.

Table 4. *Mean haematological changes ($\pm$ s.e.m.) in lactating women to six weeks of supplementation with iron, riboflavin or both supplements.* (For abbreviations see Table 1).

| | | Supplement | | |
Variable	Placebo	Riboflavin	Iron	Iron plus riboflavin
Hb (g/dl)	0.22 ± 0.26	0.34 ± 0.26	0.68 ± 0.22	0.66 ± 0.19
PCV (%)	3.19 ± 0.75	2.92 ± 0.87	2.99 ± 0.62	4.24 ± 0.65
MCV (fl)	0.07 ± 0.95	-1.63 ± 0.94	-0.93 ± 0.65	0.01 ± 0.57
RBC $(10^{12}/l)$	0.37 ± 0.10	0.47 ± 0.09	0.47 ± 0.08	0.53 ± 0.08
Plasma iron (μmol/l)	1.12 ± 1.19	-2.57 ± 1.00	3.14 ± 1.14	7.71 ± 1.58*
Plasma ferritin (ng/ml)	-4.62 ± 2.73	-1.26 ± 3.13	0.36 ± 4.90	4.81 ± 3.29*
EGRAC	0.65 ± 0.09	-0.89 ± 0.08***	0.64 ± 0.08	-0.85 ± 0.08***

Change significantly different from placebo: *$P < 0.05$, ***$P < 0.001$

status may have compromised the potential for non-haem iron absorption and have contributed to the anaemia is unclear.

Acknowledgement. The author acknowledges receipt of a post-doctoral award from F. Hoffman-La Roche and Co. Ltd., Basel.

1 Adelekan, D.A. & Thurnham, D.I. (1981): A longitudinal study on the effect of riboflavin status on aspects of iron storage in the liver of growing rats. *Proc. Nutr. Soc.* **40**, 101A.

2 Chanarin, I. (1979): *The megaloblastic anaemias*, 2nd edn, p. 193, Blackwell Scientific Publications, Oxford.

3 Dacie, J.V. & Lewis, S.M. (1975): *Practical haematology*, p. 12, Churchill Livingstone, Edinburgh.

4 Jacobs, A., Miller, F., Worwood, M., Beamish, M.R. & Woodrop, C.A. (1972): Ferritin in the serum of normal subjects and patients with iron deficiency and iron overload. *Br. Med. J.* **4**, 206–208.

5 McGregor, A., Williams, K., Billewicz, W.Z. & Thomson, A.M. (1966): Haemoglobin concentration and anaemia in young West African (Gambian) children. *Trans. Roy. Soc. Trop. Med. Hyg*, **60**, 650–667.

6 Powers, H.J., Bates, C.J., Prentice, A.M., Lamb, W.H., Jepson, M. & Bowman, H. (1983): The relative effectiveness of iron and iron with riboflavin in correcting a microcytic anaemia in men and children in rural Gambia. *Hum. Nutr.: Clin Nutr.* **37C**, 413–425.

7 Powers, H.J., Bates, C.J. & Duerden, J.M. (1983): Effects of riboflavin deficiency in rats on some aspects of iron metabolism. *Internat. J. Vit. Nutr. Res.* **53**, 371–376.

8 Powers, H.J., Bates, C.J. & Lamb, W.H. (1985): Haematological response to supplements of iron and riboflavin to pregnant and lactating women in rural Gambia. *Hum. Nutr.: Clin. Nutr.* **39C**, 117–129.

9 Romslo, I., Hasam, K., Sagen, N. & Augensen, K. (1983): Iron requirements in normal pregnancy as assessed by serum ferritin, serum transferrin saturation and erythrocyte protoporphyrin determinations. *Br. J. Obstets. and Gynaec.* **90**, 101–107.

10 Sauberlich, H.E., Dowdy, R.P. & Skala, J.H. (1977): In *Laboratory tests for the assessment of nutritional status*, CRC Press Inc. Cleveland, Ohio.

11 Thurnham, D.I. (1972): Influence of glucose-6-phosphate dehydrogenase deficiency on the glutathione reductase test for ariboflavinosis. *Ann. Trop. Med. Paras.* **66**, 505–507.

12 Topley, E. (1968): Common anaemia in rural Gambia. 1. Hookworm anaemia among men. *Trans. Roy. Soc. Trop. Med. Hyg.* **62**, 579–594.
13 WHO (1968): World Health Organization Technical Report Series No. 45. Nutritional Anaemias: WHO, Geneva.
14 Zaman, Z. & Verwilghan, R.L. (1977): Effect of riboflavin deficiency on activity of NADH-FMN oxidoreductase (ferriductase) and iron content of rat liver. *Biochem. Soc. Trans.* **5**, 306–308.

Aetiology and probable molecular basis of skin lesions in riboflavin and pyridoxine deficiencies

M. S. BAMJI
National Institute of Nutrition, Indian Council of Medical Research, Jamai Osmania PO, Hyderabad 500007, India.

Relative deficiency of vitamins can arise from selective increments in vitamin-binding proteins and increased demand for the vitamin at the cellular levels, following use of steroid hormones. Deficiency leads to a plethora of biochemical events but the molecular basis of most vitamin deficiency disorders is not understood.

Riboflavin-deficiency is amongst the most widely prevalent nutritional disorders in developing countries like India. It gives rise to skin lesions particularly of the mucocutaneous junctions. Our hypothesis is that the molecular basis of the skin lesions of riboflavin (vitamin B_2) and/or pyridoxine (B_6) deficiency may be impaired cross-linking of skin collagen.

The problem of dietary riboflavin deficiency in India. Indian diets, particularly the rice-based diets, are markedly deficient in riboflavin. The situation improves with a shift from rice as the staple to a mixed cereal millet type of diet[2]. This is understandable since the intakes of foods such as milk, vegetables and fruits which are the major sources of riboflavin in affluent communities, are very low amongst the poor in the developing countries. Cereals and millets are the major sources of nutrients in these populations.

Biochemical riboflavin-deficiency and its correlation with clinical lesions. Recent studies from our laboratory suggest that over 80 per cent of young women and children in and around Hyderabad have biochemical evidence of riboflavin-deficiency as judged by the erythrocyte glutathione reductase (E.C. 1.6.4.2.) activation test (EGR-AC)[3,4,15]. Interpretive guide-lines described in the literature[1,20] were used. EGR activity was measured by the method of Bayoumi & Rosalki[6].

The prevalence of lesions of the mouth such as angular stomatitis, glossitis and nasolabial dyssabacea which are pathognomic of riboflavin and/or pyridoxine-deficiency, varies between 10–25 per cent. In majority of the patients, these lesions respond to treatment with riboflavin, though in some cases treatment with pyridoxine helps[9,10]. A notable exception was a high incidence of angular stomatitis in a community of rural school boys, in which there was no response to vitamin therapy. The lesions healed with gentian violet, suggesting fungal infection as the aetiology[5].

In the majority of subjects with vitamin-responsive oral lesions there is biochemical evidence of riboflavin-deficiency as judged by the EGR-AC values (where EGR-AC = (EGR activity + FAD)/(EGR activity − FAD)). However, amongst the biochemically-deficient individuals clear-cut difference between subjects with and without clinical lesions is not always apparent[4,5]. This suggests that while the EGR test can identify riboflavin-deficiency it cannot further discriminate between those at risk of developing lesions. It has been observed that some individuals are at greater risk of developing the oral lesions than others and in general the energy intake of the former tends to be lower than the latter (K. Prema, unpublished). Thus, superimposed energy-deficiency may be an additional aetiological stress factor, for developing oral lesions.

Table 1. *Effects of vitamin supplements on riboflavin status frequency distribution (%).*

Subjects	Treatment	Duration	EGR-AC Values[a]			Source (Ref. no.)
			<1.2 Low risk	1.2–1.4 Medium risk	>1.4 High risk	
School boys	B-complex, therapeutic dose (viz 4 mg riboflavin)	1 month	39	29	32	(5)
School boys	B-complex low dose (viz 1.5 mg riboflavin)	1 year	17.9	32.1	50	(3)
Women	5 mg riboflavin	1 week	41.7	58.3	0	(17)
Women	B-complex low dose (viz 3 mg riboflavin)	3–6 months	39.4	24.2	36.4	Unpublished[b]

[a]where $\text{EGR-AC} = \dfrac{\text{EGR activity} + \text{FAD}}{\text{EGR activity} - \text{FAD}}$

[b]Bamji, Prema, Jacob, Rani & Samyukta

Generally, treatment with riboflavin produces a marked reduction in the EGR-AC values. However, in over 50 per cent of the women and children examined, EGR-AC values did not normalize even after supplementation with riboflavin or B-complex vitamins (Table 1). This suggests that some genetic or environmental factors interfere with the utilization of riboflavin.

Relationship between urinary riboflavin and respiratory infections. In one study among rural school boys a seasonal trend in urinary excretion of riboflavin was observed. Excretion tended to be higher in winter than in summer or monsoon. The incidence of upper respiratory tract infections also tended to be higher in winter. In the same study, 50 per cent of the boys had biochemical riboflavin deficiency, even after giving low dose B-complex supplements for one year[3] (Table 1). A tentative suggestion was that respiratory infections may impair the utilization of riboflavin.

To verify this hypothesis, Dr Bhaskaram, Mr Jacob and I are currently examining the effects of upper respiratory infections (URI) and measles on riboflavin status in children as judged by the EGR-AC test. So far 20 cases of measles, 18 cases of URI and 11 controls have been examined. All the children were in the age group 1–5 years. Urinary riboflavin was measured in 24-h collections by the fluorometric method. The mean urinary excretion of riboflavin in controls, URI patients and measles cases were found to be 0.96, 1.54 and 1.18 mg per g creatinine respectively. Though the group means were not signficantly different due to large variations, the trends were distinct, suggesting that infections such as measles and URI tend to increase the urinary excretion of riboflavin. This may deplete the body stores of the vitamin.

The EGR-AC values in the controls, URI patients and measles patients were 1.81, 1.54 and 1.24 respectively. Both the types of patients differed significantly from the controls. The reduction in the EGR-AC values in the patients, may be a transient artefact of increased mobilization of riboflavin from the tissues into the blood. However, similar change in the pyridoxal phosphate-activated enzyme aspartate aminotransferase (E.C. 2.6.1.1.) was not observed, suggesting that the effect was perhaps specific for flavoproteins. These data also suggest that EGR-AC test may be misleading in patients suffering from infections and should be interpreted with caution.

Molecular basis of skin lesions of riboflavin deficiency. Experimental deficiency of vitamin B_2 or B_6 is known to produce skin lesions, particularly of the mucocutaneous junctions in the rat and man. Lesions of the mouth such as angular stomatitis and glossitis in humans have been reported to respond to treatment with either riboflavin or pyridoxine[9,10]. Earlier it was reported that these lesions may be due to cellular deficiency of pyridoxal phosphate (PLP) since pyridoxamine phosphate oxidase (E.C. 1.4.3.5.) is a FMN-dependent enzyme. The activity of this enzyme diminishes markedly in riboflavin-deficiency[11,12,14,19] and the conversion of pyridoxine to PLP is impaired in riboflavin-deficient rats and humans. Plasma PLP levels are reduced in riboflavin-deficient as well as food-restricted rats[16]. Liver PLP levels fall in early and terminal stages of riboflavin-deficiency.

A further suggestion was that impaired collagen maturation may be the molecular basis of the skin lesions in riboflavin or pyridoxine deficiency, since the enzyme lysyl oxidase (E.C. 1.4.3.13) which is involved in the formation of collagen and elastin cross-links is believed to require PLP (as well as copper) as a cofactor[13]. Lysyl oxidase activity has been shown to diminish in the cartilage and aorta of pyridoxine-deficient chicks[7]. Collagen cross-linking is impaired in the skin of pyridoxine-deficient rats[8].

We have recently examined the effects of riboflavin or pyridoxine-deficiency on the physico-chemical and mechanical properties of the skin, such as: solubility in non-denaturing agents, denaturing agents and pronase; alpha/beta subunit ratio; tensile strength; shrinkage temperature and gel-reversibility[16]; Prasad, Lakshmi, Venkatappaiah & Bamji, unpublished (Table 2). In these experiments, *ad lib*-fed as well as weight-matched control rats were used for comparison. Marked alterations suggestive of reduced cross-linking were observed in all the above mentioned parameters in riboflavin as well as pyridoxine-deficient rats. Food restriction to limit growth had similar effects, but of lesser magnitude. However, food restriction did not affect the aldehyde content of the skin or the solubility of collagen in denaturing agents and pronase.

Table 2. *Skin collagen content and properties in vitamins B_2 and B_6-deficient growing male rats.*

	Percentage of ad lib *control rats*		
	Food restricted *(weight-matched control)*	*Vitamin B_2* *deficient*	*Vitamin B_6* *deficient*
Total collagen[a], mg per g skin	83.1	72.1	78.3
Insoluble collagen[a], %	80.7	67.4	70.3
Aldehyde content[a], μmol per g	94.9	70.8	61.8
α/β subunit ratio[b]	130	142	143

[a]Adopted from ref. no. 16. [b] Prasad, Lakshmi, Venkatappiah & Bamji, unpublished.

These data suggest that while food restriction and vitamin deficiency may both affect collagen cross-linking, the underlying biochemical site of action may differ. *In-vivo* experiments using ³H-proline suggest that in food restriction as well as vitamin-B_2 or B_6-deficiency there is an impairment in collagen synthesis as well. The magnitude of impairment tends to be greater in vitamin-deficiency. Reduction in skin collagen content and maturity may render the overlying epithelial tissue susceptible to stress and infections. Collagen is also essential for the growth of epithelium.

1 Bamji, M.S. (1981): Laboratory tests for the assessment of vitamin nutrition status. In *Vitamins in human biology and medicine* ed M. Briggs, pp. 1–27. Boca Raton: CRC Press.

2 Bamji, M.S. (1983): Vitamin deficiencies in rice rating populations. Effects of B-vitamin supplements. In *Nutritional adequacy, nutrient availability and needs*. Nestle Nutrition Research Symposium, Vevey, September, 14–15, 1982. ed J. Mauron, pp. 245–263. Basel, Boston, Stuttgart: Birkhauser Verlag.

3 Bamji, M.S., Arya, S., Rameshwar Sarma, K.V. & Radhaiah, G. (1982): Impact of long term, low dose, B-complex vitamin supplements on vitamin status and psychometor performance of rural school boys. *Nutr. Res.* **2**, 147–153.

4 Bamji, M.S. & Prema, K. (1981): Enzymatic riboflavin and pyridoxine deficiencies in young Indian women suffering from different grades of glossitis. *Nutr. Rep. Int.* **24**, 649–658.

5 Bamji, M.S., Rameshwar Sarma K.V. & Radhaiah, G. (1979): Relationship between biochemical and clinical indices of B-vitamin deficiency. A study in rural school boys. *Br. J. Nutr.* **41**, 431–441.

6 Bayoumi, R.A. & Rosalki, S.B. (1976): Evaluation of methods of coenzyme activation of erythrocyte enzymes for detection of deficiency of vitamin B_1,B_2 & B_6. *Clin Chem.* **22**, 327–331.

7 Bird, T.A. & Levene, C.I. (1982): Lysyl oxidase; Evidence that pyridoxal phosphate is a cofactor. *Biochem. Biophys. Res. Commun.* **108**, 1172–1180.

8 Fuji, K., Kajiwara, T. & Kurosu, H. (1979): Effect of vitamin B_6 deficiency on crosslink formation of collagen. *FEBS Lett.* **97**, 195–197.

9 Iyengar, L. (1973): Oral lesions in pregnancy. *Lancet* **1**, 680–681.

10 Krishnaswamy, K. (1971): Erythrocyte transaminase activity in human vitamin B_6 deficiency. *Int. J. Vitam. Nutr. Res.* **41**, 240–246.

11 Lakshmi, A.V. & Bamji, M.S. (1974): Tissue pyridoxal phosphate concentration and pyridoxine phosphate oxidase activity in riboflavin deficiency in rat and man. *Br. J. Nutr.* **32**, 249–255.

12 Lakshmi, A.V. & Bamji, M.S. (1976): Regulation of blood pyridoxal phosphate in riboflavin deficiency in man. *Nutr. Metabol.* **20**, 228–233.

13 Murray, J.C. & Levene, C.I. (1977): Evidence for the role of vitamin B_6 as a cofactor of lysyl oxidate. *Biochem. J.* **167**, 463–467.

14 Nakahara, I., Watanabe, Y., Morino, Y. & Sakamoto, Y. (1961): Enzymatic studies on pyridoxine metabolism. The influence of fat and fatty acid administration upon pyridoxine metabolism. *J. Biochem.* Tokyo **49**, 343–347.

15 Nutrition Reviews (1972): Erythrocyte glutathione reductase—A measure of riboflavin nutrition status. *Nutr. Rev.* **30**, 162–164.

16 Prasad, R., Lakshmi, A.V. & Bamji, M.S. (1983): Impaired collagen maturity in vitamins B_2 and B_6 deficiency —probably molecular basis of skin lesions. *Biochem. Med.* **30**, 333–341.

17 Prema, K., Bamji, M.S., Jacob, C. & Madhavapeddi, R. (1983): Effect of vitamin therapy on glossitis in young women. *Baroda J. Nutr.* **10**, 55–62.

18 Rameshwar Sarma, K.V., Radhiah, G. & Bamji, M.S. (1981): Impact of long term, low dose, B-complex vitamin supplements on clinical and anthropometric status of rural school boys. *Nutr. Rep. Int.* **24**, 345–352.

19 Rasmussen, K.M., Sarsa, P.M. & McCormick, D.B. (1979): Pyridoxamine 5′-phosphate oxidase activity in rat tissue during development of pyridoxine deficiency. *Proc. Soc. Exptl. Biol. Med.* **161**, 527–530.

20 Sauberlich, H.E., Dowdy, R.P. & Skala, J.H. (1973): Laboratory tests for the assessment of nutritional status. *Crit. Rev. Lab. Sci.* **4**, 215–340.

★ ★ ★

SEASONALITY AND MALNUTRITION

Modelling seasonal changes in energy balance (Africa)

A.E. DUGDALE and P.R. PAYNE
Human Nutrition Research Group, c/o Department of Child Health, University of Queensland, St Lucia Q. 4067, Australia; Department of Human Nutrition, London School of Hygiene and Tropical Medicine, Keppel Street, London WC1E 7HT, UK.

Up to now, the assessment of the state of nutrition of adults has been based on the assumption that a normal and desirable condition is approximate equilibrium between intake and expenditure of energy. However, the current interest in seasonality has focused attention on to the fact that for many people whose livelihoods depend on farms worked by human labour, the 'normal' state is one of repeated cyclic adjustments of energy balance and body weight. In order to understand the nutritional problems of peasants and to assess the viability of small farm systems, we need to develop a theoretical framework for dealing with these dynamic situations.

The model. We have described a model which simulates the regulation of energy balance in adults[5], representing the tissues of the body as four compartments linked together as shown in Fig. 1. A computer programme of the model calculates day-by-day changes in body weight and composition. After identifying initial values for body size and composition, the inputs to the computer consist of daily schedules of food energy intake and physical work output. At the end of each day, the energy needed for maintenance is calculated from the sizes of the body compartments and hence the energy balance is computed. If the balance is positive, the surplus energy is stored in the different compartments as lean tissue and fat tissue: the ratio of lean to fat stored is fixed for any particular individual. If the energy balance for the day is negative, the deficit is made up by depleting the compartments of lean and fat tissues, again in the same ratio. The model does not have any preferred value of body size, but, if provided with fixed levels of food intake and work output, will adjust its size and maintenance energy requirement upward or downward until equilibrium is again established. If intake and expenditure vary over time, for example because of seasonal effects, then the output of the model will describe the pattern and magnitude of seasonal weight fluctuations. We used this model[3] to simulate the annual weight changes observed in Gambian farmers by Fox[4].

The model farmer. We have now extended the model by linking the 'man' to a 'farm' by which he can grow food in exchange for his work. The 'harvest' from the farm is placed in a food store from

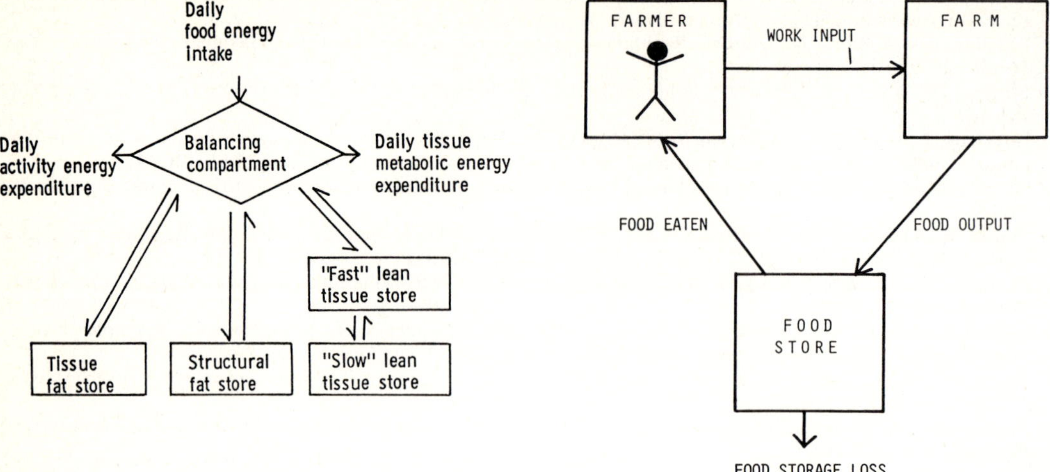

Fig. 1. *The model man showing the tissue compartments and the balancing compartment*

Fig. 2. *The model farm system. The compartments show the farmer the farm and the food store.*

which the farmer can take the food every day over the subsequent year until the next harvest comes in.

Figure 2 shows how these components of the model farm system are linked. The box containing the farmer represents the 'model man' described above. The 'farm' is restricted to a single crop production unit, which yields the same amount of food energy every year. The seasonal pattern of work input to the farm can be specified. At harvest, the total annual crop yield is transferred to the food store, after which it becomes subject to a storage loss. This loss is specified as the daily fractional rate at which the food energy contents of the store are degraded by microbiological spoilage, insect or rodent attacks etc. The farmer can take food from the store each day in various ways, so as for example to meet periods of heavy work requirements, or post-harvest feasting etc. We shall describe a number of 'runs' of the model using different food allocation patterns, all of which have been calculated so that the total amount of food available each year, ie farm production minus storage losses, is exactly used up by the farmer: there is never a surplus carried over from one year to the next. In this form, the model is self-stabilizing and after a number of simulated years (usually 10–15), settles down to an exactly repeating cycle of weight changes.

Despite the very simple nature of the model, it can be used to throw light on some interesting questions. In common with many other peasant communities, the Gambian farmers do not eat the largest amounts of food at the times when work is heaviest on land preparation and harvesting. Instead, they eat the largest amounts during the immediate post-harvest period, when their energy expenditure has fallen to a low level. The traditional pattern of post-harvest feasting is in part responsible for the seasonal weight fluctuations. Simulating various different strategies of food allocation is probably the only means of judging the rationality of the observed behaviour.

We have used the model to compare four different strategies of food allocation: (1) the time pattern of energy intakes observed by Fox for the whole Gambian farming community; (2) an exaggerated post-harvest feasting pattern, falling off rapidly to a much reduced level — this is intended to show the maximum effect of early food use on post-harvest storage losses; (3) a constant daily intake over the whole year, and (4) a feeding pattern adjusted so as to maintain constant body weight, ie intakes always balancing expenditures.

When the changes in mean weight of a group of Gambian men[4] are compared with those predicted by the model (Fig. 3), the pattern of actual and simulated weights are similar; the model shows larger seasonal swings, but these are within the range of individual variation reported by Billewicz & McGregor[1]. Figure 4 shows all four food allocation patterns together

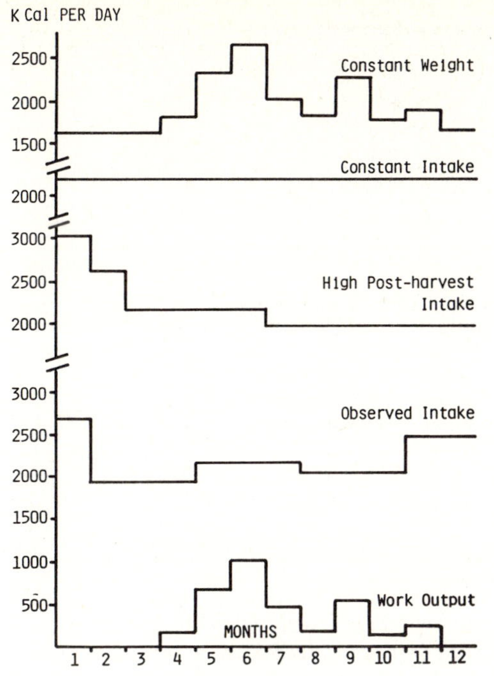

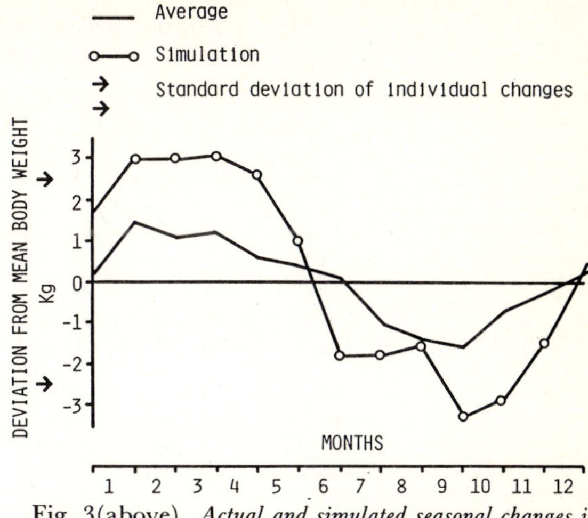

Fig. 3(above). *Actual and simulated seasonal changes in body weight of Gambian farmers. The average is that of Fox[4].*

Fig. 4(left). *Four of the possible patterns of food allocation over the year which have been tested using the model. The lower diagram shows the actual output of the Gambian farmers.*

Table 1. *Simulation of seasonal changes in body weight (kg) with different strategies of food use and different rates of storage loss.* A — average year round body weights; B — maximum body weight change.

Per cent annual storage loss (theoretical)	Observed pattern		High post-harvest		Constant intake		Constant weight	
	A	B	A	B	A	B	A	B
0	61.5	6.50	60.8	7.7	62.2	5.2	65	0
10	56.8	6.46	57.72	7.6	55.9	5.2	55.4	0
30	49.09	6.36	49.9	7.4	48.3	5.3	47.2	0

with the observed work output. Table 1 shows the average year round body weights and the maximum seasonal weight changes predicted by the model and how these are affected by the rate of storage loss.

When there are no storage losses, the 'best strategy' for food allocation seems to be that which sustains body weight at a constant level. However, as the rate of storage loss is increased, the advantages of high post-harvest consumption rates become greater, with average weights highest of all for the exaggerated post-harvest feeding schedule and lowest for the constant weight strategy.

Average year-round body weight is probably less important than the body weight at the start of the heavy work season. Table 2 shows the effects of different allocation patterns and storage loss rates on body weight at the start of the land preparation phase of farming. What is particularly striking is the relative disadvantage of attempting to maintain a constant body weight, which is the result of eating according to the conventional advice of matching intake with 'requirements'!

The relative advantage of the Gambian farmers' intake pattern over most of the others, derives partly from the fact that high body weight is sustained at the time when this is crucial for work output, but is allowed to decline and thus reduce maintenance costs during the rest of the year. But partly also because as Table 3 shows, storage losses are reduced, resulting in higher overall consumption. Table 3 also shows that the model predicts very well the effect of withdrawals for consumption on overall annual storage losses of food. Recent estimates, eg Boxall *et al.*[2], are based on long-period measurements taking account of the fact that food

Table 2. *Simulation of body weight at the start of heavy work period with different strategies of food use.*

Per cent annual storage loss (theoretical)	Observed pattern	High post-harvest	Constant intake	Constant weight
0	64.2	65.1	65.1	65.0
10	59.4	61.9	58.9	55.4
30	51.8	54.1	51.3	47.2

Table 3. *Simulation of post-harvest losses.* (per cent annual storage losses with different strategies of food use)

Theoretical loss (no food withdrawn)	Observed Gambian intake pattern	High post-harvest intake	Constant intake pattern	Intake pattern required for constant weight
10	5.1	4.9	5.3	5.5
30	16.3	15.9	16.9	17.5

10 per cent annual loss is equivalent to 0.0003 per day; 30 per cent annual loss is equivalent to 0.001 per day.

withdrawn for consumption is not subjected to further spoilage: these suggest actual annual losses in the range 4–5 per cent, ie close to those predicted by the model for an instantaneous loss rate of 10 per cent per year.

Despite its extreme simplicity, this model extends our understanding of some of the effects which seasonality imposes on energy balance and on body weight and shows the interaction between these effects and post-harvest losses of food.

The model could be elaborated so as to include other working and dependent family members, as well as more complex patterns of production and hence work requirements. In addition, the inclusion of a specific relationship between body weight and work capacity and of crop yields as a function of work inputs would make it possible to simulate and characterize critical situations which lead to progressive loss of productive capacity and the ultimate breakdown of the household food system.

1 Billewicz, W.Z. & McGregor, I.A. (1982): A birth-to-maturity longitudinal study of heights and weights in two West African (Gambian) villages, 1951–1975. *Ann. Hum. Biol.* **9**, 309–320.
2 Boxall, R., Greeley, M., Tyagr, D., Lipton, M. & Nedakarta, J. (1978): The prevention of farm-level food grain storage losses in India. A social cost benefit analysis. IDS Research Project.
3 Dugdale, A.E. & Payne, P.R. (1977): Pattern of lean and fat deposition in adults. *Nature*, London. **266**, 349–351.
4 Fox, R.H. (1953): A study of the energy expenditure of Africans engaged in various activities, with special reference to some environmental and physiological factors which may influence the efficiency of their work. PhD Thesis, London.
5 Payne, P.R. & Dugdale, A.E. (1977): A model for the prediction of energy balance and body weight. *Ann. Hum. Biol.* **4**, 525–535.

Seasonal nutritional stress in Malian agro-pastoralists, Sahel

Elizabeth DOWLER and Katherine HILDERBRAND
Department of Human Nutrition, London School of Hygiene and Tropical Medicine, Keppel Street, London WC1E 7HT, UK; Present address (KH): Save the Children Fund, BP 2145, Bamako, Mali.

The Sahelian zone of Africa has been the subject of much research, not least in response to the well-publicized droughts and famines of the early 1970s. The work reported here formed

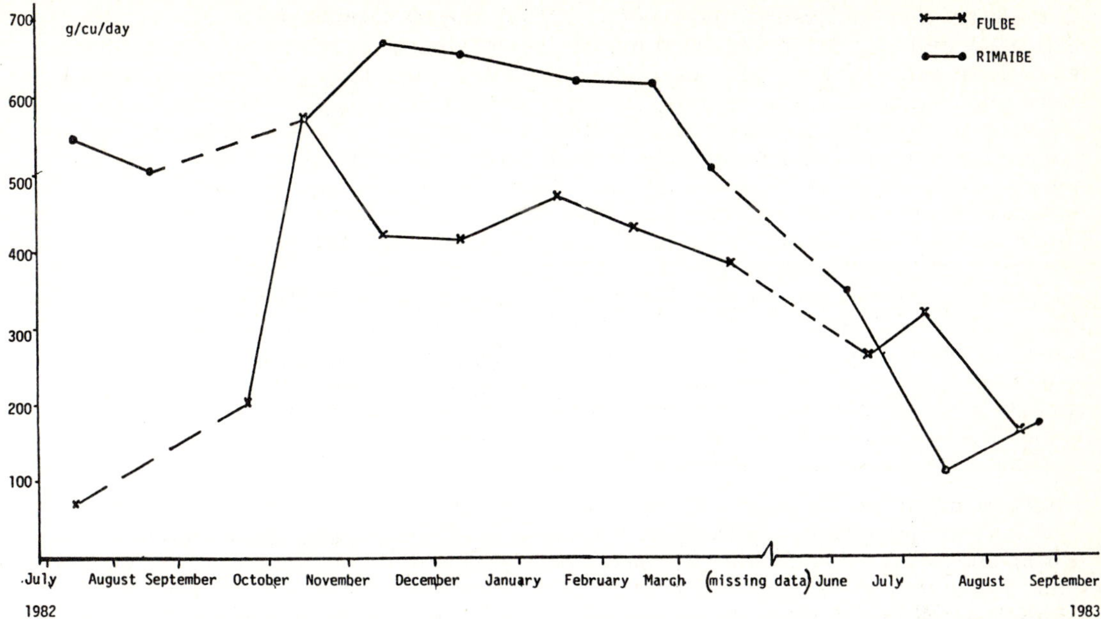

Fig. 1. *Weight of powdered millet consumed per consumption unit (cu)/d for FulBe and RimaiBe between July 1982 and September 1983.*

part of a larger study of typical Sahelian populations — their cultural and social organisation, and the various mechanisms and perceptions they have evolved for dealing with the harsh geographic environment in which they live, one of whose characteristics is pronounced seasonal stress periods consequent on climate. Sahelian rainfall, averaging 400 mm per annum, is concentrated in a short wet season some time between late June and early October. The critical factor for the inhabitants, however, is the enormous geographical and time variations between and within years.

Outline of study. This paper presents some of the data from one survey area and their interpretation, with additional observational material. The methodology and full details of results are given elsewhere[1]. The study concerned various aspects of food, work, health and nutrition in a Fulani agro-pastoral population living in the Seno-Mango region, eastern Mali. This population is totally dependent on rain-fed pastures — no migration to the Inner Niger Delta — practises dry-land millet cultivation and has strong internal social and economic links.

Three field workers lived in the villages for 15 months, enumerating the population and detailing monetary and in-kind transactions, cattle and herd sizes, grain harvest and acquisition, and population movements. Every month they recorded adult and child anthropometry, 24-h household food recall and recall of morbidity experience. However, they could never measure 100 per cent of the population in any one month because of the extreme household mobility. Households usually move from wet to dry season village sites; these were known and the field workers visited them accordingly. During the study year, the sparcity and unreliability of the wet season rains meant households moved even more than expected in search of pasture or of land suitable for sowing (some families sowed their fields four or five times) or to find work (usually weeding) on other peoples farms where rainfall had been more reliable. The problems posed for analysing and interpreting the data that were collected are described in detail elsewhere[1].

Social and cultural factors. Fulani society is made up of FulBe (the former aristocratic caste), artisans and RimaiBe (the former captives); this study concerned FulBe and RimaiBe. Although both groups live in the same place, eat similar food, speak the same language and have strong economic and social ties, there are no blood or lineage links. FulBe are traditionally pastoralists: they practise semi-transhumant herding, nowadays with associated millet cultivation, and their economy, society and diet centre around cattle and their (milk) products. RimaiBe are predominantly agriculturalists, cultivating millet primarily, with associated small ruminant breeding; they may employ FulBe to manage their cattle if they own large herds.

Two major social/economic exchanges which have nutritional signficance are the exchange of night pasturage of FulBe animals for RimaiBe water (RimaiBe tend to own water cisterns, holes dug to collect surface water) as the harvest season progresses into the cold season; and the exchange of millet for curdled milk, known as 'sippal'. FulBe women exhange curdled milk or butter from their own cows (those they brought into the marriage) for grain with RimaiBe women, in a systematic, quantitative way. The grain is mostly millet; towards the end of the hot and into the transitional-early rains season, it may be wild berries or rice. Each group thereby has access to food variety without needing to sell livestock at times of unfavourable prices. RimaiBe obtain milk for longer than the smaller herds they own might permit and FulBe acquire the grain they are reluctant to grow and have access to the wild foods their culture so strongly prevents them from collecting themselves. The relationship between the bartering women is also such that links are established and reinforced that can be drawn on in times of hardship, or when particular needs arise.

Food consumption. The main staples eaten are millet and milk; in years of bad rains, such as 1982–5, *Boscia senegalensis*, a wild berry, is collected and eaten during the hot and early rainy season, and forms the staple diet for many poorer families in both groups. (It was extremely difficult to investigate this practice because of the great shame attached). Figure 1 shows the approximate quantities of pounded millet and Fig. 2 the approximate volume of milk consumed per consumption unit[1] per day, for FulBe and RimaiBe. There were great problems initially in obtaining FulBe milk quantities. Furthermore no FulBe family admits to cereal consumption during harvest, although in practise very few have enough to exist on milk alone during the rains and harvest, despite this ideal. RimaiBe intakes were adjusted to allow for the few households with cattle and therefore access to fresh milk during the rainy season. These are shown on Fig. 2.

Millet consumption declined over the late transition and early wet season for both groups; *Boscia senegalensis* was consumed by most RimaiBe and some poorer FulBe families, other

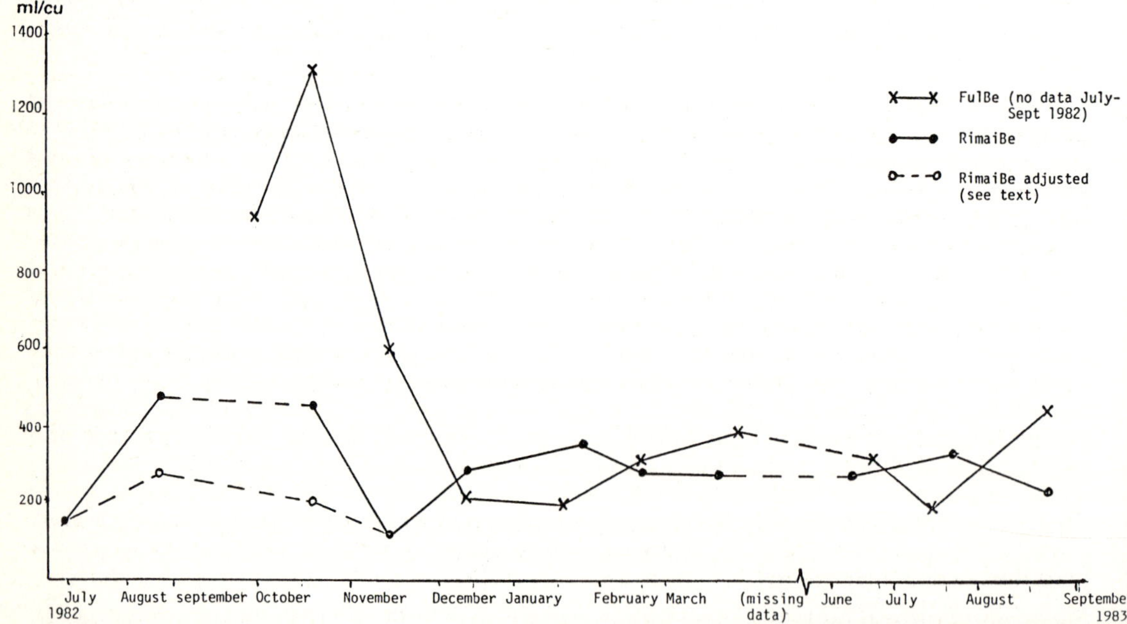

Fig. 2. *Volume of milk consumed per consumption unit (cu)/d for FulBe and RimaiBe between July 1982 and September 1983.*

Table. *Mean body weights (kg) of adult FulBe and RimaiBe from season to season.*

Group	No. subjects	Cool, dry	Hot, dry	Rains
		Season		
RimaiBe men	21	59.4***	59.4	57.7***
FulBe men	24	55.3***	53.1***	53.0
RimaiBe women	15	55.0	53.9	54.6
FulBe women	14	49.6*	48.1*	48.9**

Asterisks indicate significant of change from previous season: *$P<0.05$, **$P<0.01$, ***$P<0.001$.

households relying on stores, or animal sales and purchase of grain until the harvest period. RimaiBe millet consumption rose during the rains because families bought it for the main daily meal during weeding (*Boscia senegalensis* is said to lack sufficient 'strength'). RimaiBe millet consumption rose further with the harvest season; as the main harvest grain became available, exchange of millet began, and FulBe millet consumption therefore increased. RimaiBe milk intakes remained fairly constant over the year, probably because most of it came through sippal exchange. (Goat milk is particularly important for the RimaiBe during October to January.) FulBe milk intakes varied considerably depending on the time of year, and, in any one household, on which of their animals was lactating. Peak intakes occurred during the rains and harvest; some households maintained intakes of over 2 litres per head per day.

Health, work and nutritional status. Mean adult body weights for men and women are shown in the Table for constant samples[2]. Changes seem to be more a function of seasonal work load and food stresses than illness. The best months for both RimaiBe and FulBe were the cold dry season, despite high levels of adult diarrhoea, fevers and general infection. During these months following harvest and peak milk yields, people barter milk for millet and manure for water; it is the major time for festivals and marriages. February to May, the hot season, seemed to be healthiest time despite the temperature; however, food was increasingly in short supply, and many RimaiBe families spent long hours searching for, harvesting and processing *Boscia senegalensis*. Nonetheless, this labour was not reflected in body weight changes among the RimaiBe. Among the FulBe, however, there was massive weight loss as the dry season progressed, despite their relatively good health status because of the extremely strenuous work of watering animals. FulBe women are not involved in animal management. June/July brings the early rains/transition period, when both groups are under extreme pressure, both to pasture and water animals and to plant and replant fields. With the onset of the rains the pastoralists seemed to be better off: the FulBe lost no further weight, despite their noted susceptibility to malaria which appears with the rains, and probably started gaining weight with the slackening of heavy work and more food (from milk). The RimaiBe men lost weight massively in the wet season, in common with agriculturalists elsewhere in west Africa. The absence of wet season weight change among RimaiBe women is puzzling, since they contribute to the agricultural work and continue their demanding domestic routine. Most RimaiBe studied had regained their lost weight by November/December despite guinea worm eruptions during September.

Acknowlegement. The authors are indebted to Adam Thiam and Ced Hesse (the other two field workers), colleagues in the London School of Hygiene and Tropical Medicine and the International Livestock Centre for Africa, Mali, and most of all, to the villagers from the Seno-Mango, Mali.

1 Hilderbrand, K., Thiam, A., Tomkins, A. & Dowler, E. (1985): Food, work, health and nutrition: a comparative study of the seasonal effects in two agro-pastoralist populations in the Malian Gurma. Report to the Overseas Development Administration, UK. London and Bamako: London School of Hygiene and Tropical Medicine and International Livestock Centre for Africa, Mali. (Mimeographed).
2 Hilderbrand, K., Thiam, A., Fowler, C., Dowler, E. & Tomkins, A. (1985): Contrasting patterns of seasonal weight change within a rural community in the Sahel. *Proc. Nutr. Soc.* **44**, 13A.

Urban and rural differences in seasonal stress in The Gambia

Helen PICKERING and W.H. LAMB
*TARI Research Institue, PO Box 35, Tari, SHP, Papua New Guinea; Department of Child Health, Royal
Victoria Infirmary, University of Newcastle, Newcastle Upon Tyne, UK.*

Malnutrition is one manifestation of the complex web of poverty, ignorance, infection and inadequate food intake which is so common in developing countries. Furthermore, for subsistence farmers, poverty is often seasonally exacerbated, with peak activity in the fields coinciding with food shortages and increased levels of morbidity.

It could be argued that seasonal stresses are principally a function of agricultural cycles and are therefore less pronounced in urban areas. This paper looks at differences in levels of malnutrition and socio-economic factors in rural and urban areas of The Gambia.

The two study areas are Keneba, a rural, subsistence farming village and Bakau, a rapidly expanding peri-urban area situated 10 km from the Gambian capital, Banjul. The climate for both areas is tropical with a single rainy season between June and October and a total rainfall ranging between 600–1000 mm per annum.

Keneba. Most of Keneba's 1200 inhabitants depend on agriculture with few economic or social distinctions leading to different standards of living between individuals and families[8]. The villagers live in mud brick houses grouped together into compounds accommodating up to 130 people. Marriage is virilocal and more than half of the men practise polygamy. The co-wives, their young children and female relatives usually share rooms in a house within their husbands compounds and each wife cooks daily for her husband and family. Water for all domestic purposes is provided by six hand-drawn wells between 15 and 19 metres deep. There is little provision for sanitation.

The pattern of rainfall means that nearly all farming activities are concentrated into 6 months of the year. This period of intense activity coincides with pre-harvest food shortages and increased morbidity. During the rains all the able bodied work long hours in the fields, leaving children in the care of 5 to 9 year-old nursemaids.

Season has a marked effect on birth-weights and child growth. During the wet season most adults, including pregnant and lactating mothers, lose weight. Birth-weights are lower and young children grow slowly or not at all[2]. The combination of low food intake and increased energy expenditure in pregnancy is largely responsible for the reduction in birth-weights[6].

Infants grow well for their first 2 to 3 months in all seasons, but growth faltering occurs over the next 2 years and is especially marked in the wet seasons, when some children even show negative growth[2]. The intake of breast-milk is reduced during the rains as all but the youngest infants are left at home while the mothers work, and so are only breast-fed at night and in the early mornings. The combination of separation leading to reduced nipple stimulation and biological stress on the mother probably accounts for the lower breast-milk production also seen at this time[3]

Those young children left at home are fed watery millet gruels prepared by their mothers in the mornings. This gruel is kept throughout the day at high ambient temperatures and becomes heavily contaminated[5]. At this time of the year well water is also very polluted[1] and general environmental hygiene is at its lowest. These factors all contribute to increased levels of diarrhoea in young children which directly relates to nutritional status[4]. Therefore, in the wet season children have to cope with the emotional stress of being separated from their mothers, low levels of child care, reduced breast-milk intake and heavily contaminated nutritionally-poor supplementary foods.

Bakau. In Bakau the situation is markedly better. It has a population of nearly 10 000, two-thirds of whom are recent migrants from rural areas. Occupations vary from office and professional categories to manual labour. Some women have small kitchen gardens, growing produce for home consumption and sale. No one is dependent on subsistence farming. Adult diets are more varied than in Keneba with fresh vegetables, fish, meat and groundnuts always available. Tinned and locally soured milk is sometimes added to the gruel given to young children. Housing ranges from traditional mud brick to European style with electricity, refrigerators and flush toilets. Chlorinated water is supplied to public and private standpipes. Few mothers work away from home and nearly half have some education. In contrast to Keneba there is no seasonal increase in activity or decrease in food intake, and environmental hygiene is generally better.

Table 1. *Seasonal differences in the percentage of children underweight in Keneba[7] and Bakau (A.M. Tomkins, pers. commun.)*

	Children (%) less than 80% weight for age[a]	
	May[b]	September[c]
Keneba	30	75
Bakau	15	27

[a]In terms of standard 50th centile expected weight for age (WHO).
[b]Late dry season.
[c]Late wet season.

The incidence of childhood malnutrition is much lower than in Keneba and although less marked, seasonal factors are still important (Table 1). However, in urban communities socio-economic differences may be more important determinants of child growth than season. When over 30 social and environmental variables were analysed against child growth, four relating to the standard of living (style of house, ownership of a refrigerator, private standpipe and flush toilet in the house) were statistically associated with improved levels of child growth particularly in the wet season. Two social variables (place of residence of the father and parity of the mother) were similarly associated with child growth (A.M. Tomkins, personal communication). The most probable reason for the increased numbers of undernourished children in the wet season is the higher level of infection, particularly diarrhoea and malaria (A.M. Tomkins). The effects of infection in Bakau, however, are not nearly so marked as they are in Keneba, possibly due to the more varied diet available, the amount of time mothers have available for child care and the easy access people have to government and other facilities.

Discussion. In the Gambia we find that seasonal stresses are more pronounced in rural villages than in urban areas. Are these differences entirely due to environmental factors, or do social norms intervene in any way? Indices of poverty all point to a very precarious situation in rural areas. Infant and child mortality is very high, life expectancy is low and material possessions are minimal. During the short growing season all adults work long hours in the fields, even children are employed in weeding and bird scaring. There is little leeway for any member of the village to increase their own productivity, consumption or leisure.

In rural areas a woman's work load is increased by the necessity of cooking every day. In Bakau on the other hand over half of the mothers share cooking on a 2-day routine with other women in the compound. If this system was adopted in Keneba, allowing the woman whose turn it was to cook to be excused from farming, it would relieve mothers working in the fields of the added burden of cooking when they arrived home. It would also improve levels of child care with competent adults in the compounds to supervise and prepare fresh food for young children during the day. Soil productivity is very low and would require large investments in irrigation, fertilizer and some mechanization to increase yields sufficiently to raise consumption and income from cash crops so that standards of living in general were improved.

We can see that in Bakau, where living standards are relatively high, people have wider options making it easier to adopt new ideas. There is more sharing of domestic tasks and of consumption and increased disposable income leads to better housing and improved domestic hygiene. In societies such as Keneba where any reductions in supplies could cause serious food shortages people are understandably reluctant to experiment with new ideas until their efficiency is proven. It is therefore difficult to change social norms and modes of production to benefit child health without substantially raising living standards to the point where people have sufficient sense of security to experiment with new ideas.

1 Barrel, R.A. & Rowland, M.G.M. (1979): The relationship betwen rainfall and well water pollution in a West African (Gambian) village. *J. Hyg. (Cambridge)* **83**, 143–150.
2 McGregor, I.A., Rahman, A.K., Thompson, B., Billewicz, W.Z. & Thomson, A.A. (1968): The growth of young children in a Gambian village. *Trans Roy. Soc. Trop. Med. Hyg.* **62**, 341–352.
3 Roberts, S.B., Paul, A.A., Cole, T.J. & Whitehead, R.G. (1982): Seasonal changes in activity, birthweight and lactational performance in rural Gambia women. *Trans Roy. Soc. Trop. Med. Hyg.* **71**, 199–203.
4 Rowland, M.G.M. & McCollum, J.P.K. (1977): Malnutrition and gastro-enteritis in the Gambia. *Trans Roy. Soc. Trop. Med. Hyg.* **71**, 199–203.
5 Rowland, M.G.M. & Barrel, R.A.E. (1980): Ecological factors in gastroenteritis. In *Disease and urbanization*, ed E.J. Clegg & J.P. Garlick, pp. 21–35. London: Taylor & Francis.
6 Rowland, M.G.M., Paul, A.A., Prentice, A.M., Muller, E., Hutton, B., Barrel, R.A.E. & Whitehead, R.G. (1981): Seasonality and the growth of infants in a Gambian village. In *Seasonal dimensions to rural poverty*, ed R. Chambers, R. Longhurst, A. Pacey & F. Pinter, pp. 164–174. London: Pinter
7 Rowland, M.G.M. & Whitehead, R.G. (1979): The epidemiology of protein-energy malnutrition in children in a West African village community. 1974–78. Report of the MRC Dunn Nutrition Unit Cambridge.
8 Thompson, B. (1965): Marriage, childbirth and early childhood in a Gambian village: a sociomedical study. PhD Thesis, University of Aberdeen.

Seasonal variation in nutritional status among women of different occupational groups in Bangladesh

Najma RIZVI
International Centre for Diarrhoeal Disease Research, G.P.O. Box 128, Dhaka, Bangladesh.

People living in poverty have always known that, at certain times of the year, as food supply gets scarce diseases become more common. With the exception of a study in Matlab, Bangladesh[2], little or no detailed information is available on the impact of seasonal variation on women's nutritional status. The Matlab study showed women experiencing weight loss in the lean seasons of March–April and August–October. A recent paper (by one of the same authors[3]) on maternal nutrition and the newborn, also showed that women's body weights and arm circumference decreased during the lean period. He argued that deterioration of nutritional status occurs due to seasonal food scarcity and that lactation is not a contributory factor in the weight loss of women. A study in Gambia on seasonal changes in activity, birth weight and lactational performance[4] showed striking seasonal changes in the activity pattern of Gambian women and how the cumulative effects of intense activity and low food intake led to the birth of low-weight babies and to a striking fall in maternal weight.

The sample. The two groups of women selected for this study were lactating mothers with, either one or two, or three or more children from two occupational groups, weavers and farmers. The age range of these groups was 19–42 years. The total sample of 56 women was equally divided between farming and weaving families. Mean weight of women in weavers' households was 39.1 kg and in farmers' households 41.0 kg.

The site and methods. The study was carried out in the villages located in Karotia Union of Tangail district in rural Bangladesh. Farming comprised the major economic activity in all villages except one. About 50 per cent of the households had no agricultural land; landless and marginal landholders (<1 acre) together accounted for 75 per cent of the households.

This paper forms part of a longitudinal study on maternal and young children's food behaviour and nutritional status. Before proceeding with the collection of quantitative data, ethnographic investigation was carried out and information was collected through observation and informal interviewing. This provided qualitative data on meal patterns and rules guiding intra-household food distribution.

Food intake of women was collected using a 24-h dietary recall system. Body weights were taken monthly using a calibrated bathroom scale. The average of three measures was recorded. Careful observations were made of the activities performed in different seasons. Information on cropping pattern was gathered through observation and informal interaction with the adult members of the family.

Results and discussion. *Cropping pattern and food availability.* In examining the influence of seasonality on cropping pattern and food availability in Bangladesh it appears that the tropical wet-dry scenario characterized by farming and non-farming seasons cannot be applied without further qualifications. Three seasons are distinguished by these people: (1) summer season (March–May); (2) rainy season (June–October); (3) winter season (November–February). The crop calender shows seasonal variation in the cultivation of different crops (Fig. 1). The major food crops are rice and wheat, which together account for 70 per cent of total energy intake. Varieties of rice (Aus, Aman, Irri, Boro) are planted in all three seasons of the year. Aus summer rice is planted in April and harvested in July–August. Transplanted Aman, a wet rice, is planted during monsoon and harvested in December–January. Irri-Boro is planted in winter and harvested in May–June. With the introduction of the high-yielding variety Irri, the traditional winter Boro has been replaced by Irri-Boro, which has become an important crop in our study area. Wheat, a relatively new crop to this area, is planted in October–November and harvested in April. In discussing food availability in poor households, Irri assumes a critical position because the price of Irri rice is almost always lower than other varieties. The two lean seasons recognized by the villagers are March–April and August–October.

The available food was found to be inadequate, both in quantity and quality. Rice was the

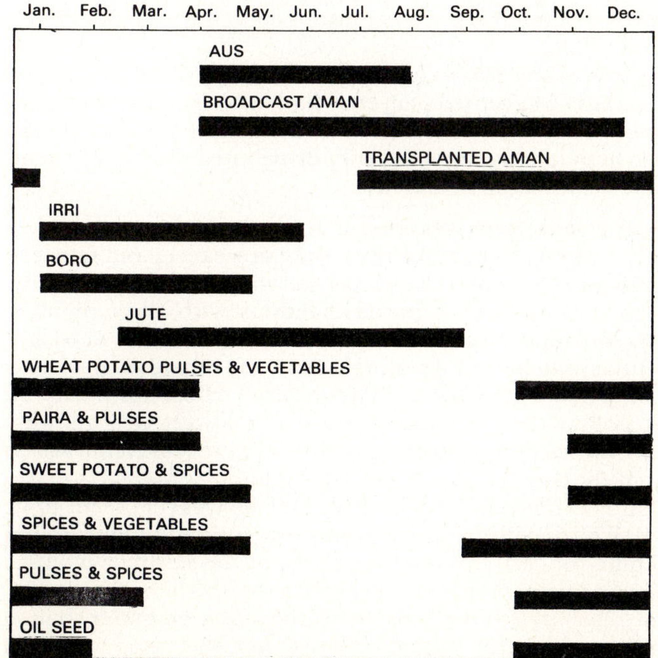

Fig. 1. *Crop calendar of Tangail rural area.*

preferred cereal; however, during the lean season of March–May, rice was supplemented with wheat and potatoes in the poorest homes. The frequency of consumption of wheat was one or two times a day. Mothers were found to eat a relatively smaller quantity of wheat than rice, because, to them, it was the least desirable food. When ill or pregnant, many mothers complained of their distaste for wheat which resulted in a lower intake.

During the preharvest seasons of Irri-Boro and Aman rice, the mothers were found to subsist on two meals a day and this was true for both landless and marginal landholders of both occupational groups. Whenever food was in short supply, it was the mother who sacrificed her own share of food for the husband and the children. The mothers were often found to go with little or no food at lunch time. Difference in gender status, coupled with the ideal image of wife and mother as the epitome of sacrifice, influenced maternal food intake.

In so far as beliefs and values guiding food practices were concerned, no difference was noticeable between women of farming and weaving households. The cultural traditions in both groups were found to be similar.

Food intake of lactating mothers in two seasons are presented in the Table. While observation of food practices and meal patterns were frequently made, quantitative information on food intake was recorded only twice: energy intake was higher for both groups in November–December than in March–April, the preharvest season.

Table. *Daily intake of energy and protein of mothers according to occupation and season.*

Season		Weaving	Farming
Nov-Dec	Energy: kcal	1411	1409
	MJ	5.90	5.90
	Protein, g	30.7	32.7
March-April	Energy: kcal	1362	1349
	MJ	5.70	5.64
	Protein, g	32.4	28.6

Activity pattern. While child-rearing, household-cleaning and food-preparation kept women engaged throughout the year, tasks related to crop-processing and weaving showed a seasonal pattern. Winter was found to be the period of intense activity for women in the weaving group, who frequently carried the baby while working.

For the farming women, winter, the harvesting season of a major rice crop, was also a period of intense activity. However, unlike landless weaver women, they had other periods of intense activity also, coinciding with the harvest of winter Irri-Boro rice, wheat and potatoes. For the farming women, the periods of intense activity were more evenly distributed during the year, whereas for the weavers, winter was the peak season of activity.

Seasonality of nutritional status. Nutritional status was measured only by body weight, taken monthly. Figure 2 shows the changes in weights from November–July in weavers and farmers. Both groups start at 41 kg but the weavers experienced a sharper fall in their weight than the farming group. Figure 3 presents weight according to parity. Mothers with three or more children weighed less than the mothers having two or fewer children. This difference in weight was maintained throughout the 9-month study period. In other words, the impact of parity on maternal weight was clearly demonstrated at all seasons. The negative effects of parity on nutritional status was not found to be offset even in good seasons. The lowest weights were recorded in April for both groups; however, weight of mothers with 3 or more children was less than the low-parity mothers throughout the 9-month study period (Fig. 3).

The impact of lean season on weight is evident in both groups, but the weavers seem to be affected more than the farmers (Fig. 2). The decline in weight of mothers from weaving families could be attributed to the low availability of cash for food purchases in the summer months. During the winter months the workload remains unusually heavy for the mothers in weavers' households, but the availability of more cash makes the household food situation better than in other seasons. Despite greater expenditure of energy in the winter season, the mean weight in

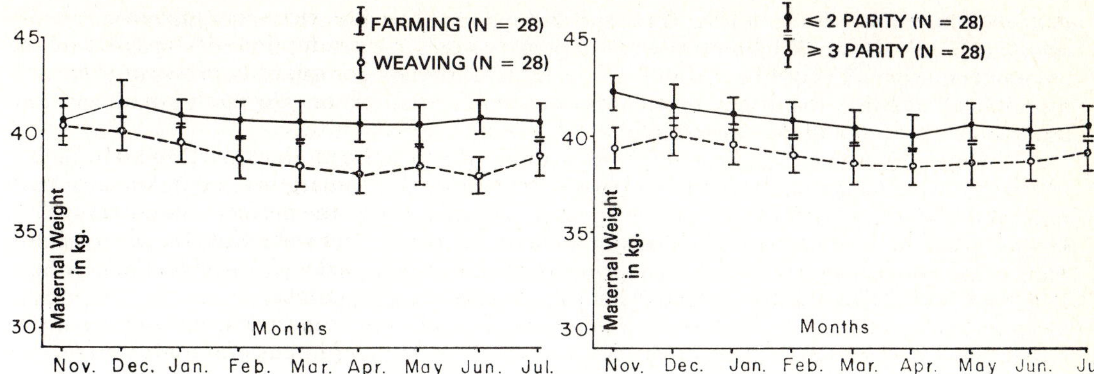

Fig. 2. *Seasonal changes in maternal weight (means ± s.e.m.) of two occupational groups in Tangail.*

Fig. 3. *Changes in maternal weight (means ± s.e.m.) according to parity in Tangail.*

the winter months remains higher than in summer and rainy seasons in the weavers' group. There is less month-to-month fluctuation in the weight of women of farming households, which can be attributed to better supplies of food. For the farming group, the December mean of 41.7 kg and the June mean of 41.4 kg were the peaks.

Monthly fluctuation in weight seems to be more pronounced in Matlab[2] than in Tangail. Even the weight curve of weaver women which shows a sharper drop than farming women appears to decline less steeply than the weight curve of Matlab women.

Since the impact of cultural tradition is similar in both occupational groups, variation in nutritional status can be attributed to seasonal nature of food intake and activity patterns. No mother was found to suffer from any major illness during our study period, and it can be safely assumed that the effects of illness among the women were minimal. The striking seasonal difference in food availability, and, in turn, nutritional status as found in many African countries is not expected in Bangladesh because the tropical wet-dry scenario as found in Gambia is not present in Bangladesh. A more varied crop calendar, coupled with the increased cultivation of HVY winter rice, wheat and potato have made the lean season of March–April less lean than before. Increased opportunities of work with a better wage rate during lean seasons can further improve the situation.

1 Abdullah, M. (1983): Dimensions of intra-household allocation of food and nutrients: a study of a Bangladeshi village. Ph.D. Thesis, London University.
2 Chen, L., Chowdhury, A.K.M.A. & Huffman, S.L. (1979): Seasonal dimensions of energy protein malnutrition in rural Bangladesh: the role of agriculture, dietary practices and infection. *Ecol. Fd Nutr.* **8**, 175–187.
3 Chowdhury, A. (1985): Maternal nutrition and newborn in rural Bangladesh. Women and health: end decade national conference publication May 2–4, 32–47.
4 Roberts, S.A., Paul, A., Cole, T.J. & Whitehead, R.G. (1981): Seasonal changes in activity, birth weight and lactation performance in rural Gambian women. *Trans. Roy. Soc. Trop. Med. Hyg.* **760**, 668–678.

Household food production and gardening for improvement of nutrition: a workshop report

L.T. TEPLY (Organizer)
UNICEF, United Nations, New York, NY 10017, USA.

The workshop consisted of three main segments. First, a number of brief presentations, interspersed with discussions, were made by participants who reviewed recent experiences in developing countries. Secondly, three sub-groups were convened to formulate recommendations and finally the workshop reconvened in plenary session to reach a general consensus on the recommendations. Forty-five individuals from 18 different countries, representing various disciplines including nutrition, horticulture, economics, anthropology and agricultural and home economics extension, participated.

J. Gershon presented the gardening programme of the Asian Vegetable Research Centre (AVRDC) which has done extensive research on home, school and community gardens in both rainy and dry seasons. From a base in Taiwan, outreach programmes have been operated in several other Asian countries. Analysis of food production, nutritional value of the food and economic value revealed favorable benefit-cost ratios. *C. Boonma* discussed a project in Thailand under AVRDC outreach. He stressed the importance of convincing government administrators, extension workers and farmers and their families of the value and importance of small plot family food production. *Aree Valyasevi* presented further information on gardening for improvement of nutrition in Thailand and *F. Solon* reported similarly on the Philippines.

Paul Sommers discussed a regional gardening project in the Western Pacific operated by UNICEF and the UN Development Programme with support from the Australian government. The mixed gardening approach based mainly on traditional practices has been described in a handbook produced by UNICEF. A regional programme is being developed through establishment of examples of successful projects in which special attention has been given to training and community activities. Administrators have welcomed the cooperation and have proved willing to provide the resources needed to promote and support the programme.

Vera Niñez, International Potato Center, Peru, summarized some of her extensive experience in Peru as well as in a number of other countries. She showed the wide variety of local conditions and approaches to gardening and pointed out a number of potential pitfalls and ways in which these can be avoided in development of programmes. A forthcoming issue of the UN University's *Food and Nutrition Bulletin* will carry a series of research reports on gardening from various countries.

Rajamal Devadas reported on a gardening programme through schools in Coimbatore, India. *Lee Debra Gelb*, CARE, is working with a similar programme (REAP) in Belize.

Barbara Underwood reported that the International Vitamin A consultative Group is developing simplified guidelines for evaluation of interventions to improve vitamin A status through dietary improvement. *Antoinette Pirie* reported on programmes extending from Madurai Medical College, India, for prevention and treatment of vitamin A deficiency through promotion of consumption of foods providing pro-vitamin A.

Albert Meisel reported on activities of the League for International Food Education (LIFE), including publication of an overview report 'Home gardening in international development —what the literature shows'. LIFE has been cooperating in training for gardening activities in a number of developing countries and is in process of establishing a 'gardening centre', which would include acting as an information clearing house.

N. Scrimshaw reported that the UN University is in a position to support research on gardening for nutrition improvement and *Blair Bybee* stated that the Thrasher Research Fund can also support work in this field.

Recommendations. (1) Ministries and Departments of Agriculture should give more serious attention to household food production and gardening and should acquaint personnel, including extension workers, with newer approaches to gardening and their adaptation to local conditions. (2) An appropriate package of services should be developed for countries, and regions within them, with due attention to seasonal problems. (3) Seeds and other planting materials of certified quality should be made available. (4) Economic motives should be sought and advantage should be taken of such motives in the promotion of gardening. (5) In many situations more attention should be given to the role of women, but the roles of other family members should not be neglected. (6) The significance of gardens in the national food supply should be determined. (7) Short courses for agricultural and nutrition planners and policy makers should be conducted on the role of food gardens in national development. (8) Short courses for trainers and field workers should be conducted on food gardens for nutritional improvement. (9) Development communications packages on the link between food gardening and nutrition should be made available. More use should be made of mass media. (10) Workshops should be arranged for non-governmental organizations on food gardening and nutrition action at the household level. (11) Special encouragement should be given to research in a number of countries. Examples of gardens effective in improving nutrition should be established. (12) Attention should be given to appraisal and evaluation of projects. There needs to be study and forethought before project implementation. There is need for simple approaches to dietary surveys for providing information as to foods that should be emphasized for improvement of the diet. The International Vitamin A Consultative Group (IVACG) is developing guidelines with respect to vitamin A. (13) Projects for evaluation should be developed in a manner that enables some determination of the disposition of the extra food produced and, where feasible, an indication of the changes produced in the diet and the effects on the nutrition and health of families and communities. (14) A directory of food gardening projects should be published. (15) International agencies and bilateral programmes should enlarge their assistance in the dissemination of home gardening technology, including communications support, among countries. For example, regional workshops could be organized. (16) It would be desirable to develop a 10-year plan of action on food gardening for improvement of nutrition. (17) The IUNS should consider establishment of a committee on food gardening for improvement of nutrition.

This workshop was attended by 45 participants from 17 countries, together with representative from FAO and other international agencies.

Nutrition as a component of farming systems research: a workshop report

M. SMITH and P. WAGNER (Organizers)
Department of Foods & Nutrition, Kansas State University, Manhattan, Kansas; Department of Food Science & Human Nutrition, Home Economics Programs, University of Florida, Gainesville, Florida, USA.

Participants. Kathryn Dewey (Department of Nutrition, University of California, Davis, California, USA); Judith McGuire (Agency for International Development; Washington, DC, USA); P. Pinstrup-Andersen (International Food Policy Research Institute; Washington, DC, USA); B. Popkin (Carolina Population Center; University of North Carolina; Chapel Hill, North Carolina; USA).

The need for increased attention to nutrition in international agricultural development and for greater involvement of nutrition scientists has been recognized[2,5]. A major goal of international agricultural research is to increase the level of food production in marginal lands of the third world[6]. An important aspect of this effort is research better to understand how to integrate appropriate technology into the farming systems utilized by limited-resource farm families in marginal areas[4]. Commercialization of traditional agricultural systems along with the introduction of new technology has been encouraged as a means of increasing productivity. However, it has become apparent that agriculture commercialization programmes which select modern farm technologies, new high yield crops, or marketing innovations solely on the basis of increased efficiency or productivity have not solved food supply problems in developing countries. Increased productivity that does not also increase food supply to the household will not affect the nutritional status of household members[5].

Awareness of the need to incorporate nutritional concerns into farming systems research represents a fairly recent development and is far from being widely accepted and supported[3,5,7,8,9]. The organizers of this workshop are nutrition scientists affiliated with United States institutions (land-grant universities) that have major leadership roles in farming systems research. The workshop was organized to provide an opportunity for participants in the XIII

International Congress of Nutrition to discuss issues related to the effect agricultural change on nutritional status of farm families in marginal areas of the developing world.

Discussion. Sound agricultural research and related policies are fundamental to long-term nutritional improvements. Ideally, this means enhancement of food quality and quantity as well as distribution to people of all socioeconomic levels. Agricultural change, especially increased commercialization, may have negative effects on nutritional status which must be identified. *Pinstrup-Andersen* cautioned that two factors about farmers must be recognized. First, regardless of how poor they are, farmers make rational decisions. Second, improving nutritional status is not likely to be a primary goal of farm households.

Although the farmer makes rational decisions, changes may have a negative impact due to: inherent risks of production such as weather, insects; price uncertainty due to policy, government intervention, export market price, input price flux; local marketing systems that are efficient at getting the cash crop out but are unable to move staple foods from one region to another; cash available which encourages new foods to enter the market, thereby increasing food choice decisions; changes in inter-household income and control of that income; changes in time allocation.

Other agricultural production factors cited earlier by Pinstrup-Andersen[5] that may influence human nutrition include; incomes acquired by households at risk of having malnourished members; cost of food commodities; nature of production systems among semisubsistence farmers; nutrient composition of foods available to households; labour demands; human energy expenditure; infectious diseases.

Dewey noted that a need for cash encourages farmers to change from subsistence agriculture to more commercial systems. This affects cash available for additional food purchases and diet diversity. In examining the impact of changing agriculture systems, the methods of cash generation must be examined also. This is not an easy task due to the variety of strategies farm families exploit to acquire cash. These strategies may affect a wider population than the target group.

The different rates at which cash and food enter the household affect food decisions. Food enters more steadily than cash which may enter and leave sporadically, in uneven sums. This may have a positive or a negative effect on nutrition, depending upon additional foods purchased and total food intake. Nutrition education may help families make better food choices although many already know which traditional foods are best. Most food decisions are economic based so that national food policy which subsidizes prices or creates an urban supply bias will have a greater effect on food choice than education.

Diet diversity and nutrition are adversely affected when land and time available for food crop production decreases[1]. This happens when the amount of land dedicated to cash crop production is increased at the expense of food crop land. Cash crops may require the same or more time as food crops, thus decreasing the proportion of time available to food production. Adjustment to this may change the type and number of foods grown or the number and preparation of meals. Dewey suggested that farming systems researchers should monitor a few key economic and dietary indicators as a strategy for preventing unintended negative effects. This information can be obtained informally through observations and key informants and does not require a large-scale formal survey. Suggested indicators are: (1) timing of cash flow; (2) ability of family to manage cash; (3) timing of crop sales in relation to market prices; (4) relative prices of purchased foods and types available; and (5) nutritional quality of diet consumed.

Popkin called attention to the need for research to quantify effects of changes in farming systems on subsistence farmers, as well as others in the target community. The assumption is often made that major nutrition problems exist among subsistence farmers. Actually it is not known if more malnutrition is found in the subsistence or in the changed sector. Also as inputs increase, land profitability may increase resulting in changes in land tenure and social structure. Farming may not be the sole activity of a given household; diverse and multiple activities to secure food and income are more typical. The effect of nutritional status on agricultural productivity of limited resource families working marginal lands is an important research question; most of the available data are from productivity studies of plantation workers. Factors that affect productivity include intensity and duration of the work as well as the choice of technology. The effect of food supplementation on increasing agricultural productivity has been difficult to measure in fixed agriculture systems due to several factors. First, households compensate for limited or inefficient labour by substituting the labour of one household member for another. Secondly, production and consumption decisions are linked so that households may expend only enough energy to produce the amount of food they perceive to be sufficient.

McGuire examined the link between nutrition and farming systems research (FSR). Successful projects attempt to help limited resource farmers increase production by better understanding of linkages between production and consumption. These linkages include: (1) seasonality of production; (2) crop mix and minor crops; (3) income; (4) role of women in production; (5) crop labour requirements; and (6) market prices and seasonality. Awareness of these linkages is important at each of the formal 'stages' of FSR project: (1) target area selection; (2) designing diagnostic baseline studies; (3) formulating recommendation domains; (4) project evaluation; and (5) extension.

Frankenberger[3] suggested that securing adequate food supplies for their families is a major goal of limited resource farmers. Therefore, *McGuire* commented, recommendation domain studies that group farmers on the basis of economic or geographic similarities should also group them on the basis of consumption demands. The unit of analysis should be the household rather than the farmer. This would bring into the diagnostic phase factors such as gathered foods, foods grown by women, womens' access to food and income, and crop labour requirements. Farming systems research uses farmers objectives. Since farmers do not value nutritional objectives, these may have to be forced into the equation.

McGuire cited several problems with the FSR approach: (1) the goal of this research is to increase production and income when it should aim to increase consumption; (2) researchers using FSR tend to adapt it to the techniques with which they are familiar rather than using it to identify new factors associated with limited resource farmers; and (3) they look primarily at the impact of changing agriculture systems on the male farmer. Males and females within the household may have different utility functions, lands, and labour patterns under different decision making concerns.

Discussion generated by the speakers reemphasized the importance of understanding existing farming systems and being aware of numerous interactions among the various components, so that potential effects of changes can be evaluated. For example, the household food garden system should be included as well as cash crops and livestock. It is also important to understand that the social system often is a major factor in the determination of the farming systems employed. Farming system researchers should develop awareness and appreciation of the types of short- and long-term survival strategies utilized by limited resource farm families, before introduction of new technologies is attempted. Effective communication between agronomists and nutritionists must involve mutual respect, as well as clarification of differing views on 'increased crop yield' alone as the major factor in bringing about sustained improvements in nutritional status.

Recommendations. (1) Strengthen linkages between farming systems researchers and nutrition scientists. (2) Demonstrate the integration of nutrition concerns in a carefully designed model project in one location. (3) Identify indicators of dietary quality and nutritional status that have practical and appropriate application within the framework of the farming systems research approach.

1 Dewey, K.G. (1979): Agricultural development, diet and nutrition. *Ecol. Fd Nutr.* **8**, 265–273.
2 Dinning, J.S. (1984): The role of the nutritionist in Third World agricultural policy planning. *J. Nutr.* **114**, 1739–40.
3 Frankenberger, T.R. (1985): *Adding a food consumption perspective to farming systems research*, p. 1–65. Washington, DC: AID and USDA.
4 Hildebrand, P.E. & Waugh, R.K. (1983): Farming systems research and development. *Farming Systems Support Project Newsletter*. **1**, 4–5.
5 Pinstrup-Andersen, P. (1984): Incorporating nutritional goals into the design of international agricultural research

— an overview. In *International agricultural research and human nutrition*, ed P. Pinstrup-Anderson, A. Berg & M. Forman, pp. 13–23. Washington DC and Rome: International Food Policy Research Institute and UN Administrative Committee on Coordination/Sub-committee on Nutrition.

6 Plucknett, D.L. & Smith, N.J.H. (1982): Agricultural research and third world food production. *Science* **217**, 215–220.

7 Smith, M.F. (1983): Nutrition in farming systems research and extension. Proceedings of Kansas State University's 1983 Farming Systems Research Symposium, Kansas State University, Manhattan, Kansas.

8 Tripp, R. (1984): On farm research and applied nutrition: some suggestions for collaboration between national institutes of nutrition and agricultural research. *Fd Nutr. Bull.* **4**(3), 49–57.

9 Wagner, P.A. (1985): Incorporation of nutrition as a component of Farming Systems Research and Extension. Institute of Food and Agricultural Sciences, University of Florida, Gainesville, Florida. (Report of workshop held on February 20, 1985).

Positive deviance in nutrition: adequate child growth in poor households: a workshop report

MARIAN F. ZEITLIN and H. GHASSEMI (Organizers)
School of Nutrition, Tufts University, Medford, Mass. 02155 and UNICEF, New York, USA.

This workshop opened with an introduction to the concept of positive deviance in nutrition, and its relevance to nutrition policy and programme development and continued with a discussion of research approaches, recent findings, and methodological problems.

Concept and policy relevance. The term 'positive deviance' is used to describe the fact that some infants and young children living in impoverished, socioeconomically depressed environments remain *adequately nourished and healthy* (deviate positively) despite pervasive malnutrition in their communities. The expression, 'positive deviance' might be replaced by the phrase, 'adaptation to nutritional stress', or 'adequate growth amidst poverty'. Successful adaptations are in part social and behavioural and in part biological. The mother and others who undertake care do a better job in managing the child's life under serious constraints. The child's body performs better in spite of chronic food and nutrient deficiencies and high exposure to infection.

Since problems of poverty are expected to prevail for the rest of this century, it is important to attempt to learn low-cost approaches to preventing malnutrition from the mothers, families and other social networks surrounding these well-adapted children. It should remain clear that this approach is no substitute for all recommended efforts to alleviate poverty in the world. It should be seen as a promising complementary effort increasing the efficiency and impact of other development policies and programmes.

Research model. The positive deviance research approach falls within traditional epidemiological methods of studying prevention. This approach is applicable to all types of disease agents and risk-factors, not only to the nutrition and health status of young children. Even now, however, most epidemiological research focuses on causes of pathology rather than prevention.

The positive deviance approach to prevention represents a second line of defence, when exposure to risk has unavoidably occurred. Accordingly, the *function of research* is to *identify protective responses* to risk-factors. These responses include both: (a) *agents or sources* of natural immunity and adaptive resistance; and (b) *pathways* of resistance. The *purpose of research* is to develop the capacity to *engineer prevention or cure* for individuals who have already been exposed to risk.

Traditional survey research in nutrition has focused on the identification of causes of malnutrition. It has tended to evaluate the correlates of nutritional status in terms of the gaps that exist between the diets and environmental conditions of low-income malnourished infants and the ideal nutrient requirements, weaning practices, sanitary conditions, and health services. This research has yielded a set of common nutritional status correlates, including education, family size, birth spacing, availability of infant care, family wealth, health services utilization, morbidity history, water supply. To the extent that these factors differ from the ideal, risk of malnutrition occurs.

By contrast, positive deviance research attempts to identify the variables associated with malnutrition versus adequate nutrition of infants living under the same less than ideal conditions of low socioeconomic status and environmental deprivation.

Recent findings. A review of the literature which produced a state-of-the-art paper on positive deviance in nutrition, for UNICEF and the WHO/UNICEF Joint Nutrition Support Programme, discovered three types of factors associated with positive deviance: (1) known malnutrition correlates, mentioned in the previous section — these correlates differ within the low-income communities, but to a lesser degree than between high and low-income groups; (2) physiological factors, such as genetically determined metabolic efficiency, good immunity and a history of good health, and (3) psychosocial and behavioural factors characterizing the mother-infant interaction, the mother's psychological characteristics, and her social support network. This third type of factor promises to yield the most new information relevant to policy-making and programmes.

A major conclusion of the state-of-the-art paper was that many of the psychosocial factors associated with adequate growth amidst poverty are not specific to nutrition alone. In resource-scarce environments, attentive and affectionate care of infants and children and a supportive social structure predict a good nutritional outcome. These factors also predict good cognitive development, health, and long-term development of the individual into a stable, productive member of society. This finding implies that action to improve infant nutrition by improving the quality of care and stimulation given to infants and young children and the social services and social support networks available in low income communities can be justified not only on nutritional grounds, but much more broadly in terms of the child's overall development and well-being. Some behavioural factors, however, are specific to nutritional outcome and these should be a focus of nutritional research.

Statements of recent research findings were presented from Thailand (*Somchai Durongdej*), Chile (*Maria Luz Alvaraz*), Pakistan (*Julian Lambert*), Malaysia (*Christine Wilson*), Mexico and Bangladesh (*Marian Zeitlin*). The Thai study of 365 children aged 0–48 months living in low-income congested areas of Bangkok found that male sex, high birth-weight, low morbidity, good appetite, antenatal care and baby clinic attendance, consumption of colostrum, and current breast-feeding differentiated between the well-nourished and malnourished.

In Chile, a study of more than 1000 families, comparing low-income families with well-nourished versus malnourished infants disclosed significant differences in the parents' own childhood history and current social support structure and marital adaptation. Mothers of the well-nourished were more likely to come from intact homes, perceive that they were loved as children, have positive parental models, and have a currently stable union, with fewer arguments and more demonstration of affection. Fathers had a more stable employment history. Mothers of the malnourished were found to need models of good parenting behaviour, which might be provided by mothers of the well-nourished. Adolescent pregnancy was a risk-factor for poor parenting.

In Pakistan, a comparison between 38 households in which all children under five were above 90 per cent of weight-for-age and 134 households having at least one child below 60 per cent, having equal income and food expenditure, found higher consumption of edible oils, dhal, eggs and rice and longer birth intervals in the well-nourished families.

In Mexico, 25 well-nourished infants, aged 8.5–20.5 months, were found to receive more physical assistance from their mothers in eating meals and snacks, than 25 age-matched malnourished infants in the same low income squatter community. The well-nourished also received more powdered milk, which was given in feeding bottles, mixed with atole.

In Bangladesh, a survey of 180 9 to 18-month-old infants in one upland and one lowland rural site, found that the mothers of well-nourished infants differed from those of the malnourished in method of cleaning infant's faeces, mother's own hand-washing after defaecation, age of introducing supplementary foods, and educational aspirations for the child. Diarrhoeal rates differed significantly between the well- and malnourished. These rates were related to the infant's contact with chicken, duck, goat, cow, and human faecal matter while playing on the ground and to the dryness of the earth surface where the baby was left to play.

In a Malay village, progress following recent off-shore oil production had rapidly altered traditional practices between 1971 and 1984 with respect to water supply, latrine use, health services, birthing practices, dietary restrictions and bottle feeding. The proportion of villagers having secondary education also had risen dramatically. This site was an example of a setting in which rapid socioeconomic development makes the study of traditional adaptations, or positive deviance, less relevant.

Methodological issues. A discussion of the methodological issues brought out the following topics and points. (1) *Measurement of nutritional status to identify positive deviants from children who are growing poorly:* very poor growth (PG) infants are easy to identify because extreme stunting and wasting are not genetic. Good growth (GG) infants, or positive deviants are harder to identify because a child in the low normal range may have been high normal earlier, with growth failure in recent months. Therefore, 6-month longitudinal data are necessary for a sensitive classification of children into PG and GG groups. Children falling into the top and bottom thirds of a weight-for-age or height-for-age distribution, based on cross-sectional data, may still be compared if longitudinal data are not available, since there still are significant differences in nutritional status between these groups. *(2) Age:* GG and PG infants must be matched for age to avoid comparing a group of malnourished children at the worst stage of weaning with younger infants, who are still well-nourished, or older children, who have recovered in nutritional status. Most studies should be limited to narrow age groups because appropriate caretaking behaviour changes greatly with the developmental stage of the young child. *(3) Sample size and unit of analysis:* in the behavioural aspects of positive deviance research, the individual behaviour frequently is the logical unit of analysis, eg method of feeding, or method of cleaning when the infant defaecates. The need to conduct detailed observations makes it difficult to cover large numbers of mother-infant pairs. Careful consultation with a statistician is necessary to avoid problems of insufficient sample size and lack of independence between behavioural events and caretakers. Unit of analysis may vary with research question, eg, the extended family, the mother-child pair and the feeding event all may be valid units. *(4) Accuracy and replicability of observational research:* much of the study of adaptive behaviours involves observation of these behaviours. Semi-structured open-ended observational methods are needed to identify the types of behaviours that exist. However, results from such observations are not strictly reproducible because of variability in the kinds and the completeness of the information recorded by different observers. Reproducible research has to be based on more structured methods of observation. Such methods can be adapted from protocols used by developmental psychologists and anthropologists. *(5) Historical versus cross-sectional perspective:* some factors contributing to positive deviance go back to the childhood of the parents or to earlier circumstances in the history of the family. Cross-sectional research approaches should not ignore these historic factors. *(6) Rationale for existing behaviours:* behaviours that appear to have negative effects on the growth and health of young children may serve other purposes related to the survival of the household; may be caused by constraints that cannot be changed; or may be caused by historical developmental disorders within the family that do not respond to short-term programme approaches. Behavioural and social factors that contribute to positive deviance must be tested for transferability before they can be incorporated into programme design. Behavioural trial methods developed by social marketing and communications professionals are suitable for tests of behaviour change messages.

Observational research and behavioural trials may be conducted simultaneously. *Zeitlin* recommended a research design currently being used in Bangladesh, in which ethnographic and other observational studies, without intervention, are conducted in one village. Simultaneously, behavioural trials are undertaken in a nearby village (separated by water from the observation village). Ideas for behavioural change are communicated from the observation to the trial village. Resistance points to change are referred back from the trial to the observational village for investigation in a natural setting.

III: Dietary fibre, gut microflora and nutrient availability

NEW APPROACHES TO THE PHYSIOLOGICAL ROLE OF DIETARY FIBRE

The chemistry of dietary fibre

R.R. SELEVENDRAN
AFRC Food Research Institute – Norwich, Norwich, NR4 7UA, UK.

Dietary fibre has been defined as the skeletal remains of plant cells in our diet that are resistant to hydrolysis by the digestive enzymes of man[19]. This implies that dietary fibre (DF) is derived primarily from plant cell walls. However, as this definition did not include polysaccharides present in some food additives, such as plant gums, algal polysaccharides, pectins, modified celluloses and modified starches, Trowell *et al.* later extended[20] the definition to include all the polysaccharides and lignin in the diet that are not digested by endogeneous secretions of the human digestive tract. Accordingly, for analytical purposes, the term DF refers mainly to non-starchy polysaccharides and lignin in the diet[13]. While the revised definition is generally accepted, it should be borne in mind that the polysaccharides of food additives generally constitute only a very small proportion (<2 per cent) of the DF component of most diets. However the food additives are commercially available and have structural features similar to those of cell wall components and have therefore served as useful model compounds in studies on the mode of action of DF. Hence, plant cell walls are the main source of DF, and most of our DF intake comes from the cell walls in food such as vegetables, fruits, cereal products and seeds (other than cereals).

The principal components of DF are complex polysaccharides some of which are associated with lignin and proteins. The non-carbohydrate components of cell walls, such as lignin, polyphenolics, protein, cutin, phenolic esters and inorganic constituents, are quantitatively minor constituents of most foods, but some of them (eg lignin and phenolic esters) have significant effects on the properties and physiological effects of DF. Although most of the DF contituents may survive digestion in the non-ruminant proximal gastrointestinal tract, a significant proportion of them are degraded by microorganisms of the human colon[7,16]

In this paper the chemistry of cell walls from various tissues of edible plant organs and some of the recent developments in this area are outlined. The chemistry of food additives is not discussed; see[9,13] for the relevant references. The main emphasis is to show that this knowledge enhances our understanding of the chemistry and composition of DF, and its possible mode of action, particularly in the large intestine.

The major constituents of the cell wall. Most food plants other than cereals are dicotyledonous. The cell walls of their parenchymatous tissues consist of the middle lamella, which cements the cells together, and the primary cell wall; the former contains mainly pectins as their calcium salts and the latter is a composite of two distinct morphological phases, a complex continuous (inter-connected) matrix of macromolecules in which are dispersed structures known as micro-fibrils. In the case of soft tissues the fibrillar and matrix polysaccharides are bathed in an aqueous medium whereas in lignified tissues the whole complex is encrusted with lignin. Lignin appears to form covalent linkages with some of the hemicelluloses and thus cements the wall polymers into a unified rigid matrix, the wall becoming stratified in the process, these walls are usually called secondary cell walls.

The matrix polysaccharides are composed of essentially linearly orientated polymers, which are present at all stages of the development of the wall, and also highly branched polysaccharides that are deposited at particular stages of growth. The fibrillar polysaccharides are made up mainly of cellulose. The α-cellulose fraction isolated from most soft tissues, however, usually contains small but significant amounts of non-glucan polysaccharides and glycoproteins associated with it. It would appear that the associated polymers serve as linking compounds for the entanglement of the cellulose microfibrils with the matrix polymers.

The detailed chemical investigations of the macromolecular constituents of the cell walls, from various tissue types, show that they can be classified into the following groups: (a) polysaccharides — cellulose, pectic substances, hemicelluloses and storage polysaccharides, eg galactomannans in guar seeds; (b) glycoproteins and proteoglycans — in the former, the protein component is substituted by one or more heterosaccharides, and in the latter the protein component carries polysaccharide substituents; (c) lignin, polyphenolics and phenolic esters; and (d) lipid complexes — waxes, cutin and suberin. Water, an important component of the cell wall, is much less abundant in secondary walls than in primary cell walls of most plant tissues other than mature dry seeds. The amount of water within the wall matrix is partly controlled by the deposition of matrix polysaccharides (which form close intermolecular associations) or of a 'hydrophobic filler' such as lignin. During secondary thickening the space occupied by water in the wall becomes progressively filled by lignin and lignin-polysaccharide complexes.

The macromolecular constituents which make up DF are summarized in Tables 1 and 2 of[10], and in Table 1 of[11], wherein the types of polymer that can be obtained from the cell walls of parenchymatous, lignified and cutinised tissues of fruits, vegetables, cereals and seeds other than cereals are listed. The parenchymatous tissues are particularly important because the walls of these tissues comprise the bulk (~90–95 per cent) of the DF from vegetables, fruits and the endosperm of cereals. The lignified tissues are of greater importance with some cereal products, eg wheat bran and bran-based products. For details on the chemistry of cell wall polymers from edible plant organs see[8,9,13]. For an account of the advances in the chemistry and biochemistry of pectic and hemicellulosic polymers, mostly from edible plant tissues, see[12]. Our increased knowledge in the above areas is mainly due to developments in the methods for the isolation and analysis of cell walls from edible plant organs[12].

The approximate compositions of the cell walls from various tissue types, on a per cent dry weight basis (in parentheses), are: *fruits and vegetables* - parenchymatous — pectic polymers (35), α-cellulose (35), hemicellulosic polymers including proteoglycans (15), glycoproteins (10) and polyphenolics (5); lignified — pectic polymers (5), α-cellulose (40), hemicellulosic polysaccharides (30), glycoproteins (<5) and lignin (20). *Cereals and products* - parenchymatous pectic polymers (<1), α-cellulose (3), hemicellulosic polysaccharides (80), proteoglycans and glycoproteins (12) and polyphenolics (5); lignified — pectic polymers (<0.5), α-cellulose (35), hemicellulosic polysaccharides (45), proteoglycans (5) and lignin + phenolic esters (15).

It should be noted: (a) the pectic polymers of the middle lamellae are highly esterified and much less branched compared with those of primary cell walls; (b) the hemicellulosic polysaccharides of parenchymatous tissues of dicotyledons (xyloglucans) are very different from those of lignified tissues (acidic xylans); (c) the cell walls of cereal endosperm are virtually devoid of pectins and have only very small amounts of cellulose microfibrils in close association with glucomannans; (d) the major hemicelluloses of cereal endosperm are either arabinoxylans (wheat) or β-D-glucans (barley and oats); and (e) the outer layers of the wheat grain (eg beeswing wheat bran) are rich in acidic arabinoxylans. Recent work in our laboratory has shown that in addition to hydroxyproline-rich glycoproteins, the cell walls of runner beans, apples and immature cabbage leaves contain small amounts of a range of polysaccharide-protein-polyphenol complexes[12]. Comparable complexes have also been isolated from the cell walls of beeswing wheat bran and de-hulled oats (R.R. Selvendran & M.S. Du Pont, unpublished results). These complexes probably serve as linking units within the wall matrix, although some of the associated proteins may be immobilized cell wall enzymes.

The DF content of some plant foods. The DF contents of potatoes, carrots, immature cabbage leaves and apples are 1.8, 2.2, 2.2 and 1.9 respectively, on a per cent fresh weight basis. The types of pectic polymers present in the products are different. The major pectic polymers of potatoes are galactans covalently associated with rhamnogalacturonans, whereas in cabbage and apples pectic arabinogalactans predominate[12]. Immature carrots are also rich in pectic arabinogalactans[18], but these appear to be somewhat different from those of cabbage. Sugar beet is also rich in pectic arabinogalactans, and some of them are cross-linked by phenolics and phenolic esters (B.J.H. Stevens & R.R. Selvendran, unpublished results;[12]. The DF contents of the following products, on a per cent dry weight basis, are given within parentheses: white flour (3.2), wholewheat flour (10.3), porridge oats (7.1), pearl barley (7.8), rye flour (13.9), wholewheat bread (9.9), corn flakes (0.7), commercial wheat bran (45), pea cotyledons (11.6), pea hull (73.0), and guar seed splits (88). These values for DF are based on the content of non-starchy polysaccharides and do not include lignin. The values are from[3], except for wheat bran, pea flour, pea hull and guar seed splits which are from[9]. The 'resistant starch' contents, on a per cent dry weight basis, of wholewheat bread and corn flakes are 0.8 and 2.9 respectively. In the listed values the following points should be noted. The DF of white flour is derived mainly from endosperm cell walls, which are rich in arabinoxylans but poor in β-glucans and cellulose. In contrast the major DF polymers of pearl barley and porridge oats are β-glucans. The rye flour used for making rye biscuits (Ryvita) is relatively rich in β-glucans, but contains significant amounts of cellulose and acidic arabinoxylans derived from the bran layers. The main DF polymers of wholewheat flour are neutral arabinoxylans, acidic arabinoxylans and cellulose.

The last two are derived from the lignified bran layers. The main non-starchy polysaccharides of wheat bran are acidic arabinoxylans and cellulose. Wheat bran also contains small but significant amounts of neutral arabinoxylans and β-glucans, derived mainly from the endosperm and aleurone layers respectively. In addition to cellulose and acidic arabinoxylans, corn flakes contain a very significant amount of starch resistant to normal enzymic hydrolysis ('resistant starch'). Pea cotyledons are rich in arabinose-containing pectic substances and cellulose, whereas the hulls are rich in cellulose, pectic acid, acidic xylan and xyloglucan. Guar seed splits are very rich in galactomannans and contain small amounts of cellulose and pectic substances.

The average intake of DF in the United Kingdon is about 20 g/person/day and, of this, about a third comes from cereal sources[1]. The approximate breakdown of DF intake is as follows: vegetables and fruits (12 g) — this could be derived from about two to three potatoes, or comparable vegetable (6 g), and three apples (6 g); cereal products (7 g); wheat–bran–based products (2–3 g), which is roughly equivalent to 1 tablespoon of wheat bran, and six slices of white bread (5 g). As yet there is no official recommendation on a desirable level of DF intake, but 30 g/person/day might be recommended. This intake is best derived equally from vegetables and fruits (15 g) and cereal sources (15 g). The intake from cereal sources could easily be enhanced by consuming more wheat-bran-based products. The above is an approximate but useful guide.

For an account of the methods available for the analysis of DF see[3–5,10,14]. In the last reference the chemical background to the analysis of DF, the problems associated with the analysis of DF including methods for determining the lignin content, and developments in the analysis of DF over the past decade are critically and objectively assessed.

Properties of DF. The properties of DF are important because they determine the mode of action and fate of DF in the human alimentary tract and some of these are listed below.

The water holding capacity of fibre, and the products derived from it on transit, modify the propulsive movement of the digesta. Pectin is thought to be an important water-binding agent[15], but our studies on the water-holding capacity of native and depectinated cell wall preparations suggest that the particle size of the preparations is an over-riding factor (B.J.H. Stevens & R.R. Selvendran, unpublished results).

The solubility characteristics of DF components (eg galactomannans, pectins and β-glucans), particularly the viscosity changes which they effect, appear to be more important than the binding characteristics of fibre in influencing the mode of action of DF in the small intestine. For example, the galactomannans of guar gum are hydrophilic and form a viscous solution, and guar appears to slow glucose absorption by interacting with intestinal mucosa[6]. The bile-salt-binding characteristics of DF probably play a smaller role in influencing serum cholesterol levels than was envisaged before.

The degradability of DF by bacteria in the large intestine determines to a large extent the contribution which undegraded fibre and bacterial flora make to faecal weight. The cell wall polymers of parenchymatous tissues appear to be far more rapidly degraded by intestinal microflora than those of lignified tissues. It has been reported that 36 per cent of wheat bran fibre was degraded and that a large increase in faecal weight was mainly due to incompletely degraded fibre and associated water[16]. On the other hand, fibre rich in pectic substances but poor in lignin and phenolic esters is more extensively degraded (92 per cent with cabbage) and stimulated microbial growth. The main increase in faecal weight is then due to the increased biomass and the water retained by it. Our detailed chemical studies on the DF preparations from wheat bran, cabbage, carrots and apples[9,17] used in clinical feeding trials by Cummings *et al.*[2] have confirmed and extended hypotheses[2,16] on the main DF component responsible for faecal bulking, and also on the fate of DF in the large intestine. Our current work on the degradation of native and chemically treated DF preparations from wheat bran, apples, sugar beet, and xylans from oat hulls and larch wood, by faecal bacteria, suggests that in addition to lignification and phenolic ester cross-links, the solubility characteristics of the polymers, which among other factors depend on the degree of branching and degree of polymerisation, play important roles in determining the mode and extent of degradation of DF (B.J.H. Stevens & R.R. Selvendran, unpublished results).

Thus it is clear that fundamental work on plant cell walls is contributing to progress in the understanding of the chemistry and analysis of DF and in investigations of its physiological roles in humans. Studies on the relationship between cell wall structure and texture, particularly on cooking, are less well advanced but are being actively pursued at the Food Research Institute — Norwich, with special reference to the potato and apple.

1 Bingham, S., Cummings, J.H. & McNeil, N.I. (1979): Intake and sources of dietary fibre in the British population. *Am. J. Clin. Nutr.* **32**, 1313–1319.
2 Cummings, J.H., Branch, W., Jenkins, D.J.A., Southgate, D.A.T., Houston, H. & James, W.P.T. (1978): Colonic response to dietary fibre from carrot, cabbage, bran and guar gum. *Lancet* **1**, 5–9.
3 Englyst, H., Wiggens, H.S. & Cummings, J.H. (1982): Determination of non-starch polysaccharides in plant foods by gas-liquid chromatography of constituent sugars as alditol acetates. *Analyst* **107**, 307–318.
4 Faulks, R.M. & Timms, S.B. (1985): A rapid method for determining the carbohydrate component of dietary fibre. *Fd Chem.* **17**, 273–287.
5 James, W.P.T. & Theander, O. (Editors) (1981): *The analysis of dietary fibre in food.* New York and Basel: Marcel Dekker.
6 Johnson, I.T. & Gee, J.M. (1981): Effect of gel-forming gums on the intestinal unstirred layer and sugar transport in vitro. *Gut* **22**, 398–403.
7 Salyers, A.A. (1979): Energy sources of major intestinal fermentative anaerobes. *Am. J. Clin. Nutr.* **32**, 1313–1319.
8 Selvendran, R.R. (1983): The chemistry of plant cell walls. In *Dietary fibre*, ed G.G. Birch & K.J. Parker, pp. 95–147. London and New York: Applied Science Publishers.
9 Selvendran, R.R. (1984): The plant cell wall as a source of dietary fibre: chemistry and structure. *Am. J. Clin. Nutr.* **39**, 320–337.
10 Selvendran, R.R. & Du Pont, M.S. (1984): Problems associated with the analysis of dietary fibre and some recent developments. In *Development in food analysis techniques-3*, ed. R.D. King, pp. 1–68. London and New York: Elsevier Applied Science Publishers.
11 Selvendran, R.R., Stevens, B.J.H. & O'Neill, M.A. (1985): Developments in the isolation and analysis of cell walls from edible plants. In *Biochemistry of plant cell walls*, ed C.T. Brett & J.R. Hillmann, pp. 39–78. Cambridge: Cambridge University Press.
12 Selvendran, R.R. (1985): Developments in the chemistry and biochemistry of pectic and hemicellulosic polymers. *J. Cell. Sci. Suppl.* **2**, 51–88.
13 Southgate, D.A.T. (1976): The chemistry of dietary fibre. In *Fibre in human nutrition*, ed G.A. Spiller & R.J. Amen, pp. 31–72. New York: Plenum Press.
14 Southgate, D.A.T., Hudson, G.J. & Englyst, H. (1978): Analysis of dietary fibre — the choices for the analyst. *J. Sci. Fd Agric.* **29**, 979–988.
15 Stephen, A.M. & Cummings, J.H. (1979): Water holding by dietary fibre *in vitro* and its relationship to faecal output in man. *Gut* **20**, 722–729.
16 Stephen, A.M. & Cummings, J.H. (1980): Mechanism of action of dietary fibre in the human colon. *Nature* **284**, 283–284.
17 Stevens, B.J.H. & Selvendran, R.R. (1981): A comparison of the compositions of dietary fibre from some cereal and vegetable products in relation to observed effects in faecal weight. *Lebensm. Wiss. Technol.* **14**, 301–305.
18 Stevens, B.J.H. & Selvendran, R.R. (1984): Structural features of cell wall polysaccharides of the carrot *Daucus carota*. *Carbohydr. Res.* **128**, 321–333.
19 Trowell, H. (1974): Definitions of fibre. *Lancet* **1**, 503.
20 Trowell, H., Southgate, D.A.T., Wolever, T.M.S., Leeds, A.R., Gassull, M.A. & Jenkins, D.J.A. (1976): Dietary fibre redefined. *Lancet* **1**, 967.

Fibre and the human foregut

K.W. HEATON
University Department of Medicine, Bristol Royal Infirmary, Bristol, BS2 8HW, UK.

The foregut and midgut co-operate in the task of making energy and nutrients available to the body in optimal amounts and at optimal speed. Therefore, they may be considered together.

Evolution by natural selection ('survival of the fittest') has ensured that the foregut and midgut can carry out their tasks of ingestion, digestion and absorption with perfect efficiency.

But they can be relied on to do this only if the job they are asked to do, that is, the food they are given to handle, is that to which they are adapted.

What is the natural diet of man? Discussion continues[5], but there can be no doubt it is devoid of fibre-depleted foods since these are inventions of civilized man. Consumption of such foods is machine-age food going into stone-age bodies and it is credibly blamed for a wide variety of machine-age diseases[3,25]. Amongst these diseases are several which are attributable, at least in part, to overnutrition — obesity, diabetes, gallstones, hyperlipidaemia and hypertension. Hyperinsulinaemia is a feature of the first four of these diseases and may be involved in their pathogenesis. I have argued elsewhere that excess energy intake and hyperinsulinaemia (due to rapid carbohydrate absorption) are inevitable consequences of consuming fibre-depleted foods especially fibre-depleted sugars[8-10]. The essence of the argument is that, in its natural state in unprocessed plant foods, dietary fibre is a physiological obstacle to the ingestion and absorption of energy-rich foodstuffs. Hence, when the fibre in foods is removed or destroyed the foods become inherently abnormal in that they are ingested, digested and absorbed too easily and quickly. The person who habitually satisfies his appetite on such foods inevitably takes in more energy than he needs and carbohydrate enters his bloodstream faster than he needs.

The effects of fibre on the human foregut and midgut are scantily documented but, when experimental data are lacking, common experience and logical reasoning often indicate the likely effects. Practically every aspect of physiology is known to be or is likely to be affected.

A physical conception of dietary fibre. To understand how fibre affects the foregut and midgut in real life it is essential to bear in mind its physical properties, that is to say, its role in the architecture and texture of plant food. To study its properties when it is concentrated or isolated as a pure product is an interesting academic exercise but it may be misleading. Studies with pectin and with gums like guar gum are pharmacological, not physiological, studies.

Dietary fibre in the sense of cell wall material is the very architecture or skeleton of plants, giving them shape, rigidity and tensile strength — in a word, solidity. This solidity is transferred intact to unprocessed plant foods, though it can be much reduced by cooking. Most unprocessed plant foods are, even in the cooked state, solid to some extent and so require to be chewed. Sometimes, as when oats are cooked into porridge, solidity is largely removed but it is replaced with stickiness or viscosity.

Another important physical fact about cell walls is, simply, that they are walls; they enclose the cell contents. The cell contents of plants provide its sugars, starches and, to a lesser extent, proteins and fats. Fibre is the wrapping or packaging around these nutrients. This wrapping limits the rate of digestion and absorption of the nutrients.

The way to identify the effects of fibre on the foregut and midgut is to compare the body's response to test meals or diets of fibre-intact and fibre-depleted foods. It is important to study not only the effects of fibre-depleted foods but also the effects of fibre-disruption (Table 1). The effects of fibre-disruption can be greater than those of fibre-depletion.

Table 1. *Examples of fibre-depletion and fibre-disruption.*

Fibre-depletion	*Fibre-disruption*
Fruit → fruit juice	Fruit → puree
Sugar beet or cane → sucrose	Vegetables → puree
Whole-meal flour → sifted flour	Grains → flour, flakes
Nuts, seeds → oils	Peanuts → peanut butter

Aspects of ingestion affected by dietary fibre. The desire to ingest may be altered. If a person who is not especially hungry is offered the choice of whole raw fruit, like apples or oranges, or the juice made from these fruits he is more likely to accept the fibre-free juice. Fibre-intact foods look bulkier and more filling.

In the mouth, solid fibre-intact food feels different and stimulates more activity. Its unyielding texture demands that it be chewed. The act of chewing evokes secretion of saliva, which washes the teeth and gums and lubricates the bolus of food so that it can be swallowed comfortably. Chewing also evokes satiety[1]. But the main effect of mastication is to slow down the ingestion of energy.

Some of these points are illustrated by our apple study[7]. When volunteers ate a meal of apples in the form of puree it took them much less time and evoked much less satiety than an equivalent meal of whole apples. Taken as juice it took even less time and was even less satiating. The same satiating effect of fibre has been observed with oranges and grapes[2].

By evoking satiety, fibre reduces the desire to go on ingesting and probably delays the reappearance of appetite. However, the latter point has not been examined systematically.

Aspects of digestion affected by fibre. Here more experimental data are available, though not all are equally appropriate. The stomach retains solids longer than liquids. Solid lumps are churned in the gastric antrum until they are reduced to a few millimetres in diameter[22]. Only then are they allowed to pass the pylorus. Hence it can be predicted that blending, milling, cooking or any other fibre-disrupting process which destroys the solidity of food will cause it to be emptied faster from the stomach.

Whether liquids are emptied more slowly when they are rendered viscous by soluble fibre is controversial. Such slowing has been found to occur with fruit juice but not with realistic meals[15,21].

There is some evidence that cereal fibre prolongs the rise in intragastric pH after a meal[16,20]. This might be relevant to peptic ulceration[19].

Pancreatic digestion is affected by dietary fibre concentrates but results vary between different concentrates[11,23]. Wheat bran reduces the activity of pancreatic enzymes *in vitro*, but the relevance of this to healthy people is uncertain. In patients with steatorrhoea due to advanced chronic pancreatitis, a very-high-fibre diet (75–80 g/d) caused a modest but significant increase in faecal weight and in faecal fat (14.7 to 19.4 g/d)[4].

Disruption of the fibrous structure of food would be expected to increase the access of pancreatic enzymes and hence increase the digestibility of starch, etc. Indeed *in vitro*, the starch in rice (white or brown) is digested much more rapidly when the rice is ground into flour (Table 2)[18]. Similarly, it has been shown the digestibility of lentils could be increased by blending and baking and then grinding them into a paste[13] (though this may have been due in part to destruction of starch-protein complexes or of amylase inhibitors during baking).

Table 2. *Effect of milling rice on plasma glucose and insulin responses to 75-g-starch-containing meals and on the rate of starch hydrolysis* in vitro *by pancreatic amylase[18].*

	Brown rice		White rice	
	Whole	*Ground*	*Whole*	*Ground*
Mean rise in plasma glucose (mmol/l)	0.92	3.33	1.51	3.65
Mean rise in plasma insulin (μU/ml)	27.3	93.7	31.9	89.5
Rate of starch hydrolysis (% of 0.2 g hydrolysed in 30 min.)	17.6	68.2	30.8	71.8

In vivo, it is very difficult to study the rate of digestion. However, the combined functions of digestion and absorption can be studied by measuring the plasma glucose and insulin responses to starch-containing test meals. The effects of fibre upon these will be considered shortly.

Effect of dietary fibre on absorption. The only practical way to study absorption as a separate entity from digestion is by perfusion techniques using multilumen tubes. Only the soluble fractions of fibre and suspensions of finely ground insoluble fibre can be studied in this way. Such studies have been done, but only with pectin or guar gum in unphysiological concentrations. The relevance of the results is doubtful.

Effect of fibre on combined digestion and absorption. Judging by the plasma insulin and glucose responses to test meals, there is no significant difference in the rate of digestion-absorption of starch between ground white rice and ground brown rice (Table 2[18]). The same is true, for plasma glucose at least, when white and brown rice, white and whole meal bread, and white and whole meal spaghetti are compared[12]. These findings could be interpreted as meaning that, in cereal foods at least, dietary fibre has no effect on the overall digestion and absorption of starch. However, this conclusion is valid only if one neglects the physical state of fibre. To do this is to ignore the very raison d'etre of dietary fibre.

Comparing the results obtain with 14 different foods, Jenkins and his colleagues have shown that there is a good correlation (r = 0.86) between the rate of digestion of starch *in vitro* and the glycaemic index *in vivo*, that is, the area under the blood glucose curve after 50 g starch from food related to the area after 50 g glucose[14]. Plasma insulin responses are a more sensitive way of revealing differences in the rate of carbohydrate absorption.

By these criteria, disruption of fibre has very definite effects on digestion-absorption. We have been encouraged to examine this systematically by several isolated observations: reduced glycaemia after wheat flakes compared with wheat bread[24]; reduced glycaemia and insulinaemia after whole compared with ground rice as shown in Table 2[18]; increased faecal fat excretion after whole peanuts compared with peanut butter[17]; and our own observation of reduced insulinaemia after whole compared with pureed apples[7]. There have also been studies showing increased recovery of undigested food from the faeces when 16 foods were swallowed without chewing[6].

We fed four wheat meals of decreasing particle size to ten healthy volunteers in random order. All meals contained 50 g carbohydrate, were made from the same batch of grain and were eaten over the same period of time. They consisted of whole-wheat grains boiled until soft, cracked wheat boiled similarly, coarse whole-wheat flour baked into a scone, and fine whole-wheat flour baked similarly. As shown in Table 3, there was a step-wise increase in glucose and, especially, insulin responses as the particle size of the wheat was reduced, that is to say, as its fibrous structure was disrupted. By analogy with rice[18] the likely reason is that with smaller particles there is increased accessibility to pancreatic amylase and so more rapid digestion of starch.

Table 3. *Effect of reducing particle size on plasma glucose and insulin responses to whole-wheat meals containing 50 g carbohydrate* (K.W. Heaton, S.N. Marcus & P.M. Emmett, unpublished data).

	Whole grains	Cracked wheat	Coarse flour	Fine flour
Rise in plasma glucose (mmol/l)	2.15 ± 0.44	2.27 ± 0.21	2.73 ± 0.16	3.03 ± 0.42
Area under glucose curve (mmol/l.min)	731 ± 31	741 ± 27	739 ± 20	777 ± 23
Rise in plasma insulin (µU/ml)	24.2 ± 2.2	26.7 ± 3.0	31.4 ± 2.2	38.6 ± 4.3
Area under insulin curve (mU/l.min)	2353 ± 220	2396 ± 456	2816 ± 302	3720 ± 293

Conclusions. Dietary fibre in its natural, intact state in food is a physiological obstacle to the ingestion and digestion of nutrients, especially carbohydrate. By rendering food more solid, it slows down both ingestion and digestion. This sets limits to energy intake and insulin responses and can be viewed as nature's built-in preventive of the diseases of overnutrition and hyperinsulinaemia. In susceptible people, such as the potentially obese and the potentially diabetic subject, disruption of fibre in food might be as detrimental to health as depletion of fibre.

1 Anand, B.K. (1974): Neurological mechanisms regulating appetite. In *Obesity symposium*, ed W.L. Burland, P.D Samuel & J. Yudkin, pp. 116–145, Edinburgh: Churchill Livingstone.
2 Bolton, R.P., Heaton, K.W. & Burroughs, L.F. (1981): The role of dietary fibre in satiety, glucose, and insulin: studies with fruit and fruit juice. *Am. J. Clin. Nutr.* **34**, 211–217.
3 Cleave, T.L. (1974): *The saccharine disease*. Bristol: John Wright.
4 Dutta, S.K. & Hlasko, J. (1985): Dietary fiber in pancreatic disease: effect of high fiber diet on fat malabsorption in pancreatic insufficiency and *in vitro* study of the interaction of dietary fiber with pancreatic enzymes. *Am. J. Clin. Nutr.* **41**, 517–525.
5 Eaton, S.B. & Konner, M. (1985): Paleolithic nutrition — a consideration of its nature and current implications. *New Engl. J. Med.* **312**, 283–289.
6 Farrel, J.H. (1956): The effect of mastication on the digestion of food. *Br. Dent. J.* **100**, 149–155.
7 Haber, G.B., Heaton, K.W., Murphy, D. & Burroughs, L. (1977): Depletion and disruption of dietary fibre. Effects on satiety, plasma-glucose, and serum-insulin. *Lancet* **2**, 679–682.
8 Heaton, K.W. (1973): Food fibre as an obstacle to energy intake. *Lancet* **2**, 1418–1421.

9   Heaton, K.W. (1978): Fibre, satiety and insulin — a new approach to overnutrition and obesity. In *Dietary fibre. Current developments of importance to health*, ed K.W. Heaton, pp. 141–149. London: Newman.

10 Heaton, K.W. (1980): Food intake regulation and fiber. In *Medical aspects of dietary fiber*, ed G.A. Spiller & R.M. Kay, pp. 223–238. New York: Plenum.

11 Isaakson, G., Lundquist, I. & Ihse, I. (1982): *In vitro* inhibition of pancreatic enzyme activities by dietary fiber. *Digestion* **24**, 54–59.

12 Jenkins, D.J.A., Wolever, T.M.S., Taylor, R.H., Barker, H.M., Fielden, H. & Gassull, M.A. (1981): Lack of effect of refining on the glycemic response to cereals. *Diabetes Care* **4**, 509–513.

13 Jenkins, D.J.A., Thorne, M.J., Camelon, K., Jenkins, A., Rao, A.V., Taylor, R.H., Thompson, L.U., Kalmusky, J., Reichert, R. & Francis, T. (1982): Effect of processing on digestibility and the blood glucose response: a study of lentils. *Am. J. Clin. Nutr.* **36**, 1093–1101.

14 Jenkins, D.J.A., Ghafari, H., Wolever, T.M.S., Taylor, R.H., Barker, H.M., Fielden, H., Jenkins, A.L. & Bowling, A.C. (1982): Relationship between the rate of digestion of foods and postprandial glycaemia. *Diabetologia* **22**, 450–455.

15 Kasper, H., Eilles, C., Reiners, C. & Schrezenmeir, J. (1985): The influence of dietary fiber on gastric transit time. *Hepatogastroenterology* **32**, 69–71.

16 Lennard-Jones, J.E., Fletcher, J. & Shaw, D.G. (1968): Effect of different foods on the acidity of the gastric contents in patients with duodenal ulcer. Part III. Effect of altering the proportions of protein and carbohydrate. *Gut* **9**, 177–182.

17 Levine, A.S. & Silvis, S.E. (1980): Absorption of whole peanuts, peanut oil, and peanut butter. *New Eng. J. Med.* **303**, 917–918.

18 O'Dea, K., Snow, P. & Nestel, P. (1981): Rate of starch hydrolysis *in vitro* as a predictor of metabolic responses to complex carbohydrate *in vivo*. *Am. J. Clin. Nutr.* **34**, 1991–1993.

19 Rydning, A., Berstad, A., Aadland, E. & Ødegaard, B. (1982): Prophylactic effect on dietary fibre in duodenal ulcer disease. *Lancet* **2**, 736–739.

20 Rydning, A., Nesland, A. & Berstad, A. (1984): Influence of fiber on postprandial intragastric juice acidity, pepsin, and bile acids in healthy subjects. *Scand. J. Gastroenterol.* **19**, 1039–1044.

21 Rydning, A., Berstad, A., Berstad, T. & Hertzenberg, L. (1985): The effect of guar gum and fiber enriched wheat bran on gastric emptying of a semisolid meal in healthy subjects. *Scand. J. Gastroenterol.* **20**, 330–334.

22 Schiller, L.R. (1983): Motor function of the stomach. In *Gastrointentinal Disease: Pathophysiology, Diagnosis, Management*, 3rd edn, ed M.H. Sleisenger & J.S. Fordtran, pp. 521–541. Philadelphia: Saunders.

23 Schneeman, B.O. (1982): Pancreatic and digestive function. In *Dietary fiber in health and disease*, ed. G.V. Vahouny & D. Kritchevsky, pp. 73–83. New York: Plenum.

24 Thomas, B. & Elchazly, M. (1976): Funktionelle wirkungen und veräanderungen der Ballastoffe des Weizens während des Verdauungsablaufes. *Qualitas Plantarum — Plant Foods for Human Nutrition*. **26**, 211–226.

25 Trowell, H.C., Burkitt, D.P. & Heaton, K.W. (1985): *Dietary fibre, fibre-depleted foods and disease*. London: Academic Press.

Fibre and the rumen

P.J. VAN SOEST
Department of Animal Science, Cornell University, Ithaca, NY 14853, USA.

Ruminants are mammals that chew their cud. This chewing (remastication) is always associated with rumen fermentation, a form of pregastric fermentation. This most fundamental feature of ruminant digestion allows grazing ruminants to be exceptional utilizers of fibre as a source of dietary energy, an adaptation which has the limitation that food intake may suffer in the interest of the retention required for digestive extraction.

The classification of ruminants and nonruminants is an oversimplification, ruminant-like capacities existing in grazing and selector types of feeding and in true ruminants and nonruminant groups. True ruminants represent a broad subfamily of artiodactyl herbivores exhibiting varied dietary adaptations. There are about 170 extant species. While all of them ruminate and have pregastric fermentation, these features are by no means exclusive to the group. Camelids, a related group, also ruminate and have pregastric fermentive digestion, and many other mammals, marsupials and birds have pregastric fermentation although they probably do not ruminate. Adaptation to pregastric fermentation may only require hypoacidity and buffering effects in the non-acid-secreting portion of the abomasum.

On the other hand, small antelope and deer, although true ruminants, are comparatively unable to utilize highly fibrous food and have adapted to selective feeding of nutritively differentiated plants (usually browsers)[11]. These species may pass unfermented food past the rumen and thus may be metabolically closer to non-ruminating species. The rumens in these animals may serve input as a detoxification system, because many alkaloids, oxalates, nitrates, cyanides can be destroyed in fermentation[23].

Virtually all ingested carbohydrate is available for fermentation in adult ruminants, and otherwise available sugars and starches are thus unavailable as sugar sources as a consequence of their fermentation. The ruminant animal is largely dependent on gluconeogenesis for maintaining blood glucose. Consequently, the division of dietary fibre into soluble and insoluble components has no meaning, since available pectins, beta-glucans and other gums have the same fate as sucrose and starch.

Pregastric digestion has required metabolic adaptations. Since most available carbohydrate is lost in fermentation, gluconeogenesis provides essential blood glucose which is only half the nonruminant level. Enzymatic adaptation to glucose sparing has caused the loss of enzymes (ATP citrate lyase and NADP malate dehydrogenase) needed to convert glucose to acetyl-CoA and fat. Blood acetate from the rumen supplies the major source of carbon for lipogenesis and general energy metabolism, glucose being reserved for essential functions. Secreted gut enzyme levels are generally lower than in nonruminants[4].

Microbes arrive alive in the abomasum where peptic digestion begins. Ruminants have evolved a special lysozyme (aspartate omitted in the peptide sequence) which is resistant to, and consequently synergistic with pepsin. It lyses cells rendering their proteins more available for hydrolysis. *In vitro* studies show ruminant lysozyme to be four to five times more effective than nonruminant enzymes for this purpose (A. Wilson, pers. comm.).

While lignification is the ultimate factor limiting the extent of digestion, all herbivores are limited in digestive capacity by finite retention times. The limits of cell wall digestion are approached only in those animals with the capability of longest retention (generally the larger ruminants) and in the case of the lowest intakes which promote the longest retentions.

The fractions most sensitive to digestive loss are the slowest moving ones, in particular cellulose, which nonruminants seem to utilize less well than hemicellulose. The correlation between mean retention and cellulose digestion in 46 species of mammals (ruminants and nonruminants) is + 0.86, ruminants representing an upper extention to the regression line[24]. Smaller animals are less able to digest fibre, because they have high metabolic requirements relative to their gastrointestinal capacities, leading to higher intakes per unit of body weight and thus short retentions[6].

The evolutionary adaptation of ruminants thus allows them to retain food for a longer time relative to body weight, and thus achieve the digestive capacity of larger nonruminant herbivores. The largest grazing nonruminant herbivores (rhinos) have the digestive capacity of grazing ruminants[6]. However, the hippo (in the large weight class) has pregastric digestion.

The organisms producing the fermentation in the rumen, caecum, large intestine and colon are an exceedingly diverse group comprising perhaps several hundred species, the numerical majority of which are obligate anaerobes of very similar type to those in the rumen[5]. Fibre-fermenting organisms are a relatively fastidious group with special nutrient requirements including carbon dioxide, ammonia, acetate, isobutyrate, 2-methylbutyrate, isovalerate, haem and various vitamins[5,12]. Some are unable to use glucose or amino acids as substrates. Methanogenic organisms require CO_2 or formate as substrate and acetate for cell synthesis of protein. All fibre-digesting and methanogenic organisms are exceedingly sensitive to oxygen and particularly so in dilute culture.

For these reasons some studies of the effects of fibre on the distribution of faecal bacteria may be distorted or lack validity. For example, the reported decrease in faecal anaerobes in humans at higher intake of dietary fibre[3] contrasts with the fact that all fibre digesters are anaerobic, and that rumen studies indicate that increased dietary fibre supports a larger fibre-digesting population. The fibre-digesting bacteria in the human gut and other monogastric species have nutrient requirements essentially identical with rumen bacteria and thus grow better on rumen fluid than on other media[5].

Factors determining the balanced proportion of end-products are the amount of methane formed and the net substrate carbon converted to cellular mass. Both of these factors are regulated by ecological conditions in the gut fermentation and the capacity of the particular species to obtain ATP from the fermented substrate. Methanogenic organisms are the most fastidious and are reduced at high rates of passage, lowered pH or by over-supply of rapidly degradable substrate. Since the methane-forming organisms serve as the hydrogen sink for balancing redox potential in the general fermentation, decrease in their production forces other organisms to rebalance their products such that oxidation and reduction equivalents remain stoichiometrically balanced relative to hydrogen. The lack of methanogenesis usually forces production of hydrogen as well.

This generally means that propionic acid increases at the expense of methane since it is the only one of the three acids that can be formed from glucose without simultaneous production of CO_2. The net effect of methanogenic suppression is to increase net acid production most of which appears in the form of propionate. The metabolic significance of this rise for the animal is in the greatly increased energy available for gluconeogenesis, as propionate is the main source. Methanogenic suppression may decrease microbial efficiency. About 50 per cent of the total carbon in fermentable fibrous carbohydrate is converted to volatile fatty acids although this value will vary inversely with microbial efficiency. Less efficient microbial growth would force a larger proportion of carbon into VFA and increase the quantitative estimate of that absorbed[27]. The amount of carbohydrates fermentable in the bowel may be greater than the sum of fermented fibre, since any starches, or other sugars, reaching the lower tract will ferment.

Nonruminants are sensitive to these factors. The feeding of starch elicits increase in the proportion of caecal propionate in the pig and pony as it does in the ruminant. This is evidence that starches can escape upper tract digestion[23]. While no data are available these factors seem likely to apply to man. People without methanogens might metabolize more propionate.

Despite the large production of fermentation acids, the pH of the lower tract remains relatively neutral[21]. This neutrality is essential for fibre digestion since most anaerobic cellulolytic bacteria are intolerant to a pH lower than 6. The ranges in concentration of acids in the caecum and/or colon of monogastrics are within the ranges observed for the rumen. Probably higher concentrations reflect a greater rate of production, a larger fermentation pool and a larger quantity of acids absorbed into the blood.

Neutral conditions are maintained by diffusion of un-ionized acids across the gut wall to the blood stream and the return flow of sodium and bicarbonate ions and urea. Urea is hydrolised to ammonium bicarbonate, also becoming a part of the buffering system[21]. The appearance of starch or lactose in the fermentation may be inhibitory to the slower fermenting fibrous carbohydrates, cellulose and hemicellulose, because the soluble carbohydrates can be rapidly fermented to the stronger lactic acid and adventitious organisms are less inhibited by lower pH. High lactic fermentation and lowered gut pH are often associated with gastrointenstinal stress in ruminants and probably in nonruminants as well, eg lactose intolerance in humans.

The portion of the fermented substrate converted to microbial cells is a major factor influencing loss of nutrients in faeces. The advantage of the ruminant with its pregastric fermentation is that available microbial protein and vitamins are digested and absorbed postgastrically, while the same products of postgastric fermentation will be largely lost in faeces.

Microbial matter forms the largest single organic fraction in the faeces of most animals, comprising in man 60–80 per cent of the dry weight of faeces. Microbial matter also comprises most (about 85 per cent) of the so-called metabolic faecal nitrogen of both ruminants and nonruminants.

Microbial cellular yield is generally proportional to the amount of substrate fermented and to the turnover in the fermentation. Thus the addition of fermentable fibrous carbohydrate increases faecal microbial loss, mainly measured as metabolic faecal nitrogen. The true digestibility of dietary proteins is often unaffected, as may be the nitrogen balance since the microbial synthesis of protein is largely at the expense of urea diffusing across the caecal or colonic wall[18]

Secondary factors influencing the distribution of cells and fermentation products involve the rate of fermentation, generation time of bacteria and the rate that they are washed out through transit and passage. Slow rates of washout relative to generation lead to cannibalism and refermentation of dead cells. The effect is to increase fermentation acids at the expense of cell yield, the total of which, plus gases, must account for net fermented carbohydrate. The addition of unfermentable fibre increases passage rate and therefore promotes increased faecal microbial losses as a proportion of fermented fibre[22].

Ruminants generally require adequate dietary fibre for normal rumen function. Feedlot cattle in the United States are not fed much fibre for economic reasons, nevertheless such recognized pathologies as acidotic conditions, rumen parakeratosis, disappear if adequate fibre is fed[7]. When dairy cattle are fed diets too low in fibre or in which fibre is too finely prepared, lowered milk fat and reduced efficiency of lactation results. The requirement for fibre as neutral detergent fibre (NDF) is about 36 per cent of the diet, providing that it is of sufficient coarseness. In fattening animals (beef or sheep) the same dietary management leads to obesity[8]. The metabolic response appears to result from excess propionic acid production and the response of the hormonal regulating system to the large increment in gluconeogenic precursors. Insulin and fat mobilizing hormones are probably involved but the phenomenon is inadequately understood. Depot fats of sheep accumulate odd carbon and methylated acids[26] some of which are also characteristic of microbial lipids[15].

The level of fibre in the diet which will provide optimum animal efficiency has been examined in several species, eg pigs[16], guinea-pigs[9] and man[20]. The feeding of lucerne to growing pigs affects gross feed efficiency and body composition. Up to a certain level (6–12 per cent NDF in total diet) fibre does not alter use of digested energy and may even improve it[16]. Feeding still more fibre generally elicits some loss in overall efficiency. However, one of the significant effects is the alteration in body composition. Fibre-fed pigs are leaner, with less fat, and have a larger gut fill and a heavier gut mucosa[14]. Fibre also stimulates caecal and colonic growth in the rat[13]. Caecal and colonic mucosal growth occurs through VFA stimulation as in the ruminant[21]. VFA are absorbed in monogastrics and in man by the same mechanisms as in the ruminant[10,19]. Butyrate is metabolized by the colonic and caecal walls as it is by the rumen wall, and is the most stimulatory of mucosal growth[2].

An increased intake of the unavailable fermentable carbohydrates leads to a greater portion of the energy being derived from VFA, leading to greater gluconeogenesis from propionate and increased metabolism of butyrate by the colonic mucosa[25]. The gluconeogenic effect of propionate may be part of the beneficial effect of high-fibre diets for diabetics[1].

The anatomical development of ruminants has metabolic relevance, since energy metabolism relies, like diabetics, upon fatty acids. In this respect all animals derive some of their energy from VFA, the portion from non carbohydrate being associated with greater intake of fermentable fibre. Caloric inefficiency in ruminants has long been associated with high-fibre diets and high ratios of acetate to propionate among the fermentation products.

The final question is whether increased intake of fibre and associated VFA will induce caloric inefficiency and provide a basis for weight control. In the aforementioned pig studies, fibre increased leanness, but not body weight, because of compensatory increases in gut weight. The argument from rumen metabolism is that acetate is inefficient relative to ATP and may also divert gluconeogenic amino acids[17] so that heat increment is elevated, although intake of energy may not have changed. This is an aspect of ruminant studies that needs application and understanding in nonruminant and human nutrition.

1 Anderson, J.W. (1983): Dietary fibre and diabetes. In *Fibre in human and animal nutrition* ed G. Wallace & L. Bell, pp. 183–187. Wellington, NZ: Royal Soc. New Zealand (Bull 20).

2 Argenzio, R.A. & Southworth, M. (1975): Sites of organic acid production and absorption in gastrointestinal tract of the pig. *Am. J. Physiol.* **228**, 454–459.

3 Aries, V., Crowther, J.S., Drasar, B.S., Hill, M.J. & Williams, R.E.O. (1969): Bacteria and the aetiology of cancer of the large bowel. *Gut* **10**, 334–335.

4 Bauman, D.E. & Currie, W.B. (1980): Partitioning of nutrients during pregnancy and lactation: A review of mechanisms involving homeostasis and homeorhesis. *J. Dairy Sci.* **63**, 1514–1529.

5 Bryant, M.P. (1978): Cellulose digesting bacteria from human feces. *Amer. J. Clin. Nutr.* **31**, (Suppl.) S113–S115.

6 Demment, M.W. & Van Soest, P.J. (1983): *Body size, digestive capacity, and feeding strategies of herbivores*, pp. 66. Morrilton, Arkansas: Winrock International.

7 Donefer, E. (1976): The importance of fibre for herbivorous animals. In *Proc. Miles Symp.* ed W.W. Hawkins. pp.

51–56. Miles Laboratories Ltd., Rexdale, Ont: Nutr. Soc. of Canada.

8 Duncan, W.R.H., Ørskov, E.R., Fraser, C. & Garton, G.A. (1974): Effect of processing of dietary barley and of supplementary cobalt and cyanocobalamin on the fatty acid composition of lamb triglycerides, with special reference to branched-chain components. *Br. J. Nutr.* **32**, 71–75.

9 Fahey, G.C., Jr., Miller, B.L. & Hadfield, H.W. (1979): Metabolic parameters affected by feeding various types of fiber to guinea pigs. *J. Nutr.* **109**, 77–83.

10 Flemming, S.E., Marthinsen, D. & Kuhnlein, H. (1983): Colonic function and fermentation in man consuming high fiber diets. *J. Nutr.* **113**, 2535–2544.

11 Hofmann, R.R. (1973): *The ruminant stomach: stomach structure and feeding habits of East African game ruminants*, pp. 354. Nairobi, Kenya: East African Literature Bureau.

12 Hungate, R.E. (1966): *The rumen and its microbes*, p. 533. New York: Academic Press.

13 Jacobs, L.R. & Schneeman, B.O. (1981): Effects of dietary wheat bran on rat colonic structure and mucosal cell growth. *J. Nutr.* **111**, 798–803.

14 Kass, M.L., Van Soest, P.J., Pond, W.G., Lewis, B.A. & McDowell, R.E. (1980): Utilization of dietary fiber from alfalfa by growing swine. I. Apparent digestibility of diet components in specific segments of the gastrointestinal tract. *J. Anim. Sci.* **50**, 175–191.

15 Keeney, M. (1970): Fat metabolism in the rumen. In *Physiology of digestion and metabolism in the ruminant*, ed A.T. Phillipson, pp. 489–503. Cambridge: Oriel Press.

16 Kornegay, E.T. (1981): Soybean hull digestibility by sows and feeding value for growing-finishing swine. *J. Anim. Sci.* **53**, 138–145.

17 MacRae, J. (In press): In *Proc. VI Internat. Ruminant Symp.* Banff, Canada.

18 Mason, V.C. (1984): Metabolism of nitrogenous compounds in the large gut. *Proc. Nutr. Soc.* **43**, 45–53.

19 McNeil, N.I., Cummings, J.H. & James, W.P.T. (1978): Short chain fatty acid absorption by the human large intestine. *Gut* **19**, 819–824.

20 Spiller, G. (1983): Dietary fibre deficiency and disease: An overview. In *Fibre in human and animal nutrition*, ed L. Wallace & G. Bell. pp. 9–10. Wellington: Royal Soc. New Zealand (Bull 20).

21 Stevens, C.E. (1977): Comparative physiology of the digestive system. In *Duke's Physiology of domestic animals*, ed M.J. Swenson, pp. 216–232. Ithaca and London: Comstock.

22 Van Soest, P.J. (1981): Some factors influencing the ecology of gut fermentation in man. In *Gastrointestinal cancer: endogenous factors*. Banbury Report 7, pp. 61–69. Cold Spring Harbor, New York: Cold Spring Harbor Laboratories.

23 Van Soest, P.J. (1982): *Nutritional ecology of the ruminant*, pp. 374. Corvallis, Oregon: O&B Books, Inc.

24 Van Soest, P.J., Jeraci, J.L., Foose, T., Wrick, K. & Ehle, F. (1983): Comparative fermentation of fibre in man and other animals. In *Fibre in human and animal nutrition*, ed L. Wallace & G. Bell, pp. 75–80. Wellington: NZ Royal Soc. New Zealand (Bull 20).

25 Von Engelhardt, W. & Rechkemmer, G. (1983): The physiological effects of short-chain fatty acids in the hind gut. In *Fibre in human and animal nutrition*, ed L. Wallace & G. Bell, pp. 149–155. Wellington: NZ. Royal Soc. New Zealand (Bull 20).

26 Wahle, K.W.J. & Paterson, S.M. (1979): The utilization of methylmalonyl-CoA for branched-chain fatty-acid synthesis by preparations from bovine (Bos taurus) adipose tissue. *J. Biochem.* **10**, 443–437.

27 Wolin, M.J. (1975): Bacterial species of the rumen: interactions between bacterial species of the rumen. In *Digestion and metabolism in the ruminant*, pp. 134–148. Armidale, Australia: The University of New England Publishing Unit.

Dietary fibre and lipid metabolism

D. KRITCHEVSKY, G.V. VAHOUNY and J.A. STORY
The Wistar Institute of Anatomy and Biology, 3601 Spruce Street, Philadelphia, Pennsylvania 19104;
George Washington Medical Center, Department of Biochemistry, 2300 Eye Street NW, Washington DC 20037; Purdue University, Department of Foods and Nutrition, Stone Hall, W. Lafayette, Indiana 47907, USA.

Effects of fibre on lipid metabolism are usually expressed as influence of fibre on serum or plasma cholesterol or lipoprotein level and, in cases of animal experiments, the data usually include liver cholesterol levels as well. This is not surprising given the preoccupation with cholesterol metabolism. However, data have been accumulated over the past 20 years which may begin to explain the mechanism(s) of action of specific types of dietary fibre and which may, ultimately, provide a rationale for developing insights into structure-function relationships.

The effect of fibre on serum and liver lipids has been reviewed in several recent books[34,35,42,43] and all data suggest that gelling fibres such as pectin or guar gum exert the greatest influence on cholesterol levels. The influence of dietary fibre on cholesterol metabolism in experimental animals has been summarized recently[16].

Binding of bile acids and other lipids. Appearance in the blood of ingested lipid depends upon the efficiency of its gastric absorption, intestinal transit and transport as lipoprotein. Dietary triglycerides are emulsified and hydrolyzed to yield monoglycerides and fatty acids which are incorporated into mixed micelles together with bile salts, phospholipids, and endogenous and exogenous cholesterol. The efficient operation of this process depends upon the availability of bile salts and phospholipids. When the diet of rats fed a (commercial) ration was changed to a laboratory-prepared semipurified ration, the rats exhibited an increase in the turnover time of cholic acid and decreased excretion of both neutral and acidic steroids[29]. That study showed that dietary fibre (as exemplified by the commercial ration) influenced steroid metabolism and suggested to future investigators that dietary fibre might exert a hypocholesterolemic effect by enhancing bile acid excretion. One of the members later showed[28] that the lipid components of the commercial ration (when added to the semipurified diet) did not affect bile acid excretion, a further suggestion that the fibre present in the ration was the component most probably responsible for the observed effects.

Table 1. *Binding of bile acids and bile salts to fibres[39]. Fibre (50 mg) and bile acid or salt (50 μmol) incubated in 5 ml phosphate buffer (pH 7.0) for 2 h at 37°C. Percentage bound calculated from material recovered from supernatant following centrifugation. Values represent means of three determinations. (Per cent bound ± SEM).*

Bile acid or bile salt	Fibre			
	Alfalfa	*Bran*	*Cellulose*	*Lignin*
Cholic	19.9 ± 0.7	10.2 ± 0.7	3.0 ± 0.9	43.7 ± 0.3
Taurocholic	6.9 ± 1.0	1.4 ± 0.7	1.0 ± 0.4	22.1 ± 0.9
Glycocholic	11.5 ± 0.5	3.8 ± 1.0	1.2 ± 0.6	22.5 ± 0.8
Chenodeoxycholic	24.8 ± 2.3	18.2 ± 0.6	1.9 ± 0.4	23.3 ± 0.3
Taurochenodeoxycholic	15.1 ± 0.7	9.8 ± 0.7	0	25.4 ± 0.7
Glycochenodeoxycholic	14.9 ± 0.9	21.4 ± 7.1	0.2 ± 0.2	25.2 ± 0.3
Deoxycholic	10.4 ± 1.3	5.4 ± 0.9	0.2 ± 0.2	17.4 ± 2.1
Taurodeoxycholic	11.4 ± 0.1	3.4 ± 1.1	0.7 ± 0.6	30.9 ± 0.6
Glycodeoxycholic	27.8 ± 0.9	7.8 ± 0.7	4.7 ± 0.3	52.6 ± 0.3

The association of bile acids with the insoluble fraction of the contents of the rat small intestine was reported[8] and it was demonstrated that cholic acid could be bound to various grains[9]. Later studies[1,4,15,39] showed that bile acids and salts were bound to fibres and that there were certain specificities in the binding (Table 1). The different binding specificities are evident. Alfalfa bound more free cholic and chenodeoxycholic acid than either salt, but more glycodeoxycholic acid than either the free bile acid or its taurine conjugate. Bran bound more of the glycine conjugates of all three bile acids and cellulose showed very little binding capacity. Lignin bound more cholic acid than its conjugates; equal amounts of all chenodeoxycholic acid derivatives and much more glycodeoxycholic than either taurodeoxycholic or deoxycholic acid. The binding is reversible to some extent[7]. Bile-acid-binding capacities of alfalfa and wheat bran were reduced by 66 and 62 per cent respectively when the lignin was extracted[40].

Fibres have been shown to interact with and bind all lipid components of micelles. Vahouny *et al.*[46,47] examined the effects of bile acid binding resins, dietary fibres and fibre-rich substances such as wheat bran and alfalfa. Their results are summarized in Table 2. The data shown that fibres have the capacity to disrupt micelles and may consequently inhibit lipid

Table 2. In-vitro *binding of micellar components by fibre preparations*[46,47]. *Micelle contained 5 mM taurocholate; 625 µM lecithin; 250 µM cholesterol; 250 µM monolein; 500 µM fatty acid. Incubations used for 40 mg fibre carried out for 2 h at 37°C. Values represent means of 6–12 incubations. (Percentage bound ± SEM).*

Test substance	Fibre				
	Alfalfa	*Bran*	*Cellulose*	*Guar Gum*	*Lignin*
Taurocholate	6.7 ± 0.5	3.6 ± 1.1	1.4 ± 0.3	35.6 ± 1.7	20.2 ± 5.7
Lecithin	3.6 ± 1.1	6.3 ± 2.0	0.5 ± 0.5	21.5 ± 1.8	8.8 ± 3.4
Cholesterol	1.1 ± 1.0	0	7.5 ± 1.9	22.7 ± 3.3	4.7 ± 5.5
Monolein	18.6 ± 1.4	11.3 ± 0.8	3.5 ± 1.0	23.1 ± 2.8	12.8 ± 1.0
Palmitic acid	14.8 ± 0.9	9.6 ± 1.1	2.3 ± 0.7	31.3 ± 1.4	10.2 ± 0.7
Oleic acid	15.2 ± 0.8	10.4 ± 1.1	5.8 ± 1.0	31.4 ± 2.1	19.5 ± 0.9
Linoleic acid	23.8 ± 0.5	13.0 ± 1.0	3.6 ± 0.6	37.0 ± 0.9	6.4 ± 0.3

absorption. The level of binding of taurocholate from micelles was similar to that seen from simple solutions. Guar gum showed surprising avidity for all the lipids and, with the exception of cholesterol, cellulose bound less of all the substrates than any of the other test substances.

While bile-acid-binding capacity may not be an infallible indicator of a fibre's effect on cholesterolemia, it is interesting that substances such as wheat bran or cellulose, which have no effect on cholesterol levels in man, bind bile acids weakly if at all.

If fibre interferes with micellar integrity, it should exert effects of lipid absorption. At the level of digestion, Schneeman and her collaborators[31–33] have shown that lipase activity in rats fed 20 per cent cellulose or 5 per cent wheat bran is similar to that seen in rats fed a fibre-free diet but lipase activity is significantly enhanced in rats fed 5 per cent pectin or 20 per cent wheat bran. In man, alfalfa, oat or wheat bran decreases lipase activity and pectin increases lipase activity, but the differences are not significant. Cellulose and xylan, however, decrease human lipase activity significantly[6].

Effects on lipid absorption. Early studies of the effects of dietary fibre on cholesterol absorption involved the use of balance techniques or faecal recovery of radioisotopes (^{3}H or ^{14}C) administered as labelled cholesterol. Pectin was found to lower plasma cholesterol in rats[21] and to result in increased excretion of bile acids, and pectin and alfalfa increased faecal steroid excretion[19,22]. Cholesterol absorption has been decreased in rats fed pectin, gum arabic or agar[12]. In studies of lymphatic absorption of cholesterol in rats fed wheat bran, alfalfa meal, yeast cell-wall glycan, cellulose or pectin, absorption (as ^{14}C recovered in lymph at 24 hours) was reduced by all of the materials fed[44,45]. Recently we have examined the effects of a number of other fibres on lymphatic absorption of cholesterol and oleic acid. In every case, cholesterol absorption was significantly lower after 4 h, but at 24 h absorption of cholesterol in rats fed cellulose or alfalfa was similar to that seen in rats maintained on a fibre-free diet (Table 3). Absorption of oleic acid followed a similar pattern, but by 24 h absorption was similar in all groups except that fed psyllium.

Table 3. *Recovery of cholesterol and oleic acid from lymph of rats fed fibres for 4 weeks. Rats given a single intraduodenal dose of lipid emulsion (1.5 ml) containing 146 mg oleic acid, 25 mg cholesterol, 144 mg taurocholate and 25 mg albumin.*

	Lipid recovered (%)				
	Cholesterol			*Oleic acid*	
Diet	*4 h*	*24 h*	*4 h*	*24 h*	
Fibre-free	19.2	51.0	47.0	69.3	
Cellulose	8.8	38.3	37.6	66.2	
Alfalfa	6.8	39.5	33.8	58.4	
Psyllium	3.3	12.6	19.8	27.0	
Pectin	4.8	19.0	25.9	54.3	
Guar gum	6.1	29.0	32.7	51.3	

Table 4. *Recovery of ^{3}H or ^{14}C cholesterol from serum and tissues of rabbits (5C, 9SP) fed commercial ration (C) or semipurified diet (SP) for 6 months[18]. SP diet: 40% carbohydrate (sucrose-starch 1:1); 25% casein; 14% coconut oil; 15% cellulose; 5% mineral mix; 1% vitamin mix. [1,2-^{3}H] cholesterol (10 μCi) and (2-^{14}C) mevalonate (0.5 Ci) injected intraperitoneally 72 h before autopsy.*

| | Group | |
Tissue	C	SP
Serum		
^{3}H dpm/mg cholesterol	676 ± 167	403 ± 31
dpm/total serum (10^{-5})	0.38 ± 0.11	4.03 ± 0.36 a
^{14}C dpm/mg cholesterol	ND	2.7
dpm/total serum	ND	2757
Liver		
^{3}H dpm/mg cholesterol ($\times 10^{-4}$)	2.52 ± 0.70	4.36 ± 0.31 b
dpm/total liver ($\times 10^{-6}$)	1.34 ± 0.4	4.41 ± 0.52 a
^{14}C dpm/mg cholesterol	465 ± 163	884 ± 106
dpm/total liver ($\times 10^{-4}$)	1.05 ± 0.28	3.99 ± 0.59 a
Aorta		
^{3}H dpm free cholesterol	800	1920
dpm ester cholesterol	120	240
^{14}C dpm free cholesterol	22	110
dpm ester cholesterol	66	88
Faecal Steroids		
^{3}H neutral (dpm $\times 10^{-6}$)	18.8 ± 10.4	3.8 ± 1.3
acidic (dpm $\times 10^{-5}$)	1.6 ± 0.9	9.5 ± 2.2 b
^{14}C neutral (dpm $\times 10^{-3}$)	10.8 ± 4.2	5.1 ± 1.8
acidic (dpm $\times 10^{-3}$)	0.04 ± 0.1	3.8 ± 1.2 c

Levels of significant difference in the values of C and of SP in one row: a, $P < 0.001$; b, $P < 0.01$; c, $P < 0.02$.

The effects of a commercial ration and a semipurified diet on the distribution of endogenous and exogenous cholesterol in the rabbit were examined (Table 4)[18]. The animals were given ^{3}H-cholesterol or ^{14}C-mevalonate 72 hours before termination of the experiment. Recovery of both tritium and carbon-14 from serum, liver and aorta was significantly lower in the rabbits fed the commercial ration. Rabbits fed commercial ration excreted 53 per cent more ^{3}H in their faeces and 13 per cent more ^{14}C than those fed the semipurified diet. Rabbits fed the semipurified diet excreted significantly more acidic steroid, probably due to slower intestinal transit time.

Soft white wheat bran has no effect on plasma cholesterol levels in man and does not affect bile acid excretion[10], whereas, bran from hard red spring wheat is hypocholesterolaemic[27,36] and causes increased excretion of bile acids[36]. Pectin has a hypocholesterolaemic effect in man and increases faecal output of bile acids[11,23]. The influence of dietary fibre on concentration of faecal steroids in rats in summarized in Table 5; concentration of faecal neutral steroids and bile acids is lowest in rats fed cellulose. The substances fed are all more hypocholesterolaemic than cellulose. Cellulose fed to rats in diets containing cholesterol often increases liver cholesterol levels above those seen in controls fed fibre-free diets[14,37,41,48]. Cellulose feeding also increases total-body cholesterol levels in rats[26]. Rabbits fed atherogenic diets containing cellulose have higher cholesterol levels and more severe atherosclerosis than those fed similar diets containing wheat straw or alfalfa[20,25].

The data show that particulate, bulking fibres such as cellulose or bran have a less marked effect on lipid metabolism than do soluble ionic (pectin) or non-ionic (guar gum) fibres. Explanations for these results include effects on bile acid formation and excretion and inhibition of absorption. Another possibility is that the volatile short chain fatty acids produced by action of the colonic microflora affect lipid metabolism. It has been shown that dietary sodium propionate lowers serum and liver cholesterol levels in rats[5].

Table 5. *Relative steroid excretion in rats: response to various sources of dietary fibre.*

	Neutral		Acidic	
Fibre (% in diet)	mg/g faeces	mg/d	mg/g faeces	mg/d
Cellulose (10)*	1.00	1.00	1.00	1.00
Wheat Bran (10)	1.64	1.02	1.08	0.67
Alfalfa (10)	1.37	0.96	1.25	0.84
Pectin (5)	2.26	0.46	1.50	0.35
Guar Gum (5)	1.89	1.07	1.08	0.61
Psyllium (5)	1.89	1.21	1.75	1.10
Fibre Free	2.39	0.66	1.94	0.55

*Values obtained from cellulose fed rats arbitrarily set at 1.00

Effects of plasma lipids and lipoproteins. Fibres which lower plasma cholesterol levels will also affect lipoprotein levels, usually the low-density lipoprotein (LDL) cholesterol ([38] for review). Oat bran has been shown to lower total cholesterol levels in man by 13 per cent, LDL levels by 13.6 per cent and high-density lipoprotein (HDL) levels by 2 per cent. The ratio of HDL-cholesterol to LDL-cholesterol was increased by 12 per cent[13]. The absolute level of HDL-cholesterol or ratio of HDL-cholesterol to total or LDL-cholesterol have all been suggested as indicators of risk of coronary disease[2,24]. When men were fed different fibres (0.75 g/2.17 MJ) for a month, cellulose had no effect on serum cholesterol level, whereas karaya gum and locust bean gum resulted in cholesterol reductions of 10 and 14 per cent, respectively[3]. The initial ratio of HDL/total cholesterol was 0.21; after feeding of cellulose, karaya gum or locust bean gum, the ratio became 0.21, 0.23 and 0.23. The ratio of HDL/total cholesterol in vegetarians was 0.34 compared to 0.27 in controls[30]. The serum lipid levels of vegetarian Seventh Day Adventists, lacto-ovo vegetarians, non-vegetarian Adventists and general public have been compared with their fibre intake. Serum cholesterol in the vegetarians was significantly lower than in the other three groups. The major difference in fibre intake was in pectin. The vegetarians ingested 7.5 g/0.02 MJ/d of this fibre, whereas the intake of the other groups was 4.0–4.5 g/d[17].

Conclusion. One aspect of lipid metabolism which has received relatively little attention is the influence of dietary fibre on assembly of lipoproteins. Although we have available data relating to influence of fibre on lipoprotein spectrum in animals and man, more work on fibre effects on apolipoprotein spectrum and on basic elements of lipoprotein release is needed.

We have advanced from considerations of fibre, without regard to structure or composition, to being able to separate effects of soluble and insoluble fibres and even ionic and non-ionic soluble fibres. Ideally we should have enough data on structure-function relationships to permit preparation of fibre mixtures to do specific metabolic tasks.

1 Balmer, J. & Zilversmit, D.B. (1974): Effects of dietary roughage on cholesterol adsorption, cholesterol turnover and steroid secretion in the rat. *J. Nutr.* **104**, 1319–1328.
2 Barr, D.P., Russ, E.M. & Eder, H.A. (1951): Protein lipid relationships in human plasma. II. Atherosclerosis and related conditions. *Am. J. Med.* **11**, 480–493.
3 Behall, K.M., Lee, K.H. & Moser, P.B. (1984): Blood lipids and lipoproteins in adult men fed refined fibers. *Am. J. Clin. Nutr.* **39**, 209–214.
4 Birkner, N.J. & Kern, F., Jr. (1974): *In vitro* adsorption of bile salts to food residues, salicylazosulfapyridine and hemicellulose. *Gastroenterology* **67**, 237–244.
5 Chen, W.J.L., Anderson, J.W. & Jennings, D. (1984): Propionate may mediate the hypocholesterolemic effects of certain soluble plant fibers in cholesterol-fed rats. *Proc. Soc. Exp. Biol. Med.* **175**, 215–218.
6 Dunaif, G. & Schneeman, B.O. (1981): The effect of dietary fiber on human pancreatic activity *in vitro*. *Am. J. Clin. Nutr.* **34**, 1034–1035.
7 Eastwood, M.A., Anderson, R., Mitchell, W.D., Robertson, J. & Pocock, S. (1976): A method to measure the adsorption of bile salts to vegetable fiber of differing water holding capacity. *J. Nutr.* **106**, 1429–1432.
8 Eastwood, M.A. & Boyd, G.S. (1967): The distribution of bile salts along the small intestine for rats. *Biochim. Biophys. Acta* **137**, 393–396.

9 Eastwood, M.A. & Hamilton, D. (1968): Studies on the adsorption of bile salts to non-absorbed components of the diet. *Biochim. Biophys. Acta* **152**, 165–173.

10 Eastwood, M.A., Kirkpatrick, J.R., Mitchell, W.D., Bone, A. & Hamilton, T. (1973): Effects of dietary supplements of wheat bran and cellulose on faeces and bowel function. *Br. Med. J.* **4**, 392–394.

11 Kay. R.M. & Truswell, A.S. (1977): Effect of citrus pectin on blood lipids and fecal excretion in man. *Am. J. Clin. Nutr.* **30**, 171–175.

12 Kelly, J.J. & Tsai, A.C. (1978): Effect of pectin, gum arabic and agar on cholesterol absorption, synthesis and turnover in rats. *J. Nutr.* **108**, 630–639.

13 Kirby, R.W., Anderson, J.W., Sieling, B., Rees, E.D., Chen, W.J.L., Miller, R.E. & Kay, R.M. (1981): Oat bran intake selectively lowers serum low density lipoprotein concentrations in hypercholesterolemic men. *Am. J. Clin. Nutr.* **34**, 824–829.

14 Kiriyama, S., Okazaki, Y. & Yoshida, A. (1969): Hypocholesterolemic effect of polysaccharides and polysaccharide-rich foodstuffs in cholesterol-fed rats. *J. Nutr.* **97**, 382–388.

15 Kritchevsky, D. & Story, J.A. (1974): Binding of bile salts *in vitro* by non-nutritive fiber. *J. Nutr.* **104**, 458–462.

16 Kritchevsky, D. & Story, J.A. (1985): Influence of dietary fiber on cholesterol metabolism in experimental animals. In *Dietary fiber in human nutrition*, ed G.A. Spiller. Boca Raton: CRC Press.

17 Kritchevsky, D., Tepper, S.A. & Goodman, G. (1984): Diet, nutrient intake and metabolism in populations at high and low risk for colon cancer. 7. Relation of diet to serum lipids. *Am. J. Clin. Nutr.* **40**, 921–926.

18 Kritchevsky, D., Tepper, S.A., Kim, H.K., Moses, D.E. & Story, J.A. (1975): Experimental atherosclerosis in rabbits fed cholesterol-free diets. 4. Investigation into the source of cholesteremia. *Exp. Molec. Pathol.* **22**, 11–19.

19 Kritchevsky, D., Tepper, S.A. & Story, J.A. (1974): Isocaloric, isogravic diets in rats. III. Effects of nonnutritive fiber (alfalfa or cellulose) on cholesterol metabolism. *Nutr. Rep. Int.* **9**, 301–308.

20 Kritchevsky, D., Tepper, S.A., Williams, D.E. & Story, J.A. (1977): Experimental atherosclerosis in rabbits fed cholesterol-free diets. 7. Interaction of animal or vegetable protein with fiber. *Atheroscler.* **26**, 397–403.

21 Leveille, G.A. & Sauberlich, H.E. (1966): Mechanism of the cholesterol depression effect of pectin in the cholesterol-fed rat. *J. Nutr.* **88**, 209–214.

22 Lin, T.M., Kim, K.S., Karvinen, E. & Ivy, A.C. (1957): Effect of dietary pectin, 'protopectin' and gum arabic on cholesterol excretion in rats. *Am. J. Physiol.* **18**, 66–70.

23 Meithinen, T.A. & Tarpila, S. (1977): Effect of pectin on serum cholesterol, fecal bile acids and biliary lipids in normolipidemic and hyperlipidemic individuals. *Clin. Chem. Acta* **79**, 471–477.

24 Miller, G.J. & Miller, N.E. (1975): Plasma high density lipoprotein concentration and development of ischaemic heart disease. *Lancet* **1**, 16–19.

25 Moore, J.H. (1967): The effect of type of roughage in the diet on plasma cholesterol levels and aortic atherosis in rabbits. *Br. J. Nutr.* **21**, 207–215.

26 Mueller, M.A., Cleary, M.P. & Kritchevsky, D. (1983): Influence of dietary fiber on lipid metabolism in meal fed rats. *J. Nutr.* **113**, 2229–2238.

27 Munoz, J.M., Sandstead, H.H., Jacob, R.A., Logan, G.M., Reck, S.J., Klevay, L.M., Dintzis, F.R., Inglett, G.F. & Shuey, W.C. (1979): Effects of some cereals and textured vegetable protein on plasma lipids. *Am. J. Clin. Nutr.* **32**, 580–592.

28 Portman, O.W. (1960): Nutritional influences on the metabolism of bile acids. *Am. J. Clin. Nutr.* **8**, 462–470.

29 Portman, O.W. & Murphy, P. (1958): Excretion of bile acids and beta-hydroxysterols by rats. *Archs Biochem. Biophys.* **76**, 367–376.

30 Sacks, F.M., Castelli, W.P., Donner, A. & Kass, E.H. (1975): Plasma lipids and lipoproteins in vegetarians and controls. *New Engl. J. Med.* **292**, 1148–1151.

31 Schneeman, B.O. & Gallaher, D. (1980): Changes in small intestinal digestive enzyme activity and bile acids with dietary cellulose in rats. *J. Nutr.* **110**, 584–590.

32 Schneeman, B.O., Jacobs, L.R. & Richter, D. (1982): Response to dietary wheat bran in the exocrine pancreas and intestine of rats. *J. Nutr.* **112**, 283–286.

33 Sheard, N.F. & Schneeman, B.O. (1980): Wheat bran's effect on digestive enzyme activity and bile acid levels in rats. *J. Fd Sci.* **45**, 1645–1648.

34 Spiller, G.A. (1985): *Dietary fiber in human nutrition*. Boca Raton: CRC Press.

35 Spiller, G.A. & Kay, R.M. (1980): *Medical aspects of dietary fiber*, New York and London: Plenum.

36 Spiller, G.A., Wong, L.G., Nunes, J.D., Story, J.A., Petor, M.S., Furumoto, E.J., Alton-Spiller, M., Whittam, J.H. & Scala, J. (1984): Effect of four levels of hard wheat bran on fecal composition and transit time in healthy young women. *Fed. Proc.* **43**, 392.

37 Story, J.A., Baldino, A., Czarnecki, S.K. & Kritchevsky, D. (1981): Modification of liver cholesterol accumulation by dietary fiber in rats. *Nutr. Rep. Int.* **24**, 1213–1219.

38 Story, J.A. & Kelley, M.J. (1982): Dietary fiber and lipoproteins. In *Dietary fiber in health and disease*, ed G.V. Vahouny and D. Kritchevsky, pp. 229–236. New York and London: Plenum Press.

39 Story, J.A. & Kritchevsky, D. (1976): Comparison of the binding of various bile acids and bile salts *in vitro* and by several types of fiber. *J. Nutr.* **106**, 1292–1294.

40 Story, J.A., White, A. & West. L.G. (1982): Absorption of bile acids by components of alfalfa and wheat bran *in vitro*. *J. Fd. Sci.* **47**, 1276–1279.

41 Tsai, A.C., Elias, J., Keeley, J.J., Lin, R.S.C. & Robson, J.R.K. (1976): Influence of certain dietary fibers on serum and tissue cholesterol levels in rats. *J. Nutr.* **106**, 118–123.

42 Vahouny, G.V. & Kritchevsky, D. (1982): *Dietary fiber in health and disease*. New York and London: Plenum Press.
43 Vahouny, G.V. & Kritchevsky, D. (1985): *Basic and clinical aspects of dietary fiber*. New York and London: Plenum Press.
44 Vahouny, G.V., Roy, T., Gallo, L.L., Story, J.A., Kritchevsky, D. & Cassidy, M.M. (1980): Dietary fibers. III. Effect of chronic intake on cholesterol absorption and metabolism in the rat. *Am. J. Clin. Nutr.* **33**, 2182–2191.
45 Vahouny, G.V., Roy, T., Gallo, L.L., Story, J.A., Kritchevsky, D., Cassidy, M.M., Grund, B. & Treadwell, C.R. (1978): Dietary fiber and lymphatic absorption of cholesterol in the rat. *Am. J. Clin. Nutr.* **31**, S208–S212.
46 Vahouny, G.V., Tombes, R., Cassidy, M.M., Kritchevsky, D. & Gallo, L.L. (1980): Dietary fibers. V. Binding of bile salts, phospholipids and cholesterol from mixed micelles by bile acid sequestrants and dietary fibers. *Lipids* **15**, 1012–1018.
47 Vahouny, G.V., Tombes, R., Cassidy, M.M., Kritchevsky, D. & Gallo, L.L. (1981): Dietary fibers. VI. Binding of fatty acids and monolein from mixed micelles containing bile salts and lecithin. *Proc. Soc. Exp. Biol. Med.* **166**, 12–16.
48 Wells, A.F. & Ershoff, B.H. (1961): Beneficial effects of pectin in prevention of hypercholesterolemia and increase in liver cholesterol in cholesterol-fed rats. *J. Nutr.* **74**, 87–92.

Dietary fibre and the colon

M.A. EASTWOOD
Wolfson Gastrointestinal Laboratories, Gastrointestinal Unit, Department of Medicine, University of Edinburgh, Western General Hospital, Edinburgh, UK.

The colon is the site of major transformation and modification of dietary fibre in the human. Colonic bacteria undertake this process[3,29]. The fibre may undergo fermentation and the metabolic byproducts, short-chain fatty acids, hydrogen and methane, may be absorbed[21,24].

Fibre appears to be the most important single determinant of stool weight[11]. Fibre is involved in three processes in the colon, fermentation, absorption of the metabolic products and determination of stool weight. There are considerable differences between different species in the importance of these three processes. The monogastric herbivores use the colon as a source of nutrition in much the same manner as the ruminant uses the foregut[26]. The carnivore has a short colon, which appears to be less important nutritionally to these animals[1]. Omnivores such as the rat and man have colons of intermediate length from which nutrient absorption may be important[5,15].

The caecum contains a large bacterial population. It is customary to attempt to classify the several hundred species of bacteria found in the colon[7]. However, the complex interrelationships between these bacteria is such[9] that it is perhaps more practical to regard the caecal bacterial population as a metabolic entity, almost as an organ in its own right, albeit biologically distinct from the host. The fermentation system created by the colon is very dependent upon the delivery of nutrition, probably coming through from the ileum. Such nutrients of import to the bacterial mass will include dietary fibre[6], starch[33] and possibly protein and fat[8]. Other sources of energy to the bacteria will be of biliary origin, eg bile acid conjugates[14], or of intestinal endogenous sources, eg mucopolysaccharides[28]. Ingested chemicals such as drugs may be of sources of bacterial energy, but little is known of this aspect of colonic physiology.

The best studied influence on bacterial mass is dietary fibre. Bacteria proliferate in the presence of certain fibres, in particular the water-soluble fibres that are found in fruit, vegetables and gums[30]. It is not known whether the increases in bacterial population are an uniform increase in all species or are restricted to certain bacterial types which benefit from, and are implicated in, the metabolism of the fibre which has stimulated the increase. The few studies described so far suggest an overall increase in bacterial population with no increase in any particular species[2]. However, there is a functional adaptation to a fibre challenge which is identifiable at 3 weeks[23] wherein breath hydrogen excretion increases. This response is probably due to an increase in bacterial enzymatic activity,[28] ie a functional change as well as a possible overall increase in bacterial mass.

In general measurements of caecal bacterial mass are indirect. In experimental animals it is possible to weigh the caecum or to measure products of bacterial fermentation. Such measurements include hydrogen[34], methane[21], and short-chain fatty acids[25]. In man such measurements are even more indirect and involve measuring faecal constituents, bacteria[32] or short-chain fatty acids[31]. There is an increase in breath hydrogen excretion when unabsorbed oligosaccharides are ingested[35]. This does not apply to the ingestion of a single amount of more complex fibres[34], although, after a period of ingestion of such complex fibres, there is a metabolic response, shown by an increase in breath hydrogen[23]. Only a proportion of human populations exhale methane in the breath[18], though most people express methane in flatus[22]. Whilst there is a relationship between breath hydrogen and the fibre content of the diet[20] the addition of fibre to the diet does not increase the excretion of methane in the breath. Adding fibre to the diet of a non-methane producer does not lead to that individual excreting methane in the breath[20]. The colon absorbs short-chain fatty acids[24], which are of particular importance to the nutrition of monogastric herbivores, such as ponies and rabbits. It has been suggested that butyrate is an important nutrient for the colonic mucosa in man[27]. Perhaps, more importantly substantial absorption of short-chain fatty acids may be of significance to the nutrition of the individual.

Wet faecal output in European men is probably about 100 g fresh material per day but is substantially greater in African populations[4]. The range of stool output varies immensely in human subjects, ranging from 15 to 280 g per day[13] and varies substantially from day to day in any individual[38]. Faeces are approximately 75 per cent water, the dry matter of stool consists of approximately 40 per cent bacteria and 40 per cent fibre[32].

Fibre appears to influence stool weight by one of two mechanisms. The water-holding capacity of that fibre which has resisted fermentation in the caecum is an important determinant of stool weight[12]. Cereal fibre is the best example of a fibre functioning through water-holding capacity, the greater the water-holding capacity the greater the effect on stool weight[10]. This is a reliable and predictable mechanism. Small particle size and cooking reduce the efficacy of this mechanism[37]. However, fibre which is readily fermented, eg pectin, gum arabic or carrot, has an indirect effect on stool weight. There is fermentation of these fibres and as the bacteria proliferate on the fibre during fermentation then there is the possibility of increased bacterial mass in the stool and hence an increase in stool weight[32]. This sequence does not always follow and therefore this is a somewhat unpredictable manner of increasing stool weight.

In experiments in the rat an increase in rat caecal bacterial mass with gum arabic ingestion can lead to an increase in faecal bacterial excretion with little or no effect on stool weight[36]. In man there is evidence of increased bacterial metabolic activity after the ingestion of gum arabic as shown by an increased breath hydrogen excretion, but there is no change in stool weight[23]. This suggests increased bacterial metabolism even bacterial growth without influencing stool weight. However, the fermentable fibres may influence sterol metabolism by increasing faecal bile-acid excretion[17]. This does not happen with wheat bran[16]. This implies that there are different mechanisms influencing stool weight and faecal constituents.

The mechanisms whereby fibre effects colonic physiology are dependent upon whether or not the fibre is fermented[19]. If the fibre, eg wheat bran, is fermented to a limited extent then association with water and increase in stool weight is the most important effect. Following prolonged ingestion of fermentable dietary fibre there are more complex effects on caecal metabolism, absorption of nutrients from the colon and sterol metabolism.

1 Alvarez, W.C. (1949): *An introduction to gastroenterology*, 4th edn. London: Heinemann.
2 Bornside, G.H. (1978): Stability of human faecal flora. *Am. J. Clin. Nutr.* **31**, S141–S144.
3 Bryant, M.P. (1978): Cellulose digesting bacteria from human feces. *Am. J. Clin. Nutr.* **31**, S113–S115.
4 Burkitt, D.P. & Trowell, H.C. (1975): *Refined carbohydrates: some implications of dietary fiber*. New York: Academic Press.
5 Cummings, J.H. (1982): Consequences of the metabolism of fiber on the human large intestine. In *Dietary fiber in health and disease* ed G. Vahouny & D. Kritchevsky, pp. 9–22. New York: Plenum Press.
6 Cummings, J.H. (1983): The colon. In *Recent advances in gastroenterology* Vol. 4, ed I.A.D. Bouchier. Edinburgh: Churchill Livingstone.
7 Drasar, B.S. & Hill, M.J. (1974): *Human intestinal flora*. London: Academic Press.

8 Eastwood, M.A. & Hamilton, D. (1969): Fatty acids in the lumen of the human small intestine following a lipid containing meal. *Scand. J. Gastroent* **5**, 225–230.

9 Eastwood, M.A. (1973): Vegetable fibre: its physical properties. *Proc. Nutr. Soc.* **32**, 137–143.

10 Eastwood, M.A., Smith, A.N. & Drummond, E. (1981): The effect of coarse and fine Canadian Red Spring wheat and French soft wheat bran in colonic motility in patients with diverticular disease. *Am. J. Clin. Nutr.* **34**, 2460–2463.

11 Eastwood, M.A. & Robertson, J.A. (1983): In *Colon structure and function*. ed L. Bustos-Fernandez, pp. 141–165, New York: Plenum.

12 Eastwood, M.A., Robertson, J.A., Brydon, W.G. & MacDonald, D. (1983): Measurement of water holding properties of fibre and their faecal bulking ability in man. *Br. J. Nutr.* **50**, 539–547.

13 Eastwood, M.A., Brydon, W.G., Baird, J.D., Elton, R.A., Helliwell, S., Smith, J.H. & Pritchard, J.L. (1984): Fecal weight and composition, serum lipids, and diet among subjects aged 18 to 80 years not seeking health care. *Am. J. Clin. Nutr.* **40**, 628–634.

14 Hofmann, A.F. (1977): The enterohepatic circulation of bile acids in man. *Clins Gastroent.* **6**, 3–24.

15 Illman, R.J., Trimble, R.P., Snoswell, A.M. & Topping, D.L. (1982): Daily variations in the concentrations of volatile fatty acids in the splanchnic blood vessels of rats fed diets high in pectin and bran. *Nutr. Rep. Int.* **26**, 439–446.

16 Kay, R.M. & Truswell, A.S. (1976): Bran and blood lipids. *Lancet* **1**, 367.

17 Kay, R.M. & Truswell, A.S. (1977): Effect of citrus pectin on blood lipids and faecal steroid excretion in man. *Am. J. Clin. Nutr.* **30**, 171–175.

18 Levitt, M.D. & Bond, J.H., Jr. (1970): Volume, composition and source of intestinal gas. *Gastroenterology* **59**, 921–929.

19 McBurney, M.I., Horevath, P.J., Jeraci, J.L. & Van Soest, P.J. (1985): Effect of *in vitro* fermentation using human faecal inoculum on the water holding capacity of dietary fibre. *Br. J. Nutr.* **53**, 17–24.

20 McKay, L.F., Brydon, W.G., Eastwood, M.A. & Smith, J.H. (1981): The influence of pentose on breath methane. *Am. J. Clin. Nutr.* **34**, 2728–2733.

21 McKay, L.F. & Eastwood, M.A. (1983): The influence of dietary fibre on caecal metabolism in the rat. *Br. J. Nutr.* **50**, 679–684.

22 McKay, L.F., Eastwood, M.A. & Brydon, W.G. (1985): Methane excretion in man — a study of breath flatus, and faeces. *Gut* **26**, 69–74.

23 McLean Ross, A.H., Eastwood, M.A., Brydon, W.G., Anderson, J.H. & Anderson, D.M.W. (1983): A study of the effect of dietary gum arabic in humans. *Am. J. Clin. Nutr.* **37**, 368–375.

24 McNeil, N.I., Cummings, J.H., James, W.P.T. (1978): Short chain fatty acid absorption by the human large intestine. *Gut* **19**, 819–822.

25 Parker, D.S. (1976): The measurement of production rates of volatile fatty acids in the caecum of the conscious rabbit. *Br. J. Nutr.* **36**, 61.

26 Parra, R. (1978): In *The ecology of arboreal folivores* ed G.G. Montgomery. Washington, DC: Smithsonian Institution Press.

27 Roediger, W.E.W. (1980): The colonic epithelium in ulcerative colitis: an energy deficiency disease. *Lancet* **2**, 712–714.

28 Salyers, A.A., West. S.E.H., Vercellotti, H. & Wilkins, T.D. (1977): Fermentation of mucins and plant polysaccharides by anaerobic bateria from the human colon. *Appl. Environment. Microbiol.* **34**, 529–533.

29 Salyers, A.A., Palmer, J.K. & Wilkins, T.D. (1978): Degradation of polysaccharides by intestinal bacterial enzymes. *Am. J. Clin. Nutr.* **31**, S128–S130.

30 Selvendran, R.R. (1984): The plant cell wall as a source of dietary fiber in chemistry and structure. *Am. J. Clin. Nutr.* **39**, 320–337.

31 Spiller, G.A., Chernoff, M.C., Hill, R.A., Gates, J.E., Nassar, J.J. & Shipley, E.A. (1980): Effect of purified cellulose, pectin and low residue diet on fecal volatile fatty aicds, transit time and faecal weight in humans. *Am. J. Clin. Nutr.* **33**, 754–759.

32 Stephen, A.M. & Cummings, J.H. (1980): Mechanism of action of dietary fibre in the human colon. *Nature, Lond.* **284**, 283–284.

33 Stephen, A.M., Haddad, A.C. & Phillips, S.F. (1983): Passage of carbohydrate into the colon. Direct measurements in humans. *Gastoenterology* **85**, 589–595.

34 Tadesse, K. & Eastwood, M.A. (1978): Metabolism of dietary fibre components in man assessed by breath hydrogen and methane. *Br. J. Nutr.* **40**, 393–396.

35 Tadesse, K., Smith, D. & Eastwood, M.A. (1980): Breath hydrogen and methane excretion patterns in normal man and in clinical practice. *Quart. J. Physiol.* **65**, 85–97.

36 Walters, D.J., Eastwood, M.A. & Brydon, W.G. (In prep): The effect of duration of feeding upon fibre fermentation when added to a fibre free diet in the male adult rat — the development of an experimental animal model.

37 Wyman, J.B., Heaton, K.W., Manning, A.P. & Wicks, A.C.B. (1976): The effect on intestinal transit and the faeces of raw and cooked bran in different doses. *Am. J. Clin. Nutr.* **29**, 1474–1479.

38 Wyman, J.B., Heaton, K.W., Manning, A.P. & Wicks, A.C.B. (1978): Variability of colonic functions in healthy subjects. *Gut* **19**, 146–150.

Dietary fibre supplements, physiological and pharmacological aspects: a workshop report

G.A. SPILLER and D.J.A. JENKINS (Organizers)
Los Altos, California, USA and Toronto, Canada.

Participants and contributors. N.-G. Asp (Lund, Sweden); C. Bonfield (Washington, DC, USA); A. Frew (Kent, UK); I. Furda (Minneapolis, Minnesota, USA); K. Heaton (Bristol, UK); H. Kasper (West Germany); Helen Klisser (Auckland, New Zealand); D. Kritchevsky (Philadelphia, Pennsylvania, USA); A. Leeds (London, UK); J. de Nadon (Paris, France) and R. Taylor (London, UK)

Introduction. Dietary fibre supplements are today being researched and/or produced in many countries. The workshop participants, from both industry and academic institutions, agreed that various points need clarification and better definition. It was also agreed that we are ready for some preliminary suggestions on what is a supplement as compared to a high fibre food.

Purpose of fibre supplements. Fibre supplements have two main purposes: (1) to add fibre to the diet of seemingly healthy people who habitually consume too little fibre; (2) to act as a pharmacological agent in the diets of constipated, hyperlipidaemic, diabetic and other patients.

Classification of fibre foods and supplements. (1) *High-fibre foods*: natural foods in which the dietary fibre portion has not been removed or to which additional fibre has not been added. Examples are typical unrefined whole grain product, beans, whole vegetables and fruits. (2) *Fibre-enriched foods*: products that are typical foods, such as bread, to which fibre concentrates have been added to increase fibre beyond the natural level. Example: a whole grain bread with extra wheat bran added. (3) *Fibre supplements for healthy individuals*. These could be called physiological supplements, and have the general function of increasing the fibre content of the diet but are not intended to have a medical or pharmacological effect. They are intended for people who are unable or unwilling to consume enough fibre in the diet. Some participants felt that these should supply a wide spectrum of fibre polymers and should contain both water soluble and insoluble components. (4) *Fibre supplements for medical use*. These are supplements with a pharmacological goal, to be recommended or prescribed by a physician to achieve a definite improvement in a pathological state, such as lowering serum cholesterol or reducing urine glucose losses in diabetic patients. Guar gum is an example of such supplements.

Need to define type of fibre. There seems to be agreement that the source and type of fibre should be precisely defined, and that it should be clearly stated on the label whether the fibre is an isolate or a natural concentrate.

Labels for fibre supplements. Statements as to amount of total dietary fibre should be mandatory on the label. Listing of individual polymers would be highly desirable (polymeric pattern of the fibre). Some of the workshop participants felt the polymeric pattern should be mandatory on a supplement label. In addition, water-soluble and insoluble fractions should be listed. The basic thrust was that labelling of supplements should be much more detailed than that of foods.

Special isolated fibres. The use of fibre products not normally used as part of the diet, such as sugar beet fibre, was discussed and the consensus was that they may fill a needed gap in supplementation, but that they should be carefully studied in a clinical setting.

Diet versus supplements. Supplement manufacturers have the responsibility to emphasize that diets high in high fibre foods are different from fibre supplemented diets. Diets high in unrefined carbohydrate not only increase fibre intake, as supplements do, but usually supply higher levels of energy from starchy foods and less from fat. Nevertheless, fibre supplements fill an important need in the modern world.

Summary. The key results of the workshop were as follows. (1) A proposed classification covering fibre foods and fibre supplements, including supplements for general or medical use; (2) A strong recommendation for specific details of fibre composition on the label, including water-soluble and insoluble fibre or fibre polymers; (3) The need to continue studies on isolated fibres for special uses. All participants agreed that fibre supplements, when properly formulated and when they supply sufficient fibre, have a place in countries where the diet is typically low in fibre.

★ ★ ★

FIBRE DEGREDATION BY BACTERIA

Polysaccharide breakdown in the human colon

J.H. CUMMINGS
MRC Dunn Clinical Nutrition Centre, 100 Tennis Court Road, Cambridge CB2 1QL, UK.

There is now substantial evidence that the polysaccharides of the plant cell wall (dietary fibre) are broken down during passage through the human gut. As long ago as 1936 Williams and Olmsted reported studies in three medical students of the digestion of insoluble fibre from a wide variety of plant substances. The most notable feature of their results is the range of digestibilities observed with fibre from carrot and cabbage being 66–74 per cent metabolized whilst that from wheat bran and pure cellulose largely survived passage through the gut (30 per cent and 10 per cent digested, respectively). More recently, similar findings were observed for cabbage and wheat bran fibre[12], with 92 per cent of cabbage and 27 per cent of wheat bran fibre being digested when fed to groups of healthy volunteers.

Factors affecting digestibility of fibre. A number of studies have been reported which deal with the digestibility of fibre in its many forms. These have been reviewed in detail elsewhere[1]. All show that there is considerable variation in the breakdown of fibre, both between sources and also between subjects. Why should this be? In ruminant nutrition a number of factors are known to affect digestibility but as yet much less information is available for man. A summary of these possible factors is shown in the Table.

Table. *Control of fibre breakdown in man*

1. Properties of the fibre source	3. Other factors
(a) Lignifications	(a) Level of intake
(b) Water solubility	(b) Other components of diet ie starch and protein
(c) Particle size	(c) Effect of food processing
(d) Molecular structure	(d) Previous diet
(e) Associated silica etc.	
2. Host factors	
(a) Characteristics of host microflora	
(b) Transit time	
(c) Colonic anatomy	

Extensive studies in ruminants have shown that the amount of lignin present in cell-wall material has marked effects on fibre digestibility whilst in man Williams & Olmsted[14] thought it important in determining digestion of various fibre sources. The relative resistance of wheat bran to digestion is probably partly explained by its high lignin content. Bran contains about 3 per cent lignin, making it one of the most highly lignified human foods.

Another intrinsic property of cell-wall polysaccharides that seems to affect their digestibility in man is water solubility. Since breakdown of fibre depends on access by the colonic microflora to these polymers, water solubility should promote rapid fermentation. In two studies of the digestion of the water-soluble polysaccharides ispaghula and pectin[4,9] their breakdown was shown to be virtually complete whilst in the same studies water-soluble non-cellulosic polysaccharides were only about 50 per cent degraded.

Particle size may also be important. In the study of Heller *et al.*[7] bran of a coarser particle size was less completely digested than fine bran milled from the same grist.

Host factors. When the same type of dietary fibre is fed to a group of human subjects a wide range of digestibilities will be observed amongst the individuals. It may be inferred from this that host factors influence fibre digestibility in addition to those intrinsic properties of fibre already discussed. One of these host factors is transit time: the time it takes material to pass through the gut.

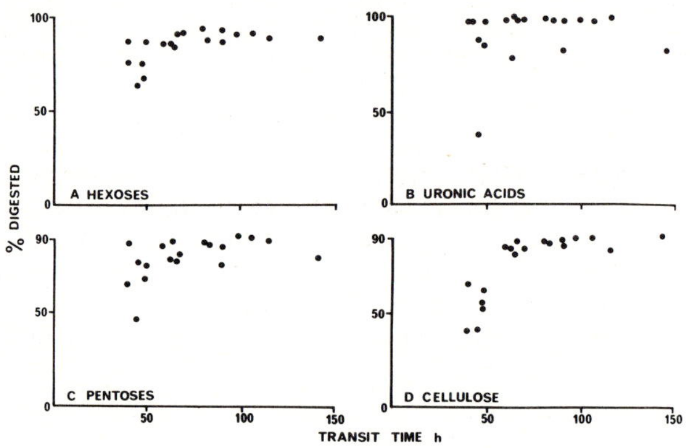

Fig. *The percentage digested* $\left[\dfrac{intake\text{-}excretion}{intake} \times 100 \right]$ *of cellulose and of the hexose, pentose and uronic acid components of the non-cellulosic polysaccharide (NCP) in the diet of five healthy subjects whilst eating either a standard UK diet or the same diet with the addition of 36 g of pectin.* Daily intakes on the control diet were cellulose 6.1 g, NCP-hexose 5.7 g, NCP-pentose 2.0 g and NCP uronic acid 1.2 g. (From[4]).

The Figure shows the digestibility of the four main fractions of fibre in a group of five healthy subjects. Subjects were given a controlled Western-style diet for 3 weeks and then 36 g of pectin was added to it for a further 6 weeks. Faeces were analysed for fibre and transit time was measured continuously. The graph of cellulose digestion shows that it has a maximum digestibility of about 90 per cent in this study, but that when transit falls below about 50 h digestibility rapidly declines. The same is true for pentoses, but it is not so evident for the hexoses and uronic acids. Similar observations have been made in the ruminant. Other factors are likely to affect fibre breakdown in man, but as yet insufficient work has been done to characterize them. The flora will almost certainly play a major role in this process, but at the present time no clear patterns of activity have emerged.

Site of breakdown. The site of breakdown of dietary fibre is undoubtedly the large intestine. In recent studies of the digestion of polysaccharides from a variety of foods it has been shown[5,6], using ileostomy subjects as a model, that the non-starch polysaccharides from oats, wheat, corn and banana all escape digestion in the small intestine. Even the highly water-soluble β-glucan in oats can be recovered completely in ileostomy effluent. Other studies have shown the complete recovery of non-starch polysaccharides from pectin and wheat bran using a similar model[10,11,13]. Of perhaps equal importance in these studies is the demonstration that not only do the non-starch polysaccharides escape breakdown in the small bowel, but that substantial amounts of starch do also.

Significance of fibre breakdown. The most important feature of fibre breakdown by the microflora of the large intestine is that it is an anaerobic process. The main end-products are the short-chain fatty acids (SCFA) (acetate, propionate, butyrate). These acids are present in high concentrations (90–130 mmol/1) in all regions of the human colon[3]. They are rapidly absorbed from the colonic lumen and once absorbed are metabolized by the colonic epithelial cells, the liver or peripheral tissues. As such they contribute to normal energy metabolism and represent 60–70 per cent of the energy available had the carbohydrate been absorbed intact in the small intestine.

The mucosal metabolism of SCFA, especially butyrate, may be of critical importance in maintaining the integrity of the colonic epithelium. Once across the colonic mucosa SCFAs enter the portal vein, but only acetate reaches peripheral tissues in significant quantities. Peripheral blood acetate levels can be linked quantitatively to fermentation of carbohydrate occurring in the large intestine[8]. Fermentation in the colon therefore makes a significant contribution to blood acetate levels in man and thus the breakdown of dietary fibre in the colon may have importance well beyond the wall of the large intestine.

Conclusion. It is now clearly established that dietary fibre is broken down in the human gut. This breakdown occurs in the large intestine by the anaerobic microflora and there is no evidence that significant breakdown occurs in any other part of the gut. Wide variation in the rate and extent of breakdown has been observed in man and some, but not all factors contributing to this have been identified. The breakdown of fibre in the large intestine is of fundamental importance both to the functioning of this organ and possibly to metabolism in general.

1 Cummings, J.H. (1981): Dietary fibre. *Br. Med. Bull.* **37**, 65–70.
2 Cummings, J.H. (1983): Fermentation in the human large intestine: evidence and implications for health. *Lancet* **1**, 1206–1209.
3 Cummings, J.H., Pomare, E.W. & Branch, W.J. (1985): Short chain fatty acids (SCFA) in human portal, hepatic and peripheral venous blood. Abstr. XIII *Int. Cong. Nutr.*, Brighton.
4 Cummings, J.H., Southgate, D.A.T., Branch, W.J., Wiggins, H., Houston, H., Jenkins, D.J.A., Jivraj, T. & Hill, M.J. (1979): The digestion of pectin in the human gut and its effect on calcium absorption and large bowel function. *Br. J. Nutr.* **41**, 477–485.
5 Englyst, H.N. & Cummings, J.H. (1985): Digestion of the polysaccharides of some cereal foods in the human small intestine. *Am. J. Clin. Nutr.* (In press).
6 Englyst, H.N. & Cummings, J.H. (1986): Digestion of the carbohydrates of banana *(Musa paradisiaca sapientum)* in the human small intestine. *Am. J. Clin. Nutr.* (In press).
7 Heller, S.N., Hackler, L.R., Rivers, J.M., Van Soest, P.J., Roe, D.A., Lewis, B.A. & Robertson, J. (1980): Dietary fibre: the effect of particle size of wheat bran on colonic function in young adult men. *Am. J. Clin. Nutr,* **33**, 1734–1744.
8 Pomare, E.W., Branch, W.J. & Cummings, J.H. (1985): Carbohydrate fermentation in the human colon and its relation to acetate concentrations in venous blood. *J. Clin. Invest.* **75**, 1448–1454.
9 Prynne, C.J. & Southgate, D.A.T. (1979): The effects of a supplement of dietary fibre on faecal excretion by human subjects. *Br. J. Nutr.* **41**, 495–503.
10 Sandberg, A.S., Andersson, H., Hallgren, B., Hasselblad, K., Isaksson, B. & Hulten, L. (1981): Experimental model for *in vivo* determination of dietary fibre and its effects on small bowel absorption of nutrients. *Br. J. Nutr.* **45**, 283–294.
11 Sandberg, A.S., Ahderinne, R., Andersson, H., Hallgren, B. & Hulten, L. (1983): The effect of citrus pectin on the absorption of nutrients in the small intestine. *Hum. Nutr.: Clin. Nutr.* **37C**, 171–183.
12 Stephen, A.M. & Cummings, J.H. (1980): Mechanism of action of dietary fibre in the human colon. *Nature, Lond.* **284**, 283–284.
13 Werch, S.C. & Ivy, A.C. (1941): On the fate of ingested pectin. *Am. J. Dig. Dis.* **8**, 101–105.
14 Williams, R.D. & Olmsted, W.H. (1936): The effect of cellulose, hemicellulose and lignin on the weight of stool. A contribution to the study of laxation in man. *J. Nutr.* **2**, 433–449.

Fibre digestion in the rumen

D.E. AKIN
*Plant Structure and Composition Research Unit, Richard B. Russell Agricultural Research Center,
ARS-USDA, Athens, Georgia 30613, USA.*

Ruminants are characterized by a massive fermentative digestion that occurs in the first two parts of the stomach, ie the rumen and reticulum[29,30]. The environmental conditions of the rumen (39 °C, −350 mV redox potential, pH 6 to 7) support a mixed population of obligate and facultative anaerobes capable of extensively catabolizing fibre in herbage.

Fibre as substrate for rumen microorganisms. Fibre contents, although variable among forages, comprise a high percentage of total dry weight of the herbage. For example, average fibre contents (determined as neutral detergent fibre) of about 66 per cent for several warm-season grasses and about 57 per cent for cool-season species have been reported[10]. Hemicellulose has been shown to comprise 24 to 38 per cent and cellulose to comprise 23 to 36 per cent of the forage dry weight[34]. Properties indigenous to these components (ie crystallinity in cellulose and branching in hemicellulose) are often reported to influence the ease of microbial degradation, but research appears to indicate that the chemical association of these polysaccharides with lignin and phenolic components is the primary factor that limits their availability for microbial degradation[13,17,32].

The phenolic components are disproportionately dispersed among plant tissues. Tissues containing high levels of lignin provide mechanical support for growing plants and are the most poorly degraded tissue in ruminants[4]. The responses of living tissues to attack by rumen microorganisms vary from slowly degraded to rapidly degraded. It is possible that variable amounts of low molecular weight phenolic compounds, perhaps present as lignin precursors, slow microbial attack on these living tissues[20]. Under conditions leading to maturity or plant stress, the phenolic and polysaccharide moieties could associate such that structural carbohydrates are then less available for microbial attack. Among the low molecular weight components, *p*-coumaric acid has been especially implicated as having a negative nutritive effect by being associated with the lower quality fibre[6,21]. Additionally, low molecular weight phenolic components, and especially *p*-coumaric acid, in their free state at levels of 0.1 per cent are known to be toxic to rumen microorganisms[3], but it is not clear if such a toxicity is exerted *in vivo*.

Attack and degradation of forage fibre by rumen microorganisms. *Protozoa.* Rumen protozoa are reported to possess enzymes (ie, cellulases and hemicellulases) active against plant polysaccharides and are able to ingest fibre fragments[16]. In particular, *Epidinium ecaudatum* appears to attack aggressively certain tissues, such as the cortex and phloem of alfalfa stems[11] and the mesophyll of cool-season grass leaves[9] (Fig. 1). Apart from its ability to degrade fibre, *E. ecaudatum* could help to disrupt the physical structure of the more fragile tissue types and increase surface area of fibre for bacterial colonization. Reports in the literature indicate that the presence of protozoa markedly enhance fibre digestion[18], but other data indicate that protozoa are not essential to fibre digestion and that their role is small when compared with that of the bacteria[23].

Fungi. Recently, primitive fungi resembling the chytrids have been shown to occupy a niche as degraders of forage fibre[26]. Results of studies in the USA indicated that populations of rumen fungi could degrade *in vitro* about 50 per cent of the neutral detergent fibre degradable by whole rumen fluid or by bacteria (Table 1,[33]). Other data from Australia indicated a more significant activity for rumen fungi[8] in that they could degrade slightly more dry matter than whole rumen fluid (62 per cent and 55 per cent respectively). Rumen fungi differ from the protozoa in that initially they colonize and degrade the lignified fibrous tissue[12]. Indeed, tissues such as

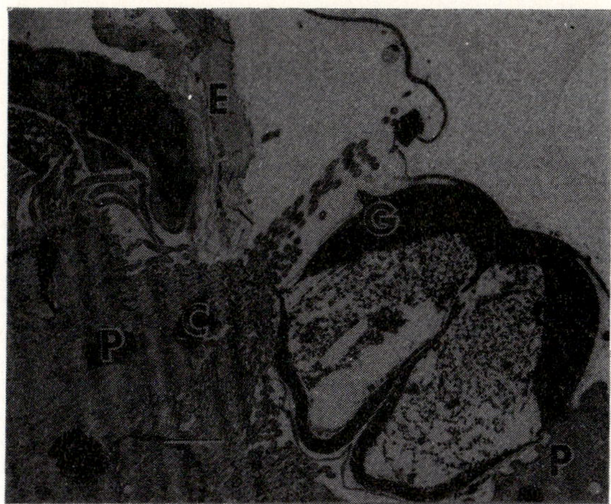

Fig. 1. *Transmission electron micrograph of a rumen protozoan attacking the rapidly degraded epidermal cells of Dactylis glomerata in the absence of fibre-digesting bacteria.* A guard cell (G) is being engulfed by the protozoan, while an epidermal cell wall (E) has been partially degraded showing plant wall disorganization. Note the protozoan (P) and cilia (C) surrounding the plant cells. Bar = 2 μm.

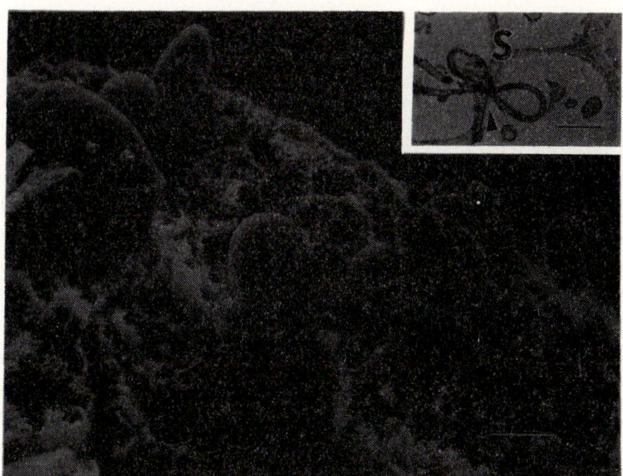

Fig. 2. *Scanning electron micrograph of a mixed population of rumen fungi colonizing a leaf blade of Cynodon datylon incubated with penicillin and streptomycon to inhibit rumen bacterial growth.* Note the particular colonization of sclerenchyma tissue (arrow). Bar = 20 μm. The inset is a transmission electron micrograph of a similarly incubated leaf blade showing the attack on the sclerenchyma cell wall (S) by fungi-like hyphae (arrow). Bar = 2 μm.

sclerenchyma and xylem cells resistant to attack by protozoa and bacteria have been shown to be degraded by rumen fungi (Fig. 2;[5,8]). These anaerobic fungi possess enzymes active against structural carbohydrates, and fungi similar to those in the rumen-solubilized lignin from grass fibre[25]. On occasion, rumen fungi can penetrate plant stomata, which provides for numerous entry sites to internal plant tissues[8]. The propensity for rumen fungi to attack and weaken lignified fibre indicates a unique role for these microbes in utilizing herbage substrates in the rumen. Their activity in sheep rumens has been stimulated by feeding the animals sulphur-fertilized *Digitaria* grass, and it is believed that the presence of the fungi contributed to a significant increase in feed intake possibly by weakening plant tissues and reducing the residence time of fibre in the rumen[12]. Stimulation of the activity of these rumen fungi to weaken lignified fibre may offer an opportunity for improving the digestibility of low quality forage *in situ*.

Table 1. *Dry weight loss of neutral detergent fibre by rumen fluid including antibiotics against microbial types in vitro[33]. WRF = whole rumen fluid diluted with buffer; WRF + S-P = inclusion of streptomycin (1.25 mg/ml) and penicillin (0.2 mg/ml) to prevent bacterial growth; WRF + C = inclusion of cycloheximide (0.5/ml) to prevent fungal growth; WRF + S-P-C = inclusion of all three antibiotics which allowed variable amounts of protozoal viability.*

Inoculum from steer fed:	Substrate	% dry weight loss in vitro			
		WRF	*WRF + S-P*	*WRF + C*	*WRF + S-P-C*
Alfalfa	Alfalfa	27.7a	14.7a	26.7a	11.2b
Alfalfa	Bermuda grass	18.0a	9.7b	15.0a	0c
Bermuda grass	Alfalfa	25.5a	9.9b	26.5a	3.9c
Bermuda grass	Bermuda grass	19.0a	8.4b	15.2a	0c

a, b, c Different superscripts within rows indicate that values differ, $P > 0.05$.

Bacteria. Anaerobic bacteria have long been considered the dominant agents that degrade herbage fibre in the rumen[22,23] (Table 1). *Ruminococcus albus, R. flavefaciens,* and *bacteroides succinogenes* are the most potent fibre-digesting bacteria in the rumen[14] and the cellulases, hemicullulases, and pectinases found in these microbes could effect a complete degradation of the plant cell wall[19,22,27]. Indeed, bacteria morphologically identical to these but in mixed populations, have shown the capacity to adhere firmly to plant cells and to penetrate through the entire cell wall[1]. A large part of the carbohydrases are cell-bound in these bacteria[23], and the bacteria firmly attached to fibre during digestion[24]. Our work has shown that often the more slowly digestible tissues in forage (eg, parenchyma bundle sheath and epidermis in warm-season grasses) are not degraded until after these bacteria adhere[1].

In contrast to rumen fungi, rumen bacteria are scarcely able to attack highly lignified tissues (eg vascular xylem) and often do not even adhere to these plant walls[7]. However, a filamentous, facultatively anaerobic bacterium isolated from rumen fluid was able to degrade partially certain lignified tissues (eg. leaf blade sclerenchyma) in forage and to grow solely on phenolic acids[2].

On the other end of the spectrum of tissue digestibility, the rapidly and extensively digested tissue (eg mesophyll) can be degraded without the necessity for bacterial attachment[7]. That such a pattern of degradation is possible is suggested by the fact that plant cell wall carbohydrases have been shown to be released from the major fibre-digesting bacteria[28,35]. These extracellular carbohydrases plus similar enzymes from many other less prevalent, non-adhering species[22] may play a significant role in rapidly degrading the least resistant plant cell walls of herbage.

In order to clarify the physical association of bacteria with fibre during digestion, research was conducted using pure cultures of bacteria and plant tissues of various digestibilities (Akin and Rigsby, unpublished data). The more resistant tissues were degraded by *R. flavefaciens* only after attachment apparently facilitated by a distinct capsule (Fig. 3), but this microbe also effected generalized clearing and disorganization of the more easily digested plant cell walls without

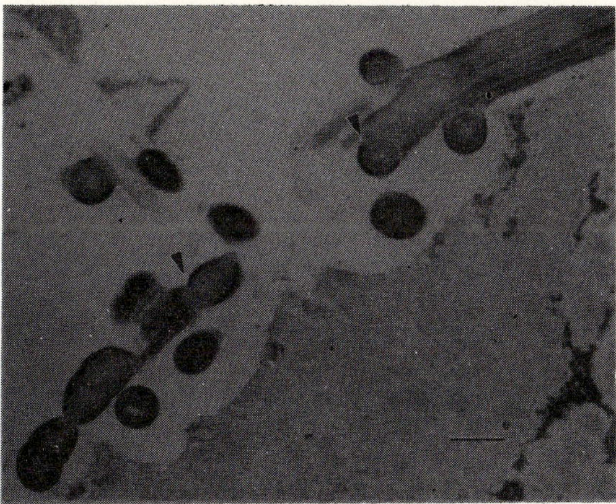

Fig. 3. *Transmission electron micrograph of attack on cell walls of the slowly digested parenchyma bundle sheath of Cynodon dactylon by a pure culture Ruminococcus flavefaciens FD-1.* Note the close adhesion facilitated by a distinct capsule (arrows); plant walls are not degraded where bacteria have not attached. Bar = 1 μm.

attachment. In our culture *Ruminococcus albus* strain 7, which was atypical in that it lacked a capsule and degraded cellulose only after an extended time, did not attach to fibre and was able to degrade portions of only the most digestible plant walls. Indeed, *R. albus* often appears to possess a less distinct capsule and to adhere less firmly to plant fibre than does *R. flavefaciens*[15]. One strain (*R. albus* 8) exhibits a relationship between increased capsule production and increased cellulolytic activity in the presence of 3-phenylpropanoic acid[31]. Degradation patterns similar to those in *R. albus* occurred with the hemicelluloytic species *Butyrivibrio*

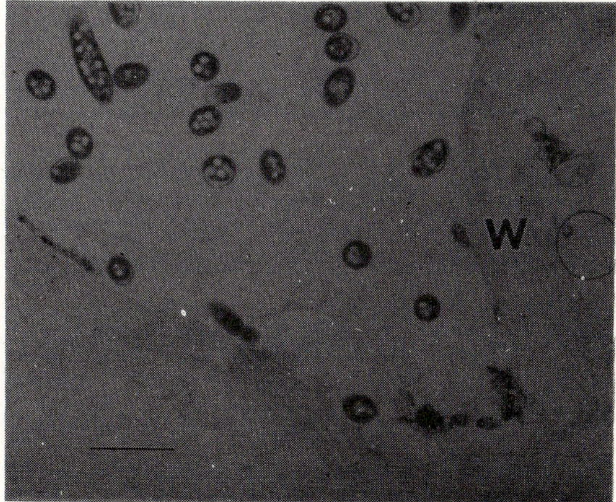

Fig. 4. *Transmission electron micrograph of attack of rapidly digested cell walls of Dactylis glomerata by a pure culture of Butyrivibrio fibrisolvens 49.* The bacteria do not have a capsule, do not adhere to the fibre but apparently release extracellular carbohydrases that cause generalized erosion and disorganization of plant walls (W). Bar = 1 μm.

fibrisolvens (Fig. 4). These data indicate that cell-free carbohydrases can degrade fragile tissues, but also suggest the importance of attachment (through a distinct capsule with ruminococci) in degrading the more resistant fibre.

1 Akin, D.E. (1976): Ultrastructure of rumen bacterial attachment to forage cell walls. *Appl. Environ. Microbiol.* **31**, 562–568.

2 Akin, D.E. (1980): Attack on lignified grass cell walls by a facultatively anaerobic bacterium. *Appl. Environ. Microbiol.* **40**, 809–820.

3 Akin, D.E. (1982). Forage cell wall degradation and *p*-coumaric, ferulic, and sinapic acids. *Agron. J.* **74**, 424–428.

4 Akin, D.E. (1982): Microbial breakdown of feed in the digestive tract. In *Nutritional limits to animal production from pastures*, ed J.B. Hacker, pp. 201–223. Farnham Royal, UK: Commonwealth Agricultural Bureaux.

5 Akin, D.E. (1983): Electron microscopic studies of fiber degradation by rumen fungi. In *Proceedings of the 41st Annual Meeting of the Electron Microscopy Society of America*, ed G.W. Bailey, pp. 814–815. San Francisco: San Francisco Press, Inc.

6 Akin, D.E. & Barton, F.E., II (1983): Forage ultrastructure and the digestion of plant cell walls by rumen microorganisms. In *Wood and agricultural residues*, ed E.J. Soltes, pp. 33–57. New York: Academic Press.

7 Akin, D.E., Burdick, D. & Michaels, G.E. (1974): Rumen bacterial interrelationships with plant tissue during degradation revealed by transmission electron microscopy. *Appl. Microbiol.* **27**, 1149–1156.

8 Akin, D.E., Gordon, G.L.R. & Hogan J.P. (1983): Rumen bacterial and fungal degradation of *Digitaria pentzii* grown with and without sulfur. *Appl. Environ. Microbiol.* **46**, 738–748.

9 Amos, H.E. & Akin, D.E. (1978): Rumen protozoal degradation of structurally intact forage tissues. *Appl. Environ. Microbiol.* **36**, 513–522.

10 Barton, F.E., II, Amos, H.E., Burdick, D. & Wilson, R.L. (1976); Relationship of chemical analysis to *in vitro* digestibility for selected tropical and temperate grasses. *J. Anim. Sci.* **43**, 504–512.

11 Bauchop, T. (1979): The rumen ciliate *Epidinium* in primary degradation of plant tissues. *Appl. Environ. Microbiol.* **37**, 1217–1223.

12 Bauchop, T. (1981): The anaerobic fungi in rumen fibre digestion. *Agric. Environ.* **6**, 339–348.

13 Brice, R.E. & Morrison, I.M. (1982): The degradation of isolated hemicelluloses and lignin-hemicellulose complexes by cell-free, rumen hemicellulases. *Carbohyd. Res.* **101**, 93–100.

14 Bryant, M.P. (1973): Nutritional requirements of the predominant rumen cellulolytic bacteria. *Federation Proc.* **32**, 1809–1813.

15 Cheng, K.J., Stewart, C.S., Dinsdale, D. & Costerton, J.W. (1983–84): Electron microscopy of bacteria involved in the digestion of plant cell walls. *Anim. Feed Sci. Technol.* **10**, 93–120.

16 Clarke, R.T.J. (1977): Protozoa in the rumen ecosystem. In *Microbial ecology of the gut.* ed R.T.J. Clarke & T. Bauchop, pp. 251–257. New York: Academic Press.

17 Dekker, R.F.H. (1976): Hemicellulose degradation in the ruminant. Misc. Paper Landbouwhogesch. Wageningen **12**, 43–54.

18 Demeyer, D.I. (1981): Rumen microbes and digestion of plant cell walls. *Agric. Environ.* **6**, 295–337.

19 Groleau, D. & Forsberg, C.W. (1983): Partial characterization of the extracellular carboxymethylcellulase activity produced by the rumen bacterium *Bacteroides succinogenes. Can. J. Microbiol.* **29**, 504–517.

20 Harris, P.J. & Hartley, R.D. (1976): Detection of bound ferulic acid in cell walls of the *Gramineae* by ultraviolet fluorescence microscopy. *Nature, Lond.* **259**, 508–510.

21 Harris, P.J., Hartley, R.D. & Lowry, K.H. (1980): Phenolic constituents of mesophyll and non-mesophyll cell walls from leaf laminae of *Lolium perenne, J. Sci. Fd. Agric,* **31**, 959–962.

22 Hungate, R.E. (1966): *The rumen and its microbes.* New York: Academic Press.

23 Hungate, R.E. (1975): The rumen microbial ecosystem. In *Annual review of ecology and systematics.* ed R.F. Johnston, pp. 39–66. Palo Alto: Annual Reviews, Inc.

24 Latham, M.J., Brooker, B.E., Pettipher, G.L. & Harris, P.J. (1978): Adhesion of *Bacteroides succinogenes* in pure culture and in the presence of *Ruminococcus flavefaciens* to cell walls in leaves of perennial ryegrass *(Lolium perenne). Appl. Environ. Microbiol.* **35**, 1166–1175.

25 Orpin, C.G. (1981): Isolation of cellulolytic phycomycete fungi from the caecum of the horse. *J. Gen. Microbiol.* **123**, 287–296.

26 Orpin, C.G. & Letcher, A.J. (1979): Utilization of cellulose, strach, xylan, and other hemicelluloses for growth by the rumen phycomycete *Neocallimastix frontalis. Curr. Microbiol.* **3**, 121–124.

27 Pettipher, G.L. & Latham, M.J. (1979): Characteristics of enzymes produced by *Ruminococcus flavefaciens* which degrade plant cell walls. *J. Gen. Microbiol.* **110**, 21–27.

28 Pettipher, G.L. & Latham, M.J. (1979): Production of enzymes degrading plant cell walls and fermentation of cellobiose by *Ruminococcus flavefaciens* in batch and continuous culture. *J. Gen. Microbiol.* **110**, 29–38.

29 Phillipson, A.T. (1977): Ruminant digestion. *Duke's Physiology of Domestric Animals, 9th edition,* ed M.J. Swenson, pp. 250–286. Ithaca: Cornell Univ. Press.

30 Reid, C.S.W. (1982): Fibre and the digestive physiology of the ruminant stomach. In *Fibre in human and animal nutrition,* ed G. Wallace & L. Bell, pp. 43–49. Wellington: The Royal Society of New Zealand.

31 Stack, R.J. & Hungate, R.E. (1984): Effect of 3-phenylpropanoic acid on capsule and cellulases of *Ruminococcus albus* 8. *Appl. Environ. Microbiol.* **48**, 218–223.

32 Van Soest, P.J. (1973): The uniformity and nutritive availability of cellulose. *Federation Proc.* **32**, 1804–1808.

33 Windham, W.R. & Akin, D.E. (1984): Rumen fungi and forage fiber degradation. *Appl. Environ. Microbiol.* **48**, 473–476.

34 Windham, W.R., Barton, F.E., II & Himmelsbach, D.S. (1983): High-pressure liquid chromatographic analysis of component sugars in neutral detergent fiber for representative warm- and cool-season grasses. *J. Agric. Fd. Chem.* **31**, 471–475.

35 Yu, I. & Hungate, R.E. (1979): The extracellular cellulases of *Ruminococcus albus*. *Ann. Rech. Vet.* **10**, 251–254.

Mechanism of bacterial attachment to dietary fibre in the rumen

C.W. FORSBERG
Department of Microbiology, University of Guelph, Guelph, Ontario N1G 2W1, Canada.

In the rumen, microbes attached to food particles may have as much as a three-fold longer retention time than those free in the fluid phase[6]. Therefore, when the ruminant receives a high forage ration (ie low carbohydrate in the liquid phase), bacteria attaching to the food particles have a competitive advantage, and furthermore, they have a central role in forage digestion. Even though bacterial attachment in the rumen ecosystem has received considerable attention, there are still gaps in our knowledge about the subject.

Bacterial populations attached to food particles. Through the use of scanning and transmission electron microscopy, the ultrastructure of the attachment of microorganisms to rumen surfaces has been characterized[1,3]. The association of microbes with food particles has been quantified with the finding that 75 per cent of the rumen microbial ATP was associated with food particles[9]. Other measures of the proportion of particle-attached microbes give values which range from 50 to 80 per cent[4,6,14] and 80 per cent of the endoglucanase activity, 70 per cent of the amylase activity and 64 per cent of the protease activity has been reported as associated with food particles[15]. It has been noted that 75 per cent of the proteolytic activity was associated with the particulate fraction[2]. In addition, it has been reported that hemicellulase, cellulase and amylase activities were higher in the attached population than in the liquid population[23]. These data demonstrate that a large proportion of the metabolically active microbial population is associated with food particles.

Two morphologically distinct types of bacteria are routinely observed attached to partially degraded plant cell walls; cocci resembling *Ruminococcus albus* and *R. flavefaciens* which appear to be attached to degraded plant cell walls via capsule-like substances, and bacilli resembling *Bacteroides succinogenes* which appear to adhere to forage with, or without, small amounts of fibrous capsular material[1]. Pure culture studies have supported this tentative identification[8,12].

Mechanism of bacterial attachment to cell wall polymers. Plant cell walls are structurally and chemically complex with numerous barriers to attachment, invasion and digestion[12], therefore, to study the mechanism of attachment, it is necessary to use purified polymers as the substrates. Bacteria in rumen fluid attach readily to crystalline cellulose powder[19]. Separate bacterial species have been tested for binding to cellulose[17]. These studies suggest that there are specific attachment sites for β-1,4-glucans on the surface of some bacterial cells and that these sites can be blocked by the modified celluloses : methylcellulose and carboxymethylcellulose (CMC).

Attachment to cellulose may be due to binding by: (1) a cell-bound cellulose, (2) a cellulose specific adhesin (ie a molecule on the surface of a bacterium which binds to a corresponding receptor, a glucan strand on a particulate molecule of cellulose), or by (3) non-specific attachment. Binding by a cell associated cellulase complex is possible for the major cellulolytic bacteria *B. succinogenes*, *R. flavefaciens* and *R. albus* because all three appear to possess surface associated cellulases[8,12,24] and bind at 38 °C, but not at 4 °C which is indicative of an enzymatic reaction. The highly cellulolytic bacterium *Clostridium polysaccharolyticum*, which is rarely found in the rumen, does not bind to cellulose[21]. This may be attributable to the fact that all cellulase activity is extracellular. It is worth noting that it has been[11] shown that the adherence of cells of the non-rumen thermophilic anaerobe *C. thermocellum* to cellulose particles is mediated by a cellulose-binding multicellulase complex composed of at least 14 distinct polypeptide subunits, many of which were shown to express endoglucanase activity. Also implicated in the complex was a cellobiohydrolase activity. Binding by proteins other than cellulases in this complex has not been precluded.

Non-cellulolytic rumen bacteria, for example *Megasphaera elsdenii*, which were found to bind to cellulose at 4 °C as well as at 38 °C and to be released by methylcellulose, must bind via a specific non-enzymatic adhesin although to date no adhesin for cellulose other than cellulase enzymes have been implicated in binding. Non-specific attachment of cells to cellulose fits best for rumen bacteria which bind at 4 °C and are not released by washing with methylcellulose. This type of binding is exemplified by that of the faecal pathogen *Escherichia coli* to cellulose. *E. coli* K12 cells suspended in a mineral solution containing either calcium or magnesium ions were reversibly retained on columns containing fibrous cellulose at 4 °C, and they were readily eluted by water[10].

Attachment to hemicellulose by *C. thermocellum* and related thermophiles has also been observed and attachment was blocked by xylose oligomers $(n_3\text{-}n_9)$[22].

Many species of rumen bacteria bind to starch granules[16,18]. The attachment of bacteria was inhibited by dextrin, amylose, and amylopectin, while glucose, maltose, maltotriose, CMC and methylcellulose had no effect. The data suggest that amylase enzymes are involved in the binding to starch, however, the information is not conclusive. In the case of the bacterium *E. coli*, it has been shown that cells bind to starch via the lambda bacteriophage receptor, which is a pore involved in the uptake of maltodextrins that is located in the outer membrane[7].

Lectins and bacterial attachment. Bacterial attachment to animal and plant cells usually involves carbohydrate lectin interactions[5,20]. Since lectins are abundant in a variety of plants[13], it would seem likely that similar attachment mechanisms will be found within the rumen.

Avenues for future research. Rumen bacteria attach readily to cellulose and starch, but are there other structural components of fibre which serve as binding components? For example, some non-rumen bacteria readily attach to hemicellulose. What are the molecular mechanisms of binding to the various polymers? Can we genetically manipulate bacteria to bind to fibre? Could the gene(s) for cellulosome production in *C. thermocellum* be transferred to *C. polysaccharolyticum*, to improve its binding to cellulose and thereby enhance its competitive nature within the rumen? Indeed, there are many fascinating and important aspects of bacterial attachment to fibre that require resolution.

1 Akin, D.E., Rigsby, L.L. & Brown, R.H. (1984): Ultrastructure of cell wall degradation in *Panicum* species differing in digestibility. *Crop. Sci.* **24**, 156–163.

2 Brock, F.M., Forsberg, C.W. & Buchanan-Smith, J.G. (1982): Proteolytic activity of rumen microorganisms and effects of proteinase inhibitors. *Appl. Environ. Microbiol.* **44**, 561–569.

3 Cheng, K.-J. & Costerton, J.W. (1980): Adherent rumen bacteria: their role in the digestion of plant material, urea and epithelial cells. In *Digestive physiology and metabolism in ruminants*, ed Y. Ruckebush & P. Thivend, pp. 227–250. Lancaster UK: MTP Press.

4 Craig, W.M., Brown, D.R., Broderick, G.A. & Ricker, B.D. (1984): Polysaccharide levels of fluid and particulate microbes. *Can. J. Anim. Sci.* **64**, 62–63.

5 Dazzo, F.B. (1984): Bacterial adhesion to plant root surfaces. In *Microbial adhesion and aggregation*, ed K.C. Marshall, pp. 85–93. Berlin, Heidelberg, New York: Springer-Verlag.

6 Falchney, G.J. (1980): Measurement in sheep of the quantity and composition of rumen digesta and the fractional outflow rates of digesta constituents. *Aust. J. Agric. Res.* **31**, 1129–1137.

7 Ferenci, T. (1983): Affinity immobilization of *Escherichia coli*: Catalysis by intact and permeable cells bound to starch. *Appl. Environ. Microbiol.* **45**, 384–388.

8 Forsberg, C.W., Beveridge, T.J. & Hellstrom, A. (1981): Cellulase and xylanase release from *Bacteroides succinogenes* and its importance in the rumen environment. *Appl. Environ. Microbiol.* **42**, 886–896.

9 Forsberg, C.W. & Lam, K. (1977): Use of adenosine 5'-triphosphate as an indicator of the microbiota biomass in rumen contents. *Appl. Environ. Microbiol.* **33**, 528–537.

10 Hwa, V. & Ferenci, T. (1984): Binding of *Escherichia coli* K-12 to cellulose. *FEMS Microbiol. Lett.* **25**, 11–15.

11 Lamed, R., Kenig, R. & Setter, E. (1985): Major characteristics of the cellulolytic system of *Clostridium thermocellum* coincide with those of the purified cellulosome. *Enzyme Microb. Technol.* **7**, 37–41.

12 Latham, M.J. (1980): Adhesion of rumen bacteria to plant cell walls. In *Microbial adhesion to surfaces*, ed R.C.W. Berkeley, J.M. Lynch, J. Melling, P.R. Rutter & B. Vincent, pp. 339–350. Chichester, UK: Ellis Horwood.

13 Liener, I.E. (1979): Protease inhibitors and lectins. *Int. Rev. Biochem: Biochem. Nutr.* 1A, 27, 98–122, ed A. Neuberger & T.H. Jukes. Baltimore: University Park Press.

14 Minato, H., Endo, A., Higuchi, M., Ootomo, Y. & Uemura, T. (1966): Ecological treatise on the rumen fermentation. I. The fractionation of bacteria attached to the rumen digesta solids. *J. Gen. Appl. Microbiol.* **12**, 39–52.

15 Minato, H., Endo, A., Ootomo, Y. & Uemura, T. (1966). Ecological treatise on the rumen fermentation. II. The amylolytic and cellulolytic activities of the fractionated bacterial portions attached to the rumen solids. *J. Gen. Appl. Microbiol.* **12**, 53–69.

16 Minato, H. & Suto, T. (1976): Technique for fractionation of bacteria in rumen microbial ecosystem. I. Attachment of rumen bacteria to starch granules and elution of bacteria attached to them. *J. Gen. Appl. Microbiol.* **22**, 259–276.

17 Minato, H. & Suto, T. (1978): Technique for fractionation of bacteria in rumen microbial ecosystem. II. Attachment of bacteria isolated from bovine rumen to cellulose powder *in vitro* and elution of bacteria attached therefrom. *J. Gen. Appl. Microbiol.* **24**, 1–16.

18 Minato, H. & Suto, T. (1979): Technique for fractionation of bacteria in rumen microbial ecosystem. III. Attachment of bacteria isolated from bovine rumen to starch granules *in vitro* and elution of bacteria attached therefrom. *J. Gen. Appl. Microbiol.* **25**, 71–93.

19 Minato, H. & Suto, T. (1981): Technique for fractionation of bacteria in rumen microbial ecosystem. IV. Attachment of rumen bacteria to cellulose powder and elution of bacteria attached to it. *J. Gen. Appl. Microbiol.* **27**, 21–31.

20 Ofek, I. & Perry, A. (1985): Molecular basis of bacterial adherence to tissues. In *Molecular basis of oral microbial adhesion*, ed S.E. Mergenhagen & B. Rosan. Washington DC: American Society for Microbiology.

21 Van Gylswyk, N.O. & Schwartz, H.M. (1984): Microbial ecology of the rumen of animals fed high-fibre diets. In *Herbivore nutrition in the subtropics and tropics*, ed F.M.C. Gilchrist & R.I. Mackie, pp. 359–377. Craighall, South Africa: The Science Press.

22 Wiegel, J. & Dykstra, M. (1984): *Clostridium thermocellum*: Adhesion and sporulation while adhered to cellulose and hemicellulose. *Appl. Microbiol. Biotechnol.* **20**, 59–65.

23 Williams, A.G. & Strachan, N.H. (1984): The distribution of polysaccharide-degrading enzymes in the bovine rumen digesta ecosystem. *Curr. Microbiol.* **10**, 215–220.

24 Wood, T.M. & Wilson, C.A. (1984): Some properties of the endo-(1,4)-β-D-glucanase synthesized by the anaerobic cellulolytic rumen bacterium *Ruminococcus albus*. *Can. J. Microbiol.* **30**, 316–321.

Catabolism of dietary fibre by human colonic bacteria

A. A. SALYERS, F. C. GHERARDINI, R. E. McCARTHY and A. P. KURITZA
Department of Microbiology, University of Illinois, Urbana, Illinois 61801, USA.

Most of the polysaccharides in the human diet are not digested appreciably during passage through the stomach and small intestine. However, these polysaccharides are degraded extensively in the colon by the bacteria that reside there[3,15]. The colon contains a very high concentration of bacteria, about 10^{11} per g dry weight[11], and these bacteria need sources of carbon and energy to sustain themselves. Most colon bacteria are carbohydrate fermenters. Since polysaccharides from the host's diet or from host secretions such as mucins and mucopolysaccharides are probably the main form of carbohydrate that is available to bacteria in the colon, the ability to digest polysaccharides is undoubtedly important for the survival of at least some colon bacteria. Many organisms are competing for available polysaccharides, thus, it is likely that colon bacteria have evolved special strategies for efficient trapping and digestion of polysaccharides. Moreover, since the mixture of polysaccharides that enters the colon is constantly changing, the ability of colon bacteria to regulate metabolic activities in response to these changes may also contribute to their survival. To understand how the colonic microflora are affected by the host's diet, we need to know: (1) what species are capable of degrading polysaccharides; (2) how they carry out this process and (3) what polysaccharides are actually being utilized in the colon.

A survey of colon isolates, representing the numerically predominant species, has shown that many colon bacteria are capable of fermenting polysaccharides[13,14]. Most of these polysaccharide-degrading bacteria were members of the genus *Bacteroides*, although other genera, notably *Bifidobacterium* and *Ruminococcus*, were also represented. These results should be interpreted with caution. In the first place, the survey was limited to bacteria that have been isolated and characterized prior to 1976. Since then, no major new groups of colonic bacteria have been reported. However, it is possible that there are still some major groups of colon organisms that have not been isolated and identified. In the second place, the polysaccharides that were used in this survey did not provide a complete representation of the polysaccharides that are found in human foods.

Despite these difficulties, it would be interesting to monitor the effect of the host's diet on the species of polysaccharide degrading bacteria. However, determining species composition by classical techniques is too cumbersome to be feasible in large studies. Recently, we have developed a method for simultaneously enumerating and identifying bacteria in faeces by using species specific DNA hybridization probes[7]. In this procedure, we are, in effect, measuring the concentration of a fragment of DNA that is unique to a particular species rather than measuring the concentration of viable organisms. The advantage of this procedure is that it does not require growth of the organisms or their isolation in pure culture. Moreover, because this procedure uses DNA hybridization, it bypasses many of the problems involved in the classical identification schemes which are based on fermentation tests. The main drawback is that, at present, this procedure can be used only to estimate the concentrations of major species of bacteria.

Detailed information on the steps involved in breakdown of polysaccharides by human colonic *Bacteroides* is available for three polysaccharides: chondroitin sulfate, polygalacturonic acid and guar gum. Chondroitin sulfate, a mucopolysaccharide that is released during the sloughing of cells from the intestinal mucosa, is an example of a host-produced polysaccharide that probably enters the colon in appreciable concentrations. Polygalacturonic acid and guar gum (a galactomannan) are both plant polysaccharides.

Breakdown of these polysaccharides by *Bacteroides* involves a number of proteins. When *B. thetaiotaomicron* is grown on chondroitin sulfate, it produces two chondroitinases which cleave chondroitin sulfate into disaccharides[8]. These enzymes are very similar with respect to molecular weight and kinetic properties and it is not clear why both are needed. These chondroitinases are not extracellular but are located inside the cell, possibly in the periplasmic space[12]. The presence of the degradative enzymes inside the cell may help to prevent loss of the products of enzyme activity to competing organisms, but it means that the organism has to solve the problem of getting a large negatively charged polymer through the outer membrane so that it can be brought into contact with the degradative enzymes. Recent work has shown that there are at least eight outer membrane polypeptides that are produced only when *B. thetaiotaomicron* is grown on chondroitin sulfate[6].

Breakdown of polygalacturonic acid by *B. thetaiotaomicron* involves a similarly complex system. There are two polygalacturonases, both of which are cell-associated rather than extracellular[10]. One of them, a polygalacturonate hydrolase, is located in the inner membrane. The other, a polygalacturonate lyase is soluble and is located either in the cytoplasm or in the periplasmic space. In addition to these enzymes there are at least six outer membrane polypeptides that are associated with growth on polygalacturonic acid[6].

Breakdown of guar gum by *B. ovatus* differs from the breakdown of chondroitin sulfate and polygalacturonic acid by *B. thetaiotaomicron* in that there appears to be an extracellular enzyme that degrades guar gum into large fragments[1]. In addition to the extracellular galactomanna-nase activity, there is a galactomannanase that is located in the outer membrane of *B. ovatus* (Gherardini, unpublished results). The products of this enzyme have not been characterized. When *B. ovatus* is grown on guar gum, it also produces an α-galactosidase that can remove galatose residues from fragments of guar gum[4]. This α-galactosidase also cleaves galactose residues from melibiose, raffinose and stachyose. However, when *B. ovatus* is grown on melibiose or raffinose, a different α-galactosidase is produced. It is not clear why two distinct enzymes are needed.

Although we can learn about the regulation of polysaccharidases and the metabolic potential of colonic organisms by studying their behaviour when they are growing as pure cultures in laboratory medium, we must be careful about using results of such experiments to draw conclusions about what is occurring in the colon. Moreover, the ability of colon bacteria to alter their metabolic activities in response to changing conditions should alert us to the probability that the equilibrium between the host's diet and the colonic microflora is probably a dynamic rather than a static one. Appreciable changes in the metabolic activities of the colonic microflora may occur without significant changes in the species composition of the colonic flora. This may explain why the species composition of the human colonic microflora appears to remain relatively constant despite changes in the host's diet[2,5].

Recently we have attempted to determine which, if any of the five colonic *Bacteroides* species that can use polygalacturonic acid is actually using this substrates in the colon[9]. All five of these species produce cell-associated polygalacturonic acid lyases. The polygalacturonic acid lyases from the different species are similar with respect to molecular weight pH optimum and calcium dependence, but they differ with respect to isoelectric point. Accordingly, we can use the isoelectric point values to determine if any polygalacturonate lyase activity that is found in recovered from faeces was produced by one of these *Bacteroides* species. Polygalacturonate lyase activity is inducible in all of the *Bacteroides* species tested. Thus an organism should be producing detectable levels of the enzyme only if it was growing on polygalacturonic acid. We were able to detect a polygalacturonate lyase in a bacterial fraction that was obtained from human faeces, but the isoelectric point and molecular weight of this activity were different from those of the enzymes that are produced by *Bacteroides* species. We do not know whether the activity in faeces is being produced by another species of bacteria or whether it is an endogenous activity present in undegraded plant cell wall material. Based on these findings, it appears that none of the five *Bacteroides* species tested are growing on polygalacturonic acid in the colon. However, we cannot rule out the possibility that they were growing on polygalacturonic acid in the ascending colon and then switched to another substrate as they moved into the lower regions of the colon. Despite its limitations, this study provides an example of the way in which information obtained from investigations of pure cultures can be used as a basis for determining what the organisms are actually doing in the colon.

Acknowledgement. This work was supported by Public Health Service grant AI 17876 from the National Institute of Allergy and Infectious Diseases.

1 Balascio, J.R., Palmer, J.K. & Salyers, A.A. (1982): Breakdown of guar gum by enzymes produced by a bacterium from the human colon. *J. Fd. Biochem.* **5**, 271–282.
2 Bornside, G.H. (1978): Stability of the human faecal flora. *Am. J. Clin. Nutr.* **31**, 521–529.
3 Ehle, F.R., Robertson, J.B. & Van Soest, P.J. (1982): Influence of dietary fibers on fermentation in the human large intestine. *J. Nutr.* **112**, 158–166.
4 Gherardini, F.C., Babcock, M. & Salyers, A.A. (1985): Purification and characterization of two alpha-galactosidases associated with catabolism of guar gum and other alpha-galactosides. *J. Bact.* **161**, 500–506.
5 Hentges, D.J. (1980): Does diet influence human faecal microflora composition? *Nutr. Rev.* **38**, 329–336.
6 Kotarski, S.F., Linz, J., Braun, D.M. & Salyers, A.A. (1985): Analysis of outer membrane polypeptides which are associated with growth of *Bacteroides thetaiotaomicron* on chondroitin sulfate. *J. Bact.* In press.
7 Kuritza, A.P. & Salyers, A.A. (1985): Use of a species specific DNA probe for enumerating *Bacteroides vulgatus* in human faeces. *Appl. Environ. Microbiol.* In press.
8 Linn, S.P., Chan. T., Lipeski, L. & Salyers, A.A. (1983): Isolation and characterization of two chondroitin lyases from *Bacteroides thetaiotaomicron.* *J. Bact.* **156**, 859–866.
9 McCarthy, R.E., Kotarski, S.F. & Salyers, A.A. (1985): Location and characteristics of enzymes involved in the breakdown of polygalacturonic acid by *Bacteroides thetaiotaomicron.* *J. Bact.* **161**, 493–499.
10 McCarthy, R.E. & Salyers, A.A. (1985): Comparison of a polygalacturonate lyase activity in human faeces with polygalacturonate lyases from five colonic *Bacteroides* species. Submitted for publication.
11 Moore, W.E.C., Cato, E.P. & Holdeman, L.V. (1978): Some current concepts in intestinal bacteriology. *Am. J. Clin. Nutr.* **31**, 933–942.

12 Salyers, A.A. & O'Brien, M. (1980): Cellular location of enzymes involved in the breakdown of chondroitin sulfate by *Bacteroides thetaiotaomicron. J. Bact.* **143**, 772–779.
13 Salyers, A.A., Vercellotti, J.R., West, S.E.H. & Wilkins, T.D. (1977): Fermentation of mucin and plant polysaccharides by *Bacteroides* from the human colon. *Appl. Environ. Microbiol.* **33**, 319–322.
14 Salyers, A.A., West, S.E.H., Vercellotti, J.R. & Wilkins, T.D. (1978): Fermentation of mucin and plant polysaccharides by anaerobic bacteria from the human colon. *Appl. Environ. Microbiol.* **34**, 529–533.
15 Van Soest, P.J. (1978): Dietary fibers: Their definition and nutritional properties. *Am. J. Clin. Nutr.* **31**, 512–520.

Influence of fibre on the gut microflora of the monogastric animal

R. DUCLUZEAU and J.P. LAPLACE
Laboratoire d'Ecologie Microbienne and Laboratoire de Physiologie de la Nutrition, INRA — CNRZ, F-78350 — Jouy en Josas, France

---

Ingestion of dietary fibre is usually·considered to be responsible for changes in the digestion and absorption in both man and monogastric animals. Numerous bacteria indeed are able to metabolize dietary fibre within the gastrointestinal (GI) tract. The resulting production of metabolites undergoes large quantitative variations, when fibre is added to the diet. Therefore it has been postulated that dietary fibre intake is able to modify the gastrointestinal flora. However, most microbiological studies performed on the human GI tract flora as a function of the fibre content of the diet, lead to the same conclusions, namely that there are very small differences, if any, between the bacterial populations considered (usually faecal flora)[1,6].

Such a discrepancy, between a common postulate and the experimental data, may be explained in several ways. First of all, the microbiological techniques used to study the composition of the faecal flora could be unsuitable for revealing small numerical changes of such bacterial species whose metabolic effects are important. It has also been suggested that dietary fibre could induce variations of the metabolic abilities of the flora, without affecting the size of the assumed bacterial populations. If these hypotheses are tenable, the characterization of the GI tract flora on the basis of specific functions or quantitative biochemical indices would be better than the counts of the various bacterial families and species. In addition it should be noted that most studies deal with the effect of additional dietary fibre, ie fibre added to a diet already containing fibre. So a total prolonged deprivation of fibre could be an interesting experimental situation to reveal changes of the GI tract flora with some certainty.

To answer these questions, the present paper will review three different experimental models.

Effect of bran ingestion on the microbial faecal flora of human donors and of recipient gnotobiotic mice, and on the barrier effects exerted by these flora against various potentially pathogenic strains. In this model, the flora were characterized by the so-called function 'barrier effect', ie the antagonistic action by some components of the GI tract flora against environmental bacteria coming into the digestive ecosystem. This barrier effect was studied in axenic mice, inoculated with faecal flora from human beings receiving or not receiving dietary bran, and reared in isolators. It was suspected that, feeding bran, or not, to these gnotobiotic mice would provide a sensitive model to reveal bran-induced variations of the barrier effect. In addition, quantitative counts of several bacterial families and species were performed on the faecal floras from human beings receiving bran or not, and on the faecal floras of the respective inoculated mice. All the methods used for these experiments have been previously published[2].

The comparison of the human faecal floras before and after 30 days of bran ingestion showed a close similarity in the bacterial families of the strictly anaerobic dominant flora: their numerical importance was in most cases identical, and at most differed by ten fold. On the other hand some occasional differences were recorded in the facultative anaerobic under-dominant flora, but they did not appear to be related to the addition of bran to the diet. Similar results were recorded when comparing the faecal flora of the recipient mice.

In the recipient mice, inoculated with the flora from three human donors, and fed or not fed bran, the barrier effect was tested against five bacteria, potentially pathogenic in the human: *Clostridium perfringens*, *Staphylococcus aureus*, *Candida albicans*, *Pseudomonas aeruginosa* and *Clostridium difficile*. Independent of the diet and of the flora of the human donor, there was a strong barrier against *C. perfringens* and *S. aureus*, and a permissive barrier against *P. aeruginosa* and *C. albicans*. As regards *C. difficile* a large variability of the barrier effect was observed, ie strong in some animals and lacking in others, but there was no relation with the diet (Table 1). On the whole, similar results were recorded in the gnotobiotic mice whether they were fed bran or not.

Table 1. *Barrier effect against five microbial strains potentially pathogenic in the digestive tract of gnotobiotic mice innoculated with the flora of three human donors (LM, SB and LZ) without bran in their diet.*

Target strain	Log$_{10}$ of number of innoculated cells			Diet[a]	Log$_{10}$ of number of viable cells[b] after:											
					1 day			3 days			6 days			9 days		
	LM	SB	LZ		LM	SB	LZ	LM	SB	LZ	LM	SB	LZ	LM	SB	LZ
C. perfringens	7.3	7.0	6.9	B	4.0	6.0	2.5	<2	<2	<2	<2	<2	<2	<2	<2	<2
				WB	4.6	<2	2.5	<2	<2	3.9	<2	<2	<2	<2	<2	<2
S. aureus	7.0	7.6	8.3	B	6.0	6.2	5.7	3.5	4.0	<2	<2	<2	<2	<2	<2	<2
				WB	4.0	5.3	5.7	<2	3.7	<2	<2	<2	<2	<2	<2	<2
C. albicans	6.4	4.0	6.7	B	6.6	5.4	5.0	4.5	3.2	4.0	4.3	<2	4.0	2.6	<2	2.5
				WB	5.5	3.0	5.0	4.7	<2	4.4	4.5	<2	4.0	4.9	<2	3.9
P. aeruginosa	7.3	7.7	7.5	B	5.7	4.0	5.3	3.6	3.0	4.8	4.0	4.5	5.3	4.7	4.2	5.0
				WB	3.8	5.0	5.0	2.5	4.0	5.9	4.0	4.0	4.6	4.7	5.4	5.9
C. difficile	7.7	6.7	6.7	B	6.7	6.5	6.0	5.7	5.0	4.5	6.5	4.0	6.0	6.0	5.5	6.2
				WB	7.0	7.0	3.3	5.6	7.0	2.7	6.5	7.0	<2	6.6	7.2	<2

[a] B = bran in diet; WB = without bran; [b] Log$_{10}$ of number of microbes in a mixture of six faecal pellets from six matched animals.

Therefore, this first experimental model confirmed that there is no clear effect of bran on the dominant flora of monogastric animals. It also pointed out that bran fails to affect an important function of this flora, its barrier effect against pathogens.

Influence of the dietary fibre intake on the amino acid composition of the faeces in the pig. The comparison of the amino acid composition of the faeces of axenic and holoxenic pigs shows large differences, mainly in THR, SER, PRO and CYS contents which are higher in the faeces from axenic pigs[3]. There is also a high proportion of these amino acids in the meconium of piglets at birth and, as a general rule, in endogenous proteins. On the other hand, the amino acid composition of the faeces from holoxenic pigs seems to be determined mainly by the amino acid composition of the dominant bacterial flora, as the proportion of bacterial proteins in the total faecal nitrogen would be around 90 per cent[3,5]. Thus it is likely that any large modification of the GI tract flora, due to a high fibre intake, might induce significant changes in the amino acid composition of the faeces.

Accordingly, we compared the amino acid composition of the faeces from holoxenic pigs fed either a semi-purified diet or a standard diet for 2 weeks before faeces collection. Nine samples were obtained and deep frozen immediately after defaecation, from two pigs (55 and 57 kg live weight) fed the standard diet, whose total neutral detergent fibre (NDF) content was 18.4 per cent of dry matter (hemicellulose 11.1, cellulose 5.9, lignin 1.4). Four samples were also collected from two pigs (47 and 48 kg) fed a semipurified diet whose total NDF content was 7.9 per cent of dry matter (hemicellulose 1.5, cellulose 6.2, lignin 0.2). In addition, the amino acid

Table 2. *Mean amino acid composition (as percentage of the sum of 17 amino acids) of the faeces (and corresponding isolates) of pigs, according to the diet(*), and sum of the 17 A.A. and diamino pimelic acid (DAP) content as percentage of freeze-dried material.*

Amino acids* Diets:	Faeces		Bacterial isolates	
	Standard	Semi-purified	Standard	Semi-purified
ASX	10.67	13.58	11.18	14.18
THR	5.40	5.04	5.47	5.06
SER	5.05	5.42	4.81	5.51
GLX	12.92	11.31	12.10	11.07
PRO	5.40	4.16	4.28	3.46
GLY	5.40	6.72	5.25	5.22
ALA	6.55	6.62	6.98	6.83
VAL	6.61	5.85	6.62	6.39
ILE	5.50	5.06	6.00	5.80
LEU	8.53	7.67	8.48	8.29
TYR	4.27	3.98	4.64	4.02
PHE	5.32	5.15	5.51	6.14
LYS	6.71	6.98	7.45	6.55
HIS	2.29	1.96	2.17	2.05
ARG	4.96	5.16	5.24	4.87
CYS	2.05	2.56	1.63	2.17
MET	2.34	2.77	2.18	2.36
Composition of freeze-dried material				
Sum 17 A.A.	14.15	9.13	35.57	25.70
DAP	0.0532	0.0264	0.1933	0.0938

composition was determined for the 13 corresponding bacterial isolates derived from the 13 faeces samples. The method used, based on several differential centrifugations allowed a final concentration of bacteria 50 times higher than that recorded in fresh faeces.

Depending on the diet fed to the pigs, there was a large difference in the quantity of amino acids in the samples (Table 2). The total amino acid content (sum of 17 amino acids, as percentage of freeze dried material; tryptophan not measured) was much lower in the faeces of pigs fed the semi-purified diet, and in the corresponding bacterial isolates, than in the corresponding homologous faeces or isolates for the standard diet. Also, the diamino pimelic acid (DAP) content was also two times lower in the 'semi-purified' samples than in the 'standard' ones. But the mean values recorded for each of the 17 individual amino acids (Table 2) did not differ according to the diet, nor between faeces samples, nor between bacterial isolates. This means that the amino acid composition of the faecal flora, and thus of the faeces, was not affected by the diet. Moreover microscopic examination suggested a reduced flora (5 times lower count and reduced number of species), but the proportions of bacterial proteins in the faecal proteins (calculated from the ratios DAP to nitrogen) were closely similar: 64.7 per cent for the standard diet and 65.7 per cent for the semi-purified diet.

Therefore, the amino acid composition of the GI tract flora determines that of the faeces, and it seems to avoid a significant dietary influence, including any fibre effect.

Effect of prolonged food deprivation on the caecal flora in the pig: the caeco-colonic bypass model. Instead of increasing the dietary fibre supplied for the fermentative processes by the flora, it may be of interest to suppress the fibre disposal, and even to suppress all exogenous dietary supplies. The procedure of the ileo-rectal end-to-end anastomosis, recently developed in the pig[4], allows a bypass of the caeco-colonic area. In this model, the large intestine is able to empty through a T-shaped simple cannula placed at its distal end, but in any case it does not receive digesta. This procedure allows the pigs to eat and grow quite normally while the caecal flora is completely deprived of exogenous materials.

Table 3. *Comparison of the bacterial counts in caecal contents of pigs collected at surgery, or at slaughter after total bypass of the caeco-colonic region for 14 to 54 days.*

Bacterial population enumerated	Number of bacteria per g of fresh contents ($log_{10} \pm SEM$)		P
	At surgery	At slaughter	
Total population in deep agar	9.02 ± 0.31[a]	9.36 ± 0.12	ns
Total population in anaerobic chamber	9.46 ± 0.15	10.02 ± 0.13	<0.01
Bacteroides	9.40 ± 0.21	9.62 ± 0.20	ns
Eubacterium	8.96 ± 0.12	9.50 ± 0.20	ns
Bifidobacterium	8.07 ± 0.35	9.16 ± 0.10	<0.02
Escherichia coli	7.24 ± 0.26	7.16 ± 0.82	ns
Streptococcus	7.46 ± 0.20	8.54 ± 0.34	<0.05
Lactobacillus	8.2 ± 0.22	<3	—

[a] Mean of five animals; [b] by Student's t test. Comparison between data at surgery and at slaughter.

Five pigs underwent such a surgical procedure at a mean live weight of 49.2 ± 0.8 kg. They were killed under deep anesthesia 14 to 54 days after the operation. Samples of caecal contents were collected on both occasions under anesthesia. The caecal flora in the digesta at surgery, and the flora in the residual contents at slaughter were compared using the previously described method of differential analysis[2]. There was no variation in the concentrations of the bacterial species, with length of time the bypass was functional. The mean values for the five pigs, independent of the bypass duration, revealed only minor changes in the bacterial numbers (Table 3). The strict anaerobes, *Bacteroides* and *Eubacterium*, remained the dominant bacteria. The *Escherichia coli* counts did not vary significantly, while *Bifidobacterium* and *Streptococcus* populations slightly increased. Only the *Lactobacillus* population fell sharply, which could be related mainly to the deprivation of easily fermentable sugars. Therefore except for this last microorganism, it seems that the deprivation of fibre, and of all exogenous nutritional supplies, does not change the equilibrium of the caecal flora.

Conclusions. The results supplied by the three experimental models confirm the statement by some authors who agree that, even under a severe control of the bacterial environment and of the diet, it is not possible to reveal any clear cut effect of the fibre content of the diet on the GI tract flora. Neither the qualitative or quantitative composition of the flora, as assessed by the present techniques, nor the barrier effect against pathogens, nor the amino acid composition of digesta, seem to be affected by the addition or by the lack of fibre. It must be admitted that the bacteriological techniques used do not permit detection of small changes in the flora and some of the various biochemical functions of the flora are probably affected. Nevertheless, our results support the view that fibre in the diet does not strongly modify the equilibrium and overall function of the GI tract flora.

1 Drasar, B.S., Jenkins, D.J.A. & Cummings, J.H. (1976): The influence of a diet rich in wheat fibre on the human faecal flora. *J. med. Microbiol.* **9**, 425–431.
2 Ducluzeau, R., Ladire, M. & Raibaud, P. (1984): Effet de l'ingestion de son de blé sur la flore microbienne fécale de donneurs humains et de souris gnotoxéniques receveuses, et sur les effets de barrière exercés par ces flores à l'égard de divers microorganismes potentiellement pathogènes. *Ann. Microbiol. (Inst. Pasteur).* **135A**, 303–318.

3 Laplace, J.P., Darcy-Vrillon, B., Duval, Y. & Raibaud, P. (1985): Comparison of the amino acid composition of pure endogenous and microbial proteins in the G.I. tract of the pig. In *Digestive physiology in the pig*, ed A. Just, H. Jorgensen, J.A. Fernandez, pp. 296–299. Report 580 National Inst. Anim. Sci. Copenhagen.

4 Laplace, J.P., Darcy-Vrillon, B. & Picard, M. (1985): Evaluation de la disponibilité des acides aminés: choix raisonné d'une méthode. In *Journées Rech. Porcine en Frnace*. pp. 353–370. Paris: INRA-ITP.

5 Mason, V.C., Just, A. & Bech-Andersen, S. (1976): Bacterial activity in the hind gut of pigs. 2. Its influence on the apparent digestibility of nitrogen and amino acids. *Z. Tierphysiol. Tierernähr. Futtermittelkde* **36**, 310–324.

6 Moore, W.E.C., Cato, E.P. & Holdeman, L.V. (1978): Some current concepts in intestinal bacteriology. *Am. J. Clin. Nutr.* **31**, S33–S42.

Use of ionophores to increase meat production by ruminants: a workshop report

G.T. SCHELLING (Organizer)
Texas A & M University, College Station, Texas 77843, USA.

This workshop was conceived with the idea of assessing the current role, and exploring the future potential, of the ionophores for the enhancement of meat production by ruminants. The currently approved ionophores have been commercially successful and have significantly contributed to the efficiency of utilization for meat production. There is considerable interest in using other ionophores with different properties in order to further improve animal responses. The development of delivery systems to support greater ionophore use with grazing animals is of interest. The longer-term role of ionophores as a research tool to gain more insight into biological concepts will eventually pay rewards in animal production. A group of scientists presented the following summaries of their work on the fundamental and applied aspects of feeding ionophores to ruminants.

Fundamental mode of action of ionophores at the cellular level. (*Werner G Bergen* and *Douglas B Bates*, Michigan State University, E. Lansing and University of Florida, Gainesville, FL, USA.). Carboxylic polyether ionophores have a myriad of effects on both the rumen fermentation and animal physiology. The underlying mode of action of ionophores is on transmembrane ion fluxes and the dissipation of proton and cation gradients. Cells will respond to this metabolic insult by maintaining proton extrusion (primary transport) by expending metabolic energy, thus depleting ATP stores. The dissipation of the proton (ΔpH) gradient appears to lower intracellular pH. This in turn affects the midpoint potential of the redox couple and hence the activity profile of many enzymes. Proton (cation) gradient dissipation also interferes with secondary solute uptake (eg amino acids) coupled to primary transport. If a cell can maintain adequate ATP levels, these adverse effects can be partially overcome. Anaerobes not strictly dependent on substrate level phosphorylation for ATP synthesis have a decided survival advantage. In the rumen, propionate-succinate producers have such an advantage. The inhibition by ionophores of amino acid deamination by ruminal bacteria is apparently linked to cellular amino acid uptake mechanisms. The process of microbial adaptation to ionophores is currently not understood.

Ionophore effects in the digestive tract. (*G. T. Schelling* and *F. M. Byers*, Texas A&M University, College Station, Texas, 77843, USA.). The basic ionophore mode of action of modifying the movement of ions across the membranes of specific cells results in several system modes of action which can have positive effects on productivity by ruminants. Many biological responses associated with the digestive tract due to ionophores have been reported, and they can be grouped into seven categories (system modes of action). The modification of volatile fatty acid production is one widely recognized category of importance. Modified feed intake is the second category of significance. A change in gas production probably represents a definite, but small, saving in energy. Modified digestibilities, the fourth category, may be somewhat variable, but appear to be of significance with several nutrient classes. The fifth category is a change in protein utilization in the digestive tract, and seems to result in several factors that occur simultaneously. Modification of rumen fill and rate of passage can occur, and may be the cause of some of the previously mentioned system modes of action. The seventh category includes several responses more indirect to the rumen and more sporadic in nature. Increased animal productivity due to ionophores probably results directly or indirectly from several of these system modes of action acting in concert. The relative importance of each category appears to change with different dietary conditions, thus it is difficult to accurately assess the contribution of each category. The various characteristics ascribed to different ionophores provide potential for further exploiting these compounds to enhance further productivity.

Influence of ionophores on energy utilization and maintenance energy requirements. (*F. M. Byers* and *G. T. Schelling*, Texas A&M University, College Station, Texas 77843, USA.). An extensive volume of research published in the past decade clearly indicates that ionophores impact on animal productivity and result in a reduction in feed required for comparable production. Energy utilization reflects these effects and is modified in several areas and through several mechanisms. Digestibility of energy is usually enhanced; the response varies from 0 to 6 per cent depending on level of intake and forage/grain level. Diet ME is usually increased more than DE, depending on the degree of impact on methane production. ME/DE ratio is increased and ME is increased from 0 to 10 per cent, with greater response at low levels of intake and with high-forage diets. A dichotomy in response is evident in energetics of maintenance vs growth. Most research indicates a reduction in DM and ME for maintenance and/or enhanced utilization of ME for maintenance. While the magnitude of this response is variable and ranges from 2 to 10 per cent, a positive effect on maintenance requirements or efficiency of diet use for maintenance is noted in all studies. However little or no effect of ionophore is evident in the efficiency of DM or of ME use for growth (RE/ME), indicating that ionophores do not alter energetic efficiency of growth. Ionophores enhance digestibility, metabolism, and use of diet energy for maintenance with little or no impact on energetics of growth.

Response of grazing cattle to ionophores. (*James A. Boling*. Department of Animal Sciences, University of Kentucky, Lexington, KY, 40546, USA.). The quantity of an ionophore consumed, frequency of consumption and forage composition are factors contributing to the performance response of grazing cattle. Seventy-two Angus steers averaging 211 kg were allotted to four treatments and hand-fed (1) no monensin-control, (2) 25 mg, (3) 50 mg, or (4) 100 mg monensin per head daily in 0.91 kg ground corn. Calves grazed Kentucky bluegrass-clover pastures throughout the 140-day study (4 May-23 October). Average daily gains were 0.55, 0.55, 0.73 and 0.68 kg, respectively. The molar percentages of ruminal propionate (day 56) were 18.8, 19.3, 20.3 and 20.5 and increased ($P<0.05$) due to monensin feeding. Daily hand-feeding of other ionophores at or exceeding the threshold level for efficacy results in similar performance and ruminal responses. A less labor intensive practice is to feed the ionophore in a mineral mixture offered ad libitum. Performance responses in these management systems have been variable due to reduced consumption of some ionophore-containing mineral mixtures. Sequential rumen sampling showed that ruminal responses (volatile fatty acids and monensin-resistant bacteria) continued for several days after monensin feeding was terminated. Also, several strains of rumen bacteria were more resistant to higher concentrations of monensin and lasalocid at elevated potassium levels. Since many cool season grasses are high in potassium (>3.0 percent of dry matter) in the spring, animal performance and ruminal metabolism may be altered at specific (mg/d) ionophore intakes during such grazing periods. Further data are needed concerning this aspect of feeding ionophores to grazing growing calves and lactating beef cows.

Response of cattle fed forage and grain to ionophores. (*R. D. Goodrich and J. E. Garrett*. University of Minnesota, St. Paul, Minnesota, 55108, USA.). Data from over 15 000 head of cattle were summarized to determine the response of cattle fed monensin (an ionophore). Performance data were analysed by comparing the response of cattle fed monensin-containing diets to cattle fed the same diet without monensin. Monensin concentration in the trials summarized was 31.8 ± 7.5 mg/kg diet dry matter (DM). Cattle fed diets containing monensin gained faster (1.6 per cent), consumed less feed DM (6.4 per cent) and required less feed DM/100 kg gain (7.5 per cent). Influence of monensin on daily gain decreased as rate of gain increased. Maximum reduction in feed DM intake occurred at a monensin concentration of 35.5 mg/kg diet DM. Improvement in feed/gain due to monensin was greatest when metabolizable energy (ME) concentration was 2.9 Mcal/kg diet DM. High monensin concentration did not significantly improve feed/gain over that obtained from lower concentrations. Carcass characteristics were not influenced by monensin. Effect of monensin and implants on cattle performance were additive. Sex and weight of cattle did not influence response to monensin. Monensin appears to improve performance by improving DM digestibility, reducing fasting heat production and increasing dietary net energy. Trials (4) comparing response of cattle fed different amounts of monensin (200 to 300 mg/d) or lasalocid (300 to 450 mg/d) showed faster gains, reduced feed DM intakes and improved feed/gains (1.0 and 5.9 per cent, 4.1 and 4.6 per cent, and 6.7 and 10.3 per cent respectively) for cattle fed ionophore-containing diets.

Animal response to various ionophores. (*L. L. Berger*, Department of Animal Sciences, University of Illinois, Urbana, IL 61801 USA.). In the USA over 90 per cent of feedlot cattle are fed either monensin or lasalocid. Salinomycin is awaiting Food and Drug Administration approval and should be available within a year. Relatively few data have been published in scientific literature comparing effects of these ionophores. Factors such as dietary energy level, differences in optimum dosage, prior nutritional status, environmental stress, sex of cattle and length of trial make it difficult to compare ionophores when fed in separate trials. To avoid these confounding effects, all response data will be expressed relative to controls. Data used for these comparisons were restricted to animals fed in confinement. Data from 35 (monensin), 23 (lasalocid) and 10 (salinomycin) trials involving approximately 7100 cattle were summarized. When more than one dosage was fed, performance responses were averaged across dosages. Average percentage changes in daily gain, feed intake and feed/gain for monensin, lasalocid and salinomycin were: 2.4, -4.9, -6.8; 6.8, -4.3, -9.9; 4.9, -2.6 and -6.3 per cent, respectively. The optimum dosage of each ionophore will give a greater performance response than averages listed here. Relative economic improvement in performance was calculated by multiplying the feed/gain response by 2.5 and adding the gain response for various dosages of monensin and lasalocid. Adjusting for ionophore cost, the optimum concentration of monensin and lasalocid was 22 and 33 mg/kg diet respectively.

International potential of ionophores. (*J. I. D. Wilkinson*, Lilly Research Centre Ltd., Erl Wood Manor, Windlesham, Surrey, GU20 6PH, UK.). Monensin has been used commercially to improve the efficiency of beef production in the USA since 1975 and in Europe since 1978. Ninety-one beef production trials have been carried out in the USA and in nine European countries. They involved bulls, heifers and steers of most of the major breeds, in a broad variety of production systems:

Description	No. of Trials	Monensin dosage	Liveweight gain	Feed/gain
			Improvements (%)	
European confined, total:	35	40 mg/kg	4.8	10.2
Barley beef	(12)	30–40 mg/kg	7.5	9.7
Maize silage	(8)	30 mg/kg	4.7	8.3
European pasture	13	200 mg/d	14.7	—
US feedlot	19	33 mg/kg	0	10.6
US high roughage	19	33 mg/kg	14.1	15.3
US pasture	12	200 mg/d	20.3	—

West European beef production is characterized by small family farms often lacking in home feed-mixing facilities, dependency on farm-grown feedstuffs and the close interdependence of beef and dairy production. Bulls are the preferred animal purpose-grown for beef, but cull-cows make-up a substantial part of total beef produced.

The use of any feed additive depends on being able to incorporate it into feeds. The use of ionophores is limited by the lack of suitable treatment carriers on some farms. The successful development of a ruminal delivery device could significantly extend the use of these compounds.

In Western Europe, growth of state support of agriculture will slow and the farmers opportunity to defray increasing costs by increasing output will be restricted. He will be forced to reduce production costs to maintain income. The improvement in feed utilization provided by ionophores, with a high ratio of benefit to cost, can play an important part in this.

★ ★ ★

GUT MICROFLORA AND INTESTINAL PHYSIOLOGY

Anatomical adaptations of the gut promoting microbial digestion

R.R. HOFMANN
Institut für Veterinär-Anatomie, -Histologie, -Embryologie Abt. Vergleichende Anatomie der Haus- und Wildtiere, Justus Liebig-Universität Giessen, Frankfurterstraße 98, D-6300 Giessen, FRG.

Many comparative studies have shown that the gut structure of vertebrates reflects the nutritional separation and specialization of animals.

Starck[20] voices doubts concerning the general rule that carnivores have short guts and herbivores long guts when a broad, comparative view is adopted. Different morphological variations along the gut have differing physiological consequences. Obvious divergence in ecological niching and feeding behaviour may have little influence upon gut structure as observed, eg in rodents[3].

The morpho-physiological adaptation to microbial cellulolytic activity, however, appears to be a distinct though variable feature in all those species which depend entirely on plant material (herbivores) or which utilize vegetable matter as the occasion arises, (omnivores). Many of them, including man, derive nutrients mainly from plant cell contents.

As soon as plant cell walls (cellulose and similar plant structural polymers) are used as a source of nutrition, the necessity for providing a suitable cellulase arises. In consequence, whenever a species derives its energy from cellulose, it has to host cellulolytic bacteria, frequently in addition to specific ciliates and fungi. The anatomical precondition is to provide a suitable environment for these microbes.

Structural variations and specialization of the gut which facilitate and promote microbial digestion must: (1) reduce the passage rate of ingesta in order to enhance the slow process of cellulolysis during an increased mean retention time; (2) provide conditions optimal for the undisturbed activity and reproduction of anaerobic microbes releasing enzymes capable of breaking down plant cell walls[13]; (3) include adaptive mechanisms which prevent excessive congestion (and thus promote new intake) and which protect from loss the nutrients formed during microbial fermentation.

The primitive gut of all vertebrate embryos is initially a tube of even calibre with a ventral (umbilical) flexure. Its foregut portion is determined very early by the gastric spindle. The second pouch formed demarcates the primordial caecum on the border between midgut and hindgut. The mid-gut portion does not show any substantial anatomical adaptation to microbial digestion but foregut and hindgut are the sites of remarkable anatomical variations.

Microbial digestion of plant cell wall remains ineffective and wasteful unless mechanical breakdown permits enzymatic penetration. The preconditions are: (a) incongruence of the temporo-mandibular joint, permitting lateral grinding movement of the cheek teeth; (b) transformation of the cheek teeth into instruments for splitting, grinding and crushing. This is achieved to a great extent by the tuberculate (bunodont) teeth of omnivores (man, monkeys, pigs). The optimal adaptation is found in herbivores with extremely complicated systems of enamel infolding and lamellation (lophodont or, in ruminants, selenodont teeth, which can reduce plant fibre to less than 0.1 mm particle size); (c) specific development of those masticatory muscles which facilitate grinding actions (masseter and pterygoideus). There is a gradation in the relative development of these muscles amongst ruminants of different feeding types. Concentrate selectors (CS) preferring 'soft' plant material rich in cell contents have less pronounced masticatory muscles (Fig. 1) than grass and roughage eaters (GR). Their mandibles, with their different shape and angulation, offer a larger muscle attachment surface resulting in more effective grinding actions.

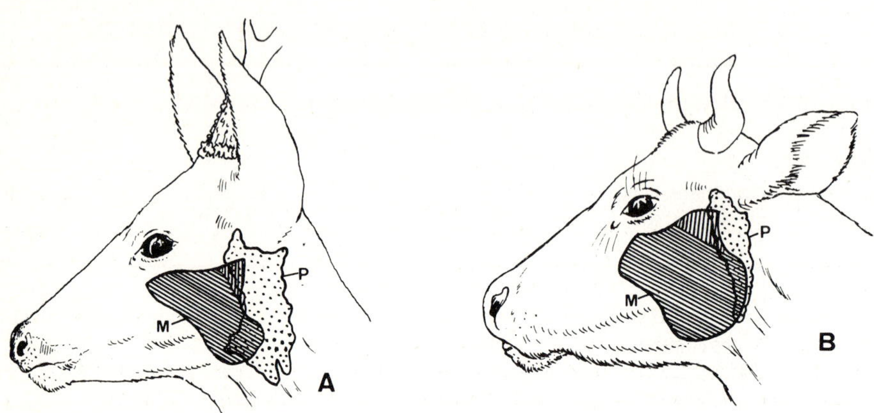

Fig. 1. *Relative size differences of M. masseter (M) and Gl. parotis (P) in ruminants with predominantly amylolytic microbial digestion (A) and cellulolytic microbial digestion (B); relatively weak masseter and large parotid in fruit and/foliage digesting concentrate selectors (A: roe deer 30 kg); relatively strong masseter and small parotid in fibre digesting grass eaters (B: cattle 500 kg).*

Rumination has the primary effect of reducing particle size for microbial fermentation. Adaptations cranial to the specific stomach of ruminating animals are cranial and caudal oesophageal sphincters, an oesophageal muscular tunic composed entirely of striated (voluntary) muscle tissue permitting antiperistalsis, and a funnel-shaped widening of the caudalmost portion of the oesophagus situated in the underpressurized mediastinal space.

Mechanical mixing and maceration are also important factors. This is reflected in the differentiated development of the interal oblique muscle fibres of the ruminant forestomachs. They form the ruminal pillars which are simple wall infoldings in CS-ruminants, but thick and powerful bulges in GR-ruminants which digest plants with high fibre contents[5,15]. Propelling ingesta in the rumino-reticular chamber during a well-coordinated sequence of motor events (and comparable variations of peristalsis in non-ruminants) appears to be directly related to microbial digestion. As has been suggested[23], these motor events are linked to rumination, onward transport and the separation of sinkable (small) and floating (coarser) particles.

Peristaltic muscular propulsion in the widened or sacculated portions of the gut fermentation chambers should also contribute to the physical breakdown of plant particles which are contained in a liquid pool. Although all acids including volatile fatty acids (VFA) have an obvious macerating effect upon plant fibre, this may require passage through the glandular (low pH) stomach even in forestomach fermenters[22]. Several hemicelluloses, the structural carbohydrates of many dicotyledonous plants, resist ruminal breakdown. CS-ruminants which select foliage primarily because of its readily available cell contents, have proportionally more HCl-producing parietal cells in their abomasum than GR-ruminants[6,8] possibly to aid microbial hindgut fermentation.

In order to accommodate cellulolytic bacteria, the digestive tube must: (a) increase in diameter and capacity over a distance, to be followed by a constriction (congestion effect); (b) form blindsacs, pouches or cul-de-sac segments, or (c) provide sacculations due to muscular taenia and/or a sequence of semicircular or circular folds. They compartmentalize the gut into peripheral delay sections and a common central stream tube, usually permitting rapid flow or back flow. The suborder Ruminantia are a perfect model for studying the evolutionary 'switch-over' from microbial hindgut to foregut fermentation[9].

Several mammalian orders include species which have transformed foregut portions into the principal site for microbial digestion: Marsupialia, Edentata, Artiodactyla and Primates. A substantial part of the proventricular portion of their stomach is lined by a nonglandular cutaneous mucosa, the stratified squamous epithelium of which shows adaptations to a microbial association and to absorption.

Theoretically, foregut fermenters have to subject all nutrients to microbial breakdown — unless selective by-pass or through-pass mechanisms have evolved.

In a broad comparative study, Langer[15,16] has compiled the remarkable diversity of adaptive anatomical variations in this portion of the gut. He points to the complex system of valve-like folds, blind-sacs and sacculations in the Hippopotamidae and to the different, not less complex transit-regulating and delaying structures of the stomachs of Macropodidae and Colobidae and to the astounding variety of macro-anatomical adaptations in the mammalian foregut portion, of which about 90 per cent have been converted into anaerobic fermentation chambers.

That it is the cellulolytic microbes, and increasing proportions of plant fibre in the diet, which have driven evolutionary processes to develop the most voluminous forestomachs with more effective structures for passage delay (and absorption of microbial products like VFA) can be shown for the ruminants as a very diversified group[7]. The view that the relative volume of fermentation chambers tends to increase with the body size of a species has been disputed[6,7] since large CS-ruminant species which select in the wild for plant cell content rather than for cell wall (eg giraffe, kudu, moose) have a relatively small ruminoreticulum with weak pillars and wide openings. They are distinguished by high proportions of amylolytic bacteria, high fermentation rates and evenly distributed absorptive papillae. Their mucosa shows a greater surface enlargement (SE) than grass-eaters. The more fibrous food GR-ruminant species have adapted to, the more voluminous is their ruminoreticulum, the stronger its pillars, the narrower its openings. Slower fermentation, in combination with a distinct stratification of fibrous food, has reduced the SE to the centrally placed liquid phase of the ingesta (atrium ruminis, pouches and niches next to the ruminal pillars). The dorsal wall of the rumen can be used as an indicative area of anatomical adaptation, some of which is evolutionary, some a direct result of VFA-stimulation, or lacking stimulation[11]. These differences are rooted in the vascular system of the ruminal mucosa[1,6,10,17]. Ruminal bacteria, by producing more butyrate and propionate stimulate ruminal blood flow which in turn stimulates vascular loop formation, epithelial mitotic index and thus papillary growth, ie absorptive SE.

In areas of constant bacterial activity the ruminal epithelium shows specific adaptations. Its superficial horn cells become transformed into balloon cells[18] which break open to accommodate rumen bacteria; the inner fibrillar substructures of these cells have been recognised[4] as glycocalyx and there is an epithelial barrier layer between stratum granulosum and stratum corneum. However rapid selective absorption of fermentation products is a precondition for maintaining an optimal microbial environment and pH in the rumen or any other fermentation vat. In areas of reduced microbial activity the stratum corneum consists of several if not many layers of flat horn scales — here, the protective function of this layer supercedes its absorptive adaptation.

Microbial anaerobic activity depends upon a stable substrate pH about the neutral point. Foregut fermenters have the immediate benefit of large salivary glands providing alkaline HCO_3^- secretions (for neutralization and buffering of short-chain fatty acids released by the microbes).

There is a direct relationship between a ruminant's position within the flexible system of morpho-physiological feeding types and its salivary glands: the relative weight of saliva-producing tissue, especially parotid, decreases with increasing adaptation to fibre digestion. CS have 3 to 4 times more saliva-producing tissue than GR[9,14].

Hindgut fermenters have no such salivary buffer influx. A neutral liquid phase is produced by the secretions of the crypts of Lieberkühn, but mainly by the intestinal goblet cells. The enteric bacterial adherence system in the luminal mucin layer (LML) and bacterial attachment to membrane glycoproteins is currently the subject of intensive research. It has been shown that the LML represents a special microclimate for bacteria in the large intestine of several rodents (differences in the thickness, compactness and histochemistry).

The hindgut, the principal site of microbial production of nutrients, shows anatomical adaptations in herbivorous reptiles, birds and many mammalian species. A multiplicity of form variations serves basically the same physiological purpose. Widespread generalisations which simply refer to 'caecal' fermentation are incorrect as the colon ascendens is frequently or exclusively involved.

Anatomical adaptations of the hindgut promoting microbial digestion are always distinguished by taenia, sacculations and semilumas folds[16] but frequently added to by merely distended gut portions (as in Perissodactyls and Hyracoids). Sacculation on its own may not be a sufficiently effective anatomical device for ingesta passage delay, as can be seen in man and other primates. The human colon is relatively long and furnished with taenia and sacculations, yet unlike the pig, it remains evenly wide along its entire course up to the widening of the ampulla recti. It appears that the abrupt formation of one or even a series of permanent constrictions (bottlenecks) along the hindgut is the anatomical precondition for the desired congestion permitting microbial cellulolysis.

Perissodactyls (eg horse) have enormous colonic fermentation chambers, with the addition of a huge caecum. Between the ileal orifice into the caecum and the relatively thin, sacculated descending colon, there are four distinct bottlenecks: caecocolonic, pelvic flexure, and two transverse colonic. Their congestive, delaying effect is also expressed in well-known malfunctions (eg bloat, volvulus). The alternation of distended and constricted gut portions is even more pronounced in the small hyraxes (Fig. 2) where in addition to a caecum (with sacculations and several blind-sacs), one short and two long, pointed colonic blind-sacs, one observes also four constrictions of the gut lumen (see arrows).

A specific morpho-physiological differentiation of the caecum[19] is found in the rabbit and other caecotrophic hindgut fermenters leading to separation of fermentable solutes and small digesta particles from rapidly expelled coarse particles rich in fibre and lignin. A number of species have evolved fermentation vats in more than one portion of their digestive tube[16] eg Macropus, Potorous and Colobus.

Phylogenetically, the hindgut-fermenting Suidae have been followed by the Ruminantia. It has been postulated that hindgut fermentation is the 'older' development and 'all foregut fermenters should have some fermentation in the hindgut'[12]. This applies to Colobidae, Potorinae, Macropodinae and certainly to the Ruminantia. A comparative table giving the net weight of hindgut contents as a percentage of body weight, with a range from about 0.5 per cent in man and dog to 13 per cent in elephant and horse, has been drawn up[2]. Ruminants show great variations, wild species included. Cattle, sheep and other GR-ruminants with voluminous forestomachs are perfectly adapted to cellulolytic microbes. The distended initial portion of their hindgut, however, is comparatively short and tight, Its capacity has a ratio to ruminorecticular capacity of 1:15–30 (Fig. 3). There is a gradually tightening transition into the short colonic spiral which has but few turns.

CS-ruminants, apparently still rely much more on hindgut fermentation. The anatomical adaptation of CS like giraffe, moose, kudu or roe deer clearly points in this direction. Our current investigations of so far 26 ruminant species reveal a 'switch-over' development: the smaller the ruminoreticulum and the poorer its passage delay structures, the larger the caeco-colonic (distal) fermentation chamber (DFC) at a ratio of 1 : 6–10. Although without semilunar folds and sacculations, it is distended and long, has a more abrupt tightening, followed by more numerous, longer tight spiral coils. This offers a considerable resistance to the digesta. Cellulolytic microbial activity centres more on dicotyledonous hemicelluloses. The

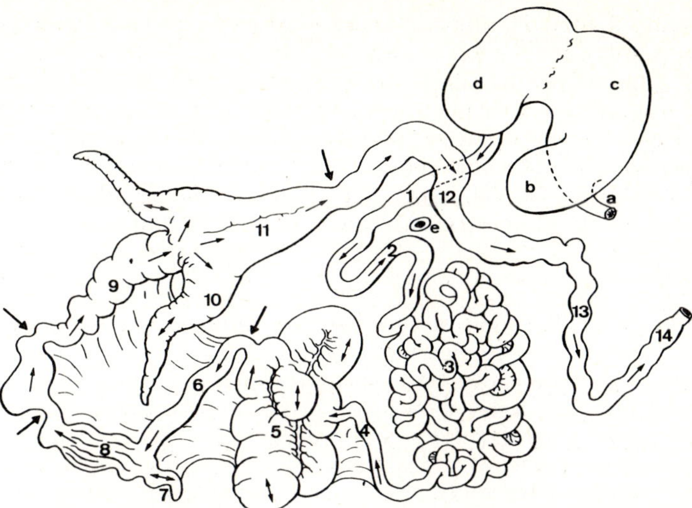

Fig. 2. *Stomach and intestine of Heterohyrax syriacus (from Hofmann and Lackhoff, in prep.).* a = oesophagus; b = blindsac (proventricular portion); c = fundus; d = pyloric portion of stomach; e = cut surface of cranial mesenteric artery. 1,2 = duodenum; 3 = jejunum; 4 = ileum, 5 = caecum (with blindsacs, haustra and taeniae); 6 − 11 = ascending colon (6 = thickwalled, tight portion, 7 = unpaired blindsac, 8 = thinwalled, wide proximal portion, 9 = thinwalled, wide distal portion, 10 = paired colonic blindsacs, 11 = stomachlike colonic dilatation); 12 = transverse colon; 13 = descending colon; 14 = rectum. Thin arrows indicate flow of ingesta, thick arrows: anatomical constrictions.

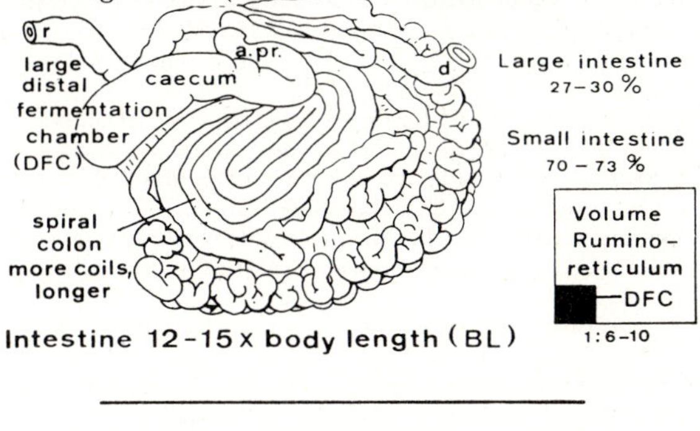

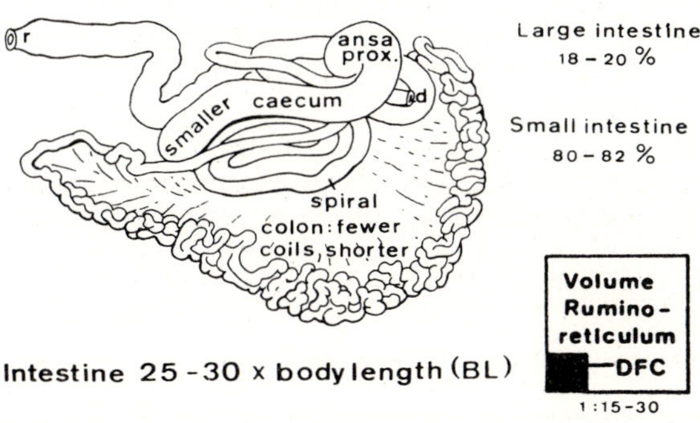

Fig. 3. *Anatomical differences of ruminant mid- and hindgut according to feeding type — concentrate selector, low fibre (cell content) on top and grass eater, high fibre (cell wall) above — schematic; from Hofmann (1985).* d = duodenum; r = rectum.

morphological-evolutionary relationship of this gradually regressing structure in ruminants to the spiral colonic cone of the Suidae is obvious. These adaptations to an increased microbial digestion in the hindgut may have survival importance during periods of poor or one-sided food availability. Attention has been drawn to the surface area available for absorption[21], to the greater efficiency of the large intestine in conserving Na, Cl, and HCO_3^- and their multiple inderdependencies with VFA produced by the intestinal microbes.

In a broad comparison, CS-ruminants show an anatomical adaptation to a fractionated microbial digestion which is functionally well comparable to that of the rabbit.

Conclusions. Microbial digestion of cellulose has induced a great number of anatomical adaptations which reveal homologies, analogies and convergences in different classes and orders. The adaptive variations of a basic structural plan reflect co-evolutionary processes in animals and plants, but they rarely show an all-or-nothing principle. Examples are ruminants and marsupials which show extremes and intermediate. Nutritional studies can benefit immensely from comparative work and will suffer from uncritical extrapolations, especially to man. Anatomical methods are more than ever a reliable means to establish the basis of nutritional adaptations.

 1 Amasaki, H. & Daigo, M. (1984): Morphogenesis of the ruminal microvasculature in bovine fetuses. *Can. J. Anim. Sci.* **64**, (Suppl.), 257–258.
 2 Engelhardt, W. von & Rechkemmer, G. (1983): The physiological effects of short-chain fatty acids in the hind gut. In *Fibre in human and animal nutrition*, ed G. Wallace & L. Bell, pp. 149–155. Wellington: Royal Society of New Zealand Bulletin 20.
 3 Gorgas, M. (1967): Vergleichend anatomische Untersuchungen am Magen-Darm-Kanal der Sciurumorpha, Hystricomorpha und Caviamorpha (Rodentia). *Z. Wiss. Zool.* **175**, 237–404.
 4 Henrikson, R. (1970): Developmental changes in the structure of perinatal ruminal epithelium. *Z. Zellforsch.* **109**, 15–19.
 5 Hofmann, R.R. (1969): Zur Topographie und Morphologie des Wiederkäuermagens im Hinblick auf seine Funktion. *Zbl. Vet. Med.* Beiheft 10, 1–180. Berlin und Hamburg: Paul Parey Verlag.
 6 Hofmann, R.R. (1973): *The ruminant stomach.* Stomach structure and feeding habits of East African game ruminants. *E.A. Monogr. Biol.* Vol. 2, 1–354. Nairobi: Kenya Literature Bureau.
 7 Hofmann, R.R. (1983): Adaptive changes of gastric and intestinal morphology in response to different fibre contents in ruminant diets. In *Fibre in human and animal nutrition*, ed G. Wallace & L. Bell, pp. 51–58. Wellington: Royal Society of New Zealand Bulletin 20.
 8 Hofmann, R.R. (1984): Comparative anatomical studies imply adaptive variations of ruminant digestive physiology. *Can. J. Anim. Sci.* **64**, (Suppl.), 203–205.
 9 Hofmann, R.R. (1985): Digestive physiology of the deer — their morpho-physiological specialisation and adaptation. In *Proc. Int. Conf. Biol. Deer Production*, ed K. Drew, P. Fennessy & P. Volz, pp. Wellington: Royal Society of New Zealand Bulletin 22.
10 Hofmann, R.R., Geiger, G. & König, R. (1976): Vergleichend-anatomische Untersuchungen an der Vormagen-schleimhaut von Rehwild (Capreolus capreolus) und Rotwild (Cervus elaphus). *Z. Säugetierkunde* **41**, 167–193.
11 Hofmann, R.R. & Schnorr, B. (1982): *Die funktionelle Morphologie des Wiederkäuer-Magens*, pp. 1–76. Stuttgart: Ferdinand Enke Verlag.
12 Hume, I.D. & Warner, A.C.I. (1980): Evolution of microbial digestion in mammals. In *Digestive physiology and metabolism in ruminants*, ed Y. Ruckebusch & P. Thivend, pp. 665–684. Lancaster: MTP-Press.
13 Hungate, R.E. (1975): The rumen microbial ecosystem. *Ann. Rev. Ecol. & Systematics* **6**, 39–64.
14 Kay, R.N.B., v. Engelhardt, W. & White, R.G. (1980): The digestive physiology of wild ruminants. In *Digestive physiology and metabolism in ruminants*, ed Y. Ruckebusch & P. Thivend, pp. 743–761. Lancaster: MTP-Press.
15 Langer, P. (1973): Vergleichend-anatomische Untersuchungen am Magen der Artiodactyla (Owen, 1848), II. Teil. *Gegenbaurs Morph. Jahrb., Leipzig* **119**, 633–695.
16 Langer, P. (1984): Comparative anatomy of the stomach in mammalian herbivores. *Quart. J. Exp. Physiol.* **69**, 615–625.
17 Sakata, T. & Tamate, H. (1978): Influence of butyrate on the microscopic structure of ruminal mucosa in adult sheep. *Jap. J. Zootechn. Sci.* **49**, 687–696.
18 Schnorr, B. & Vollmerhaus, B. (1967): Die Feinstruktur des Pansenepithels von Ziege und Rind. *Zbl. Vet. Med. A* **14**, 789–818.

19 Snipes, R.L. (1978): Anatomy of the rabbit colon. *Anat. Embryol.* **155**, 57–80.
20 Starck, D. (1982): *Vergleichende Anatomie der Wirbeltiere auf evolutionsbiologischer Grundlage.* Band 3. Berlin, Heidelberg, New York: Springer Verlag.
21 Stevens, C.E., Argenzio, R.A. & Clemens, E.T. (1980): Microbial digestion: rumen versus large intestine. In *Digestive physiology and metabolism in ruminants*, ed Y. Ruckebusch & P. Thivend, pp. 685–706. Lancaster: MTP Press.
22 Ulyatt, M.J., Dellow, D.W., Reid, C.S.W. & Bauchop, T. (1975): Structure and function of the large intestine of ruminants. In *Digestion and metabolism in the ruminant*, ed I.W. Mc Donald & A.C.I. Warner, pp. 119–133. Armidale: New England Publishing Unit.
23 Wyburn, R.S. (1980): The mixing and propulsion of the stomach contents of ruminants. In *Digestive physiology and metabolism in ruminants*, ed Y. Ruckebusch & P. Thivend, pp. 35–51. Lancaster: MTP Press.

Symbiosis between gut microbes and animals

R.E. HUNGATE
Department of Bacteriology, University of California, Davis, California 95616, USA.

In the guts of carnivorous vertebrates the action of the host's digestive enzymes releases abundant soluble food, and with the favourable moisture, temperature and neutral acidity, dense microbial populations would develop, except that the animal secretes enough hydrochloric acid to kill the bacteria before host enzymes act. But herbivorous animals have a different problem. They cannot digest the complex carbohydrates in the cell walls of higher plants.

Soluble carbohydrate became an important food because of its superiority for accomplishing the chemical work of cell synthesis under anaerobic conditions[5], with simultaneous rearrangement of its atoms plus N and others to form the components of primordial aquatic protoplasts. But, in addition, the polymerized carbohydrate, cellulose, appeared in freshwater plants as a strengthener of cell envelopes against plasmoptysis. When photosynthetic reduction of CO_2 with water evolved, cellulose became as cheap as air, light and water, and was extensively incorporated into cell walls of land plants.

Numerous gut microbe-animal symbioses evolved as a mechanism to exploit the microbial muralytic (plant cell wall digesting) enzymes. A portion of the gut is much enlarged, slowing the passage of digesta to a rate less than the growth rate of the muralytic population. The enlarged portion of the gut serves as a continuous fermentation chamber to which the vertebrate supplies consumed macerated plant bodies, inorganic foods, moisture and favourable temperature, and from which the animal removes the undigested residues.

In ruminants, herbivorous marsupials, the hippopotamus, some primates and some rodents, the digesta are subjected to microbial fermentation before entering the acid region of the gut where the microbes are killed. In subsequent regions the latter are digested, the products absorbed, and used to supply an important part of the protein, vitamin and lipid, and a minor part of the carbohydrate requirement of the host. These animals we class as fore-gut fermenters.

Not only carbohydrates, but also proteins and amino acids, in their feed are fermented in the fore-gut, releasing ammonia, the chief nitrogenous food for other microbial symbionts[2]. Since protein cannot anaerobically accomplish nearly as much metabolic work as can carbohydrate, it is uneconomic to feed protein as a source of protein to fore-gut fermenters unless it bypasses the fermentation process and enters the acid gut directly. Fermentable polysaccharides plus inorganic and trace organic nutrients are the feed of choice for fore-gut fermenters, preferably plant cell wall polysaccharides.

In most rodents, the horse and its relatives, elephants, termites and the dugong and manatee, the digesta enter the microbial fermentation chamber only after passage through the acidified portion of the gut and after the animal has removed from the digesta the foods solubilized by its own enzymes. These animals we class as hind-gut fermenters. The microbes formed in the hind-gut fermentation are voided through the anus, and would be lost to the host animal except that many hind-gut fermenters practice coprophagy: selected faeces rich in microbial bodies are eaten whereas other faecal pellets containing primarily indigestible plant residues are not refected.

In even relatively small metazoa, such as insects, the rate of utilization of dioxygen by the animal and its gut population exceeds the rate of diffusion of atmospheric oxygen into the lumen of the gut, and gut habitats are anaerobic, or more specifically, adioxic, since air contains several gases besides O_2. The concentration of dioxygen in the gut is normally so minute that gut microbes must be able to grow in its complete absence. Not only are most of them unable to use O_2, but they are killed by even trace concentrations.

Obligatory anaerobic gut microbes greatly outnumber those able to use O_2. Microbes adapted to a wider range of growth conditions and substrates must contain more metabolic machinery, and consequently require a greater amount of metabolic work in growing new cells, a handicap in competition with less burdened species. In spite of their relatively small numbers, microbes able to use O_2 or grow without it play an essential role in the gut. They reduce the dioxygen concentration to the low level required by even the most adioxic microbes, unable alone to create their required anaerobiosis. This emphasizes that the animal symbiosis is really with the entire gut population. Although for its complete understanding we need to define and quantify the detailed relationships of each gut species to the host and to other microbes, and from the standpoint of autecology this is a fascinating task, it is no prerequisite for many nutritional studies in which the gut contents can be considered as a whole.

The fermentation hypothesis to explain gut microbe-animal symbioses envisions that the plant cell walls are digested by muralytic microbes which ferment the solubilized carbohydrates to wastes such as CO_2, CH_4, and acetic, propionic and butyric acids, with some energy degradation, but via metabolic reactions with surprising efficiency in synthesizing new cells. The waste acids, relatively poor reactants for accomplishing work under anaerobic conditions, are absorbed by the animal and oxidized to CO_2 and H_2O.

Many microbial species can assimilate inorganic nitrogen and other elements into protein when carbohydrate is available. In order to exploit this a thorough knowledge of the nutrients required by symbiotic muralytic species is needed. Studies over many years[2] have disclosed a most intriguing cycling of the amino acids, for example valine and isoleucine. Certain gut bacteria deaminate and decarboxylate them to form isobutyric and 2-methylbutyric acids, respectively, as waste products, accomplishing cell synthesis in the process. The wastes are required nutrients for other gut microbes which reverse the decarboxylation and deamination, using high energy molecules derived through carbohydrate fermentation, and assimilate the reformed valine and isoleucine.

Much more information is needed on factors increasing *de-novo* synthesis of microbial protein from plant cell wall material and inorganic nutrients. Also, factors increasing the microbial digestibility of the great quantities of plant cell walls annually produced on earth need to be explored, and are currently receiving much attention, but the problems are formidable, particularly the digestion of lignin under anaerobic conditions. Also aerobic processes for the conversion of plant cell walls into protein need study, since the yield of protein per unit of carbohydrate metabolized aerobically is significantly greater than for anaerobic conversions.

The nitrogen nutrition of the fore-gut fermenter is like that of a plankton-feeder, except that the continuous food supply and waste services support production in a confined space of sufficient microbial cells to supply the major part of the animal's protein needs, and this in substrates not suitable for direct use as animal food.

Animals without symbionts, if supplied with carbohydrates their enzymes can metabolize, can conserve more food in the form of animal growth than can be conserved in the symbiotic animal. To illustrate this, the free energy of the complete anaerobic conversion of carbohydrate to the anaerobically stable end products, CO_2 and CH_4, is 393 kJ, as compared with 2650 kJ when carbohydrate is dehydrogenated to CO_2 and the hydrogen combined with O_2 to form water. The difference between these values, 2257 kJ, available to the symbiotic host animal through oxidation of the acetic, propionic and butyric acids, is sufficient to assimilate significantly more protein than the symbiotic microbes can produce with the 393 kJ available to them anaerobically. For the host, energy is in excess but protein is limiting. This handicap in the forestomach fermentation is offset by its utilization of cellulose, hemicellulose and pectin, foods unusable by humans without microbial aid.

The hind-gut fermentation is similarly limited in the microbial protein it can produce but the host animal's ability to digest the feed proteins and absorb the amino acids before the plant cell walls are fermented, can provide additional protein, assimilable with the energy available through oxidation of the fermentation acids. A greater efficiency of the mammalian hind-gut symbiosis and of carnivores as compared to fore-gut symbiosis is indicated by the fact that the two former groups contain representatives smaller than the smallest fore-gut symbiote. Since the energy requirement of mammals is approximately proportional to the body weight to the 3/4 power, the energy needed per unit body weight is greatest for the smallest animals. An African suni, perhaps the smallest fore-gut fermenter weighed 3700 g as compared to the carnivorous shrew and hind-gut fermenting mice with weights as small as 10 g. The latter bodies are too small to accommodate a fermenter large enough to supply their nutritional needs through microbial symbiosis alone.

The lower termites are one of the most interesting examples of a hind-gut microbial symbiosis, evolved in parallel with a highly differentiated and complex social organization containing many individuals in colonies composed of morphologically distinct castes, each differentiated for performance of certain functions and linked into an organized unit by nutrients (hormones) licked from other individuals during oral grooming and feeding. The king and queen each produce a hormone inhibiting maleness and femaleness, respectively, and the first egg develops into a soldier which then produces a hormone inhibiting differentiation into soldier. It is less effective than the sexual hormones and after several dozen young termites molt through several instars another individual differentiates into a soldier, keeping the ratio of soldiers to workers constant as the colony grows. Ultimately, the sex hormones are insufficient to inhibit the many young, and the eggs develop into winged royalty, potential founders of new colonies.

The workers, inhibited from differentiating into royalty and soldiers, remain morphologically less specialized though with strong mandibles capable of comminuting plant cell walls into extremely small particles which are ingested, soluble carbohydrates and starches are digested and absorbed in the fore-gut, proteins in the mid-gut, and cellulose, hemicellulose and some lignin are fermented by protozoa in the hind-gut. The workers are solicited by members of the colony to give off almost liquid faecal pellets containing microbial symbionts which are consumed by the solicitor. Analyses of the fore-, mid-, and hind-gut contents of workers in natural colonies as compared to workers isolated on wood in individual vials show[3] that pellets constitute about three-fourths of the material ingested by the workers in the natural colony, an indication of the extent of proctodeal feeding. This refection increases the period of exposure of digesta to muralytic enzymes.

The nitrogen nutrition of termites is extremely economical. The western dampwood termite can grow on wood containing as little as 0.03 per cent w/w nitrogen, yet assimilate as much as half of it into termites while digesting as much as 60 per cent of the weight of the wood. In a primitive termite, fungal activity in the wood can concentrate the nitrogen by assimilating it while oxidizing much of the carbohydrate-lignin complex and growing toward the termite burrows in response to the metabolic water from termite respiration[4]. Uric acid is the chief nitrogenous waste of the termite, secreted by the Malpighian tubules into the hind-gut at its junction with the mid-gut, and shown[1] to be fermented chiefly to acetic acid, NH_3 and CO_2 by certain bacteria, with the ammonia then assimilated by many elements in the population. Nitrogen in the colony is also conserved by consumption of chitinous exoskeletons shed when an instar molts, and by cannibalism of moribund individuals. Also, in some termites significant quantities of atmospheric nitrogen appear to be fixed[1].

The termite symbiosis is particularly interesting because there appears to be a greater fraction of the lignin digested than occurs in most other symbiotic systems. Termites thus appear to have exploited to an advanced degree the potentials for using symbiotic microbes for the utilization of plant cell walls.

We have omitted thus far any specifics regarding the kinds of microbes concerned in symbiotic gut fermentations, and there is insufficient time to allow their proper description. The major groups are bacteria (broad sense) and protozoa but a few species of primitive phycomycetous fungi are sufficiently numerous in the rumen to be nutritionally important, and are of particular interest because they may be more effective than rumen protozoa and bacteria in digesting lignified plant tissues.

Ciliate protozoa are a prominent component of the gut microbiota of ruminants and marsupials and occur also in the sea urchins, whereas flagellate protozoa predominate in the primitive termites in which protozoa occur. Some of the gut ciliates and flagellates have a structure more complex than that of any other representatives of their respective protozoal classes.

A role in cellulose digestion and fermentation has been established definitely for certain of the termite flagellates and rumen ciliates but is by no means restricted to them. Many muralytic bacteria have been identified in the rumen and other gut habitats, including humans. There has been much speculation on the possibility that the protozoal cellulases are elaborated by intracellular bacteria. Yamin[8] could find no evidence for this, and instances have been cited[6] in which higher termites contain muralytic enzymes but very few microbial symbionts, interpreted as indicating possible enzyme formation by the termite itself. This may be explained by a report that *Macrotermes*, a fungus-cultivating African termite, ingests enough of the fungus to obtain enzyme sufficient to digest the plant polymers consumed, and digests them in the mid-gut. The symbiont in this case does not reside in the gut, and the same is true of the symbiotic cellulose digestion recently discovered[7]. It was found that, in the teredo, a wood-boring mollusc, the cellulase is produced on the gills in the gland of Deshaye by an aerobic symbiotic bacterium able to grow on cellulose plus inorganic salts, and to fix N_2 if conditions are microaerophilic. Ducts connect the gland to the oesophagus.

These examples indicate that animals may form non-gut symbiotic associations with microbes, growing them aerobically elsewhere than in the gut, and harvesting their enzymes produced. They encourage further search for intracellular muralytic symbionts in animals digesting plant cell walls but for which no muralytic symbiont has been found, eg the garden snail.

1 Breznak, J.A. (1982): Intestinal microbiota of termites and other xylophagous insects. *Ann. Rev. Microbiol.* **36**, 323–343.

2 Bryant, M.P. (1973): Nutritional requirements of the predominant rumen cellulolytic bacteria. *Fed. Proc.* **32**, 1809–1813.

3 Hungate, R.E. (1983): Studies on the nutrition of *Zootermopsis*. II. The relative importance of the termite and the protozoa in wood digestion. *Ecology* **19**, 1–25.

4 Hungate, R.E. (1944): Termite growth and nitrogen utilization in laboratory cultures. *Proc. Texas Acad. Sci.* **27**, 91–98.

5 Hungate, R.E. (1955): Why carbohydrates? Appendix II In *Biochemistry and physiology of the protozoa*, ed S.H. Hutner & A. Lwoff, pp. 195–197. New York: Academic Press.

6 O'Brien, R.W. & Slaytor, M. (1982): Role of microorganisms in the metabolism of termites. *Aust. J. Biol. Sci.* **35**, 239–262.

7 Waterbury, J.B., Calloway, C.B. & Turner, R.D. (1983): A cellulolytic nitrogen-fixing bacterium cultured from the gland of Deshayes in shipworms (Bivalvia: Teredinidae). *Science* **221**, 1401–1403.

8 Yamin, M.A. (1981): Cellulose metabolism by the flagellate *Trichoympha* from a termite is independent of endosymbiotic bacteria. *Science* **211**, 58–59.

Rumen microbial metabolism and its manipulation

R.J. WALLACE
Rowett Research Institute, Bucksburn, Aberdeen AB2 9SB, UK.

The rumen can be considered to be a microbiological fermenter, controlled to some extent in flow rate and pH by the host animal, but in which all of the metabolic reactions are carried out by vast numbers of bacteria, ciliate protozoa and phycomycetous fungi. The rumen fermentation can potentially be altered deliberately to benefit ruminant nutrition, by giving faster or more efficient breakdown of feedstuffs or by producing a different, nutritionally more effective mixture of fermentation products.

Rumen microbial metabolism. *Microbial carbohydrate metabolism.* A group of converging reactions converts many different polysaccharides and sugars in the ingested food to a smaller number of monosaccharides which then enter the common metabolic route of glycolysis, the Embden-Meyerhof-Parnas pathway. In this pathway, much of the ATP required for microbial growth is formed. From pyruvic acid, the pathways diverge once more to form the fermentation end-products. The NAD^+ converted to NADH as a result of glycolysis is regenerated during the divergent pathways, and additional ATP is produced[39]. The most abundant products of metabolism are the volatile fatty acids (VFA), — mainly acetic, propionic and butyric acids, which are absorbed through the rumen wall and provide both carbon skeletons and energy for the host's biosynthetic reactions — and methane.

The relative simplicity of these fermentation products conceals a much more detailed and complex group of reactions that occurs within and between species. Many rumen bacteria produce one or more of the VFA, as seen in the mixed population, but products not seen in the rumen, such as H_2, formate, ethanol, lactate and succinate are equally prevalent (Table 1).

Table. *Sensitivity of different species of rumen bacteria to chemical manipulating agents[a].*

Organism	Fermentation products[b]	Cell wall type	Monensin /lasalocid[c]	Avoparcin[d]	Synperonic NP9[e]	Trichloroethanol[e]	DIC[e]
Streptococcus bovis	L	+	S	S	R	R	R
Butyrivibrio fibrisolvens	F,B,L,H$_2$	+	S	S	S	R	R
Ruminococcus albus	F,A,E,H$_2$	+	S	S	S	R	R
Lachnospira multiparus	F,A,L,E	+	ND	S	S	R	R
Bacteroides succinogenes	F,A,S	−	(R)	S	S	R	R
Bacteroides ruminicola	F,A,S	−	R	R	R	R	S
Selenomonas ruminantium	A,P,L	−	R	R	R	R	R
Methanobrevibacterium ruminantium	CH$_4$	−	R	R	R	S	R

[a]S-sensitive; R-resistant; ND-not determined; DIC-diphenyliodonium chloride;
[b]F-formate; A-acetate; P-propionate; B-butyrate; L-lactate; E-ethanol; S-succinate;
[c]From Chen & Wolin (1979), Henderson *et al.*, (1981);
[d]From Stewart *et al.*, (1983);
[e]Author, unpublished results.

H_2 and formate do not accumulate *in vivo* because they are utlised by methanogenic bacteria as soon as they are formed. Ethanol, which is produced in pure cultures by bacteria such as *Ruminococcus albus* as an alternative electron sink product only when H_2 accumulates, is then no longer formed[14]. Succinate and lactate are utilised rapidly in the rumen by a secondary population of succinate and lactate fermenters. In any case, lactate production *in vivo* is much less than its predominance in some pure cultures might suggest, due to the influence of bacterial growth rate on its production. Even *Streptococcus bovis*, usually regarded as a homolactic fermenter, produces different products when its growth rate is restricted to the range found for rumen bacteria *in vivo*[24].

Microbial N metabolism. Urea which enters the rumen in saliva and by diffusion through the rumen wall is rapidly broken down to ammonia, which can then be incorporated into microbial amino acids and protein. This can be of great importance to the N economy of animals grazing on poor quality tropical grasses where the protein content of the food is low[19]. On the other hand, the hydrolysis of feed proteins entering the rumen introduces an inefficiency to ruminant N metabolism under higher planes of nutrition. The peptides and amino acids released are for the most part not incorporated directly into bacteria, but are firstly broken down forming ammonia. Thus the biological value of the original amino acids is considerably reduced by microbial metabolism[34].

Manipulation. *Objectives.* The aim of manipulation is to improve the efficiency of ruminant animal production, by inducing the animal to gain weight more quickly, or by developing a higher weight gain/food consumption ratio, or sometimes by introducing new, cheaper or improved foodstuffs. Increased weight gain and feed efficiency can be achieved by anabolic hormone implants, but these do not affect rumen microbial metabolism directly and will not be considered here. The other main method of improving the nutrition of ruminants is to manipulate the rumen fermentation.

Several inefficiencies and potential areas for improvement have been identified. (a) Plant cell walls are incompletely degraded in the rumen. (b) Protein degradation generally exceeds microbial N requirements and leads to NH_3 overflow, as does ureolysis. Decreases in proteolysis, amino acid catabolism or ureolysis would therefore be expected to be beneficial. (c) Propionate is the only VFA which is glucogenic when metabolised by the host, so a change in VFA stoichiometry to improve the relative production of propionate should lead to improved feed efficiency. (d) Methane production involves the waste of potentially useful chemical energy. (e) An increased growth yield of microorganisms would give an increased protein flow to the abomasum. (f) Nutritional disorders with a rumen microbiological aetiology, such as lactic acidosis and bloat, can cause major problems. (g) Microbial enzymes may enable cheap materials, indigestible by monogastrics, to be used in ruminant feeding.

These objectives may be achieved in different ways, and it will become clear that the improvement of one particular objective often results in improvements in others too, because of interrelationships within the microbial community.

Physical and chemical treatment of feeds; development of alternative feedstuffs. A full discussion of these aspects will not be given here, but more details can be found in recent reviews. The main physical treatments of feeds are in creating different particle sizes of forages[35] and protection of protein supplements by heat treatment and packaging[16]. Chemical treatments include alkali treatment of straw[15] and modification of proteins and amino acids[16]. New feedstuffs include both new, better (for ruminants) varieties of plants[12] and urea and other synthetic products.

The microbial physiologist's approach. The conditions prevailing in any industrial or laboratory fermenter are controlled very strictly so that microorganisms are in optimal physiological condition for the desired process. The rumen fermenter is no different in principle, but success in manipulating the fermentation on microbial physiological principles has been limited. Factors regulated by the operator in fermenter technology include substrate concentration, agitation rate, pH, E_h, temperature, gas composition, surface area and dilution rate (D). At least some of these offer scope for manipulation of the rumen fermentation.

When energy yielding nutrient is in transient excess in pure bacterial cultures 'energy spillage' occurs, which results in a depressed microbial growth yield[21]. One might expect this to occur in the rumen immediately after feeding and predict that if the transient nutrient excess could be decreased by more frequent feeding the microbial growth yield should be higher. Growth efficiency does indeed appear to increase with increased feeding frequency[7], although it has not been established if this is due to an improved microbial yield. The effect is more pronounced with concentrates[7], suggesting that it may indeed be. A decreased residence time and degradability may offset this benefit with forages[33].

pH has an important influence on the rumen fermentation, because cellulolytic rumen bacteria do not grow at pH's less than 6[30]. Thus, when roughages and concentrates are fed together and the pH falls as a result of the rapid fermentation of the concentrate, fibre digestion is depressed. This associative effect can be largely overcome if the pH is maintained above 6 by addition of bicarbonate[20].

Increasing D increases the growth yield of bacteria by reducing the proportion of energy devoted to maintenance[22], and again a similar effect is seen *in vivo*[9]. As before, this beneficial effect on yield may be lost, however, if the faster turnover of solids results in a decreased degradability (eg[18]).

The nutritional benefit of altering D therefore depends on the type of diet used. A possible manipulation strategy might be to select genetically animals with small rumens (and high D) for some intended applications, and animals with large rumens (and slow D) for others that would benefit from longer retention times.

Chemical manipulation. The commercial potential of compounds which when added to ruminant feeds given improved feed efficiency or increased intake has not unexpectedly attracted a great deal of research interest. Many chemicals have proved to have interesting properties, including the inhibition of deamination, methanogenesis and lactate production by some diaryliodonium compounds, halogenated hydrocarbons and thiopeptin antibiotics respectively, and the suppression of protozoa by surface-active agents and other chemicals[2]. However, the compounds that have been found to be most effective and to be of greatest practical usefulness are the propionate-enhancing antibiotics and ionophores, notably monensin (Rumensin, Lilly), lasalocid (Bovatec, Hoffmann LaRoche) and avoparcin (Avoton, Cyanamid).

Monensin, lasalocid and avoparcin produce an economically valuable improvement in feed efficiency[2,8,27] and, although there is some adaptation of the rumen flora to their application[4,31], their effect on fermentation stoichiometry persists for several weeks or months, sufficient for their use in growing and finishing cattle.

Patterns in manipulation. Experiments in manipulation, particularly chemical manipulation, have revealed a number of interesting patterns. Methanogenesis and propionate production are closely related thermodynamically and mechanistically and although inhibitors of methanogenesis and propionate enhancers may have very different modes of action, they have quite similar net effects. It has been shown precisely how the switch of electron flow from methanogenesis must lead to increased propionate production[5,13], and it has been demonstrated[10] that methane rather than propionate was the usual fate of metabolic H_2 because the methanogens' hydrogenase has a lower $K_m(H_2)$ than that of propionate and succinate producing bacteria.

Other, less readily explained, patterns occur, however. Monensin is usually regarded as a propionate inhancer, and its influence on feed efficiency is usually highly significant, yet its effect on propionate production *in vivo* often does not reach statistical significance. Monensin has also been reported to inhibit proteolysis, ureolysis, amino acid catabolism, lactate production and to have many other effects, as well as its indirect effect on methane production, and it must be concluded that these play an important part in its overall efficacy[27]. This is a pattern seen to a lesser extent with lasalocid, avoparcin and other compounds. Antimethanogenic halogenated hydrocarbons appear to inhibit proteolysis as well as increasing propionate production[28]. The absence of protozoa, caused by defaunating chemicals or by isolation of animals, leads to improved microbial yields and to increased propionate and decreased methane production[17,38]. Diaryliodonium compounds inhibit amino acid catabolism principally, but can also lead to decreased methanogenesis and increased propionate production[1]. Some other cross-reactions occur[2], and these tend to be a normal consequence of manipulating compounds rather than exceptions.

The microbial ecology of chemical manipulation. The basis of all of these effects on rumen metabolic activity is, of course, the effect of the compounds on the microorganisms. The mode of action of monensin has received most attention.

Effects of monensin on protozoa have sometimes been noted[23,36], but these do not always occur[6], and the main effect is on rumen bacteria. Monensin selectively inhibits the growth of Gram positive organisms, including the acetate and H_2-producing ruminococci, and lactate-producing *Streptococcus bovis* (Table). Thus acetate, methane (from H_2 and formate) and lactate production would be expected to be suppressed, with increased propionate production a secondary consequence. The methanogenic bacteria are not significantly affected. The decrease in deamination due to monensin is presumably due to decreased numbers of Gram-positive *Eubacterium* and *Streptococcus* species[26], and some inhibition of proteolysis would be expected by the suppression of *S. bovis*[25,37]. Lasalocid and avoparcin, which share many of the effects of monensin, have similar, but not identical, patterns of toxicity to different bacterial species (Table). A defaunating agent, nonyl phenol ethoxylate (Synperonic NP9; ICI) had a quite similar spectrum of antibacterial effects (Table), whereas the methane inhibitor trichloroethanol specifically inhibited the growth of the methanogen and diphenyliodonium chloride (DIC) appeared to be most toxic to *Bacteroides ruminicola* (Table).

The microbiological effects of other chemicals are generally not known, but in view of their overlapping spectrum of effects *in vivo*, there would be expected to be some overlap in their effects on the rumen microbial population, despite their having quite different primary targets. The degree of overlap can be discerned from the results obtained by mixing different chemicals. For example, combination of monensin with amicloral (an inhibitor of methanogenesis) or 4,4'-dimethyldiphenyliodonium chloride (amino acid catabolism) produces additive effects[2], because they have different primary sites of action. An appreciation of the mode of action of chemicals and their consequences for the rumen microbial population is therefore vital in forming a strategy for chemical manipulation.

Potential future areas of manipulation. It is a salutary lesson for rumen microbiologists that the efficacy of monensin was discovered in a fairly empirical way by incorporating into ruminant diets a compound already well established as a coccidiostat in poultry. How might future developments occur?

A new generation of ionophores will have properties superior to those of the presently used compounds, and better methods of administering them and ways of extending their application (to dairy cows or grazing animals, for example) may be found. Successes may also occur in areas discussed earlier, such as control of proteolysis or ureolysis. However, the greatest promise arguably lies in the new technology that has grown from advances in molecular genetics over the last decade.

This work has already begun in many laboratories around the world. An excellent provocative article has discussed[29] the prospects for applying genetic engineering to the rumen fermentation and how it could benefit the recognised problem areas such as controlled degradation of feedstuffs, propionate/methane stoichiometry, the control of undesirable bacteria and so on. It also pointed out that the main significance of recombinant DNA technology may not, in fact, be in the presently recognised areas of manipulation at all, and concluded that 'The potential for genetic engineering to improve ruminal digestion and efficiency is great and bounded only by the limits of one's imagination'.

Few would quarrel with such a projection, although one shares the concern expressed by these authors that, as has occurred in other areas of biotechnology, our fundamental understanding of microbial metabolism and ecology might impose a greater limit to potential improvements than does the technology now available.

1 Chalupa, W. (1977): Manipulating rumen fermentation. *J. Anim. Sci.* **45**, 585–599.

2 Chalupa, W. (1980): Chemical control of rumen microbial metabolism. In *Digestive physiology and metabolism in ruminants*, ed Y. Ruckebusch & P. Thivend, pp. 325–347. Lancaster: MTP Press.

3 Chen, M. & Wolin, M.J. (1979): Effect of monensin and lasalocid-sodium on the growth of methanogenic and rumen saccharolytic bacteria. *Appl. Environ. Microbiol.* **38**, 72–77.

4 Dawson, K.A. & Boling, J.A. (1983): Monensin-resistant bacteria in the rumens of calves on monensin-containing and unmedicated diets. *Appl. Environ. Microbiol.* **46**, 160–164.

5 Demeyer, D.I. & Van Nevel, C.J. (1975): Methanogenesis, an integrated part of carbohydrate fermentation, and its

control. In *Digestion and metabolism in the ruminant*, ed I.W. McDonald & A.C.I. Warner, pp. 366–382, Armidale, Australia: University of New England Publishing Unit.

6 Dinius, D.A., Simpson, M.S. & Marsh, P.B. (1976): Effect of monensin fed with forage on digestion and the ruminal ecosystem of steers. *J. Anim. Sci.* **42**, 229–234.

7 Gibson, J.P. (1981): The effects of feeding frequency on the growth and efficiency of food utilisation of ruminants: an analysis of published results. *Anim. Prod.* **32**, 275–283.

8 Goodrich, R.D., Garrett, J.E., Gast, D.R., Kirick, M.A., Larson, D.A. & Meiske, J.C. (1984): Influence of monensin on the performance of cattle. *J. Anim. Sci.* **58**, 1484–1498.

9 Harrison, D.G. & McAllan, A.B. (1980): Factors affecting microbial growth yields in the reticulo-rumen. In *Digestive physiology and metabolism in ruminants*, ed Y. Ruckebusch & P. Thivend, pp. 205–226. Lancaster: MTP Press.

10 Henderson, C. (1980): The influence of extracellular hydrogen on the metabolism of *Bacteroides ruminicola*, *Anaerovibrio lipolytica* and *Selenomonas ruminantium*. *J. Gen. Microbiol.* **119**, 485–491.

11 Henderson, C., Stewart, C.S. & Nekrep, F.V. (1981): The effect of monensin on pure and mixed cultures of rumen bacteria. *J. Appl. Bacteriol.* **51**, 159–169.

12 Howarth, R.E., Cheng, K.-J., Majak, W. & Costerton, J.W. (1985): Ruminant bloat. In *Control of digestion and metabolism in ruminants* (In press).

13 Hungate, R.E. (1966): *The rumen and its microbes*. Academic Press: London.

14 Iannotti, E.L., Kafkewitz, D., Wolin, M.J. & Bryant, M.P. (1973): Glucose fermentation of *Ruminococcus albus* grown in continuous culture with *Vibrio succinogenes*: changes caused by interspecies transfer of H_2. *J. Bacteriol.* **114**, 1231–1240.

15 Jackson, M.G. (1977): Review article: the alkali treatment of straws. *Anim. Fd Sci. Technol.* **2**, 105–130.

16 Kaufmann, W. & Lupping, W. (1982): Protected proteins and protected amino acids for ruminants. In *Protein contribution of feedstuffs for ruminants*, ed E.L. Miller, I.H. Pike & A.J.H. Van Es, pp. 36–75. London: Butterworths.

17 Kayouli, C., Demeyer, D.I. Van Nevel, C.J. & Dendooven, R. (1984): Effect of defaunation on straw digestion *in sacco* and on particle retention in the rumen. *Anim. Fd Sci. Technol.* **10**, 165–172.

18 Kennedy, P.M. & Milligan, L.P. (1978): Effects of cold exposure on digestion, microbial synthesis and nitrogen transformations in sheep. *Br. J. Nutr.* **39**, 105–117.

19 Kennedy, P.M. & Milligan, L.P. (1980): The degradation and utilization of endogenous urea in the gastrointestinal tract of ruminants: a review. *Can. J. Anim. Sci.* **60**, 205–221.

20 Mould, F.L. & Ørskov, E.R. (1983): Manipulation of rumen fluid pH and its influence on cellulolysis in sacco, dry matter degradation and the rumen microflora of sheep offered either hay or concentrate. *Anim. Feed Sci. Technol.* **10**, 1–14.

21 Neijssel, O.M. & Tempest, D.W. (1976): The role of energy-spilling reactions in the growth of *Klebsiella aerogenes* in aerobic chemostat culture. *Archs Microbiol.* **110**, 305–311.

22 Pirt, S.J. (1965): The maintenance energy of bacteria in growing cultures. *Proc. R. Soc. B* **163**, 224–231.

23 Richardson, L.F., Potter, E.L. & Cooley, C.O. (1978): Effect of monensin on ruminal protozoa and volatile fatty acids. *J. Anim. Sci.* **47**, (Suppl. 1), 45.

24 Russell, J.B. & Baldwin, R.L. (1979): Comparison of maintenance energy expenditures and growth yields among several rumen bacteria grown on continuous culture. *Appl. Environ. Microbiol.* **37**, 537–543.

25 Russell, J.B. , Bottje, W.G. & Cotta, M.A. (1981): Degradation of protein by mixed cultures of rumen bacteria: identification of *Streptococcus bovis* as an actively proteolytic rumen bacterium. *J. Anim. Sci.* **53**, 242–252.

26 Scheifinger, C., Russell, N. & Chalupa, W. (1976): Degradation of amino acids by pure cultures of rumen bacteria. *J. Anim. Sci.* **43**, 821–827.

27 Schelling, G.T. (1984): Monensin mode of action in the rumen. *J. Anim. Sci.* **58**, 1518–1527.

28 Singh, Y.K. & Trei, J.E. (1971): Ruminal NH_3 concentrations as influenced by methane inhibitors. *Fed. Proc.* **30**, 404.

29 Smith, C.J. & Hespell, R.B. (1983): Prospects for development and use of recombinant deoxyribonucleic acid techniques with ruminal bacteria. *J. Dairy Sci.* **66**, 1536–1546.

30 Stewart, C.S. (1977): Factors affecting the cellulolytic activity of rumen contents. *Appl. Environ. Microbiol.* **33**, 497–502.

31 Stewart, C.S. & Duncan, S.H. (1985): The effect of avoparcin on cellulolytic bacteria of the ovine rumen. *J. Gen. Microbiol.* **131**, 427–435.

32 Stewart, C.S., Crossley, M.V. & Garrow, S.H. (1983): The effect of avoparcin on laboratory cultures of rumen bacteria. *Eur. J. Appl. Microbiol. Biotechnol.* **17**, 292–297.

33 Sutton, J.D. (1980): Digestion and end-product formation in the rumen from production rations. In *Digestive physiology and metabolism in ruminants*, ed Y. Ruckebusch & P. Thivend, pp. 271–290. Lancaster: MTP Press.

34 Tamminga, S. (1979): Protein degradation in the forestomachs of ruminants. *J. Anim. Sci.* **49**, 1615–1630.

35 Thomson, D.J. & Beever, D.E. (1980): The effect of conservation and processing on the digestion of forages by ruminants. In *Digestive physiology and metabolism in ruminants*, ed Y. Ruckebusch & P. Thivend, pp. 291–308. Lancaster: MTP Press.

36 Wallace, R.J., Czerkawski, J.W. & Breckenridge, G. (1981): Effect of monensin on the fermentation of basal rations in the Rumen Simulation Technique (Rusitec). *Br. J. Nutr.* **46**, 131–148.

37 Wallace, R.J. & Brammall, M.L. (1985): The role of different species of bacteria in the hydrolysis of protein in the rumen. *J. Gen. Microbiol.* **131**, 821–832.

38 Whitelaw, F.G., Eadie, J.M., Bruce, L.A. & Shand, W.J. (1984): Methane formation in faunated and ciliate-free cattle and its relationship with rumen volatile fatty acid proportions. *Br. J. Nutr.* **52**, 261–275.
39 Wolin, M.J. (1981): Fermentation in the rumen and human large intestine. *Science* **213**, 1463–1468.

Elemental diets in gut physiology

R.I. RUSSELL
Gastroenterology Unit, Royal Infirmary, Glasgow G4 0SF, UK.

'Elemental diets' or predigested-chemically-defined-diets contain basic nutritional components — purified L-amino acids alone or with oligopeptides, simple carbohydrates, essential lipids, vitamins, minerals and trace elements. These nutrients are rapidly and almost completely absorbed in the upper gastrointestinal tract without the requirements of full digestive processes[21]. The principal elemental diets at present available in the UK are Vivonex and Vivonex HN (Eaton), Flexical (Mead-Johnson), Nutranel (Roussel), and Elemental 028 (Scientific Hospital Supplies).

The intrinsic properties of elemental diets are adequate nutritional efficacy, minimal digestion requirements, almost complete absorption in the upper gastrointestinal tract, minimal residue and hypoallergenicity.

The original formulas were shown to maintain normal nutritional indices in normal subjects[25] and recent studies have confirmed this[14,26]. Nutrients from elemental diets appear to be efficiently absorbed in the upper gastrointestinal tract without the requirements of full digestive process. Early studies demonstrated that this was so in normal subjects, and the absorption of nutrients from Vivonex has been shown to be comparable with that from a crushed food homogenate in normal healthy subjects, using a small intestinal perfusion system[11]. The minimal residue nature of elemental diets has recently been confirmed in a well-controlled study in rats[15] and is of potential value in the provision of bowel rest, as for fistula healing, when nutritional improvement and minimal residue are important. Elemental diets, particularly Vivonex, have been shown to be hypoallergenic[7-9]. This suggests a possible basis for the use of elemental diets in allergic and immunological conditions such as food allergy, and possibly Crohn's disease.

The use of elemental diets is likely to affect gastrointestinal microflora and have other wide-ranging effects on gastrointestinal physiology, structure and function. These are important in determining how the gastrointestinal tract alters or adapts to their use. These have been recently reviewed[22] and a study of these effects together with the effects on the microflora provide guidance towards the rational clinical use of these preparations.

Effect of elemental diets on gut microflora. Many factors determine the composition and activity of gut microflora; these include host-mediated factors (intestinal secretions, motility and mucin), bacterial interference and interreactions, environmental pathology and the diet itself[13].

Colonic bacteria metabolize carbohydrate to obtain energy for growth and maintenance. Fermentation stimulates microbial growth in the colon and the faecal microbial mass increases when there is an increase in fermentable carbohydrate in the diet. The stimulation of microbial growth is partly responsible for the increase in stool mass due to fermentable carbohydrate such as dietary fibre.

Elemental diets are likely to affect the microflora in various parts of the alimentary tract in different ways and some studies have been performed on the effect by subsite of these preparations in healthy subjects. *Mouth.* Elemental diets are almost entirely available to oral bacteria because of the nature of their composition, and thus there is a tendency for total anaerobic and aerobic bacteria in the mouth to increase when elemental diets are used. *Stomach.* Bacteria may increase due to a reduced rate of acid secretion associated wth the use of some elemental diets, an increased buffering effect and the presence of increased oral bacteria. *Small Intestine.* Bacteria which may survive the stomach may not be killed because of reduced bile and pancreatic secretions. However, reduction of small intestinal overgrowth of enterobacteriaceae, streptococci, staphylococci, yeasts and fusobacteria was reported in one patient[5]. Abnormal duodenal flora was 'normalized' in four of six patients with gastrointestinal conditions, including three with ulcerative colitis[2]. The faecal flora, was, however, unchanged. *Colon and faeces.* Early studies on glucose and sucrose-based elemental diets[25] showed that the glucose-based diets caused a marked decrease in the number of all types of organisms per gram, but with the sucrose-based diets, the decrease occurred particularly in the entero and lactobacilli groups. Using a glucose-based diet some decrease in enterococci and anaerobes[1] was found, and others found[4] little change in the faecal flora, although study of specific organisms showed some decrease in enterococci and lactobacilli. Thus variable effects have been reported with respect to colon and faeces. Reduced residue may mean reduced nutrients available to the flora and may explain a reduction in the total number of organisms if diet is the main source of nutrient. However, mucus and desquamated cells are also nutritive. Some reduction of colonic bile acid concentration may determine the relative proportions of strict anaerobes in the flora and it is to be noted that bacteroides are stimulated by bile acids.

Elemental diets do not have a profound effect on the types of bacteria present in the alimentary tract but appear to reduce the overall bacterial mass present in intestinal content. It is to be noted, however, that the metabolites of the microflora are reduced during elemental diet therapy. If dietary residue is the principal cause of the numbers of organisms, the decrease would be greatest in saccharolytic organisms which depend on dietary fibre. If the effect is secondary to reduction of mucosal cell desquamation, the proteolytic organisms would be more affected. The results with elemental diets show mixed effects. The alterations of gastrointestinal microflora with the use of elemental diets are somewhat similar to those obtained in germ-free rats[10], although to a lesser extent. Some other alterations of gastrointestinal physiology follow the same pattern as are found with germ-free rats.

Effects of elemental diets on gastrointestinal structure and function. *Stomach.* Gastric emptying has been shown to be delayed by both Vivonex and Flexical when given by bolus-feeding through a nasogastric tube, compared with blenderised food of similar nutritional content[3]. Some reduction of gastric acid secretion may also occur, although this may not be of great clinical significance in man[20]. *Small intestine.* Studies on the small intestine in rats have shown that both Flexical and Vivonex significantly increase villous height and decrease the ratio crypt height : villous height in both jejunum and ileum, suggesting a possible reduction of cell turnover[19]; few significant changes in intestinal function have been observed, as assessed by enzyme activity and by intestinal absorption measured by a perfusion system.

When the effect of isoenergetic amounts of Vivonex, oral solid food and an equivalent diet given i.v., on intestinal mass was compared[16] it was found that it was well maintained by Vivonex in the proximal small intestine but less well than by solid food provided orally. The distal small intestine and colon in rats given Vivonex atrophied and became similar to those given intravenous feeding within the time course of the study. When the effect of Vivonex on the intestinal mucosa after jejuno-ileal bypass in rats was studied it was found that, after two weeks, hypertrophy of the functioning part of the small bowel occurred, together with atrophy of the blind loop[6]. The changes seem to be unrelated to the composition of the elemental diet and confirm that these preparations are as effective as normal diets in inducing intestinal adaptive changes. They provide a basis for the possible use of elemental diets in the management of the short bowel syndrome in man.

Exocrine pancreatic function. Elemental diets require minimal digestion and thus absorption can occur in the absence of normal pancreatic exocrine secretion. However there have been conflicting results on the effect of the preparations on pancreatic function. Comparison of the effect of Vivonex HN with that of intravenous feeding on pancreatic proteolytic activity and ultrastructure, showed that the synthesis and release of proteolytic enzymes was reduced by the elemental diet and that this reduction was equivalent to that which occurs with i.v. feeding[23]. When Vivonex and isoenergetic crushed-food homogenate was infused into the normal human jejunum, and lipase and chymotrypsin in the jejunal fluid were measured, it was found that the homogenate induced greater pancreatic enzyme secretion than Vivonex and that this secretion increased in relation to the energy and nitrogen content of the feed[24]. These results suggest a basis for the use of elemental diets in chronic pancreatic insufficiency and cystic fibrosis, when adequate absorption of nutrients can be achieved in the absence of full digestive function. They may also be of value in healing pancreatic fistulas because of reduced exocrine pancreatic stimulation, in addition to minimal residue.

Bile acid metabolism. The effect of Vivonex and Flexical on faecal bile acid excretion and cholic acid half life in rats has been studied[17]. Total faecal bile acids were significantly reduced by both preparations and cholic acid half life increased, without alteration of the bile acid pool. These results are similar to those obtained in germ-free rats[10]. The changes were more marked with Vivonex than with Flexical but were not significant. The alterations may be related to a longer transit time in animals receiving the elemental diet. A similar reduction in faecal bile acid excretion with Vivonex has been reported in man in patients suffering from cholerheic diarrhoea[18] and Vivonex may be of some value in managing these patients, some of whom are unable to take cholestyramine. Bile acid reduction together with pancreatic enzyme production can also be helpful in the healing of ileal fistulas[12].

During these studies in animals it was found that elemental diets (notably Vivonex) increased total liver lipid content, and hepatic histology showed marked fatty changes in animals fed Vivonex and slight changes in those given Flexical.

Conclusions. The essential properties of elemental diets are nutritional efficacy, minimal digestion requirement, rapid and effective absorption, minimal residue and hypoallergenicity.

Their use leads to alterations in gut microflora and physiology. They reduce the overall bacterial content in colon and faeces, although individual types of bacteria are not altered, induce small intestinal adaptation, reduce pancreatic stimulation compared with normal food, reduce bile production and faecal bile acid excretion, but lead to increased fat deposition in the liver.

These findings lead to rational clinical uses of elemental diets. In addition to providing nutritional support, they may be of value in healing fistulas, in the management of the short bowel syndrome, chronic pancreatic insufficiency, cystic fibrosis, pancreatic fistulas, bile acid-induced diarrhoea and ileal fistulas, and diagnosis and management of food allergy and sensitivity, and may possibly be of value in treating Crohn's disease.

1 Attebury, H.R., Sutter, V.L. & Finegold, S.M. (1972): Effect of a partially chemically defined diet on normal human faecal flora. *Am. J. Clin. Nutr.* **25**, 1391–1398.
2 Axelsson, C.K. & Justesen, T. (1977): Studies of the duodenal and faecal flora in gastrointestinal disorders during treatment with an elemental diet. *Gastroenterology* **72**, 397–401.
3 Bury, K.D. & Jambunathan, G. (1974): Effects of elemental diet on gastric emptying and gastric secretion in man. *Am. J. Surg.* **127**, 59–64.

4 Crowther, J.S., Drasar, B.S., Goddard, P., Hill, M.J. & Johnson, K. (1973): The effect of a chemically defined diet on the faecal flora and faecal steroid concentration. *Gut* **14**, 790–793.

5 Dickman, M.D., Chappelka, A.R. & Schaedler, R.W. (1975): Evaluation of gut microflora during administration of an elemental diet in a patient with an ileoproctostomy. *Am. J. Dig. Dis.* **20**, 377–380.

6 Fenyo, G. & Hallberg, D. (1976): The influence of a chemical diet on the intestinal mucosa after jejuno-ileal bypass in the rat. *Acta Chirurg. Scand.* **142**, 270–274.

7 Ferguson, A., Logan, R.F.A. & MacDonald, T.T. (1980): Increased mucosal damage during parasite infection in mice fed on elemental diet *Gut* **21**, 37–43.

8 Ferguson, A., Paul, G. & MacDonald, T.T. (1978): Immunodeficiency and fatty liver in mice reared on an elemental diet. *Arch. Gastroent. Sao Paolo* **15**, 11–15.

9 Galant, S.P., Franz, M.L., Walker, P., Wells, I.D. & Lundak, R.L. (1977): A potential diagnostic method for food allergy; clinical application and immunogenicity evaluation of an elemental diet. *Am. J. Clin. Nutr.* **30**, 512–514.

10 Gustafsson, B.E. & Norman, A. (1969): Influence of the diet on the turnover of bile acids in germ free and conventional rats. *Br. J. Nutr.* **23**, 429–442.

11 Hecketsweiler, P., Vidon, N., Emouts, P. & Bernier, J.J. (1979): Absorption of elemental and complex nutritional solutions during a continuous jejunal perfusion in man. *Digestion* **19**, 213–217.

12 Hill, G.L., Meyer, W.S.J., Edwards, J.S., Morgan, G.D. & Goligher, J.C. (1975): Effect of a chemically defined liquid elemental diet on the composition and volume of ileo fistula drainage. *Gastroenterology* **68**, 676–682.

13 Hudson, M.J., Boriello, S.P. & Hill, M.J. (1981): Elemental diets and the bacterial flora of the gastrointestinal tract. In *Elemental diets*, ed R.I. Russell, pp. 105–125, Boca Raton Florida: CRC Press.

14 Jones, B.J.M., Lees, R., Andrews, J., Frost, P. & Silk, D.B.A. (1983): Comparison of an elemental and polymeric enteral diet in patients with normal gastrointestinal function. *Gut* **24**, 78–84.

15 Main, A.N.H., Nelson, L.M., East, W., Preston, T., Mitchell, G., Cummings, J.A. & Russell, R.I. (1984): Comparative effects of enteral liquid diets on growth, nitrogen (N) balance, whole body N, N wastage and faecal residue in rats. *Gut* **25**, A1158.

16 Morin, C.L., Ling, B. & Bourassa, D. (1980): Small intestinal and colonic changes induced by a chemically defined diet. *Dig. Dis. Sci.* **25**, 123–128.

17 Nelson, L.M. (1979): Effects of elemental diet feeding on bile acid metabolism and small intestinal structure and function. PhD Thesis, University of Glasgow.

18 Nelson, L.M., Carmichael, H.A., Russell, R.I. & Atherton, S.T. (1977): Use of an elemental diet (Vivonex) in the management of bile acid induced diarrhoea. *Gut* **18**, 792–794.

19 Nelson, L.M., Carmichael, H.A., Russell, R.I. & Lee, F.D. (1978): Small intestinal changes induced by an elemental diet (Vivonex) in normal rats. *Clin. Sci. Molec. Med.* **55**, 509–511.

20 Rivilis, J., McArdle, H., Wolodek, J.K. & Gurd, F.N. (1972): The effect of an elemental diet on gastric secretion. *Ann. R. Coll. Surg. Can.* **5**, 57–60.

21 Russell, R.I. (1975): Elemental diets. *Gut* **16**, 68–69.

22 Russell, R.I. (1985): Intestinal adaptation to an elemental diet. *Proc. Nutr. Soc.* **44**, 87–93.

23 Traverso, L.W., Abou-Zamzam, A.M., Maxwell, D.S., Lacy, S.M. & Tompkins, R.K. (1981): The effect of total parenteral nutrition or elemental diet on pancreatic proteolytic activity and ultrastructure. *J. Parent. Ent. Nutr.* **5**, 496–500.

24 Vidon, N., Hecketsweiler, P., Butel, J. & Bernier, J.J. (1978): Effect of continuous jejunal perfusion of elemental and complex nutrition solutions on pancreatic enzyme secretion in human subjects. *Gut* **19**. 194–198.

25 Winitz, M., Adams, R.F., Geedman, D.A., Davies, P.N., Jayko, L.G. & Hamilton, J.A. (1970): Studies in metabolic nutrition employing chemically defined diets. Effects on gut microflora populations. *Am. J. Clin. Nutr.* **23**, 546–559.

26 Yeung, C.K., Smith, R.C. & Hill, G.L. (1979): The effect of an elemental diet on body composition. A comparison with intravenous nutrition. *Gastroenterology* **77**, 652–657.

Colonic metabolism and absorption

L. BUSTOS-FERNANDEZ
Instituto de Gastroenterologia, Dr. Jorge Perez Companc, Potosi 4240–(1199), Buenos Aires, Argentina

Most studies on human colon physiology have been limited to the investigation of mucosal functions, (absorption, secretion and motility)[11] excluding the activity of the luminal content, ie the bacterial flora. From a functional standpoint, the colon can be considered as a single unit made up of four components (Fig. 1): ileal input, intraluminal bacterial metabolism, clearance of nutrients (transparietal colonic absorption), and faecal output.

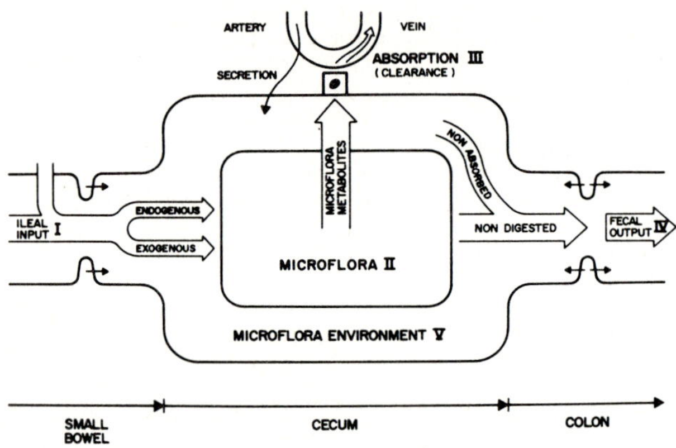

Fig. 1. *Colonic physiology*

There is a balance between the amount of substances entering the colon and its capacity for clearing those end-products arising from intraluminal bacterial metabolism. In order to maintain a symbiotic intraluminal bacterial flora, this metabolic equilibrium must be achieved without modifying the stability of the chemical composition or the concentration of the intraluminal colonic medium.

Ileal input. Ileum motility must adapt to normal intraluminal bacterial digestion and to absorption through the gut wall[15].

Since the biochemical aspects of fermentation processes, both in the animal rumen and in human gut, are dealt with in detail elsewhere in this book, greater emphasis will be given here to clearance of nutrients and faecal output.

The ileal input consists of nutrients, biliary pigments, bile acids, pancreatic enzymes, steroid hormones, amines and peptides, prostaglandins, bacteria and other microorganisms, growth factors and carbon dioxide. The ileal input is enriched by additional nutrients derived from the colonic wall itself (mucus, electrolytes, immunoglobulins, etc.), which are incorporated into the luminal medium.

Because 99 per cent of microorganisms within the large intestine live under anaerobic conditions, the major energy source arises from polysaccharide and oligosaccharide fermentation, proteins and fats participating to a lesser extent in this energy break-down[13,17]. The bacterial cell protein matrix is derived mainly from serum urea, entering the lumen by diffusion from the bloodstream. Ureolytic bacterial enzymes break down the urea into ammonia which is employed in protein synthesis. The surplus is absorbed in the colon and recycled through the liver to return to the gut as urea[20].

Further investigations are necessary in order to establish the effect of other components on ileal input and on the metabolic activity of the microorganisms towards bile acids, steroid hormones, amines, peptides, growth factors such as branched fatty acids, pancreatic enzymes and electrolytes[2,3].

Bacterial metabolism. All substrates entering the colon are not broken down by the flora to the same degree, for this reason the faeces are rich in nutrients not subject to enzyme action such as lignin, and have small amounts or lack those subject to intense hydrolysis such as pectins; other substances such as hemicellulose occupy an intermediate position[6] — Fig. 2.

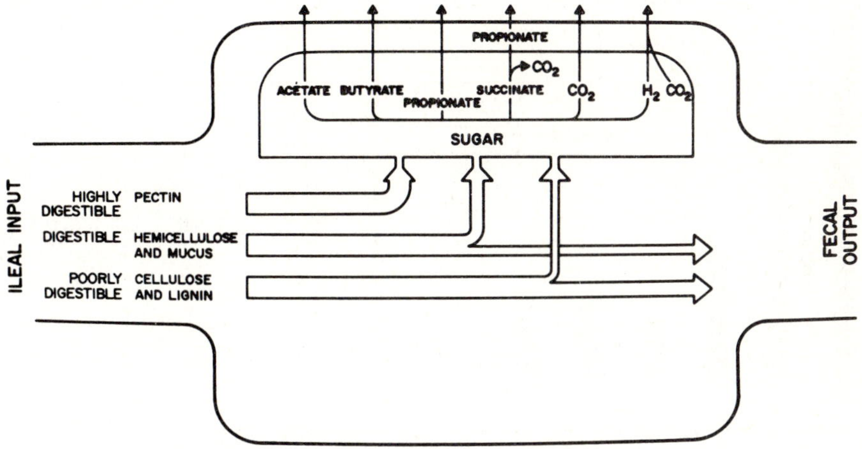

Fig. 2. *Intraluminal colonic metabolism.*

Bacterial action on substances entering the lumen is conducted through the complex mechanisms involved in enzyme activity which follow a chain-reaction involving the coordinated participation of several microorganisms[21]. One example illustrating the metabolic interrelationship existing amongst bacteria, is that of anaerobic microorganisms representing 99 per cent of the flora population, which cannot develop without the cooperation of aerobic organisms consuming the small amounts of oxygen drawn from the blood[19].

Carbohydrate metabolism is initiated by certain microorganisms possessing mucolytic[9] and cellulolytic[4] enzymes which remove long carbohydrate side-chains; shorter chains of water-soluble oligo- and polysaccharides are further broken down in a second step, with the ultimate formation of new metabolites. A third group of enzymes produce methane from hydrogen and CO_2[21]. Another example of enzyme chain reactions is represented by bile pigment metabolism[8]. It has been shown that a reduced number of microorganisms isolated from the colon are insufficient to modify bilirubin structure; the whole flora must be present, together with an adequate environment for changes in the pigment to occur, just as in the normal animal.

Clearance (colonic absorption). A fundamental difference exists between the absorptive function of the small intestine and that of the colon. In the former, absorption benefits the host exclusively, whereas the colonocyte has an added role apart from the one it shares with the enterocyte; which is to maintain a stable intraluminal medium in order to secure the metabolic and growth requirements of the microorganisms within the lumen.

The brilliant studies carried out by Demigné and colleagues from the French school have brought to light this subtle metabolic function of the colon[7]. Employing comparative studies conducted in rats given two different diets for 20 days, one free of fibre and the other of high fibre content, they were able to prove that in both cases the concentration of substances present in the caecum remains constant. Simultaneously, however, transparietal caecal flux is highly variable depending directly upon diet composition (Fig. 3). These investigations show how the colon adapts its absorption rate to ileal input on the basis of maintaining the composition of the intracaecal medium. The experiments also indicate how, after 20 days of fibre-rich diet, caecal wall weight and vascular flow increase. These findings suggest that an abrupt overload in ileal input would be subject to complete clearance after only a few days have elapsed, ie after the necessary adaptation has occurred.

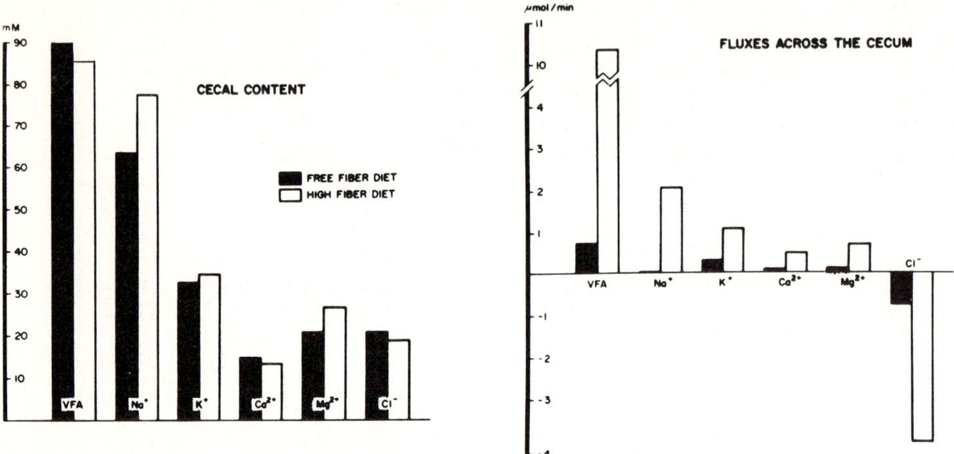

Fig. 3. *Fibre-free and high-fibre diet: colonic absorption and caecal homoeostasis.*

Faecal output. The faeces have three components; undigested matter, incompletely absorbed substances, and substances synthesized by bacteria within the colon. Lignin is an example of an undigested substance.

The second component mentioned is of little importance under physiological conditions, but may play a greater role in pathological circumstances. Phillips has experimentally demonstrated the high absorptive capacity of the human colon to be 600 mEq/day for Na, and 6 l/d for water[14]. These figures are only surpassed when the ileal input greatly exceeds the aforementioned amounts as in the case of cholera and Vernier Morrison Syndrome, when excessive amounts of unabsorbed water and sodium will be excreted in the faeces producing diarrhoea.

Several investigators have questioned our assumption[5] that excessive amounts of unabsorbed carbohydrates could reach the distal segments of the colon and after transformation into organic acids through bacterial action surpass colonic absorption capacity. Our work shows that in severe digestive pathologies such as pancreatic disorders, sprue, disaccharidase deficiency and massive small intestine resections abundant colonic accumulation of volatile fatty acids can occur, which judging by the enormous surplus which must be excreted in the faeces, far surpasses the absorption capacity of the colonocytes (viz isolated epithelial cells). In cases of massive resection of the small intestine, daily organic anion (volatile fatty acids) faecal output which is normally about 10 mEq/day, can reach 100 mEq.

The third component of the faecal output is those nutrients which instead of being absorbed, are incorporated into the intraluminal bacteria; thus bacteria can contribute to the excretion of substances from the body. Nephrologists have suggested this route as an alternative pathway for the excretion of nitrogen metabolites, replacing the renal pathway in cases of terminal renal failure.

Intracolonic homoeostasis regulation. If the intracolonic medium remains biologically stable, factors affecting its regulation should therefore be analysed. There are four main control mechanisms which secure colon homoeostasis. (*A*) *Variations in ileo-caecal inflow.* The flow of nutrients entering the colon from the small intestine varies in relation to caecal functional digestive and absorption capacity. Terminal ileum motor response (phase-III-migrating-motility complexes) is directed mainly towards fluid propulsion, solid residues can remain within the distal ileum for several hours, probably protecting the colon from massive nutrient overload[15]. Although motor response in the ileocaecal region has not been studied in detail, it could be similar to that of the antro-pyloric-duodenal region. In both cases, nutrient transit from the proximal to the distal organ would occur only when the latter is fully prepared to carry out normal digestive and absorption functions. (*B*) *Variations in bacterial enzymes.* An appreciable amount of bacteria (75 g) is excreted together with the faeces nevertheless this loss is replenished, the colon remaining remarkably constant[10]. The great variability in nutrient composition of the input accounts for the existence of regulating substances which stimulate bacterial growth such as: carbohydrates, volatile fatty acids, CO_2, NH_3, and others which inhibit it such as: O_2, bile acids, and all the metabolites accumulated after nutrients break-down[18]. (*C*) *Variations in colon clearance mechanisms.* Absorption can vary according to modification in the regulating capacity of: (i) the number of absorptive cells, (ii) the metabolic mechanisms of the epithelial cell itself, (iii) the quantity and quality of the mucus barrier[1], and

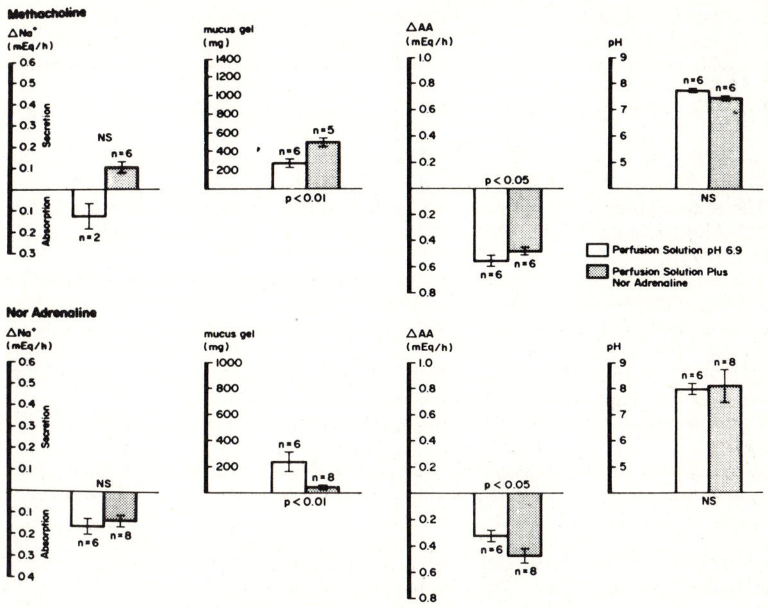

Fig. 4. *Adrenergic and cholinergic influence on colonic absorption and secretion.* (AA = acetate anion).

(iv) the vascular flow[12]. Studies conducted in our laboratory (Fig. 4) to establish neuroregulatory influence on absorption mechanisms in the colon have allowed us to demonstrate that organic anion absorption increases due to nonadrenergic action with a fall in mucus secretion; conversely, methacholine administration leads to a decrease in organic anion[5] absorption coinciding with increased mucus secretion. These examples illustrate how colon clearing mechanisms could be subject to neuroendocrine control. (*D*) *Variations in colon motor activity.* The importance of motor function cannot be excluded from an analysis of the mechanisms regulating colon metabolic activity. In healthy individuals with an occidental type of diet, food residues remain two or three days, on average, within the colonic lumen[16]. This prolonged period appears to be mandatory for adequate substrate contact with bacterial enzymes, as well as for the absorption of colon metabolites. A delay or an acceleration in transit velocity could affect both metabolic and absorptive functions in the colon.

Conclusion and bases for future studies on pathophysiology. Future studies on colon pathophysiology should be based on physiological concepts, ie possible alterations in the four regulating mechanisms: ileal flow characteristics, modifications in the metabolic capacity of the flora, variations in colonocyte absorption capacity and colon propulsion velocity.

Another aspect of colon pathophysiology which has yet to be clarified and requires careful investigation relates to the necessity of maintaining barriers between the contents of the colon and the blood.

There are marked differences in composition between the colon and blood compartments regarding, for example, sodium, potassium, chloride and volatile fatty acids thanks to the efficient mucosal barrier which separates them. Perhaps in this organ as in the stomach, the loss of the barrier can affect both compartments, but in the case of the colon not only is damage to mucosa provoked, but there is also a loss of bacterial homoeostasis of great risk for the host.

1 Allen, A. (1983): The structure of colonic mucus. In *Colon: structure and function*, ed L. Bustos-Fernández, pp. 45–77. New York: Plenum.

2 Allison, M.J., Bryant, M.P. & Doetsch, R.N. (1962): Studies on the metabolic function of branched -chain volatile fatty acids, growth factors for Ruminococci. I. Incorporation of isovalerate into leucine. *J. Bact.* **83**, 523–532.

3 Allison, M.J., Bryant, M.P., Katz, I., & Keeney, M. (1962): Metabolic function of branched -chain fatty acids growth factors for Ruminococci. II. Biosynthesis of higher branched-chain fatty acids and aldehydes. *J. Bact.* **83**, 1084–1093.

4 Bryant, M.P. (1973): Nutritional requirements of the predominant rumen cellulolytic bacteria. *Fed. Proc.* **32**, 1809–1813.

5 Bustos-Fernández, L., Gonzalez, E., Marzi, A. & Ledesma de Paolo, M.I. (1971): Fecal acidorrhea. *New Engl. J. Med.* **284**, 295–298.

6 Cummings, J.H., Southgate, D.A.T., Branch, W.J., Wiggins, H.S., Houston, H., Jenkins, D.J.A., Jivraj, T. & Hill, M.J. (1979): The digestion of pectin in the human gut and its effect on calcium absorption and large bowel function. *Br. J. Nutr.* **41**, 447–485.

7 Demigné, C. & Rémesy, C. (1985): Stimulation of absorption of volatile fatty acids and mineral in the cecum of rats adapted to very high fiber diet. *J. Nutr.* **115**, 53–60.

8 Gustafsson, B.E. (1982): The physiological importance of the colonic microflora. *Scand. J. Gastroenterol.* **17**, Suppl. 77, 117–131.

9 Hoskins, L.C. (1978): Degradation of mucus glycoproteins in the gastrointestinal tract. In *The glyconjugates II.* ed M.I. Horowitz, W. Pigman, pp. 235–253. New York: Academic Press.

10 Høverstad, T. & Bjørneklett, A. (1984): Short-chain fatty acids and bowel functions in man. *Scand. J. Gastroent.* **19**, 1059–1065.

11 Johnson, L.R. (1981): *Physiology of the gastrointestinal tract. Vol. I & Vol. II.* New York: Raven Press.

12 Lundgren, O. & Jodal, M. (1983): Circulation of the colon. In *Colon: structure and function*, ed L. Bustos-Fernández, pp. 211–231. New York: Plenum.

13 McNeil, N.I. (1984): The contribution of the large intestine to energy supplies in man. *Am. J. Clin. Nutr.* **39**, 338–342.

14 Phillips, S.F. & Kerlin, P. (1983): Absorption and secretion of electrolytes by the human colon. In *Colon: structure and function*, ed L. Bustos-Fernández, pp. 17–44, New York: Plenum.

15 Phillips, S.F. (1983): Diarrhea: Role of the ileo–cecal sphincter. In *International symposium on gastroenterology. New trends in pathophysiology and therapy of the large bowel* (Abstract book), pp. 33. Bologna: Fondazione Giovanni Lorenzini.

16 Read, N.W. (1981): The relationship between colonic motility and transport. *Scand, J. Gastroent.* **19**, Suppl. 93, 35–42.

17 Salyers, A.A. & Leedle, J.A. (1983): Carbohydrate metabolism in the human colon. In *Human intestinal microflora in health and disease.* ed D.J. Hentges, pp. 129–146. New York: Academic Press.

18 Savage, D.C. (1977): Microbial ecology of the gastrointestinal tract. *Ann. Rev. Microbiol.* **31**, 107–133.

19 Savage, D.C. (1981): The microbial flora in the gastrointestinal flora. In *Nutrition in health and disease and international development: symposia from XII Int. Cong. Nutr.* pp. 893–908. New York: Alan R. Liss.

20 Visek, W.J. (1972): Effects of urea hydrolysis on cell life -span and metabolism. *Fed. Proc.* **31**, 1178–1193.

21 Wollin, M.J. (1974): Metabolic interactions among intestinal microorganisms. *Am. J. Nutr.* **27**, 1320.

Methods for estimating ruminal degradation of feed proteins: a workshop report

G.A. BRODERICK (Organizer)
U.S. Dairy Forage Research Centre, University of Wisconsin, Madison, WI 53706, USA.

Ruminants depend upon microbial protein plus feed protein which escapes the rumen for their amino acid supply. The N requirements of rumen organisms are quite simple, and microbial protein synthesis is proportional to fermentability of the diet. Degradation of dietary protein is independent of microbial protein synthesis. Hence, the value of feed protein to the animal depends largely on its ruminal escape.

Natural feed proteins vary greatly in ruminal degradability. Proteins with greater ruminal escape are valuable to ruminants with high protein requirements such as lactating dairy cows or rapidly growing calves and lambs. However, there are specialized situations where ruminants at low levels of production will respond to additional escaped protein: wool production and growing cattle being fed high non-protein nitrogen (NPN) diets containing little preformed protein. Amino acid pattern or total supply is inadequate to meet requirements of these animals.

Methods for estimating ruminal protein degradation then have applicability for identifying resistant proteins and for developing ways of protecting proteins. Also, several new feeding systems require data on protein degradability. Hence, there is a substantial need for improved methods to rapidly assess ruminal degradability of feed proteins.

Enzymology and microbiology of ruminal protein degradation (*G.P. Hazlewood*, AFRC, Institute for Animal Physiology, Babraham, Cambridge, CB2 4AT, UK). It was shown in studies with soluble proteins that protein degradation in the rumen follows typical Michaelis-Menten kinetics and is first-order with respect to protein concentration[9]. Degradation of fraction 1 protein was increased 3 to 9 fold by feeding a diet of fresh lucerne, vs feeding a dry diet of hay plus concentrate — suggesting that proteolytic enzymes can be induced in rumen microbes[4,9]. Other work indicated rapid adsorption of protein to microbes preceded proteolysis[13], and proteolysis rather than clearance of peptides, limited overall protein degradation[9].

Protein solubility is only one of several factors determining protein degradation. There is large variation among soluble proteins in degradability, apparently related to tertiary structure. Globular proteins were degraded slowly, but these rates were increased by breaking disulphide bonds[8]. Although little is known about what controls their degradation, insoluble proteins vary greatly in degradability.

The majority of research has been done with microbes isolated from the fluid phase; however, most of the microbial population is associated with the particulates[3]. In mixed rumen organisms, more than 90 per cent of proteolytic activity is present with the microbial pellet, and not as free enzyme. Specific activity of bacterial proteases is 10 times greater than protozoa; hence, bacteria are more important in proteolysis. Proteases are largely associated with the bacterial cell envelope and easily released by blending or detergent treatment[5].

Inhibitor studies indicate most bacterial endopeptidases fall into one of four classes: (1) serine proteases; (2) cysteine proteases; (3) metal-ion-dependent proteases, and (4) aspartate proteases. The most important proteolytic bacteria isolated from the rumen are: (1) *Bacteroides amylophilus* (first isolated); (2) *Ba. ruminicola*; (3) *Butyrivibrio spp*; (4) Selenomonads; (5) Clostridia; and (6) Streptococci Type 2 is most important, and types 3–6 are important if present in the rumen in large numbers.

Use of commercial proteases and microwave techniques (*M.B. Assoumani*, Sanders 17, Quai de l'Industrie, 91200 Athis Mons, France). This method was developed from work with pronase, an active commercial protease[6]. However, pronase was found to over-estimate ruminal degradation, possibly due to specificity which is much broader than that of rumen microbes. Several other commercial proteases, including neutral fungal protease, have been found to give more reliable results. A neutral protease from *Bacillus subtilis* was adapted to study protein degradation.

Results indicated that the pH of the medium influenced degradation through alteration of protein solubility. Unphysiologically high pH's solubilize more than normal amounts of protein. Complex carbohydrates physically protect feed proteins from proteolytic attack. Hence, estimation of ruminal protein degradation of high carbohydrate feeds may be improved by supplementing the medium with amylases and similar enzymes to mimic digestion by rumen organisms in exposing proteins to continuing proteolytic attack.

Heat-treatment is one of the most effective means of protecting proteins, but the effects of heating are difficult to characterise. Novel procedures were developed to assess extent of protein-carbohydrate interaction, with the goal of identifying 'ideal' heat-treatments. Microwave scanning of the heat-treated feed assessed the extent of Maillard reaction by relating microwave frequency and absorbed energy to available-lysine and estimated ruminal degradability. This technique also provides information on the most appropriate wavelengths to use in protein-treatment by microwave heating.

Labelling proteins to assess degradability (*R.J. Wallace*, Rowett Research Institute, Bucksburn, Aberdeen, AB2 9SB, UK). Some proteins are naturally labelled such that their disappearance can be followed in the presence of other proteins (eg the alkali-labile phosphorus bound to casein). However, these natural labels are of course not applicable to the majority of feed proteins. Therefore, exogenous 'tags' have been developed to label proteins. These include the azo-dye method[8] and a reductive methylation procedure[12].

Reductive methylation[12] involves protein treatment with a small amount of ^{14}C-formaldehyde of high specific activity, followed by reduction with sodium borohydride. This mild procedure methylated about 1/200 of the lysine residues, and did not alter the rate of proteolysis. ^{14}C-monomethyl lysine released during degradation was stable in rumen fluid for many hours, while azo-dye begins disappearing in minutes. The problem of microbial reduction of azo-dye can be overcome by quantifying dye bound to undegraded protein[8]; however, diazotization alters protein degradability. An alternative to radioactivity would be use of fluorescent dyes. Although these may also be unstable in rumen fluid, inherent sensitivity of fluorescent methods would require only minor modification to adequately label proteins.

Experience with tagging of soluble proteins has been satisfactory, but successful application of these methods to feed proteins which are largely insoluble remains to be seen. Physical limitations to reaction of much of the protein in intact feeds may prevent homogeneous labelling, and hence, restrict use of these techniques to soluble proteins.

In situ bag procedures (*E.R. Ørskov*, Rowett Research Institute, Bucksburn, Aberdeen, AB2 9SB, UK; *P. Thivend*, INRA, Laboratoire de la Digestion des Ruminants, Theix, 63122 Ceyrat, France). This method has been adequately described in the literature (eg,[10]) and extensively applied, forming the basis by which many *in vitro* procedures are evaluated. Known amounts of protein are sealed in small nylon or dacron bags, suspended in the rumen, then removed after specific intervals and residual N quantified. Usually there is rapid, early loss of soluble N, followed by exponential disappearance of remaining N. The general scheme for dealing with this pattern is to assume all of the rapidly lost protein is degraded, and to combine the exponential disappearance rate with ruminal passage to estimate the fraction of the remaining protein which escapes the rumen. Ruminal passage has been estimated using chromium mordanted proteins[10].

There are several important considerations in application of *in-situ* procedures. (1) It is essential to use bags of controlled porosity, with pores ranging from 35 to 60 microns. (2) Washing procedures are required to remove microbial and feed N which adheres to the outside of the bags. While washing is necessary, it also introduces variability into the method. (3) There is considerable effect of diet on observed *in-situ* rates of protein degradation. One suggestion is to suspend *in-situ* bags routinely in animals fed both concentrate and roughage diets. (4) There is substantial animal variation in observed *in-situ* degradations, possibly due to differences among animals in ruminal turnover.

Correlations between *in-situ* degradation and pronase digestibilities[6] have been excellent. In estimating ruminal protein escape using *in-situ* techniques, the effect of rate of passage is generally greater than that of *in-situ* degradation. *In-situ* procedures are restricted to proteins which are largely insoluble. Completely soluble proteins will of course appear to be completely degradable, even though some soluble proteins (eg the albumins) are known to be slowly degraded in the rumen.

Incubations using pure cultures of proteolytic rumen bacteria (*E.L. Miller*, Department of Applied Biology, Cambridge University, Cambridge, CB2 3DX, UK). This procedure[7] was developed because of problems with the pronase method described earlier[6] and the need for more rapid and less labour-intensive techniques than *in-situ* methods. Pure cultures of proteolytic rumen bacteria isolated from the rumen (either *Butyrivibrio spp.* or *Streptococcus bovis*) were incubated with the test protein. Protein degradation is computed from amount of solubilized N plus N incorporated into growing cells (collected by filtration). The observed pattern of soya-bean meal degradation was a 2–4 h lag, followed by rapid degradation for 6–8 h, then a plateau for the remaining time up to 24 h. The pattern was similar to that observed *in situ* by the same workers[7], but others have not found a lag in degradation of soya-bean meal *in-situ*[10].

Substrates were sterilised using gamma-irradiation (to prevent contamination of the pure cultures). Use of protein precipitants (eg TCA) reduced estimated degradation. Maximal extent of degradation by *Butyrivibrio spp.* was greater than that obtained using *Streptococcus bovis*. However, degradation using either organism was only about 50–60 per cent of that obtained *in-situ*. This interesting procedure is worthy of further investigation, possibly employing combinations of pure cultures of proteolytic rumen bacteria.

Use of gas production to correct *in vitro* ammonia release (*K.H. Memke*, Institut für Tierernahrung, University of Hohenheim, 7000 Stuttgart 70, West Germany). A method was developed to correct for ammonia uptake by ruminal microbes using gas production as the index of microbial growth[11]. This correction was developed from regressions of ammonia concentration on gas production, where starch or other carbohydrates were the energy sources. Net ammonia formation (plus-protein minus blank), corrected for ammonia loss based on gas production, was converted to proportion of total N degraded. Typical extents of degradation at 24 h ranged from 100 per cent and 94 per cent for casein and soya-bean meal, respectively, to 17 per cent for feather meal.

At least two potential problems are inherent in this approach. (1) As typically applied, the method required 12 replicate vessels plus blanks for each protein at each time interval. (2) Of greater concern was that N liberation from cell lysis in incubations longer than 12 h represented a source of non-feed ammonia which cannot be corrected for using blanks. Nevertheless, this novel procedure has yielded *in vitro* estimates of degradability that are similar to those determined *in vivo* using[15]N techniques.

An inhibitor *in vitro* system to estimate protein degradability (*G.A. Broderick*, US Dairy Forage Research Centre, University of Wisconsin, Madison, WI 53706, USA). This method was based on use of mixed rumen organisms to which inhibitors were added to prevent N incorporation by growing microbes[1], allowing quantitative recovery of protein degradation products. Inhibitors now being used are 1 mM hydrazine (an inhibitor of ammonia uptake) plus 30 µg/ml chloramphenicol (an inhibitor of amino acid utilisation). Although microbial growth does not occur, protein degradation proceeds normally for up to 6 hours. The inoculum was enriched with particle-associated microbes[2]. Extents of degradation were computed from the proportion of added N released in the form of ammonia and amino acids. Fractional degradation rates were sloped from regressions on time of log of fraction undegraded. Degradation rates were used in conjunction with rates of passage to estimate ruminal degradation and escape.

In typical incubations with 16 vessels and duplicate samples at eight times over 4 h, 256 samples plus recoveries and standards must be analyzed for ammonia and total amino acids. Analyses were done using an autoanalyzer system equipped with micro-computer data collection. Degradations of solvent and expeller soya-bean meals determined using this system were similar to *in vivo* results obtained using cannulated cows.

This method is well-adapted only to laboratories with extensive sample analysis and data handling equipment. Results with silages have been unreliable because additional release of ammonia and amino acids must be measured against very high backgrounds. Incomplete recoveries were observed with low concentrations of amino acids, such as would be found with slowly degraded proteins. However, this problem appears to have been obviated by addition of chloramphenicol to the inoculum.

Summary. N-solubility and uncorrected ammonia release can no longer be considered adequate indices of ruminal degradability when used across unrelated classes of feed proteins. Care must be exercised in application of *in vitro* methods based on commercial proteases because proteases elaborated by rumen microbes have rather specific characteristics. Limited work with pure cultures has yielded degradations similar in pattern to *in-situ* results, but of lower magnitude. Difficulty in quantifying undegraded feed protein has been circumvented by 'tagging' protein, correcting for N-uptake from gas production, and using inhibitors to prevent microbial removal of protein degradation products. All three approaches show promise as well as unresolved problems. In *in-situ* method, when conducted under standard conditions, yields apparently reliable estimates of *in vivo* ruminal protein degradation.

1 Broderick, G.A. (1984): In vitro determination of rates of ruminal protein degradation. *Canadian J. Anim. Sci.* **64**, (suppl.), 31–32.
2 Craig, W.M., Hong, B.J., Broderick, G.A. & Bula, R.J. (1984): In vitro inoculum enriched with particle-associated microorganisms for determining rates of fiber digestion and protein degradation. *J. Dairy Sci.* **67**, 2902–2909.
3 Forsberg, C.W. & Lam, K. (1977): Use of adenosine 5'-triphosphate as an indicator of microbiota biomass in rumen contents. *Appl. Environ. Microbiol.* **33**, 528–537.
4 Hazlewood, G.P., Orpin, C.G., Greenwood, Y. & Black, M.E. (1983): Isolation of proteolytic rumen bacteria by use of selective medium containing leaf fraction 1 protein (ribulosebisphosphate carboxylase). *Appl. Environ. Microbiol.* **45**, 1780–1784.
5 Kopecny, J. & Wallace, R.J. (1982): Cellular location and some properties of proteolytic enzymes of rumen bacteria. *Appl. Environ. Microbiol.* **43**, 1026–1033.
6 Krishnamoorthy, U., Sniffen, C.J., Stern, M.D. & Van Soest, P.J. (1983): Evaluation of a mathematical model of rumen digestion and an in vitro simulation of rumen proteolysis to estimate the rumen-undegraded nitrogen content of feedstuffs. *Br. J. Nutr.* **50**, 555–568.
7 Laycock, K.A., Hazlewood, G.P. & Miller, E.R. (1985): Potential use of proteolytic rumen bacteria for assessing feed protein degradability in vitro. *Proc. Nutr. Soc.* **44**, 54A.
8 Mahadevan, S., Erfle, J.D. & Sauer, F.D. (1980): Degradation of soluble and insoluble proteins by *Bacteroides amylophilus* protease and by rumen microorganisms. *J. Anim. Sci.* **50**, 723–728.
9 Nugent, J.H.A. & Mangan, J.L. (1981): Characteristics of the rumen proteolysis of fraction 1 (18S) leaf protein from lucerne (Medicago sativa L.). *Br. J. Nutr.* **46**, 39–58.
10 Orskov, E.R. & McDonald, I. (1979): The estimation of protein degradability in the rumen from incubation measurements weighted according to rate of passage. *J. Agric. Sci. (Camb).* **92**, 499–503.
11 Raab, L., Cafantaris, B., Jilg, T. & Menke, K.H. (1983): Rumen protein degradation and biosynthesis. 1. A new method for determination of protein degradation in rumen fluid in vitro. *Br. J. Nutr.* **50**, 569–582.
12 Wallace, R.J. (1983): Hydrolysis of ^{14}C-labelled proteins by rumen micro-organisms and by proteolytic enzymes prepared from rumen bacteria. *Br. J. Nutr.* **50**, 345–355.
13 Wallace, R.J. (1985): Adsorption of soluble proteins to rumen bacteria and the role of adsorption in proteolysis. *Br. J. Nutr.* **53**, 399–408.

★ ★ ★

ASSESSMENT OF NUTRIENT AVAILABILITY

A concept of availability and its technical implications

N.F. SUTTLE
Moredun Research Institute, 408 Gilmerton Road, Edinburgh EH17 7JH, UK.

Few natural phenomena have been assessed in as many diverse ways and studied so intensely with so little progress towards a practical objective as the availability of nutrients. This is doubly unfortunate because availability is synonymous with nutrient value, the key to matching

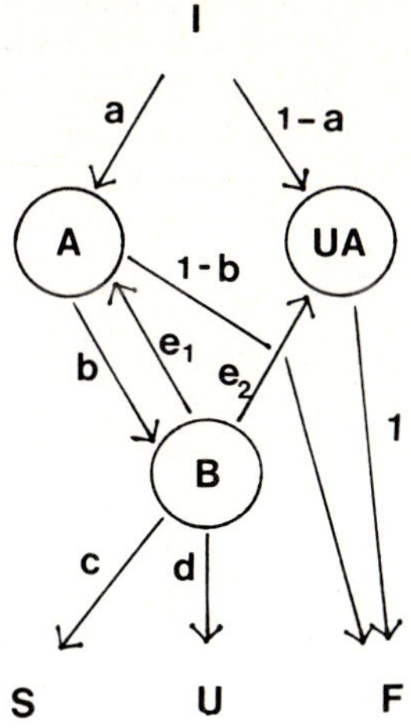

Fig. *A model of nutrient flows to and from the body tissues.* The dietary nutrient input (I) is partitioned between two pools in the gut lumen, absorbable (A) and unabsorbable (UA). Nutrient is absorbed from A into the tissue pool (B) and is lost via the body surface (S), urine (U) and faeces (F): faecal losses contain nutrient of endogenous origin (e) which has moved from B to A and UA. Small letters denote fractional flow rates. B can change in size within physiological limits and nutrients (eg carbohydrates and amino acids) change in form.

Table. *Principal methods for measuring nutrient 'availability' grouped by the concept implied – gastro-intestinal (GI) or whole body (WB) – and the principal nutrient flows and outputs (see Fig.) which they measure or predict quantitatively (+) or qualitatively (−).*

Concept	Group	Flows/pools	Description of technique	Quantitative/qualitative
GI	1	$a\,I$	*In vitro* (eg microbial or chemical assay, solvent extraction)	±
GI	2	$ab\,I$	(a) Faecal monitoring ⎫ with correction (b) Whole body/counting ⎬ for endogenous loss (c) Entry rates of tracer of nutrient into circulation	+ + ±
WB	3	$I(1-a)$ $+e_1B(1-b)+e_2B$	Faecal monitoring	+
WB	4	$I-(U+S+F)$	Retention (eg balance study, growth assay, whole body counting)	±
WB	5	$\dfrac{I-(U+S+F)}{\times}$	Partial retention (eg as haemoglobin; organ analysis or counting) relative to standard.	−

nutrient supply and consumer need, and we know relatively little about it. A simple model of the flows of a nutrient through the body (Fig.) enables the techniques for assessing nutrient availability to be classified by what they measure or predict (Table): it's clear that our techniques often measure different things with neither a common concept nor a quantitative result. Progress will remain slow until we find a common concept and then use appropriate techniques to obtain absolute values for the availability of nutrients.

A unifying concept of availability. To merit universal acceptance our concept of availability must satisfy five conditions: it must be definable, distinct from terms already accepted, appropriate to all nutrients, measurable and above all useful. The model (Fig.) shows that of the nutrient ingested (I), only a proportion may be absorbable (a) and only a part of this may be absorbed (b). The product ab gives the proportion of the ingested nutrient which flows to the tissues and its *maximal* value (the need for that qualification will become apparent later) should in my view be universally regarded as availability. I describe this as a 'gastrointestinal' (GI) concept of availability and the two coefficients as its dietary (a) and consumer (b) components. The dietary component will largely be determined by chemical composition and in particular by: (1) the form in which the nutrient is present, (2) the digestibility of the matrix in which the nutrient is consumed, and (3) other constituents affecting the proportion which remains absorbable.

The consumer component b will be influenced mainly by the genetically determined efficiency of the absorptive process and the need for the capacity to absorb the nutrient. There may also be interactions between the diet and the consumer, caused by nutrient or non-nutrient factors in the diet which influence b. The consumer factors mostly influence b when the supply of nutrient from the diet exceeds the requirement: when there is no excess and no genetic variation, availability in the healthy individual becomes essentially a dietary attribute.

Availability as ab Max is distinct from the widely used terms 'digestibility'; 'metabolizability' and the many reflecting 'efficiency of utilization' (eg energy use for fattening, biological value of protein, metabolic efficiency of zinc utilization): it is second only to intake as an important determinant of the response of the consumer to carbohydrates, amino acids, vitamins and minerals (macro- and trace).

The alternative concept is that availability should relate to the form suitable for digestion, absorption *and* utilization, shifting the emphasis to the proportion of the nutrient retained (eg amino acids[2]). The object of this whole-body (WB) concept is to completely describe the response to a particular nutrient source. However, changes in body content can be influenced by factors which have nothing to do with the nutrient assessed: response to energy input may be determined by the maturity of the consumer species; responses to an amino acid may be determined by the supply of other amino acids; responses to all nutrients may be influenced by growth inhibitors. Furthermore, nutrients differ widely in their post-absorptive metabolism, increasing the difficulty of embracing them in a common definition.

Implications for the measurement of availability. Nutrient availability can be measured by several *in vivo* techniques which adhere to a GI concept although they are not all easy to apply (Table). Among those that reflect the WB concept by measuring the net outcome of absorptive, excretory and secretory processes is the commonly used method of faecal monitoring: its popularity stems from the simplicity and non-invasiveness of the technique but simplicity is no substitute for veracity. The first technical implication of the GI concept of availability is that the right type of method should be used (ie those from Group 2 in the Table). Before a particular GI technique is taken up, however, there are a number of additional technical implications to be considered to avoid the intrusion of factors which have nothing to do with availability (as ab), some introduced by the consumer species, others by the researcher.

Many minerals are absorbed in amounts closely related to the consumer's need for them and the proportion which is absorbed (b) will fall as the absorbable supply (aI) increases: most species use this device to control their Ca, Fe and Zn status to some degree. Thus the absorptive efficiency of Zn in adult sheep fell from 80 to 3 per cent as Zn intake increased from 8 to 200 mg/d[18]. If young and old animals are given the same diets, the young will absorb a greater proportion of the Ca[10], Zn[5], and Fe[6] from the diet than the old simply because they need more of each element for growth. For such elements, no technique will give true estimates of availability if the diet provides an excess of the minerals and a large proportion of values cited in the literature for their so called 'availabilities' can be discarded for this reason: only the maximum obtainable value in normal animals is relevant.

All methods use small groups of consumers to characterize nutrient availability and assume they are representative of a wider population, ie that there is no genetic variation: this may not be true. Thus some sheep breeds absorb Cu more efficiently than others[19] and there are individual sheep within breeds which absorb P more efficiently than others[8]. Between-species differences may also be important. Comparisons of availability between the weanling rat and chick using a similar technique have given contrasting values for the availability of Zn^{13}, Fe^9 and lysine[2] in plant or animal foodstuffs: although the techniques used were of the WB concept, they nevertheless, emphasise the dangers of extrapolating from the sample tested. Wherever possible assessments should be made in genotypes which are representative of those to whom the data will be extrapolated.

Assessments of nutrient availability are usually made on food constituents and the investigator chooses a basal diet, often highly purified, in which to test the constituent: two examples (involving WB methods but not specific to them) illustrate the profound effect which this choice can make. Using the test-meal method to measure Fe 'availability' in wholewheat flour, it was found that it fell logarithmically from 0.60 to 0.09 as Fe in the pre-test diet increased from 8 to 1270 mg/kg: only 24 h exposure to the pre-test diets was needed to elicit the effect[6]. The assessment reflected the need for the consumer to absorb Fe from the pre-test diet rather than availability of Fe in the test diet. The second example relates to the assessment of Zn availability which is highly dependent on the level of Ca selected for the basal diet because of the Ca × Zn × phytate interaction. The common use of Ca-rich diets is justified in studies pertaining to poultry because of their high requirements for Ca, but underestimates the normal availability of Zn from phytate rich foods for species (including man) whose Ca requirements are much lower. The assessment of nutrient availability should be largely independent of the choice of basal diet.

The use of the test-meal generally involves an overnight fast to avoid the confounding effects of the basal diet and to ensure complete and rapid consumption of the test meal. Fasting itself may, however, have confounding effects: it enhances the uptake of minerals such as Fe^3 and Pb^{14} possibly by stimulating the production of mucin by the intestinal mucosa which in turn enhances absorption. Fasting is not a desirable prelude to the assessment of availability because it is likely to exaggerate the consumer's influence.

Extrinsic labels are often used in assessments of nutrient availability to simplify the task of tracing the flow of nutrient through the consumer but differences in mineral availability between extrinsically and intrinsically labelled foods are not uncommon[17]. The margin of disagreement reflects the inability of the tracer to exchange completely with the tracee and is likely to increase as the availability of the nutrient decreases. If there is good agreement, availability of the nutrient is probably not affected by the form or matrix in which it is presented. If a nutrient does vary in availability from one foodstuff to another, however, extrinsic labels are unlikely to indicate the true extent of the variation.

GI techniques for measuring nutrient availability. The techniques which give absolute estimates of nutrient availability (relative values have little use in terms of applied nutrition) while avoiding most of the above complications are many and varied though they have rarely been used to assess natural diets or constituents. In animals, radioisotopes are often essential to correct balance or retention data for faecal endogenous loss, and convert the method to one of GI concept. In the comparative balance method the excretion of tracer is measured after both i.v. and oral administration (eg[11]), but the oral tracer may not be a valid marker. The isotope dilution technique is preferable because it uses a combination of stable and radioisotope balance methods following a parenteral does of tracer and the tracer need only equilibrate with the endogenously secreted nutrient to give valid data (eg[12]). Thus, the availability of P in eight plant sources to sheep has been measured[8] and the availability of Zn in hay determined[18]: no other such estimates exist.

The isotope dilution principle can be used to estimate entry rates for a nutrient into the bloodstream following i.v. injection of tracer. The rates of change in enrichment of body pools (plasma or milk) between 3 to 6 weeks after dosing have been simply measured using the stable isotope ^{65}Cu to assess the availability of Cu in silage to cattle[4]; what is one of the few valid estimates of the availability of any mineral nutrient in this species was thus obtained. A similar application of stable isotopes to the study of nutrient availability in man is urgently required.

Valid measurements of availability can be obtained without radioisotopes. The availabilities of all amino acids can be derived simultaneously from their digestibility at the ileum, measured by the use of indigestible markers, with an appropriate correction for endogenous excretion[1]. If the endogenous loss is small and constant as it is for Ca in ruminants, balance data can be corrected to given measures of available Ca. Another approach is to measure nutrient absorption as the product of portal blood flow and arteriovenous differences in nutrient concentration: portal blood flow is not easily measured, however, and corrections for recycled nutrient are still required.

If the principal route of partition for a nutrient absorbed in excess of needs is to the urine, the slope of the relationship between amount ingested and excreted in urine can be a measure of availability (eg of Mg to cattle[7]): if it is to a body store then the relationship with amount stored gives an availability figure (eg of Cu to sheep[19]). With both methods corrections may be needed to deal with curvature in the response due to reduction in b and increases in e_1 and e_2 (Fig.) at high intakes.

When availabilities are less than 0.10, all balance methods are unlikely to be sensitive enough to measure quantitatively important variations in I-F (Fig.) in deriving availability values. Measurements of abI overcome this difficulty and it has been shown[16] that the repletion method can be used for such purposes. The relative rates of recovery in plasma Cu concentrations in hypocupraemic ewes given continuous intravenous or dietary supplies of Cu indicated the entry rates of absorbed Cu into the bloodstream, ie availability.

In-vitro methods. While *in-vivo* techniques are essential in the initial studies of nutrient availability, to provide a reference base, it is impractical to use them routinely for the purposes of dietary assessment and formulation because of the complexity and slowness. *In-vitro* methods can measure the (a) component of availability and this is often more important than the (b) component as a source of variation in availability (Fig.). The *in-vitro* approach is widely used to predict the availability of fermentable carbohydrate and degradable nitrogen for rumen microorganisms, the prime determinants of the host's response to energy and nitrogen: ultimately, it will have to be perfected for other nutrients and species. Microbial assays have been used widely, but they merely use microbes as crude detection devices: it would be surprising if they could not be improved upon. For example HPLC could be used to determine the amino acid and peptide profile of protein sources subjected to simulated digestion to give a simultaneous assessment of the availability of all the essential amino acids. Isotope dilution methods are being used to study the exchangeability of tracer and nutrient under conditions of simulated digestion[15] in the hope that there could be a good correlation between *in-vitro* exchangeability and aI. Another approach is to accumulate information on the most likely chemical determinants of nutrient availability in foodstuffs tested by valid *in-vivo* methods and to derive equations whereby availability can be predicted subsequently from the chemical analysis of the food. For example, the availability of Cu to sheep is determined largely by the Mo and S concentrations in the diet and these were found to account for 78 per cent of the variation in Cu availability in grazed herbage[17].

Application of availability data. The final requisite of a universal concept of availability (with its appropriate technology) is that it should generate useful information. The product of an availability coefficient (obtained by valid GI methods) and nutrient input gives almost a complete statement of dietary potential with respect to the nutrient: coupled with a coefficient for the efficiency of utilisation it can give a prediction of performance. The valid availability coefficient also allows gross nutrient requirements to be derived from the net requirements calculated by factorial methods: the same cannot be said of the relative measures of availability given by some methods of the WB concept (Table). The availability coefficient for a nutrient is a powerful and useful statistic, yet there are surprisingly few situations in which we can confidently say what the average value for a particular foodstuff is and whether there is significant variation about the mean.

Conclusions. We know little about nutrient availability because we have used unhelpful concepts and inappropriate techniques in trying to measure it. The concept of availability as largely a dietary attribute, determined by chemical composition, focuses attention on past errors. It is time to stop burdening the literature with invalid, relative or unusable values and to adopt techniques which yield valid, absolute and usable measurements of availability as a dietary attribute. Thus, the next international nutrition congress may be able to focus attention on the strengths and weaknesses of foods as nutrient sources rather than the same attributes of our techniques.

1 Austic, R.E. (1983): The availability of amino acids as an attribute of feeds. In *Proc. 2nd Symp. Int. Network Feed Information Centres*, ed G.E. Robards & R.G. Packham, pp. 175–189. Slough: Commonwealth Agricultural Bureaux.
2 Batterham, E.S. (1983): Species differences in ability to utilize lysine from different sources. In *Proc. 2nd Symp. Int. Network Feed Information Centres*, ed G.E. Robards & R.G. Packham, Ibid, pp. 291–298. Slough: Commonwealth Agricultural Bureaux.
3 Brise, H. (1962): Influence of meals on iron absorption in oral iron therapy. *Acta Med. Scand.* Suppl. 376 **59**, 39–45.
4 Buckley, W.T., Huckin, S.N. & Eigendorf, G.K. (1985): Stable isotope tracer methods for determining absorption of dietary copper in dairy cattle. In *Proc. 5th Int. Symp. on Trace element metabolism in man and animals*, ed C.F. Mills, I. Bremner & J.K. Chesters. Slough: Commonwealth Agricultural Bureaux. (In press).
5 Evans, G.W., Johnson, C.E. & Johnson, P.E. (1979): Zinc absorption in the rat determined by radioisotope dilution. *J. Nutr.* **109**, 1258–1264.
6 Fairweather-Tait, S.J. & Wright, A.J.A. (1984): The influence of previous iron intake on the estimation of bioavailability of Fe from a test meal given to rats. *Br. J. Nutr.* **51**, 185–191.
7 Field, A.C. & Suttle, N.F. (1979): Effect of high potassium and low magnesium intakes on the mineral metabolism of monozygotic twin cows. *J. Comp. Path.* **89**, 431–439.
8 Field, A.C., Woolliams, J.A., Dingwall, R.A. & Munro, C.S. (1984): Animal and dietary variation in the absorption and metabolism of phosphorus by sheep. *J. Agric. Sci. Camb.* **103**, 283–291.
9 Fritz, J.D., Pla, G.W., Roberts, T., Boehne, J.W. & Hove, E.L. (1970): Biological availability in animals of iron from common dietary sources. *J. Agric. Fd Chem.* **18**, 647–651.
10 Hansard, S.L., Crowder, H.M. & Lyke, W.A. (1957): The biological availability of calcium in feeds for cattle. *J. Anim. Sci.* **16**, 437–443.
11 Heth, D.A. & Hoekstra, W.G. (1965): Zinc 65 absorption and turnover in rats. 1. A procedure to determine ^{65}Zn absorption and the antagonistic effect of calcium in a practical diet. *J. Nutr.* **85**, 367–374.
12 House, W.A., Welch, R.M. & Van Campen, D.R. (1982): Effect of phytic acid on the absorption, distribution and endogenous excretion of zinc in rats. *J. Nutr.* **112**, 941–953.
13 O'Dell, B.L., Burpo, C.E. & Savage, J.E. (1972): Evaluation of zinc availability in foodstuffs of plant and animal origin. *J. Nutr.* **102**, 653–660.
14 Quarterman, J. & Morrison, E. (1981): Effects of short fasts on heavy metal absorption in the rat. In *Industrial and environmental xenobiotics*, ed I. Gut, M. Cikrt & G.L. Plaa. pp. 37–43. Heidelberg: Springer.
15 Schwarz, R., Belko, A.Z. & Wien, E.M. (1982): An *in-vitro* system for measuring intrinsic dietary mineral exchangeability: alternative to intrinsic isotopic labelling. *J. Nutr.* **112**, 497–504.
16 Suttle, NF. (1974): A technique for measuring the biological availability of copper to sheep using initially hypocupraemic ewes. *Br. J. Nutr.* **12**, 395–405.
17 Suttle, N.F. (1983): Assessment of the mineral and trace element status of feeds. In *Proc. 2nd Symp. Int. Network/Feed Information Centres*, ed G.E. Robards & R.G. Packham, pp. 211–237. Slough: Commonwealth Agricultural Bureaux.
18 Suttle, N.F., Lloyd Davies, H. & Field, A.C. (1982): A model for zinc metabolism in sheep given a diet of hay. *Br. J. Nutr.* **47**, 105–112.
19 Woolliams, J.A., Suttle, N.F., Wiener, G., Field, A.C. & Woolliams, C. (1983): Long term accumulation and depletion of copper in the liver of different breeds of sheep and fed diets of differing copper content. *J. Agric. Sci. Camb.* **100**, 441–449.

Availability of energy

R.L. BALDWIN
Department of Animal Science, University of California, Davis, California 95616, USA.

Investigation of the availability and usefulness of dietary energy to animals and man was initiated in the late 1800s. These investigations were based upon the foundation created by, among others, Lavoisier, von Liebig, Regnault and von Voit. These workers had established the essential relationships among combustion, heat production, the chemical composition of foods, respiratory exchange, and nitrogen excretion which culminated in establishment of the theoretical bases of direct and indirect calorimetry and demonstration, by Rubner, that the first law of thermodynamics — conservation of energy — applies to animal systems[10]. Prominent workers during the late 1800s included Rubner, Armsby, Atwater and Kellner[2]. Although they used somewhat different terms, these workers established the basic classification of energetic relationships we use today to describe availability of energy[16] — see Figure.

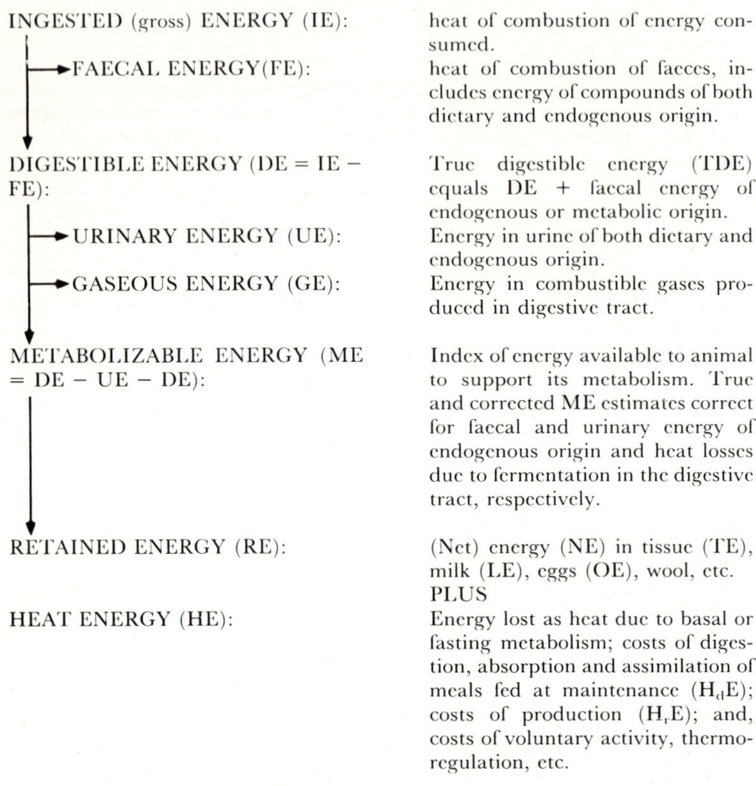

Figure. *Basic classification of energetic relationships*

Use of heats of combustion of feeds or foods consumed (IE) as an index of availability was discarded by these workers because of large differences among foods in their digestibilities. Use of ME as an index was preferred over DE because of variation in losses due to combustible gases and incomplete combustion of, largely, protein. Correction of ME estimates for endogenous energy losses in faeces and urine and for heat of fermentation were (are), generally, not applied because of difficulties with routine measurement of these. Differences of opinion arose with regard to application of this scheme. Armsby (1917)[2] and Atwater & Bryant (1900)[3] took the view that availability of a feed or food should be assessed in terms of energy delivered to and metabolizable by the animal (ME). This view led to development of the physiological fuel value (PFV) and total digestible nutrient (TDN) systems which found wide acceptance and are still in use today. Kellner[2] took the alternate view that feeds should be assessed in terms not only of energy delivered to the animal, but also in terms of usefulness to the animal, ie net conversion to product. This led to development of the starch equivalent (SE) system which also found wide acceptance and is still in use today.

Analytical aspects. At the turn of the century, methods for analysis of all components of the major nutrient fractions of foods — carbohydrate, protein and lipid — were not available. As a result, estimates of ME values of foods were based upon proximate composition, coefficients of digestibility, heats of combustion and energy loss in urine.

Fat was determined after extraction using ether and was thus, largely, triacylglycerol with a heat of combustion of about 39 kJ/g (9.4 kcal/g). Application of an average digestion coefficient for fat determined for a wide variety of foods led to the 'generalized' factor of 37.6 kJ/g (9.0 kcal) for the ME value of fat[3]. Actual values for heat of combustion of triacylglycerols vary from 37.9 to 39.7 kJ/g (9.1 to 9.5 kcal/g) leading to some error when the generalized factor is used but, more important, is the fact that the more polar solvents used for lipid extraction today, chloroform-methanol for example, achieve a more complete extraction than attained with ether[8]. The additional lipids extracted are, largely, phospholipids which have a heat of combustion of 29 kJ/g (6.9 kcal/g) and more variable digestibilities than triacylglycerol[12]. Consideration of the chemical nature of extracted lipids leads to more accurate estimates of metabolizability.

Protein is estimated from nitrogen content and a factor — usually 6.25. More recently, factors specific to the percentage nitrogen in proteins of individual foods have been utlized[7,14]. Generally, no corrections are applied for non-protein nitrogen compounds in foods. Errors in estimates of ME values incurred due to use of inappropriate factors and failure to account for non-protein nitrogen are small, because, after correction of DE values of protein for energy losses in urine, the 'generalized' factor of 16.7 kJ/g (4 kcal/g) obtained for protein is the same as the 'generalized' factor for carbohydrate. Since carbohydrate contents of foods are (most) often calculated by difference, errors in estimates of protein content are incorporated into estimates of carbohydrate content and, from an energetic point of view, the errors cancel. Development and application of specific and direct methods for analysis of carbohydrates in foods[19] eliminate compensatory errors and require more specific consideration of proteins and non-protein nitrogen in foods. Most adjustments of the apparent digestibility coefficient of 93.5 per cent applied by Atwater & Bryant[3] for proteins in mixed diets have been small. However, the digestibility values of protein of animal and plant origin differ significantly leading to physiological fuel values of 17.9 kJ/g (4.28 kcal/g) and 15.0 kJ/g (3.58 kcal/g), respectively. Thus, the generalized factor of 16.7 kJ/g (4.0 kcal/g) represents respective contributions of animal and plant protein to total protein intake of 60 and 40 per cent[11]. When groups consume considerably less protein of animal origin a lower factor should be applied.

Based upon heats of combustion of mixed carbohydrates and digestion coefficients averaged across foods, Atwater & Bryant[3] set the 'generalized' factor for carbohydrate at 16.7 kJ/g or (4 kcal/g). At the turn of the century, methods alternative to estimation of carbohydrate by difference were not available. For food commonly consumed by humans the generalized factor for carbohydrate has worked well and is in widespread, current use. For diets commonly consumed by livestock, which contain considerably more fibre, it was recognized early that application of the generalized factor of 1.0 for carbohydrate used in the TDN system led to considerable error. This led to separation of carbohydrate into a (weak) acid soluble and/or hydrolyzable fraction (nitrogen-free extract) and an insoluble, not-acid-hydrolyzable fraction (crude fibre). After application of (measured) digestion coefficients for these in a feed, TDN content is calculated using a generalized factor of 1.0.

Suggested changes in existing systems have taken two directions: simplified, more highly aggregated and empirical approaches; and, approaches requiring less empiricism and deaggregation. A premise underlying the latter approach is that explicit consideration of a greater number of sources of variance will reduce coefficients of variation in comparisons of observed compared with predicted responses while aggregation usually leads to greater coefficients of variation. However, both approaches must be considered because accuracy achieved with highly aggregated systems is often sufficient for many purposes. Also, implementation of deaggregated systems requires a great many more measurements, data and expense.

In the direction of aggregation, estimation of ME values (MJ/kg) from estimates of the gross energy (GE; MJ/kg) and total nitrogen content (g/kg) of (human) diet composites has been proposed[9] using the equation $ME = 0.976GE - 33.3N - 250.2$. The following relationship was proposed for human diets[13]: $ME = 0.95GE - 31.4N$. The equation $ME = 0.977GE - 27.6N - $

16.7UC was presented for human diets where UC = unavailable carbohydrate (g/kg diet)[20]. The following relationship was proposed to estimate feed conversion to fat (NEF) by ruminants[18]: NEF = 10.5DCP + 36.9D fat + 7.0DCF + 13.6NFE, where DCP = digestible crude protein, DCF = digestible crude fibre and NFE = nitrogen free extract (all expressed in g/100 g diet). A compendium of equations for estimating DE and ME values for feeds from proximate composition has also been presented[6].

In the direction of deaggregation, or more explicit consideration of causes of variation in energy availability, consider the UK system wherein 'available carbohydrate' is estimated from direct determinations of specific carbohydrates in foods[19], the extensive work on the chemical composition of feeds carried out by Van Soest and colleagues[21], the New Zealand system for feed analysis in which the 'carbohydrate' fraction is partitioned into sugars, organic acids, pectins, starch, hemicellulose and cellulose[5], and definition of the products formed from each carbohydrate fraction during fermentation in the rumen[15]. In view of increasing use of fructose in place of sucrose and current interest in 'complex' carbohydrates and dietary fibre, more exact definition seems appropriate. Also, these efforts are leading toward more exact definition of not only energy available from foods but also quantitative estimates of amounts of each nutrient absorbed. Since individual nutrients differ significantly in efficiencies with which they support work and productive processes[4], estimates of amounts of nutrients absorbed might be considered superior to simple definition of availability of energy.

Improvement of old and development of new systems. Impetus to develop new systems for assessments of nutritive value arise either from observations that predictions made using a current system deviate greatly and/or systematically from reality; or, from significant advances in understanding which partially invalidate concepts which underlie an existing system. In either case, adoption of a new system should be based upon a clear demonstration of superiority, ie average error of prediction is reduced. This requirement has not always been fulfilled in practice since perception of superiority has often been sufficient to justify adoption of a new system. Herein, we will make the assumption that newer systems are better than older ones and that systems currently under development will be still better.

Systematic errors of prediction are most easily identified and addressed. The PFV and TDN systems were based upon measurements of digestibility at maintenance level intakes. Two problems arise from this. First, digestibility decreases as feed intake increases such that energy availability can be seriously overestimated in animals consuming 2 to 5 times their maintenance requirement. For example, in cattle the respective digestibilities of concentrate feeds and forages decrease two and four percentage units for each multiple of intake above maintenance. The second problem is that at maintenance level feeding, dietary protein is used as an energy source and has an energy value equal to carbohydrate. In rapidly growing animals, protein provided above maintenance is incorporated into tissue and has a energetic value about 30 per cent greater than carbohydrate. In humans, these problems are not important because food intake by humans rarely exceeds 1.1 — 1.15 times maintenance. In other species, with intakes of 2 to 3 times maintenance during growth and 3 to 5 times maintenance during lactation, corrections for changes in digestibility and energy values assigned protein are appropriate.

Another systematic error was noted in application of early systems to farm animals, particularly, ruminants: a unit of TDN derived from cereals yields greater performance than a unit of TDN from forage. In the starch equivalent system, the value of corn relative to forage is greater for fattening than for maintenance. These errors are due to differences in efficiencies of utlization of the differing products of digestion from cereals and forages. The current ARC system[1] for ruminant feeding corrects for this systematic error by changing efficiency estimates for ME use for maintenance and production as a function of energy contents (MJ of ME/kg) of diets.

The starch equivalent system is based upon net rather than metabolizable energy concepts[12]. In this system, feeds are assigned a value relative to starch based upon the amount of fattening they support in adult animals fed above maintenance. Systematic errors in predicting performance using this system were alluded to above and arise from the fact that differing nutrients are used at differing efficiencies for different functions even when evaluated on a relative (to starch) scale. The current NRC system[17] accommodates this type of error by assigning feeds multiple net energy values: net energy for maintenance value based upon the amount of body energy spared by a kg of feed in animals fed below maintenance; and, a net energy for gain value based upon the incremental increase in retained energy resulting from consumption of a kg of feed by growing animals. This approach is highly analogous to the ARC approach in which varying efficiencies of ME use for maintenance, gain, lactation, etc are used.

Concluding statements. Some, but not all, errors encountered with the early systems of feed and food evaluation were identified and changes made to correct these during evolution of newer systems were alluded to. To date, emphasis has been placed upon evolving systems based upon the energy classification scheme developed at the turn of the century and progress has been good. Many current systems evaluate energy availability from foods and feeds with excellent accuracy and lead to excellent predictions of animal performance. Not all types of errors have been accommodated, however. Some of these can be addressed within the classical framework but others may not be. Examples are that 118 MJ (28 Mcal) of acetate must be oxidized to provide the same amount of ATP for use in work supplied by oxidation of 100 MJ (23.9 Mcal) of glucose; and, that the relative efficiencies of use of acetate, glucose and diet fat for fattening are 60–70 per cent, 75–80 per cent and 92–96 per cent, respectively[4]. Thus, the true availability of energy for use by an animal considered in terms of amount of work that can be done, growth attained or milk produced varies dependent upon the chemical form of the energy provided. Current systems account for this implicitly and perhaps this is often sufficient. On the other hand, considerable data now exist which indicate that pattern of nutrients (energy sources) absorbed can affect how nutrients are partitioned among functions. Might we not consider, at least at the research level, assessing availabilities of diets not only in terms of total energy provided but also in terms of amounts of specific nutrients provided?

1 Agricultural Research Council. (1980): *The nutrient requirements of ruminant livestock*, pp. 24–117. London: HMSO.

2 Armsby, H.P. (1917): *The nutrition of farm animals*. New York: The Macmillan Company.

3 Atwater, W.O. & Bryant, A.P. (1900): *The availability and fuel value of food materials*, pp. 73–110. 12th Annual Report (1899) of the Storrs, CT Agricultural Experiment Station.

4 Baldwin, R.L. & Smith, N.E. (1979): Regulation of energy metabolism in ruminants. In *Advances in nutritional research*, Vol. 2, ed H.H. Draper, pp. 1–27. New York: Plenum Press.

5 Butler, G.W. & Bailey, R.W. (1973): *Chemistry and biochemistry of herbage*. London: Academic Press.

6 Fonnesbeck, P.V., Wardeh, M.F. & Harris, L.E. (1984): *Mathematical models for estimating energy and protein utilization of feedstuffs*. Bull. 508. International Feedstuffs Institute, Utah State University, Logan UT.

7 Jones, D.B. (1931): *Factors for converting percentages of nitrogen in foods and feeds into percentages of proteins*, pp. 1–22. US Department of Agriculture Circular No. 183.

8 Kinsella, J.E., Posati, L., Weihrauch, J. & Anderson, B. (1975): Lipids in foods: problems and procedures in collating data. *CRC Crit. Rev. Food Technol.* **5**, 299–324.

9 Levy, L.M., Bernstein, L.M. & Grossman, M.I. (1958): *The caloric content of urine of human beings and the estimation of metabolizable energy of foodstuffs*, pp. 1–61. Report No. 226. US Army Medical Research and Nutrition Laboratory. Denver: Fitzsimons Army Hospital.

10 Lusk, G. (1922): A history of metabolism. *Endocrinol. Metabol.* **3**, 3–78

11 Merrill, A.L. & Watt, B.K. (1973): *Energy values of foods: basics and derivation*, pp. 1–105. US Department of Agriculture Handbook No. 74.

12 Miles, C.W., Hardison, N., Weihrauch, J.L., Bodwell, C.E. & Prather, E.S. (1984): Heats of combustion of chemically different lipids. *J. Am. Diet. Ass.* **84**, 659–664.

13 Miller, D.S. & Payne, P.R. (1959): A ballistic bomb calorimeter. *Br. J. Nutr.* **13**, 501–508.

14 Morr, C.V. (1981): Nitrogen conversion factors for several soybean protein products. *J. Fd Sci.* **46**, 1362–1367.

15 Murphy, M.R., Baldwin, R.L. & Koong, L.J. (1982): Estimation of stoichiometric parameters for rumen fermentation of roughage and concentrate diets. *J. Anim. Sci.* **55**, 411–421.

16 National Research Council. (1981): *Nutritional energetics of domestic animals and glossary of energy terms*, pp. 1–54. Washington DC: National Academy Press.

17 National Research Council. (1984): *Nutrient requirements of beef cattle*, pp. 2–6. Washington DC: National Academy Press.

18 Nehring, K. & Haenlein, G.F.W. (1973): Feed evaluation and ration calculation based on net energy. *J. Anim. Sci.* **36**, 949–964.

19 Paul, A.A. & Southgate, D.A.T. (1978): *McCance and Widdowson's 'The composition of foods'*, 4th edn. New York: Elsevier/North Holland.

20 Southgate, D.A.T. (1975): Fiber and other unavailable carbohydrates and energy effects in the diet. In *Proceedings of the Western Hemisphere Nutrition Congress IV*, pp. 51–55. ed P.L. White & N Selvey. Acton, MA: Publishing Sciences Group.

21 Van Soest, P.J. (1982): *Nutritional ecology of the ruminant*, pp. 1–344. Portland, OR: Durham and Downey.

Variations in the availability of carbohydrates

D.J.A. JENKINS, Alexandra L. JENKINS, T.M.S. WOLEVER, Lilian U. THOMPSON and A. Venkat RAO
Department of Nutritional Sciences, Faculty of Medicine, Division of Endocrinology and Metabolism, St. Michael's Hospital, University of Toronto, Toronto, Ontario, Canada M5S 1A8.

The issue of carbohydrate availability is a broad one with many important implications. Some types of carbohydrate which are totally unavailable in the small intestine may be salvaged as short-chain fatty acids (SCFA) in the colon. Of overall importance in this respect is the rate at which the carbohydrate is digested and absorbed for this will determine both the fraction which is truly available and the form in which it is absorbed.

Absorption along the gut and the factors involved. A model for carbohydrate availability is shown in the Fig. When a mixture of carbohydrates is eaten, in general, the sugars are available for absorption as soon as the food enters the duodenum. The starches are digested in the lumen by pancreatic amylase to liberate glucose, maltose, maltotriose and oligosaccharides which are then cleaved to glucose at the brush border and absorbed. Depending on the nature of the starch and the other factors present in the food the efficiency of this process is reduced and a proportion of the starch, perhaps as much as 10–20 per cent, may enter the colon[1,29]. Also entering the colon together with this starch will, by definition, be that fraction of the total food carbohydrate which is classed as dietary fibre. Once in the colon the starch, most of the hemicellulosic material and a smaller proportion of the cellulose will be fermented to SCFA and gases by colonic bacteria and the SCFA rapidly absorbed[5]. These will thus become available to contribute to the energy requirements of the host. The unfermented carbohydrate will contribute to faecal bulk and be eliminated.

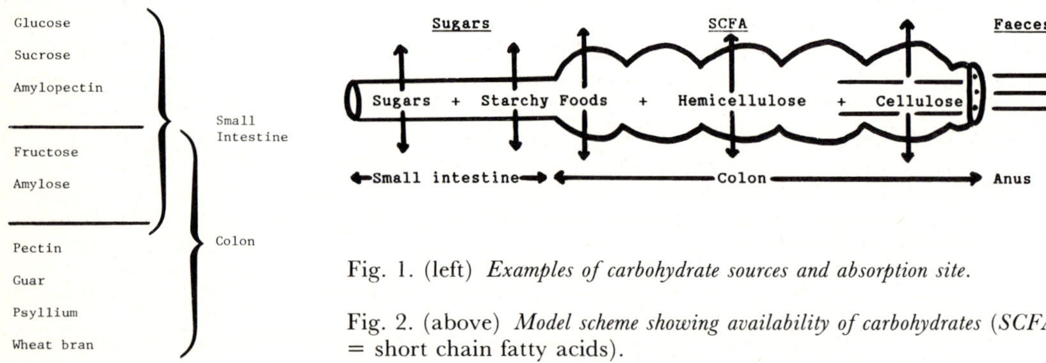

Fig. 1. (left) *Examples of carbohydrate sources and absorption site.*

Fig. 2. (above) *Model scheme showing availability of carbohydrates (SCFA = short chain fatty acids).*

There is thus a partitioning of carbohydrate into that which is available as sugars in the small intestine and that which is available as SCFA in the colon. However, the other and simpler classification of carbohydrates as simple sugars as opposed to complex carbohydrates is not helpful in this respect. As shown starches will tend to be absorbed in the small intestine, a process favoured by a high amylopectin/amylose ratio, while certain sugars, eg fructose and sorbitol, which are slowly absorbed, may enter the colon, the amount depending on the dose taken.

Differences in rates of digestion and glycaemic response. Undoubtedly much interest has focused on carbohydrate availability, the rate of carbohydrate assimilation and the metabolic consequences of manipulating these variables, and on the glycaemic response to foods. Because of the many factors involved it is not surprising that over the past half decade it has become clear that different starchy foods are digested at different rates[12]. The rates of digestion *in vitro* using pooled human digestive juices also appear to relate well to the glycaemic responses observed *in vivo* after feeding equicarbohydrate portions of these foods to normal[12] and diabetic[18] volunteers. Certain foods, especially the legumes, were digested slowly *in vitro* and also produced some of the flattest glycaemic responses *in vivo*[19,20]. As much as three-fold differences were observed in rates of digestion and degree of blood glucose rise between different starchy foods[26].

Food factors affecting digestion. Many food factors and food components play a major role in determining the rate of digestion and hence the rate, site and amount of carbohydrate absorbed. These include the food form, fibre content, starch-nutrient (protein or fat) interactions and the presence of the so-called antinutrients such as phytates, lectins, tannins, saponins and enzyme inhibitors.

Thus, for example, in relation to food form, white spaghetti is digested more slowly and gives half the glycaemic response of white bread. Although the use of durum wheat in spaghetti may be important, the compact structure of spaghetti may retard penetration of enzymes and be a determining factor in reducing the rate of digestion. Particle size also plays a major role. Whole rice is more slowly digested and raises the blood glucose less than ground rice. Pumpernickel bread made with whole rye kernels results in a flatter blood glucose response curve than whole meal rye bread made from ground flour[21].

In addition, the higher the amylose content of a starch the less rapidly it is digested and the less it raises the blood glucose. This probably relates to the ease of access to enzymatic attack of the open branched structure of amylopectin starch as opposed to the compact nature of the amylose starch. Thus legumes are digested less rapidly than bread and release more maltose and glucose and less maltotriose than bread, an indication of their higher amylose content[16]. Rice with a high amylose content raises the blood glucose less than rice with a higher amylopectin content[8].

Processing, such as cooking, or modification of the starch will alter digestibility[31] as will the natural starch nutrient interactions present in the food. Thus although blending cooked lentils or cooking them to 60 min (three times as long as necessary) had little effect on digestibility or glycaemic response, heating and drying them for 12 h enhanced both the rate of digestion and the postprandial blood glucose rise[16].

The non-nutrient components in foods appear to be potentially important determinants of absorption and subsequent metabolic events. Fibre, especially viscous fibre, has been shown to alter the activity of enzymes involved in luminal digestion[10] and was shown early on to reduce the postprandial glycaemic and insulin responses of healthy volunteers[13] and diabetics[14]. In the longer term fibre was demonstrated to improve many aspects of diabetic control[2,22,28] in addition to reducing serum lipids[2,15,22,24,28].

The effects of the so-called antinutrients which are often associated with dietary fibre may exert a powerful influence on digestion, absorption and subsequent postprandial nutrient and endocrine fluxes. Thus lectins, although heat-labile, are found in appreciable concentrations in many starchy foods[25] and have been shown to relate well to the glycaemic responses to the foods tested in both normal and diabetic volunteers[27]. When added to bread, kidney bean lectin (but not concanavalin A) reduced the rate of digestion *in vitro*[2]. Similarly, phytic acid added to bread in the quantities found in beans reduced the rate of digestion *in vitro* and the glycaemic response *in vivo*. The effect could be minimised by addition of Ca^{++}[32].

Physiological mechanisms which may alter the rate of absorption. There has been considerable debate as to whether the effect of food factors in modifying absorption has been the result of their actions on gastric emptying or small intestinal absorption. Initially, studies focused on gastric emptying as the mechanism by which absorption could be delayed[9,23]. Food studies, such as the comparison between potatoes, whole and ground rice, had demonstrated that there was a good correlation between gastric emptying rate and postprandial glycaemia[30]. However, detailed studies with viscous fibres, guar and pectin have failed to confirm the originally established correlation between delayed gastric emptying and flattened glycaemic response[3] but rather emphasized the importance of small intestinal events as explored in jejunal perfusion studies[3,7]. In these an increase in the thickness of the unstirred water layer was seen with pectin[7] while with guar an overall impedence of luminal diffusion was demonstrated in elegant studies, which also demonstrated the impedence of luminal diffusion was demonstrated in elegant studies, which also demonstrated the impedance to uptake of Na^+ and Cl^- in the presence of viscous fibre[3]. In dealing with foods it is also likely that small intestinal effects are of great importance since, with legumes, delayed gastric emptying does not relate to their marked effect in flattening the glycaemic response[30].

Thus the balance between the rate of gastric emptying and small intestinal absorption is likely to influence the site and amount of carbohydrate absorbed. However, the position is not always clear cut. Pectin which delays the rate of absorption in healthy volunteers[3], reduces the loss of glucose to the colon when given to patients with dumping syndrome[11]. This is probably related to the increased small intestinal transit time seen with pectin which allows more efficient absorption.

Colonic recovery of carbohydrate. All the dietary fibre, some sugars such as raffinose and stachyose, and a proportion of the starch escape absorption in the small intestine and enter the colon. Breath H_2 and ileostomy studies[29] indicate that 7–20 per cent of the starch in bread enters the colon. With other foods, such as legumes, the percentage lost may be higher[16]. In the colon, carbohydrates are fermented by colonic bacteria to the short-chain fatty acids (SCFA) acetate, propionate and butyrate which may be used for bacterial cell synthesis, to nourish the colonic mucosa (butyrate) and to take part in whole body metabolism after absorption (acetate and propionate)[6].

Studies in man have indicated that the appearance of labelled $^{14}CO_2$ is as rapid when labelled glucose is given by caecal intubation as when the same amount of labelled glucose was taken by mouth[4]. In studies with germ-free rats the same workers demonstrated that while labelled $^{14}CO_2$ was rapidly evolved after caecal instillation of labelled acetate and lactate none was produced after glucose, a clear indication of the need for bacteria to produce SCFA from glucose to allow absorption.

Subsequent studies have indicated the differential uptake and utilization of SCFAs in man from fresh post mortem specimens. Little butyrate is found in portal blood despite substantial amounts in the gut lumen. Propionate levels fall dramatically across the liver suggesting significant uptake by that organ. Acetate is reported as the dominant SCFA in peripheral blood[6].

The carbohydrate substrates for colonic SCFA production include malabsorbed starch, unabsorbable sugars (such as raffinose and stachyose), pectins and gums and other hemicellulosic dietary fibres, the majority of which are completely fermented. In addition, a proportion of the cellulose component of dietary fibre is broken down depending on the plant source.

Conclusion. To a very large extent the energy from carbohydrate foods is made available after absorption at some point along the gastrointestinal tract either as sugars (eg glucose, fructose, galactose) in the small intestine or as SCFA (together with alcohol and lactate) in the colon. The distinction between dietary fibre and 'available carbohydrate', although of great importance, must be seen in these terms. Thus some starch and sugars (fructose, sorbitol) are not absorbed in the small intestine but are retrieved as SCFA from the colon along with the SCFAs from a large proportion of certain rapidly degraded dietary fibre (eg pectins and gums).

The rate of digestion determines both the site of absorption and the metabolic effect of the carbohydrate. Many factors in foods influence this including the nature of the carbohydrate, the food form and the presence of so-called antinutrients.

In turn, those carbohydrates which are released slowly in the small intestine have attracted much interest in the treatment of diabetes and raised blood lipids. The carbohydrate fermented in the colon may have a value in nourishing colonic mucosa, contributing to energy balance and regulating aspects of intermediary metabolism of the host and cell types and numbers of colonic bacteria. That carbohydrate which is truly unavailable will contribute to faecal bulk. Availability in terms of carbohydrate is thus a multifaceted subject.

Acknowledgements. The authors studies in relation with this work have been supported by Strategic and Operating Grants of the Canadian Natural Sciences and Engineering Research Council.

1 Anderson, I.H., Levine, A.S. & Levitt, M.D. (1981): Incomplete absorption of the carbohydrate in all-purpose wheat flour. *New Engl. J. Med.* **304**, 891–892.

2 Aro, A., Uusitupa, M., Vontilainen, E., Hersio, K., Korhonen, T. & Siitonen, O. (1981): Improved diabetic control and hypocholesterolemic effect induced by long term dietary supplementation with guar gum in Type 2 (insulin-dependent) diabetes. *Diabetologia* **21**, 29–33.

3 Blackburn, N.A., Redfern, J.S., Jarjis, H., Holgate, A.M., Hanning, I., Scarpello, J.H.B., Johnson, I.T. & Read, N.W. (1984): The mechanism of action of guar gum in improving glucose tolerance in man. *Clin. Sci.* **66**, 329–336.

4 Bond, J.H. & Levitt, M.D. (1976): Fate of soluble carbohydrate in the colon of rats and man. *J. Clin. Invest.* **57**, 1158–1164.

5 Cummings, J.A. (1981): Short chain fatty acids in the human colon. *Gut* **22**, 763–779.

6 Cummings, J.H. (1985): *Fiber and short chain fatty acids (SCFA) in dietary fiber: basic and clinical aspects*, ed G. Vahonny & D. Kritchevsky. New York: Plenum.

7 Flourie, B., Vidor, N., Florent, C.H. & Berrier, J.J. (1984): Effect of pectin on jejunal glucose absorption and unstirred layer thickness in normal man. *Gut* **25**, 936–941.

8 Goddard, M.S., Young, G. & Marcus, R. (1984): The effect of amylose content on insulin and glucose responses to ingested rice. *Am. J. Clin. Nutr.* **39**, 388–392.

9 Holt, S., Heading, R.C., Carter, D.C., Prescott, L.F. & Tothill, P. (1979): Effect of gel fibre on gastric emptying and absorption of glucose and paracetamol. *Lancet* **1**, 636–639.

10 Isaksson, G., Lundquist, I. & Ihse, I. (1982): Effect of dietary fiber on pancreatic enzyme activity *in vitro*: the importance of viscosity, pH, ionic strength, absorption, and time of incubation. *Gastroenterology* **82**, 918–924.

11 Jenkins, D.J.A., Gassull, M.A., Leeds, A.R. *et al.* (1977): Effect of dietary fiber on complications of gastric surgery: prevention of postprandial hypoglycemia by pectin. *Gastroenterology* **73**, 215–217.

12 Jenkins, D.J.A., Ghafari, H., Wolever, T.M.S., Taylor, R.H., Barker, H.M., Fielden, H., Jenkins, A.L. & Bowling, A.C. (1982): Relationship between the rate of digestion of foods and postprandial glycaemia. *Diabetologia* **22**, 450–455.

13 Jenkins, D.J.A., Leeds, A.R., Gassull, M.A., Cochet, B. & Alberti, K.G.M.M. (1977): Decrease in postprandial insulin and glucose concentrations by guar and pectin. *Ann. Int. Med.* **36**, 20–23.

14 Jenkins, D.J.A., Leeds, A.R., Gassull, M.A., Wolever, T.M.S., Goff, D.V., Alberti, A.G.M.M. & Hockaday, T.D.R. (1976): Unabsorbable carbohydrates and diabetes: Decreased postprandial hyperglycaemia. *Lancet* **2**, 172–174.

15 Jenkins, D.J.A., Reynolds, D., Slavin, B., Leeds, A.R., Jenkins, A.L. & Jepson, E.M. (1980): Dietary fiber and blood lipids: treatment of hypercholesterolemia with guar crispbread. *Am. J. Clin. Nutr.* **33**, 575–581.

16 Jenkins, D.J.A., Thorne, M.J., Camelon, K., Jenkins, A.L., Rao, A.V., Taylor, R.H., Thompson, L.U., Kalmusky, J., Reichert, R. & Francis, T. (1982): Effect of processing on digestibility and the blood glucose response: A study of lentils. *Am J. Clin. Nutr.* **36**, 1093–1101.

18 Jenkins, D.J.A., Wolever, T.M.S., Thorne, M.J., Jenkins, A.L., Wong, G.S., Josse, R.G. & Csima, A. (1984): The relationship between glycemic response, digestibility, and factors influencing the dietary habits of diabetics. *Am. J. Clin. Nutr.* **40**, 1175–1191.

19 Jenkins, D.J.A., Wolever, T.M.S., Taylor, R.H., Barker, H.M., Rielden, H. & Gassull, M.A. (1981): Lack of effect of refining on the glycemic response to cereals. *Diabetes Care* **4**, 509–513.

20 Jenkins, D.J.A., Wolever, T.M.S., Jenkins, A.L., Lee, R., Wong, G.S. & Josse, R. (1983): Glycemic response to wheat products: reduced response to pasta but no effect of fiber. *Diabetes Care* **6**, 155–159.
21 Jenkins, D.J.A., Wolever, T.M.S., Jenkins, A.L., Kalmusky, J., Giordana, C., Thompson, L.U., Wong, G.S. & Josse, R.G. (1985): The glycemic indices of rye breads of rye kernels. Submitted for publication.
22 Jenkins, D.J.A., Wolever, T.M.S., Taylor, R., Reynolds, D., Nineham, R. & Hockaday, T.D.R. (1980): Diabetic glucose control, lipids, and trace elements on long term guar. *Br. Med. J.* **1**, 1353–1354.
23 Leeds, A.R., Ralphs, D.N., Boulos, P., Ebied, F., Metz, G.L., Dilawari, J., Elliott, A. & Jenkins, D.J.A. (1978): Pectin and gastric emptying in the dumping syndrome. *Proc. Nutr. Soc.* **37**, 23A.
24 Miettinen, T.A. & Tarpila, S. (1977): Effect of pectin on serum cholesterol, fecal bile acids, and biliary lipids in normolipidemic and hyperlipidemic individuals. *Clin. Chim. Acta* **79**, 471.
25 Nachbar, M.S. & Oppenheim, J.D. (1980): Lectins in the United States diet: a survey of lectins in commonly consumed foods and a review of the literature. *Am. J. Clin. Nutr.* **33**, 2338.
26 O'Dea, K., Nestel, P.J. & Antonoff, L. (1980): Physical factors influencing postprandial glucose and insulin responses to starch. *Am. J. Clin. Nutr.* **33**, 760–765.
27 Rae, R., Thompson, L.U. & Jenkins, D.J.A. (1985): Effect of lectins on digestibility *in vitro* and on the glycemic response to foods. *Nutr. Res.* (In press).
28 Smith, U. & Holm, G. (1982): Effect of a modified guar gum preparation on glucose and lipid levels in diabetics and healthy volunteers. *Atherosclerosis* **45**, 1–10.
29 Stephen, A.M., Haddad, A.C. & Phillips, S.E. (1983): Passage of carbohydrate into the colon: direct measurements in humans. *Gastroenterology* **85**, 589–595.
30 Torsdottir, I., Alpsten, M., Andersson, D., Brummer, R.J.M. & Anderson, H. (1984): Effect of different starchy foods in composite meals on gastric emptying rate and glucose metabolism. In comparisons between potatoes, rice and white beans. *Hum. Nutr.: Clin. Nutr.* **38C**, 329–338.
31 Wurzburg, O. (1985): Nutritional aspects and safety of modified food starches. In *The nutritional re-emergence of starchy foods*. Marabou Symposium 12, (In press).
32 Yoon, J.H., Thompson, L.U. & Jenkins, D.J.A. (1983): The effect of phytic acid on *in vitro* rate of starch digestibility and blood glucose response. *Am. J. Clin. Nutr.* **38**, 835–842.

Availability of amino acids

E.S. BATTERHAM
Department of Agriculture, Agricultural Research Centre, Wollongbar, NSW 2480, Australia.

The search for techniques to assess protein quality and subsequently amino-acid availability can be characterized by three main phases. In the first, up until the late 1950s, emphasis was directed towards techniques for assessing protein quality: biological value, net protein utilization, and protein efficiency ratio. With the advances in amino acid technology in the early 1960s, the emphasis changed to developing techniques for assessing individual amino-acid availability. This phase was one of considerable activity and substantial progress was made. From the mid 1970s until now, there appears to have been a decline in interest in this field with most activity concentrating on refining the advances made in the 1960s to mid 1970s. This decline in interest in part appears to stem from the belief that the major problems in the field have been solved and that the availability of amino acids is no longer a major problem.

This complacency appears misplaced, and the development of suitable techniques for estimating availability remains as elusive as ever.

Definition of availability. There has been considerable confusion created by the lack of a generally accepted definition of 'availability'. The word 'available' has been assigned to a host of *in vitro* and *in vivo* techniques, ranging from simple dye-binding tests to more complex biological assays. The Little Oxford Dictionary defines 'availability' as 'capable of being used' and in this context the word 'availability' is applied to amino acids to mean 'an amino acid is in a form suitable for digestion, absorption and utilization'. Thus 'availability' is a measure of potential 'usability' of an amino acid.

Determining amino-acid availability. Availability can only be measured by techniques that taken into account the amount of an amino acid that is digested, absorbed and utlized by an animal when fed a diet containing the test amino acid as the limiting amino acid. The techniques used are called growth assays, or more precisely, slope-ratio or parallel assays, depending on the design of the treatments. With these techniques, the animal is given a control diet adequate in all nutrients except the test amino acid, and the response to graded additions of the test amino acid is assessed. The test protein is also incorporated into the control diet, to supply graded levels of the test amino acid and the animal's response expressed as a proportion or ratio of the response to the test amino acid. There are a number of criteria which must be applied to ensure the statistical validity of the assay[6].

Obviously, slope-ratio assays are time consuming, relatively expensive, and limited in through-put as only one amino acid can be assessed at a time. Being based on biological responses, they also have inherently higher standard errors than those associated with many analytical techniques. Considerable care has also to be taken with dietary formulations to minimize the effects of other nutrients contributed by the test protein source. Despite these limitations, slope-ratio assays are the only techniques currently available for assessing the proportion of an amino acid in a food which is usable by the animal.

Techniques for estimating availability. A considerable number of techniques have been proposed for estimating amino-acid availability. Of these, chemical tests for reactive lysine[7] and more recently, ileal digestibility assays, have been the most widely adopted.

Relevance of the techniques for estimating availability. Only a limited number of experiments have been conducted to assess the ability of the different techniques to predict availability for a wide range of protein sources and for different species. Most comparisons indicate little relationship between these techniques and lysine availability, particularly for pigs and rats.

Pigs. The development of a slope-ratio assay to determine lysine availability in protein concentrates, and for assessing the usefulness of other *in vivo* and *in vitro* assays for estimating availability, has been reported[2]. The availability of lysine in a number of protein concentrates, and comparisons with the direct- and indirect-1-fluoro-2,4-dinitrobenzene (FDNB) chemical assays are presented in Table 1.These results show that availability varied considerably and these differences were not detected by the chemical assays. This suggests that the reductions in availabilities were not associated with Maillard-type reactions and presumably indicate reactions between amino acids within the protein molecule. It seems likely that Maillard-type reactions are more likely to occur in proteins rich in reducing sugars, such as milk products. Similar observations that the FDNB assays may over-estimate availability were made by others[5].

With pigs, the majority of comparative work on the ileum has been with faecal digestibility assays. There is only limited information on the relationship between ileal digestibility values and availability. In Table 2, a comparison is made between ileal digestibility and lysine availability for two lupin-seed meals. The results indicate that the low lysine availabilities were not due to reduced digestibility at the terminal ileum.

Clearly, there is a need for additional information on the degree to which reductions in ileal digestibility contributes to reduced availability of amino acids over a wider range of protein sources and degress of availability.

Rats. A slope-ratio assay was developed with rats to determine if they could be used to predict pig response[3]. A comparison of results (Table 3) indicates that for some meals (cottonseed, soyabean and sunflower meals) there was good agreement. For others (blood meal, lupin-seed meals and meat and bone meals) there was little agreement. The reason for this species

Table 1. *Availability of lysine (proportion of total) in protein concentrates for growing pigs and comparisons with chemical tests (FDNB-reactive lysine) for estimating availability. From Batterham et al. (1979); Batterham et al. (1981); Batterham et al. (1984) and unpublished values.*

Protein concentrate	Lysine availability	FDNB-reactive lysine Direct	FDNB-reactive lysine Indirect
Blood meal (ring dried)	1.03	0.97	0.91
Cottonseed meal			
Pre-press solvent	0.43	0.65	0.93
Expeller	0.39	0.83	0.87
Field peas	0.93	0.83	0.98
Fish meal	0.89	0.90	0.89
Lupin-seed meal			
L. albus	0.53	–	0.96
L. angustifolius	0.54	0.76	0.97
Meat and bone meal			
No. 1	0.42	–	0.80
No. 2	0.66	0.79	0.78
No. 3	0.88	0.84	0.82
Peanut meal	0.57	0.80	0.91
Skim-milk powder	0.85	0.79	0.96
Sunflower meal			
Pre-press solvent	0.59	0.46	0.92
Expeller	0.66	0.71	0.87
Soyabean meal	0.84	0.77	0.93

Table 2. *Comparison of the digestibility of lysine at the terminal ileum and availability of lysine for growing pigs (proportion of total).*

Protein concentrate	Digestibility at the terminal ileum[a]	Lysine availability[b]
Lupinseed-seed meal		
L. albus	0.82	0.57
L. angustifolius	0.86	0.37

[a] From Taverner (1982) and personal communication;
[b] From Batterham *et al.* (1981) and unpublished results.

difference is not clear but it indicates that caution is needed when applying the results from rat assays to pigs.

Limited information on the relationship between ileal digestibility of nitrogen (and lysine) and nutritive value indicates that for the rat, with some meals, reduced ileal digestibility accounts for only part of the fall in nutritive value[8].

Chicks. A slope-ratio assay was developed with chicks to compare lysine availabilities on the same meals with pigs. The results in Table 4 indicate that availability was less of a problem for chicks, as high availabilities were determined for the different meals.

The reason for the species difference in lysine availability may reflect in part an ability of the chick to utilize derivatives of lysine more efficiently than the other species. For example, ε-N-propionyl-L-lysine can be utilized by chicks[12] whereas it has no nutritional value for rats[4]. Both species absorb the lysine derivative but only the chick possesses the necessary enzyme (ε-N-lysine acylase) in the kidneys which enables them to release the lysine molecule.

There was closer agreement between lysine availabilities for the chick and the chemical tests for reactive lysine, but a wider range of lysine availabilities is needed before more valid conclusions can be made.

There has been considerable interest in using faecal or ileal digestibility assays as estimates of amino-acid availability for the chick[10,13]. In view of the more rapid transit time of digesta in chicks, and its greater ability to utilize lysine from different sources, it is possible that reductions in digestibility contribute to a greater extent to reductions in availability than in the rat or pig.

Man. Slope-ratio assays are not applicable for use with humans, thus the rat is normally used to provide a biological assessment of the quality of foods. In view of the differences in response between species in lysine availability, a positive relationship between the rat and man for all foods cannot be assumed.

Most assays of foods involve an assessment of protein quality, rather than an assessment of amino-acid availability. Currently protein efficiency ratios (PER) are normally used. However,

Table 3. *Comparison of availability of lysine (proportion of total) in protein concentrates for growing rats and pigs. From Batterham et al. (1981); Batterham et al. (1984) and unpublished results.*

Protein concentrate	Lysine availability	
	Rat	Pig
Blood meal	0.81	1.03
Cottonseed meal	0.35	0.39
Lupin-seed meal		
No. 1	0.70	0.54
No. 2	0.81	0.37
Meat and bone meal		
No. 1	0.49	0.87
No. 2	0.68	0.48
No. 3	0.78	0.74
Sunflower meal		
No. 1	0.68	0.66
No. 2	0.49	0.54
Soyabean meal		
No. 1	0.89	0.89
No. 2	0.91	0.98

Table 4. *Comparison of the availability of lysine in protein concentrates for chicks with growing pigs and with chemical techniques for reactive lysine (proportion of total). From Major & Batterham (1981) and unpublished results.*

Protein concentrate	Lysine availability		FDNB-reactive lysine	
	Chick	Pig	Direct	Indirect
Blood meal	1.07	1.03	0.97	0.91
Cottonseed meal	0.79	0.43	0.65	0.93
Fish meal	0.94	0.89	0.90	0.89
Lupin-seed meal	0.93	0.54	0.76	0.97
Meat and bone meal	0.86	0.49	0.79	0.84
Soyabean meal	0.93	0.84	0.77	0.93
Sunflower meal	1.01	0.54	0.88	0.94

PERs are a characteristic of an individual protein, are not additive in dietary formulations, and are only appropriate if the test protein is the sole source of dietary protein.

PERs have most application to proteins with a good balance of amino acids. In this case, the value reflects the availability of the limiting amino acid. For cereals, and other proteins of poor amino-acid balance, the low PER value is only a confirmation of the total amino acid analysis.

An alternative approach, using the rat as the biological model, would be to determine the total amino-acid profile by chemical analysis and determine the availability of one amino acid (lysine) by slope-ratio analysis and use the value obtained to estimate the availability of all essential amino acids is similar. This appears reasonable, especially as non-Maillard reactions appear to account for losses in availability for most protein sources.

This approach would provide information on the estimated amino-acid availability of foods, which would allow more meaningful dietary formulations. The main weakness would be the applicability of the rat results to man, a problem common to the current use of PERs.

Development of alternative techniques for assessing availability. There is also the need for the development of more rapid tests for the routine monitoring of the processing of foods and for the rapid estimation of amino-acid availability. However, there is a need for a greater understanding of the factors affecting availability in the wide range of foods for the different species before such techniques can be developed.

Conclusions. (1) Slope-ratio assays are the only techniques capable of determining amino acid availability (the summation of digestion, absorption and utilization). At present, there is no technique that could be recommended for the routine estimation of availability in foods. There is a need for further research to define the causes of reduced availability, particularly the relationship between ileal digestibility and availability, over a wide range of protein sources. (2) Considerable species differences exist in their ability to utilize amino acids from different sources, with the chick being more efficient with a number of protein sources than the pig or rat. These differences limits the application of availability values from one species to another. (3) For man, a measurement of total amino acids, together with a determination of amino-acid availability with the rat would provide more useful information for recommended dietary intakes than that provided by protein efficiency ratios. (4) There is a need for more careful use of terminology in the literature. The term 'availability' should be restricted to techniques capable of assessing the summation of digestion, absorption and utilization. Prefixes should be used to identify more clearly the techniques used in estimating availability.

1 Batterham, E.S., Murison, R.D. & Anderson, L.M. (1984): Availability of lysine in vegetable protein concentrates as determined by the slope-ratio assay with growing pigs and rats and by chemical techniques. *Br. J. Nutr.* **51**, 85–99.
2 Batterham, E.S., Murison, R.D. & Lewis, C.E. (1979): Availability of lysine in protein concentrates as determined by the slope-ratio assay with growing pigs and rats and by chemical techniques. *Br. J. Nutr.* **41**, 383–391.
3 Batterham, E.S., Murison, R.D. & Lowe, R.F. (1981): Availability of lysine in vegetable protein concentrates as determined by the slope-ratio assay with growing pigs and rats and by chemical techniques. *Br. J. Nutr.* **45**, 401–410.
4 Bjarnason, J. & Carpenter, K.J. (1969): Mechanisms of heat damage in proteins. 1. Models with acylated lysine units. *Br. J. Nutr.* **23**, 859–868.
5 Carpenter, K.J. & Booth, V.H. (1973): Damage to lysine in food processing: its measurement and its significance. *Nutr. Abst. Rev.* **43**, 423–451.
6 Finney, D.J. (1964): *Statistical method in biological assay*, 2nd edn. London: Griffin.
7 Friedman, M. (1982): Chemically reactive and unreactive lysine as an index of browning. *Diabetes* **31**, 5–14.
8 Hurrell, R.F., Carpenter, K.J., Sinclair, W.J., Otterburn, M.S. & Asquith, R.S. (1976): Mechanisms of heat damage in proteins 7. The significance of lysine-containing isopeptides and lanthionine in heated proteins. *Br. J. Nutr.* **35**, 383–395.
9 Major, E.J. & Batterham, E.S. (1981): Availability of lysine in protein concentrates as determined by the slope-ratio assay with chicks and comparisons with rat, pig and chemical assays. *Br. J. Nutr.* **46**, 513–519.
10 Nordheim, J.P. & Coon, C.N. (1984): A comparison of four method for determining available lysine in animal protein meals. *Poult. Sci.* **63**, 1040–1051.
11 Taverner, M.R. (1982): Nutritive value for pigs of white lupins (*L. albus* cv. Hamburg): *Proc. Aust. Soc. Anim. Prod.* **14**, 667.
12 Varnish, S.A. & Carpenter, K.J. (1975): Mechanisms of heat damage in proteins 5. The nutritional values of heat-damaged and propionylated proteins as sources of lysine, methionine and tryptophan. *Br. J. Nutr.* **34**, 325–337.
13 Wallis, I.R. & Balnave, D. (1984): A comparison of amino acid digestibility bioassays for broilers. *Br. Poult. Sci.* **25**, 389–399.

Bioavailability of vitamins

G.B. BRUBACHER
Department of Vitamin and Nutrition Research, F. Hoffmann-La Roche & Co. Ltd., Grenzacherstrasse 124, CH-Basle, Switzerland.

Everson *et al.*, (1948) studied the availability of the riboflavin in ice cream, peas, and almonds as judged by urinary excretion of the vitamin by women subjects and observed that compared with a test dose of 1 mg pure riboflavin, 90.4 per cent, 41.5 per cent and 38.7 per cent of the vitamin B_2 activity of ice cream, green peas, and almonds, respectively, as determined microbiologically, was available to young women when measured by the above-mentioned urinary excretion method. Also at this time, similar observations were made for vitamin B_1, biotin, and ascorbic acid. The authors concluded 'that knowing the content of the diet is only one step toward knowing whether the individual consuming it is well-fed'.

This statement of 1948 is still valid. Besides knowing its analytical value, we need for each vitamin data on its chemical nature, ie its bioavailability, as well as needing to know of the requirement of the individual, in order to decide whether a food item can be considered as a rich source of the vitamin in question.

When discussing the bioavailability of vitamins it has to be kept in mind that the term vitamin has a physiological rather than a chemical meaning. Different chemical compounds may correspond to the same kind of physiological activity; such compounds are often called vitamers, of which two classes may be distinguished: (1) compounds which can be easily converted by more or less simple chemical or biochemical reactions into the active form, that is vitamin A-palmitate may be saponified to retinol or dehydroascorbic acid may be reduced to ascorbic acid; (2) compounds which cannot be inter-converted by simple means, as for example α-, β-, γ-, δ-tocopherol, or α-, β-carotene. It is clear that for compounds of the second class the specific molar vitamin activity may differ considerably between the various compounds. It is also clear that within this class of chemical compounds only animal models can be used to measure the vitamin activity. (For details see for instance[1]).

It is generally assumed that vitamers belonging to the first class of compounds have the same biological activity on a molecular weight basis. Most methods for chemical determination of vitamins in foods are based on this assumption. For example, in the course of the determination of retinol, retinylpalmitate and retinyl acetate are converted to retinol and the result of the analysis is given as weight units of retinol per 100 g. In the case of riboflavin, riboflavin-5′-phosphate, and riboflavin adenine dinucleotide are converted to riboflavin and the result of the analysis is given as weight units of riboflavin per 100 g. The assumption mentioned above may generally be true, but cases are reported where on a molecular basis the biological activity of such compounds was found to be significantly different when measured in animal assay. Thus it has been reported[6] that free α-tocopherol has only 62 per cent of the theoretically expected vitamen E activity compared to α-tocopheryl acetate measured in the so-called rat resorption gestation test. These results have been confirmed, in principle, using, besides the rat resorption gestation test, the blood cell haemolysis test and the rat liver storage test[9]. Similar results using the rat resorption gestation test and the rat myopathia test have been recently found (H. Weiser, R. Maurer & H. Brunner, Pers. Communic.). Thus, the biological activity of free α-tocopherol is probably only 1 i.u./mg, whereas by stoichiometric conversion 1.49 i.u./mg results, a value which corresponds to the conversion factor recommended by the USP. We do not know why α-tocopherol has this irregular behaviour. It is possible that a part of the free tocopherol is destroyed during the intestinal passage, whereas α-tocopherol acetate remains stable.

Another example is the biological activity of stereoisomers of vitamin A. Despite the fact that a thermic equilibrium exists between all-trans retinol and 13-cis-retinol, the biological activity of these two compounds differs by about 20 per cent[5]. With regard to the two stereoisomers, precholecalciferol and cholecalciferol the difference in biological activity is even higher.

We can assume that in humans similar differences in biological activity exist. Yet, when only the vitamin content of a food is given, without any specification of the method used for determination of the vitamin and, moreover, a biological activity for this food is observed, which is lower than expected, this fact may be explained not only by lower bioavailability of these compounds, but also by the presence of compounds in the food with lower biological activity.

In the case of vitamers belonging to the second class of compounds it is desirable to assay food for each single vitamer and to take into consideration its biological activity. However, food analysis is often carried out in a more pragmatic way. In the case of vitamin E, for instance, often only the main component, that is α-tocopherol, is determined. In this case the analytical result gives too low a value for the vitamin E activity, which may lead to the false conclusion as to a high bioavailability. The analysis may also be performed in a manner where all the vitamers of the vitamin E groups, that is α-, β-, γ-, and δ-tocopherol are determined together without being separated. In this case the analytical value is higher than the biological activity, which in this case would lead to the false conclusion of a low bioavailability. A similar situation exists with the naturally occurring provitamins A.

We do not know whether the biological activities found in animals can also be applied in humans. However, we have to accept these values since we have no practical means of testing them in humans.

Vitamers of both classes may occur in food bound to other food components. The most striking example is that of some niacin derivatives. It has been shown that the major part of the nicotinic acid in cereal grains is in a bound form that is practically unavailable as a source of the vitamin[7] and it was found that bound niacin in cereals is as an ester with glucose and this is embedded in a glycopeptide macromolecule[10,11]. Since the ester linkage is alkali labile, nicotinic acid may be liberated by treatment with alkali. This is what occurs in the traditional Central American food practice, whereas in the maize-growing parts of the old world this practice has not been introduced, subsequently resulting in endemic pellagra in regions where maize was the only staple food consumed.

Not all models are as clear cut as niacin: free niacin seems to be fully available, whereas it is not at all available with bound niacin. In such cases even with analytical methods it is possible to distinguish between the available and the total amount of a vitamin simply by using acidic and alkaline extraction, respectively.

In many cases the bound vitamers cannot be isolated and assayed as pure chemical compounds. The animal assay for testing bioavailability of such compounds has therefore to be performed with the food item itself. But there not only does the vitamer to be tested differ from the standard substance but the whole test diet is different from the standard diet; this makes the evaluation of such trials extremely difficult. For this reason an animal growth test was developed[4] in which the influence of different diets was minimized. With the help of this test the author investigated the bioavailability of biotin in different feed ingredients for the chicken. Some of the results obtained are given in Table 1. From this table it can be seen that depending on the nature of feed ingredient a growth-response in the chicken is found which corresponds to values ranging from zero to 100 per cent of the microbiologically determined biotin content. Strictly speaking, the values in Table 1 do not represent the bioavailability of single chemical compounds, but rather the sum effect of the biological activities of some unknown biotin derivatives which can be converted to microbiologically determinable biotin and their bioavailability. In principle, reduced bioavailability can be caused by two different factors. Since biotin is linked by a lysyl group to food proteins, only as far as this linkage is split during digestion, is free biotin available to the body. At the same time food may contain some proteins or other ingredients with a higher affinity for biotin than the mucosa cell and these compounds may therefore impair the absorption. One of the best known of such compounds in the case of biotin is avidin, present in raw egg-white.

Table 1. *Microbiologically analysed and available biotin content in various feed ingredients (Frigg, 1984). Available biotin*

$$(\%) = \frac{(Estimate\ by\ standard\ curve \times 100)}{Microbiological\ estimate}$$

Ingredient	Mean % availability ± s.d.
Whey powder	117.0 ± 18.8
Skim milk powder	64.8 ± 15.5
Peanut meal	52.8 ± 5.0
Oats	40.5 ± 2.8
Sorghum	24.8 ± 1.7
Barley	21.6 ± 4.1
Wheat middlings	6.4 ± 8.7

Table 2. *Conversion rate of β-carotene of food (Brubacher & Weiser, 1985).*

β-Carotene intake (μg)	Conversion of β-carotene Amounts equivalent to 1 μg retinol	
	β-Carotene in oily solution	β-Carotene in vegetables
< 1500	1.87 μg	< 6.0 μg
1500 – 4000	3.33 μg	6.0 μg
> 4000	> 3.33 μg	> 6.0 μg

Factors enhancing or diminishing vitamin absorption are found in all kinds of foods. The absorption of β-carotene and its conversion to vitamin A for instance depends on a diversity of factors, among which the physical chemical state and the presence of oil are of great importance. β-Carotene in raw carrots is very poorly absorbed, whereas β-carotene in an oily solution has a high absorption and conversion rate.

Another factor which may influence the bioavailability of vitamins may be the amount of the vitamin ingested. Only small percentages of very high dosages of vitamin B_1, B_{12} or vitamin C are absorbed. In this connection the conversion rate of β-carotene in the rat and chicken, using three different kinds of biological tests, has been studied[2]. It was possible to demonstrate that with low dosage levels the vitamin A activity of β-carotene equals 100 per cent of the theoretical value, assuming that one mol β-carotene equals 1 mol retinol in activity. With higher dosage levels the percentage conversion rate becomes smaller and smaller. On a logarithmic scale there is a linear relationship between conversion rate and dosage level, which suggests a saturation kinetic for the conversion of β-carotene to vitamin A. Based on these findings, we suggest acceptance for practical purposes the conversion rates for β-carotene given in Table 2. Below a dose of 1500 µg β-carotene in oily solution, which may occur by ingestion of butter, margarine or red palm oil, 1.87 µg β-carotene equals 1 µg retinol in biological activity. With a higher intake of β-carotene or with an intake of β-carotene in the form of vegetables a greater amount of β-carotene has to be taken to give a value equal to 1 µg retinol. Thus, it is not possible to assign a fixed value of retinol equivalents to 1 mg of β-carotene and it would be more appropriate not to express analytical data on β-carotene content of food in retinol equivalents, but rather to use weight units.

There is only a restricted number of possibilities for measurement of bioavailability of vitamins in man. The classical procedure is still the one used by Everson *et al.* (1984)[3] in the case of vitamin B_2, as mentioned above and which had been suggested by Melnick *et al.*[12]. This method can be used in all cases where an appreciable part of the ingested vitamin is excreted as a single vitamer or a metabolite thereof.

Since most vitamins are not synthesized in our body and are in this respect similar to pharmaceuticals, pharmacokinetic methods could be applied. However, such methods have to be used with caution, for two reasons: first, some vitamins are synthesized to an appreciable extent by our intestinal flora and this unknown part may disturb the interpretation of the observed curves; secondly, since it is not possible to deplete human beings to point zero and since in pharmaceutical research the starting point is in general an organism free of the pharmaceutical in question, normal pharmacokinetic equations have to be modified. By means of this methodology the bioavailability of β-carotene has been measured and it has been found that 5 mg of β-carotene emulsified with linseed oil and diluted with milk is absorbed to about 10 per cent, of which about one-half is converted to vitamin A[8]. It is hoped that these investigations will be taken up again.

From a practical point of view, some priority should be given to the investigation of the following problems. *Vitamin A*: since vitamin-A-deficiency is one of the major deficiency diseases of the world's population as a whole, and since vitamin A provitamins are the main sources of vitamin A activity for the world population, simple, analytical methods should be developed to separate the main vitamin A precursors in food. Vitamin A activity should not be listed in retinol equivalents but rather as weight units of each of the vitamin A precursors in food composition tables. Moreover, estimates should be made of their bioavailability, taking into account the various situations occurring in the field. *Vitamin B_2*: vitamin-B_2-deficiency is also one of the principal deficiency diseases of the world population, mainly in regions with a short supply of animal proteins. We still have no better knowledge on the bioavailability of vitamers with regard to vitamin B_2 and their bound forms than had Gladys Everson 40 years ago. It is of great importance to know whether bound forms of vitamin B_2 could be converted to a more assimilable vitamin B_2-form during food preparation. *Folic acid*: not only in developing countries does marginal folic-acid-deficiency seem to be widespread but also in industrialized ones. Folic acid itself does not occur naturally in food, but is used for enrichment. Most of the naturally-occurring folates are derivatives of 5, 6, 7, 8-tetrahydrofolic acid and exist in monoglutamate and polyglutamate forms. It seems that the bioavailability of free folic acid is highest and that of polyglutamates several times lower. For the time being there exists no commonly used method for the separation of folic acid active compounds and subsequent separate assay. There is also no ideal method to convert all folic acid active compounds to folic acid without loss, in the course of the analytical procedure. Finally, there is no good method to assess the bioavailability of folic acid active compounds in humans. *Vitamin B_6*: there are some indications that at least in certain situations borderline vitamin-B_6-deficiency exists in humans. Vitamin B_6 occurs in at least six different forms in nature. We do not know whether all of these vitamers show the same biological activity, but it is generally assumed that on a molar basis their activity is equal. Modern analytical methods[1] allow one to separate at least pyridoxol, pyridoxamine and pyridoxal. As long as we do not have exact knowledge of the biological activity of these compounds of their bioavailability nor of their bound forms, it would be desirable to indicate the amount of these vitamers separately in food composition tables.

Of further scientific interest are investigations of the bioavailability of vitamins which are partly synthesized in our intestinal tract, such as vitamin K, vitamin B_2, biotin and folic acid. A more profound knowledge of bioavailability of these vitamins would allow us to judge the importance of intestinal synthesis. There is no good methodology at the moment to tackle this question. Finally, in connection with the question of quantitative aspects of the biosynthesis of nicotinic acid from tryptophan, bioavailability of the various bound forms of nicotinic acid should be re-investigated.

1 Brubacher, G., Müller-Mullot, W. & Southgate, D.A.T. (1985): *Methods for the determination of vitamins in food.* London, New York: Elsevier Applied Science Publishers.
2 Brubacher, G. & Weiser, H. (1985): The vitamin A activity of β-carotene. *Int. J. Vit. Nutr. Res.* **55**, 5–15.
3 Everson, Gladys, Wheeler, Elizabeth, Walker, Helen & Caulfield, W.J. (1948): Availability of riboflavin of ice cream, peas, and almonds judged by urinary excretion of the vitamin by women subjects. *J. Nutr.* **35**, 209–223.
4 Frigg, M. (1984): Available biotin content of various feed ingredients. *Poultry Sci.* **63**, 750–753.
5 Harris, P.L., Ames, S.R. & Brinkman, J.H. (1951): Biopotency of Neovitamin A in the rat. *J. Am. Chem. Soc.* **73**, 1252–1254.
6 Harris, P.L. & Ludwig, M.I. (1949): Vitamin E potency of α-tocopherol and α-tocopherol esters. *J. biol. Chem.* **180**, 611–614.
7 Kodicek, E. (1962): Nicotinic acid and the pellagra problem. Bibliotheca *Nutr. Diet.* **4**, 109–127.
8 Kübler, W. (1963): Die Carotine in der Säuglingsernährung. In *Carotine und Carotinoide*, ed K. Lang, pp. 222–234. Darmstadt: Steinkopff.
9 Leth, T. & Søndergaard, H. (1983): Biological activity of all-rac-α-tocopherol and RRR-α-tocopherol determined by three different rat bioassays. *Int. J. Vit. Nutr. Res.* **54**, 297–311.
10 Mason, J.B., Gibson, N. & Kodicek, E. (1973): The chemical nature of the bound nicotinic acid of wheat bran: nicotinic acid containing macromolecules. *Br. J. Nutr.* **30**, 297–311.
11 Mason, J.B. & Kodicek, E. (1973): The chemical nature of the bound nicotinic acid of wheat bran: studies of partial hydrolysis products. *Cereal Chem.* **50**, 637–647.
12 Melnick, D., Hochberg, M. & Oser, B.L. (1945): Physiological availability of the vitamins. I. The human bioassay technic. *J. Nutr.* **30**, 67–79.

Availability of minerals — with special reference to iron

L. HALLBERG
Department of Medicine, University of Göteborg, Sahlgren's Hospital, Göteborg, Sweden.

More is known about the bioavailability of iron than about that of most other minerals. The reasons are that (1) iron is almost completely retained in the body after its absorption, (2) iron has two radio-iron isotopes with suitable half-lives and suitable energies which allow the use of good experimental designs, and (3) the extrinsic tag technique to label food iron was first developed and validated for iron.

There are two main forms of iron in the diet — haem iron derived from haemoglobin and myoglobin and non-haem iron derived mainly from cereals, vegetables and fruits[1]. Haem iron forms a relatively minor part of the dietary iron intake — even in diets with a high meat intake it accounts for only 10–15 per cent of the total iron intake. Non-haem iron is thus the main part of the dietary iron and differs from haem iron in two important respects: first, the bioavailability of non-haem iron is markedly influenced by a number of dietary factors and secondly it is also markedly influenced by iron status, whereas the absorption of haem iron is only slightly affected by iron status, and less affected by other dietary factors. This discussion will be limited to non-haem iron.

The amount of non-haem iron absorbed from a particular meal is determined both by dietary factors and by individual factors. An iron-deficient subject may absorb ten times or more iron from a meal than a subject who is iron replete. When we want to compare the bioavailability of iron from different meals we must therefore refer the absorption to a defined iron status.

Individual factors influencing the bioavailability of iron. When differences in iron absorption are observed between different meals studied in different groups of subject it is difficult to determine if these differences relate to properties of the meals or to the iron status of the subjects. A model using a reference dose of an inorganic iron salt (3 mg Fe) labelled with radio-iron and given under standardized conditions to each subject has been introduced[6]. In each subject the absorption of iron from various foods is then expressed as the ratio: food iron absorption/reference dose absorption. In a group of subjects with varying iron status given a particular meal a relationship is obtained which is a measure of the bioavailability of the iron in that meal.

Usually, we want to express the iron absorption from a meal in relation to a particular iron status. We must then translate reference dose absorption to iron status. In large groups of subjects we have studied several parameters of iron status and the absorption of iron from the reference dose. Our results imply that a reference dose absorption of 40 per cent roughly corresponds to the absorption in subjects who are borderline iron-deficient, that means subjects with individually optimal haemoglobin values but who have no iron stores[7]. Such hypothetical subjects are of great interest in all iron balance calculations and consideration. In studies on the bioavailability of iron from meals served to groups of subjects the reference dose absorption is thus used as a basis of comparison. For each type of meal the bioavailability is expressed as the amount of iron absorbed or the fraction absorbed in subjects who would have absorbed 40 per cent from the reference dose of 3 mg ferrous iron given in a fasting state.

Dietary factors influencing the bioavailability of non-haem iron. The development of the technique of extrinsic labelling of non-haem iron in a composite meal by simply adding a radioiron tracer in the form of an inorganic salt made it possible for the first time to measure the absorption of non-haem iron from a whole meal.

The concept of the common non-haem iron pool that was uniformly labelled by the extrinsic tracer, implied that there were two main factors in the diet influencing the absorption of iron: (1) the amount of iron in the pool, and (2) the balance between factors that enhanced or inhibited the absorption from the pool. That means that the final results of these factors can be considered as some kind of chemical net effect of all ligands in the gastrointestinal lumen that affected the iron or rather compete in binding iron ions, in relation to the affinity of the total amount of mucosal receptors for iron.

The first condition for absorption according to this concept is that the non-haem iron has joined the non-haem iron pool. We know that this is valid for almost all native non-haem iron in most foods. The main exceptions are: some of the iron in common compounds used in iron fortification; *and* a great part of so-called contamination iron. The latter forms a considerable part of the dietary iron intake in many developing countries and originates mainly from soil residues on vegetables and cereals or dust that has settled on the surface of foods during air drying. Drinking water and water used for cooking may also be contaminated with iron.

Some contamination iron is not available, for example some of the iron-rich red soil (laterite) seen in various parts of the world. The iron in some other soil samples we have examined, such as clay, varied markedly in availability. We have studied the potential availability of contamination iron using an *in-vitro* method[3]. The exchangeability of the soil iron with an inorganic radioiron tracer is measured using conditions similar to those prevailing in the gastrointestinal tract. The extent of isotopic exchange is considered to be a measure of the potential availability. The properties of the soil iron can affect the bioavailability of the iron from the non-haem iron pool but that can then be measured by the absorption of the tracer and the extent of isotopic exchange. The observed exchangeability of iron in clay varied between 20 and 35 per cent. This exchangeability or relative potential bioavailability is not low considering the rather high content of such soil iron in many diets. The Ethiopian teff is famous for its high iron content originating from the soil. In a sample we studied we found 36.2 mg contamination iron per 100 g teff. About 2.5 per cent of this iron (0.9 mg/100 g) joined the non-haem iron pool.

In rice flour samples in South East Asia we have found a fairly high iron content, about 30 mg/100 g flour which is about 20 times more than in unmilled but polished rice from the same area. About 60 per cent of the iron is in particles that can easily be removed by a magnet. More than one-third of the total iron in the rice flour was exchangeable with the radio-iron tracer and the main part (80 per cent) was derived from contamination. We have examined meals and foods from Africa and Asia and as a rule found considerable amount of contamination iron with varying degrees of exchangeability (ie iron that joins the non-haem iron pool and becomes potential bioavailability)[4].

Fortification iron. Easily soluble iron salts such as ferrous sulphate join the non-haem iron pool and can thus be considered to have an absorbability or a relative bioavailability of 100 per cent. The high solubility, however, at the same time causes severe technical problems such as rancidity and discoloration. Metallic iron in various forms has therefore been extensively used especially to fortify flour. Unfortunately no studies have been reported on the bioavailability in man of commercially available products. We have recently studied the absorbability in man of one of the most used and probably one of the best iron powders — carbonyl iron[5]. The carbonyl iron was labelled by neutron irradiation to obtain a ^{55}Fe-labelled product. No change in chemical properties of the carbonyl iron could be detected by the irradiation or storage. We found that only 5–25 per cent of the carbonyl iron joined the non-haem iron pool. The variation was related to the composition of the meals to which the labelled fortified bread was served.

Ferric phosphates are much used to fortify infant foods and other products because they are insoluble in water and thus cause no technical problems. Ferric orthophosphate is not a uniform compound and various analogues may be synthesized with different chemical properties. We have recently examined a newly developed ferric orthophosphate with interesting properties as it is insoluble in water yet still showed a high absorbability (relative bioavailability) of 63 per cent when baked into bread and served with a continental type of breakfast.

It can thus be concluded that not all non-haem iron compounds in a meal join the non-haem iron pool. To measure the bioavailability it is necessary to determine not only the total iron intake but rather the size of the non-haem iron pool (the amount of absorbable iron) especially when the meals are fortified with iron or when the presence of contamination cannot be excluded. In the next stage the factors that enhance or inhibit the non-haem iron absorption will act on the iron that is present *in* this pool. (For a review see[1]).

The main dietary factors enhancing non-haem iron absorption are as follows. (1) *Ascorbic acid*. The effect is determined both by the amount of ascorbic acid included in a meal and by properties of the meal such as the content of inhibitors. (2) *Meat, poultry, fish, seafood* also regularly increase the iron absorption. Roughly 1–2 g of meat induce the same absorption promotion as 1 mg of ascorbic acid. The mechanism for the effect of meat is not fully understood but is probably additive to the effect of ascorbic acid. (3) *Organic acids*. There is no doubt that some organic acids such as lactic acid, malic acid and succinic acid improve iron absorption. Still, however, there are considerable gaps in our knowledge of how and when they act. Just as an example I will mention that in meals served with Sauerkraut we have obtained average absorption figures around 45 per cent ie higher than the 40 per cent absorption from the reference dose of ferrous ascorbate given to a subject in a fasting state.

The main dietary factors inhibiting non-haem iron absorption are as follows. (1) *Polyphenols/tannins* -the most well known example is tea but there are also vegetables and cereals with a high content of tannins. (2) *Phytates* have long been known to interfere with the absorption of non-haem iron. There are some divergent results about their mechanism of action and their role in explaining the inhibitory effect of bran[8]. Recent data from our laboratory, however, show that phytates are mainly responsible for the bran effect (unpublished observations). (3) *Various fibres* beside bran have little effect on the absorption of iron in man. On the other hand there is evidence that starch from different cereals influence the absorption of iron very differently. Iron absorption is high from meals based on wheat starch but markedly lower from rice or maize starches.

The term available iron has been used for the iron that joins the non-haem iron pool. A fraction of this potentially available iron will then be absorbed and become bioavailable. Bioavailability of iron is then the fraction of iron absorbed from the diet by subjects with a particular iron status. For iron it is fairly meaningless to speak about bioavailability of iron in different *foods* as it is not so much the properties of single foods, but rather the composition of the meals in which the foods are included, that determines the bioavailability of the iron in the foods.

Comments about the bioavailability of some other minerals. The absorption of dietary zinc is more difficult to study than the absorption of iron for several reasons: an unknown fraction of the absorbed zinc is not retained in the body, there is for example, only one suitable radio-zinc isotope. In spite of that it has been clearly shown, just as for iron, that phytates strongly inhibit the zinc absorption. It has also been shown that certain proteins favour the absorption of zinc. It is not known, however, whether a deficiency or an excess of zinc in the body affects the bioavailability of dietary zinc. It may well be so, but a serious problem is that there is no reliable, quantitative method to assess the zinc status.

For calcium there is good evidence that the active transport of this mineral is regulated in a way similar to that of iron to meet the calcium needs of the body. The calcium absorption is thus increased when the needs are great as during pregnancy and growth spurts. The vitamin D hormone system is involved in this active calcium absorption. Dietary components and digestibility also affect the bioavailability of dietary clacium. It has been shown, just as for iron and zinc, that, for example, phytates bind calcium and reduce the absorption. Dietary oxalate also reduces the calcium absorption as calcium oxalate is a poorly soluble compound. Similarly, excess of unabsorbed fatty acids will also bind calcium by forming calcium soaps. The net retention of iron is almost exclusively determined by its absorption. For calcium, as for many other minerals, the net retention is determined not only by variations in absorption but also by variations in losses. The intake of for example protein and phosphorus markedly affects the urinary calcium losses. It is therefore much more difficult to find a useful definition of bioavailability for calcium than it is for iron.

Another difficulty in studying the bioavailability of minerals, and especially of trace minerals, is the interaction between mineral elements. Calcium may affect the absorption of zinc and copper. A deficiency of iron may increase the absorption not only of iron, but also of other elements such as manganese and cadmium.

These examples are mentioned to illustrate the difficulties in designing studies on bioavailability of minerals and in the interpretation of the results. It is important, however, not only to mention the difficulties in measuring bioavailability but also the potential achievements. It is important that we are aware of the difficulties and that we define what we want to know and how we want to use the information.

It is of course important to know that the absorption of iron varies very much between different meals but to get a really useful measure of the bioavailability of iron we want to relate it to something — what is normal, what is acceptable? A primary nutritional problem today, especially in industrialized countries is to absorb sufficient amounts of essential nutrients at the present low energy intake. A meaningful measure of bioavailability is thus the amount of the nutrient absorbed in relation to the energy content of a meal. That was the reason for the introduction of the concept bioavailable nutrient density in iron nutrition which has turned out to be very useful in evaluating both meals and diets[2]. This concept can of course be applied to all nutrients and not only to minerals.

Finally, I would suggest that we examine the possibility of reaching agreement about the terminology. My suggestion would be that the term 'absorbable' is used to describe the amount of a nutrient that is in such a form in the meal that it is potentially available for absorption whereas the term 'bioavailable' is used to describe the amount of a nutrient that is absorbed from the meal by subjects with a defined nutritional status.

1 Hallberg, L. (1981): Bioavailability of dietary iron in man. *Ann. Rev. Nutr.* **1**, 123–47.
2 Hallberg, L. (1981): Bioavailability nutrient density: a new concept applied in the interpretation of food iron absorption data. *Am. J. Clin. Nutr.* **34**, 2242–47.
3 Hallberg, L. & Björn-Rasmussen, E. (1981): Measurement of iron absorption from meals contaminated with iron. *Am. J. Clin. Nutr.* **34**, 2808–15.

4 Hallberg, L., Björn-Rasmussen, E., Rossander, L., Suwanik, R., Pleehachinda, R. & Tuntawiron, M. (1983): Iron absorption from some Asian meals containing contamination iron. *Am. J. Clin. Nutr.* **37**, 272–77.

5 Hallberg, L., Brune, M. & Rossander, L. (1986): Low bioavailability of carbonyl iron in man: studies on iron fortification of wheat flour. *Am. J. Clin. Nutr.* (In press).

6 Layrisse, M., Cook. J.D., Martinez, C., Roche, M., Kuhn, I.N., Walter, R.B. & Finch, C.A. (1969): Food iron absorption; a comparison of vegetable and animal foods. *Blood* **33**, 430–33.

7 Magnusson, B., Björn-Rasmussen, E., Hallberg, L. & Rossander, L. (1981): Iron absorption in relation to iron stores. Model proposed to express results of food iron absorption measurements. *Scand. J. Haematol.* **27**, 201–208.

8 Simpson, K.M., Morris, E.R. & Cook, J.D. (1981): The inhibitory effect of bran on iron absorption in man. *Am. J. Clin. Nutr.* **34**, 1469–78.

IV: Nutritional status and body composition

New methods of measuring body composition

L. BURKINSHAW and C.B. OXBY
Department of Medical Physics, University of Leeds, The General Infirmary, Leeds LS1 3EX, UK

Nutritional problems are essentially those of energy balance, ie of disadvantageous changes in the energy stores of the body, fat, protein and carbohydrate, and investigations of nutritional problems should, ideally, include measurements of all three stores. In practice, the most commonly used methods of measuring body composition divide the body into fat and the fat-free mass (FFM)[1]; if the protein content of the fat-free tissues is assumed to be constant, then the FFM is a measure of total body protein. Alternatively, total body protein can be estimated more directly from total body nitrogen (TBN) measured by *in-vivo* neutron activation analysis (IVNAA)[1]. Total body carbohydrate cannot yet be determined. New methods of measuring body composition are continually being proposed because accurate measurements are so important in nutritional studies. Three recent proposals are described here.

Measurement of total body carbon. Fat contains no constituent that is measurable *in-vivo* and is not present in other tissues. However, in a healthy subject, more than half the carbon in the body is in fat, the remainder being in protein and other non-fat tissues[8]. Therefore total body carbon (TBC), corrected for the carbon in non-fat tissues, should be a measure of total body fat (TBF). To investigate this possibility we are adapting our technique of multi-element IVNAA,[7] to measure TBC also.

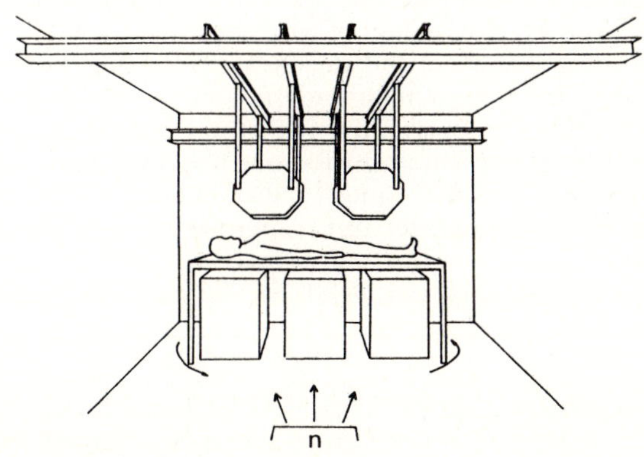

The Figure shows the apparatus, in which the subject lies supine while being irradiated from the right and left sides in turn with a horizontal beam of 14 Mev neutrons. The beam is designed to irradiate the whole body without directly irradiating the five scintillation counters that are positioned two above and three below the couch. The counters have sodium iodide crystals 150 mm in diameter and 130 mm thick. They are housed in shields of steel, boric acid and lead which exclude scattered neutrons and unwanted gamma radiation while admitting gamma rays from the patient through suitably placed apertures. The amplitude spectrum of the electrical signals from the counters contains a peak corresponding to a quantum energy of 4.43 Mev, due to gamma rays emitted when neutrons are scattered inelastically by carbon nuclei in the body. The net counting-rate within this peak is the required measure of TBC. The net counting-rate is converted to a mass of carbon by multiplying by a factor derived from experiments with phantoms of known composition[3].

Not all the scintillation counters have yet been installed. However, a preliminary estimate of the precision of the method, ie the standard deviation of repeated measurements of a subject of constant composition, has been obtained by irradiating and counting an anthropomorphic phantom five times with a single detector placed in each of the five shielded housings in turn. The results show that, if a typical subject containing 16 kg of carbon[8], is given a dose equivalent of 1 mSv, the estimate of carbon will have a precision of approximately 480 g, ie 3 per cent of the carbon content.

To calculate TBF from TBC, carbon is assumed to reside entirely in fat, protein and bone, forming 77 per cent of fat and 52 per cent of protein, and being present in bone in the proportion of 740 g/kg of calcium[8]. A separate measurement by multi-element IVNAA gives total body calcium (TBCa) and TBN; multiplying the latter by 6.25 gives an estimate of total body protein. Then TBF can be calculated from the equation[1]:

$$TBF = 1.30TBC - 4.22TBN - 0.96TBCa$$

The precision of TBF will be approximately 0.7 kg, or 5 per cent of a typical fat content of 13.5 kg[8]. This is similar to the precision of alternative methods such as whole-body densitometry, anthropometry or dilution of tracer substances[1]. Unlike most methods, the body carbon method does not assume that the fat-free tissues as a whole are of constant composition, but assumes only that fat, protein and mineral contain known, constant concentrations of carbon. Disease may change the proportions of these components in the body, but is unlikely to change their chemical compositions. Therefore the carbon method should measure the fat content of patients of abnormal composition more accurately than alternative methods.

Measurement of the electrical impedance of the body. Cellular tissue has higher electrical conductivity and permittivity than fat at frequencies above 1 MHz[5]; therefore the overall conductivity and permittivity of the whole body depend on the proportions of fat and cellular tissue present. An apparatus described for measuring total body electrical conductivity (TOBEC)[6] consists of a large solenoidal coil of wire carrying a 5 MHz radiofrequency current. TOBEC is deduced from the change in the electrical impedance of the coil when a patient is placed within it. Measurements of four men and 15 women, mostly overweight but otherwise healthy, showed that TOBEC was correlated with total body potassium (TBK), total body water (TBW) and FFM estimated from anthropometrics, correlation coefficients ranging from 0.69 to 0.87. Others[4] reported a rather simpler system which uses an electrical impedance plethysmograph to measure resistance (R) and reactance between arm and leg in a group of 37 healthy young men. These authors found[4] that (body height)^2/R was correlated with TBK, TBW and FFM determined by underwater weighing, with correlation coefficients between 0.95 and 0.98.

Measurement of infrared interactance. This method depends on the differential absorption of infrared light by fat and water[2]. The skin at five sites is irradiated with monochromatic infrared radiation of variable wavelength between 600 and 2500 nm; the intensity of reflected radiation, I, is measured at each wavelength and standardized against the signal from a reference block of teflon measured in the same way. Next, the second derivative of log (1/I) with respect to wavelength is computed. Finally the ratio of these second derivatives at wavelengths of 916 and 1026 nm is calculated; this ratio is the infrared interactance (IRI). In a study of 20 male and 33 female volunteers, IRI was highly correlated ($r = 0.94$) with TBF, estimated from measured TBW and expressed as a percentage of total body mass. The percentage of fat in an individual could be estimated from measured IRI with a standard error of 3 percentile units.

Conclusions. The electrical and infrared methods are quick, non-invasive methods of estimating fat and FFM. However, they have to be standardized against methods which assume a fat-free body of invariant composition, and that assumption may not be valid for wasted or obese patients. IVNAA measures fat and protein more directly, but is time-consuming and involves irradiating the patient with neutrons. There remains a need for cheap, simple, non-invasive methods of measuring total body fat, protein and carbohydrate in nutritional studies.

Acknowledgements. We are grateful for the contributions of our colleagues B. Dean, B. Oldroyd, D.W. Krupowicz, K. Brooks and S.C. Moore to the development of the method of measuring total body carbon. Author L.B. is a member of the External Scientific Staff of the Medical Research Council, who have supported the development of IVNAA with a series of grants.

1. Burkinshaw, L. (1985): Measurement of human body composition *in-vivo*. In *Progress in medical radiation physics*, 2, ed C.G. Orton, pp 113–137. New York: Plenum.
2. Conway, J.M., Norris, K.H. & Bodwell, C.E. (1984): A new approach for the estimation of body composition: infrared interactance. *A. J. Clin. Nutr.* **40**, 1123–1130.
3. Kyere K., Oldroyd B., Oxby C.B., Burkinshaw L., Ellis R.E. & Hill G.L. (1982): The feasibility of measuring total body carbon by counting neutron inelastic scatter gamma rays. *Phys, Med. Biol.* **27**, 805–817.
4. Lukaski, H.C., Johnson, P.E., Bolonchuk, W.W. & Lykken, G.I. (1985): Assessment of fat-free mass using bioelectrical impedance measurements of the human body. *Am. J. Clin. Nutr.* **41**, 810–817.
5. Pethig, R. (1979): *Dielectric and electronic properties of biological materials*. Chichester: John Wiley.
6. Presta, E., Wang, J., Harrison, G.G., Björntorp, P., Harker, W.H. & VanItallie, T.B. (1983): Measurement of total body electrical conductivity: a new method for estimation of body composition. *Am. J. Clin. Nutr.* **37**, 735–739.
7. Sharafi, A., Pearson, D., Oxby, C.B., Oldroyd, B., Krupowicz, D.W., Brooks, K. & Ellis, R.E. (1983): Multi-element analysis of the human body using neutron activation. *Phys, Med. Biol.* **28**, 203–214.
8. Snyder, W.S., Cook, M.J., Nasset, E.S., Karhausen, L.R., Parry Howells, G. & Tipton, I.H. (1975): *Rep. Task Group on Reference Man. I.C.R.P. Rep. No 23*. Oxford: Pergamon Press.

Validation of methods for estimating body composition in man

J.S. GARROW
Nutrition Research Group, Clinical Research Centre, Watford Road, Harrow, HA1 3UJ, UK.

The desire to measure body composition in man may arise for different reasons, and the appropriate validation procedure will vary correspondingly. The first effective measurements of body composition in living human subjects related to very muscular athletes who were overweight, and hence deemed unfit for military service[1], and to subjects who were grossly undernourished as a result of wartime privations[16], or volunteers undergoing experimental semistarvation[15]. These investigators wanted to distinguish between fat and non-fat weight, and in the case of the undernourished subjects to investigate the change in composition of the fat-free tissues.

The ultimate validation for this type of measurement is carcass analysis, but obviously this is not possible with living subjects. However, between 1945 and 1956 analyses were made of six adult cadavers[6,7,9,17,22]. The results are summarized in Table 1, and Table 2 shows the

Table 1. *The age and composition of six fat-free bodies, determined by chemical analysis.*

Age (yr)	Sex	Water (g/kg)	Protein (g/kg)	Remainder (g/kg)	Density (g/ml)	Potassium (mmol/kg)
25	m	728	195	77	1.120	71.5
35	m	775	165	60	1.083	—
42	f	733	192	75	1.013	73.0
46	m	674	234	92	1.131	66.5
48	m	730	206	64	1.099	—
60	m	704	238	58	1.104	66.6
mean		724	205	71	1.106	69.4
s.d.		34	28	13	0.017	3.3

Table 2. *Chemical composition of selected organs in adult man*

	Water (g/kg)	Protein (g/kg)	Remainder (g/kg)	Potassium (mmol/kg)	K:N ratio (mmol/g)
Skin	694	300	6	23.7	0.45
Heart	827	143	30	66.5	2.90
Liver	711	176	113	75.0	2.66
Kidney	810	153	37	57.0	2.33
Brain	774	107	119	84.6	4.96
Muscle	792	192	16	92.2	2.99

chemical composition of selected tissues[5,21]. Particular attention has been given to the density of the tissues, and their water and potassium content, since all these can be measured in living subjects. It is fortunate that potassium contains a natural radioactive isotope and therefore emits radiation which can be measured with very sensitive detecting systems[2]. The density of the fat-free bodies in Table 1 was not measured directly: it was calculated on the assumption that all the 'remainder' was mineral, with a density of 3.00 g/ml, and that the density of water, protein and fat were 0.993, 1.340 and 0.900 g/ml respectively.

The fat-free body is made up from a mixture of tissues in varying proportions. The composition of tissues which make up the majority of the fat-free body is shown in Table 2, and it is evident that these tissues vary widely in water and potassium content. It is not possible to calculate the density of the fat-free tissues from the data given, since the remainder column in Table 2 includes fat.

Validation of *in vivo* estimates of body composition. It is possible to measure a component of body composition such as potassium in a dead body, and then to check the answer by chemical analysis. This has been done in the case of malnourished children, and good agreement was found between the two methods for estimating body potassium[11]. Another approach is to measure potassium balance over a period of about a month, and to observe the change in potassium calculated by [40]K counting: comparisons of this sort tend to show a greater apparent retention by balance than by [40]K counting[8]. The errors in any balance experiment tend to exaggerate retention.

However, the important problem is not to demonstrate that an estimate of total body potassium by whole body counting gives an answer which agrees with the actual amount of potassium in the body: it is to demonstrate that total fat-free mass (or fat) calculated from total body potassium corresponds to actual fat-free mass (or fat). The two problems are not the same. For example the ratio of potassium to water is higher than normal in anorectic patients[4], and lower than normal in obese subjects[12], so clearly the same constants cannot apply to estimates of fat-free mass based on potassium or water in both anorectic and obese subjects.

With estimates based on measurements of density there is evidence on racial differences: the density of the fat-free mass in Blacks is about 1.113 g/ml compared with 1.100 g/ml in Whites[18].

Comparison of energy balance, nitrogen balance and indirect estimates of body composition in obese patients before and after weight loss. It is possible to measure energy balance and nitrogen balance in patients kept under strict control in a metabolic ward[13]. If body composition is measured by density, water and potassium at the start and finish of the balance period estimates of change in fat and in fat-free mass can be compared with the losses calculated from the balance data. A study of this sort had been reported[14] on 19 obese women in whom the mean estimated fat loss (kg) over a period of about 3 weeks was 2.77, 2.69, 2.83, 2.37 and 2.90 by energy balance, nitrogen balance, density, water and potassium respectively. The general agreement between the different methods in estimating mean fat loss indicates that the assumed values for the energy, nitrogen, density, water and potassium in fat-free tissue was roughly correct. However it is more informative to examine the standard deviations associated with these mean values, namely 0.71, 1.23, 2.32, 2.38 and 3.54 kg respectively. Clearly the 19 women would not all lose exactly the same amount of fat, so if the measurements had been made by an infinitely accurate method the values for fat loss among the 19 women would have shown some variation about the mean value. It is also obvious that if the women had in fact lost exactly the same amount of fat an inaccurate method would tend to cause apparent variation within the group. Thus the error in the method is reflected in an increasing magnitude in the standard deviation, and the methods are listed above in order of increasing error. If we assume the energy balance data to give a true estimate of fat loss the errors of the other methods are 1.00, 2.17, 2.27 and 3.47 kg for nitrogen balance, density, water and potassium respectively.

It must be noted, however, that these are estimates of the error in estimating change in body composition, which is not necessarily the same as the error in estimating the absolute quantity present at any time. During weight loss the fat-free tissue lost probably differs in composition from the fat-free tissue of the whole body[3].

Body composition versus degree of obesity. It is well known that obese human subjects, unlike some obese rodents, have an increase in both fat and fat-free tissue[10]. Thus it is possible to compare methods for estimating body composition by applying them to a range of people from very thin to very fat. We have done this on a series of 104 women, and have found that the slope of the line relating fat to weight (each divided by height^2) is 1.21, 1.24 and 1.20 for density, water and potassium respectively with a correlation coefficient of 0.93[20]. This suggests that the increase in fat-free tissues for unit increase in fat is smaller when measured by the three methods. However if creatinine excretion is used as the measure of fat-free tissue associated with increased fat the correlation is only 0.40[19], because creatinine excretion reflects muscle mass, and much of the fat-free tissue gained in obesity is not muscle.

1 Behnke, A.R., Feen, B.G. & Welham, W.C. (1942): The specific gravity of healthy men: body weight and volume as an index of obesity. *J. Am. Med. Ass.* **118**, 495–498.
2 Burch, P.R.J. & Spiers, F.W. (1953): Measurement of the gamma radiation from the human body. *Nature* (Lond) **172**, 519–521.
3 Burkinshaw, L. & Morgan, D.B. (1985): Mass and composition of the fat-free tissues of patients with weight loss. *Clin. Sci.* **68**, 455–462.
4 Dempsey, D.T., Crosby, L.O., Lusk, E., Oberlander, J.L., Pertsschuck, M.J. & Mullen, J.L. (1984): Total body water and total body potassium in anorexia nervosa. *Am. J. Clin. Nutr.* **40**, 260–269.
5 Dickerson, J.W.T. & Widdowson, E.M. (1960): Chemical changes in skeletal muscle during growth. *Biochem. J.* **74**, 247–257.
6 Forbes, R.M., Cooper, A.R. & Mitchell H.H. (1953): The composition of the adult human body as determined by chemical analysis. *J. Biol. Chem.* **203**, 359–366.
7 Forbes, R.M., Cooper A.R. & Mitchell, H.H. (1956): Further studies on the gross composition and mineral elements of the adult human body. *J. Biol. Chem.* **223**, 969–975.
8 Forbes, G.B., Kreipe, R.E., Lipinski, B.A. & Hodgman, C.H. (1984): Body composition changes during recovery from anorexia nervosa: comparison of two dietary regimes. *Am. J. Clin. Nutr.* **40**, 1137–1145.
9 Forbes, G.B. & Lewis, A.M. (1956): Total sodium, potassium and chloride in adult man. *J. Clin. Invest.* **35**, 596–600.
10 Forbes, G.B. & Welle, S.L. (1983): Lean body mass in obesity. *Int. J. Obesity* **7**, 99–107.
11 Garrow, J.S. (1965): The use and calibration of a small whole body counter for measurement of total body potassium in malnourished infants. *W. Ind. Med. J.* **24**, 73–81.
12 Garrow, J.S. (1978): *Energy balance and obesity in man*, (2nd edn), p.130. Amsterdam: Elsevier/North-Holland Biomedical Press.
13 Garrow, J.S., Durrant, M.L., Mann, S., Stalley, S.F. & Warwick, P. (1978): Factors determining weight loss in obese patients in a metabolic ward. *Int. J. Obesity.* **2**, 441–447.

14 Garrow, J.S., Stalley, S., Diethelm, R., Pittet, P.H., Hesp, R. & Halliday, D. (1979): A new method for measuring the body density of obese adults. *Br. J. Nutr.* **42**, 173–183.

15 Keys, A., Brozek, J., Hanschel, A., Mickelson, O. & Taylor H.L. (1950): *The biology of human starvation.* Minneapolis: University of Minnesota Press.

16 McCance, R.A. & Widdowson, E.M. (1951): A method of breaking down the body weights of living persons into terms of extracellular fluid, cell mass and fat, and some applications to physiology and medicine. *Proc. Roy. Soc. B.* **138**, 115–130.

17 Mitchell, H.H., Hamilton, T.S., Steggerda, F.R. & Bean, H.W. (1945): The chemical composition of the adult human body and its bearing on the biochemistry of growth. *J. Biol. Chem.* **158**, 625–637.

18 Schutte, J.E., Townsend, E.J., Hugg, J., Shoup, R.F., Malina, R.M., Blomqvist, C.G., (1984): Density of lean body mass is greater in blacks than whites. *J. Appl. Physiol.* **56**, 1647–1649.

19 Webster, J.D. & Garrow, J.S. (1985): Creatinine excretion over 24 hours as a measure of body compositions or of completeness of urine collection. *Hum. Nutr. Clin. Nutr.* **39C**, 101–106.

20 Webster, J.D., Hesp, R. & Garrow, J.S. (1984): The composition of excess weight in obese women estimated by body density, total body water and total body potassium. *Hum. Nutr. Clin. Nutr.* **38C**, 299–306.

21 Widdowson, E.M., Dickerson, J.W.T. (1960): The effect of growth and function on the chemical composition of soft tissues. *Biochem. J.* **77**, 30–43.

22 Widdowson, E.M., McCance, R.A. & Spray, C.M. (1951): The chemical composition of the human body. *Clin. Sci.* **10**, 113–125.

Fat distribution and its metabolic associations

Margaret ASHWELL
MRC Dunn Nutrition Unit, Milton Road, Cambridge CB4 1XJ, UK.

Evidence relating fat distribution to metabolic abnormalities. The metabolic implications of body fat distribution have recently received considerable attention[2,3]. Vague[16] was the first to point out that 'android' or centralised obesity was more closely associated with diabetes, gout and atherosclerosis than the more peripheral 'gynaecoid' obesity. Researchers in Wisconsin[6,8,9] classified fat distribution in women on the basis of the waist to hip circumference ratio (WHR). They found that WHR was a significant predictor of plasma triglyceride, glucose and insulin and correlated with an 'in vivo' index of insulin resistance[6]. In Gothenburg, Krotkiewski *et al*[11] also found that it was the women with high values of WHR who were most likely to suffer these metabolic abnormalities of obesity while prospective studies of risk factors for ischaemic heart disease (IHD) in men[14] and women[13] found that WHR was a better predictor for IHD than the degree of adiposity.

A recent conference devoted to metabolic complications of human obesities[4] further emphasized the overwhelming evidence associating centralised obesity with the risk of metabolic abnormality.

How does 'centralised obesity' relate to fat distribution? Until recently, classification of body fat distribution into 'centralised' obesity ('apples') and peripheral obesity ('pears') has been derived mainly from anthropometry. It was not known how centralised obesity related to intra-abdominal fat content. Do 'apples' and 'pears' have similar proportions of intra-abdominal fat, differing only in the placement of their subcutaneous fat or do 'apples' and 'pears' differ in their proportions of intraabdominal and subcutaneous fat? To answer this question, we[1] used the technique of computer tomography which has recently allowed a direct assessment of the two fat compartments[5,7,15].

Twenty eight women presenting for routine computed tomography (CT) scans had circumference measurements taken at the level of waist, hips and thighs. The ratio of the area of intra-abdominal fat to the area of subcutaneous fat in the CT scan taken at the umbilical level was calculated (ABDO–SUBCUT). This ratio was found to correlate highly significantly with the waist to hip circumference ratio (WHR) (see Fig. 1). The correlation between WHR and the

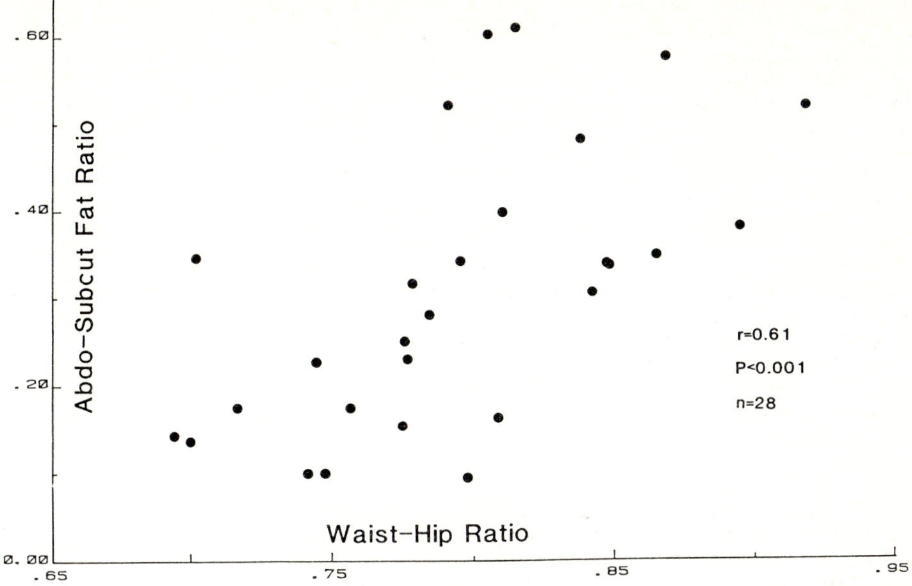

Fig. 1. *The relationship between the ratio of intra-abdominal to subcutaneous fat (ABDO-SUBCUT) determined by computed tomography to the waist to hip circumference ratio ([1] for details).*

ABDO–SUBCUT ratio remained significant after allowing for the degree of obesity ($^W/_H{}^2$) and age, whereas there was no significant correlation between the ABDO–SUBCUT ratio and ($^W/_H{}^2$).

What is the nature of the association between the accumulation of intra-abdominal fat and metabolic disturbances? An association between the ratio of abdominal to subcutaneous fat to various metabolic abnormalities can have at least three interpretations: (1) the enlarged intra-abdominal fat depot might be a direct consequence of the metabolic abnormalities, (2) the metabolic abnormalities might be a direct consequence of the enlarged intra-abdominal fat depot, and (3) both the metabolic abnormalities and the enlarged intra-abdominal fat depot could be consequences of a third, independent, factor.

Interpretation (1) is probably the least likely of the three to be correct. Vague[17] has analysed the role of android obesity in the appearance of non-insulin dependent diabetes (NIDDM) and has documented cases where the diabetes emerges 20 years after the appearance of android obesity. He considers it much more likely that a genetic predisposition to NIDDM acts synergistically with the presence of android obesity to unmask NIDDM.

Interpretation (2) is the one which was suggested originally by the Swedish group[4]: a large, lipolytically sensitive collection of intra-abdominal fat cells would empty excessive free fatty acids (FFA) directly into the portral vein. This could cause not only an elevated synthesis of liver triglycerides but also an inhibition of liver insulin uptake leading to peripheral hyper-insulinaemia followed by insulin resistance. Diabetes, hypertension, or hypertriglyceridemia could therefore follow.

Interpretation (3) has recently been advanced[10] with the proposition that an imbalance in androgenic/oestrogenic activity could play an important role in fat distribution and in the associated metabolic abnormalities. Increased values of WHR were shown to be associated with increased levels of plasma free testosterone (FT) and decreased levels of sex-hormone-binding globulin (SHBG). Furthermore, the degree of androgenic activity (SHBG and FT) correlated with the metabolic profile. SHBG was inversely correlated with fasting insulin whilst FT correlated directly with fasting postprandial insulin levels.

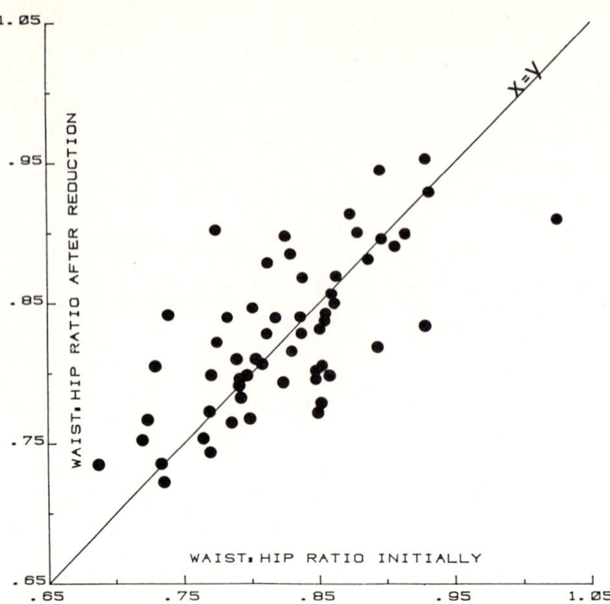

Fig. 2. *The effect of weight reduction on the waist to hip circumference ratio (WHR)*. Fifty-eight women were measured before and after an average weight reduction of 11.7 kg (range = 1.8 to 38.2 kg). There was no significant change in WHR (from Ashwell, Cole & Garrow, in preparation).

In order to substantiate this particular hypothesis, it is obviously essential to show that the increased exposure to unbound androgens precedes the changes in fat distribution (FD) and the associated metabolic abnormalities. It would also be important to explain why no consistent sex-related differences in the distribution of fat between internal and external depots have ever been found in other mammals (C. Pond, personal communication).

On the other hand, further evidence for interpretation (3) has come from a study[12] of muscle fibre types and FD. Men have a different distribution of muscle fibre types to women; they have a relatively greater number of fast twitch Type B 'body builder' fibres whereas women have a relatively greater number of slow twitch 'endurance type' fibres. However, if women are classified as 'apples' or 'pears' according to their WHR value 'apples' show a typical 'male' profile of muscle fibre distribution. Since it is extremely unlikely that changes in muscle fibre types could occur as a consequence of changes in FD, this particular observation would also seem to indicate that interpretation (3) is perhaps the most likely one to be correct.

How can the new knowledge about fat distribution and metabolic abnormalities influence the treatment of obesity? Since it is very clear that 'apples' are much more likely than 'pears' to suffer from the metabolic complications of obesity, it would seem reasonable to identify 'apples' as a high risk group and to suggest that they are examined more liberally for complicating disorders and should be given preferential treatment for weight reduction[4].

This seems an obvious step until one examines the present confusion in the literature relating metabolic risk to FD and to degree of obesity. It has been concluded that the effects of centralised obesity are independent of, and additive to, those of obesity level[10]. On the other hand, a longitudinal study of Swedish men revealed that the group with the greater risk of developing CHD were not the most obese group with the highest values of WHR. Furthermore, the longitudinal study of Swedish women[13] showed that lean and obese women with high WHR were equally likely to develop CHD.

It would seem, therefore, that the safest way to decrease risk of developing any metabolic complication is to reduce the value of WHR at the same time as reducing the degree of obesity. Unfortunately, measurements of waist and hip girth on a group of 58 obese women before and after weight reduction (Fig. 2) suggest that although there are significant decreases in both waist and hip measurements, their ratio (WHR) shows no significant downward trend. Even if a miracle drug were found which could preferentially mobilise intra-abdominal fat deposits and thus reduce values of WHR as well as reducing weight, it could only help to reduce the metabolic abnormalities associated with FD if the intra-abdominal fat depots had been the primary cause of the abnormalities.

Conclusions. The strong associations between fat distribution and the metabolic abnormalities of obesity certainly warrant further exploration. However, this research can only stimulate novel approaches to the treatment of obesity if it can be proved that the abnormalities are direct consequences of a supra-normal accumulation of internal fat. Otherwise, the importance of the association can only be used to identify and treat a high risk group of obese people and to hope that a reduction in the degree of obesity even in the absence of a reduction in WHR may improve their prospects of a healthy life.

1 Ashwell, M., Cole, T.J. & Dixon, A.K. (1985): Obesity: new insight into anthropometric classification of fat distribution shown by computed tomography. *Br. Med. J.* **290**, 1692–1694.
2 Anon (1984): The shape of fatness. *Lancet.* **1**, 889.
3 Björntorp, P. (1984): Hazards in subgroups of human obesity. *Eur. J. Clin. Invest.* **14**, 239–241.
4 Björntorp, P. ed (1985): *Metabolic complications of human obesities.* Amsterdam: Elsevier.
5 Dixon, A.K. (1983): Abdominal fat assessed by computed tomography: sex difference in distribution. *Clin. Radiol.* **34**, 189–191.
6 Evans, D.J., Hoffman, R.G., Kalkhoff, R.K. & Kissebah, A.H. (1984): Relationship of body fat topography to insulin sensitivity and metabolic profiles in premenopausal women. *Metabolism* **33**, 68–75.
7 Grauer, W.O., Moss, A.A., Cann, C.E. & Goldberg, H.I. (1984): Quantification of body fat distribution in the abdomen using computed tomography. *Am. J. Clin. Nutr.* **39**, 631–637
8 Kalkhoff, R.K., Hartz, A.H., Rupley, D., Kissebah, A.H. & Kelber, S. (1983): Relationship of body fat distribution to blood pressure, carbohydrate tolerance, and plasma lipids in healthy obese women. *J. Lab. Clin. Med.* **102**, 621–627.
9 Kissebah, A.H., Vydelingum, N., Murray, R., Evans, D.J., Hartz, A.J., Kalkhoff, R.K. & Adams, P.W. (1982): Relation of body fat distribution to metabolic complications of obesity. *J. Clin. Endocrinol. Metab.* **54**, 254–260.
10 Kissebah, A. (1985): Endocrine characteristics in regional obesities: role of sex steroids. In *Metabolic complications of the human obesities*, ed Evans, D.J., Peiris, A. & Wilson, C.R. Amsterdam: Elsevier.
11 Krotkiewski, M., Björntorp, P., Sjostrom, L. & Smith, U. (1983): Impact of obesity on metabolism in men and women. *J. Clin. Invest.* **72**, 1150–1162.
12 Krotkiewski, M. & Björntorp, P. (1985): The effects of physical training in obese women and men and in apple-and pear-shaped obesity. In *Metabolic complications of the human obesities*, ed P. Björntorp, Amsterdam: Elsevier.
13 Lapidus, L., Bengtsson, C., Larsson, B., Pennert, K., Rybo, E. & Sjostrom, L. (1984): Distribution of adipose tissue and risk of cardiovascular disease and death: a 12 year follow up of participants in the population study of women in Gothenburg, Sweden. *Br. Med. J.* **288**, 1257–1261.
14 Larsson, B., Svardsudd, K., Welin, L., Wilhelmsen, L., Björntorp, P. & Tibblin, G. (1984): Abdominal adipose tissue distribution, obesity and risk of cardiovascular disease and death: 13 year follow up of participants in the study of men born in 1913. *Br. Med. J.* **288**, 1401–1404.
15 Tokunaga, K., Matsuzawa, Y., Ishakawa, K. & Tarui, S. (1983): A novel technique for the determination of body fat by computed tomography. *Int. J. Obesity* **7**, 437–445.
16 Vague, J. (1953): *La differenciation sexuelle humaine: ses incidences en pathologie.* Paris: Masson.
17 Vague, P. (1985): Adipose tissue distribution in type II diabetes mellitus, and relationship to insulin resistance. In *Metabolic complications of the human obesities*. Amsterdam: Elsevier.

Immunological methods for assessment of nutritional status

R. DIONIGI and L. DOMINIONI
Department of Surgery, Sezione di Patologia Chirurgica, University of Pavia, Italy

---

It is well known that malnutrition is one of the major causes of increased morbidity and mortality among hospitalized patients. There are many indirect and direct methods of assessing nutritional status. These include history of dietary intake, physical examination for signs of deficiency syndromes, anthropometry, biochemical, physical and radiosotope measurement of body composition, immunological tests and miscellaneous procedures. However, the relative value of these measurements has not been clearly defined. This is especially true for the immunological parameters, where abnormalities are often observed in clinical and subclinical malnutrition.

The demonstration of consistent changes in immunological responses in PEM and in deficit of specific nutrients led to the hypothesis that immunocompetence can be used as a functional index of nutritional status. We will briefly review the alterations caused by malnutrition on the immune system and will discuss the clinical relevance of the immunological parameters more commonly used to evaluate nutritional status.

Effects of malnutrition on the immune system. Many studies have shown that nearly every aspect of the body's defense can be damaged by inadequate nutrition. Immunoglobulin levels, antibody production, phagocytic function, inflammatory responses, complement function, secretory and mucosal immunity, and other defence mechanisms may all be impaired by the absence of biologically essential nutrients.

Effects of lymphocytes. In malnutrition the primary lymphoid structures of the immune system, notably the thymus, as well as such secondary structures as the spleen and lymph nodes, are significantly altered in size, weight, architecture and cellular components[7,18]. The thymic-dependent areas are especially affected and germinal centres are usually reduced in number. In addition lymphocyte depletion becomes evident in the blood. On the basis of these observations, which were confirmed experimentally[5], it has been recognized that one of the most simple and reliable immunological measurements of nutritional status is the blood lymphocyte count. It has been shown[2] that the percentage of T-cells in the peripheral blood is reduced in malnutrition. The reduction parallels the severity of weight loss, impaired cutaneous delayed hypersensitivity response to dinitrochlorobenzene (DNCB) and decreased DNA synthesis by lymphocytes stimulated with phytohaemagglutinin (PHA). The abnormalities were quickly and completely reversed with nutritional improvement, thereby ruling out any primary defect of the thymus. Lymphocyte blastogenic response to PHA has been studied during malnutrition and found to be reduced[4,5]. The percentage of B-lymphocytes in the peripheral blood in malnutrition is normal or increased. An increase is often seen in those children who have an obvious infection associated with nutritional deficiency[1].

Effects on immunoglobulins and complement. Hypogammaglobulinaemia is usually associated with severe uncomplicated undernutrition, but children with malnutrition may have elevated levels of immunoglobulins as a consequence of repeated infections. In general, IgM levels are higher than in age-matched normal controls. Levels of IgA are variable, but often elevated with concomitant infection, and IgE is frequently markedly elevated as a result of parasitic infections. Results obtained in our laboratory showed that the average IgG levels slowly and constantly decrease during a malnutrition period, reaching a significantly low concentration after 5 weeks of undernutrition. Malnutrition caused a statistically non-significant reduction in IgM concentration, whereas levels of the third complement component showed a marked fall[5]. Patients with kwashiorkor[19] have depressed haemolytic complement levels, as well as depressed levels of all complement components, except C4, but including Factor B. In a clinical study performed in patients with oesophageal carcinoma, suffering from PEM and shown to be in negative nitrogen balance, there were no significant differences in the levels of C3, C4 and Factor B between these patients and controls[10]. This apparently seems to be contrary to our findings from experimental work performed in dogs[11]; however, the neoplastic process acts as a stimulus to the synthesis of acute phase proteins, which include complement components[8], and this may explain the conflicting results.

Effect of delayed hypersensitivity response (DHR). Studies employing a battery of antigens have confirmed the frequent occurrence of depression of DHR during undernutrition[3]. Nutrition-related cutaneous anergy is not confined to the severe deficiency syndromes observed in the developing countries. Delayed hypersensitivity skin testing on more than 500 surgical patients demonstrated that anergy and relative anergy were associated with malnutrition, sepsis, shock and trauma[11]; in these studies the maintenance of body cell mass by the use of total parenteral nutrition was associated with reversal of the anergic state and an improved prognosis. In our centre the DHR of preoperative patients has been studied to evaluate possible relationships between DHR, malnutrition and postoperative infections[6]. The incidence of infections in anergic patients was found to be significantly higher than that in normoergic or hypoergic individuals. Serum albumin concentration was significantly lower in anergic than in normoergic patients. This study also indicated that nutritional deficiency may influence some aspects of the immunological processes which may contribute to the development of infection or its progression.

The evidence supporting the determination of DHR for the purpose of nutritional assessment however is not completely satisfactory, and problems often arise in the interpretation of the results of skin tests[20]. There is little doubt that the cause of depressed DHR is multifactorial, especially in cancer patients, and at least five possible causative conditions have been identified[9]: (1) preexisting primary or acquired immunodeficiency, (2) the presence of cancer *per se*, (3) malnutrition (either primitive or cancer-induced cachexia), (4) advance aged, (5) previous immunosuppresive therapy.

Effects on neutrophils and phagocytes. A decreased bactericidal activity of nutrophils was observed in children with kwashiorkor[17] and it was also reported that leucocytes of children with PEM presented an impaired phagocytosis and a metabolic defect[16]. It should be noted that tests of neutrophil phagocytosis are not easy to perform, probably explaining why they have not been widely used for the purpose of nutritional assessment. However, there are some simpler tests of leucocyte function, such as cytochemical reactions for polysaccharides, alkaline and acid phosphatases, peroxidases, esterases and lipase, and Arneth's formula, which could be used to document alterations occurring in undernutrition; we are currently exploring this possible application[12].

Conclusions. From the data reviewed above it can be observed that a very large number of tests of immunological functions could theoretically be used for the purpose of nutritional assessment. However many of these tests require specialized laboratory skills, take time and probably provide few data to the clinician, in terms of nutritional assessment, in addition to the basic information that can be obtained just by performing a few simple, selected immunological measurements, In fact, many clinical studies carried out during the past decade have shown that only a few immunological tests are simple, reproducible and reliable enough as indicators of nutritional assessment, in addition to the other non-immunological indices. They are (1) blood total lymphocyte count[14,15], and (2) DHR[13]. At present all the other immunological measurements which have been reviewed above should be considered as research tools in the field of nutritional assessment; obviously they can be used in selected patients to document specific alterations related to nutrition. Moreover it must be underlined that immunological tests can be affected by many clinical variables unrelated to nutrition, such as specific pathological conditions, immunodepressive therapy, accidental or surgical trauma, infection. This should always be taken into consideration in interpreting immunological results from the nutritional point of view.

1 Bang, B.G., Mahalanabis, D. & Mukherjee, K.L. (1975): T and B lymphocyte rosetting in undernourished children. *Proc. Soc. Exp. Biol. Med.* **149**, 199–205.

2 Chandra, R.K. (1974): Rosette-forming T-lymphocytes and cell-mediated immunity in malnutrition. *Br. Med. J.* **3**, 608–609.

3 Chandra, R.K. (1974): *Progress in immunology, Vol. 4. Clinical aspects*, p.355, ed L. Brent & F. Holborow. New York: Elsevier-North Holland.

4 Chandra, R.K. (1975): Immunocompetence in undernutrition. *J. Pediatrics* **81**, 1184–1190.

5 Dionigi, R., Zonta, A., Dominioni, L., Gnes, F. & Ballabio, A. (1977): The effects of total parenteral nutrition on immunodepression caused by malnutrition. *Ann. Surg.* **185**, 467–474.

6 Dionigi, R., Gnes, F., Boner, A., Dominioni, L. & Fossati, G.S. (1979): Delayed hypersensitivity response (DHR) and infections in surgical cancer patients. *Br. J. Surg.* **66**, 900.

7 Dominioni, L., Gnes, F., Dionigi, R., Zonta, A. & Prati, U. (1976): Histopathological studies on dog lymphoid structures during malnutrition and total parenteral nutrition. *Boll. Ist. Sieroter. Milanese* **55**, 311–316.

8 Dominioni, L., Dionigi, R. & Jemos, V. (1981): The acute phase response of plasma proteins in surgical patients. In *Clinical nutrition '81*, ed Wesdorp R.I.C. & Soeters P.B., p.239–259, Edinburgh: Churchill-Livingstone.

9 Dominioni, L., Dionigi, R., Dionigi, P., Nazari, S., Fossati, G.S., Prati, U., Tibaldeschi, C. & Pavesi, F. (1981): Evaluation of possible causes of delayed hypersensitivity impairment in cancer patients. *J. Parent, Ent. Nutr.* **5**, 300–306.

10 Haffejee, A.A. & Angorn, I.B. (1979): Nutritional status and the nonspecific cellular and humoral immune response in oesophageal carcinoma. *Ann. Surg.* **189**, 475–479.

11 Meakins, J.L., Pietsch, J.B., Bubenick, O., Kelly, R., Rode, H., Gordon, J. & MacLean, L.D. (1977): Delayed hypersensitivity: indicator of acquired failure of host defenses in sepsis and trauma. *Ann. Surg.* **186**, 241–249.

12 Monico, R., Manelli, A., Michienzi, M. & Perseghin, P. (1985): Cytochemical and functional leucocyte tests in undernourished surgical patients. *Procs. Int. Workshop* on 'Nutritional assessment in hospital malnutrition', p.9, Venice Lido, Italy, Apr. 26–27.

13 Mullen, J.L., Buzby, G.P., Waldman, M.T., Gertner, M.H., Hobbs, C.L., Rosato, E.F. (1979): Prediction of operative morbidity and mortality by preoperative nutritional assessment. *Surg. Forum* **30**, 80–82.

14 Nazari, S., Comincioli, V., Dionigi, R., Capelo, A., Dionigi, P., Comodi, I., Tibaldeschi, C. & Bonoldi, A.P. (1980): Cluster analysis of nutritional and immunological indicators for identification of high risk surgical patients. *IRCS Surg. Sci.* **8**, 866–867.

15 Seltzer, M.H., Bastidas, J.A., Cooper, D.M., Engler, P., Slocum, B. & Fletcher, H.S. (1979): Instant nutritional assessment. *J. Parent, Ent. Nutr.* **3**, 157–159.

16 Selvaraj, R.J. & Bhat, K.S. (1972): Metabolic and bactericidal activities of leucocytes in protein-calorie malnutrition. *Am J. Clin. Nutr.* **25**, 166–174.

17 Shousha, S. & Kamel K. (1972): Nitro blue tetrazolium test in children with kwashiorkor with a comment on the use of latex particles in the test. *J. Clin. Path.* **25**, 494–497.

18 Smythe, P.M., Schonland, M., Brereton-Stiles, G.G., Coovadia, H.M., Grace, H.J., Loening, W.E.K., Mafoyane, A., Parent, M.A. & Vos, G.H. (1971): Thymolymphatic deficiency and depression of cell-mediated immunity in protein-calorie malnutrition. *Lancet* **2**, 939–943.

19 Suskind, R., Edelman, R. & Kulapongs, P. (1976): Complement studies in children with kwashiorkor. *Am. J. Clin. Nutr.* **29**, 1089–1092.

20 Twomey, P., Ziegler, D. & Rombeau, J. (1982): Utility of skin testing in nutritional assessment: a critical review. *J. Parent. Ent. Nutr.* **6**, 50–58.

Pitfalls of anthropometry

J. O. MORA
International Nutrition Unit, OIH/DHHS. 121 Congressional Lane, Suite 304, Rockville, Maryland 20852 USA

Physical growth is the best available indicator of overall nutritional status[4,6,14]. Anthropometry represents a relatively simple, objective and valid means to assess physical growth and it is used in health and nutrition programmes worldwide, as a means of identifying children at risk or already affected by PEM, and as a source of information on the general health and nutritional status of the population.

To what extent do physical growth measurements provide useful and valid indicators of the nutritional status of children? This may have important practical implications for the use and interpretation of anthropometry. Two major types of pitfalls are discussed.

Ascertaining abnormal growth. A major limitation of anthropometry is the difficulty of ascertaining the extent to which apparent deviations in growth are only the result of genetic variation or whether they can be attributed to environmental action or to genetic/environmental interaction. Allowing for the effect of genetic factors is a critical problem in interpreting anthropometric indicators. Only by estimating the growth potential of the individual within an acceptable degree of accuracy can deviations from such potential be reasonably attributed to the influence of adverse environmental factors. An additional problem is establishing whether a given deviation from a mean reference value is functionally abnormal or merely the result of a normal physiological adaptation to sub-optimal conditions.

Two major related issues are relevant to the interpretation of single observations. First, abnormality can only be established by comparisons with patterns of normality or reference values; second, the choice of cut-off points for normality/abnormality has become a controversial issue.

Reference values. The use of international reference values has been proposed by WHO[16] and convincingly justified[3,5,13]. Reference values are used to set up normality boundaries based on the estimated probability that a given anthropometric value belongs to the normal distribution of the reference population. The use of appropriate local reference values may be adequate, but there is an obvious pitfall involved in using local norms based on whole mixed populations living under a wide range of environmental conditions where malnutrition is a significant problem.

A single anthropometric measurement at a given point in time is usually not enough for the individual assessment of the normality of growth. This always requires a series of measurements over time to observe the tendency of the growth curve[11]. The simple rule is: steady growth with a sustained slope is probably normal and is always desirable, no growth or a flattening of the curve is a warning sign, and a declining growth curve is a serious signal of abnormal growth. Notice that this interpretation of growth monitoring curves, as in the road-to-health charts, does not require the use of reference values. These are particularly important for estimating indicators based on single observations, such as in cross-sectional prevalence studies, which brings out the problem of cut-off points.

Cut-off points. Two of the three approaches used in clinical epidemiology for selecting measurements and setting cut-off points for diagnostic or screening purposes are applicable to anthropometry: (a) probability estimations based on the statistical properties of the normal distribution of values from a supposedly healthy reference population; (b) identification of breaking (threshold) points for significant changes in the risk of disease, disability or death associated with changes in the values obtained by the diagnostic/screening instrument. The third approach, based on the observed response to a treatment, is not applicable to anthropometry, since there is practically no breaking point for such response.

The two approaches are complementary in that the cut-off points set up on statistical grounds may be validated in functional terms by using the risk approach. Unfortunately, validating anthropometric cut-off points is extremely difficult due to the lack of reliable external criteria, eg true direct measures of nutritional status. Thus investigators have relied on predictive validity using non-specific outcomes such as morbidity and mortality[2,7].

The cut-off points of anthropometric indicators for prevalence assessments should be standardized, not only for comparison purposes, but also because true prevalence figures can only be obtained when a clear-cut and well defined criterion for abnormality is used[10]. Besides its statistical justification, the use of -2s.d. or the third percentile of the reference population as proposed by WHO[15], is supported by studies indicating a sharp increase in the risk of death and a decreased immune response when weight-for-age drops below these points[2,7,12]. A reasonable alternative approach suggested by WHO[16] to estimate prevalence figures in population studies uses 1s.d. as the cut-off point, but the resulting prevalence is adjusted by subtracting 16.9 per cent, the proportion of cases under this point in the normal distribution.

Prevalence figures vary depending upon the cut-off point used (Table 1). The so-call Gomez classification with its 90 per cent weight-for-age cut-off point (about 1s.d. below the mean) has tended to overestimate the prevalence of child malnutrition in developing countries by including a sizeable amount of false positives whose weights are within the normal range of the reference population distribution. This may contribute to increase the awareness of the problem, but it may also generate a feeling of scepticism about the feasibility of measurable improvements, in part due to the difficulty in detecting significant changes in the population at greatest risk. This problem has been approached by taking only second and third degree malnutrition (below 75 per cent weight-for-age).

When targetting nutritional rehabilitation interventions or evaluating changes in the nutritional status of population groups over time, cut-off points far enough from the reference median so as to select the truly malnourished individuals, with few false positives (high specificity), are more likely to detect significant changes. The magnitude of the positive change

Table 1. *Prevalence (per cent) PEM in Colombian children under 5 years, using different weight-for-age cut-off points.* (Colombia National Health Survey, 1977–80).

		Weight-for-age cut-off points	
Age group (months)	90% (Gomez)	75% (Gomez II & III)	3rd percentile (WHO)
0–5	21.9	2.2	3.0
6–11	28.6	11.6	14.9
12–23	45.1	12.1	26.9
24–60	50.2	7.5	21.0
Total	43.4	8.3	19.4

Table 2. *Percentage change in the total prevalence of PEM in Colombian children under 5 years over a 15 year period, using different weight-for-age cut-off points.* (Colombia National Health Surveys, 1965–66 and 1977–80).

		Weight-for-age cut-off points	
Age group (months)	90% (Gomez)	75% (Gomez II & III)	3rd percentile (WHO)
0–5	+23.6	−62.1	−26.8
6–11	−37.6	−42.3	−33.5
12–23	− 5.3	−27.5	− 5.6
24–60	− 3.8	−53.5	−23.4
Total	− 7.3	−47.1	−20.5

occurring over a 15-year period in the prevalence of PEM in the Colombian population below five years varies according to the cut-off point used (Table 2).

Assessing the environmental determinants of abnormal growth. After an abnormal deviation from the growth potential is established beyond any doubt, the problem of determining the environmental determinants of this deviation remains. Unfortunately, anthropometric indicators are sensitive to changes in a number of environmental conditions thus having *low specificity*. This has triggered the controversy of the relative importance of dietary inadequacies versus infectious diseases in the causation of physical growth retardation in young children in developing countries. Dietary inadequacies may have been overemphasized, and infection may play a more important role as a cause of retarded growth in many children[9]. Indeed, both are capable of impairing physical growth. An important question is whether some anthropometric indicators may be more sensitive than others to changes in specific environmental conditions; similarly, the identification of specific adverse environmental factors associated with the onset of growth failure would be useful, if feasible.

Since the so called nutritional anthropometry indicators are influenced not only by dietary factors but also by genetics and disease, strictly speaking they do not specifically assess energy-protein nutritional status. The practical implications of their poor specificity would not be so serious, however, if growth retardation (PEM) were not often regarded and treated as caused by primary dietary deficiencies. This has resulted in a general tendency to treat and prevent growth retardation through only dietary measures, ignoring other major environmental influences such as diarrhoeal and other infectious diseases.

A reciprocal relationship between diarrhoeal diseases and growth has been documented. Diarrhoeal disease severity and duration, but not incidence, tend to be greater in children with retarded growth[1] and, conversely, incremental growth is lower as the incidence of diarrhoea increases[8]. In our longitudinal studies in Bogota, Colombia we found a significant negative association between days ill with diarrhoea and concurrent gain in weight and length, and also, though less consistently, between physical growth achieved at a given time and the subsequent

Table 3. *Covariance analysis of periodic diarrhoeal incidence by initial weight and length attained.* Covariate: The incidence of diarrhoea in the preceding period. (n.s. = not significant).

Incidence Period (months)		Source of variance			F-ratio	P
9–12	Diarrhoea	6–9	months		30.5	0.001
	Weight	9	months		1.6	n.s.
	Length	9	months		2.5	n.s.
12–18	Diarrhoea	9–12	months		33.9	0.001
	Weight	12	months		1.9	n.s.
	Lenght	12	months		1.5	n.s.
18–24	Diarrhoea	12–18	months		51.5	0.001
	Weight	18	months		2.4	n.s.
	Length	18	months		2.5	n.s.

incidence of diarrhoeal diseases. Interestingly, highly significant positive correlations were found between the incidence rates of diarrhoeal diseases occurring in successive periods of observation, suggesting diarrhoeal incidence disappeared when the previous incidence of diarrhoea was first taken into account in an analysis of covariance (Table 3).

These findings suggest that the eventual relation between nutritional status and subsequent diarrhoeal disease may be mostly accounted for by the association between the incidence of diarrhoea and both the concurrent incremental growth and the subsequent diarrhoeal incidence. It appears that diarrhoea leads to growth retardation and it is just those growth retarded children who continue to experience high incidence rates of the disease.

1 Black, R.E., Brown, K.H. & Becker, S. (1984): Malnutrition is a determining factor in diarrhoeal duration, but not incidence, among young children in a longitudinal study in rural Bangladesh. *Am. J. Clin. Nutr.* **37**, 87–94.
2 Chen, L.C., Chowdhury, A. & Huffman, S.L. (1980): Anthropometric assessment of energy-protein malnutrition and subsequent risk of mortality among preschool aged children. *Am. J. Clin. Nutr.* **33**, 1836–1845.
3 Graitcer, L.P. & Gentry, E.M. (1981): One reference for all, *Lancet.* **1**, 297–299.
4 Griffiths, M. (1981): *Growth monitoring*, Primary Health Care Issues Series I, No. 3. Washington DC: American Public Health Association, International Health Programs.
5 Habicht, J.P., Martorell, R., Yarbrough, C., Malina, R.M. & Klein, R.E. (1974): Height and weight standards for preschool children. How relevant are ethnic differences in growth potential? *Lancet* **1**, 611–615.
6 Keller, W., Donoso, G. & DeMaeyer, E.M. (1976): Anthropometry in nutritional surveillance: A review based on results of the WHO collaborative study on nutritional anthropometry. *Nutr. Abstr. Rev.* **46**, 591–609.
7 Kielman, A.A. & McCord, C. (1978): Weight-for-age as an index of risk of death in children. *Lancet.* **1**, 1247–1250.
8 Martorell, R., Yarbrough, C., Lechtig, A., Habicht, J.P. & Klein, R. (1975): Diarrhoeal diseases and growth retardation in preschool Guatemalan children. *Am. J. Phys. Anthrop.* **43**, 341–346.
9 Mata, L.J., Kromal, R.A., Urrutia, J.J. & Garcia, B. (1977): Effect of infection on food intake and the nutritional state: perspectives as viewed from the village. *Am. J. Clin. Nutr.* **30**, 1215–1227.
10 Mora, J.O. (1984): Assessment of anthropometry in prevalence studies. In *Malnutrition and behaviour: critical assessment of key issues*, eds J. Brozek & B. Schurch, pp.98–106. Nestlé Nutrition Publication Series No. 4.
11 Morley, D. & Woodland, M. (1979): *See how they grow. Monitoring child growth for appropriate health care in developing countries*. New York: Oxford University Press.
12 Reddy, V., Jagadeesan, V., Ragharamulu, N., Bhaskaram, C., & Srikantia, S.G. (1976): Functional significance of growth retardation in malnutrition. *Am. J. Clin. Nutr.* **29**, 3–7.
13 Waterlow, J.C. (1980): Child growth standards. *Lancet.* **1**, 717–719.
14 Waterlow, J.C., Buzina, R., Keller, W., Lane, J.M., Nichaman, M.Z. & Tanner, J.M. (1977): The presentation and use of height and weight data for comparing the nutritional status of groups of children under the age of 10 years. *Bull. WHO* **55**, 489–498.
15 WHO (1978): A growth chart for international use in maternal and child health care. Guidelines for primary health care personnel. Geneva: World Health Organization non-serial publication.
16 WHO (1979): *Measurement of nutritional impact*. Geneva: World Health Organization.

Nutritional studies in the field

D. NABARRO
*Department of International Community Health, Liverpool School of Tropical Medicine, Pembroke Place,
Liverpool L3 5QA, UK.*

Three nutritional field studies undertaken in Nepal since 1977 are described. The purpose for which each study was undertaken and the circumstances under which they were established influenced the design and conduct of the studies and the results they yielded. The lessons learnt from the conduct of these studies are discussed: they may have application in countries other than Nepal.

The studies. *Chuliban longitudinal study.* A mother-and-child health-care programme was established in Dhankuta district, East Nepal (pop. 160 000) in 1977 by Save the Children Fund and the Nepal Children's Organisation. Since the start of the programme its staff have wanted to obtain information about influences on the growth and development of the children in the district in order to decide the most suitable strategies for tackling their nutritional problems. As a part of the service programme, field staff were making regular visits to homes in the settlement of Chuliban, (pop. 3000; one of the district's poorest communities), close to Dhankuta Bazaar, the district capital. During these visits staff assessed children's health and nutrition (weighing and measuring the children at each visit) and offered preventive and curative care. Field workers' records were used to provide data on the growth of children, the illnesses they experienced, and the data were later analysed[5] to explore relationships between illnesses, seasons, child age and growth patterns.

The data collected were not easily analysed. The value of the data was limited both by errors in data collection and by missing values. For example, field workers found it difficult to measure heights precisely using a height-stick (one month all the children under study appeared to shrink by about three centimetres!). To overcome this problem a portable stadiometer was manufactured, and a weight-for-height chart was painted onto it to permit the rapid identification of wasted children[6]. This innovation was not popular with the field workers who had to carry the heavy stadiometer up and down steep hills. Missing values resulted from seasonal movement of mothers and their children into and out of their villages and with problems of identifying individual children.

The Chuliban data were analysed by hand, and then on a mainframe computer in London: a great deal of specialist assistance was needed to get the work done. Results[3] revealed that young children were most likely to lose weight and become wasted during the summer months (the monsoon season) and that this weight loss was usually triggered by an illness (particularly measles, diarrhoea or whooping cough).

Qualitative data, collected from the case studies[9], emphasized the importance of the time available to mothers in determining their ability to maintain children's food intake during, and immediately after, episodes of illness. Data from cross-sectional studies, undertaken simultaneously, revealed that children from poorer households were more likely to have slowed skeletal growth and to become stunted at an early age[4]. The results have been incorporated into a slide programme on malnutrition in Nepal[8]. 'dBase2' microcomputer Software (Ashton Tate Ltd, Milton Keynes) has been adapted to permit the further analysis of these data on microcomputer systems[1].

Khardep impact study. In 1979 the Nepal Government's Ministry of Panchayat and Local Development initiated an integrated rural development programme in four hill districts in eastern Nepal. These districts (Terathum, Bhojpur, Sankhuasabbha and Dhankuta) have a combined population of over 500 000. It was proposed that the impact of the Kosi Hill Area

Development Programme (KHARDEP) be assessed through the study of changes in the well-being of households likely to be affected by KHARDEP funded development initiatives (irrigation schemes, small farmer credit programmes and agricultural extension service centres). Earlier cross-sectional studies had suggested that children from poorer households were more likely both to be wasted and stunted during the monsoon months, so children's nutritional status and growth rates were chosen as indicators of household well-being.

The impact studies were started in 1980 and were expected to continue at least until 1985, the end of the implementation of KHARDEP phase 2[5]. Because of the dramatic seasonal variations in growth rate and nutritional status of children, data were obtained from households in the KHARDEP area at least twice each year during the 5 years that the programme was being implemented. Two teams each with three skilled surveyors were assembled (teams also included porters, to carry equipment and surveyors' food, and cooks). Team members were trained to collect data on a variety of subjects — including land area cultivated by households, crop production, animal holding, consumption of food items, births and deaths of household members, weights of adults and weights, heights and arm circumference of children. Team members were involved in the development of the questionnaires and pretested them at one of the study sites before the studies were intiated. They were taught to collect additional information if there had been a noticeable change in the circumstances of any household that they visited. The data collected was subjected to regular review by the team members, the KHARDEP co-ordinator and planning officers and by ODA's technical advisers working with KHARDEP.

The need to visit households at defined times each year and the time taken for surveyors to travel through the hills meant that only a limited number of households could be visited by each team. This restricted the number of sites where households could be studied. It was decided that the minimum number of households to be selected for study at each site was 30 (each with a child under the age of 3 years); seven study sites were selected — four that were likely to be influenced by KHARDEP funded initiatives and three — in similar locations — that were less likely to be so influenced.

It was planned that the size of the sample for study would be increased after the first year of data collection but an increase in sample size was not possible before 1983 because of limited staff availability. The system for data analysis was devised at the time the study was designed, in 1980[5]. Data from the surveyors' record forms were to be listed on specially printed forms — one row for each household, and over a hundred columns for each of the variables studied. The structures of tables to be produced from the data were decided in advance: some merely described (using frequencies, means and measures of dispersion) the data collected for each variable from the different study sites. Other tables analysed study variables (nutritional status or changes in weights of adults and children) with respect to predictor variables — such as indicators of household economic status. It proved possible to computerise this system for data analysis using a microcomputer installed in Nepal during 1983. The computer uses dBase2 software which has been adapted to handle KHARDEP Impact Studies' data. Nepalese personnel can both run the programmes and adapt them for data handling purposes. The computer is also used to produce the reports of the data analyses, again in a format which was decided during the first year of the studies[7].

To date the results have revealed little evidence of a difference in the nutritional status of adults and children in sites close to KHARDEP-funded development initiatives as compared with those distant from them. This is not surprising as the implementation of KHARDEP has been rather slower than expected. The impact studies will need to be continued for several more years to demonstrate a nutritional impact of KHARDEP.

Outcomes of the Chautara mother child health programme. The Save the Children Fund established its fourth mother and child health programme in Nepal during 1982 at Chautara, capital of Sindhupalchok District (pop. 200 000), in the central development region. The programme was established in cooperation with the Nepalese Government's Department of Health Services with the aim of providing in-service training to field workers from both government and non-governmental organisations.

The field workers who had been trained were encouraged to keep careful records of the children they saw in their communities. It was not possible for them to carry weighing scales and an alternative anthropometric measure of children's nutritional status was needed. They have been using three-coloured arm circumference tapes to identify malnourished children aged between 1 and 5 years. Studies in Bangladesh reveal that the absolute value of the arm circumference of a child aged between one and five years is a sensitive and specific indicator of the child's risk of death in succeeding months (Briend and Zimicki, 1985; personal communication). If field staff are taught to make arm circumference measurements correctly, they will obtain valuable information about a child's nutritional status. The Chautara trainees also collect data on children's health status and their use of locally available services.

Field workers' data are returned to the Chautara programme headquarters at quarterly intervals and are analysed to reveal the percentages of children with differing arm circumference and immunisation status, the percentages of children with symptoms and registered in the MCH centre, the percentages of households using family planning measures.

The results are used to provide information for field workers (and District health personnel) and to assess workers' performance. They also reveal the outcome of mother and child health services throughout the District. Analyses of a field workers' data are returned to them throughout their supervisory staff and changes from quarter to quarter are discussed with them.

It has again proved possible to computerise both data analysis and the preparation of reports, using dBase2 software.

The study has been underway for two years. In early 1985, 29 field workers were collecting data from upwards of 2500 children; changes in immunisation coverage and nutritional status of children in the population have occurred more rapidly than changes in their parents' acceptance of family planning measures[2].

Lessons that we have learnt from our studies. It is vital that any data collection activity is planned in advance and that the circumstances under which data are to be collected, as well as the purposes for data collection, are taken into consideration. This advance planning has to be divided into stages: (1) The reasons for which data are being collected must be thought through in advance, with care, as they will influence decisions about both the types of data to be collected and the collection methods. Such advance planning is needed whatever the purposes of collection. The data to be collected should be only those items needed to address the questions under study. (2) Practical details of the data collection also need careful advance planning. Many pitfalls can be overcome through pilot studies and through carefully conducted case-studies (family profiles) of selected families. These preliminary steps will help investigators to identify those data items, required for the study, which cannot be collected without additional facilities (staff, equipment) or training. (3) Those collecting data must be carefully supervised to ensure that errors are minimal and that they use simple equipment well. Poor quality data are likely to prove hard to analyse and may lead to erroneous results. Well-collected qualitative data are often more useful than volumes of unreliable figures. (4) If the data for analysis are being collected routinely by field workers as part of their service activities, study managers should anticipate possible conflicts between the programme's needs for staff to deliver services and their needs for reliable data. (5) Whether the study to be undertaken is a simple assessment of field-workers' performance or a more complex analysis of influences on nutritional status, the system for data analysis should be decided as the study is designed. The analysis system should take into account the likelihood that there will be missing values and, in a longitudinal study, that it will prove difficult to link together data collected from the same household at different visits. (6) The use of a computer should only be considered once the analysis system has been finalised or else a great deal of time-wasting and confusion will result. The system chosen for analysis determines the software needed to control data entry, storage, sorting and analysis, Commercially available software packages are extremely useful but usually need adaptation. (7). Lengthy reports are seldom read by those we want to read them. Short 'executive summaries' backed up by clear diagrams, illustrations and brief case-studies have more impact than journal articles (though the latter are important for our credibility). The clear presentation of results and their implications for programme planners is important and requires both time and money. (8) Every opportunity should be taken to present the results in seminars, meetings of professional groups or audiences with government officers or politicians. We should only make those recommendations that are supported by our results.

Acknowledgements. The work described in this presentation has been undertaken by the personnel from His Majesty's Government Department of Health Services, Ministry of Health and Department of Local Development, Ministry of Panchayat and Local Development, Kingdom of Nepal. Others involved in the work include direct employees (both Nepal and expatriate) of Save the Children Fund (UK), the UK Government Overseas Development Administration Technical Co-operation Office, Nepal and staff and postgraduate students at the London School of Hygiene and Tropical Medicine. Save the Children Fund works in Nepal under a direct agreement with His Majesty's Government's Ministry of Health; in Chautara under an additional agreement with the Institute of Medicine, Tribhuvan University, Kathmandu. A large number of individuals have had responsibility for different aspects of the studies: without their efforts the studies could not have been accomplished:
Chuliban: Ann Brister, Miguel Campas, Ann Dalrymple Smith, Devindra Dewan, Blodwen Edwards, Marion Goddaeus, Wendy McLean, Shiraz Ramji.
Karrdep; John Dunsmore, Jonathan Innes, Dick Jenkin, Dan Marsh, Claudia McConnell, Mahesh Pant.
Chautara; Susanna Graham-Jones, Ramji Dhakal, Renuka Munakarmi, Kedarnath Uprety.
We would like to acknowledge the generous financial support for these studies provided by UK Government Overseas Development Administration and Save the Children Fund (UK), and the long term encouragement received from Professor U. Malla (Member, National Planning Commission, Kathmandu), Mrs Chandra Kala Kiran (Acting Secretary, Ministry of Health, Kathmandu), Dr T.B. Khatri (Chief, Nepal Mother and Child Health and Family Planning Project), Dr Savitri Pahadi (lately Chief, Nutrition Section, Ministry of Health, Kathmandu), Professor J.C. Waterlow (lately Nutrition Adviser, UK, ODA), Dr N.A. Ward (Principal Medical Adviser, ODA), Col Hugh Mackay (Overseas Director, SCF), Dr John Seaman (Senior Overseas Medical Officer, SCF) and Rose Deakin (Transam Microsystems). Rajendra Bal and B.K. Aryal provided clerical and administrative assistance.
The work described in this presentation was undertaken while the author worked as ODA-funded Technical co-operation Lecturer at the London School of Hygiene and Tropical Medicine Department of Human Nutrition: from 1982 to 1985 he was seconded to work as Save the Children Fund Regional Medical Adviser for South Asia. Views expressed in the presentation are solely those of the author.

1 Deakin, R. (1984): dBaseII explored. London: Century Communications.
2 Graham-Jones, S. (1985): Save the Children Fund (UK) Nepal Chautara Project. Half-yearly reports, July 1984 and February 1985.
3 Nabarro, D. (1983): Influences on the growth of children (observations from Nepal). *J. Nepal Paed. Ass.* **2**, 137–205.
4 Nabarro, D. (1984): Social economic, health and environmental determinants of nutritional status. WHO *UNU Fd Nutr. Bull.* **6**, 18–32.
5 Nabarro, D.N. & Innes, J.B. (1982): Monitoring and evaluating the Kosi Hill area rural development programme: Report 1: methods and procedures used in the study of the programme's impact. Dhankuta, Nepal: KHARDEP Co-ordinator's Office.
6 Nabarro, D. & McNab, S. (1980): A simple new technique for identifying thin children *J. Trop. Med. Hyg.* **83**, 21–33.
7 Nabarro, D. & Pant, M. (1984): Monitoring and Evaluation of the Kosi Hill Area Rural Development Programme: Report 3: The Impact of the Kosi Hill Area Rural Development Programme: Description of Data collected in the Second Year of the KHARDEP Impact Studies — 2038/039 (1981/82) Dhankuta, Nepal: KHARDEP Co-ordinator's Office.
8 Nabarro, D., Verney, J., Clugston, G. & McNab, S. (1984): Child malnutrition in Nepal: causes and consequences. Teaching slide set prepared for National Nutrition Cell, Kathmandu, Nepal. Kathmandu: Save the Children Fund (UK) South Asia Office.
9 Roberts, N.C.E. (1981): Programmes and studies M Phil Thesis, University of Reading.

V: Energy metabolism

Regulation of energy balance in animals and man

Nutrition and endurance performance: a challenge to energy balance

Brown adipose tissue

REGULATION OF ENERGY BALANCE IN ANIMALS AND MAN

Energy metabolism in man and animals

A.J.H. van ES
Institute for Livestock Feeding and Nutrition Research, 6 Runderweg, 8219 PK Lelystad and Department of Animal Physiology, Agricultural University, 10 Haarweg, 6709 PJ Wageningen, the Netherlands

---

More than 120 years ago Pettenkofer[35] studied energy metabolism of man and animals and performed 24-h measurements of respiratory gas exchange in both. Because of their economic importance work with *farm animals* got by far the most attention from 1890–1912, 1920–1940, and especially after 1960. After the famous experiments of Atwater & Benedict[3] —with only five men! — it took till 1970 before *man*'s 24-h energy metabolism was studied thoroughly again and at the moment the subject receives more attention[22]. Moreover, the new doubly-labelled water technique is coming into use permitting measurement of man's energy expenditure for periods up to 14 d under circumstances of every-day life[22]. Specialized symposia on work with *farm animals* were organized under the auspices of the European Association for Animal Production from 1958 onwards every 3rd year[16]; one on *man* was held last autumn with support of the European Community[22]. These symposia were attended by members of most research groups involved in this work.

Energy studies in *farm animals* aim at evaluating the nutritional value of the various feeds used for production of milk, meat, eggs and wool, at assessing energy requirements of the animals, and at finding optimal climatic conditions for their housing. Young, healthy animals are used, fairly well adapted to the experimental procedures and diet. The main interest in energy studies in *man* comes from the obesity problem and questions about food-energy needs during every-day life (also in relation to world food-consumption) and during pregnancy and lactation. Most energy balances are performed on students and other young adults, few involve children and elderly persons. For obvious reasons preliminary and collection periods and calorimeter runs are much shorter than in animals, diets have far more variation and the adaptation to diet and experimental routines is not always optimal[19].

In *farm animals*, energy needed for maintenance is an economic disadvantage, and is kept relatively low by aiming at high rates of production, so that energy for maintenance is 50 per cent or less of total energy required. In *man*, especially when physical activity is low, food energy is nearly completely used to maintain the body in a good state. Even during pregnancy, lactation or growth the major part of food energy is used for maintenance.

In view of the differences in interests, in methods used and in background of research workers, it is not surprising that until recently research on man's energy metabolism, developed with little contact with similar studies on farm animals although sometimes using rats. In the next sections the main results of both types of research will be described and compared.

Biochemical approach of energy metabolism. In *animal* energetics a biochemical approach is usually followed[1,2,5,18,20,38]. Requirements for maintenance and work are seen as requirements for ATP, those for retention of body fat, and for fat, lactose and protein in milk and eggs, as requirements for both building blocks, ATP and in some cases NADPH. Mature rats, pigs and poultry were in general found to utilize their nutrients for maintenance according to the biochemical potential for ATP of these nutrients[2,11]. Evidence for this was less clear for young, growing monogastrics because of the difficulty of assessing their maintenance needs. Also with regard to the conversion of nutrients into body fat in mature monogastrics the actual energetic efficiency was only slightly below the one expected from biochemistry. There is some evidence that fat is used with some preference for fat deposition rather than for maintenance[38].

Protein deposition during growth was found to require more food energy than biochemically expected, probably due to increased protein turnover[18]. Estimates of the energetic efficiency of the use of metabolizable energy (ME) for pregnancy and lactation in the pig still lack precision, mainly due to the difficulty of correcting accurately for the sow's maintenance requirements[2,12,29].

In ruminants, biochemically expected and measured energetic efficiencies of ME utilization show considerable gaps, especially as to pregnancy and fattening[1,20]. Neither can the influence of the type of ration on energy conversion be fully explained biochemically. There exists fair agreement among research groups on 60 per cent efficiency for the conversion of ME above maintenance into milk energy. Extrapolated to humans this suggests an energetic efficiency of ME utilization for lactation of at least 80 per cent.

Soon after the renewed interest in *human* energy metabolism in the seventies Flatt's paper[23] on its biochemical aspects appeared and is often cited. Essentially Flatt's views do not differ much from those of Blaxter[5] and Schiemann *et al.*[38] for animals, mentioned above. Also recent studies with man confirm that, in general, the biochemical approach is correct. ME of starch is[15], as expected, more efficiently used for maintenance than ME of protein. Conversion of carbohydrate-ME into body-energy retention was indeed found to be less efficient and thus giving a higher heat production[3,4] than conversion of fat-ME[13]. Results of our own experiments[21] with a diet with about 40 per cent of the ME from fat were in agreement with these studies. A protein test-meal increased 24-h heat production as expected in non-obese persons; however, there was no increase in some obese subjects[39].

In *man*, heat production resulting from ordinary biochemical conversions is often called 'obligatory thermogenesis'. The words 'regulatory thermogenesis' are used for heat produced by the body to a greater or smaller extent with the aim of preventing excessive body energy retention or loss[25].

Maintenance. Kleiber concluded[28] from several studies that basal metabolic rate of mature *animals* of various species in a postabsorptive condition, in a comfortable microclimate and at rest, is related to metabolic body mass, live weight in kg raised to the power[0.75]. For mature fed animals in energy equilibrium this relationship was also used with reasonable success. The probable cause of the lower metabolic rate, of larger animal species, per kg body mass, is their relatively lower proportion of organs and tissues with a high metabolic rate (heart, liver, gastrointestinal tract, kidney, brain)[10].

Within animal species it is also usual to express basal or maintenance energy needs per $kg^{0.75}$ body mass. One would expect that animals with much fat, a metabolically less active tissue, would have lower maintenance needs per $kg^{0.75}$ than lean ones. This, however, was not found. Blaxter fattened some sheep for 3 years[6] and McNiven fattened sheep of the same weight to various degrees of fatness[31]. In both studies fasting metabolism, as well as maintenance energy needs in the second, were closely related to metabolic body mass ($kg^{0.75}$). Earlier studies suggested that correlation with fat-free mass gave a closer fit than with total mass. On this McNiven's remark is interesting, she mentions that in these earlier studies lean and fat animals were selected from the same large group of animals. Thus, the degree of fatness might have been due to their genetic variation in maintenance needs because in a herd animals with low maintenance requirements might have become fattest. In her own experiments she fattened animals of similar weight and fatness to various degrees and then measured basal and maintenance metabolism, and so largely excluding the influence of genetic variation.

Problems arose when the relationship between maintenance metabolism and metabolic weight was applied to young, growing animals in which case a much lower power, 0.6 or less, was calculated[2,17], thus suggesting a much higher metabolism per kg body weight of young animals than of more mature ones. However, it was not fully realised that Kleiber's relationship was not to be used in this case. Unequal animals are compared: the younger animals are more easily stressed, show a higher physical activity, and have a higher protein to fat ratio than the more mature animals. Moreover, their rate of protein turnover, a process requiring much energy, is higher than in slowly growing animals[18].

In studies on *man*'s energy metabolism, energy needs for maintenance as in every-day life, including some but not more than a few hours light physical activity — are seldom expressed on a metabolic body mass ($kg^{0.75}$) basis. Instead the energy needs are given per kg body mass, or preferably per kg fat-free mass[25,41], as it is argued that fatty tissue has a low metabolic rate. In many studies with humans, subjects with a higher fat content were found to have a higher total maintenance requirement because they were heavier than non-obese subjects. Per kg or $kg^{0.75}$, however, their maintenance needs were usually lower than for the non-obese[8,21,25,26,34]. This suggests a low metabolic rate of fatty tissue and/or low energy needs per kg or $kg^{0.75}$ due to reduced activity and/or low genetic requirements for maintenance.

Little information exists on the size of between-animal variation in energy requirements for maintenance, within a breed, for monogastric farm animals and rats. In the studies performed it is repeatedly stated that this size was clearly larger than between-animal variation in the efficiency of the utilization of ME for body-fat deposition[32,38]. More data are available on between-animal variation of maintenance energy requirements of mature ruminants within a breed, which was found to have a coefficient of variation of 8–10 per cent[1,17].

In our studies[8,21] in men and women with standardized light physical activity we found coefficients of variation in maintenance requirements between persons of about 15 per cent for total requirement, and about 10 per cent for requirement per metabolic body mass. In the first study, maintenance requirements per kg body mass differed much more between subjects than did efficiencies of the utilization of ME for maintenance of fat production.

Evidence for regulatory changes in energy metabolis. Experiments with nearly mature or mature *animals* (rats, pigs, steers and dairy cows) have shown that the conversion of the ME available above maintenance into energy in body-fat deposition or milk does not decrease at higher intake levels[1,11,32,33,38]. Body fat was deposited with efficiencies close to those expected from biochemistry. Growing farm animals at a continuous high feeding level show an increase in the ME utilization for energy deposition rather than a decrease. This is to some extent due to a shift from protein to fat deposition, less protein turnover and lower physical activity and excitability. Neither example supports the theory of a regulatory change in energy metabolism to prevent high fat deposition.

In our own studies in *man* two volunteers ate the same diet in quantities of 50 per cent above maintenance needs for 3 weeks. ME utilization in the 1st week did not differ from that in the 3rd week[21]. Nor was evidence found[42] for a change toward higher heat production with time during prolonged food intake. Evidence for its existence from cafetaria-fed rodents[36] is for technical reasons still weakly based[24,30]. In chickens[43] determination of physical activity in such cases is a necessity, because method of feed application influences behaviour.

In *animals*, there exists some evidence for regulatory reduction of heat production at low feed intake. Animals with little or no feed adapt in a few days to the new situation and often show less physical activity thereafter. Low feed and low N intake[40] decrease their rate of N-turnover, which very probably lowers energy needs. Studies from the Oskar-Kellner Institute at Rostock[11,32,33,37,38] showed that the basal energy needs of undernourished animals were more variable than, and usually lower than, those of well-nourished animals.

In *man*, most studies mention a 10–15 per cent lower basal metabolic rate during fasting compared to the situation of sufficient energy intake[25]. Few data on 24-h heat production during fasting or marked undernutrition are available. Dauncey[14] found a 6 per cent decrease in total heat production, not corrected for possible body weight changes, for a diet supplying about 4 MJ per day. Her subjects were not adapted to a low food intake. We found[21] in a similar situation no significant change in heat production per kg or $kg^{0.75}$ body mass in subjects that were adapted to the diet and low ME intake for 5 days. Our recent results show about 10 per cent and 15 per cent lower heat production per kg or $kg^{0.75}$ body mass at similar low ME intake after 5 days and 8 weeks, respectively[9].

Theoretically, one would expect that irregular food intake, eg 150 per cent and 50 per cent of a maintenance diet, respectively, on successive days, would lead to more (obligatory) heat production than a daily intake of 100 per cent. On the high-intake day fat probably is deposited, a process which for carbohydrates and fats would have an obligatory heat production of about 20 and 5 per cent respectively, if the excess ME is used for fat synthesis. When mature *pigs* were fed 25 per cent and 175 per cent of a maintenance diet on alternate days[27] the same heat production and energy utilization was found as during a constant daily intake of 100 per cent. We compared, in *man*, the 150/50 regimen with the 100 per cent regimen and also failed to find a significant difference[7]. Most nutrients are efficiently stored temporarily before utilization without conversion of carbohydrate into body fat.

Conclusion. Clear indications that basic aspects of energy metabolism of humans and monogastric homoeotherm animals differ, were not found. Both the studies with animals and those with humans can improve our understanding of the principles of energy metabolism. However, extrapolation of results obtained with one of these two kinds of subjects to the other should be made only with caution. Energy studies in humans have other objectives than those in (farm) animals which are usually younger and fed at higher level than humans. Furthermore, the human diets contain considerably more fat than the rations of most animals.

Acknowledgement. The author thanks the Netherland Heart Foundation for financial support for his studies in humans.

1 ARC (1980): *The nutrient requirements of ruminant livestock*, pp. 73–119. Slough: Commonw. Agric. Bureau.

2 ARC (1981): *The nutrient requirements of pigs.* p. 1–65. Slough: Commonw. Agric. Bureau.

3 Atwater, W.O. & Benedict, F.G. (1905): A respiration calorimeter with appliances for the direct determination of oxygen. *Carnegie Inst. Washington, Publ. 42.*

4 Bisdee, J.T. & James, W.P.T (1984): Carbohydrate-induced thermogenesis in man. *Proc. Nutr. Soc.* **43**, 149A

5 Blaxter, K.L. (1962): *The energy metabolism of ruminants*, London: Hutchinson.

6 Blaxter, K.L. (1976): Experimental obesity in farm animals. In *Proc. 7th EAAP Symp. Energy Metabolism*, pp. 129–132.

7 Boer, J.O. de, Es, A.J.H. van, Raay, J.M.A. van & Hautvast, J.G.A.J. (In prep): Energy balance of 16 subjects with either daily constant levels of energy intake or daily alternating levels of energy intake.

8 Boer, J.O. de, Es, A.J.H. van, Raay, J.M.A. van & Hautvast, J.G.A.J. (In prep): Twenty-four-hour energy expenditure in lean and overweight women, simulating a sedentary working-day in a whole body indirect calorimeter.

9 Boer, J.O. de, Es, A.J.H. van, Roovers, L.M., Raay, J.M.A. van & Hautvast, J.G.A.J. (In prep): Adaptation of energy metabolism to low energy intake in overweight women.

10 Brody, S. (1945): *Bioenergetics and growth*. New York: Reinhold.

11 Chudy, A. & Schiemann, R. (1969): Zur energetischen Verwertung der Nähr- und Futterstoffe für Erhaltung und Fettbildung. 1. Mitt. Die energetische Verwertung der Nährstoffe für Erhaltung oberhalb der kritischen Temperatur nach Modellversuchen an Ratten. *Arch. Tierernähr.* **19**, 231–247.

12 Close, W.H., Noblet, J. & Heavens, R.P. (1985): Studies on energy metabolism of the pregnant sow, 2. *Br. J. Nutr.* **53**, 267–279

13 Dallosso, H.M. & James, W.P.T. (1984): Whole-body calorimetry studies in adult men. *Br. J. Nutr.* **52**, 49–64 and 65–72.

14 Dauncey, M.J. (1980): Metabolic effects of altering the 24 h energy intake in man, using direct and indirect calorimetry. *Br. J. Nutr.* **43**, 257–269.

15 Dauncey, M.J. & Bingham, S.A. (1983): Dependence of 24 h energy expenditure in man on the composition of the nutrient intake. *Br. J.Nutr.* **50**, 1–13.

16 EAAP (European Association for Animal Production): Proc. Symposia on Energy Metabolism — Publications **8** (1958), **10** (1961), **11** (1965), **12** (1967), **13** (1970), **14** (1973), **19** (1976), **26** (1979), **29** (1982).

17 Es, A.J.H. van (1972): Maintenance. In *Handbuch der Tierernährung* II, ed W. Lenkeit & K. Breirem, pp. 1–54. Hamburg: Parey.

18 Es, A.J.H. van (1980): Energy costs of protein deposition. In *Protein deposition in animals*, ed P.J. Buttery & D.B. Lindsay, pp. 215–224. London: Butterworths.

19 Es, A.J.H. van & Boer, J.O. de (1985): Energy metabolism of man and animals. In *Proc. Dreiländertagung*, St. Gallen, Switzerland, September 1984.

20 Es, A.J.H. van & Honing, Y. van der (1979): Energy utilization. In *Feeding strategy for the high yielding dairy cow*, ed. W.H. Broster & H. Swan, pp. 68–89. London: Granada.

21 Es, A.J.H. van, Vogt, J.E., Niessen, C., Veth, J., Rodenburg, L., Teeuwse, V., Dhuyvetter, J., Deurenberg, P., Hautvast, J.G.A.J. & Beek, E. van der (1984): Human energy metabolism below, near and above energy equilibrium. *Br. J. Nutr.* **52**, 429–442.

22 Euro-Nut (1985): *Human energy metabolism: physical activity and energy expenditure measurements in epidemiological research based upon direct and indirect calorimetry*. Report 5, ed A.J.H. van Es, pp. 121–152. Wageningen, Netherlands.

23 Flatt, J.P. (1978): The biochemistry of energy expenditure in man. In *Recent advances in obesity research II*, ed G.A. Bray, pp. 211–288. London: Newman.

24 Hervey, G.R. & Tobin, G. (1982): The part played by variation of energy expenditure in the regulation of energy balance. *Proc. Nutr. Soc.* **41**, 137–153.

25 James, W.P.T. (1983): Energy requirements and obesity. *Lancet* **2**, 386–389.

26 Jéquier, E. & Schutz, Y. (1983): Long-term measurements of energy expenditure in humans using a respiration chamber. *Am. J. Clin. Nutr.* **38**, 989–998.

27 Kirchgessner, M. & Müller, H. L. (1981): Einfluss einer einmalig erhöhten Energiezufuhr innerhalb von 2 Tagen auf Wärmeproducktion und Energieverwertung bei ausgewachsenen Sauen. *Ann. Nutr. Metab.* **25**, 362–370.

28 Kleiber, M. (1961): *The fire of life*. New York: Wiley.

29 Lange, P.G.B. de, Kempen, G.J.M. van, Klaver, J. & Verstegen, M.W.A. (1980): Effect of condition of sows on energy balances during 7 days before and 7 days after parturition. *J. Anim. Sci.* **50**, 886–891.

30 McCracken, K.J. & Barr, H.G. (1985): Reply to letter by Rothwell and Stock. *Br. J. Nutr.* **53**, 192.

31 McNiven, M.A. (1984): The effect of body fatness on energetic efficiency and fasting heat production in adult sheep. *Br. J. Nutr.* **51**, 297–304.

32 Nehring, K., Hoffman, L. & Schiemann, R. (1959): Die Verwertung der Futterenergie in Abhängigkeit vom Ernährungsniveau. 1. Mitt. Versuche mit Kaninchen und Ratten. *Arch. Tierernähr.* **9**, 85–139.

33 Nehring, K., Schiemann, R., Hoffmann, L. & Klippel, W. (1960): Die Verwertung der Futterenergie in Abhängigkeit vom Ernährungsniveau. 2. Mitt. Versuche mit Schweinen. *Arch. Tierernähr.* **10**, 275–320.

34 Noack, R., Aust, L., Karst, H., Eschrich, H. & Zahn, L. (1983): Effizienz der Energieverwertung und Adipositas. *Arch. Tierernähr.* **33**, 515–516.

35 Pettenkofer, M. (1862): Uber die Respiration. *Ann. Chemie und Pharm.* Suppl. 2, 1–52.

36 Rothwell, N.J. & Stock, M.J. (1985): Is diet-induced thermogenesis an experimental artefact? *Br. J. Nutr.* **53**, 191.

37 Schiemann, R., Hoffmann, L. & Nehring, K. (1960): Die Verwertung reiner Nährstoffe. 2. Mitt. Versuche mit Schweinen. *Arch. Tierernähr.* **11**, 265–283.

38 Schiemann, R., Nehring, K., Hoffmann, L., Jentsch, W. & Chudy, A. (1971): *Energetische Futterbewertung und Energienormen*. VEB Deutscher Landwirtsch Verlag.

39 Steiniger, J., Karst, H., Janietz, K. & Noack, R. (1983): Tagesenergieumsatz und nahrungsinduzierte Thermogenese bei Normalgewichtigen und Adipösen. *Arch. Tierernähr.* **33**, 516.

40 Waterlow, J.C., Garlick, P.J. & Millward, D.J. (1978): *Protein turnover in mammalian tissues and in the whole body*. Amsterdam: North-Holland.

41 Webb, P. (1981): Energy expenditure and fat-free mass in men and women. *Am. J. Clin. Nutr.* **34**, 1816–1826.

42 Webb, P. & Annis, J.F. (1983): Adaptation to overeating in lean and overweight men and women. *Human Nutr.: Clin. Nutr.* **37C**, 117–131.

43 Wenk, C. & Es, A.J.H. van (1976): Energy metabolism of growing chickens as related to their physical activity. In *Proc. 7th EAAP Symp. on Energy Metab.*, pp. 189–192.

The regulation of food intake

G.A. BRAY and Susan BRAY
Section of Diabetes and Clinical Nutrition, University of Southern California, USC School of Medicine, 2025 Zonal Avenue, Los Angeles, CA 90033, USA.

The average American eats nearly 400 kg (about 1000 lb) weight of food in a year, providing an energy intake of roughly 4200 MJ (a million calories, assuming 4.2 kcal = 1 kJ). A net storage of only 0.4 MJ/d (100 kcal) would result in a weight gain, for the year, of 4.5 kg (about 10 lb), ie from 36 500 'excess' calories. Yet such a cumulative rate of weight gain is experienced by only a very tiny fraction of the adult human population. While the body weight of the normal individual may show small fluctuations from time to time, generally it will remain relatively stable. By implication then, food intake and energy expenditure are fairly well regulated in most of the population.

Unfortunately, not all individuals are able to regulate food intake this well, as witnessed by the large numbers of obese persons. The magnitude of this problem has been graphically illustrated by calculations on the total amount of fossil fuel[13] that would be equivalent to the food calories saved by reducing overweight individuals to optimal weight. These calculations go as follows: adult Americans carry an excess of 2.3 billion lb of fat. If these calories were used for daily metabolic needs, the reduced intake of food would be equivalent to 1–3 billion gallons of petrol. Such a saving in energy would more than supply the electrical demands of residences in all of Boston, Chicago, San Francisco, and Washington DC!

This paper will deal with food intake in both normal and obese subjects. In addition to describing methods for measuring food intake, the various factors which influence it and some alleged differences between lean and obese subjects will be described.

Methods of measuring food intake. Methods vary from quantitative administration of nutrients, whose energy content has been analysed by bomb calorimetry, to estimates of food intake using dietary histories and the subject's memory.

Weighed or quantitative diets. Several different approaches have been used to obtain quantitative information about food intake. Liquid energy intake can be provided intravenously in patients on total parenteral nutrition, enabling the investigator to be in complete control of all nutrient intake. Less rigid, but equally quantitative, are systems where food during specified meals is dispensed from liquid dispensers or, in solid form, from mechanical machines. In this same category are the metabolic diets dispensed on a metabolic ward. We will consider each of these briefly.

Liquid diets. Jordan *et al.*[14] and Pudel[26] were among the first to utilize liquid diets dispensed during a lunch period to identify some of the characteristics of the meal. This approach has been used to develop a quantitative estimate of food intake, the rate of eating a single meal in a laboratory setting being described by a decelerating curve[17]. That is, the rate of ingestion is greater at the start of a meal and decreases with passing time. From an analysis of single meals in non-obese men and women, it has been concluded that the simplest model for description of single meals is a quadratic function[18]. The use of quantitative liquid diets has also been employed for studies of preloading, that is, for examination of the effects of introducing food into the stomach at defined intervals prior to the actual meal[22,27].

Solid fuel. Since most people do not live on liquid diets, attempts to estimate food intake from solid food dispensed quantitatively has been a desirable research goal. This has been achieved by providing weighed quantities of biscuits in a box[29], or by providing sandwiches and other known quantities of food[28], or by providing food dispensed from an electrically operated apparatus. The latter technique has been used to study preference for snack food of different compositions selected by normal and obese individuals[35].

Weighed diets on metabolic wards. Preparation of normal foods on metabolic wards for patients eating fixed intakes can be done in several ways. The most accurate is to provide individuals with standardized meals, keeping an identical weighed portion for subsequent quantitative analysis. Thus eight meals identical in weight and composition are prepared and fed to a subject over 7 days with the eighth portion held back for quantitative analysis. Less accurate but widely used is the technique of preparing diets and estimating their nutrient value from food tables. Since the food values may vary from time to time, the reliability of such techniques is questionable.

Observational techniques. To gain insight into spontaneous eating behaviour, several investigators have observed individuals eating in restaurants. This technique has the advantage of spontaneity on the part of the subject in selecting the quantities and qualities of food chosen, but is limited in terms of quantitative analysis by the portion sizes of the foods selected, since an identical duplicate is not available. A similar approach has been made by observing subjects in their homes and in school[4].

Diet histories. The technique of dietary histories is one of the most widely used means of analysing food intake, but is clearly the least reliable. The technique involves asking an individual to recall what he has eaten during the previous 24 hours or 3 days. A variation on this method is to give individuals forms and ask them to record what they eat during the next several days. But, with awareness that they are being recorded, individuals may alter their food consumption during the period of self-monitoring, or they may simply fail accurately to record all food intake. In a recent study, 12 men and 12 women recorded their caloric intakes for 7 days, and then their records were compared with the levels of energy consumption previously documented during an 18-week controlled dietary study in which body weight was maintained. The men on average reported consuming 3.8 MJ/d (905 kcal) less and the women 2.1 MJ/d (500 kcal) less than they had in fact consumed to maintain weight. Similar discrepancies between estimated intake from the first, second and third replicate measurement on a group of obese subjects has been reported[6,12]. Three studies on food records showed that, in the laboratory, obese individuals make large errors in estimating the energy values of food, and make similar errors in their daily self-monitoring record form[20]. However, comparisons of 1-day and 3-day records show that there was little difference in the mean intakes[24].

A final approach to looking at the structure of meals may be to use labelled nutrient excretion or labelled food, or to measure the act of chewing and swallowing. Instruments designed to quantitate chewing and swallowing have been employed[3]. Measurement of nitrogen excretion or of the dilution of doubly-labelled water ($^2H_2{}^{18}O$) provides a measure of the estimate of energy expenditure.

Estimates of food intake. The relationship between energy expenditure and intake of five subjects over a period of 13 days led to the conclusion[25] that the measurement of energy expenditure and intake were reasonably satisfactory over this period of time. The estimated intake ranged from a low of 150 MJ (35 700 kcal) to a high of 223 MJ (53 110 kcal), with an estimated imbalance ranging from a deficit of 13 MJ (3100 kcal) to a surfeit of 21 MJ (5000 kcal). An estimate of day-to-day intake among a group of Army recruits[8] showed considerable day-to-day variation in food intake. Intakes ranged from a low of 5 MJ (1200 kcal) to a high of over 25 MJ (6000 kcal) per day. For groups ranging from six to 12 in number recorded at six different centers, the daily food intake ranged from 15 MJ/d (3600 kcal) to 20 MJ/d (4800 kcal). Thus substantial variations in day-to-day food intake can be found in normal subjects under observed experimental conditions, and similar variations in estimated food intake have been reported for obese subjects.

Despite these limitations on estimates of intake and the variability from day to day, there have been studies on food intake in the population which were in suprisingly good agreement[1,4,21]. The peaks levels of energy intake occur in the first and second decades of life, with the peak intake for males being approximately 50 per cent higher than the peak for females. Following the peaks, there is a gradual decline in successive decades.

Interestingly, the estimates of fat intake from the Lipid Research Clinics study[21] are significantly lower at all ages than the data from the Nationwide Food Consumption Survey (NFCS)[24]. A correspondingly greater intake of carbohydrates recorded by the Lipid Research

Clinics made up the difference. Differences in recorded intakes probably reflect the different ways in which data were collected. For the National Health and Nutrition Examination Survey (HANES)[1] and the Lipid Research Clinics studies[21], dietary recall was the method. For the NFCS[24], however, food disappearance was measured. Since fat on purchased foods may be discarded before eating, the technique used for the food disappearance data may well overestimate total fat intake.

Net energy changes. In spite of the decrease in food intake with age depicted above, all evidence indicates that Americans are now fatter than in earlier decades[5]. Life insurance statistics[30], the longitudinal prospective data from Framingham[15], and the cross-sectional data from the HANES[1] have shown an increase in body weight for most heights. As shown in existing cross-sectional and longitudinal data, this rise in body weight almost certainly reflects an increase in body fat. We must conclude therefore that the decline in food intake is more than compensated for by a decline in energy expenditure with age.

Factors influencing food intake. Males on average eat significantly more than females as shown in all of these cross-sectional studies and essentially in all other published studies. There is also a clear inverse relationship between environmental temperature and average food intake for these various groups of individuals. Food intake can also be influenced by various drugs. For example, increased quantities of insulin or phenothiazine-related drugs can produce increased food intake, and any number of anorectic drugs can reduce appetite and intake.

Obesity and food intake. Do the obese ingest more calories than the lean? Two general techniques have been used in attempting to answer this question. The first of these involves retrospective nutritional histories as discussed above[4]. The other has been the use of observational methods on in food choices in natural settings, which hopefully remain unaltered by the reviewer's presence[31]. In most epidemiologic studies using nutritional histories, the food intake of obese subjects is lower than that of lean subjects. For example, the early data of Beaudoin & Mayer[2] estimated that caloric intakes were significantly lower in overweight subjects than in normal weight ones. Similar data have been obtained from Nutrition Canada[23], a survey by the FAO/WHO[9], Thomson *et al*[33], HANES[1], The Zutphen study from the Netherlands[19], and an English study[16]. The validity of such data is open to question in light of the serious errors found with the technique of dietary histories. However, interestingly enough, Stunkard & Waxman[32] have reported good agreements between self-reports of food intake and more objective measurements, although the accuracy of reporting may have been influenced by the subjects' knowledge that their intake was being recorded. As noted in the section on diet histories above marked discrepancies have been reported between prior records of weight-maintaining levels of energy intake and an individual's subsequent food intake. It has also been suggested that food intake measured in periods of little change in body weight may differ from food intake obtained from subjects who are actively gaining weight.

Direct observations of food intake reveal a somewhat different story from dietary records. In a controlled setting, three facts have usually emerged from independent studies. First, there is a deceleration in the rate of food ingestion for both young and old subjects whether obese or of normal weight. Another now-documented fact is that oral and gastric preloads of all three major macronutrients will depress food intake of both obese and lean subjects as a function of the size as well as the timing of the preload[11]. Unfortunately, depression of food intake is not sufficient to compensate for the size of the preload, and many subjects eat more than their baseline quantity during one-meal test situations. Finally, the studies of adjustments in energy intake due to chronic changes in dietary energy concentration have produced a nearly uniform pattern—a general failure of the obese individual to compensate for such changes[10].

A review of several studies on food choices[31] found relative uniformity among studies measuring the size of meals chosen in naturalistic settings. Obese persons chose and/or ate larger meals than lean persons. In a survey of 720 meals, conducted in a university cafeteria, obese persons chose more food than did non-obese individuals of the same gender, height and age. There are two other variables that have also been observed to influence the amount of food which was selected. Men, as noted above, ate more than women, and tall subjects ate more than short ones. In a second study of 2731 meals at two cafeterias, it was noted that obese subjects ate more frequently in the cafeteria serving fancier food, and at the same time tended to eat larger quantities of food. Nonetheless, attempts to document an obese eating style have been conflicting. Obese persons do consume more food per minute than non-obese persons. However, in a study of 5000 separate food choices[7] showed that the major influence was where individuals chose to eat, both energy content and total intake being variable from site to site—and most studies have agreed with this. In one study[34] obese adolescent boys ate more than their lean siblings at school, but not at home, and there was a great deal of variability in the amount eaten at any one site.

1 Abraham, S., Johnson, C.L. & Najjor, M.F. (1974): Weight and height of adults 18–74 Years of age in the United States. In *Advance data from vital health statistics*, Series 11, No. 211. DHEW Publication No. (PHS)79–1659. Washington DC: US Government Printing Office.
2 Beaudoin, R. & Mayer, J. (1953): Food intakes of obese and non-obese women. *J. Am. Diet. Ass.* **29**, 29–33.
3 Bellisle, F. & Le Magnen, J. (1981): The structure of meals in humans: Eating and drinking patterns in lean and obese subjects. *Physiol. Behav.* **27** 649–658,
4 Bray, G.A. (1981): Obesity: A human energy problem. In *Beltsville symposia in agricultural research*, vol. 4, ed G.R. Beecher, pp. 95–112. Granada: Allanheld, Osmun.
5 Bray, G.A. (1976): *The obese patient*, pp. 1–450. *Major problems in internal medicine*, vol. 9. Philadelphia: W.B. Saunders.
6 Bray, G.A., Zachary, B., Dahms, W.T., Atkinson, R.L. & Oddie, T.H. (1978): Eating patterns of the massively obese individual. *J. Am. Diet. Ass.* **72**, 24–27.
7 Coll, M., Meyer, A. & Stunkard, A.J. (1979): Obesity and food choices in public places. *Archs Gen. Phychiatry* **36**, 795–797.
8 Edholm, O.G., Adam, J.M., Healy, M.J.R., Wolff, H.S., Goldsmith, R. & Best, T.W. (1970): Food intake and energy expenditure of army recruits. *Br. J. Nutr.* **24**, 1091–1107.
9 FAO/WHO (1973): *Energy and protein requirements*. Report on a joint FAO/WHO Ad Hoc Expert Committee. FAO Nutr. Mtgs Rep. Ser. No. 41. Geneva, Switzerland: WHO Tech. Rep. Ser.
10 Garrow, J. (1974): *Energy balance and obesity in man*, pp. 1–243. New York: Elsevier.
11 Geleibter, A.A. (1979): Effect of equicaloric loads of protein, fat and carbohydrate on food intake in the rat and man. *Physiol. Behav.* **22**, 267–273.
12 Hallfrisch, J., Steele, P. & Cohen, L. (1982): Comparison of seven-day diet record with measured food intake of twenty-four subjects. *Nutr. Res.* **2**, 263–273.
13 Hannon, B.M. & Lohman, T.G. (1978): The energy cost of overweight in the United States. *Am. J. Publ. Hlth* **68**, 765–767.
14 Jordan, H.A., Weiland, W.F., Zebley, S.P., Stellar, E. & Stunkard, A.J. (1966): The direct measurement of food intake in man: a method for the objective study of eating behavior. *Psychosomat. Med.* **28**, 836–842.
15 Kannel, W.B., Gordon, T. & Castelli, W.B. (1979): Obesity, lipids and glucose intolerance: in Framingham Study. *Am. J. Clin. Nutr.* **32**, 1238–1245.
16 Keen, H., Thomas, B.J., Jarrett, R.J. & Fuller, J.H. (1979): Nutrient intake, adiposity, and diabetes. *Br. Med. J.* **1**, 655–658.
17 Kissileff, H.R. (1982): Universal eating monitor for continuous recording of solid or liquid consumption in man. *Am. J. Physiol.* **238**, R14–R22.
18 Kissileff, H.R., Thornton, J, & Becker, E. (1982): A quadratic equation adequately describes the cumulative food intake curve in man. *Appetite* **3**, 255–272.
19 Kromhout, J. (1983): Changes in energy and macronutrients in 871 middle-aged men during 10 years of follow-up (the Zutphen study). *Am. J. Clin. Nutr.* **37**, 287–294.
20 Lansky, D. & Brownell, K.D. (1982): Estimates of food quantity and calories: Errors in self-report among obese patients. *Am. J. Clin. Nutr.* **35**, 727–732.
21 Lipid Research Clinics Program Epidemiology Committee (1979): Plasma lipid distributions in selected North American populations: the Lipid Research Clinics program prevalence study. *Circ.* **60**, 427–439.
22 Mayer, J.E. & Pudel, V. (1972): Experimental studies on food intake in obese and normal weight subjects. *J. Psychosomat. Res.* **16**, 305–308.
23 Nutrition Canada (1973): *Nutrition—a national priority*, pp. 1–136. Ottawa: Department of National Health and Welfare.
24 Pao, E.M., Mickle, S.J. & Burk, M.C. (1985): One-day and 3-day nutrient intakes by individuals—Nationwide Food Consumption Survey findings, spring 1977. *J. Am. Diet. Ass.* **85**, 313–324.
25 Passmore, R. (1971): The regulation of body weight in man. *Proc. Nutr. Soc.*, **30**, 122–127.
26 Pudel, V. (1971): Food dispenser. Eine Methode zur Untersuchung des spontanen appetitverhaltens. *Z. Ernähr Wiss.* **10**, 382–393.
27 Pudel, V.E. & Oetting, M. (1977): Eating in the laboratory: behavioral aspects of positive energy balance. *Int. J. Obesity* **1**, 369–386.

28 Rolls, B.J., Rowe, E.A., Rolls, E.T., Kingston, B., Megson, A. & Gunary, R. (1981): Variety in a meal enhances food intake in man. *Physiol. Behav,* **26**, 215–221.
29 Schachter, S. (1968): Obesity and eating. *Science* **161**, 751–756.
30 Seltzer, C.C. (1966): Some re-evaluations of the Build and Blood Pressure Study, 1959, as related to ponderal index, somatotype, and mortality. *New Engl. J. Med.* **274**, 254.
31 Stunkard, A.J. & Kaplan, D. (1977): Eating in public places: A review of reports of the direct observation of eating behavior. *Int. J. Obesity* **1**, 89–101.
32 Stunkard, A.J. & Waxman, M. (1981): Accuracy of self-reports of food intake: A review of the literature and report of a very small series. *J. Am. Diet. Ass.* **79**, 547–551.
33 Thomson, A.M., Billewicz,. W.Z. & Passmore, R. (1961): The relation between calorie intake and body-weight in man. *Lancet* **1**, 1027–1028.
34 Waxman, M. & Stunkard, A.J. (1980): Calorie intake and expenditure of obese boys. *J. Pediatrics.* **96**, 187–193.
35 Wurtman, J.J. & Wurtman, R.J. (1983): Studies on the appetite for carbohydrates in rats and humans. *Psychiat. Res.* **17**, 213–221.

Efficiency of energy deposition in growth and fattening

A.J.F. WEBSTER
Deparment of Animal Husbandry, University of Bristol, Langford House, Langford, Bristol BS18 7DU, UK.

The efficiency with which food energy may be deposited in the tissues of the animal that eats it depends on: (i) interactions between food chemistry and digestive physiology that together determine the proportion of food energy that is absorbed from the gut and utilized in metabolism—conventionally this is defined as metabolizable energy (ME); (ii) the gross efficiency of deposition of the metabolizable energy which is defined as [energy retention (RE)/ME]. $RE = (ME - H)$ when H is metabolic heat production—net efficiency of utilization of increments of ME is given by $\Delta RE/\Delta ME$; (iii) the relationship of RE to gains in body mass which is defined by EV_g, the energy value of body gains. This depends upon the relative proportions of water, ash (both having zero energy content), protein (23.5 kJ/g) and fat (39 kJ/g). This paper deals with those matters of anatomy and physiology that determine RE, EV_g and thus ME conversion to body mass.

Energy value of body gain. The body composition of any animal, and thus its energy content (MJ/kg), is the consequence of the effect of nutrition over a period of time on the genetic and physiological factors that, together with nutrition, determine its phenotype. Information relating to the composition of the body and body gains is, for obvious reasons, most complete for the meat animals. Both the nutrition scientist and the practical animal feeder require to be able to estimate EV_g with some precision *in vivo* in order not only to select the optimal slaughter weight for any individual animal, but also to interpret properly, trials designed to compare feeds, breeds, systems of management and their various interactions. Because systems for the production of pig meat and poultry have become very uniform both in terms of genetic make-up of the animals and their systems of feeding and management, EV_g during growth can be estimated with an acceptable degree of precision. However, beef production is beset by considerable uncertainties as to EV_g. The most important factors determining EV_g are as follows.

1. Stage of maturity. During continuous growth on a high quality diet the proportion of fat in the body gains of mammals increases from the time of weaning to maturity, although EV_g before weaning often exceeds that which occurs thereafter because of the very high quality of mother's milk. Other things being equal, when two meat animals grown similarly are examined at the same weight, the fatter animal will be that which is closer to its mature size.

2. Plane of nutrition. At a given stage of maturity, the more an animal eats (ie the greater ME exceeds H) the greater the proportion of RE as fat and therefore the greater becomes EV_g.

3. Genotype. The most obvious difference between genotype is in mature size. The Charolais is, on average, larger than the Hereford breed although the variation between individuals within each breed is in fact far greater than that which exists between mean values for the two breeds[1]. In the UK., genetic comparisons between different beef animals are now made at a constant body fat content estimated ultrasonically[8]. This goes some way towards standardizing EV_g but cannot fully account for genetic difference in the distribution of fat between subcutaneous, intermuscular and intra-abdominal depots. There is a real need for improved methods for estimating the body composition of beef animals *in vivo*[10]. New techniques emerging from medical physics such as X-ray computed tomography and nuclear magnetic resonance can be used with pigs, poultry and sheep, but cannot cope with the size of cattle.

4. Hormonal factors. As a general rule, intact males are leaner than castrate males or females. Treatment of castrates and females with exogenous hormones is designed mainly to achieve the growth and carcass characteristics of the intact male. The commercial success of anabolic steroids is well documented but the interpretation of their effects is not always clear. Body composition has recently been compared in twin cattle, mostly of the Fresian breed[5]. Differences between bulls and steers in subcutaneous and intermuscular fat were as expected. Implanting steers with trenbolone acetate and oestradiol-17β also increased food intake and growth rate in accordance with commercial expectations, but the proportions of protein, water and fat in their carcass remained essentially those of a steer.

5. Environmental factors. Cold conditions increase H and thus decrease RE. Since EV_g is proportional to RE it follows that cold stress tends to decrease EV_g at a given ME. Prolonged cold and hot conditions also affect the shape and composition of the body in pigs, this being mediated in part by hormones and in part by redistribution of blood flow between deep and superficial tissue[4].

Photoperiod affects the ratio of protein to fat deposition in sheep and cattle, the effect being mediated at least in part by prolactin[19]. In natural daylight, prolactin levels decrease sharply at the beginning of autumn[20] and sheep and cattle appear to shift partition of retained nutrients from further lean tissue growth towards fat deposition.

Retention of ME within the individual animal. The overall efficiency of any energy deposition is determined by food intake and heat production.

ME intake. The most obvious way to regulate energy deposition during growth or avoid it altogether at maturity is to regulate ME intake. In the case of farm animals, man usually regulates ME and thus RE and EV_g according to the economic dictates of the time. More interesting and profound is the perennial physiological question, 'Do animals, in the long-term, regulate ME and thus RE or is appetite no more than simply a response to a series of relatively short-term signals emanating from the gut and tissues?' In the case of man, one might assume that our food intake is regulated by a sense of self-awareness. I consider this to be an inadequate explanation. Consider two adults, one who manages to gain only 5 kg body weight between the ages of 20 and 40 years. Such an individual will have a balanced ME with H with a precision better than 1 : 1000. The second adult has paid no apparent concern to his body composition and increased weight from 80–120 kg over 20 years. In this extreme example ME/H is only 1.013. This indicates either a very precise control of ME intake even in the most extreme circumstances or a form of adaptive diet-induced thermogenesis designed to regulate H to match ME. This is a beguiling hypothesis but not one that has yet been supported by any hard evidence.

Most studies of food intake control have involved the rat. There is no doubt that when given a regular supply of a nutritionally balanced diet the laboratory rat regulates ME intake very precisely during growth and at maturity and does not lay down excess fat. This precise control can be upset by the technique of cafeteria-feeding[18]. Effects of cafeteria-feeding on H, and thus RE, are the subject of considerable controversy[2,18]. It is also not clear why the animals overeat. The successful induction of hyperphagia by cafeteria-feeding requires not only that a wide range of feeds be provided but that no feed be provided on a regular basis. This suggests the possibility that hyperphagia may be due at least in part to the fact that the rats are unable to interpret the consequences of eating any particular food.

This interpretation is reinforced by the studies of Radcliffe & Webster[13–15] who investigated growth and body composition in congenitally obese and lean Zucker rats offered, *ad libitum* during growth, a wide range of diets varying in protein concentration and quality, carbohydrate quality and proportion of ME in the form of fat, and measured protein and fat retention between 34 and 66 days in rats given diets that did not impair normal rate of lean tissue growth for either sex or phenotype. This study may be summarized as follows. (1) Food intake was precisely regulated in each sex and phenotype so as to sustain a constant, maximum rate of protein deposition which may be called the target for that phenotype. (2) Rates of lipid deposition (and weight gain) varied enormously within phenotype in a way that reflected the ratio of ME to protein in the diet: ie fat deposition was increased by increasing dietary fat from 40 to 200 mg/g and reduced by increasing dietary cellulose from 0 to 300 mg/g. In rats (at least), it appears there is a target for lean tissue growth which dominates the control of food intake. During this time the animal pays little, if any, attention to body fat content.

This precise long-term control of food intake may not extend to herbivores. It has been shown that[3] in sheep given *ad libitum* access to food, ME greatly exceeded H even at maturity. This may in part have been due to the use of castrates who cannot truly be said to mature, but it is also likely that natural selection has favoured over-eating in herbivores so that they may conserve as much food energy as possible from grass during the growing season in the highly concentrated form of fat to last them through the period when the food is scarce.

Analysis of heat production. The nutritionist conventionally analyses H according to (i) body size; (ii) the heat increment of feeding (HIF); (iii) activity and (iv) the work of thermoregulation. The latter two components may be discounted for an animal at rest in a thermoneutral environment. The effect of size on H is conventionally determined by measuring H when ME = zero. This makes arithmetic sense but can be criticised on biological grounds[23].

As a first approximation, fasting metabolism (F) in mammals is about 300 kJ/kg body weight per day[22]. The main source of variation in measured F or predicted F^1 [23] can be attributed primarily to anatomy. Fat individuals tend to have lower values for F^1 expressed per unit of total body weight than lean individuals of the same species. This can often be attributed entirely to the fact that in adequately fed individuals the metabolic rate of the fat mass is considerably less than that of the protein mass. Values for F^1 expressed as a function of lean mass tend to be similar in lean and fat individuals even when the differences are as large as those seen in the congenitally obese Zucker rat[21]. Elaborating this argument, it is possible to interpret H as the sum of the metabolic rates of the individual tissues: liver, gut wall, muscle, skin, nervous tissue, fat[22]. This anatomical approach is able to account for quite large differences in H between animals and avoids the necessity to invoke subtle differences between individuals in metabolism at the cellular level in order to explain overall differences in H. There do, however, appear to be some residual differences in F that are not simply related to anatomy and may reflect differences in physiological state. For example, F in bulls is about 15 per cent higher than in castrate males (steers)[24]. This may be due to differences in endocrinology or simply due to increased activity by the intact males. G.E. Lobley (personal communication) reports that implantation of steers with anabolic steroids does not affect F^1. This is consistent with observations[5] that anabolic steroids did not affect EV_g, ie implanted steers retain more fat and produce less heat than intact bulls.

Net efficiency of protein and fat deposition. Kielanowski[9] first attempted to partition, by multiple regression analysis, the utilization of ME by growing pigs into that associated with protein deposition RE_p, fat deposition RE_f and maintenance aW^n. His approach is described by the equation $ME = aW^n + bRE_p + cRE_f$. Acknowledging the theoretical limitations of this approach, Kielanowski concluded that the net efficiencies of utilisation of ME for protein and fat deposition in simple-stomached animals like the rat and pig were 0.45 and 0.75 respectively. Energy balance has been measured[12] during growth in lean and congenitally obese Zucker rats which differ markedly in the way that they partition ME between H, RE_p and RE_f at the same age or body weight and ME intake. This approach permits the exploration of variations between individuals in H that are reasonably independent of the major determinants ME and W. Efficiencies of protein and fat deposition calculated in this way are 0.44 and 0.75 respectively. The agreement between this trial and the preferred figures of Kielanowski[9] indicates that these values may be used with confidence to predict the energy costs of protein and fat deposition in simple-stomached animals given balanced diets based largely on protein and carbohydrate. The amounts of ME required to deposit 1 g of protein and fat are therefore 2.25 and 1.36 kJ respectively. Since the energy value of protein and fat are 23.5 and 39.3 kJ ME/g, the ME requirements for deposition of 1 g protein or 1 g fat are similar at 53 kJ/g.

Protein and fat synthesis. The energy costs of protein and fat deposition are useful for predicting the energy costs of growth in simple-stomached animals, but they do not reveal how much thermogenesis is associated with the total synthesis of protein and fat in the body. The amount of heat liberated during the synthesis of a mole of fat can be calculated with high precision from a knowledge of its precursors. The energy cost of protein synthesis (H_p) is less certain but is probably about 4.5 kJ/g protein[11]. Combining data for Zucker rats[12] with estimates of protein synthesis based on the difference between leucine flux and the rate of leucine oxidation[16] gave a remarkably consistent relationship between the estimated energy cost of protein synthesis and total H for rats on a low plane of nutrition, H_p/H being 0.18 irrespective of phenotype or body size[22]. On a high plane of nutrition, H_p/H was more variable, ranging from 0.22 to 0.31 but the ratio increased in each case with increasing food intake. The increase in H_p with increasing ME was on average 20 kJ: the increase in H on average was 28 kJ. These results suggest that the energy cost of protein synthesis makes a minor but significant contribution to total H for rats growing slowly on restricted amounts of feed (ie about 20 per cent), but a major contribution to HIF above maintenance (ie 20/28 or 72 per cent). From observations by Reeds *et al.*[17] one can predict that the contribution of the energy costs of fat synthesis to H was trivial, being about 1 per cent in lean rats and 4 per cent in fatties. There was no suggestion in these experiments that increases in H associated with increasing ME involved any form of regulatory dietary induced thermogenesis in brown fat or any other tissue. Our experiments differ from those of Rothwell & Stock[18] or Barr & McCracken[2] in that our rats were not made to overeat by cafeteria or forced-feeding. Rothwell & Stock[18] have consistently managed to increase synthesis and catabolism of brown adipose tissue in rats by cafeteria-feeding and in consequence increase H and so reduce the efficiency of energy deposition. Other workers[2,7] have equally consistently failed to reproduce their findings. The controversy remains. It may not however be very important since the phenomenon relates only to a species containing significant amounts of brown adipose tissue in adult life and seduced into a very abnormal form of feeding behaviour. One cannot seriously contemplate extrapolating from this situation to the control of energy balance in adult man. However, the extraordinarily close agreement between H and ME in adult man and the observation that human individuals of comparable size show very large differences in ME intake over very long periods[6] make it very difficult to reject outright the hypothesis that adult man equates ME and H at least in part by regulating H. How this is achieved, if this is achieved, no-one knows.

1 Allen, D. & Kilkenny, B. (1980): *Planned beef production.* London: Granada

2 Barr, H.G. & McCracken, K.J. (1984): High efficiency of energy utilisation in 'cafeteria' and force-fed rats kept at 28°C. *Br. J. Nutr.* **51**, 379–387.

3 Blaxter, K.L., Fowler, V.R. & Gill, J.C. (1982): A study of the growth of sheep to maturity. *J. Agric. Sci., Camb.* **98**, 405–420.

4 Dauncey, M.J. & Ingram, D.L. (1983): Evaluation of the effects of environmental temperature and nutrition on body composition. *J. Agric. Sci., Camb.* **101**, 351–358.

5 Fisher, A.V., Wood, J.D. & Whelehan, O.P. (1985): The effects of a combined androgenic-oestrogenic anabolic agent in steers and bulls. 1. Growth and carcass composition. *Anim. Prod.* (In press)

6 Garrow. J.S. (1978): *Energy balance and obesity in man.* Amsterdam: Elsevier.

7 Hervey, G.R. & Tobin, G. (1982): The part played by variation of energy expenditure in the regulation of energy balance. *Proc. Nutr. Soc.* **41**, 137–154.

8 Kempster, A.J., Cook, G.L. & Southgate, J.R. (1982): A comparison of the progeny of British Friesian dams of different sire breeds in 16– and 24–month beef production systems. *Anim. Prod.* **34**, 167–178.

9 Kielanowski, J. (1976): Energy cost of protein deposition. In *Protein metabolism and nutrition*, ed. D.J.A. Cole, pp. 207–216. EAAP Publ. No. 16. London: Butterworths.

10 Lister, D. (1984): *In vivo measurement of body composition in animals.* Amsterdam: Elsevier.

11 Millward, D.J., Garlick, P.J. & Reeds, P.J. (1976): The energy cost of growth. *Proc. Nutr. Soc.* **35**, 339–349.

12 Pullar, J.D. & Webster, A.J.F. (1977): The energy cost of protein and fat deposition in the rat. *Br. J. Nutr.* **37**, 355–363.

13 Radcliffe, J.D. & Webster, A.J.F. (1976): Regulation of food intake during growth in fatty and lean female Zucker rats given diets of different protein content. *Br. J. Nutr.* **36**, 451–469.
14 Radcliffe, J.D. & Webster, A.J.F. (1978): Sex, body composition and the regulation of food intake during growth in the Zucker rat. *Br. J. Nutr.* **39**, 483–492.
15 Radcliffe, J.D. & Webster, A.J.F. (1979): The effect of varying the quality of dietary protein on food intake and growth in the Zucker rat. *Br. J. Nutr.* **41**, 111–124.
16 Reeds, P.J. & Lobley, G.E. (1980): Protein synthesis, are there real species differences? *Proc. Nutr. Soc.* **39**, 43–51.
17 Reeds, P.J., Wahle, K.W.J. & Haggerty, P. (1982): Energy costs of protein and fatty acid synthesis. *Proc. Nutr. Soc.* **41**, 155–161.
18 Rothwell, N.J. & Stock, M.J. (1984): Diet induced thermogenesis. In *Mammalian thermogenesis*, ed L. Girardier & M.J. Stock, pp. 208–233. London: Chapman & Hall.
19 Schanbacher, B. & Crouse, J.D. (1980): Growth and performance of lambs exposed to long or short photo-periods. *J. Anim. Sci.* **51**, 943–948.
20 Schams, D. (1972): Prolactin levels in bovine blood. *Acta Endocrinol.* **71**, 684–696.
21 Webster, A.J.F. (1981): The energetic efficiency of metabolism. *Proc. Nutr. Soc.* **40**, 121–128.
22 Webster, A.J.F. (1984): Energetics of maintenance and growth. In *Mammalian thermogenesis*, ed L. Girardier & M.J. Stock, pp. 178–207. London: Chapman & Hall.
23 Webster, A.J.F., Brockway, J.M. & Smith, J.S. (1974): Prediction of the energy requirements for growth in beef cattle. 1. The irrelevance of fasting metabolism. *Anim. Prod.* **19**, 127–139.
24 Webster, A.J.F., Smith, J.S. & Mollison, G.S. (1977): Prediction of the energy requirements for growth in beef cattle. 3. Body weight and heat production in Hereford × Friesian bulls and steers. *Anim. Prod.* **24**, 237–244.

Energy balance and obesity in man

E. JÉQUIER
Institut de Physiologie, Rue du Bugnon 7, CH-1005 Lausanne, Switzerland.

Obesity arises when energy intake chronically exceeds energy expenditure. It is usually admitted that the control of food intake plays a major role in the regulation of energy balance. The renewed interest in considering that obesity may not be entirely due to a chronic excess of energy intake, but that a failure of the regulation of energy expenditure may also contribute to weight gain, stems from studies on energy balance in animals. Weanling rats induced to eat a highly palatable diet (cafeteria diet) increase their food intake by 50 to 60 per cent without gaining excess weight, thanks to a marked stimulation of diet-induced thermogenesis[16], which results mainly from the stimulation of brown adipose tissue metabolism. Conversely, in genetic models of obesity (*ob/ob* mice and *db/db* mice), an excessive gain in body weight can occur even if hyperphagia is prevented[3,23]. In these animals, a defective diet-induced thermogenesis seems to play an important role in the development of obesity; a mitochondrial defect has been described in the brown adipose tissue of these animals, which favours energy retention and thus weight gain[7].

In man, the role of a defect in the regulation of energy expenditure, which may favour the development of obesity, is less clearly demonstrated than in animal models of genetic obesity. Since I have recently published a review article on this topic[10], only a short summary will be presented here.

The two components of diet-induced thermogenesis. The main factor which stimulates energy expenditure in man at rest is food intake. The postprandial increase in energy expenditure includes two components: the 'obligatory' and the 'facultative thermogenesis'. The 'obligatory thermogenesis' is explained by the energetic cost of absorbing and processing the nutrients, while the 'faculatative thermogenesis' represents a dissipation of energy which cannot be accounted for by these 'obligatory' processes[1]. The sympathetic nervous system plays a role in modulating the 'facultative thermogenesis' as shown by the stimulation of noradrenaline turnover in the rat heart[25] after carbohydrate ingestion, and the increase in plasma noradrenaline levels in man during glucose administration[17]. While sympathetic-mediated activation of brown adipose tissue metabolism is an important mechanism for dissipating heat in cafeteria-fed rats[15], there is no convincing evidence that this tissue is functional in man. The tissues which are responsible for the 'facultative thermogenesis' are not known in man. However, the activation of β-adrenergic receptors during glucose/insulin i.v. administration in man is indirectly supported by the fact that propranolol, a β-receptor antagonist, partially inhibits the thermogenic response induced by glucose[1]. This finding further supports the concept of a sympathetic-mediated component of thermogenesis in man.

Diet-induced thermogenesis in obese subjects. Conflicting results have been published on the thermogenic responses to glucose-feeding or to mixed meals in obese individuals. Some investigators have reported decreased thermogenic responses[6,12,13,18,20,22], whereas others have shown unaltered responses[4,21,24]. The reasons for these conflicting results are not known, but it is likely that human obesity is a heterogeneous syndrome, with some individuals presenting a defective thermogenetic response to meal ingestion, whereas other obese subjects exhibit unaltered responses[10].

The overall importance of a thermogenetic defect in the aetiology of human obesity has been questioned, because obese people generally have a higher energy expenditure than the lean, even in those situations in which a low thermogenic response is produced[5]. After food ingestion, the overall energy expenditure is usually found to be higher in the obese than in lean subjects, in spite of a lower postprandial thermogenic response in the former. This is due to the higher basal metabolic rate in the obese than that in lean individuals[8,14]. In addition, obese subjects living in a respiration chamber expend more energy than lean control subjects[14,19].

The practical consequence of these findings is that the mean daily energy intake which is needed to maintain a constant body weight and body composition is elevated more in obese individuals than in sedentary lean control subjects. These results also indicate that an energy intake of 8300 kJ (2000 kcal) per day represents the lower limit for maintenance energy requirements of obese subjects[14]; a mean daily energy intake lower than 8300 kJ (2000 kcal) will induce weight loss in obese subjects.

Studies on the effect of weight loss on energy expenditure. Until now, we have considered only the static phase of obesity, which is usually characterized by an elevated resting energy expenditure. The possibility that a thermogenic defect is involved during the dynamic phase of weight gain has caused much interest recently[10]. Studies of the postprandial thermogenic responses in obese subjects after weight loss have shown that the thermogenic defect does not disappear[2,19]. Thus, the thermogenic defect in these individuals does not seem to be a consequence of their excessive body weight; it could represent a constitutive factor of genetic origin which favours energy retention and weight gain. It is of interest to note that when obese subjects have been able to reduce their excessive body weight to close to normal values by dieting, their overall postprandial energy expenditure can be significantly lower than that of lean controls (Golay, personal communication). If these 'post-obese' individuals were to ingest the same mean daily energy intake as the lean control subjects, they would be in positive energy balance and would gain weight. This shows that a defective thermogenic response to feed can lead to weight gain. It can be shown, however, that the weight gain resulting from a defect in energy expenditure alone is about 10 kg[11]. Greater weight gains must include a component of 'excessive food intake' since it cannot be explained solely on the basis of a defective thermogenesis.

For the obese individual, the practical implications of these studies on the effect of weight loss on energy expenditure is the need to adopt a new maintenance energy intake after weight loss, in order to avoid the relapse to increasing body weight. Thus, after a weight loss of 25 kg, a 'post-obese' individual should decrease his habitual maintenance energy intake by approximately 2100 kJ/d (500 kcal/d) when compared with the previous maintenance energy intake of the obese state (ie before weight loss). Failure to reset food intake to a lower level after weight loss accounts for the very frequent relapse to increasing body weight.

In conclusion, abnormalities in the regulatory control of both appetite and thermogenesis are involved in obesity[9]. Although the obvious treatment of this condition is to limit energy intake, increasing energy expenditure may contribute to weight loss. Exercise is certainly useful;

thermogenic drugs which stimulate β-adrenergic receptors are presently developed and are of potential interest in obese patients with a thermogenic defect. Further work is needed to assess the effects of increasing energy expenditure in the treatment of human obesity.

Acknowledgements. The main concepts presented in this paper were developed with the active contribution of Dr Y. Schutz, Dr K. Acheson and Dr A. Golay whose help is gratefully acknowledged. This work was supported by research grants from Nestlé, Vevey, Switzerland.

1 Acheson, K., Jéquier, E. & Wahren, J. (1983): Influence of beta-adrenergic blockade on glucose-induced thermogenesis in man. *J. Clin. Invest.* **72**, 981–986.

2 Bessard, T., Schutz, Y. & Jéquier, E. (1983): Energy expenditure and postprandial thermogenesis in obese women before and after weight loss. *Am. J. Clin. Nutr.* **38**, 680–693.

3 Cox, J.E. & Powley, T.L. (1977): Development of obesity in diabetic mice pair-fed with lean siblings. *J. Comp. Physiol. Psychol.* **91**, 347–358.

4 Felig, P., Cunningham, J., Levitt, M., Hendler, R. & Nadel, E. (1983): Energy expenditure in obesity in fasting and postprandial state. *Am. J. Physiol.* **244**, E45–E51.

5 Garrow, J.S. (1981): Thermogenesis and obesity in man. In *Recent Advances in obesity research*, III. ed P. Björntorp, M. Cairella, & A.N. Howard, pp. 208–215. London: John Libbey.

6 Golay, A., Schutz, Y., Meyer, H.U., Thiébaud, D., Curchod, B., Maeder, E., Felber, J.P. & Jéquier, E. (1982): Glucose induced thermogenesis in non-diabetic and diabetic obese subjects. *Diabetes* **31**, 1023–1028.

7 Himms-Hagen, J. & Desautels, M. (1978): A mitochondrial defect in brown adipose tissue of obese (ob/ob) mouse: reduced binding of purine nucleotides and a failure to respond to cold by an increase in binding. *Biochem. Biophys. Res. Comm.* **83**, 628–634.

8 James, W.P.T., Bailes, J., Davies, H.L. & Dauncey, M.J. (1978): Elevated metabolic rates in obesity. *Lancet* **1**, 1122–1125.

9 James, W.P.T. (1983): Energy requirements and obesity. *Lancet* **2**, 386–389.

10 Jéquier, E. (1984): Energy expenditure in obesity. *Clin. Endocr. Metab.* **13**, 563–580.

11 Jéquier, E. (1985): Thermogenèse induite par les nutriments chez l'homme: son rôle dans la régulation pondérale. *J. Physiol. Paris* **80**, 129–140.

12 Kaplan, M.L. & Leveillé, G.A. (1976): Calorigenic response in obese and nonobese women. *Am. J. Clin. Nutr.* **29**, 1108–1113.

13 Pittet, P.L., Chappuis, P.L., Acheson, K., de Techtermann, F. & Jéquier, E. (1976): Thermic effect of glucose in obese subjects studied by direct or indirect calorimetry. *Br. J. Nutr.* **35**, 281–292.

14 Ravussin, E., Burnand, B., Schutz, Y. & Jéquier, E. (1982): Twenty-four-hour energy expenditure and resting metabolic rate in obese, moderately obese, and control subjects. *Am. J. Clin. Nutr.* **35**, 566–573.

15 Rothwell, N.J. & Stock, M.J. (1979): A role for brown adipose tissue in diet-induced thermogenesis. *Nature* **281**, 31–55.

16 Rothwell, N.J. & Stock, M.J. (1980): Thermogenesis induced by cafeteria feeding in young growing rats. *Proc. Nutr. Soc.* **39**, 5A.

17 Rowe, J.W., Young, J.B., Minaker, K.L., Stevens, A.L., Pallotta, J. & Landsberg, L. (1981): Effect of insulin and glucose infusions on sympathetic nervous system activity in normal man. *Diabetes* **30**, 219–225.

18 Shutz, Y., Bessard, T. & Jéquier, E. (1984): Diet induced thermogenesis measured over a whole day in obese and nonobese women. *Am. J. Clin. Nutr.* **40**, 542–552.

19 Schutz, Y., Golay, A., Felber, J.P. & Jéquier, E. (1984): Decreased glucose-induced thermogenesis after weight loss in obese subjects: a predisposing factor for relapse of obesity? *Am. J. Clin. Nutr.* **39**, 380–387.

20 Schwartz, R.S., Halter, J.B. & Bierman, E. (1983): Reduced thermic effect of feeding in obesity: role of norepinephrine. *Metabolism* **32**, 114–117.

21 Sharief, N.N. & MacDonald,. I (1982): Differences in dietary-induced thermogenesis with various carbohydrates in normal and overweight men. *Am. J. Clin. Nutr.* **35**, 267–272.

22 Shetty, P.S., Jung, R.T., James, W.P.T., Barrand, M.A. & Callingham, B.A. (1981): Postprandial thermogenesis in obesity. *Clin. Sci.* **60**, 519–525.

23 Thurlby, P.L. & Trayhurn, P. (1979): The role of thermoregulatory thermogenesis in the development of obesity in genetically obese (ob/ob) mice pair fed with lean siblings. *Br. J. Nutr.* **42**, 377–385.

24 Welle, S.L. & Campbell, R.G. (1983): Normal thermic effect of glucose in obese women. *Am. J. Clin. Nutr.* **37**, 87–92.

25 Young, J.B. & Landsberg, L. (1977): Stimulation of the sympathetic nervous system during sucrose feeding. *Nature* **269**, 615–617.

Very-low-calorie diets: a workshop report

A.N. HOWARD (Organizer)
Department of Medicine, University of Cambridge, Addenbrooke's Hospital, Hills Road, Cambridge, CB2 2QQ.

Background to the criticism of very low calorie diets *(Howard)*. Very-low-calorie diets have been used for the treatment of obesity for at least 50 years. The earlier diets containing normal food have now been replaced by formula diets which have the advantage of containing the RDAs of vitamins and minerals, and adequate levels of other nutrients. In addition to protein (33–70 g/d) all formulas contain at least 25 g carbohydrate which moderate ketosis and retain electrolytes. The Cambridge Diet (CD) contains only 330 kcal (1.38 MJ)/d (33 g protein, 44 g carbohydrates, 3 g fat, US-RDAs of essential vitamins and minerals), and has been severely criticized on the grounds that it is inadequate in electrolytes, causes loss of lean body mass (LBM) and is less safe than conventional diets.

Two groups of five inpatients were given in sequence either CD or a conventional hospital diet (HD) containing 800 kcal (50 g protein, 54 g carbohydrate and 39 g fat) for two periods of four weeks. During the first four weeks the mean weight loss was, CD: 9.3 kg, HD: 6.6 kg; during the second four weeks, CD: 7.0 kg, HD: 4.8 kg. On analysis the HD was found to contain only 8 mg iron, 6 mg zinc, 1.5 mg manganese, 130 mg magnesium and 1 mg copper. These volumes are well below the US-RDAs. It is concluded that there is no basis to claim the HD is theoretically safer than CD.

Lean body mass accounts for 25–33 per cent of the increased body weight in obese people. Since the body composition of the obese who achieve normal weight becomes normal, then this large quantity of nitrogen has to be utilized for metabolism and must cause an apparent negative nitrogen balance during weight reduction whatever the diet employed. For example, men on the CD lose about 2.2 kg body weight per week and women 1.8 kg/week (correcting for dehydration and loss of body contents). If the protein contribution produced by this weight loss is added on to that present in the diet (33 g) the total new available protein for metabolism is 61 g/day for men and 54 g/day for women. This is, incidentally, well above the US-RDA for protein which is intended for people on a weight-maintenance diet. On weight reduction using CD, it is estimated that the additional nitrogen (N) available to the metabolic pool ranges from 2.1 to 3.6 g N/day. This is more than sufficient to account for the small negative N balance. It is concluded that the loss of LBM is of the same magnitude as would be expected from the decrease in body weight, that CD is fundamentally safe in healthy obese subjects and much more effective than HD.

The United States experience *(S.N. Kreitzman,* Emory University School of Dentistry, 1462 Clifton Road, N.E., Atlanta, GA 30322, USA.). The two overriding issues in the use of very-low-calorie diets (VLCD) for weight control are safety and effectiveness. Risk associated with dieting must be viewed against the risks associated with overweight, the high morbidity and mortality associated with surgical methods of weight control, the ineffectiveness of standard dietetics, diets or behaviour modification programmes, and the risks associated with starvation or liquid protein diets that claimed the lives of 59 individuals/hundred thousand users. This unacceptable number was compared by the FDA with 2 deaths/hundred thousand in healthy non-dieting white women between the ages of 22 and 45, the background level of unexplained cardiovascular deaths.

Twenty-seven obese subjects were studied before, during and after four weeks of VLCD. Each subject was asked to consume the 330 kcal (1.38 MJ)/d liquid formula CD for a period of 28 d as their sole source of food. Mean weight loss was approximately 9 kg with the largest single weight loss at 19 kg. Each subject was assigned to one of six physicians for pre-diet and subsequent weekly physicals including ECGs, height, weight and blood pressure. Blood

(SMA-22) and urine were also evaluated at the beginning of the diet and then weekly. Eight subjects also used 24 h continuous cardiac monitors before and after the diet. Despite considerable weight loss, no evidence of biochemical or clinical abnormalities or cardiac changes were observed. In several subjects blood pressures were normalized during the study period and cholesterol and triglyceride values fell substantially in all subjects.

Serum potassium levels were maintained at normal levels except for those subjects being treated with diuretics. These individuals were taken off their diuretics with no further difficulty. Several subjects exhibited transient elevations in serum uric acid. This potentially could pose some difficulty for those with gout; however, none of our subjects experienced any problems.

The results of this investigation suggest that substantial weight loss is possible with VLCD and that the diets are safe for overweight but otherwise healthy people. The results emphasize the need for pre-diet medication to identify systemic disease, cardiovascular problems, diabetes, gout, etc. The value of constant and expensive medical monitoring in otherwise healthy subjects, however, can be questioned in the light of the benign effect of the diet on any observable parameter.

Long-term studies of electrolyte and nitrogen balance. (*V. Wynn*, Alexander Simpson Laboratory for Metabolic Research, St Mary's Hospital Medical School, London, UK.). VLCD
are commercially available in a variety of powdered or liquid forms and variously constituted to provide adequate nutrition in terms of protein, carbohydrate, minerals, trace elements and vitamins. At the Metabolic Unit we have been using a 650–750 VLCD formula providing approximately 53–55 g protein and 70–75 g carbohydrate in a liquid formula[1]. We have carried out continuous metabolic studies involving N and electrolyte balance and this has enabled us to determine daily rates of fat loss and protein loss from the daily change in weight. The method assumes that fluid balance can be assessed from electrolyte balance[2]. We have found this method is effective in monitoring patient compliance with the treatment. Our studies show that the rate of fat loss is constant for up to 120 d and that the 'plateau phenomenon' so widely believed to be a bar to continuous effective weight loss on low-calorie diets is due to fluid retention and not to a metabolic adaption significantly reducing energy output. Negative nitrogen balance has not proved to be a problem in female patients. In males nitrogen balance is persistently negative reaching an equilibrium figure of about -2 g N/d after about 28 d of continuous dieting. There have been no untoward clinical or electrocardiographic changes in our subjects so far.

1 Abraham, R.R., Densem, J.W., Davie, M.W.J. Wynn, V. (1985): Factors that influence nitrogen loss in obese patients on calorie restricted diets *Am. J. Clin. Nutr.* (in press)
2 Wynn, V., Abraham, R.R. & Densem, J.W. (1985): Method for estimating rate of fat loss during treatment of obesity by calorie restriction. *Lancet* **1**, 482–486.

Cardiac rhythms in obese females not dieting and on very-low-calorie diets. (*I. McLean Baird*, West Middlesex Hospital, Isleworth, Middlesex, UK.) There have been several ambulatory monitoring studies in young subjects but none have described an obese group. The present study was an investigation of 36 obese females not on a diet. The normal range of heart rhythm in this group is important because of the reports of ventricular tachycardias in some patients who had been on VLCD for several months.

For comparison, two groups of non-dieting subjects had two 24 h ECG recordings using an Oxford Medilog recorder. Statistical evaluation using contingency χ^2 tables with Yates correction showed significantly higher ventricular premature beats in the > 35-year-old group. One young subject had a second degree A-V block. There were three patients over the age of 35 years with ventricular tachycardias and three with supraventricular tachycardias.

Twelve obese females with no clinical or electrocardiographic abnormality underwent ambulatory monitoring under hospital conditions for one month on a 330 kcal (1.38 MJ) formula diet and on a 800 kcal (3.35 MJ) conventional diet. No patients developed ventricular tachycardias on either diet, although two patients had transient A-V block at night both on the diet of lower energy content.

There was no evidence in the present study of dieting patients of any trend towards serious arrhythmias on VLCD and previous ambulatory monitoring 'abnormalities' may have been within the normal range of findings which are dependent on age.

The response of plasma lipoproteins and clotting factors to low-energy diets in obese women. (*G.J. Miller*, MRC Epidemiology and Medical Care Unit, Northwick Park Hospital, Harrow, Middlesex, UK). The effects of the two low-energy diets on cardiovascular risk-factor status were studied in 11 obese women. A two-period crossover trial was used to determine whether the responses observed were related primarily to the low energy intake or the loss of body weight.

Patients were given a 1000 kcal (4.18 MJ) diet for 7 d. Six were then allotted at random to Gp 1, and five to Gp 2. No statistically significant group-differences were observed at baseline, indicating that randomization had been satisfactory. Overall means were body weight, 102 kg; height, 1.63 m; low-density lipoprotein cholesterol (LDL_{ch}), 4.7 mmol/l; high-density lipoprotein cholesterol (HDL_{ch}), 0.99 mmol/l; serum triglyceride, 1.54 mmol/l; plasma-fibrinogen, 437 mg/dl; clotting factor activities as per cent of standard: II, 133 per cent; VII_c, 104 per cent; VIII_c, 141 per cent; X_c, 98 per cent.

Group 1 then took an 800 kcal (3.35 MJ) diet for 4 weeks while Gp 2 took a 330 kcal (1.38 MJ) liquid formula. Diets were then exchanged and continued for a further 4 weeks. Risk-factors were measured at change-over and at completion of the trial. When examined with respect to energy intake, no significant difference in body weight was observed after completion of the two diets because of the crossover method of administration (overall mean, 91 kg). Nevertheless, all other measurements were lower after 330 kcal than after 800 kcal, differences being statistically significant ($P < 0.01$) for LDL_{ch} (3.26 v 4.25 mmol/l), HDL_{ch} (0.80 v 0.94 mmol/l), VII_c (80 per cent v 98 per cent) and X_c (73 per cent v 90 per cent). Respective means for LDL_{ch}/HDL_{ch} were 4.3 and 4.9.

A different pattern was found when results were related to time. Mean weight at the end of the trial (88 kg) was significantly less than at its midpoint (94 kg). Despite this difference, no differences were observed between time points for any other variable except fibrinogen and VII_c, both of which were significantly higher ($P < 0.05$) at the end of the trial than at changeover (fibrinogen, 440 v 414 mg/dl; VII_c, 92 per cent v 86 per cent). Thus changes observed were in the inverse direction to change in body weight.

The results indicated that short-term use of low-energy diet was associated with improvement of cardiovascular risk-factor status in obese women. This improvement was related more to change in energy intake than on the accompanying reduction in body weight. The decrease in HDL_{ch} was thought unlikely to have been disadvantageous because no increase in LDL_{ch}/HDL_{ch} occurred.

Methods of inducing hyperphagia — advantages and disadvantages: a workshop report

K.J. McCRACKEN (Organizer)
Department of Agricultural & Food Chemistry, The Queen's University of Belfast and Department of Agriculture for Northern Ireland, Newforge Lane, Belfast, BT9 5PX, UK.

This Workshop in which approx. 40 people took part, concentrated on examining a range of procedures used to induce hyperphagia in the growing adult rat though some mention of other species was made. It had been the intention of the organizer that the workshop should address in some detail the question of the relevence of rat models to the subject of regulation of energy intake and obesity in the human but little progress was made in that direction. However, a number of aspects of this problem were raised during the discussion and should be borne in mind by anyone tempted to directly apply results obtained in the rat to the human situation. Firstly, most of the problems of human obesity relate to the adult and develop over a period of months or years as a result of a relatively small difference between energy intake and expenditure. The anatomical and metabolic consequences may not necessarily be the same as those observed when relatively large degrees of hyperphagia are induced experimentally over short periods of time. Secondly, much of the literature relates to hyperphagia induced in the young growing rat and the considerable differences in relative food intake and relative growth rate of rats and humans must be recognised. Thirdly, the rat is a nocturnal animal which eats a large number of small meals (nibbler) mainly at night in contrast to the human situation. Fourthly, almost all studies conducted on hyperphagic rat models have been done at temperatures well below thermoneutrality and this has obvious consequences for the interpretation of sympathetically-mediated alterations in metabolism.

It was generally accepted that, leaving aside the problem of extrapolation from one species to another, each of the model approaches which had been adopted with the rat provide an insight into some aspect of one or more of four subject areas, viz the regulation of food intake, changes in energy expenditure, the metabolic causes of obesity and the metabolic consequences of obesity. Each of the models has its strengths and weaknesses and most of the discussion centred on these.

Introductory comments on specific topics were provided by a number of invited speakers and the discussion was led by *H.G. Barr, A.J.F. Webster* and the organizer.

High-fat diets (*R.A. Schemmel*). High-fat diets can be used to initiate obesity at various stages of the life-span of the rat including nursing pups by feeding a high-fat diet to the dam. The obesity is mainly the result of increased energy intake (hyperphagia), but is probably related in part to the high efficiency of incorporation of dietary fat into body lipid. Although very high levels of fat (600 g/kg diet) have been used in some studies, hyperphagia (15 to 20 per cent) has been induced in growing and adult rats with pelleted diets containing 220 g fat/kg diet. Thus high-fat diets can be used to simulate the chemical composition of diets consumed by Western man and provide close control over other dietary variables. The effects of specific fats, eg long-chain saturated, polyunsaturated or medium-chain triglycerides, can be evaluated in relation to the effects on energy intake, expenditure and the metabolic consequences of high-fat diets. A problem with the existing literature is the lack of information given about the nature of the fat sources used in some studies and the chemical composition of the final diets. However, this problem is not confined to studies using high-fat diets and it was agreed that interpretation of results would be enhanced by careful descriptions of the physical and chemical composition of diets in all studies using hyperphagic models.

It was noted that a number of the metabolic consequences of high-fat-induced obesity in the rat parallel the situation observed in the obese human, eg blood lipid and blood pressure changes. Since it is normally only possible to examine the end-effect of obesity in the human, one area in which the high-fat diet model could be more fully exploited is the examination of the time-course of anatomical and metabolic changes during hyperphagic-induced obesity under standardized conditions.

Tube-feeding (*M.J. Stock*). In view of the metabolic differences observed in several species and particularly the rat as a result of a shift from 'nibbling' to 'meal-feeding' it would appear that the rat model might be improved by altering the feeding pattern towards that normally adopted by humans. However, voluntary consumption is normally reduced when a rat is forced to become a 'meal-feeder'. Hence the only effective means of achieving above-normal intakes on a meal-feeding regimen is to resort to tube-feeding. This provides precise control over food intake and meal frequency and large energy intakes can be achieved. Adult rats have been fed energy intakes in excess of twice the maintenance requirement for several months and have become extremely obese. However the range of physical and chemical compositions of diets which are suitable for tube-feeding, especially to young animals, is somewhat limited and problems of electrolyte balance can arise. The most serious criticism of tube-feeding is that it appears to result in alterations in intermediary metabolism which differ from those observed with voluntary meal-feeding. The changes observed include a reduction in the rate of protein deposition in growing animals, increased efficiency of energy utilization and hence elevated fat deposition. It is probable therefore that tube-feeding will exacerbate the effects which occur under conditions of voluntary hyperphagia. The hormonal aspects have not been fully elucidated though it would appear that stress associated with tube-feeding is the primary cause of the changes, some of which are similar to those induced by oral treatment with corticosteroids. In view of these problems the dangers inherent in extrapolation from the tube-feeding model are emphasized. However, further elucidation of the effects of diet composition, feeding frequency and energy intake on the hormonal changes associated with tube-feeding may provide useful fundamental information to assist in our understanding of the metabolic causes and consequences of hyperphagic obesity.

Cafeteria-feeding (*N.J. Rothwell*). Offering a range of palatable human foods in addition to laboratory chow (cafeteria-feeding) is an effective means of inducing hyperphagia. Average increases of 30 per cent above the voluntary consumption of controls offered stock diet *ad libitum* have frequently been observed and in some cases the mean increase has been considerably higher than this. A 7-d menu of four palatable ingredients per day has proved satisfactory in achieving sustained hyperphagia for several weeks and it is probable that a less complicated menu would suffice. Although cafeteria diets have frequently resulted in relatively high fat intakes the degree of hyperphagia appears to be related to variety rather than energy density since 28 per cent hyperphagia occurred on a cafeteria diet containing only 30 g fat/kg compared with 15–20 per cent achieved with a high-fat pelleted diet.

The major problems of cafeteria-feeding are those associated with accurate measurement of energy intake, individual variations in nutrient consumption and possible nutrient deficiencies. Variations in individual nutrient intake can be considerable depending on the range of palatable foods used and the composition of the stock diet. Some degree of nutrient deficiency is almost inevitable since consumption of the stock diet usually amounts to only 10 to 20 per cent of the energy intake. Many of the studies reported in the literature have failed to take adequate account of these problems and it is recommended that greater attention be paid to them in designing experiments and during preparation for publication. A particular area for concern in long-term studies would be the low calcium content of many cafeteria diets. An additional problem associated with cafeteria-feeding is the increased consumption of food during the day thus exacerbating the 'nibbling' pattern. These problems apart, cafeteria-feeding is an effective natural means of inducing hyperphagia in rats and the diet composition can be manipulated by appropriate choice of stock diet and palatable foods. One interesting aspect of this model is the degree of individual variation observed in terms of food preference and degree of hyperphagia. It is recommended that closer attention be paid to this in future studies in view of the increased interest in psychological and behavioural aspects of regulation of food intake in the human. It is further recommended that protocols should be designed to permit analysis of complete bulked samples of the cafeteria diets offered, of total food spilled or refused and of faeces, thus permitting accurate definition of the nutrients consumed by individual animals.

Sucrose-induced hyperphagia (*D. York*). Sucrose offered as a liquid supplement (up to 320 g/l) is an effective means of inducing hyperphagia and can be a useful adjunct in a low-fat cafeteria model. Normally a reduction in intake of stock diet occurs and this can lead to problems of reduced intakes of protein, minerals and vitamins in studies on growing animals. Recent results from USA suggest that the high intakes of sucrose are not directly related to the sweetness of sucrose since a greater degree of hyperphagia was attained by offering a bland polysaccharide (Polycox) in place of sucrose. The use of such compounds in place of sucrose will provide an opportunity to examine the effects of excess carbohydrate consumption uncomplicated by the contribution of the unique hepatic pathway for conversion of fructose to acetyl CoA.

Genetic obesity (*O. Tulp*). Discussion centred on two strains of rat, the Zucker (*fa/fa*) and the LA/N-corpulent. The underlying metabolic causes of genetic obesity can be examined by studying the pre-obese pups prior to the onset of hyperphagia. For example, hypersecretion of insulin and glucagon have been observed *in vivo* in response to glucose or arginine load. Comparisons of the lean and obese strains during the development of hyperphagic obesity or under conditions of imposed food restriction on the obese group should provide an effective means of establishing metabolic differences. This approach, coupled with techniques such as adrenalectomy and hypothalamic lesion, forms the basis for differentiation of the factors predisposing to hyperphagia from those predisposing to obesity in the absence of hyperphagia or from the metabolic consequences of obesity. There would appear to be considerable scope for further integration of some of the nutritional means of inducing hyperphagia in conjunction with studies on lean/obese strains.

★　★　★

NUTRITION AND ENDURANCE PERFORMANCE

Carbohydrate and endurance performance

D.L. COSTILL
Human Performance Laboratory, Ball State University, Muncie, Indiana 47306, USA.

Muscle and liver glycogen serve as the principal fuel for energy production during intense muscular activity. In long-term exercise bouts, however, limited glycogen stores may be unable to meet the energy demands associated with ≥ 2 h effort. Carbohydrate (CHO) ingestion before and during such activity has been used to enhance muscle and liver glycogen storage and to maintain the blood glucose concentration.

Endurance-trained subjects generally demonstrate a lesser hyperglycaemia and a lower insulin response to a given oral glucose load than do normally active men and women[7,13]. It appears that endurance-training alters the tissue sensitivity to insulin and the controls on blood insulin and glucose. Thus, the responses to sugar-feedings before, during and after exercise will, to some extent, be dependent on the training status of the subject. Likewise, the intensity of exercise has a bearing on the glycaemic and insulin responses to CHO feedings. Studies of glucose uptake during 60 min of exercise and at rest demonstrate a marked reduction in blood glucose and insulin as a result of the activity[5]. In light of these interactions between exercise and the hormone responses to CHO feedings, it is not surprising that the metabolic responses to sugar ingestion are dramatically different when taken at varied times before and during exercise. The absorption and ultimate assimilation of oral CHO feedings depends, also, on the rate of gastric emptying.

Dietary preparation for exercise. Carbohydrate intake in the days, hours and minutes before exercise has a significant effect on substrate utilization and performance[1,8,12]. Feeding CHO-rich diets to subjects for 3–5 days results in elevated liver and muscle glycogen storage, provided such a regimen is preceded by prolonged, severe exercise[9]. In contrast to mixed and CHO-poor diets, subjects tend to oxidize more CHO at rest and during exercise following days on the CHO intake[11]. There is evidence[12] suggesting that the rate of CHO metabolism is reduced following a high-fat-protein diet as a result of increased intramuscular citrate production, with a subsequent inhibition of the phosphofructokinase reaction. Although this response would tend to spare the limited muscle glycogen reserves, it does not diminish the demands on liver glycogen depots that are expectedly low as a consequence of the low-CHO diet. Thus, the diet rich in CHO suffices to keep muscle and liver glycogen normalized, and results in higher blood glucose levels during exercise. It has been shown[9] that when liver glycogen stores are high, as following the CHO-rich diet, hepatic glucose production is derived principally from glycogenolysis. When liver glycogen is low, as in the low-CHO diet regimen, the availability of blood glucose depends on gluconeogenesis, a relatively slow process that generally cannot match the rate of glucose uptake by the exercising muscles[9].

Evidence to date has clearly shown that performance in prolonged, severe exercise is improved by eating a CHO-rich diet to elevate the liver and muscle glycogen stores. Bergstrom *et al.*[3] and Astrand[2] proposed that an optimal plan to maximize muscle glycogen storage should involve exhaustive exercise followed by 3 days of low dietary CHO consumption, with three additional days of high CHO intake. This regimen was reported to increase leg muscle glycogen by roughly two-fold (100 to 220 mmol/kg wet muscle). More recent studies[14] have tested the effectiveness of different dietary regimens on muscle glycogen storage. This research demonstrated that it was unnecessary to introduce a high-fat-protein diet for 3 days in order to attain very high muscle-glycogen depots. On the contrary, following exhaustive exercise, similar muscle-glycogen values were achieved when 3 days of either a mixed (353 g CHO/d) or a low CHO diet (104 g CHO/d) was followed by 3 days of rich CHO intake (542 g CHO/d).

Diet also plays an important role in preparing the liver for the demands of endurance exercise. It has been shown[10] that, when subjects are deprived of carbohydrates for only 24 h, the glycogen stores of the liver will decrease rapidly to values below 10 g/kg wet tissue. As a result of strenuous exercise lasting 60 min, liver glycogen was reported to decrease from a mean of 44 g/kg tissue to 20 g/kg. In combination with a low CHO diet, hard physical activity will likely empty the liver glycogen stores. It is interesting to note, however, that when the period of CHO-starvation was followed by 2 days of a carbohydrate-rich diet normal in its content of total energy (400 g CHO/d), liver glycogen increased rapidly to 78–102 g/kg tissue. Thus, the inclusion of CHO in the diet and rest during the days preceding prolonged, severe (60–70 per cent $\dot{V}O_2$ max) exercise will expand liver and muscle glycogen reserves, and minimise the threat of premature exhaustion associated with exertional hypoglycaemia and/or glycogen depletion.

Although the ingestion of carbohydrates in the days before exercise has demonstrated a positive influence on performance, the uptake of sugar solutions in the last 30–60 min before the activity may reduce the subject's exercise tolerance[6]. Ingesting glucose and/or sucrose before exercise elevates blood glucose and insulin, and stimulates CHO oxidation. It has been demonstrated[1] that glucose ingestion 50 min before exercise increased arterial glucose levels by 30–40 per cent, whereas glucose uptake by the exercising legs was 40–100 per cent greater than when no CHO was taken before the activity. Under these conditions blood-borne glucose accounted for 48–58 per cent of the total oxidation fuel consumption as compared to 27–41 per cent in the control treatment. Although such CHO feedings result in elevated blood glucose (6.5–7.0 mmol/l) at the initiation of the exercise, there is a rapid decline in the first 10–15 min of activity, reaching levels of less than 2.5 mmol/l[4]. Despite their state of hypoglycaemia, the subjects experienced no greater fatigue than during the exercise when their blood glucose averaged 4.6–5.8 mmol/l. This would suggest that hypoglycaemia, *per se*, may not be responsible for the fatigue associated with long-term activity. It is interesting to note, however, that two of the subjects who were found to have the lowest blood glucose values following the glucose-exercise regimen, also utilized 71–100 per cent more muscle glycogen than when no sugar was ingested before the exercise[6]. This would suggest that when blood glucose concentrations are very low, the exercising muscles may adjust their rate of glycogen utilization to compensate for the lack of available glucose, provided muscle-glycogen stores are high. It has been suggested that the hyperinsulinaemia accompanying the glucose-feeding is responsible for the increased muscle-glucose utilization during exercise. The greater dependence on muscle glycogen results in a more rapid depletion of these reserves and an earlier onset of exhaustion[6].

Recent studies using pre-exercise (45 min before) feedings of sucrose, fructose or water (control) show that the blood glucose and insulin levels are related to the rate of CHO metabolism and glycogen utilization during subsequent exercise (unpublished). When fed 50 g of sucrose, the blood glucose of eight resting subjects in this study increased from 4.4 to 6.2 mmol/l in 45 min. A similar fructose feeding (ie, 50 g) resulted in a rise from 4.3 to 5.0 mmol/l in the same time period. After 20 min of exercise, blood glucose declined to 3.8, 3.1 and 4.0 mmol/l in the fructose, sucrose and control trials, respectively. The blood insulin levels at the start of exercise averaged 8.8 (control), 13.4 (fructose), and 17.9 uU/ml (sucrose). As a result of 30 min of cycling at approximately 75 per cent of $\dot{V}O_2$ max, glycogen concentration in the vastus lateralis muscle decreased 42.8 mmol/kg in the control trial, and 45.6 and 55.4 mmol/kg in the fructose and sucrose trials, respectively. Similar patterns of total CHO oxidation were calculated from the respiratory exchange data. That is, 64.1, 65.3 and 79.1 g of CHO were metabolized during the 30 min of exercise in the control, fructose, and sucrose trials, respectively. Thus it appears that fructose consumption before exercise will not induce the same order of stimulation for carbohydrate oxidation and glycogen use observed following the intake of glucose and/or sucrose.

1 Ahlborg, G. & Felig, P. (1977): Substrate utilization during prolonged exercise preceded by ingestion of glucose. *Am. J. Physiol.* **233**, E188–E194.
2 Astrand, P.O. (1967): Diet and athletic performance. *Fed. Proc.* **26**, 1772–1777.
3 Bergstrom, J., Hermansen, L. & Hultman, E. (1967): Diet muscle glycogen and physical performance. *Acta Physiol. Scand.* **71**, 140–150.
4 Bonen, A., Malcolm, S.A., Kilgour, R.D., MacIntyre, K.P. & Belcastro, A.N. (1981): *J. Appl. Physiol.: Respirat Environ. Exercise Physiol.* **50**, 766–771.
5 Costill, D.L., Bennett, A., Branam, G. & Eddy, D.O. (1973): Glucose ingestion at rest and during prolonged exercise. *J. Appl. Physiol.* **34**, 764–769.
6 Costill, D.L., Coyle, E., Dalsky, G. & Fink, W. (1977): Effects of elevated plasma FFA and insulin on muscle glycogen usage during exercise. *J. Appl. Physiol.* **43**, 695–699.
7 Costill, D.L. & Miller, J.M. (1980): Nutrition for endurance sports: carbohydrate and fluid balance. *Int. J. Sports Med.* **1**, 2014.
8 Foster, C., Costill, D.L. & Fink, W.J. (1979): Effects of preexercise feedings on endurance performance. *Med. Sci. Sports.* **11**, 1–5.
9 Hultman, E. (1978): Liver as glucose supplying source during rest and exercise, with special reference to diet. *Nutritional, physical fitness, and health*, ed J. Parizkova and V.A. Rogzkin, pp. 9–30. Baltimore: University Park Press.
10 Hultman, E., & Nilsson, L.H. (1971): Liver glycogen in man: Effect of different diets and muscular exercise. In *Muscle metabolism during exercise*, ed B. Pernow & B. Saltin, pp. 143–151. New York: Plenum Press.
11 Jacobs, I. (1981): Lactate concentrations after short, maximal exercise at various glycogen levels. *Acta Physiol. Scand.* **111**, 465–469.
12 Jansson, E. (1980): Diet and muscle metabolism in man. *Acta Physiol. Scand.* Suppl. 487, 24.
13 Lohmann, D., Liebdd, F. & Heilmann, W. (1978): Diminished insulin response in highly trained athletes. *Metabolism* **27**, 521–524.
14 Sherman, W.M., Costill, D.L., Fink, W.J. & Miller, J.M. (1981): Effects of exercise-diet manipulation on muscle glycogen and its subsequent utilization during performance. *Int. J. Sports Med.* **2**, 1–15.
15 Van Handel, P.J., Fink, W.J., Branam, G. & Costill, D.L. (1980): Fate of ^{14}C glucose ingested during prolonged exercise. *Int. J. Sports Medicine.* **1**, 127–131.

Nutrition for glycogen repletion during exercise

M. SUZUKI
Laboratory of Biochemistry of Exercise and Nutrition, Institute of Health and Sports Sciences, University of Tsukuba, Sakura-mura, Niihari-gun, Ibaraki 305, Japan.

There is considerable evidence that depletion of liver and muscle glycogen is one of the major factors in the development of exhaustion during prolonged strenuous exercise[2]. There is also strong evidence that endurance performance can be increased by raising, and diminished by lowering, body glycogen stores[1].

The increase in endurance performance with exercise training is partially mediated by the exercise-adapted increase in the lipolytic activity of adipose tissue[5] and also in the capacity of muscle to oxidize fatty acids[3], with utilization of more fat and proportionately less glycogen during exercise.

Therefore the development of nutritional regimens useful for increasing glycogen accumulation in liver and muscle prior to exercise and stimulation of adipose tissue lipolytic activity during exercise is much needed to promote endurance performance.

Increase in glycogen stores in liver and lipolytic activity of adipose tissue with decreased meal frequency. It has been reported that liver glycogen stores are much greater in meal-fed rats as compared with rats fed *ad libitum*. For instance it has been shown[12] in rats fed *ad* *libitum* or meal-fed one, two or three meals per day that liver glycogen stores become greater as meal frequency is decreased. It has also been demonstrated[9] that lipolytic activity of adipose tissue is significantly increased with meal-feeding, due to an elevated lipolytic responsiveness of fat cells to adrenaline and theophylline.

Diurnal changes of glycogen stores in liver and muscle. Diurnal changes have been demonstrated[10] in glycogen stores in liver and muscle in meal-fed rats. Rats were fed a diet containing 35 per cent sucrose in the evening and a basal diet in the morning or the same diets at the reversed time for 7 weeks. Glycogen stores in liver and muscle showed sharp increases over 8 h after the sucrose meal, regardless of its timing. In contrast, glycogen stores in the tissues did not show any marked increase after the basal diet. Thus, in order to promote bigger glycogen stores in liver and muscle prior to exercise, the timing of a meal as well as its composition are very important.

Enhancement of glycogen repletion in liver and muscle with citrate after exhaustive exercise. In most sports events two competitions are held in a day, morning and afternoon, and training exercise is also usually conducted twice a day. Therefore, a rapid recovery of liver and muscle glycogen stores, of which larger parts might be utilized with the first exercise, is necessary to achieve good results in the second exercise.

It has been demonstrated[7] in exercise-trained rats that, as compared with a single feeding of 3.3 g of glucose per kg body weight, a feeding of 3.0 g of glucose with 0.5 g of citrate following exhaustive exercise can significantly increase the rate of glycogen repletion in liver and muscle. This dietary regimen has been reported to inhibit phosphofructokinase (PFK) *in vitro*[13,14].

Further increase in glycogen repletion in liver and muscle with a high-carbohydrate meal containing dextrin following citrate and glucose administration after exhaustive exercise. In order to achieve further glycogen repletion in liver and muscle after the citrate and glucose administration, the composition of the meal to be fed after the first exercise has been investigated[11]. Rats were adapted to meal feeding three times a day and trained with light swimming. On the final day, rats received citrate and glucose immediately after exhaustive exercise, and 2 h later they were fed on diets with different energy patterns or carbohydrate types. Results showed that a high-carbohydrate diet (carbohydrate, fat, protein = 80, 5, 15 per cent of energy) is more effective than a high-fat diet (45, 40, 15 per cent) for promoting further glycogen repletion in liver and muscle during 4 h of recovery. In addition, dextrin is revealed as superior to starch as a carbohydrate source in tissue-glycogen repletion.

Replenishment of liver and muscle glycogen with fructose and arginine during exercise without inhibiting lipolysis. A rapid repletion of glycogen stores during exercise is required in endurance types of sports such as the marathon, Nordic skiing, ball games. It has been agreed that endurance performance can be increased by sparing glycogen utlization by keeping a high availability of FFA during exercise. Therefore the development of nutritional regimens which can promote liver and muscle glycogen repletion without inhibiting fat metabolism during exercise would be of great value.

Glucose itself, and any other sugars which yield glucose molecules on hydrolysis, are highly glycogenic substrates and also bring about a favourable physiological conditions for glycogen synthesis by stimulating insulin secretion. However, the administration of such sugars is not always desirable for endurance exercise, because glucose inhibits lipolysis.

It has been demonstrated in rats[8] that arginine, which is known to stimulate insulin secretion *in vivo*[4], given after an exhaustive exercise does not inhibit lipolysis. On the other hand, fructose is a poor stimulant of insulin secretion as compared with glucose but one of the sugars available as a glycogen substrate. Fructose has been reported[6] not to inhibit lipolysis *in vivo*.

The effect of fructose and arginine given together on the repletion of glycogen stores in liver and skeletal muscle and on lipolysis in exercise-trained rats during a bout of endurance exercise has been examined[8]. The question of whether citrate can stimulate the tissue glycogen repletion with fructose and arginine has also been examined.

Rats were adapted to meal feeding twice a day and trained with treadmill running. On the final day, after the first 1.5 h during a 3-h running, rats were given one of three types of drinks; 3.3 g of fructose plus 0.5 g of arginine, 3.3 g of glucose plus 0.5 g of arginine and water or 3.3 g of fructose plus 0.5 g of arginine plus 0.5 g of citrate per kg body weight.

There was a significant reduction in liver and muscle-glycogen stores during the second half of the exercise period after water administration, whereas the administration of either fructose plus arginine or glucose plus arginine prevented liver glycogen depletion and increased muscle glycogen stores. The addition of citrate to fructose plus arginine spared muscle glycogen stores during the latter half period of exercise more significantly than the administration of glucose plus arginine.

The administration of glucose plus arginine significantly decreased lipolytic activity of adipose tissue and serum FFA levels, as compared with the administration of either fructose plus arginine or water.

Conclusion. We have investigated the nutritional regimens which can rapidly replenish the tissue glycogen stores after or during exercise. Our series of studies have demonstrated that: (1) citrate is a good stimulant for glycogen repletion in liver and muscle; (2) a high-carbohydrate meal containing dextrin taken during the recovery period is favourable for the tissue glycogen repletion, and (3) the administration of fructose plus arginine plus citrate during exercise is able to spare liver glycogen store and replenish muscle glycogen in the latter period of exercise without inhibiting lipolysis.

We have also suggested the importance of taking the matter of meal frequency into account and the diurnal rhythms of tissue-glycogen stores in relation to meal timing to achieve maximum glycogen stores in liver and muscle prior to exercise and a high lipolytic activity of adipose tissue during exercise.

1 Bergstrom, J., Hermansen, L., Hultman, E. & Saltin, B. (1967): Diet, muscle glycogen and physical performance. *Acta Physiol. Scand.* **71**, 140–150.
2 Hermansen, L., Hultman, E. & Saltin, B. (1967): Muscle glycogen during prolonged severe exercise. *Acta Physiol. Scand.* **71**, 129–139.
3 Holloszy, J.O. & Booth, F.W. (1976): Biochemical adaptations to endurance exercise in muscle. *Ann. Rev. Physiol.* **38**, 273–291.
4 Levin, S.R., Karam, J.H., Hane, S., Grodsky, G.M. & Forsham, P.H. (1971): Enhancement of arginine-induced insulin secretion in man by prior administration of glucose. *Diabetes* **20**, 171–176.
5 Parizková, J. & Stanková, L. (1964): Influence of physical activity on a treadmill on the metabolism of adipose tissue in rat. *Br. J. Nutr.* **18**, 325–332.
6 Rozen, P. & Shafrir, E. (1972): Comparison of changes in plasma free fatty acids, glycogen and insulin following glucose and fructose loads. *Israel J. Med. Sci.* **8**, 838–840.
7 Saitoh, S., Yoshitake, Y. & Suzuki, M. (1983): Enhanced glycogen replation in liver and skeletal muscle with citrate orally fed after exhaustive treadmill running and swimming. *J. Nutr. Sci. Vitaminol.* **29**, 45–52.
8 Saitoh, S. & Suzuki, M. (1985): Nutritional design of a sports drink administered during endurance exercise for repletion of liver and muscle glycogen without inhibiting lipolysis. *J. Nutr. Sci. Vitaminol.* (In press).
9 Suzuki, M., Shimomura, Y. & Satoh, Y. (1983): Diurnal changes in lipolytic activity of isolated fat cells and their increased responsiveness to epinephrine and theophylline with meal feeding in rats. *J. Nutr. Sci. Vitaminol.* **29**, 399–411.
10 Suzuki, M., Ide, K. & Saitoh, S. (1983): Diurnal changes in glycogen stores in liver and skeletal muscle of rats in relation to the feed timing of sucrose. *J. Nutr. Sci. Vitaminol.* **29**, 545–552.
11 Suzuki, M., Saitoh, S., Yashiro, M. & Hariu, J. (1984): Dietary effects on liver and muscle glycogen repletion in exhaustively exercised rats; energy composition and type of complex carbohydrates. *J. Nutr. Sci. Vitaminol.* **30**, 453–466.
12 Suzuki, M. & Chiba, K. (1983): Effects of feeding patterns on food intake and body composition of rats. *J. Jpn. Soc. Nutr. Fd Sci.* **36**, 175–183.
13 Tornheim, K. & Lowenstein, J.M. (1976): Control of phosphofructokinase from rat skeletal muscle. *J. biol. Chem.* **251**, 7322–7328.
14 Underwood, A.H. & Newsholme, E.A. (1965): Properties of phosphofructokinase from rat liver and their relation to the control of glycolysis and gluconeogenesis. *Biochem. J.* **95**, 868–875.

Diet and physical performance in the horse

D.H. SNOW
Physiology Unit of The Animal Health Trust, Balaton Lodge, Snailwell Road, Newmarket, Suffolk CB8 7DW, UK.

The decline of the horse as an agricultural animal led to a hiatus in earlier research activity in this field (eg[1]) until the last decade. A renewed impetus is related to the resurgence of this species for leisure activities and the considerable sums invested, especially on racehorses, in their purchase and upkeep. Unfortunately, scientific studies into the nutritional requirements of the exercising horse have lagged behind the numerous preparations placed on the market with usually unsubstantiated claims on how they improve performance. Nutritional requirements of the exercising horse have been reviewed[9], and some recent work is described in this paper. Not only are studies in the horse of interest for application to that species, but the athletic eliteness of many breeds, eg $\dot{V}O_2$max in excess of 130 ml/kg/min, is of comparative interest[21].

Prolonged exercise. At present prolonged activity in the horse is largely confined to leisure sports. These may entail long-distance rides which may vary from 80–160 km performed over varying terrain and environmental conditions as rapidly as possible, to longer rides spread over several days; marathon races (42 km) for Arab horses, and approximately 25 km involved in day 2 of a 3-day horse trials competition. This latter event involves periods of slow aerobic work with two periods of additional anaerobic activity in the steeplechase and cross-country phases.

Recently a number of studies have been undertaken to study fuel utilization during these prolonged periods of aerobic work. As would be expected, the pattern of utilization is very similar to that seen in man. Glucose (blood-borne and from muscle glycogen) and free fatty acids (FFA) are the major fuel supplies. Studies on muscle biopsy material taken before, during, and after endurance competitions, have shown a selective recruitment of fibres with IIB fibres, which are not normally recruited during such work, being recruited as type I and IIA fibres become depleted[6,10,22]. In extreme circumstances, as shown in the Figure, the horse is able to undergo almost complete glycogen depletion. In this study of complete glycogen depletion, mean blood glucose at this time was reduced to 1.9 mmol/l, with one animal having a concentration as low as 0.7 mmol/l without showing any clinical manifestations attributable to hypoglycaemia. This ability of the horse to tolerate extremely low blood-glucose concentrations has also been seen following insulin administration (Snow, unpublished data). Glycogen depletion patterns following day 2 of a 3-day horse trial have been reported[12]. Although there was only about a 55 per cent utilization, a glycogen decrease had occurred in all fibre types, due to both the aerobic and aerobic/anaerobic components of the competition.

The utilization of free fatty acids is also an important energy source, as indicated by studies using C-labelled palmitate[2], and changes in plasma FFA concentration and composition, and marked increases in plasma glycerol[15,18,23,28]. Although FFAs increase markedly during prolonged exercise and FFA-degradative enzymes, eg 3-hydroxyacyl CoA dehydrogenase, increase with training, the ability to use FFAs as an energy source may be more limited than in man. This is because plasma albumin concentrations are lower in the horse than in man, being in the range of 28–36 and 35–42 g/l respectively. Consequently maximal plasma FFAs reported after prolonged exercise and starvation in man are of the order of 1.8 mmol/l[17], and in the horse after prolonged exercise 1.4 mmol/l[27] and 0.7 mmol/l after 96 hours starvation[18].

A point of comparative interest is that, despite the high mobilization of FFAs, only very small changes in ketone bodies, ie acetoacetate and β-hydroxybutyrate, are found following either prolonged exercise or starvation[4,15,18]. This has led to the suggestion that the ketone pathway is relatively unimportant in the horse[18].

The importance of protein catabolism as an energy source during prolonged exercise has not

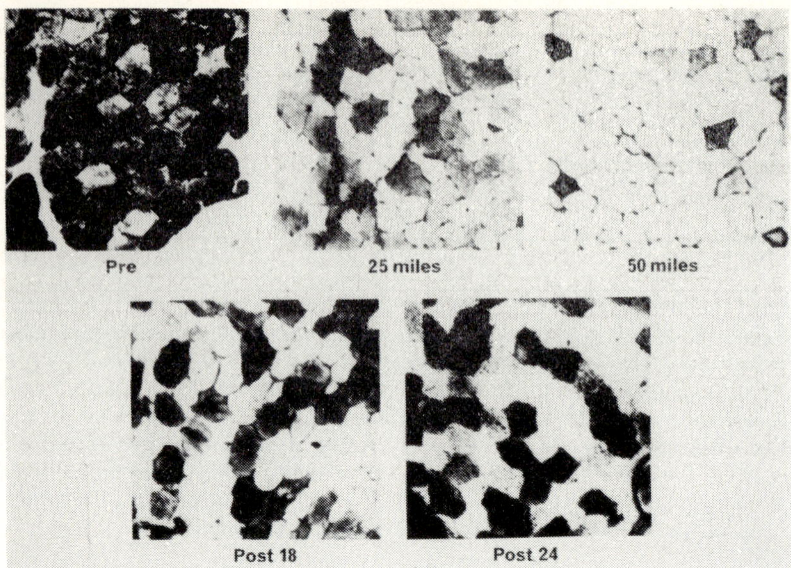

Figure. *The effects of an 80 km exercise on glycogen depletion and repletion.* Samples taken from the middle gluteal muscle. The darker the fibre the higher the glycogen content.

been studied in detail. However, increases in plasma urea during endurance exercise (eg[27]) suggest that gluconeogenesis from amino acids occurs.

Studies on dietary manipulation that may permit more sustained periods of aerobic exercise in the horse are virtually non-existent. Although dietary/exercise schedules are available for glycogen supercompensation in man, there is no adequate documentation of similar successful attempts in the horse. In the author's opinion, in a horse on a normal high energy ration, it is unlikely that attempts at carbohydrate-loading will be successful. The horse, through its natural diet and the effects of training[7], has a high muscle-glycogen content. Normal values in fit horses are of the order of 500–700 mmol glycosyl units/kg muscle dry weight, whilst in man it is 300–350. It is also unlikely that the horse could tolerate the more severe regimen used, eg glycogen depletion/high-protein low-carbohydrate/high carbohydrate. In addition any loading, if possible, above the high concentrations seen in the horse may be deleterious due to extra weight imposed on the muscle.

Of more importance is the best method of repleting muscle glycogen stores, especially in situations when peak performance is expected over several days. Using normal diets it has been found that up to 48 hours may be required for glycogen repletion, with replacement occurring in the reverse order to depletion[10,27].

Although traditionally horses are fed low-fat diets, recent evidence indicates that diets as high as 16 per cent fat can be well tolerated[8]. It has been suggested that using high-fat diets is a means of providing concentrated energy for the long-distance horse, and such diets have been made commercially available. However, whether these have any beneficial effect in increasing performance speed or time to fatigue, has not been well documented. Horses fed a diet of 12 per cent fat, and ridden over 67 km over mountainous terrain for 8–10 hours, performed better and had higher blood glucose levels at the end of the ride, than horses fed a control diet (3 per cent fat)[19].

Maximal exercise. It is well known that the racehorse is an elite speed animal attaining speeds in excess of 1000 m/min. Racing distances vary from galloping events over 400 m (quarterhorse) to 1000–3600 m on the flat to longer distances over jumps (thoroughbreds) and trotting races over 1600–3200 m (standardbreds). All these place large demands on both aerobic and anaerobic supplies of energy. The anaerobic capacity for lactate formation is greater in the horse than man, although phosphocreatine stores are similar[24]. In contrast to conventional ideas, it has been shown that maximal exercise in the horse results in large decreases in ATP as well as phosphocreatine and glycogen[26]. From studies on maximal exercise over distances of 800 and 2000 m, it appears that most of the glycogen is utilised during the initial stages of the exercise[11,25]. However, despite the lower utilization of glycogen over the latter stages of the longer distance, muscle lactate content continues to rise suggesting that blood-borne glucose is now an important substrate for aerobic and anaerobic energy supply. It has been suggested[23] that FFAs may contribute approximately 15 per cent of the energy supply.

As a result of the very high lactate production in racing and its important role in fatigue, as in man, there have been numerous preparations marketed as supplements that may either reduce the formation of lactate or enhance buffering capacity. In the former category, the compound known as dimethylglycine and the related substance pangamic acid (vitamin B_{15}) have been claimed to have a beneficial effect on performance[14]. Unfortunately the evidence for such claims is rather unconvincing. The administration of bicarbonate and even Tris-buffer has been used by a number of trainers for many years. These have been given by both oral and i.v. routes. Whether the amount of compound used, and the time of administration prior to exercise is correct, and any possible effects on performance have not been ascertained.

Thermoregulation. As horses can attain very high speeds and also maintain relatively high workloads for prolonged periods, large quantities of heat are produced, For example, at 60 per cent. $\dot{V}O_2$max, ie approximately 80 ml/kg/min, a total of 756 kJ (180 kcal) is produced in a 450-kg horse. In the horse, as in man, most of this heat is dissipated via sweating. Under favourable climatic conditions sweat loss can be of the order of 7–8 l/hour in long-distance rides[27], but in hot humid conditions where sweating is partially ineffective, it can be as high as 10–12 l/hour[3]. In addition to the problems that can be encountered due to this large fluid loss, in contrast to man (Table) sweating results in a high loss of sodium, potassium and chloride[13]. Therefore, replacement of these electrolytes by either salt licks or addition to the feed is important during prolonged exercise. This is especially important for sodium as the diet is naturally low in this electrolyte, with a negative balance occurring even for 1 hour of moderate exercise.

Table. *Concentration (mmol/l) of major electrolytes in sweat.*

	Sodium	Potassium	Chloride
Plasma	140	3.5 − 4.5	100
Human sweat	10 − 60	4.0 − 5.0	10 − 60
Equine sweat	130 − 190	20 − 50	160 − 190

Since 1890[20] it has been known that horse sweat contains protein which is responsible for the lathering of the coat seen with exercise. It has been suggested that this protein loss in sweat should be considered when formulating protein requirements for the working horse. However, it has been shown[13] that this protein content is high only in the initial stages of sweating, with a progressive decrease to concentrations below lg/litre. Protein concentration is highest in the unfit animal, with concentrations of the order of 7g/l being measured, whilst in the fit animal lower concentration are seen, explaining the empirical observation of a more watery sweat with increasing fitness. This protein has been found to consist of two similar glycoproteins of relatively low molecular weight, with only low levels of sulphur containing amino acids and histidine. Ultrastructural studies indicate[16] that these proteins are found within secretory vesicles in the sweat gland. The surfactant properties of the glycoproteins have led to the suggestion that they cause dispersion of sweat droplets on the coat and therefore aid in evaporation[5]. The initial concentration of magnesium in sweat is of the order of 8.5 mmol/l, but falls in parallel with protein concentration. The magnesium is not bound to the protein[13], but may be involved in its active secretion.

Conclusions. I have tried to highlight here the metabolic changes associated with different intensities of exercise. A knowledge of these is required before the planning of suitable diets can be undertaken. This may become more important as substitutes for traditional feeds will be necessary, as the latter escalate in cost. Although there are many similarities in the alterations seen with exercise in horse and man, differences exist that often invalidate extrapolation from findings in man.

1 Brody, S. (1945): *Bioenergetics and growth*. New York: Reinhold.
2 Carlson, L.A., Froberg, S. & Persson, S. (1965): Concentration and turnover of the free fatty acids of plasma and concentration of blood glucose during exercise in horses. *Acta Physiol. Scand.* **63**, 434–441.
3 Carlson, G.P. (1983): Thermoregulation, fluid and electrolyte balance. In *Equine exercise physiology*, ed D.H. Snow, S.G.B. Persson & R.J. Rose, pp. 291–309. Cambridge: Granta Editions.
4 Dybdal, N.O., Gribble, D., Madigan, J.E. & Stabenfeldt, G.H. (1980): Alterations in plasma corticosteroids, insulin and selected metabolites in horses. *Equine Vet. J.* **12**, 137–140.
5 Eckersall, P.D., Beeley, J.G., Snow, D.H. & Thomas, A. (1984): Characterisation of glycoproteins in the sweat of the horse (*Equus caballus*). *Res. Vet. Sci.* **36**, 231–234.
6 Essén-Gustavsson, B., Karlström, K. & Lindholm, A. (1984): Fibre types, enzyme activities and substrate utilisation in skeletal muscles of horses competing in endurance rides. *Equine Vet. J.* **16**, 197–202.
7 Guy, P.S. & Snow, D.H. (1977): The effect of training and detraining on muscle composition in the horse. *J. Physiol.* **269**, 33–51.
8 Hambleton, P.L., Slade, L.M., Hamar, D.W., Kienholz, E.W. & Lewis, L.D. (1980): Dietary fat and exercise conditioning effect on metabolic parameters in the horse. *J. Anim. Sci.* **51**, 1330–1339.
9 Hintz, H.F. (1983): Nutritional requirements of the exercising horse — a review. In *Equine exercise physiology*, ed D.H. Snow, S.G.B. Persson & R.J. Rose, pp. 275–290. Cambridge: Granta Editions.
10 Hodgson, D.R., Rose, R.J. & Allen, J.R. (1983): Muscle glycogen depletion and repletion patterns in horses performing various distances of endurance exercise. In *Equine exercise physiology*, ed D.H. Snow, S.G.B. Persson & R.J. Rose, pp. 229–236. Cambridge: Granta Editions.
11 Hodgson, D.R., Rose, R.J., Allen, J.R. & DiMauro, J. (1984): Glycogen depletion patterns in horses performing maximal exercise. *Res. Vet. Sci.* **36**, 169–173.
12 Hodgson, D.R., Rose, R.J., Allen, J.R. & Di Mauro, J. (1985): Glycogen depletion patterns in horses competing in day 2 of a three day event. *Cornell Vet.* **75**, 366–374.
13 Kerr, M.G. & Snow, D.H. (1982): Composition of sweat of the horse during prolonged epinephrine (adrenaline) infusion, heat exposure and exercise. *Am. J. Vet. Res.* **44**, 1571–1577.
14 Levine, S.B., Myhre, G.D., Smith, G.L. & Burns, J.G. (1982): Effect of a nutritional supplement containing N_1 N-dimethylglycine (DMG) on the racing standardbred. *Equine Practice* **4**, 17–20.
15 Lucke, J.N. & Hall, G.M. (1980): Long distance exercise in the horse. Golden Horseshoe Ride 1978. *Vet. Rec.* **106**, 405–407.
16 Montgomery, I., Jenkinson, D. McE. & Elder, H.Y. (1982): The effects of thermal stimulation on the ultrastructure of the fundus and duct of the equine sweat gland. *J. Anat.* **135**, 13–28.
17 Newsholme, E.A. (1983): Control of metabolism and the integration of fuel supply for the marathon runner. In *Biochemistry of exercise*, ed H.G. Knuttgen, J.A. Vogel & J. Poortmans, pp. 144–150. Champaign, Illinois: Human Kinetics Publishers.
18 Rose, R.J. & Sampson, D. (1982): Changes in certain metabolic parameters in horses associated with food deprivation and endurance exercise. *Res. Vet. Sci.* **32**, 198–202.
19 Slade, L.M., Lewis, L.D., Quinn, C.R. & Chandler, M.L. (1975): Nutritional adaptations of horses for endurance performance. *Proc. Equine Nutritional Physiol. Soc.* 114–128.
20 Smith, F. (1890): Note on the composition of the sweat of the horse. *J. Physiol.* **11**, 497–503.
21 Snow, D.H. (1985): The horse and dog, elite athletes, why and how? *Proc. Nutr. Soc.* (In press).
22 Snow, D.H., Baxter, P. & Rose, R.J. (1981): Muscle fibre composition and glycogen depletion in horses competing in an endurance ride. *Vet. Rec.* **108**, 374–378.
23 Snow, D.H., Fixter, L.M., Kerr, M.G. & Cutmore, C.M.M. (1983): Alterations in composition of venous plasma FFA pool during prolonged and spring exercises in the horse. In *Biochemistry of exercise*, ed H.G. Knuttgen, J.A. Vogel & J. Poortmans, pp. 336–342. Champaign, Illinois: Human Kinetics Publishers.
24 Snow, D.H. & Harris, R.C. (1985): Thoroughbreds and greyhounds: biochemical adaptations in creatures of nature and man. In *Proc. 1st Int. Congress of Comp. Physiol. Biochem.*, ed R. Gilles. Berlin: Springer Verlag (In press).
25 Snow, D.H. & Harris, R.C. (1985): Limitations to maximal performance in the racing thoroughbred. In *Proc. 6th Int. Symposium on Biochem. of Exercise*, ed B. Saltin. Champaign, Illinois: Human Kinetics Publishers (In press).
26 Snow, D.H., Harris, R.C. & Gash, S. (1985): Metabolic responses of equine muscle to intermittent maximal exercise. *J. Appl. Physiol.* **58**, 1689–1697.
27 Snow, D.H., Kerr, M.G., Nimmo, M.A. & Abbott, E.A. (1982): Alterations in blood, sweat, urine and muscle composition during prolonged exercise in the horse. *Vet. Rec.* **110**, 377–384.
28 Snow, D.H. & Mackenzie, G. (1977): The metabolic effects of maximal exercise in the horse and adaptations with training. *Equine Vet. J.* **9**, 134–140.

Body composition and nutrition of different types of athlete

Jana PAŘÍZKOVÁ
*Research Institute for Physical Education, Charles University, Újezd 450, 118 07 Prague 1,
Czechoslovakia.*

Studies on athletes during past decades have shown a great variety of adaptations in energy intake, nutrient selection and the resulting nutritional status, including such characteristics as absolute and relative weights, various body weight indices, subcutaneous and total body fat, and lean body mass evaluated by various methodological approaches[5–7].

Body composition reflects various energy balance and turnover situations during different exercise regimens in a characteristic way and is moreover related to various functional and metabolic parameters of the organism. This can be seen first of all, from the comparison of champion athletes in contrasting sports. Weight-lifters and swimmers have the highest body weight and fat proportion, but vary in body height. Thus the highest relative body weight values are seen in weight-lifters. The fat percentage is the same in these two groups and in the controls (students with usual sporting activity). The lowest proportion of fat is found in long-distance runners and gymnasts, who vary markedly in body height and relative weight. The differences mentioned are paralleled by differences in various levels of aerobic power (maximal oxygen uptake — $\dot{V}O_2$max), which are always highest in endurance runners and lowest in weight lifters, typical of dynamic and static work loads, respectively. Adaptation to various work loads based on suitable genetic predispositions is the cause of these morphological and functional differences. According to previous observations there appear to be more marked changes in the absolute and relative amounts of depot fat (which is significantly lower) than in lean body mass, which increases in the absolute values mainly in static sports such as weight-lifting[2,5].

A certain type of body composition seems to run parallel, not only with a certain aerobic power, but also with other functional variables such as anaerobic threshold (AT) and mechanical efficiency. In another study, champion long-distance and marathon runners, canoeists and football players aged approximately 24 years were followed up. Long-distance and marathon runners (adapted to long lasting uninterrupted exercise) were significantly lower in height, weight, body mass index and fat percentage than canoeists and football players (adapted to intermittent exercise). Relative aerobic power ($\dot{V}O_2$max/kg B.Wt or lean body mass) was significantly lower in the canoeists and football players. Functional variables at the level of the anaerobic threshold ($\dot{V}O_2$ measured in terms of min; or ml/kg/per min) in all groups showed similar differences. Long distance runners had more favourable, ie higher, values of the functional variables than canoeists and footballers. The energy cost of work, ie the energy necessary for the transfer of 1 kg along a distance of 1 m (W_{AT}), was significantly lower in long-distance runners compared with canoeists and football players. Mechanical efficiency was therefore significantly higher in long-distance and marathon runners than in the other two groups. All these characteristics enhance running performance during prolonged periods in subjects adapted to this type of exercise, compared with those adapted to intermittent or other types of exercise[1].

Studies that combine measurements of food intake as well as body size and composition, aerobic power, anaerobic threshold, energy cost of work, and mechanical efficiency are relatively rare. Attention was therefore focused on other groups of long-distance and marathon runners of similar height and weight and food intake. The fat percentage was significantly lower in marathon runners, who were older and had longer training. $\dot{V}O_2$max per kg B.Wt did not differ between the two groups. Control men of the same height had a significantly higher weight and fat percentage and significantly lower $\dot{V}O_2$max per kg B.Wt. Considerable variations in fat percentage were observed in all groups. The assessment of food intake in one week, using the inventory method[3] in both groups of runners, showed a slightly higher energy intake compared with the recommended allowances (RA) for the normal population of men, and markedly lower energy intake compared with the RA (23–25 per cent) for this particular sport. This was due to a lower intake of proteins (mostly animal) especially in long-distance runners. Fat intake was 16–25 per cent higher[6]. This has also been found quite frequently in a control Czechoslovak population. The intake of carbohydrates was even lower than the RA for normal population, and markedly lower (ie approximately 40 per cent) compared with the RA for this sports discipline. The intake of minerals and vitamins roughly corresponded to the RA with the exception of a slight deficit in vitamins B_2 and C in long-distance runners. Inter-individual differences were large, indicating even greater discrepancies compared to RA in certain individuals. Nevertheless, the performance in training and competitions was adequate in all runners. Individual athletic achievements were not related to energy or individual nutrient intakes.

Low deposition of fat in endurance runners, which is advantageous for the energy cost of their performance, does not result only from a relatively low energy intake in comparison with energy output, but also from a high level of lipid turnover and high utilization of lipids in athletes adapted to this type of exercise. Champion ski runners (national performance class — NPC) compared with those of a low performance class were measured in our laboratory at the end of their competition period. Fat percentage was lower and relative aerobic power was higher in the NPC group. Significantly higher levels were also observed in this group in the activity of most important mitochondrial enzymes such as hydroxyacyl-CoA-dehydrogenase (HOADH, involved in beta-oxidation of fatty acids), malate dehydrogenase (MDH), and citrate synthetase (CS) in biopsy samples of the vastus lateralis muscle. The activity of these enzymes was always highest in the best-adapted champion-class ski runners. Correlation analysis in another group of champion ski runners showed significant positive relationships between the activities of CS, MDH and HOADH and $\dot{V}O_2$max, max O_2, pulse, and laboratory performance. The reverse was true of the relationships between these enzymes and maximal pulse frequency and fat percentage[4]. Similar relationships were shown in another study on skiers and marathon runners performed in our laboratory.

Another sport for which a very low percentage of fat and low weight is indispensable is gymnastics, which is non-cyclic exercise requiring the development of skill and strength rather than endurance. According to the character and energy cost of gymnastic training, the aerobic power is relatively low compared with that in other sports disciplines, and also in untrained controls. In a group of growing gymnasts, the values of $\dot{V}O_2$max were at the lower limit of (or below) standard values. Longitudinal measurements of total blood lipids during the 3 years of training did not show any significant changes, but mean values were significantly higher than in controls, ie untrained girls of the same age. Furthermore, high- and low- density lipoprotein (HDL and LDL) levels did not vary during the 3 year period of gymnastic training. There were no changes in total blood lipid levels after a work load. The level of FFA increased significantly after a work load, but this was not the case in untrained controls (Krausová *et al.* 1978 cited in[6]).

Repeated measurements of food intake showed very low values in girl gymnasts, which did not seem to correspond at all with the estimated energy output[6]. This discrepancy was more apparent when the food intake was compared with the RA for the normal population. Even when the somatic development of gymnasts corresponded only to the 3rd–50th percentile according to our growth grids, it was still comparable with that of many girls of the same age, without any training, but with a higher food intake. Adaptation to this type of exercise, ie gymnastics, again results in more efficient energy metabolism, which enhances the desirable performance in this sport discipline, also due to suitable physique and body composition (Table).

The examples mentioned above seem to indicate certain problems arising from the apparent disproportion between energy input and output. As methods for the measurement of energy output are still inadequate, it is very possible that the theoretical estimations of energy output based mostly on short-term measurements, do not reflect reality. Results of morphological, functional and biochemical measurements show marked adaptive changes at all levels of the

Table. *Somatic characteristics and nutritional and metabolic parameters in girl gymnasts: mean values with s.d. in parentheses.*

Age (years): 12.818 (1.081) Lean body mass (kg): 32.9 (3.6) Protein (g intake/d): 74.1 (9.7)
Height (cm): 144.4 (5.2) Basal metabolism rate (MJ/day); 4.456 (0.333) Fat (g intake/d): 100.2 (17.5)
Weight (kg): 34.3 (3.9) Energy expenditure — training (MJ/d): ~ 4.5 Carbohydrate (g intake/d): 193.6 (32.4)
Fat (%): 3.8 (2.0) Energy intake (MJ/d): 8.157 (1.182)

organism, which may economize the energy. Thus, more efficient economy of the energy metabolism seems to be one of the important prerequisites of successful performance in the sports discussed.

Previous studies on children and/or on experimental models with laboratory animals seem to indicate that even more profound changes can be expected when adaptational processes to adequately increased work loads, superimposed on genetic predispositions are initiated very early in growth. For example spontaneously increased physical activity is paralleled by trends towards lower weight, lower fat percentage, increased cardiorespiratory efficiency, and more favourable blood lipids level (ie higher HDL) not only in adults but also in children of pre-school age (Pařízková *et al.* submitted for publication). When such a situation is developed by training during adolescence and adulthood, even more marked and more favourable changes can be expected, as has been shown by many successful athletes throughout the world.

1 Bunc, V., Šprynarová, Š., Pařízková, J. & Leso, J. (1984): Effects of adaptation on the mechanical efficiency and energy cost of physical work. *Human Nutr.: Clin. Nutr.* **38C**, 317–319.
2 Forbes, G.B. (1985): Body composition as affected by physical activity and nutrition. *Fed. Proc.* **44**, 343–347.
3 Hejda, S. & Ošancová, K. (1981): Recommended allowances for Czechoslovak population. Prague: Association for Rational Nutrition. (In Czech).
4 Macková, E., Bass, A., Šprynarová, Š., Teisinger, J., Vondra, K. & Bojanovsky, I. (1981): Enzyme activity patterns of energy metabolism in skiers of different performance levels. *Eur. J. Appl. Physiol.* **48**, 315–322.
5 Pařízková, J. (1977): Body fat and physical fitness. The Hague: Martinus Nijhoff, B.V./Medical Division.
6 Pařízková, J. (1985): Adaptation to functional capacity and exercise. In *Nutritional adaptation in man*, ed Sir Kenneth Blaxter & J.C. Waterlow, pp. 127–139. London & Paris: John Libbey.
7 Wilmore, J.H. & Freund, B.J. (1984): Nutritional enhancement of athletic performance. *Nutr. Abstr. Rev.* **54**, 1–16.

★ ★ ★

BROWN ADIPOSE TISSUE

Mechanisms of thermogenesis in brown adipose tissue

D. NICHOLLS, Sonia CUNNINGHAM and E. RIAL
Neurochemistry Laboratory, Ninewells Medical School, University of Dundee, Dundee DD1 9SY, Scotland, UK.

Although the mechanisms by which energy intake and expenditure are balanced in the homoeostatic adult remain controversial, for the past 7 years the possible involvement of brown fat has been vigorously debated. In experimental animals such as the cold-adapted rat, brown fat accounts for only 1.5 per cent of body weight, and yet can respond to sympathetic stimulation with an oxygen consumption which can exceed that of all the other tissues combined[3]. We shall summarize here the molecular mechanisms responsible for this thermogenesis, and discuss recent evidence from our laboratory as to the quantitative importance of brown fat in adult man.

The brown adipocyte is sympathetically innervated. The cell possesses atypical beta-receptors which are distinct from the classical beta subtypes[1]. Noradrenaline raises the cyclic AMP in the cell, and this in turn activates a hormone-sensitive lipase which liberates FFA from the triglyceride stores within the cell (reviewed in[9]). While it is frequently found that these cells contain many small fat droplets, rather than one large droplet filling nearly the whole cytosol, this multilocular appearance of the cell is not reliable as a diagnostic aid since brown adipocytes from thermogenically inactive tissue may have a unilocular appearance similar under the light microscope to white adipocytes.

Brown adipocytes contain a high concentration of mitochondria, and it is the behaviour of these organelles, and in particular their response to the fatty acids liberated by lipolysis, which provide the key to the enormous thermogenic capacity of the tissue *in vivo*. Electron flow through the mitochondrial respiratory chain is linked to the pumping of protons out of the mitochondria (reviewed in[8]). In a conventional cell, a circuit of protons is completed by their re-entry through the ATP synthase to generate the ATP required by the cell. Regardless of the rate of substrate supply, respiration will only proceed sufficiently to replenish the ATP utilized by extra-mitochondrial energy-requiring reactions. In the brown fat mitochondrion an alternative pathway of proton re-entry exists, which is not linked to ATP synthesis and which thus allows the rate of respiration to be 'uncoupled' from the rate of ATP turnover in the cell (reviewed in[9]). This pathway is catalysed by a unique 'uncoupling protein'[4] which may function as a dimer of identical 32 kDa polypeptide subunits[5]. The uncoupling protein binds purine nucleotide such as GDP or ATP[7], and this is a convenient means of identifying and quantifying the protein. With the aid of the uncoupling protein brown fat mitochondria are able to oxidize the fatty acids liberated by lipolysis without the constraints of respiratory control.

The maximal capacity of brown fat thermogenesis is not constant, but varies in response to the animal's demand for non-shivering thermogenesis (reviewed in[9]). Thus in experimental animals it is high at birth, declines as the animal develops in the thermoneutral environment, and can be restored by acclimation to cold. Thermogenic capacity also decreases during lactation, and increases when experimental animals are fed high-energy diets under thermoneutral conditions. These changes in brown fat non-shivering thermogenesis are reflected in the mitochondrial content of uncoupling protein. In a fully thermogenic animal, the mitochondria may bind up to 0.7 nmol of GDP per mg protein, and this value may be decreased by an order of magnitude in mitochondria from thermogenically inactive brown fat (see, eg[11]).

Chronic stimulation of the brown adipocyte beta-receptor appears to be sufficient to induce the uncoupling protein. Thus it has been shown[6] that rats maintained in the warm, but chronically infused with noradrenaline from an implanted osmotic pump, show an increase in GDP-binding capacity comparable to that seen with mitochondria from a parallel group of rats adapted to the cold.

Brown fat cells. The most physiologically relevant preparation with which to study the biochemical mechanisms of brown fat thermogenesis is the isolated brown adipocyte. Isolated cells may be prepared from the tissue by collagenase digestion. The Dunkin-Hartley guinea-pig is a suitable source of cells from both warm- and cold-adapted animals. Figure 1 shows the typical respiratory response to added noradrenaline of cells from warm- and cold-adapted guinea-pigs[10]. In the absence of lipolysis (or added fatty acid) even the cells from the cold animals show respiratory control (ie the uncoupling protein is inactive) — Figure 1a. Following beta-adrenergic stimulation both warm (Figure 1c) and cold (Figure 1b) cell respiration is increased. However, it is apparent that the cold-adapted cells show a much larger thermogenic response to the neurotransmitter.

In the case of the cold cells (containing mitochondria with uncoupling protein) there are two aspects to this increased respiration. The first is that lipolysis provides an additional substrate for the mitochondria (on top of the pyruvate generated by glycolysis). Thus even when additional pyruvate is added to the incubation lipolysis can increase respiration in the presence of a synthetic 'uncoupler' from 1250 to 1850 nmol O per min per million cells (Fig. 1a). However, the most dramatic effect is due to the ability of noradrenaline to activate the uncoupling protein in the cold cell mitochondria. Thus, in the absence of added synthetic uncoupler, noradrenaline can increase cell respiration from 230 to 1823 nmol O per min per million cells (Fig. 1b). In this case the beta-agonist is acting as both activator of lipolysis and as activator of the uncoupling protein. When the beta-antagonist propranolol is added to the incubation respiration is greatly inhibited. This is due to the re-induction of respiratory control (ie the inhibition of the uncoupling protein) rather than the limitation of substrate supply, as shown by the stimulation

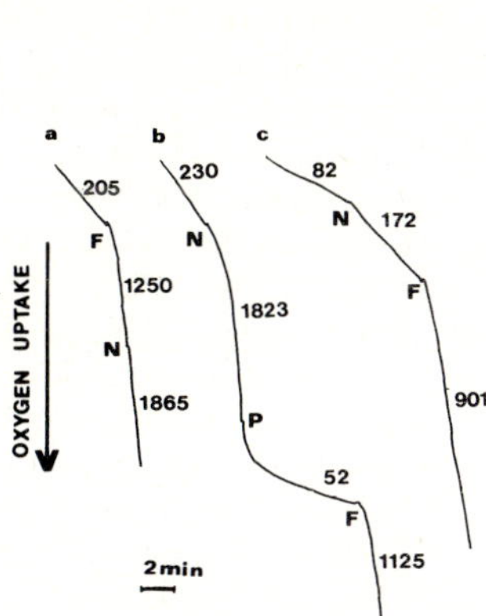

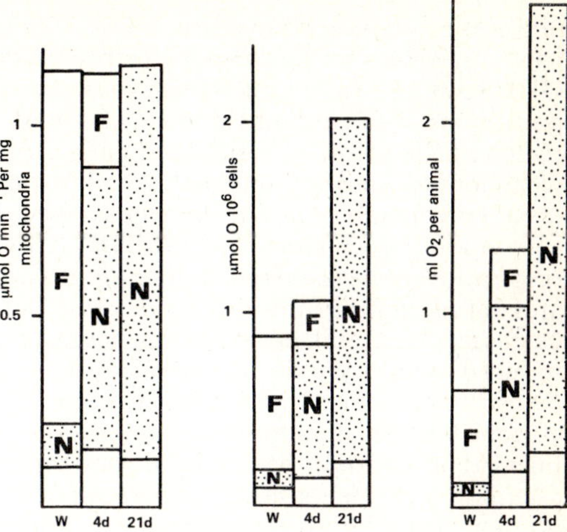

Fig. 1. *Respiration of isolated brown adipocytes from cold-adapted and warm-adapted guinea-pigs.* (a,b) 47 000 'cold' cells per ml were incubated at 37 °C in the presence of 10 mM pyruvate. Where indicated a synthetic mitochondrial uncoupler 'F' (10 μM-FCCP), 2 μM (±) noradrenaline ('N') or 10 μM-propranolol ('P') were added. (c) 49 000 'warm' cells per ml were incubated at 37 °C with additions as above. Values are respiratory rates (nmol O per min per 10^6 cells). For further details see[10].

Fig. 2. *Comparison of the thermogenic parameters of brown fat from warm- and cold-adapted guinea-pigs.* Basal (blank); noradrenaline-stimulated (N) and uncoupler- releasable (F) respiration is plotted related to mitochondria, cells and total tissue for warm-adapted (W), 4-day cold-exposed (4d) and 21-day cold-adapted (21d) guinea-pigs. Data from[10].

when the synthetic uncoupler FCCP is added, allowing uncontrolled oxidation of the pyruvate present in the incubation (Fig. 1b).

Thus pyruvate supplies substrate to the mitochondria without activating the uncoupling protein whereas noradrenaline does both. From experiments with isolated mitochondria there is good evidence that the fatty acids liberated by lipolysis act not only as the immediate substrate of the mitochondria, but also interact with the uncoupling protein to activate it into a conducting conformation[12].

Relative to the warm control, the cold-adapted cells are doubled in number, each adipocyte has twice the mitochondrial protein[10] and each mitochondrion has seven times the complement of uncoupling protein[11]. The total uncoupling protein in the animal is thus increased some 28-fold, and this correlates well with the 30 to 40-fold increase in noradrenaline stimulated respiration seen for the total brown adipocytes of cold — compared to warm — guinea-pigs (Fig. 2). There would thus appear to be some experimental basis for the assumption that the capacity of an animal's brown fat for non-shivering thermogenesis can be estimated from the content of uncoupling protein in the tissue.

Brown fat in man. There are many ethical and practical constraints to the investigation of brown fat in man. The approach our laboratory has taken has been to examine the perirenal fat of 23 subjects from 3 months to 74 years. Perirenal adipose tissue has long been considered one of the most promising sites for the detection of brown fat. In each of our subjects under the age of 50 from which the total perinephric fat could be obtained it was possible to observe by eye regions with a distinctly darker appearance compared with the surrounding tissue. Only one of the five subjects over the age of 51 showed such areas. That these represented brown fat was confirmed by light and electron microscopy and by determination of mitochondrial one of the five subjects over the age of 51 showed such areas. That these represented brown fat was confirmed by light and electron microscopy and by determination of mitochondrial GDP-binding[2]. In the case of the youngest subject, it was possible to prepare functional brown adipocytes which responded to noradrenaline with a respiratory stimulation comparable to that seen with cells from cold-adapted guinea-pigs (S. Cunningham, unpublished data). However, when marker enzymes were measured to quantify the maximal response to noradrenaline of the total mitochondria in the perirenal tissue, it was found that in no case could the tissue surrounding both kidneys contribute more than 0.15 ml oxygen per min to the whole body respiration[2]. The basal metabolic rate of a healthy adult is of the order of 200 ml oxygen per min, and noradrenaline infusion can increase this value by about 30 ml per min[2]. Thus, even in the best case, the total perirenal fat could contribute 0.5 per cent towards the noradrenaline-induced thermogenesis in normal adult man. In the rat, which has prominent and well-defined deposits of brown fat throughout the thoracic region, the perirenal brown fat accounts for about 10 per cent of the total tissue[3]. In man, where the perirenal site is the most apparent upon visual inspection, it would be expected that this proportion would be a minimal estimate. On this assumption, a best-case analysis would be that brown fat in normal adult man could contribute no more than 5 per cent towards the observed noradrenaline-induced non-shivering thermo-genesis.

Conclusions. While the case for brown fat in the regulation of nutritional balance in the normal adult seems weak, the adaptive powers of the tissue should be borne in mind. Thus, if selective pharmacological activation of the human brown fat beta-receptor could be maintained, and a 30-fold increase in thermogenic capacity obtained (as for the guinea-pig) then this pharmacolo-gically-induced thermogenic capacity of brown fat could become a significant factor in aiding the regulation of human obesity in cases where the normal, if obscure, homoeostatic mechanisms are defective.

Acknowledgements. Research from our laboratory is supported by the Medical Research Council and by the Scottish Home and Health Department.

1 Arch, J.R.S., Ainsworth, A.T., Cawthorne, M.A., Piercy, V., Sennitt, M.V., Thody, V.E., Wilson, C. & Wilson, S. (1984): Atypical beta-receptor on brown adipocytes as target for anti-obesity drugs. *Nature, Lond.* **309**, 163–165.

2 Cunningham, S., Leslie, P., Hopwood, D., Illingworth, P., Jung, R.T., Nicholls, D.G., Peden, N., Rafael, J. & Rial, E. (1985): The characterization and energetic potential of brown adipose tissue in man. *Clin. Sci.* (In press).

3 Foster, D.O. & Frydman, M.L. (1978): Non-shivering thermogenesis in the rat. II. *Can. J. Physiol. Pharmacol.* **56**, 110–122.

4 Heaton, J.M., Wagenvoord, R., Kemp, A. & Nicholls, D.G. (1978): Brown adipose tissue mitochondria: photoaffinity labelling of the regulatory site for energy dissipation. *Eur. J. Biochem.* **82**, 515–521.

5 Lin, C.S., Hackenberg, H. & Klingenberg, M. (1980): The uncoupling protein from brown adipose tissue mitochondria is a dimer: a hydrodynamic study. *FEBS Lett.* **113**, 304–306.

6 Mory, G., Bouillaud, F., Combes-George, M. & Ricquier, D. (1984): Noradrenaline controls the concentration of the uncoupling protein in brown adipose tissue. *FEBS Lett.* **166**, 393–397.

7 Nicholls, D.G. (1976): Hamster brown adipose tissue mitochondria: purine nucleotide control of the ionic conductance of the inner membrane, the nature of the nucleotide-binding site. *Eur. J. Biochem.* **62**, 223–228.

8 Nicholls, D.G. (1982): *Bioenergetics: an introduction to the chemiosmotic theory.* London: Academic Press.

9 Nicholls, D.G. & Locke, R.M. (1984): Brown adipose tissue. *Physiol. Rev.* **64**, 1–64.

10 Rafael, J., Fesser, W. & Nicholls, D.G. (1985): Cold-adaptation in the guinea-pig at the level of the isolated brown adipocyte. *Am. J. Physiol.* (In press).

11 Rial, E. & Nicholls, D.G. (1984): The uncoupling protein from guinea-pig brown adipose tissue mitochondria: synchronous increase in structural and functional parameters during cold-adaptation. *Biochem. J.* **222**, 685–693.

12 Rial, E., Poustie, A. & Nicholls, D.G. (1983): Brown adipose tissue mitochondria: the regulation of the 32,000 Mr uncoupling protein by fatty acids and purine nucleotides. *Eur. J. Biochem.* **137**, 197–203.

Features of 'recruitment' in brown adipose tissue

Barbara CANNON and J. NEDERGAARD
The Wenner-Gren Institute, University of Stockholm, Biologihus F3, S-106 91 Stockholm, Sweden.

A few years ago, we considered that we had a rather clear picture of the cellular biology of the brown fat cell. The picture then accepted consisted of a cell endowed with β-adrenergic receptors only, the stimulation of which, through an increase in cyclic AMP, led to an increased activity of hormone-sensitive lipase. This lipase in its turn degraded the intracellularly-stored triglycerides into FFA, which proceeded via β-oxidation in the mitochondria and which were finally converted into water, CO_2 and heat.

Today we know that this picture is much simplified, The brown fat cell has a large number of α_1-receptors. Not only intracellular, but also circulating triglycerides are broken down. β-Oxidation occurs not only in mitochondria but also in peroxisomes. We shall review some of these features in more detail, and especially we shall examine whether they are found in all recruitment situations — ie in animals acclimated to cold, adapted to certain types of diet, and during perinatal development. The evidence for the activation of each of these 'new' pathways is compiled in the Table.

Table. *Pathways and characteristics in studies cited.*

		Characteristics		
Pathways	*Cold*	*Young*	*Diet*	*Obese[a]*
Lipoprotein lipase activation	Radomski & Orme (1971)[r] Carneheim et al. (1984)[r]	Cryer & Jones (1978)[r]	Carneheim et al. (unpubl.)	Boulangé et al. (1981)[r]
Peroxisomal proliferation	Nedergaard et al. (1980)[r]	Seccombe & Hahn (1980)	Alexson et al. (unpubl.)	Bas et al. (1983)[m]
Increase in thermogenin	Lean et al. (1983)[r] Nedergaard & Cannon (1985)[r] Trayhurn et al. (1983)[h] Sundin et al. (1985)[h]	?	Nedergaard et al. (1984)[r] Ashwell et al. (1984)[r]	Ashwell et al. (1983)[m]
Alpha-adrenergic activation	Raasmaja et al. (1985)[r,h]	?	Raasmaja et al. (1984)	?

References to thermogenin increase only refer to demonstrations of the immunologically active component. Superscripts r, m and h indicate examinations on rats, mice, and hamsters, respectively. [a]:- denotes decrease.

Activation of lipoprotein lipase. The fatty acids stored within the cells in the form of triglycerides constitute only a limited supply of substrate for thermogenesis, and this supply is fully exhausted within a few hours of intense cold stress[19]. For prolonged thermogenic functioning of the tissue, fuel for combustion must be extracted from the circulation. This may occur by the activation of lipoprotein lipase.

Lipoprotein lipase is activated both in a cold-stress situation[9] and postnatally[13]. We have now also examined whether this is the case in diet-induced thermogenesis. As seen in Fig. 1, the activity in general follows the growth of the tissue, but when the animals received a high-fat diet (here Intralipid), there is also a large increase in lipoprotein-lipase activity.

The increase seen in the cold-stressed situation is clearly a β-adrenergic effect; insulin is without effect[9]. The molecular events behind the activation are presently being investigated[10].

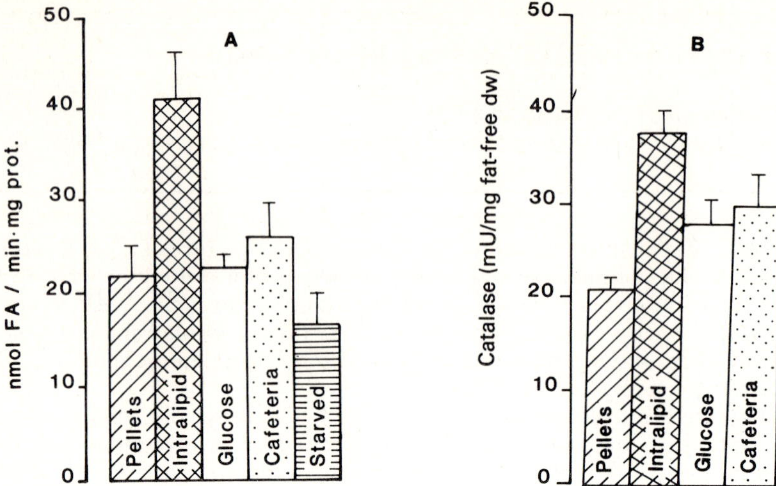

Fig. 1. *Activation of lipoprotein lipase (A) and peroxisomal activity (B) by different diets.* For lipoprotein lipase (LPL) activity, rats had been offered the indicated diets 8 h per day for 4 d; they were then examined 4 h after the food was made accessible to them on the last day (Carneheim *et al.*, unpublished observations). For peroxisomal activity, rats were examined after having had free access to the indicated diets for 14 d (Alexson *et al.*, unpublished observations).

In the cold-stressed situation, the half-life of the lipase is unchanged (about 2 h); thus the increase in activity seen in the cold is not caused by a decrease in degradation rate. From studies with the mRNA-synthesis inhibitor actinomycin-D, we have concluded that the activation of the enzyme is caused fully by an increased transcription of the gene coding for the lipase. The mRNA synthesized has apparently a half-life of about 8 h. The activation can be mimicked by cholera toxin, confirming that this increased gene expression is a cyclic-AMP-dependent process. The molecular steps leading from cyclic-AMP synthesis to increased transcription of specific genes are, however, presently unknown.

Activation of peroxisomal β-oxidation. During acclimation to cold, peroxisomal β-oxidation, which can be found in brown fat, is increased more than the mitochondrial oxidative capacity[24]. Also in the new-born, both ultrastructural[1] and enzymatic (catalase[30]) data indicate an activation of peroxisomes, although peroxisomal β-oxidation has not been followed in this situation. We have now also examined whether certain diets can activate peroxisomes, and, as seen in Fig. 1B, all cafeteria-type diets have this ability.

The molecular mechanisms underlying peroxisomal recruitment are totally unknown, and the function of peroxisomal β-oxidation in thermogenesis is not clear. However, it is noteworthy that the peroxisomes have a greater affinity and capacity for β-oxidation of middle-chain and very-long-chain acyl esters than have mitochondria[2,7].

Increase on thermogenin. An increase in thermogenin (the 'uncoupling' protein) is the traditional parameter for recruitment of brown adipose tissue. By development of an enzyme-linked immuno-sorbent assay (ELISA) for thermogenin[8], we have been able to quantify the amounts of thermogenin in a mitochondrial preparation. In Fig. 2, we have collected some scores of combined determinations by the ELISA technique and the traditional

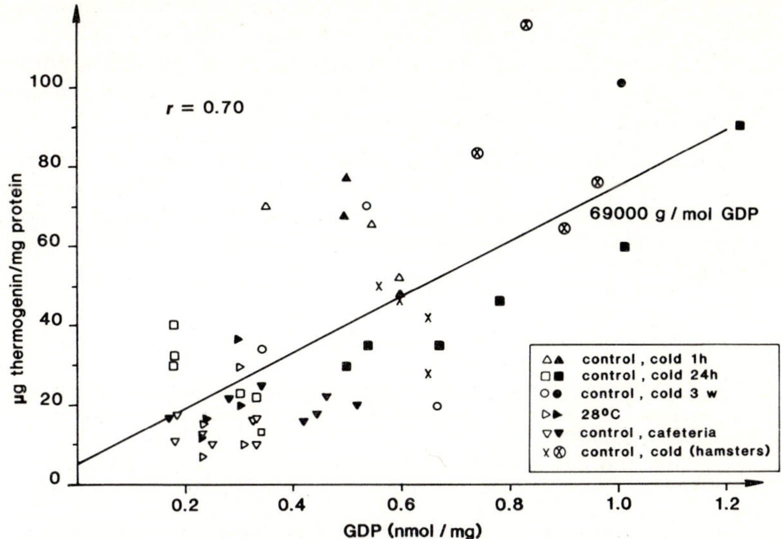

Fig. 2. *Correlation between thermogenin content and (^{3}H)GDP binding.* Data consist of results from individual preparations, where the mean values have earlier been published[25,26,31], together with some hitherto unpublished measurements. The 95% confidence intervals of the slope of the line are 49 000 and 90 000 g thermogenin per mol GDP bound (the intercept with the y-axis is thus not significantly different from the origin).

(^{3}H)GDP-binding technique, performed on the same preparations in our laboratory. From this compilation, several features are evident.

First, the scatter is quite large. However, when results from many preparations are compiled, a clear relationship between the amount of (^{3}H)GDP-binding and the amount of thermogenin detected is observed — indicated by the very significant line drawn after least-square analysis of the data. Both characteristics of the line are physiologically important: the slope is 69 000 g per mol (^{3}H)GDP bound — this is very close to what would be predicted (64 000) if thermogenin indeed binds only one GDP molecule per dimer[18] — and the intercept is very close to the origin, indicating that there is no (^{3}H)GDP-binding which does not represent thermogenin, and, similarly, that there is no thermogenin which does not bind GDP. Further, there is no 'outside grouping' of points; all points fall fairly symmetrically along the line drawn, independent of temperature (28, 22 or 5° C), acclimation period (1 h, 24 h, or 3 weeks), cafeteria-feeding, or species (rat or hamster). We therefore conclude that an increased amount of thermogenin protein can be observed in all the recruitment situations studied.

Activation of α-adrenergic responses. Perhaps the most engimatic new aspect of the metabolism of the brown fat cell is the discovery that it is very well endowed with an α_1-adrenergic pathway. This α_1-adrenergic pathway encompasses the following components. There is an increased phosphatidyl-inositol metabolism[14,21] and an increased formation of inositol-*tris*-phosphate[23]. There is also an increased formation of prostaglandins, probably from the arachidonic acid released from diglyceride produced from phosphatidyl-inositol breakdown (Henschen *et al.*, unpublished observations). There is an α-adrenergic membrane depolarisation[15], and an adrenergic increase in Na^+ permeability, both when measured electrically[16] and as an ion flux[12]. There is an α_1-adrenergic mobilization of Ca^{2+} from intracellular stores[11], and as one of its functions, this Ca^{2+} activates K^+-channels in the cell membrane[22].

The direct significance of the α_1-adrenergic pathway for thermogenesis is quite small[20], but in other tissues many of the events mentioned above are associated with cell proliferation and differentiation, and it is possible that the α_1-adrenergic pathways in brown adipose tissue are associated with the acquisition of the recruited state. It is in the context noteworthy that an increased α_1-receptor density is associated with the recruited state[27,28].

Conclusions. Recruitment of brown fat is apparently associated with a concerted activation and increased relative expression of many different genes, coding for proteins as different as lipoprotein lipase, peroxisomal oxidases, thermogenin and α_1-adrenergic receptors. Some of these increased transcriptions may be initiated by increased cyclic-AMP levels, in a way presently unexplored.

1 Ahlabo, I. & Barnard, T. (1971): Observations on peroxisomes in brown adipose tissue of the rat. *J. Histochem. Cytochem.* **19**, 670–675.

2 Alexson, S. & Cannon, B. (1984): A direct comparison between peroxisomal and mitochondrial preferences for fatty acyl beta-oxidation predicts channelling of medium-chain and very-long-chain unsaturated fatty acids to peroxisomes. *Biochim. Biophys. Acta* **796**, 1–10.

3 Ashwell, M., Jennings, G. & Trayhurn, P. (1983): Evidence from radioimmunoassay for a decreased concentration of mitochondrial 'uncoupling' protein from brown adipose tissue of genetically obese (ob/ob) mice. *Biochem. Soc. Trans.* **11**, 727–728.

4 Ashwell, M., Rothwell, N.J., Stirling, D., Stock, M.J. & Winter, P.D. (1984): Changes in mitochondrial uncoupling protein and GDP-binding in brown adipose tissue of cafeteria-fed rats. *Proc. Nutr. Soc.* **43**, 148A–148A.

5 Bas, S., Imesch, E., Ricquier, D., Assimacopoulos-Jeannet, F., Seydoux, J. & Giacobino, J.-P. (1983): Fatty acid utilization and purine nucleotide binding in brown adipose tissue of genetically obese (ob/ob) mice. *Life Sci.* **32**, 2123–2130.

6 Boulangé, A., Planche, E. & de Gasquet, P. (1981): Onset and development of hypertriglyceridemia in the Zucker rat (fa/fa). *Metabolism* **30**, 1045–1052.

7 Cannon, B., Alexson, S. & Nedergaard, J. (1982): Peroxisomal beta-oxidation in brown fat. *Ann. N.Y. Acad. Sci.* **386**, 40–58.

8 Cannon, B., Hedin, A. & Nedergaard, J. (1982): Exclusive occurrence of thermogenin antigen in brown adipose tissue. *FEBS Lett.* **150**, 129–132.

9 Carneheim, C., Nedergaard, J. & Cannon, B. (1984): Beta-adrenergic stimulation of lipoprotein lipase activity in rat brown adipose tissue during acclimation to cold. *Am. J. Physiol.* **246**, E327–E333.

10 Carneheim, C., Nedergaard, J. & Cannon, B. (In prep): Protein synthesis dependent increase in lipoprotein lipase activity in rats.

11 Connolly, E., Nånberg, E. & Nedergaard, J. (1984): Na$^+$ dependent, alpha-adrenergic mobilization of intracellular (mitochondrial) Ca^{2+} in brown adipocytes. *Eur. J. Biochem.* **141**, 187–193.

12 Connolly, E., Nånberg, E. & Nedergaard, J. (In prep): Norepinephrine-induced Na$^+$ influx in brown fat cells.

13 Cryer, A. & Jones, H.M. (1978): Development changes in the activity of lipoprotein lipase (clearing factor lipase) in rat lung, cardiac muscle, skeletal muscle and brown adipose tissue. *Biochem. J.* **174**, 447–452.

14 Garcia-Sainz, J.A., Hasler, A.K. & Fain, J.N. (1980): Alpha$_1$-adrenergic activation of phosphatidylinositol labeling in isolated brown fat cells. *Biochem. Pharmacol.* **29**, 3330–3333.

15 Girardier, L. & Schneider-Picard, G. (1983): Alpha- and beta-adrenergic mediation of membrane potential changes and metabolism in rat brown adipose tissue. *J. Physiol.* **335**, 629–641.

16 Horowitz, J.M., Horwitz, B.A. & Smith, R.E. (1971): Effect *in vivo* of norepinephrine on the membrane resistance of brown rat cells. *Experientia* **27**, 1419–1421.

17 Lean, M.E.J., Branch, W.J., James, W.P.T., Jennings, G. & Ashwell, M. (1983): Measurement of rat brown adipose tissue mitochondrial uncoupling protein by radioimmunoassay: increased concentration after cold acclimation. *Biosci. Rep.* **3**, 61–71.

18 Lin, C.S. & Klingenberg, M. (1982): Characteristics of the isolated purine nucleotide binding protein from brown fat mitochondria. *Biochemistry* **21**, 2950–2956.

19 Lindbergm O., Bieber, L.L. & Houstek, J. (1976): Brown adipose tissue metabolism: an attempt to apply results from *in vitro* experiments on tissue *in vivo*. In *Regulation of depressed metabolism and thermogenesis* ed L. Jansky & X.J. Musacchia pp. 117–136. Springfield, Ohio: Thomas.

20 Mohell, N., Nedergaard, J. & Cannon, B. (1983): Quantitative differentiation of alpha- and beta-adrenergic respiratory responses in isolated hamster brown fat cells: evidence for the presence of an alpha$_1$-adrenergic component. *Eur. J. Pharmacol.* **93**, 183–193.

21 Mohell, N., Wallace, M. & Fain, J.N. (1984): Alpha$_1$-adrenergic stimulation of phosphatidylinositol turnover and respiration of brown fat cells. *Mol. Pharmacol.* **25**, 64–69.

22 Nånberg, E., Connolly, E. & Nedergaard, J. (1985): Presence of a Ca^{2+}-dependent K$^+$ channel in brown adipocytes. Possible role in maintenance of alpha$_1$-adrenergic stimulation. *Biochim. Biophys. Acta* **844**, 42–49.

23 Nånberg, E. & Putney, Jr., J.W. (In prep): Formation of IP$_3$ by alpha$_1$-adrenergic stimulation of brown fat cells.

24 Nedergaard, J., Alexson, S. & Cannon, B. (1980): Cold adaptation in the rat: increased brown fat peroxisomal beta-oxidation relative to maximal mitochondrial oxidative capacity. *Am. J. Physiol.* **239**, C208–C216.

25 Nedergaard, J. & Cannon, B. (1985): (^{3}H) GDP binding and thermogenin amount in brown adipose tissue mitochondria from cold-exposed rats. *Am. J. Physiol.* **248**, C365–C371.

26 Nedergaard, J., Raasmaja, A. & Cannon, B. (1984): Parallel increases of amount of (^{3}H)GDP binding and thermogenin antigen in brown-adipose-tissue mitochondria of cafeteria-fed rats. *Biochem. Biophys. Res. Commun.* **122**, 1328–1336.

27 Raasmaja, A., Mohell, N. & Nedergaard, J. (1984): Increased alpha$_1$-adrenergic receptor density in brown adipose tissue of cafeteria-fed rats. *Biosci. Rep.* **4**, 851–859.

28 Raasmaja, A., Mohell, N. & Nedergaard, J. (1985): Increased alpha$_1$-adrenergic receptor density in brown adipose tissue of cold-acclimated rats and hamsters. *Eur. J. Pharmacol.* **106**, 489–498.

29 Radomski, M.W. & Orme, T. (1971): Response to lipoprotein lipase in various tissues to cold exposure. *Am. J. Physiol.* **220**, 1852–1856.

30 Seccombe, D.W. & Hahn, P. (1980): Carnitine acyltransferase in developing mammals. *Biol. Neonate* **38**, 90–95.

31 Sundin, U., Moore, G. & Cannon, B. (In prep): Parallel increases of brown-adipose-tissue mitochondrial thermogenin protein content, GDP binding, halide permeability and thermogenetic capacity during cold acclimation of golden hamsters.

32 Trayhurn, P., Richard, D., Jennings, G. & Ashwell, M. (1983): Adaptive change in the concentration of the mitochondrial 'uncoupling' protein in brown adipose tissue of hamsters acclimated at different temperatures. *Biosci. Rep.* **3**, 1077–1084.

Substrate metabolism in brown adipose tissue

P. TRAYHURN
Dunn Nutrition Laboratory, Medical Research Council and University of Cambridge, Downham's Lane, Milton Road, Cambridge CB4 1XJ, UK.

The extremely high rates of thermogenesis that can occur in brown adipose tissue (BAT), particularly in cold-adapted animals, impose a considerable substrate requirement. In principle, thermogenesis can be fuelled either by the utilization of the endogenous triacylglycerol stores or by the direct uptake of circulating substrates. If the former are used then clearly they have to be replenished from the circulation. Apart from the endogenous lipid, there are several circulating substrates which may serve as fuels for thermogenesis, including triacylglycerols, FFA, glucose, ketone bodies, and even lactate, acetate and certain amino acids[15]. Most of these substrates could be oxidized directly, or they might be used as precursors for the synthesis of fatty acids.

In recent years there have been two key areas of interest relating to the fuel supply for BAT — the extent to which the tissue synthesizes its own fatty acids, and the importance of glucose as a direct fuel for thermogenesis.

Fatty acid synthesis. Early studies suggested that the capacity for lipogenesis in BAT was low, but this view was largely based on *in vitro* experiments and the use of specific lipogenic substrates[6]. The position was altered radically, however, with the advent of *in vivo* studies using tritiated water as a precursor[7]. Since BAT yields a poor *in vitro* preparation (particularly in the form of tissue slices or tissue pieces) for assessing the true rates of metabolic pathways[6], the advantages of *in vivo* studies are particularly strong with this tissue. Studies with tritiated water have the considerable advantage of giving rates of lipogenesis that are independent of the carbon source, and in the case of *in vivo* studies the specific activity of the precursor pool is essentially constant over the course of an experiment.

BAT is now established as having a considerable capacity for lipogenesis in rats and mice[1,7,10,12]. On a 'per g wet weight' or a 'per cell' basis, the lipogenic capacity of the tissue is very much higher than that of white adipose tissue or of the liver. The rate of lipogenesis in BAT varies greatly with the environmental temperature to which the animals are adapted, the lower the temperature the greater being the rate[12]. In mice, for example, the rate of lipogenesis in the interscapular brown fat pad (on a whole tissue basis) is approximately 16-fold higher for animals adapted at 4 °C than for those at the thermoneutral temperature of 33 °C[12]. This compares with a 6-fold increase for the epididymal white adipose tissue and no increase for the liver, over the same temperature range[12].

In the cold-adapted rat or mouse, BAT is a major site of the conversion of carbohydrate to lipid[7,12]. Taking the mouse again as an example, the total BAT has been estimated to account for at least 30 per cent of whole-body lipogenesis in animals adapted to the cold. The liver accounts for only 10 per cent of total lipogenesis in these animals. In contrast, for mice adapted at a thermoneutral temperature, the liver accounts for a third of whole-body lipogenesis and BAT only some 5 per cent[12]. Thus not only does adaptation temperature have a substantial effect on the relative importance of BAT as a site of lipogenesis, but the importance of the liver also changes markedly.

The data described relate to adult animals fed a normal low-fat/high-carbohydrate diet. However, lipogenesis in BAT, as in other lipogenic tissues, is influenced by the level of dietary lipid. Feeding a high-fat diet to cold-adapted mice results in a substantial reduction in the rate of lipogenesis in BAT, the reduction being greater than in other tissues, particularly in animals fed a maize-oil diet[14]. This suggests that in the cold-adapted animal there is a preferential channelling of dietary lipid to BAT. Feeding rats a 'cafeteria diet' (which is generally high in fat) also reduces the rate of lipogenesis in BAT[9]. Additionally, rates of lipogenesis in the tissue are very low in sucking animals, and this presumably relates to the suppressive effect of the high lipid content of milk[12].

Lipogenesis in BAT is stimulated by insulin, and as in white adipose tissue this involves a parallel activation of two key enzymes, pyruvate dehydrogenase and acetyl-CoA carboxylase[7]. It should be noted that the importance of BAT as a site of lipogenesis varies according to species. The lipogenic capacity of the tissue is lower in the golden hamster (*Mesocricetus auratus*) and the Mongolian gerbil (*Meriones unquiculatus*) than in rats and mice — even in cold-adapted animals[11,13].

Glucose utilization. The recent interest in glucose as a direct substrate for thermogenesis in BAT stems from the studies on lipogenesis. It now seems that glucose is a major precursor for fatty acid synthesis in BAT[6], implying that the tissue is likely to have a major glucose requirement. High activities of two key glycolytic enzymes, hexokinase and 6-phosphofructokinase, have been found in BAT of the rat, and in the case of hexokinase the activity in brown fat of the cold-adapted animal is greater than in any other tissue[2,3]. From the measurements of enzyme activity it has been suggested that BAT could be a quantitatively important site of glucose removal from plasma after carbohydrate load, and thereby play a role in overall glucose homoeostasis[3].

Recent studies using the 2-deoxyglucose technique for measuring glucose utilization *in vivo* are certainly consistent with this general proposition[4,8,16]. Insulin has been shown to stimulate glucose uptake into BAT *in vivo*, and both acute cold exposure or the administration of noradrenaline have similar effects[4,8]. The marked stimulation of glucose uptake by cold exposure and noradrenaline clearly suggests that glucose is required as a substrate for thermogenesis, at least in acute situations. This possibility is strongly supported by the observation that noradrenaline decreases the rate of lipogenesis and the activity of acetyl-CoA carboxylase in BAT, while increasing the proportion of pyruvate dehydrogenase in the active form[5]. Thus noradrenaline produces a stimulation of glucose uptake into BAT, and channels it towards oxidation rather than lipogenesis.

The importance of glucose as a substrate for BAT is also suggested by studies on the thermogenic responsiveness of *ob/ob* mice to cold. These animals develop insulin resistance in BAT during the 5th week of life (*ob* gene on the 'Aston' background), coinciding with the development of an impaired thermogenic response to acute cold exposure[8]. Studies with 2-deoxyglucose have indicated that insulin resistance in BAT is linked to the thermogenic abnormality through its effects on the uptake of glucose, insulin resistance resulting in a loss of the cold-induced increase in glucose uptake by the tissue[8].

Conclusions. In rats and mice the lipogenic capacity of BAT is very high, and in cold-adapted animals in particular it is an important site for the conversion of carbohydrate to lipid.

Lipogenesis in the tissue is stimulated by insulin, and is subject to long-term regulation by the level of dietary fat. BAT also has a high rate of glucose utilization, and glucose may be an important direct fuel for thermogenesis. The insulin sensitivity of BAT appears increasingly to be a key element in thermogenic responsiveness.

1 Agius, L. & Williamson, D.H. (1980): Lipogenesis in interscapular brown adipose tissue of virgin, pregnant and lactating rats. The effects of intragastric feeding. *Biochem. J.* **190**, 477–480.
2 Cooney, G.J. & Newsholme, E.A. (1982): The maximum capacity of glycolysis in brown adipose tissue and its relationship to control of the blood glucose concentration. *FEBS Lett.* **148**, 198–200.
3 Cooney, G.J. & Newsholme, E.A. (1984): Does brown adipose tissue have a metabolic role in the rat? *Trends Biochem. Sci.* **9**, 303–305.
4 Cooney, G.J., Caterson, I.D. & Newsholme, E.A. (1985): The effect of insulin and noradrenaline on the uptake of 2-[1-^{14}C]deoxyglucose *in vivo* by brown adipose tissue and other glucose-utilising tissues of the mouse. *FEBS Lett.* **188**, 257–261.
5 Gibbons, J.M., Denton, R.M. & McCormack, J.G. (1985): Evidence that noradrenaline increases pyruvate dehydrogenase activity and decreases acetyl-CoA carboxylase activity in rat interscapular brown adipose tissue *in vivo*. *Biochem. J.* **228**, 751–755.
6 McCormack, J.G. (1982): The regulation of fatty acid synthesis in brown adipose tissue by insulin. *Prog. Lipid Res.* **21**, 195–223.
7 McCormack, J.G. & Denton, R.M. (1977): Evidence that fatty acid synthesis in the interscapular brown adipose tissue of cold-adapted rats is increased *in vivo* by insulin by mechanisms involving parallel activation of pyruvate dehydrogenase and acetyl-coenzyme A carboxylase. *Biochem. J.* **166**, 627–630.
8 Mercer, S.W. & Trayhurn, P. (1984): The development of insulin resistance in brown adipose tissue may impair the acute cold-induced activation of thermogenesis in genetically obese (ob/ob) mice. *Biosci. Rep.* **4**, 933–940.
9 Rothwell, N.J., Stock, M.J. & Trayhurn, P. (1983): Reduced lipogenesis in cafeteria-fed rats exhibiting diet-induced thermogenesis. *Biosci. Rep.* **3**, 217–224.
10 Trayhurn, P. (1979): Fatty acid synthesis *in vivo* in brown adipose tissue, liver and white adipose tissue of the cold-acclimated rat. *FEBS Lett.* **104**, 13–16.
11 Trayhurn, P. (1980): Fatty acid synthesis in brown adipose tissue in relation to whole body synthesis in the cold-acclimated golden hamster (*Mesocricetus auratus*). *Biochim. Biophys. Acta* **620**, 10–17.
12 Trayhurn, P. (1981): Fatty acid synthesis in mouse brown adipose tissue: the influence of environmental temperature on the proportion of whole-body synthesis in brown adipose tissue and the liver. *Biochim. Biophys. Acta* **664**, 549–560.
13 Trayhurn, P. & Douglas, J.B. (1984): Fatty acid synthesis in brown adipose tissue of the Mongolian gerbil (*Meriones unguiculatus*): influence of acclimation temperature on synthesis in brown adipose tissue and the liver in relation to whole-body synthesis. *Comp. Biochem. Physiol. B* **78**, 601–607.
14 Van den Brandt, P.A. & Trayhurn, P. (1981): Suppression of fatty acid synthesis in brown adipose tissue of mice fed diets rich in long chain fatty acids. *Biochim. Biophys. Acta* **665**, 602–607.
15 Williamson, D.H. (1986): Fuel supply to brown adipose tissue. *Biochem. Soc. Trans.* **14**, in press.
16 Young, P., Cawthorne, M.A., Levy, A.L. & Wilson, K. (1984): Reduced maximum capacity of glycolysis in brown adipose tissue of genetically obese, diabetic (db/db) mice and its restoration following treatment with a thermogenic B-adrenoceptor agonist. *FEBS Lett.* **176**, 16–20.

Diet-induced thermogenesis and energy flux through brown adipose tissue

M.J. STOCK and Nancy J. ROTHWELL
Department of Physiology, St. George's Hospital Medical School, Cranmer Terrace, London SW17 0RE, UK.

Regulation of energy balance and body composition in mammals appears to be achieved by controls operating on both food intake and energy expenditure[9]. The importance and magnitude of regulatory changes in energy expenditure have been fully realized only recently, and advances in this area have depended to a large extent on overfeeding studies in laboratory rodents.

The ingestion of food usually produces an increase in metabolic rate, which may result from a number of obligatory or adaptive processes. However, terminology is confusing since these increases in heat production after feeding or hyperphagia have been variously labelled by groups of workers. For example, there exist 'specific dynamic action', 'heat increment of feeding', 'luxoskonsumption', 'thermic effect'. In spite of this plethora of terms, an increasing number of workers consistently use the term 'diet-induced thermogenesis' (DIT) to describe changes in heat production due to dietary stimuli, in the same way as 'cold-induced (or thermoregulatory) thermogenesis' is used to describe responses to environmental temperature. However, DIT can be sub-divided into obligatory and adaptive forms — the former describing the inevitable heat production (ie chemical work) associated with the assimilation of nutrients and with synthesis of body tissue and energy stores. Obligatory DIT depends on the amount and nature of the diet consumed and the purpose to which it is put in the body (eg production of muscle, fat, milk, progeny).

The adaptive component of DIT is much more variable and unpredictable, but probably has two main functions. First, it allows animals consuming poor quality (eg protein-deficient) diets to metabolize non-essential energy whilst increasing food intake to obtain sufficient essential nutrients. Secondly, adaptive DIT provides a mechanism for adjusting energy balance to counteract errors in appetite control. Clearly, this is most obvious in hyperphagic animals which is why developments in this area required the introduction of simple, non-invasive and non-stressful methods for inducing voluntary hyperphagia.

Overfeeding and DIT.   Most laboratory rodents can be induced to overeat voluntarily simply by presenting them with a choice of varied and highly palatable human food items, ofter referred to as the 'cafeteria diet'. This feeding regimen results in increases in energy intake of up to 80 per cent, but in young animals causes no change in body weight and only small increases in fat and energy content. The hyperphagia of these animals is associated with marked increases in energy expenditure (up to 100 per cent) and reduced levels of energetic efficiency[9,17]. Increases in DIT in response to overfeeding have been demonstrated in several species (eg, mouse, guinea-pig, pig, dog, man) and in many strains of rats, including wild ones[21] Initially, some questions arose over the quantitative significance of DIT in cafeteria-fed rats, so we assessed food intakes and body composition by two different methods[13] and determined energy expenditure both from carcass energy balance and directly from acute and chronic measurements of oxygen consumption[14]. These studies confirmed the large potential for DIT in young animals, and showed that energy equivalent to the entire maintenance requirement (450–$650kJ/W^{0.75}/d$) can be dissipated as heat via this adaptive phenomenon.

Only a very small proportion of this increased energy expenditure can be ascribed to the extra energy costs (ie obligatory DIT) of assimilating nutrients and depositing body protein and fat. However, like most physiological systems, the magnitude of the DIT is variable and dependent on many factors, such as the level of hyperphagia, composition of the diet, season, temperature, feeding frequency and the age, sex and genetic background of the animals[10]. Thus, modest increases in energy intake (less than 30 per cent) of a high-fat diet can produce little or no change in energy expenditure, particularly in older animals, or those with a genetic predisposition to obesity. DIT declines rapidly with age in many laboratory rodents[18] and it has been suggested that similar changes in thermogenesis in middle-aged human subjects could be responsible for their greater propensity to obesity.

Mechanisms of DIT. Increases in energy expenditure resulting from hyperphagia appear to be mediated by the sympathetic nervous system, which causes activation of heat production in brown adipose tissue (BAT). The distribution of BAT within the rat is shown in the Figure, but the locations are very similar in other species (including man), although the relative size of each depot and the contribution to total body mass varies considerably. The small amounts of BAT should not allow its thermogenic potential to be underestimated. When stimulated, it has one of the highest blood flows and oxygen extraction of any tissue, and its capacity for aerobic heat production has been estimated to be as much as 500 watt/kg — this should be compared with the maximal aerobic capacity of skeletal muscle, which is only 60–70 watt/kg.

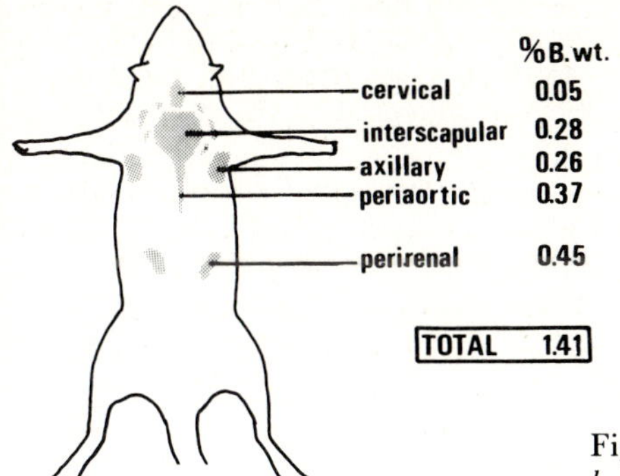

Figure. *Distribution and relative size (per cent of body weight) of brown adipose tissue in the rat.*

Adaptive DIT can be inhibited by pharmacological or surgical blockade of the sympathetic nervous system, mimicked by injection of sympathetic agonists, and is accompanied by increased tissue turnover rates of noradrenaline, particularly in BAT[5]. The quantitative importance of BAT in non-shivering thermogenesis has been established from measurements of *in vivo* metabolic rate of the tissue[3]. The same techniques have now been applied to hyperphagic cafeteria-fed rats and have shown that the enhanced thermogenic capacity of these animals can be almost entirely ascribed to BAT[11]. These very high rates of heat production in brown fat are due to a physiological uncoupling of oxidative phosphorylation, involving a proton conductance pathway in the inner mitochondrial membrane[7]. The activity of this pathway is enhanced by overfeeding, which also causes hypertrophy and, in young animals, hyperplasia of BAT[2]. Conversely, the activity of the sympathetic nervous system and BAT are depressed in animals with reduced levels of DIT, such as food-restricted rats[15] or genetically obese rodents[27].

Hormonal control of DIT and BAT. Noradrenaline appears to be the primary activator of BAT, with other neural systems possibly exerting minor effects on the tissue (eg dopaminergic, serotonergic, histaminergic). However, heat production in BAT, and the metabolic rate and energy balance of the whole animal, can be modified by a number of hormonal systems.

Circulating levels of triiodothyronine (T3) are usually elevated in overfed animals and depressed by food restriction[4]. Despite the marked thermogenic actions of thyroid hormones, it is generally accepted that their role in non-shivering and diet-induced thermogenesis is largely permissive, and they may be required only to maintain sensitivity to noradrenaline. However, a rise in T3 levels does appear essential for the delayed thermogenic response to refeeding in fasted animals[22], and the recent report of high levels of the 5′-deiodinase enzyme in BAT[26] could indicate a close relationship between thyroid hormones and DIT.

Insulin has generally been considered an anabolic hormone which acts mainly to promote fat deposition and a positive energy balance. However, recent evidence has suggested that insulin is required for DIT and may even activate thermogenesis. Experimental diabetes inhibits BAT activity and impairs DIT, while supplementation of animals with insulin can result in lower weight gains and dramatic increases in BAT thermogenesis[9,12,17,25]. Furthermore, the acute thermogenic response to a carbohydrate meal is suppressed by inhibition of insulin release with diazoxide[23], or by subdiaphragmatic vagotomy[1], while responses to fat are unaffected. It is not known whether insulin exerts direct effects on BAT, but a more likely site of action may be the ventromedial hypothalamus, which is known to be insulin-sensitive and appears to be involved in the activation of brown fat thermogenesis[8].

Surgical adrenalectomy can arrest or prevent the development of obesity in genetically obese rodents and older rats fed a cafeteria diet[6,28]. This effect is achieved not only by a reduction in food intake, but also by lower levels of energetic efficiency and stimulation of DIT and brown fat activity[6,24]. The effects of adrenalectomy can be reversed by treatment with corticosterone or by surgical denervation of brown fat[19], indicating that this steroid inhibits brown fat by suppression of the sympathetic nervous system. However, changes in circulating levels of ACTH may partly be responsible for the effects of adrenalectomy on energy balance[20].

In addition to the hormones discussed above, many others such as glucagon, melatonin, TSH, endorphins and sex hormones have in some way been implicated in the regulation of energy balance or the control of thermogenesis.

The evolutionary significance of DIT and brown adipose tissue metabolism has been discussed elsewhere[16], particularly with reference to the advantages of DIT for animals consuming poor quality (eg low-protein) diets. However, sympathetic control of brown fat heat production may also be involved in some of the alterations in energetic efficiency seen in other physiological or pathological conditions such as pregnancy, lactation, fever, injury and cancer cachexia[16].

1 Andrews, P.L.R., Rothwell, N.J. & Stock, M.J. (1985): Effects of sub-diaphragmatic vagotomy on energy balance and thermogenesis in the rat. *J. Physiol.* **362**, 1–12.

2 Brooks, S.L., Rothwell, N.J. & Stock, M.J. (1982): Effects of diet and acute noradrenaline treatment on brown adipose tissue development and mitochondrial purine nucleotide binding. *Q. J. Exp. Physiol.* **67**, 259–268.

3 Foster, D.O. & Frydman, M.L. (1978): Nonshivering thermogenesis in the rat. II Measurements of blood flow with microspheres point to brown adipose tissue as the dominant site of the calorigenesis induced by noradrenaline. *Can. J. Physiol. Pharmacol.* **56**, 110–22.

4 Himms-Hagen, J. (1983): Thyroid hormones and thermogenesis. In *Mammalian thermogenesis*, ed L. Girardier & M.J. Stock, pp. 141–177. London: Chapman & Hall.

5 Landsberg, L. & Young, J.B. (1983): Autonomic regulation of thermogenesis. In *Mammalian thermogenesis*, ed L. Girardier & M.J. Stock, pp. 99–140. London: Chapman & Hall.

6 Marchington, D., Rothwell, N.J., Stock, M.J. & York, D.A. (1983): Energy balance, diet-induced thermogenesis and brown adipose tissue in lean and obese (fa/fa) Zucker rats after adrenalectomy. *J. Nutr.* **113**, 1395–1402.

7 Nicholls, D.G. & Locke, R. (1983): Thermogenic mechanisms in brown fat. *Physiol. Rev.* **64**, 1–64.

8 Perkins, M.N., Rothwell, N.J., Stock, M.J. & Stone, T.W. (1981): Activation of brown adipose tissue thermogenesis by the ventromedial hypothalamus. *Nature.* **289**, 401–402.

9 Rothwell, N.J. & Stock, M.J. (1981): Regulation of energy balance. *Ann. Rev. Nutr.* **1**, 235–256.

10 Rothwell, N.J. & Stock, M.J. (1981): Thermogenesis: Comparative and evolutionary considerations. In *The body weight regulatory system: normal and disturbed mechanisms*, L.A. Cioffi, W.P.T. James & T.B. Van Itallie, pp. 335–343. New York: Raven Press.

11 Rothwell, N.J. & Stock, M.J. (1981): Influence of noradrenaline on blood flow to brown adipose tissue in rats exhibiting diet-induced thermogenesis. *Pflugers Arch.* **389**, 237–242.

12 Rothwell, N.J. & Stock, M.J. (1981): A role for insulin in the diet-induced thermogenesis of cafeteria fed rats. *Metabolism* **30**, 673–678.

13 Rothwell, N.J. & Stock, M.J. (1982): Effects of feeding a palatable 'cafeteria' diet on energy balance in young and adult lean (+/?) Zucker rats. *Br. J. Nutr.* **47**, 461–471.

14 Rothwell, N.J. & Stock, M.J. (1982): Energy expenditure of 'cafeteria-fed' rats determined from measurements of energy balance and indirect calorimetry. *J. Physiol.* **328**, 371–377.

15 Rothwell, N.J. & Stock, M.J. (1982): Effect of chronic food restriction on energy balance, thermogenic capacity, and brown adipose tissue activity in the rat. *Bioscience Rep.* **2**, 543–549.

16 Rothwell, N.J. & Stock, M.J. (1982): *Obesity and leanness*. London: John Libbey.

17 Rothwell, N.J. & Stock, M.J. (1983): Diet-induced thermogenesis. In *Mammalian Thermogenesis*, ed L. Girardier & M.J. Stock, pp. 208–233. London: Chapman & Hall.

18 Rothwell, N.J. & Stock, M.J. (1983): Effects of age of diet-induced thermogenesis and brown adipose tissue metabolism in the rat. *Int. J. Obesity* **7**, 583–589.

19 Rothwell, N.J. & Stock, M.J. (1984): Sympathetic and adrenocorticoid influences on diet-induced thermogenesis and brown fat activity in the rat. *Comp. Biochem. Physiol.* **79A**, 575–579.

20 Rothwell, N.J. & Stock, M.J. (1985): Acute and chronic effects of ACTH on thermogenesis and brown adipose tissue in the rat. *Comp. Biochem. Physiol.* **81A**, 99–102.

21 Rothwell, N.J., Saville, M.E. & Stock, M.J. (1982): Effect of feeding a 'cafeteria' diet on energy balance and diet-induced thermogenesis in four strains of rat. *J. Nutr.* **112**, 1515–1524.

22 Rothwell, N.J., Saville, M.E. & Stock, M.J. (1982): Sympathetic and thyroid influences on metabolic rate in fed, fasted and refed rats. *Am. J. Physiol.* **243**, R339–346.

23 Rothwell, N.J., Stock, M.J. & Warwick, B.P. (1984): Involvement of insulin in the acute thermogenic responses to food and non-metabolisable substances. *Metabolism* **34**, 43–47.

24 Rothwell, N.J., Stock, M.J. & York, D.A. (1984): Effects of adrenalectomy on energy balance, diet-induced thermogenesis and brown adipose tissue in adult cafeteria-fed rats. *Comp. Biochem. Physiol.* **78A**, 565–569.

25 Seydoux, J., Trimble, E.R., Bouillaud, F., Assumacopoulos-Jeannet, F., Bas, S., Ricquer, D., Giacobino, J.P. & Girardier, L. (1984): Modulation of β-oxidation and proton conductance pathway of brown adipose tissue in hypo and hyperinsulinaemic states. *FEBS Letters* **166**, 141–145.

26 Silva, J.E. & Larsen, P.R. (1983): Adrenergic activation of triiodothyronine production in brown adipose tissue. *Nature* **305**, 712–713.

27 Trayhurn, P. & James, W.P.T. (1983): Thermogenesis and obesity. In *Mammalian Thermogenesis*, ed L. Girardier & M.J. Stock. pp. 234–258. London: Chapman & Hall.

28 Yukimura, Y. & Bray, G.A. (1978): Effect of adrenalectomy on body weight and the size and number of fat cells in the Zucker (fatty) rat. *Endocrinol. Res. Commun.* **5**, 189–193.

Brown adipose tissue and obesity

Jean HIMMS-HAGEN
Department of Biochemistry, University of Ottawa, Faculty of Health Sciences, 451 Smyth Road, Ottawa, Ontario, Canada K1H 8M5.

Thermogenesis in brown adipose tissue (BAT) induced by cold or by diet can, under certain conditions, be a major component of overall energy expenditure. One or another type of defect in control of thermogenesis in BAT has been identified in most animal models of obesity. The consequent deficit in energy expenditure is believed to contribute to a high metabolic efficiency and thus to the development of obesity in these animals (for review see[3,4]). It is at present unclear to what extent the concept of defective energy buffering by BAT is a causal factor in obesity applies to humans.

Normal control of thermogenic and trophic responses of BAT. Thermogenesis in BAT is switched on by noradrenaline released from its sympathetic innervation. Both β- and α_1-adrenergic receptors are intimately involved in this sympathetic nervous control. Other hormones, such as thyroid hormone and insulin, play a permissive role in the response. Long-term stimulation of BAT results in a trophic response. In addition to hyperplasia, this comprises selective increases in certain components of BAT that are important in the thermogenic response, such as the concentration of uncoupling protein in the mitochondria and the activities of such enzymes in the plasma membrane as lipoprotein lipase and thyroxine 5′-deiodinase. Although BAT thyroxine 5′-deiodinase is known to be stimulated when thermogenesis is induced by noradrenaline, the role of endogenous production of 3,5,3′-triiodothyronine in the thermogenic response is not clear.

Any stimulus which increases the activity of the sympathetic nervous system will increase thermogenesis in BAT and, if sustained, will produce a trophic response. Stimuli to the sympathetic nervous system that are important in control of BAT include diet and environmental temperatures below thermoneutrality. Animal room temperatures are commonly maintained at 20–24 °C. Because this is well below the thermoneutral temperature for rats and mice, sympathetic nervous system activity, BAT thermogenesis, and growth of BAT, are already above the level seen at thermoneutrality; in these animals, therefore, BAT is in a partially cold-acclimated state.

Brown adipose tissue and thermogenesis in obese animals. *Hypothalamic obesity.* Medical hypothalamic lesions, induced in rats by radiofrequency or electrolytic lesions or by parasagittal knife cuts, result in an inhibition of diet-induced thermogenesis (DIT) in BAT without interfering with cold-induced non-shivering thermogenesis in this tissue (see[2–4,8]). Goldthioglucose-induced ventromedial hypothalamic lesions in mice also interfere with DIT but not with cold-induced non-shivering thermogenesis in BAT[7]. Lateral hypothalamic lesions do not interfere with either process (Park, Himms-Hagen & Coscina, unpublished results). Thermoregulation is normal in hypothalamic-lesioned rats, but goldthioglucose-lesioned mice thermoregulate at a body temperature below normal (Eley & Himms-Hagen, unpublished results) and this also contributes to their high metabolic efficiency. The ventromedial region of the hypothalamus is apparently required for dietary influences on BAT tissue but is not essential for thermal influences.

In contrast, mice with monosodium glutamate-induced hypothalamic lesions can activate thermogenesis in their BAT in response to either diet or cold; their high metabolic efficiency that leads to the development of obesity in the absence of hyperphagia is associated with thermoregulation at a lower than normal body temperature and suppression of BAT thermogenesis (Tokuyama & Himms-Hagen, unpublished results).

Genetic obesity. The young genetically fatty (*fa/fa*) rat resembles the rat with a hypothalamic lesion, in that it is unable to respond to diet by activation of BAT thermogenesis, but is able to activate BAT thermogenesis in the cold. In the aging fatty rat, BAT atrophies, the concentration of uncoupling protein in its mitochondria decreases[1], its sympathetic innervation disappears and the tissue becomes entirely non-functional.

BAT of the adult *ob/ob* mouse is likewise atrophied. It has a low concentration of the mitochondria uncoupling protein[1] and is refractory to noradrenaline. Thus, the cold-exposed obese *ob/ob* mouse fails to activate thermogenesis in its BAT[6] and fails to increase the activity of thyroxine 5′-deiodinase in this tissue[9] despite adequately increased cold-induced activity of the sympathetic nervous innervation to its BAT[10]. When exposed to cold, the *ob/ob* mouse becomes hypothermic and dies. The atrophy of its BAT is probably secondary to the chronically low activity of the tissue's sympathetic nervous innervation at usual animal room temperature. The *ob/ob* mouse is in a state of almost continual torpor, ie it regulates its body temperature at a lower than normal level. Torpor is a normal physiological occurrence in lean mice that is induced on a daily basis when food supply is restricted. However, the *ob/ob* mouse enters torpor even when fed, probably because of a faulty hypothalamic control of this process. Procedures that can prevent torpor, such as acclimation to mild cold (14 °C) or feeding a cafeteria diet, are those that chronically increase synpathetic nervous system activity. BAT of the *ob/ob* mouse can respond to such procedures by growth and thermogenesis. Even food restriction, by inducing daily arousal from torpor and thereby stimulating thermogenesis in BAT, improves the thermogenic function of BAT of the *ob/ob* mouse[5]. Thus, in this obese animal there is no inherent defect in the BAT, only in the central control mechanism.

Brown adipose tissue and thermogenesis in obese humans. It has not yet proved possible to assess the quantitative contribution of BAT thermogenesis to overall energy expenditure in humans because techniques currently used in animal studies are inapplicable. There is no doubt that BAT is present and that sympathetic nervous system activity is modified by diet and by temperature as it is in the animals. There is, however, no direct evidence that defective thermogenesis in BAT can play a role in human obesity.

Conclusions. The principal conclusion from studies of obese experimental animals is that suppression of the thermogenic function of BAT occurs in all types and is secondary to defective central control of this process. No inherent defect in BAT itself has as yet been identified. The suppression of the thermogenic activity of BAT contributes to the high metabolic efficiency of these animals and, together with their usual hyperphagia, to the development of their obesity. The applicability of the concept of BAT thermogenesis as an energy buffer to humans is not yet established. Assessment of the thermogenic function of BAT in humans, and of a possible defect in it in obese humans, must await the development of new experimental approaches[3,4].

1 Ashwell, M., Holt, S., Jennings, G., Stirling, D.M., Trayhurn, P. & York, D.A. (1985): Measurement by radioimmunoassay of the mitochondrial uncoupling protein from brown adipose tissue of obese (*ob/ob*) mice and Zucker (*fa/fa*) rats at different ages. *FEBS Lett.* **179**, 233–237.
2 Coscina, D.V., Chambers, J.W., Park, I.R.A., Hogan, S. & Himms-Hagen, J. (1985): Impaired diet-induced thermogenesis in brown adipose tissue of rats made obese with parasagittal knife cuts. *Brain Res. Bull.* **14**, in press.
3 Himms-Hagen, J. (1984): Thermogenesis in brown adipose tissue as an energy buffer. Implications for obesity. *New Engl. J. Med.* **311**. 1549–1558.
4 Himms-Hagen, J. (1985): Brown adipose tissue metabolism and thermogenesis. *Ann. Rev. Nutr.* **5**, 69–94.
5 Himms-Hagen, J. (1985): Food restriction increases torpor and improves brown adipose tissue thermogenesis in *ob/ob* mice. *Am. J. Physiol.* **248**, E531–E539.

6 Hogan, S. & Himms-Hagen, J. (1980):Abnormal brown adipose tissue in obese (*ob/ob*) mice: response to acclimation to cold. *Am. J. Physiol.* **239**, E301–E309.

7 Hogan, S. & Himms-Hagen, J. (1983): Brown adipose tissue of mice with goldthioglucose-induced obesity: effect of cold and diet. *Am. J. Physiol.* **244**, E581–E588.

8 Hogan, S., Himms-Hagen, J. & Coscina, D.V. (1985): Lack of diet-induced thermogenesis in brown adipose tissue of obese medial hypothalamic-lesioned rats. *Physiol. Behav.* **35**, in press.

9 Kates, A-L. & Himms-Hagen, J. (1985): Defective cold-induced stimulation of thyroxine 5'-deiodinase in brown adipose tissue of the genetically obese (*ob/ob*) mouse. *Biochem. Biophys. Res. Commun.* **130**, 188–193.

10 Zaror-Behrens, G. & Himms-Hagen, J. (1983): Cold-stimulated sympathetic activity in brown adipose tissue of obese (*ob/ob*) mice. *Am. J. Physiol.* **244**, E361–E366.

VI: Lipid metabolism

WHITE ADIPOSE TISSUE

Fundamental aspects of development of fat cells in man and animals

P. BJÖRNTORP
Department of Medicine I, Sahlgren's Hospital, University of Göteborg, 41345 Göteborg, Sweden.

Obesity is a condition in which the adipose tissue in the body increases in size. In moderate cases this may occur simply by an increase in the triglyceride content of the fat cells. In more severe cases, however, the number of adipocytes in adipose tissue also increases. Such a condition seems to be associated with a poor prognosis for treatment[6]. Furthermore, when adipose tissue enlargement, including adipocyte hyperplasia, occurs in certain regions of adipose tissue, an increased risk of complicating diseases is a consequence[1]. This clinical background demonstrates the importance of studying factors that regulate hyperplastic growth of adipose tissue, particularly since this seems to be an irreversible condition.

The mature, monovacuolar adipocyte does not multiply. It is therefore necessary to study the lipid-poor adipocyte precursor cells by isolating and characterizing them and by trying to elucidate the regulatory factors involved in the growth of adipose tissue during positive energy balance that result in obesity.

Methods. The methods utilized in this project have all been described in detail[2,4,5].

Adipose tissue is digested with collagenase and free fat cells separated from the stromal-vascular cells by flotation and filtration procedures. The latter cells are then cultured in monolayer or in suspension cultures. In the former system, cells attach themselves to the bottom of the culture disk and multiply, until they reach confluence. Here an irreversible differentiation of the cells occurs, resulting in morphological and functional changes. Eventually the differentiated cells fill with triglyceride to become mature adipocytes. In the suspension culture system, however, multiplication is prevented during lipid filling, effectively until the mature adipocytes formed are identifiable.

These methods make it possible to obtain a series of adipocyte cells at different stages of development. First, mature adipocytes are obtained from collagenase digestion. The stromal-vascular cells during multiplication in the monolayer culture consist mainly of non-differentiated adipose precursor cells, adipoblasts. When differentiated preadipocytes are formed, they are fully equipped with the functions of mature adipocytes, but do not yet contain their full load of triglycerides. In the suspension culture system essentially no multiplication of cells occurs. Cells already differentiated when removed from the host animal fill up with lipid, and can be identified. This then is a way to follow, at least semi-quantitatively, how adipose precursor cells have been differentiated to preadipocytes in the host animal *in vivo*. It is then possible to identify 'lipid-free' adipocytes by this method.

With these methods adipose tissue from adult rats subjected to different feeding regimens has been studied.

Results and discussion. In a first study male Sprague-Dawley and Osborne-Mendel rats were examined after various periods of prolonged overfeeding. It was observed that an increased rate of multiplication of cells in the stromal-vascular fraction occurred after only a few days of overfeeding. This was shown by measuring the rate of incorporation of labelled thymidine into DNA. An increase in the triglyceride contents of the adipocytes also occurred very early. When the adipocyte enlargement had reached a 'critical' level of about 0.6–0.8 µg triglyceride per cell we began to find an increased number of preadipocytes in the suspension cultures, indicating that differentiation of precursor cells had now started. At this time, or slightly later, new adipocytes appeared in the adipose tissue[3].

This series of events occurred in both strains of rats and in both epididymal and retroperitoneal adipose tissue, but was observed earlier in Osborne-Mendel rats than in Sprague-Dawley rats and in the retroperitoneal than the epididymal fat pad.

These results were in accordance with the following chain of events leading to adipose tissue expansion. Adipoblasts and probably other cells in the stromal-vascular fraction of cells, including capillary endothelium start to multiply very soon after overfeeding (G. Sypniewska & P. Björntorp, unpublished results). This seems to be a generalized phenomenon in various adipose tissue depots. When all available fat cells in the depot concerned are full, as indicated by a critical adipocyte size, adipoblasts are differentiated to preadipocytes, which quickly fill and form new adipocytes. This occurs at different times in various depots, depending on the rate of filling of these depots. This chain of events is summarized schematically in the Figure.

Several points of regulation of this series of events can be imagined. First, the increased adipoblast multiplication apparently occurring generally, is probably regulated by factor(s) in circulation round the body. Second, differentiation of these adipoblasts is probably regulated by local factors, because it occurs in a region which has been filled up to the capacity of the available adipocytes. The latter event is dependent on the inflow of triglyceride from the circulation into that particular adipose tissue depot. Available evidence indicates that this inflow is regulated by the local activity of lipoprotein lipase. This enzyme is synthesized in the adipocytes in the fat depot, but is actively attached to an adjacent capillary wall, where glucose-aminoglycans catch circulating triglyceride particles. The triglyceride is then hydrolyzed by the enzyme and transported into the adipocytes. Clearly, this regional regulation of lipoprotein-lipase activity then becomes important for the local capture of triglyceride, in turn responsible for the rate of growth of adipocytes in that adipose tissue region. This, in turn, will have decisive importance for the formation of new adipocytes. Thus, three regulatory points may be visualized. These will be discussed in the following paragraphs.

Plasma factors. The first regulatory point, presumably caused by circulating factor(s), has been examined by measuring rate of replication, differentiation and lipid filling of adipoblasts in the presence of plasma from rats of different nutritional status. Neither replication, nor differentiation of the cells, was dependent on the nutritional status of the rats, which included control rats eating chow *ad libitum*, rats starved for 4 days and rats overfed with a high-sucrose, high-fat diet for up to about 3 weeks. The rate of lipid filling of the differentiated cells was, however, highly dependent on the nutritional status of the rats. A closer analysis revealed that the triglyceride, or very-low-density lipoprotein contents, controlled the rate of lipid filling. In other words, the more substrate available for filling of the adipocytes, the more rapidly did this occur, which might be expected (Björntorp 1985, submitted for publication).

This study then has not provided a complete understanding of the increased multiplication of adipoblasts during the early phases of overfeeding. More work is needed to try to reveal what is causing this to occur. The most impressive result of the studies referred to above was the high level of mitogenic and differentiation activity of plasma under all nutritional regimes, including a long period of starvation where, clearly, no formation of new fat cells is occurring.

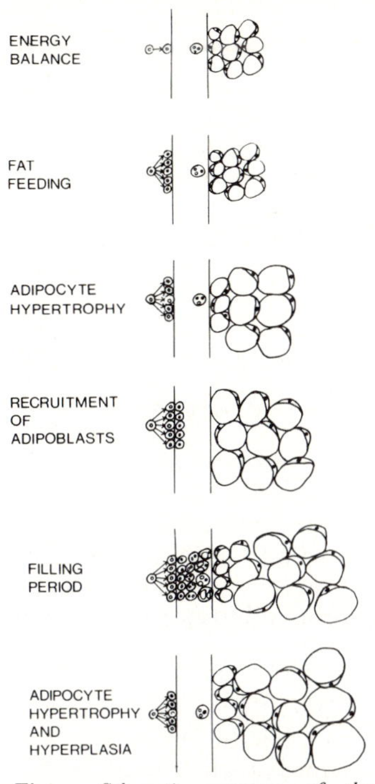

Figure. *Schematic summary of the chain of events leading to the development of lipid-filled adipocytes in fat depot tissue.* From: Björntorp *et al.* Metabolism 1982, 31: 366–373 by permission.

Regulation of regional triglyceride influx. of triglyceride. In another series of experiments the regulation of local lipoprotein lipase activity has been examined. These investigations have been performed mainly in humans, where lipoprotein lipase activity has been estimated in biopsies from different adipose tissue regions in subjects with precisely defined endocrine status. The following results have been obtained[7].

In women with intact sex steroid production the femoral region has a high activity of lipoprotein lipase. This disappears with the menopause, and can be restored by administration of steroid sex hormones. Men do not show such an increase in femoral lipoprotein lipase activity. These data indicate a function of female sex steroid hormones crucial to the local activity of lipoprotein lipase activity. Whether this is due to local differences of hormone binding to adipocytes is not known, but that appears to be an attractive possibility.

Regional regulatory factors of cellular determination. Finally studies have been performed aiming at elucidation of a possible local regulation of adipoblast differentiation. These studies started out from the observation described above that a high level of cell activity leading to differentiation was detected under all feeding treatments, including chronic starvation. Because of this it was proposed that the regional regulation of adipoblast differentiation was caused by a local inhibition of the excess of factors inducing differentiation circulating in the body. This hypothesis was tested in the culture systems developed, by following adipoblast differentiation in monolayer cultures in the presence of adipose tissue or fractions thereof to see whether regulatory factors were the cause or were affected by these additions. In addition, the tissues added were obtained from rats with different previous feeding regimes.

In the presence of plasma, differentiation of the cultured adipoblasts occurred swiftly within a few days. When adipose tissue was added, this differentiation was strongly inhibited to an extent proportional to the amount of tissue added. Also when isolated adipocytes were added inhibition resulted but was apparently less pronounced when adipocytes from overfed animals were used. Medium exposed to adipocytes had reduced differentiating activity. This was apparently not due to the production of an inhibitory factor, but rather to absorption of a factor from the medium or more precisely from the plasma constituents added.

These experiments, which are still rather preliminary, indicate that regulation of local differentiation of adipoblasts is actually occurring by the inhibition of an excess of a circulating differentiating factor.

1 Björntorp, P. (1985): Hazards in subgroups of human obesity. *Eur. J. Clin. Invest.* **14**, 239–241.

2 Björntorp, P., Karlsson, M., Gustafsson, L., Smith, U., Sjöström, L., Cigolini, M., Storck, G. & Pettersson, P. (1979): Quantitation of different cells in the epididymal fat pad of the rat. *J. Lipid Res.* **20**, 97–106.

3 Björntorp, P., Karlsson, M. & Pettersson, P. (1982): Expansion of adipose tissue storage capacity at different ages in rats. *Metabolism* **31**, 366–373.

4 Björntorp, P., Karlsson, M., Pettersson, P. & Sypniewska, G. (1980): Differentiation and function of rat adipocyte precursor cells in primary culture: *J. Lipid Res.* **21**, 714–723.

5 Björntorp, P., Karlsson, M., Perloft, H., Pettersson, P., Sjöström, L. & Smith, U. (1978): Isolation and characterization of cells from rat adipose tissue developing into adipocytes. *J. Lipid Res.* **19**, 316–324.
6 Krotkiewski, M., Sjöström, L., Björntorp, P., Carlgren, G., Garellick, G. & Smith, U. (1978): Adipose tissue cellularity in relation to prognosis for weight reduction. *Int. J. Obesity* **1**, 395–416.
7 Rebuffé-Scrive, M., Enk. L., Crona, N., Lönnroth, P., Abrahamsson, L., Smith, U. & Björntorp, P. (1985): Fat cell metabolism in different regions in women. Effect of menstrual cycle, pregnancy and lactation. *J. Clin. Invest.* **75** (In press).

Growth and development of fat depots in animals and birds of agricultural importance

R.L. HOOD
CSIRO Division of Food Research, PO Box 52, North Ryde, NSW 2113, Australia.

In contrast to its inert appearance, adipose tissue is in a state of flux in response to fluctuating nutritional, hormonal and neural influences. The extent of fat deposition in animals and birds of agricultural importance is related to differences in the partitioning of nutrients between fat and muscle. Knowledge of the partitioning of energy during growth and development is of practical significance in the production of lean animals and birds. This review will emphasize cellular aspects of growth and discuss mechanisms by which growth of adipose tissue can be limited.

Growth and body composition. The size to which animals grow before they attain a similar body composition depends on heredity. It was concluded that differences in body composition between strains of Australian merino sheep compared at the same weight were due to differences in maturity[6]. When compared at any given body weight, animals that are large at maturity will be leaner than animals that are small at maturity. Besides genetic influences, partitioning of nutrients is influenced by physical activity, appetite, gonadal hormones, dietary regimen and balance of nutrients, particularly energy and protein.

Genetic factors are also important in determining the distribution of fat depots. Species and strain account for differences in relative sizes of fat depots at different ages. For example, 'beef' breeds of cattle have lower proportions of internal fat depots than 'dairy' breeds of cattle[40]. The rat is not a suitable model for adiposity of meat animals since the perirenal fat depot of the rat grows at a rate faster than the subcutaneous fat depots[5], which is in contrast to most animals of agricultural importance. The extent of fat deposition at different anatomical locations is also reflected in the metabolic activity of the adipose tissue at these sites[18].

Genetic control of fat deposition. The propensity of animals and birds to deposit fat can be decreased by genetic selection. The broiler chicken can be used as an example; in a study on its body composition, selection for improved food conversion efficiency (FCE) resulted in a marked reduction in total body fat, whereas selection for increased food consumption had the opposite effect[35]. Selection had a similar effect on fat deposited in the abdominal fat pad[21].

Selective breeding can result in lean chickens[25,41]; by selecting birds for high and low contents of abdominal fat two diverse genetic lines were produced[25]. Changes in the ratio of abdominal fat to body weight in the two lines were very rapid, reaching a plateau in the fat line in the third generation whereas the lean line continued to become leaner. Differences were less pronounced in females, suggesting that sex hormones, by modulating other hormones important in lipid metabolism, influence genetic control of fattening. Two recent reviews have detailed differences in body composition[24] and plasma parameters[26] between the two lines.

A simple assay for plasma concentration of very-low-density lipoprotein (VLDL) in fed birds[13] has provided a good indicator of body lipid content of live broilers. The assay has been used as a selection parameter in a breeding programme[41] and after three generations, correlated responses to selection for low plasma VLDL (heritability coefficient = 0.50 ± 0.11) resulted in a decreased abdominal and total body fat content along with an improved FCE. The response of FCE to selection for plasma VLDL is consistent with observations that VLDL concentration is correlated with FCE and body fat content[42].

These two examples, applicable to the broiler chicken industry, indicate the scope of genetic selection as a long-term method of producing avian carcasses with desirable body compositions.

Cellular aspects of fat deposition. Accretion of fat in adipose tissue is due to an increase in the number of adipocytes by cell differentiation and multiplication (hyperplasia) and/or lipid accumulation in existing cells (hypertrophy). These processes begin in the fetus[15] and continue during postnatal development. The estimated age at which hyperplasia appears to be complete varies among species and tissue sites and is influenced by the method used to count adipocytes[17]. Hyperplasia, however, is generally confined to early stages of postnatal development and, at maturity, cellular hypertrophy is the dominant mechanism for increase in depot fat.

The importance of cellular hypertrophy is well documented for cattle[19], sheep[14,22], pigs[1,10,20] and birds[16,33]. In one study a difference of 16 per cent was noted[20] in the weight of extramuscular fat between 109-kg pigs of two breeds. The obese pigs had 20 per cent fewer adipocytes than the muscular pigs, therefore differences in adiposity were related solely to the volume of adipocytes present in the fat depots. Differences in fatness of littermates were explained on the basis of adipocyte volume since the number of adipocytes was similar for pigs within a litter. In contrast to extramuscular fat depots, adipocyte number makes an important contribution to the accumulation of interfascicular fat (marbling) in cattle[19] and pigs[27].

Recent studies indicate the re-initiation of adipocyte hyperplasia in mature obese animals[11,34,38]. When the Coulter Counter is used to size osmium-fixed adipocytes from fat animals a bimodal distribution is often obtained, this distribution should be verified by alternative procedures since it may be artefactual[17]. The appearance of genuine small adipocytes in fat depots from mature animals is due either to a turnover of adipocytes or re-initiation of precursor adipocyte differentiation and multiplication.

In young chickens, rate of incorporation of lipid into adipocytes increases with adipocyte volume (Hood, unpublished results). In the adult bird, significant incorporation of radioactivity, derived from intravenous infusion of labelled glucose, was observed in small adipocytes (Figure) providing evidence of precursor adipocyte differentiation and multiplication in adult chickens with large abdominal fat pads. Despite a bimodal pattern of incorporation of radioactive substrate, the presence of a large population of newly formed adipocytes was not identified with a Coulter Counter.

Control of adipocyte differentiation. Studies on cultured preadipocytes suggest that it may be possible to manipulate adipose tissue growth. For example, dexamethasone, insulin and fibroblast growth factor induce lipogenesis in fibroblasts, but only if they are obtained from adipose tissue[3]. The importance of these factors *in vivo* is not clear. Although the triggering mechanisms are unknown, it has been suggested[4] that an approach, similar to one using azacytidine infusions[28], may be adopted at specific times in the development of sheep in order to alter the number of preadipocytes available for differentiation and multiplication. It has been proposed that animals be immunized against specific hormones involved in growth and development (sex hormones and somatostatin) as a means of regulating regional distribution of fat depots[43].

Repartitioning agents. Repartitioning agents are β-adrenergic agonists which stimulate muscle production while limiting synthesis of lipid in all fat depots. When animals are fed these agents, nutrient utilization and deposition is repartitioned and animals become efficient in converting feed to weight gain. If repartitioning agents are approved as feed additives or as subcutaneous implants, they offer the opportunity of altering body composition at a rate greater than can be achieved by nutritional and genetic management.

Clenbuterol (benzylalcohol,4-amino-α-[t-butyl-amino] methyl-3,5-dichloro) and cimaterol (AC 263,780) (5-[1-hydroxy-2-(isopropylamino)ethyl]-anthranilonitrile) are examples of repartitioning agents which have been evaluated in meat animals and birds. Both compounds are structurally similar to natural catecholamines such as adrenaline, and both effectively repartition energy at low concentrations. The use of these compounds has been most effective in feedlot studies with sheep and cattle.

Table. *Carcass characteristics of lambs fed clenbuterol for 8 weeks* (Baker et al., 1984).

	Clenbuterol in diet ppm	
Observation	0	2
Number of lambs	10	10
Live weight, kg	53.7	54.0
Dressing, %	54.6	57.2*
Semitendinosis muscle weight, g	143.8	176.9**
Longissimus muscle area, cm^2	16.9	23.9**
Kidney and pelvic fat weight, g	998	664**
Fat depth (12th rib), mm	5.9	3.7**
USDA yield grade (1–5)	3.5	2.5**

* $P<0.05$, differs from control; ** $P<0.01$, differs from control.

The Table outlines the effect of clenbuterol on performance and body composition of finishing crossbred wethers. Treatment with 2 ppm clenbuterol resulted in an improvement of 24 per cent in average daily gain and feed per gain[2]. Data on body composition characteristics demonstrated that clenbuterol increased muscle mass and decreased subcutaneous and kidney/pelvic fat. Similar results were obtained when crossbred lambs were injected subcutaneously with clenbuterol at a dose of 2.5 μg/kg liveweight per day[39]. In this study, growth rate for clenbuterol-treated lambs was similar to that of controls and a 30 per cent reduction in the size of fat depots was accounted for by an equivalent weight of lean tissue.

Performance improvements were not observed when Hereford steers were fed clenbuterol at a

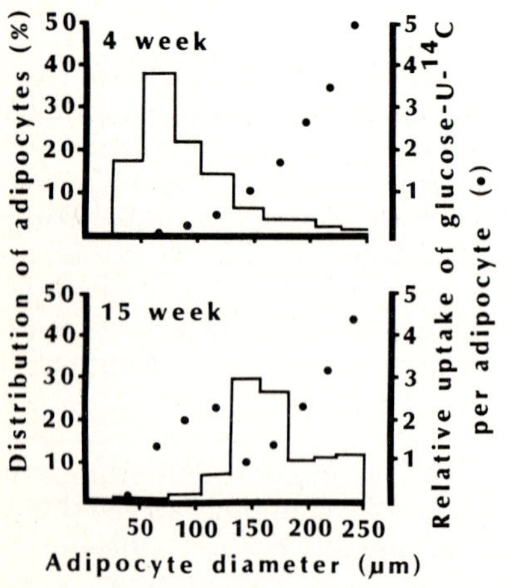

Figure. *Relationship between the incorporation of radioactive substrate, derived from the i.v. infusion of labelled glucose, and adipocyte diameter in the abdominal fat pad of 4 and 15 week-old female broiler chickens. Incorporation of radioactive substrate into individual adipocytes was determined by the method of Hood & Thornton (1980) and the distribution of adipocytes measured with a Coulter Counter. The uptakes of radioactivity, derived from labelled glucose, are expressed relative to the uptake in the 130–153 μm diameter group.*

dose of 500 mg per animal per day[36]. Carcass evaluation, however, showed that the treated group had 42 per cent less fat depth at the 12th rib and 33 per cent less kidney, pelvic and heart fat. Chemical analysis of the 9th to 11th rib section from the carcasses indicated that the steers treated with clenbuterol had a 14 per cent higher protein content and 30 per cent less fat than ribs from control steers.

For broiler chickens, repartitioning agents need only be administered during the finishing period to produce a maximum effect. When fed to broiler chickens at 1 ppm, significant improvements in performance were observed, however, alterations in carcass composition in favour of repartitioning were only small[7].

Several trials including β-adrenergic agonists in the feed of pigs have given equivocal results[8,32,37]. The efficacy of repartitioning agents in pigs is not as high as in ruminant animals. It has been noted that several potential β-adrenergic agonists were not active in swine adipose tissue, but were active in rat adipose tissue[31].

Clenbuterol and other β-agonists have been examined as human anti-obesity agents since in obese rodents they trigger a dramatic reduction in fat depots with little effect on lean body mass[30]. This effect is achieved by β-adrenergic-mediated stimulation of lipolysis and enhanced oxidation of released fatty acids in brown adipose tissue[12]. Although the mode of action of β-agonists is not clear, it appears they mediate the loss of energy by thermogenesis in futile cycles and divert mobilised fatty acids for use as an efficient energy source for protein synthesis. Certain β-agonists are known to limit muscle protein catabolism[29] and increase *in vivo* muscle protein anabolism in chronically-treated rats[9].

1 Anderson, D.B., Kauffman, R.G. & Kastenschmidt, L.L. (1972): Lipogenic enzyme activities and cellularity of porcine adipose tissue from various anatomical locations. *J. Lipid Res.* **13**, 593–599.

2 Baker, P.K., Dalrymple, R.H., Ingle, D.L. & Ricks, C.A. (1984): Use of a β-adrenergic agonist to alter muscle and fat deposition in lambs. *J. Anim. Sci.* **59**, 1256–1261.

3 Broad, T.E. & Ham, R.G. (1983): Growth and adipose differentiation of sheep preadipocyte fibroblasts in serum-free medium. *Eur. J. Biochem.* **135**, 73–79.

4 Broad, T.E. & Harris, P.M. (In press) Control of distribution of fat — is there a cellular basis? *Proc. Nutr. Soc. N.Z.* **8**.

5 Broad, T.E., Sedcole, J.R. & Ngan, A.S. (1983): Incorporation of glucose into lipid of perirenal and subcutaneous adipocytes of rats and sheep. *Aust. J. Biol. Sci.* **36**, 147–156.

6 Butterfield, R.M., Griffiths, D.A., Thompson, J.M., Zamora, J. & James, A.M. (1983): Changes in body composition relative to weight and maturity in large and small strains of Australian Merino rams. I. Muscle, Bone and fat. *Anim. Prod.* **36**, 29–37.

7 Dalrymple, R.H., Ricks, C.A., Baker, P.K., Pensack, J.M., Gingher, P.E. & Ingle, D.L. (1983): Use of the beta-agonist clenbuterol to alter carcass composition in poultry. *Fed. Proc. Fed. Am. Soc. Exp. Biol.* **42**, 668.

8 Dalrymple, R.H., Baker, P.K., Doscher, M.E., Ingle, D.L., Pankavich, J.A. & Ricks, C.A. (1984): Effect of repartitioning agent AC 263,780 on muscle and fat accretion in finishing swine. *J. Anim. Sci.* **59**, 212.

9 Emery, P.W., Rothwell, N.J., Stock, M.J. & Winter, P.D. (1984): Chronic effects of beta-agonists on body composition and protein synthesis in the rat. *Biosci. Rep.* **4**, 83–91.

10 Etherton, T.D. (1980): Subcutaneous adipose tissue cellularity of swine with different propensities for adipose tissue growth. *Growth* **44**, 182–191.

11 Etherton, T.D., Wangsness, P.J., Hammers, V.M. & Ziegler, J.H. (1982): Effect of dietary restriction on carcass composition and adipocyte cellularity of swine with different propensities of obesity. *J. Nutr.* **112**, 2314–2323.

12 Fain, J.N. & Garcia-Sainz, J.A. (1983): Adrenergic regulation of adipocyte metabolism. *J. Lipid Res.* **24**, 945–966.

13 Griffin, H.D. & Whitehead, C.C. (1982): Plasma lipoprotein concentration as an indicator of fatness in broilers: development and use of a simple assay for plasma very low density lipoproteins. *Br. Poult. Sci.* **23**. 307–313.

14 Haugebak, C.D., Hedrick, H.B. & Asplund, J.M. (1974): Adipose tissue accumulation and cellularity in growing and fattening lambs. *J. Anim. Sci.* **39**, 1016–1025.

15 Hausman, G.J., Campion, D.R. & Martin, R.J. (1980): Search for the adipocyte precursor cell and factors that promote its differentiation. *J. Lipid Res.* **21**, 657–670.

16 Hood, R.L. (1980): The cellular basis for growth of the abdominal fat pad in broiler-type chickens. *Poult. Sci.* **61**, 117–121.

17 Hood, R.L. (1982): Relationships among growth, adipose cell size, and lipid metabolism in ruminant adipose tissue. *Fed. Proc. Fed. Am. Soc. Exp. Biol.* **41**, 2555–2561.

18 Hood, R.L. (1983): Changes in fatty acid synthesis associated with growth and fattening. *Proc. Nutr. Soc,* **42**, 303–313.

19 Hood, R.L. & Allen, C.E. (1973): Cellularity of bovine adipose tissue. *J. Lipid Res.* **14**, 605–610.
20 Hood, R.L. & Allen, C.E. (1977): Cellularity of porcine adipose tissue: effects of growth and adiposity. *J. Lipid Res.* **18**, 275–284.
21 Hood, R.L. & Pym, R.A.E. (1982): Correlated responses for lipogenesis and adipose tissue cellularity in chickens selected for body weight gain, food consumption, and food conversion efficiency. *Poult. Sci.* **61**, 122–127.
22 Hood, R.L. & Thornton, R.F. (1979): The cellularity of ovine adipose tissue. *Aust. J. Agric. Res.* **30**, 153–161.
23 Hood, R.L. & Thornton, R.F. (1980): A technique to study the relationship between adipose cell size and lipogenesis in a heterogeneous population of adipose cells. *J. Lipid Res.* **21**, 1132–1136.
24 Leclercq, B. (1984): Adipose tissue metabolism and its control in birds. *Poult. Sci.* **63**, 2044–2054.
25 Leclercq, B., Blum, J.C. & Boyer, J.P. (1980): Selecting broilers for low or high abdominal fat: initial observations. *Brit. Poult. Sci.* **21**, 107–113.
26 Leclercq, B., Hermier, D. & Salichon, M.R. (1984): Effects of age and diet on plasma lipid and glucose concentrations in genetically lean or fat chickens. *Reprod. Nutr. Dev.* **24**, 53–61.
27 Lee, Y.B. & Kauffman, R.G. (1974): Cellular and enzymatic changes with animal growth in porcine intramuscular adipose tissue. *J. Anim. Sci.* **38**, 532–537.
28 Ley. T.J., De Simone, J., Anagnou, N.P., Keller, G.H., Humphries, R.K., Turner, P.H., Young, N.S., Hecler, P. & Nienhuis, A.W. (1982): 5-Azacytidine selectively increases γ-globin synthesis in a patient with B^{+} thalassemia. *New. Engl. J. Med.* **307**, 1469–1475.
29 Li, J.B. & Jefferson, L.S. (1977): Effects of isoproterenol on amino acid levels and protein turnover in skeletal muscle. *Am. J. Physiol.* **232**, E243–E249.
30 Massoudi, M., Evans, E. & Miller, D.S. (1983): Thermogenic drugs for the treatment of obesity, screening using obese rats and mice. *Ann. Nutr. Metab.* **27**, 26–37.
31 Mersmann, H.J. (1984): Adrenergic control of lipolysis in swine adipose tissue. *Comp. Biochem. Physiol.* **77**, 43–53.
32 Moser, R.L., Dalrymple, R.H., Cornelius, S.G., Pettigrew, S.G. & Allen, C.E. (1984): Evaluation of repartitioning agent on the performance and carcass traits of finishing pigs. *J. Anim. Sci.* **59**, 255.
33 Pfaff, F.E., Jr. & Austic, R.E. (1976): Influence of diet on development of the abdominal fat pad in the pullet. *J. Nutr.* **106**, 443–450.
34 Powell, S.E. & Aberle, E.D. (1981): Skeletal muscle and adipose tissue cellularity in runt and normal birth weight swine. *J. Anim. Sci.* **52**, 748–756.
35 Pym, R.A.E. & Solvyns, A.J. (1979): Selection for food conversion in broilers: body composition of birds selected for increased body weight gain, food consumption and food conversion ratio. *Br. Poult. Sci.* **20**, 87–97.
36 Ricks, C.A., Dalrymple, R.H., Baker, P.K. & Ingle, D.L. (1984): Use of a β-agonist to alter fat and muscle deposition in steers. *J. Anim. Sci.* **59**, 1247–1255.
37 Ricks, C.A., Baker, P.K., Dalrymple, R.H., Doscher, M.E., Ingle, D.L. & Pankavich, J.A. (1984): Use of clenbuterol to alter muscle and fat accretion in swine. *Fed. Proc. Fed. Am. Soc. Exp. Biol.* **43**, 857.
38 Robelin, J. (1981): Cellularity of bovine adipose tissues: developmental changes from 15 to 65 percent mature weight. *J. Lipid Res.* **22**, 452–457.
39 Thornton, R.F., Tume, R.K., Payne, G., Larsen, T.W., Johnson, G.W. & Hohenhaus, M.A. (1985): The influence of the β_2-adrenergic agonist, clenbuterol, on lipid metabolism and carcass composition of sheep. *Proc. N.Z. Soc. Anim. Prod.* **45** (In press).
40 Truscott, T.G., Wood, J.D. & Macfie, H.J.H. (1983): Fat deposition in Hereford and Friesian steers. I. Body composition and partitioning of fat between depots. *J. Agric. Sci. Camb.* **100**, 257–270.
41 Whitehead, C.C. & Griffin, H.D. (1984): Development of divergent lines of lean and fat broilers using plasma very low density lipoprotein concentration as selected criterion: the first three generations. *Br. Poult. Sci.* **25**, 572–582.
42 Whitehead, C.C., Hood, R.L., Heard, G.S. & Pym, R.A.E. (1984): Comparison of plasma very low density lipoproteins and lipogenic enzymes as predictors of body fat content and food conversion efficiency in selected lines of broiler chickens. *Br. Poult. Sci.* **25**, 277–286.
43 Wood, J.D. (1982): Factors controlling fat deposition in meat animals. *Proc. N.Z. Soc. Anim. Prod.* **42**, 113–116.

Fat cell size and number : relevance to obesity

D. LEMONNIER
Unité de Recherches sur la Nutrition et l'Alimentation INSERM, Unité 1, Hôpital Bichat, 170 Bd. Ney, 75877 PARIS Cedex 18, France.

S tudies using animal models permit exact measurement of the weight of a given adipose tissue depot and the determination of the total number of fat cells contained within that depot. Such studies aid the understanding of adipose tissue development and abnormalities. This is particularly so in the case of long-term nutritional studies.

In this review, the term fat cell or adipocyte concerns a cell filled with one large lipid droplet. For practical reasons, most of the studies have been performed in male mice and rats and concern one site, the epididymal fat pad. Development of this site is well-documented; cell size and number increase up to about 3 months of age[9–12]. By measuring the incorporation of tritiated thymidine into adipocyte DNA following a pulse injection, it was established that in the normal rat this pad grows largely by an increase in adipocyte number until the 3rd postnatal week[8]. After this, further increases in pad weight are due only to fat cell enlargement. Thus the apparent increase in cell number observed during the 2nd and 3rd month resulted from the filling of preexisting cells with lipid. Fat cell number at this site appeared to be fixed in the young adult male mouse and rat, although it is not excluded that in middle age, fat cell number increases. Such biphasic changes in adipocyte number occurs in bovine animals[17].

Yet several data are now available indicating that the constancy of fat cell numbers in young adult animals is not a general rule: adipose tissue growth changes from site to site. For example, in normal rats fed a control diet we have observed a two to three-fold increase in cell number in both sexes at the perirenal site from the 5th to the 18th month[13]. No changes in the epididymal fat cell number were observed in these animals. The authors concluded that when a maximum cell size was observed for a given diet, the perirenal adipose tissue grew by an increase in fat cell number and that this phenomenon may be of importance for fat storage in adult or aging animals. Such results have been recently confirmed[2]. Similar patterns of development have been also reported in other animal species fed a control diet. In the guinea-pig the expansion of the epididymal fat pad between 6 weeks to 1 year of age is mainly attributable to an increase in cell number[6]. In the rabbit, growth of perirenal and interscapular fat pads until month 6 is due to an increase in both adipocyte number and site. Then between 6 and 10 months of age these fat pads double in weight due to a continuous increase in fat cell number[15].

Heterogeneity in the development of the adipose tissues has been also demonstrated in experimental obesities. All experimental obesities show adipocyte hypertrophy and most of them show fat cell hyperplasia. It is important to note that hyperplasia appears in young animals or in adults, depending on the site and sex. Hypoplasia has been found in young obese animals but hypertrophy of the fat cells seems to occur first. This pattern of development is observed whatever the aetiology of the obesity: dietary-induced obesity, obesity of central origin, or genetic obesities. It is also observed in these obesities that hyperplasia appears in the sites where fat cell number is not fixed in the adult, lean animals. This is clearly demonstrated in the perirenal fat. In young as well as in adult animals a high-fat diet produces cell enlargement and hyperplasia in this site[4,7,13]. This dietary-induced hyperplasia is observed in lean as well as in genetically obese animals: *ob ob* mice or *fa fa* rats[14]. Obesity induced by a high-fat diet is proportional to the amount of fat in the diet, but an increase in fat cell number is not necessarily related to hyperphagia[5,12]. Thus, the first effect of obesity on the adipocyte cellularity is an increase in fat cell size, when size is at its maximum level. Hyperplasia appears at least in some sites and a hypertrophic hyperplastic obesity is observed in most experimental obesities in young adult animals. In middle age rats rendered obese by a high-fat diet, hypertrophy tends to disappear while hyperplasia increases. For example, in 18-month-old rats the excess of adipose tissue weight is mainly due to hyperplasia (Table). Another interesting demonstration of the

Table. *Number and volume of cells in perirenal adipose tissue (PRAT) of male Wistar rats fed a control or a high-fat diet for 18 months.* (Values are means ± s.e.m. for five animals per group).

			Fat cell	
Diet	*Body wt (g)*	*PRAT wt (g)*	*Volume (pl)*	*Total number ($\times 10^6$)*
High-fat	653 ± 34**	84 ± 11**	1214 ± 165	78 ± 11**
Control	520 ± 13	17 ± 1.1	887 ± 92	22 ± 2.6

** Significantly greater than control values (P<0.01)

heterogeneity of adipose tissues is supported by the studies on fat tissue regeneration. Surgical removal of fat tissue induces regeneration in some sites but not in others. This regeneration is observed in young and adult animals; in the rabbit regeneration is observed in the perirenal site but not in inguinal, omental and other sites[16]. In some experiments a compensatory hypertrophy is observed[13] but not in others.

There are few data in the literature on the effect of energy restriction on adipose tissue cellularity in obese animals. An attempt was made to answer this question in the following experiment. Several 11-week-old male *fa/fa* rats were subjected to food restriction at three different levels for 15 weeks. It can be seen that, surprisingly, fat cells enlarged when food intake was reduced by 25 and 50 per cent ad libitum intake (Figure). This was attributable to the

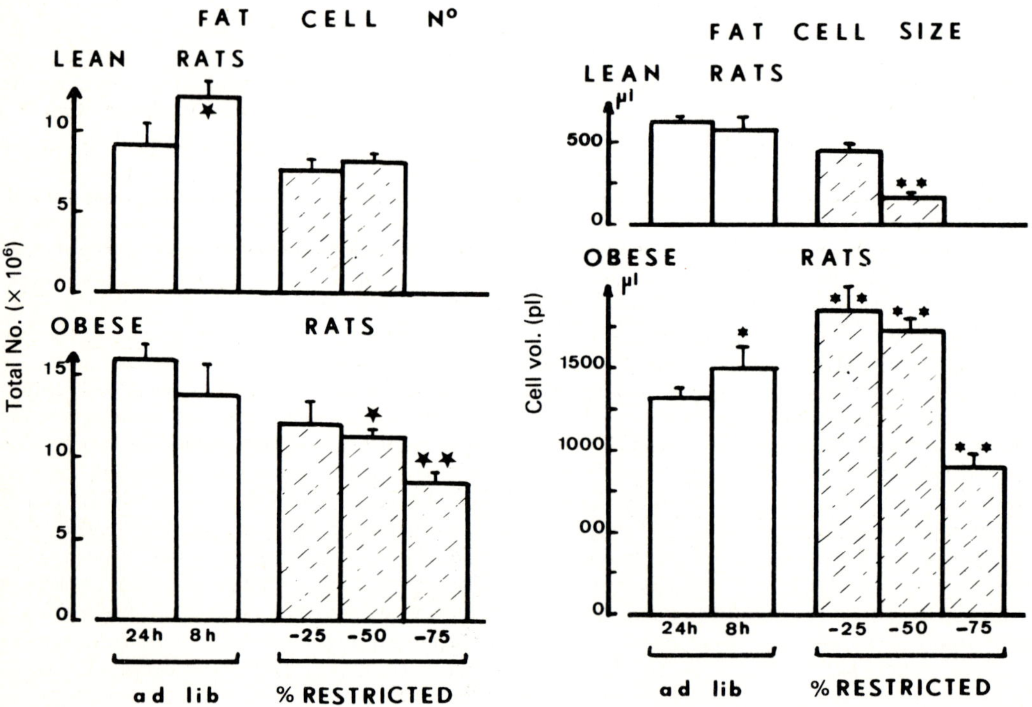

Figure. *Number and volume of cells in perirenal adipose tissue (PRAT) of lean Fa/- and genetically obese fafa rats fed ad-lib 24 h or 8 h per 24 h, or restricted by 25, 50 and 75 per cent of their ad lib intake.* *significantly different (P<0.05) and **very significantly different (P<0.01) from corresponding control (fed *ad lib* 24 h) mean.

meal-eating pattern of food intake in these rats which induced a rise in lipoprotein lipase activity and in serum insulin (unpublished data). All restricted groups showed a reduction in fat cell number. Thus hyperplasia was reduced but not suppressed, total cell number being 7.2×10^6 at the beginning of the experiment in both groups. When the rats were refed for 5 weeks, fat cell size returned to normal and cell number increased significantly (14×10^6 adipocytes for the *fa/fa* rats). Whether this was due to the proliferation or to the filling of preadipocytes has not been established. Since fat cell hypertrophy was maintained even in the most severely restricted group, it is unlikely that fat cells were too small to be counted or had disappeared after lipid depletion.

Food restriction in lean animals prevents the normal increase in fat cell number in young[1] and in adult animals[3].

In conclusion, experimental obesities in animals have demonstrated the high sensitivity of adipose tissue cellularity to the diet. They have also revealed that fat tissues are not identical in their cellular responses: the changes observed in one site cannot be extrapolated to another site. The plasticity of fat cell number is an important phenomenon which is observed in lean and obese animals whatever their age.

1 Aubert, R., Suquet, J.P. & Lemonnier, D. (1980): Long term morphologic and metabolic effects of early under-and overnutrition in mice. *J. Nutr.* **110**, 649–661.
2 Bertrand, H.A., Masoro, E.J. & Yu, B.P. (1978): Increasing adipocyte number as a basis for perirenal depot growth in adult rats. *Science* **201**, 1234–1235.
3 Bertrand, H.A., Stacy, C., Masoro, E.J., Yu, B.P., Murata, I. & Maeda, H. (1984): Plasticity of fat cell number. *J. Nutr.* **114**, 127–131.
4 Björntorp, P., Karlsson, M. & Pettersson, P. (1982): Expansion of adipose tissue storage capacity at different ages in rats. *Metabolism* **31**, 366–373.
5 Bourgeois, F., Alexiu, A. & Lemonnier, D. (1983): Dietary-induced obesity: effect of dietary fats on adipose tissue cellularity in mice. *Br. J. Nutr.* **49**, 17–26.
6 Di Girolamo, M. & Mendlinger, S. (1971): Role of fat cell size and number in the enlargement of epididymal fat pads in three species. *Am. J. Physiol,* **221**, 859–864.
7 Faust, I.M., Johnson, P.R., Stern, J. & Hirsch, J. (1978): Diet-induced adipocyte number increase in adult rats; a new model of obesity. *Am. J. Physiol.* **235**, E279–286.
8 Greenwood, M.R.C. & Hirsch, J. (1974): Postnatal development of adipocyte cellularity in the normal rat. *J. Lipid Res.* **15**, 474–483.
9 Hellman, B., Thelander, L. & Taljedal, I.B. (1963): Postnatal growth epididymal adipose tissue in yellow obese mice. *Acta Anat.* **55**, 286–294.
10 Hirsch, J. & Han. P.W. (1977): Cellularity of rat adipose tissue: effects of growth, starvation and obesity. *J. Lipid Res.* **18**, 275–284.
11 Hollenberg, C.H. & Vost, A. (1968): Regulation of DNA synthesis in fat cells and stromal elements from rat adipose tissue. *J. Clin. Invest.* **47**, 2485–2498.
12 Lemonnier, D. (1972): Effect of age, sex and site on the cellularity of the adipose tissue in mice and rats rendered obese by a high fat diet. *J. Clin. Invest.* **51**, 2907–2915.
13 Lemonnier, D. & Alexiu, A. (1974): Nutritional, genetic, and hormonal aspects of adipose tissue cellularity. In *The regulation of the adipose tissue mass*, ed J. Vague, and J. Boyer, p. 158. Amsterdam: Excerpta Medica.
14 Lemonnier, D. (1981): Adipose tissue development in normal and obese animals. In *Adipose tissue in childhood*, ed E.D. Bonnett, p. 57. Boca Raton, Fl: CRC Press.
15 Vougues, J. & Vezinhet, A. (1977): Evolution, pendant la croissance, de la cellularité du tissu adipeux chez le lapin et l'agneau. *Ann. Biol. Anim. Bioch. Biophys.,* **17**, 799–805.
16 Reyne, Y., Nougues, J. & Vezinhet, A. (1983): Adipose tissue regeneration in 6-month old and adult rabbits following lipectomy. *Proc. Soc. Exp. Biol. Med.* **174**, 258–264.
17 Robelin, J. (1985): Cellularité des différents dépôts adipeux des bovins en croissance. *Reprod. Nutr. Dévelop.* **25**, 211–215.

Regulation of fatty acid synthesis in white and brown adipose tissue

R.M. DENTON, J.G. McCORMACK, Janine M. GIBBINS and R.W. BROWNSEY
Department of Biochemistry, University of Bristol Medical School, University Walk, Bristol BS8 1TD, UK; Present address (JGMcC): Department of Biochemistry, University of Leeds, Leeds LS2 9JT, UK; Present address (RWB): Department of Biochemistry, University of British Columbia, Vancouver BC, Canada V6T 1W5.

In mammals the principal sites of fatty acid synthesis are white and brown adipose tissue together with liver and the lactating mammary gland. Rates of fatty acid synthesis in these tissues alter greatly according to the nutritional and hormonal status of the animal. In part these changes are brought about by long-term changes in the concentrations of enzymes in the pathway[2,26]. For example, tissue from starved animals has a greatly diminshed capacity for converting glucose to fatty acids and this is largely due to a large reduction in the amount of many of the enzymes involved in fatty acid synthesis. On refeeding, there are parallel increases in both fatty acid synthesis and in the amounts of the enzymes and these can attain levels greater than fed controls. Similar repression of enzymes in fatty acid synthesis is observed in diabetes (reversed by insulin treatment) and following feeding with a fat-rich diet (reversed by a high-carbohydrate diet). However, in addition to these long-term means of regulating fatty acid synthesis through changes in specific gene expression, rates of fatty acid synthesis can also be altered by hormones in the short-term (ie within minutes) through changes in the catalytic properties of two enzymes catalysing key steps in the pathway whereby glucose is converted to fatty acids. These enzymes are the mitochondrial enzyme, pyruvate dehydrogenase, and the cytoplasmic enzyme, acetyl-CoA carboxylase; both enzymes have interconvertible active and inactive forms. For fuller accounts of the work reported here the reader should consult[6,7,11,12].

Effects of insulin and catecholamines on rates of fatty acid synthesis in rat white and brown adipose tissue. The Table gives some typical values for the rates of fatty acid synthesis from glucose found in fat cells isolated from rat white epididymal adipose tissue by collagenase digestion and incubated *in vitro*. It is clear that insulin greatly stimulates the conversion of glucose to fatty acids whereas adrenaline inhibits the process, especially in the presence of insulin. Similar changes in fatty acid synthesis in rat epididymal adipose tissue were also found in studies *in vivo* in which the circulating insulin level was varied within the physiological range by injections of glucose or anti-insulin serum. This same technique has also been used to demonstrate the stimulatory effects of insulin on fatty acid synthesis in rat interscapular brown adipose tissue. In contrast, injection of noradrenaline results in a marked decrease in fatty acid synthesis. The magnitude of the effects in brown adipose tissue are similar to those found in white adipose tissue but it should be noted that rates of fatty acid synthesis on a wet weight basis are much greater in brown than white adipose tissue.

Short-term effects of insulin and catecholamines on the activities of pyruvate dehydrogenase and acetyl-CoA carboxylase in rat white and brown adipose tissue. Both insulin and adrenaline increase glucose uptake into rat epididymal fat cells and it is very likely that both insulin and noradrenaline increase glucose uptake into brown fat cells. It is thus to be expected that these hormones bring about their contrasting effects on fatty acid synthesis through causing opposing changes in the activities of key enzymes which determine the rate of fatty acid synthesis within fat cells. Strong candidates are pyruvate dehydrogenase and acetyl-CoA carboxylase and marked changes in the activity of both these two enzymes are found in fresh extracts of cells or tissues previously exposed *in vitro* or *in vivo* to the presence or absence of insulin and/or catecholamines (Table).

In white adipose tissue, insulin increases the proportion of both enzymes in their respective active forms whereas adrenaline decreases this proportion (especially in the presence of insulin). In this tissue, it seems reasonable to conclude that changes in the activity of both

Table. *Short-term effects of insulin and catecholamines on rates of fatty acid synthesis and proportions of pyruvate dehydrogenase and acetyl-CoA carboxylase in their respective active forms in rat white fat cells in vitro and white brown adipose tissue in vivo.*

	Fatty acid synthesis (μmol fatty acid/g/h)	Enzyme activities (as % of maximum)	
		Pyruvate dehydrogenase	Acetyl-CoA carboxylase
(a): Rat epididiymal fat cells (*in vitro*) during incubation with glucose plus:			
no hormone	0.2	20	14
insulin	1.8	55	35
adrenaline	0.14	15	6
insulin + adrenaline	0.7	35	10
(b): Rat epididymal white adipose tissue (*in vivo*) following injection with:			
anti-insulin serum	0.5	17	18
glucose	2.3	40	32
(c): Rat interscapular brown adipose tissue (*in vivo*) following injection with:			
anti-insulin serum	1.8	13	18
glucose	9.5	31	50
glucose + propranolol	6.0	3	22
glucose + nor-adrenaline	1.6	28	8

Rates of fatty acid synthesis were calculated from the incorporation of either ^{14}C from (U-^{14}C) glucose (*in-vitro* studies) or ^{3}H from ^{3}H$_2$O (*in-vivo* studies). Initial enzyme activities were measured in fresh extracts of tissue or cells previously rapidly frozen in liquid N_2 after treatment with hormones. These activities are expressed as per cent of the maximum activity (observed after treatment of control tissue extracts with pyruvate dehydrogenase phosphatase for pyruvate dehydrogenase and with citrate for acetyl-CoA carboxylase). Data has been taken from the following sources (where additional details can be obtained):- (a) Denton & Halperin, 1968; Martin *et al.*, 1972; Brownsey *et al.*, 1979 and unpublished observations: (b) Stansbie *et al.*, 1976: (c) McCormack & Denton, 1977; Gibbins *et al.*, 1985.

enzymes are important in the short-term hormonal regulation of fatty acid synthesis. The situation in brown adipose tissue is similar but with one important difference; noradrenaline results in a striking activation of pyruvate dehydrogenase in contrast to the modest inactivation observed with adrenaline in white adipose tissue.

Comment on the mechanism involved in the effects of insulin and catecholamines on pyruvate dehydrogenase in white and brown adipose tissue. Pyruvate dehydrogenase from mammalian tissues is regulated by reversible phosphorylation. A specific kinase introduces phosphate into three different sites of the α-subunits of the complex and this results in the near complete loss of catalytic activity. Reactivation is brought about by a specific protein phosphatase which is activated by Ca^{2+}. The changes in activity shown in the Table are almost certainly due to changes in the proportion of the enzyme in its active non-phosphorylated form since all the hormone effects are lost on treatment of the extracts with phosphatase. In the case of the effect of insulin on white fat cells it has been demonstrated directly that insulin results in the dephosphorylation of all three sites on the α-subunits[19].

In theory, the effects of insulin could be brought about by activation of the phosphatase or inhibition of the kinase. It has proved possible to show that the first mechanism is correct by making use of the persistence of the effects of insulin during the preparation and subsequent incubation of intact mitochondria from both white and brown adipose tissue[13,18,23]. It seemed possible that insulin might increase phosphatase activity by increasing the intramitochondrial concentration of Ca^{2+} but recent work has shown that this hypothesis is incorrect[24]. On the other hand evidence has been obtained that insulin results in a decrease in the K_a of the phosphatase for Mg^{2+} (Thomas & Denton, unpublished observations). This change is similar to that observed with the polyamine spermine[8] which raises the intriguing possibility that insulin action on pyruvate dehydrogenase and perhaps other processes may involve changes in the concentration of spermine or more likely another polybasic molecule whose actions are mimicked by spermine.

Much less is known about the mechanisms involved in the effects of catecholamines on adipose tissue pyruvate dehydrogenase activity. It is possible that the inhibitory effects seen in white fat cells are the result of increased fatty acid oxidation. In heart muscle, it is well-established that this is associated with activation of the kinase and hence a loss of pyruvate dehydrogenase activity. The marked activation in brown adipose tissue is reminiscent of the effects of catecholamines on pyruvate dehydrogenase on heart muscle acting through β-receptors[15,22] and in liver acting through α-receptors[1,27]. In both these situations it has become evident that the increases in pyruvate dehydrogenase activity are the result of activation of pyruvate dehydrogenase phosphate phosphatase brought about by increases in intramitochondrial concentration of Ca^{2+}. It seems reasonable to suggest that the activation in brown adipose tissue is also brought about through an increase in the intramitochondrial concentration of Ca^{2+}. Such an increase would be expected to also lead to the activation of NAD-isocitrate dehydrogenase and oxoglutarate dehydrogenase[10,21] and hence may be important in the observed increase in citrate cycle flux which occurs when brown adipose tissue is stimulated by noradrenaline[14].

Comments on the mechanisms involved in the effects of insulin and catecholamines on acetyl-CoA carboxylase activity in white and brown adipose tissue. Acetyl-CoA carboxylase from mammalian tissues is, like pyruvate dehydrogenase, regulated by reversible phosphorylation (see[6,7,12]). It is now well-established that the inhibition of fatty acid synthesis observed in liver and white fat cells exposed to hormones which increase cyclic AMP is the result of increased phosphorylation of the enzyme by cyclic AMP-dependent protein kinase[3,4,16,17]. This kinase phosphorylates specific serines on acetyl-CoA carboxylase and this results in a marked decrease in catalytic activity which is evident even when the enzyme is incubated with high concentrations of citrate. Although it has yet to be demonstrated directly it seems likely that the inhibitory effect of noradrenaline on acetyl-CoA carboxylase activity and fatty acid synthesis in brown adipose tissue is the result of increased phosphorylation of the enzyme by cyclic AMP-dependent protein kinase.[14].

The activation of acetyl-CoA carboxylase by insulin, at least in white fat cells, is not due to dephosphorylation of the enzyme as might be expected from the inhibitory effects of phosphorylation discussed above. In fact insulin results in an actual increase in phosphorylation of the enzyme[4]. However, this increase is due to the phosphorylation of apparently a single site quite distinct from those exhibiting increased phosphorylation in cells exposed to adrenaline[4]. Some progress has been made in characterising the kinase involved[6,7]. In particular, an increase in acetyl-CoA carboxylase kinase activity has been found in the cytoplasmic fraction of fat cells previously exposed to insulin[5] and it is possible that this increase is the result of the release of the kinase from sites on the plasma membrane following the binding of insulin to its receptor[11]. Recently it has also been shown that triton extracts of human placenta membranes contain substantial serine protein kinase activity apparently capable of phosphorylating the same site as that exhibiting increased phosphorylation in cells exposed to insulin. Moreover, evidence has been obtained for increases, albeit rather variable, in the rate of acetyl-CoA carboxylase phosphorylation on addition of insulin to the triton extracts[29].

Some conclusions. Under conditions of high circulating insulin, brown adipose tissue, at least in the rat fed a high carbohydrate diet, is an important site of fatty acid synthesis. However, under conditions of catecholamine-induced thermogenesis fatty acid synthesis is inhibited while fuel oxidation is greatly stimulated. The fuel would appear to be a combination of both fatty acids and glucose. We suggest that Ca^{2+} ions may play an important role in the stimulation of mitochondrial metabolism under these conditions.

Acknowledgement. These studies have been supported by grants from the Medical Research Council, the British Diabetic Association and the Percival Waite Salmond Bequest. JMG holds a Medical Research Council Postgraduate Studentship.

1 Assimacopoulos-Jeannet, F., McCormack, J.G. & Jeanrenaud, B. (1983): Effect of phenylephrine on PDH activity in rat hepatocytes and its interaction with insulin plus glucagon. *FEBS Lett.* **159**, 83–88.
2 Block, K. & Vance, D. (1977): Control mechanisms in the synthesis of fatty acids. *Ann. Rev. Biochem* **46**, 263–298.
3 Brownsey, R.W., Hughes, W.H. & Denton, R.M. (1979): Adrenaline and the regulation of acetyl-CoA carboxylase in rat epididymal adipose tissue. Inactivation of the enzyme is associated with phosphorylation and can be reversed by dephosphorylation. *Biochem. J.* **184**, 23–32.
4 Brownsey, R.W. & Denton, R.M. (1982): Evidence that insulin activates acetyl-CoA carboxylase by increased phosphorylation of a specific site. *Biochem. J.* **202**, 77–86.

5 Brownsey, R.W., Edgell, N.J., Hopkirk, T.J. & Denton, R.M. (1984): Studies on insulin-stimulated phosphorylation of acetyl-CoA carboxylase, ATP-citrate lyase and other proteins in rat epididymal adipose tissue. Evidence for activation of a cyclic AMP independent protein kinase. *Biochem. J.* **218**, 733–743.

6 Brownsey, R.W. & Denton, R.W. (1985): Role of phosphorylation in the regulation of acetyl-CoA carboxylase activity by insulin. In *Molecular basis of insulin action*, ed M. Czech, pp. 297–314. New York: Plenum Press.

7 Brownsey, R.W. & Denton, R.M. (1985): Acetyl-CoA carboxylase. In *Enzyme control by phosphorylation*, (3rd edn of *The Enzymes*), ed P.D. Boyer & E.G. Krebs, New York: Academic Press (In press).

8 Damuni, Z., Humphreys, J.S. & Reed, L.J. (1984): Stimulation of pyruvate dehydrogenase phosphatase activity by polyamines. *Biochem. Biophys. Res. Commun.* **124**, 95–99.

9 Denton, R.M. & Halperin, M.L. (1968): The control of fatty acid and triglyceride synthesis in rat epididymal adipose tissue. *Biochem. J.* **110**, 27–38.

10 Denton, R.M. & McCormack, J.G. (1980): Review letter. On the role of the calcium transport cycle in heart and other mammalian mitochondria. *FEBS Lett.* **119**, 1–8.

11 Denton, R.M., Brownsey, R.W. & Belsham, G.J. (1981): Invited review: A partial view of the mechanism of insulin action. *Diabetologia* **21**, 347–363.

12 Denton, R.M. & Brownsey, R.W. (1983): The role of phosphorylation in the regulation of fatty acid synthesis by insulin and other hormones. *Phil. Trans. R. Soc. Lond. B.* **302**, 33–45.

13 Denton, R.M., McCormack, J.G. & Marshall, S.E. (1984): Persistence of the effect of insulin on pyruvate dehydrogenase activity in rat white and brown adipose tissue during the preparation and subsequent incubation of mitochondria. *Biochem. J.* **217**, 441–452.

14 Gibbins, J.M., Denton, R.M. & McCormack, J.G. (1985): Evidence that noradrenaline increases pyruvate dehydrogenase activity and decreases acetyl-CoA carboxylase activity in rat interscapular brown adipose tissue *in vivo*. *Biochem. J.* (In press).

15 Hiraoka, T., Debuysere, M. & Olson, M.S. (1980): Studies of the effects of β-adrenergic agonists on the regulation of PDH in the perfused rat heart. *J. Biol. Chem.* **225**, 7604–7609.

16 Holland, R., Witters, L.A. & Hardie, D.G. (1984): Glucagon inhibits fatty acid synthesis in isolated hepatocytes via phosphorylation of acetyl-CoA carboxylase by cyclic AMP-dependent protein kinase. *Eur. J. Biochem.* **140**, 325–333.

17 Holland, R., Hardie, D.G., Clegg, R.A. & Zammit, V.A. (1985): Evidence that glucagon-mediated inhibition of acetyl-CoA carboxylase in isolated adipocytes involves increased phosphorylation of the enzyme by cyclic AMP dependent protein kinase. *Biochem. J.* **226**, 139–145.

18 Hughes, W.A. & Denton, R.M. (1976): Incorporation of ^{32}P$_i$ into pyruvate dehydrogenase in mitochondria from control and insulin-treated adipose tissue. *Nature, Lond.* **264**, 471–473.

19 Hughes, W.A., Brownsey, R.W. & Denton, R.M. (1980): Studies on the incorporation of ^{32}P-phosphate into pyruvate dehydrogenase in intact rat fat cells. Effects of insulin. *Biochem. J.* **192**, 469–481.

20 McCormack, J.G. & Denton, R.M. (1977): Evidence that fatty acid synthesis in the interscapular brown adipose tissue of cold-adapted rats is increased *in vivo* by insulin by mechanisms involving parallel activation of pyruvate dehydrogenase and acetyl-CoA carboxylase. *Biochem J.* **166**, 627–630.

21 McCormack, J.G. & Denton, R.M. (1980): Role of calcium ions in the regulation of intramitochondrial metabolism. Properties of the Ca^{2+} sensitive dehydrogenases within intact uncoupled mitochondria from the white and brown adipose tissue of the rat. *Biochem. J.* **190**, 95–105.

22 McCormack, J.G. & Denton, R.M. (1981): Activation of pyruvate dehydrogenase in the perfused rat heart by adrenaline and other isotropic agents. *Biochem. J.* **194**, 639–643.

23 McCormack, J.G. (1982): The regulation of fatty acid synthesis in brown adipose tissue by insulin. *Prog. Lipid Res.* **21**, 195–223.

24 Marshall, S.E., McCormack, J.G. & Denton, R.M. (1984): Role of Ca^{2+} ions in the regulation of intramitochondrial metabolism in rat epididymal adipose tissue. Evidence against a role for Ca^{2+} in the activation of pyruvate dehydrogenase by insulin. *Biochem. J.* **218**, 249–260.

25 Martin, B.R.., Denton, R.M., Pask, H. & Randle, P.J. (1972): Mechanisms regulating adipose tissue pyruvate dehydrogenase. *Biochem. J.* **129**, 763–773.

26 Numa, S. & Tanabe, T. (1984): Acetyl-CoA carboxylase and its regulation. In *Fatty acid metabolism and its regulation*, ed S. Numa, pp. 1–27. (New Comprehensive Biochemistry, Vol. 7) Amsterdam: Elsevier.

27 Oviasu, O.A. & Whitton, P.D. (1984): Hormonal control of pyruvate dehydrogenase activity in rat liver. *Biochem. J.* **224**, 181–186.

28 Stansbie, D., Brownsey, R.W., Crettaz, M. & Denton, R.M. (1976): Acute effects *in vivo* of anti-insulin serum on rates of fatty acid synthesis and activities of acetyl-CoA carboxylase and pyruvate dehydrogenase in liver and epididymal adipose tissue of fed rats. *Biochem. J.* **160**, 413–416.

29 Tavaré, J.M., Smyth, J.E., Borthwick, A.C., Brownsey, R.W. & Denton, R.M. (1985): Insulin activated acetyl-CoA carboxylase kinase in triton extracts of human placenta membranes. *Biochem. Soc. Trans.* (In press).

Distinction between white and brown adipose tissue

Myriam NECHAD
*Laboratoire de Physiologie Comparée, CNRS UA 307, Université P. et M. Curie, 4, place Jussieu, F-75230
Paris Cedex 05, France.*

It is well established that there are two kinds of adipose tissue: the familiar white adipose tissue
(WAT) and brown adipose tissue (BAT). With the exception of hibernators and some other
small mammals, BAT is generally prominent only in the new-born and, later on, it progressively
takes on the appearance of WAT (review in[21]). This, together with some other similarities
between the two tissues, has led to the contention that BAT and WAT were nothing more than
two different forms of the same tissue and therefore were capable of interconversion. However,
such an interpretation is hardly reconcilable with the fact that BAT is a potent thermogenic
effector (review in[10,13]). The recognition of this function about 20 years ago has been followed by
a very rapid progress in BAT research and it will be shown here that BAT is now known to
possess a number of structural, functional and developmental characteristics which together
designate it as a tissue quite different from WAT.

Structural features. The discrimination between BAT and WAT is very easy when these
tissues are in their typical form. Besides its colour, the most obvious feature of BAT is the
multilocularity of its lipid deposits: functional brown adipocytes store triglycerides in the form
of several fat droplets dispersed throughout their cytoplasm. Therefore, BAT is still often called
multilocular adipose tissue in contrast with the unilocular WAT. However, such a method of
distinction between BAT and WAT is very misleading and should be abandoned since
differentiating white adipocytes are also multilocular before transforming into signet-ring cells.
Furthermore, the multilocularity of the fat stores is far from being a permanent characteristic of
BAT: it is entirely dependent on the metabolic activity of the tissue.

The structure of the mitochondria is undoubtedly a much better criterion to distinguish
between WAT and BAT. In BAT, these organelles are very abundant and their mean volume is
about four times larger than that of WAT mitochondria[18]. Their cristae generally are parallel,
tightly packed and extend across the whole width of the organelle. Thus, the concentration of
respiratory enzymes and electron transport components is much higher in BAT than in WAT
(review in[13]). Typically, the amount of ATP synthetase in BAT mitochondrial inner membrane
is small compared with the amount of respiratory chain enzymes. Therefore, contrary to what
occurs in other tissues, the chemical energy released by substrate oxidation is converted only to
a small extent into ATP. Most of it is dissipated as heat, due to an inner membrane protein
called 'uncoupling protein' or 'thermogenin', which appears to be specific for BAT (review
in[3,17]). Attempts to demonstrate its presence in WAT mitochondria were negative[2].

BAT and WAT can be distinguished from each other further by comparison of their
vascularization and innervation. Both tissues are supplied by a dense capillary network which
surrounds each adipocyte, but the blood flow in BAT is very much higher than in WAT[7,8,20].
Both are innervated by the sympathetic nervous system but, as illustrated by the very large
difference in noradrenaline content between the two tissues, this innervation is much denser in
BAT[9,14,22]. Vessels and adipocytes receive noradrenergic terminals, and this was earlier
thought to be a distinguishing characteristic of BAT[5]. Such a double innervation has now been
shown to occur also in WAT, but to a much smaller extent (review in[9,20]).

Functional features. Whereas the structure of a tissue generally varies with the functional
activity of this tissue, its function is a permanent feature and therefore is the best criterion to
characterize the tissue considered. The primary function of WAT is to store food energy in order
to maintain a stable fuel supply for all other tissues. Lipolysis is activated and fatty acids
released in all situations when other tissues need substrate. On the contrary, the function of
BAT is to combust food energy and to dissipate it as heat.

In good agreement with this, while the anatomical localization of WAT is diffuse and mainly superficial, BAT occurs at specific sites (around the major blood vessels and the vital organs) which are mainly internal (review in[13,21]). It has recently been shown to be a dominant site of both cold-induced nonshivering thermogenesis and diet-induced thermogenesis in rodents. Fatty acids released by lipolysis in response to the activation of BAT by cold or overeating are very rapidly oxidized by the mitochondria which thus produce heat. The oxygen consumption rate and the thermogenic potential of BAT cells are tremendous, compared with that of WAT cells, and this requires a sustained supply of substrate to the mitochondria. Consistent with this, lipoprotein lipase activity is stimulated by the sympathetic activity in the tissue; it appears to be unchanged by insulin, while the opposite seems to occur in WAT[1,4]. Furthermore, fatty acid synthesis is much higher in BAT than in WAT (review in[16,17]).

Developmental features. The similarities between the developmental features of BAT and WAT are the main reason for the hesitation in regarding these tissues as two distinct entities. Indeed, brown and white adipocytes originate from morphologically similar precursors, perivascular mesenchymal cells (review in[11]). As described above, functional BAT is structurally very different from WAT but, in the absence of sympathetic activation, the metabolic activity of BAT and the blood flow perfusing it decrease rapidly, the adipocytes accumulate fat, become unilocular and their mitochondria involute. BAT is then morphologically indistinguishable from WAT.

However, there is now good evidence that these similarities between the two tissues are merely morphological. Indeed, BAT and WAT precursor cells cultured in parallel in identical conditions show different developmental patterns: after one week *in vitro*, the BAT cells contain many more mitochondria than the WAT cells and are multilocular, whereas the WAT cells show a clear tendency to unilocularity[15]. This indicates that BAT and WAT precursors are committed to develop differently. Therefore, the structural differences observed between white and brown adipocytes result from an early determination of their precursors, and not simply from differences in their neurohumoral microenvironment, as was suggested[6]. This fundamental difference between the two tissues persists even when BAT shows a WAT-like appearance: the inactive BAT which occurs in the perirenal region in adult humans is induced by chromaffin tumours to redifferentiate, while the mesenteric WAT of these patients keeps its WAT characteristics[19]. Data supporting the same line of evidence have been reported concerning the unilocular BAT of adult rabbits[12].

Conclusion. The presently available data clearly demonstrate that BAT and WAT are two different tissues. While WAT is primarily an energy store, the function of BAT is the opposite: to dissipate energy as heat. Its structure is highly specialized for this function and contrasts with that of WAT. When subject to disuse, BAT becomes morphologically similar to WAT but remains inherently different from it and capable to show BAT responses in case of stimulation.

1 Ashby, P. & Robinson, D.S. (1980: Effects of insulin, glucocorticoids and adrenalin on the activity of rat adipose-tissue lipoprotein lipase. *Biochem. J.* **188**, 185–192.

2 Cannon, B., Hedin, A. & Nedergaard, J. (1982): Exclusive occurrence of thermogenin antigen in brown adipose tissue. *FEBS Lett.* **150**, 129–132.

3 Cannon, B. & Nedergaard, J. (1985): The biochemistry of an 'inefficient' tissue: brown adipose tissue. *Essays Biochem.* **20**, 110–164.

4 Carneheim, C., Nedergaard, J. & Cannon, B. (1984): Beta-adrenergic stimulation of lipoprotein lipase activity in rat brown adipose tissue during acclimation to cold. *Am. J. Physiol.* **246**, E327–E333.

5 Daniel, H. & Derry, D.M. (1969): Criteria for differentiation of brown and white fat in the rat. *Can. J. Physiol. Pharmacol.* **47**, 941–945.

6 Derry, D.M., Morrow, E., Sadre, N. & Flattery, K.V. (1972): Brown and white fat during the life of the rabbit. *Dev. Biol.* **27**, 204–216.

7 Fawcett, D.W. (1952): A comparison of the histological organization and cytochemical reactions of brown and white adipose tissues. *J. Morphol.* **90**, 363–405.

8 Foster, D.O. & Frydman, M.L. (1979): Tissue distribution of cold-induced thermogenesis in conscious warm- or cold-acclimated rats reevaluated from changes in tissue blood flow: The dominant role of brown adipose tissue in the replacement of shivering by nonshivering thermogenesis. *Can. J. Physiol. Pharmacol.* **57**, 257–270.

9 Fredholm, B.B. (1985): Nervous control of circulation and metabolism in white adipose tissue. In *New perspectives in adipose tissue*, ed R. Van & A. Cryer, pp. 45–64. London: Butterworth.

10 Girardier, L. (1983): Brown fat: an energy dissipating tissue. In *Mammalian thermogenesis*, ed L. Girardier & M.J. Stock, pp. 50–98. London: Chapman & Hall.

11 Hausman, G.J., Campion, D.R. & Martin, R.J. (1980): Search for the adipocyte precursor cell and factors that promote its differentiation. *J. Lipid Res.* **21**, 657–670.

12 Kumon, A., Hara, T. & Takahashi, A. (1976): Effects of catecholamines on the lipolysis of two kinds of fat cells from adult rabbit. *J. Lipid Res.* **17**, 559–564.

13 Lindberg, O. (ed) (1970): *Brown adipose tissue*. New York: American Elsevier.

14 Mory, G., Combes-George, M. & Néchad, M. (1983): Localization of serotonin and dopamine in the brown adipose tissue of the rat and their variations during cold exposure. *Biol. Cell* **48**, 159–166.

15 Néchad, M., Kuusela, P., Carneheim, C. Björntorp, P., Nedergaard, J. & Cannon, B. (1983): Development of brown fat cells in monolayer culture. I. Morphological and biochemical distinction from white fat cells in culture. *Exp. Cell Res.* **149**, 105–118.

16 Nedergaard, J. & Lindberg, O. (1982): The brown fat cell. *Int. Rev. Cytol.* **74**, 187–286.

17 Nicholls, D.G. & Locke, R.M. (1984): Thermogenic mechanisms in brown fat. *Physiol. Rev.* **64**, 1–64.

18 Rafael, J., Huesh, M., Stratmann, D. & Hohorst, H.-J. (1970): Mitochondrien aus braunem und weissem Fettgewebe: Struktur, Enzymprofil und oxidative Phosphoryluerung. *Hoppe Seylers Z. Physiol. Chem.* **351**, 1513–1523.

19 Ricquier, D., Néchad, M. & Mory, G. (1982): Ultrastructural and biochemical characterization of human brown adipose tissue in pheochromocytoma. *J. Clin. Endocrinol. Metab.* **54**, 803–807.

20 Rosell, S. & Belfrage, E. (1979): Blood circulation in adipose tissue. *Physiol. Rev.* **59**, 1078–1104.

21 Smith, R.E. & Horwitz, B.A. (1969): Brown fat and thermogenesis. *Physiol. Rev.* **49**, 330–425.

22 Young, J.B., Saville, E., Rothwell, N.J., Stock, M.J. & Landsberg, L. (1982): Effect of diet and cold exposure on norepinephrine turnover in brown adipose tissue of the rat. *J. Clin. Invest.* **69**, 1061–1071.

★ ★ ★

ESSENTIAL FATTY ACIDS

Functions of the n-6 and n-3 polyunsaturated fatty acids

J.F. MEAD
Laboratory of Biomedical and Environmental Sciences, University of California, Los Angeles, 900 Veteran Avenue, Los Angeles, California 90024, USA.

Certain members of both families of polyunsaturated fatty acids (PUFA) act as precursors of the eicosanoids. This function involves largely the 20-carbon members of each family: 20:3ω6, 20:4ω6 and 20:5ω3 (Fig. 1). Arachidonic acid is the precursor of the most active and most thoroughly investigated members of this class of substances and some of the reactions and types of compounds formed are shown in Fig. 2. The ω3 family of PUFA may serve to control not only the interconversions of the members of the other families[26] but also the formation of the eicosanoid products of the other families[4,13] and some of their actions, notably platelet aggregation, since TXA_3 is a weak stimulator of aggregation whereas prostacyclin, PGI_3, is an active antiaggregation effector[4].

The ω6 and ω3 PUFA have some functions in common since members of both families can lower the melting points of fatty acid mixtures and, by the same token, the liquid crystal-gel

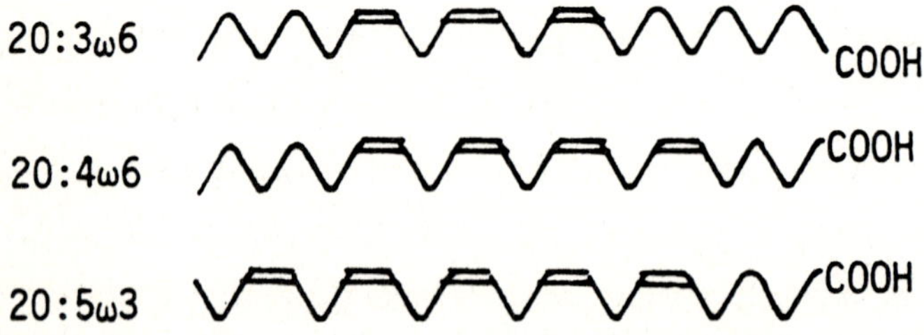

Fig. 1. *Eicosanoid precursors*

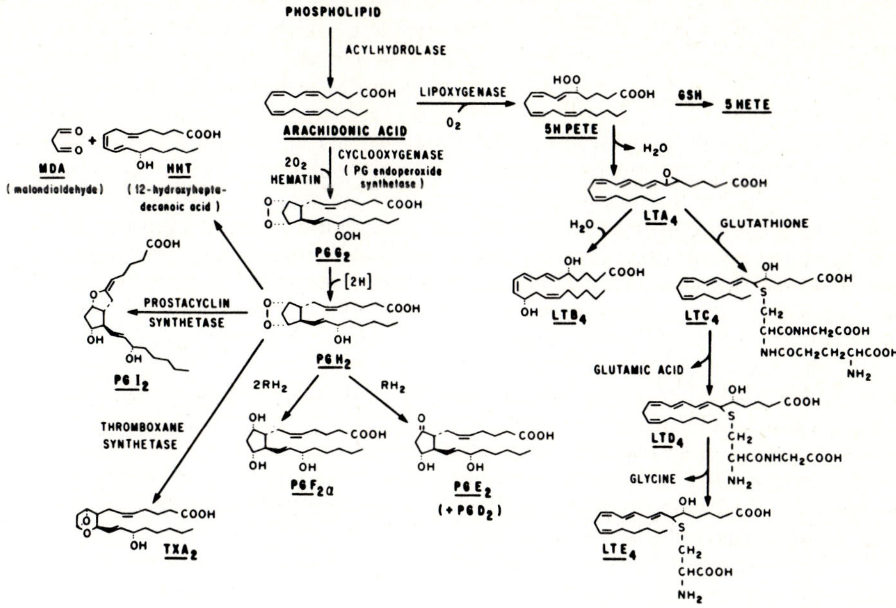

Fig. 2. *Arachidonic acid — some reactions and compounds*

transition points of membrane bilayers. The question that arises from this action is why it should be associated with a specific family of fatty acids since, presumably, any low-melting fatty acids, when incorporated into the membrane bilayer phosphoglycerides, should have the same effect. The important point is that, for most mammalian systems, polyunsaturated fatty acids are largely derived from the major dietary precursor, linoleate. Marine organisms, on the other hand, derive their PUFA largely from linolenate. Oleate is not a good PUFA precursor since its further desaturation is largely suppressed. In any event, the very important function of regulation of the viscotropic properties of membranes[7,10,29] is carried out by the unsaturated fatty acids available to the organism involved.

The assembly of the blood lipoproteins involves the same considerations and thus transport also depends, to a large extent, on the availability of the proper mix of unsaturated fatty acids[24,34].

The integrity of the skin and other membranes, as indicated by increased water passage[23], by dermatitis, and by fragility of mitochondrial and other cellular membranes in fat deficiency, appears to be prevented or cured largely by the ω6 family of PUFA and not by the ω3 family[4,14,22]. Moreover, careful study of the effects of both ω6 and ω3 PUFA on testicular development have revealed that only ω6 PUFA can prevent degeneration or restore normal development[21]. For these reasons the ω3 family has not been termed essential by most investigators even though some of its members may have important, if not vital, functions[3]. It is interesting that columbinic acid (5E,9Z,12Z-octadecatrienoic acid) can mimic most of these effects even though it is not converted to a C_{20} PUFA and does not form an active product with cyclooxygenase, in fact inhibiting it[17]. Recently, it has been reported that both columbinic acid (Fig. 3) and a lipoxygenase product, 13-hydroxy-5E-9Z-11E-octadecatrienoic acid, can reverse the scaley dermatitis of EFA deficiency[9]. The mechanism of this action, however, is not clear nor has it been shown that the oxidized product can restore normal water transport. Thus, it appears that columbinic acid can distinguish between those EFA activities that depend on conversion to prostaglandins and those that appear to be structural. A comparison of structures of columbinic and arachidonic acids reveals that they are strikingly similar.

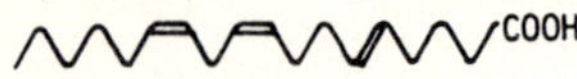

Fig. 3. *Columbinic acid*

A best guess, at the moment, is that these fatty acids, particularly arachidonic, serve as components of certain membrane lipids that act as regulators of pores or channels which facilitate the transport of water and small electrolytes or non-electrolytes across the membranes. The inner surface of the pore is hydrophilic and is provided by specific *trans*membrane proteins that carry out this function as dimers or higher oligomers[30,33]. The outer surface must, by virtue of its contact with the lipid bilayer, be hydrophobic and is in close contact with a more or less specific boundary lipid which can change its nature around the gel-liquid crystal transition point and thus control the conformation of the protein and its ability to permit or prevent access to the channels[27,31]. If the fit of the boundary lipids and transmembrane proteins is more favourable for certain phosphoglycerides and their component fatty acids, an explanation may be on hand for the specific nature of the essential fatty acids, particularly arachidonic[39].

The ω3 PUFA are required in the diet of some fish and may carry out structural functions in these organisms similar to those of the ω6 PUFA in terrestrial animals[6,40]. This difference might be partially because the more highly unsaturated members of this family have the ability to form a mixture of membrane lipids with a lower melting point than do those of the ω6 family. A more likely explanation stems from the fact that the dietary source of PUFA available to most marine organisms consists largely of the ω3 family.

They do, however, appear to have an important function in mammals even though they have not been shown to be required in the diet to prevent or cure most symptoms of fat deficiency[35,37]. Hints of the nature of this function stem first from the many analyses demonstrating that the ω3 PUFA are in unusually high concentration in the brain particularly in retinal phosphoglycerides (largely EPG[1,8,32]) and, second, the reports from several laboratories that at very low tissue concentrations of 22:6ω3 stemming from low dietary 18:3ω3, visual acuity[2,5,18,36] and, in some cases, mental abilities[19] have been impaired. Why these fatty acids should have such specific functions is not apparent at this time but it may be significant that in the retinal rod outer membranes, a GPE has been reported with the hazardous composition of 1,2-di 22:6[12]. Apparently, the properties imparted to the membranes by a phosphoglyceride of this composition are sufficiently vital to risk the ready susceptibility of the lipid to peroxidation. One report has implicated linolenic acid as a participant of photosynthetic reactions in plants[38] but it is a large jump from a function of 18:3 in plants to one of 22:6 in mammalian retinal rods. As is always the case when functions of a substance are unclear, there have been many reports ascribing typical EFA properties to the ω3 PUFA[11,16,28]. However, since there have also been several reports denying these properties[20,25], a definitive answer to the question of ω3 PUFA essentiality in mammals has not been decided[3].

1 Alling, C., Bruce, A., Karlson, I. & Svennerholm, L. (1974): Effect of different dietary levels of essential fatty acids on lipids of rat cerebrum during maturation. *J. Neurochem.* **23**, 1265–1270.
2 Anonymous (1974): Essential fatty acid deficiency and the photoreceptors. *Nutr. Rev.* **32**, 342–345.
3 Anonymous (1979): Linolenic acid, an essential fatty acid? *Nutr. Rev.* **37**, 296–297.
4 Anonymous (1979): Does eicosapentaenoic acid prevent thrombosis and atherosclerosis? *Nutr. Rev.* **37**, 316–317.
5 Benoiken, R.M., Anderson, R.E. & Wheeler, T.G. (1973): Membrane fatty acids associated with the electrical response in visual excitation. *Science* **182**, 1253–1254.
6 Castell, J.D., Lee, D.J. & Wales, J.H. (1972): Essential fatty acids in the diet of the rainbow trout (*Salmo gairdneri*): growth, feed conversion and some gross deficiency symptoms. *J. Nutr.* **102**, 77–86.
7 Cornwell, D.G. & Patil, G.S. (1977): Surface chemistry and the physical properties of polyunsaturated fatty acid-containing lipids. In *Symposium of polyunsaturated fatty acids*, ed W.H. Kunau & R.T. Holman, Chapter 7. Champaign, IL: Am. Oil Chem. Soc.
8 Dhopeshwarkar, G.A. & Subramanian, C. (1975): Metabolism of linolenic acid in developing brain: Incorporation of radioactivity from [1-¹⁴C] linolenic acid into (1) Brain fatty acids; (2) Brain lipids. *Lipids* **10**, 238–241; 241–247.
9 Elliott, W.J., Morrison, A.R., Sprecher, H.W. & Needleman, P. (1985): The metabolic transformations of columbinic acid and the effect of topical application of the major metabolites on rat skin. *J. Biol. Chem.* **260**, 987–992.
10 Esfahani, M. & Devlin, T.M. (1982): Effects of lipid fluidity on quenching characteristics of tryptophan fluorescence in yeast plasma membranes. *J. Biol. Chem.* **257**, 9919–9921.

11 Fiennes, R.N., Sinclair, A.J. & Crawford, M.A. (1973): Essential fatty acid studies in primates. Linolenic acid requirements in capuchins. *J. Med. Prim.* **2**, 155–169.

12 Galli, C., Agradi, E. & Paoletti, R. (1974): The (n-6) pentaene: (n-3) Hexaene fatty acid ratio as an index of linolenic acid deficiency. *Biochim. Biophys. Acta* **369**, 142–145.

13 Hansen, H.S. & Jensen, B. (1983): Urinary prostaglandin E_2 and vasopressin excretion in essential fatty acid-deficient rats: Effect of linolenic acid supplementation. *Lipids* **18**, 682–690.

14 Holman, R.T. (1971): Biological activities of and requirements for polyunsaturated fatty acids. In *Progress in the chemistry of fats and other lipids*, ed R.T. Holman, pp. 611–682, Vol. 9. Oxford: Pergamon Press.

15 Holman, R.T. (1971): Essential fatty acid deficiency. In *Progress in the chemistry of fats and other lipids*, R.T. Holman, pp. 279–348, Vol. 9. Oxford, Pergamon Press.

16 Holman, R.T., Johnson, S.B. & Hatch, T.F. (1982): Linolenic acid deficiency in man. *Nutr. Rev.* **40**, 144–147.

17 Houtsmuller, U.M.T. (1981): Columbinic acid, a new type of essential fatty acid. In *Progress in lipid research*, ed R.T. Holman, pp. 889–896, Vol. 20. Oxford: Pergamon Press.

18 Hyman, B.T. & Spector, A.A. (1981): Accumulation of n-3 polyunsaturated fatty acids by cultured human y79 retinoblastoma cells. *J. Neurochem.* **37**, 60–69.

19 Lamptey, M.S. & Walker, B.L. (1976): A possible role for dietary linolenic acid in the development of the young rat. *J. Nutr.* **106**, 86–93.

20 Leat, W.M.F. & Northrup, C.A. (1981): Effect of dietary linoleic and linolenic acids on gestation and parturition in the rat. *Quant. J. Exp. Physiol.* **66**, 99–103.

21 Leat, W.M.F., Northrup, C.A., Davidson, K. & Harrison, F.A. (1984): The effect of n-6 and n-3 polyunsaturated fatty acids on testicular development in the rat. *Proc. Nutr. Soc.* **43**, 50A.

22 Levin, E., Johnson, R.M. & Albert, S. (1957): Mitochondrial changes associated with essential fatty acid deficiency in rats. *J. Biol. Chem.* **228**, 15–21.

23 MacMillan, A.L. & Sinclair, H.M. (1958): *Essential fatty acids*, p. 208. New York: Academic Press.

24 Massey, J.B., Gotto, A.M., Jr. & Pownall, H.J. (1981): Thermodynamics of lipid-protein interactions: interaction of apolipoprotein A-II from human plasma high-density lipoproteins with dimyristoylphosphatidylcholine. *Biochemistry* **20**, 1575–1581.

25 Meng, H.C. (1983): A case of human linolenic acid deficiency involving neurological abnormalities. *Am. J. Clin. Nutr.* **37**, 157–159.

26 Mohrhauer, H. & Holman, R.T. (1963): Effect of linolenic acid upon the metabolism of linoleic acid. *J. Nutr.* **81**, 67–74.

27 Read, B.D. & McElhaney, R.N. (1976): Influence of membrane lipid fluidity on glucose and uridine facilitated diffusion in human erythrocytes. *Biochim. Biophys. Acta* **419**, 331–341.

28 Rudin, D.O. (1982): The dominant diseases of modernized societies as omega-3-essential fatty acid deficiency syndrome: substrate beriberi. *Med. Hypotheses* **8**, 17–47.

29 Sandermann, H., Jr. (1978): Regulation of membrane enzymes by lipids. *Biochim. Biophys. Acta* **515**, 209–237.

30 Schindler, H. & Nelson, N. (1982): Proteolipid of adenosinephosphatase from yeast mitochondria forms proton-selective channels in planar lipid bilayers. *Biochemistry* **21**, 5785–5794.

31 Silvius, M.R. & McElhaney, R.N. (1980): Membrane lipid physical state and modulation of the Na^+,Mg^{2+}-ATPase activity in *Acholeplasma laidlawii B*. *Proc. Natl. Acad. Sci. USA* **77**, 1255–1259.

32 Sinclair, A.J. & Crawford, M.A. (1972): Accumulation of arachidonate and docosahexaenoate in the developing rat brain. *J. Neurochem.* **19**, 1753–1758.

33 Solomon, A.K., Chasan, B., Dix, J.A. & Lukacovik, M.F. (1983): The aqueous pore in the red cell membrane. Band 3 as a channel for anions, cations, non-electrolytes and water. *Ann. NY Acad. Sci.* **44**, 97–124.

34 Thilo, L., Trauble, H. & Overath, R. (1977): Mechanistic interpretation of the influence of lipid phase transitions in transport functions. *Biochemistry* **16**, 1283–1289.

35 Tinoco, J., Williams, M.A., Hincenbergs, I. & Lyman, R.L. (1971): Evidence for the nonessentiality of linolenic acid in the diet of the rat. *J. Nutr.* **101**, 937–946.

36 Tinoco, J., Miljanich, P. & Medwadowski, B. (1977): Depletion of docosahexaenoic acid in retinal lipids of rats fed a linolenic acid-deficient, linoleic acid-containing diet. *Biochem. Biophys. Acta* **486**, 575–578.

37 Tinoco, J., Babcok, R., Hincenbergs, I., Medwadowsky, B., Miljanich, P. & Williams, M.A. (1979): Linolenic acid deficiency. *Lipids* **14**, 166–173.

38 Vereschchagn, A.G. & Novitskaya, G.V. (1964): Anomalous ionization of methyl linolenate by metastable argon atoms: possible linolenic acid participation in photosynthetic reactions. *Nature* **203**, 1384–1385.

39 Yorek, M.A., Strom, D.K. & Spector, A.A. (1984): Effect of membrane polyunsaturation on carrier-mediated transport in cultured retinoblastoma cells: alterations in taurine uptake. *J. Neurochem.* **42**, 254–261.

40 Yu, T.C. & Sinnhuber, R.O. (1975): Effect of dietary linolenic and linoleic acids upon growth and lipid metabolism of rainbow trout (*Salmo gairdneri*). *Lipids* **10**, 63–66.

Assessment of essential fatty acid status

J.G. McLEAN and A.J. SINCLAIR
School of Veterinary Science, The University of Melbourne, Parkville, Victoria 3052; Veterinary Research Institute, Department of Agriculture of Victoria, Park Drive, Parkville, Victoria 3052, Australia.

The early assessments of essential fatty acid (EFA) status based on growth rate and severity of skin lesions were imprecise and highlighted the need for biochemical techniques which could be used to measure EFA status. The first technique applied was the measurement of the ratio of triene to tetraene fatty acids in the plasma using alkaline isomerization[19].

With the advent of gas-liquid chromatography (GLC) the triene and tetraene fatty acid fractions were partially resolved using packed columns and the ratio of 20:3(n-9) to arachidonate became the indicator of EFA status. However, with the introduction of capillary columns it was found that 20:2(n-6), 20:3(n-6) and 22:0 could contaminate the 20:3(n-9) fraction whilst 20:3(n-3) and 22:1 could cause errors in the estimation of arachidonate. A value of 0.4 was originally suggested as the upper limit for normality for the triene to tetraene ratio. This corresponded to about 1 per cent of the dietary energy as linoleic acid, for most of the species studied[10]. As analytical techniques were refined this ratio was defined as 20:3(n-9) to arachidonate and the upper limit of normality reduced to 0.2[12].

Despite the usefulness of the 20:3(n-9) to arachidonate ratio for assessment of EFA status a number of problems still remain. It has been customary to express individual fatty acids as a percentage of the total fatty acids present, but this is subject to considerable variation because it is common to arbitrarily exclude some short or long chain fatty acids from the total. In addition many of the early studies were carried out on the rat and human infant, but it is now known that there are considerable species variations in the 20:3(n-9) to arachidonate ratio and in polyunsaturated fatty acid metabolism[5] as exemplified by studies in the cat[33] and fetal and neonatal lamb[28].

Other methods have been proposed for assessing EFA status and these include measurement of total (n-6) fatty acids in tissue lipids, multiple regression techniques to relate tissue fatty acid levels to linoleic acid intake and ratios of various fatty acids in phospholipid fractions[11,30].

Although alpha-linolenic has now a well-established role as an EFA, there have been few studies which attempt to quantitatively assess its status[34]. It has been suggested that a triene to pentaene or a 20:3(n-9) to 20:5(n-3) ratio may be used as a measure of linolenic acid status[24]. A value of 0.4 for this ratio corresponded to about 0.5–1 per cent of the total dietary energy as linolenic acid and resulted in the synthesis of sufficient (n-3) long-chain polyunsaturated fatty acids (LCP) to suppress the production of 20:3(n-9)[27]. It has been shown that a characteristic feature of a linolenic acid deficiency in capuchin monkeys was an elevation in the levels of 22:4(n-6) and 22:5(n-6) relative to 22:5(n-3) and 22:6(n-3) in erythrocyte and liver phospholipids[8]. This was also found[13] in a case of linolenic acid deficiency in a human.

The EFA are now the only major nutrients the status of which is determined in such an indirect way. It is only recently that precise measurements of concentrations of EFA and LCP in food and body tissues has become more common, but there is still a need to determine optimum levels and relate these to the deficiency state. The accurate estimation of small amounts of LCP in food is important because they are readily absorbed and efficiently incorporated into tissues including the plasma and have a marked effect in alleviating EFA deficiency[24,32]. Conversely, EFA deficiency results in different tissues being depleted at varying rates and this must be quantified[20].

A standardized technique is necessary to enable comparison of results from different laboratories. The basis of this technique should include the use of suitable internal standard which is readily available, stable and reasonably priced and its use should not prolong the time taken for analyses. It was recommended that the standard fatty acid should chromatograph near the fatty acid of interest, but this introduces difficulties when all of the LCP are considered important and many are present in very small amounts[1]. Heptadecanoic acid (C17:0) is a suitable standard, although it is possible that low levels of this acid may already be present in certain extracts[2]. A heneicosanoate (C21:0) standard has been used to estimate the fatty acid content of meat[23], however this standard does not separate from arachidonate on all columns. Other methods of determining fatty acids are available, but these are unduly time consuming and hence not suitable for routine analyses[18]. Therefore, despite certain reservations, heptadecanoic is probably the only suitable standard which meets the requirements previously outlined.

The broad biological expression of EFA deficiency such as weight loss, skin and hair condition, water loss, fatty liver, impaired wound healing and resistance to infection are too non-specific to be applied to assessment of EFA status. Because tissue EFA and LCP are depleted in EFA deficiency, it has been shown that there is a significant decrease in prostaglandin level[22], and such observations indicated the possibility of using prostaglandin levels for assessment of EFA status. However, a number of factors have emerged which have made this approach unsatisfactory. The eicosanoids are present in very small amounts, are unstable and difficult to analyse. Dietary lipid manipulations can cause substantial changes in prostaglandin levels[9,17]. It has also been shown that 20:3(n-9) may be metabolised to compounds with eicosanoid-like activity and which interfere with platelet function[19]. The observation that columbinic acid (t5, c9,c12–18:3) was about as effective as arachidonic acid in alleviating most of the clinical signs of EFA deficiency, but was not converted into any eicosanoids further, complicated any use of eicosanoid measurements for assessment of EFA status[15].

Deficiencies have been recognised in the ability to desaturate dietary EFA into LCP in the cat[29], turbot[25] and cultured mammalian cells[6,21]. When investigating the EFA status of different species including man, the possibility of at least reduced ability to desaturate should not be overlooked, especially if it is associated with such factors as iron deficiency[31], hypothyroidism[7], amino acid content of the diet[26], pyridoxine deficiency[3], dietary cholesterol levels[16] and race[14].

The use of non-invasive techniques, such as metabolic studies using peripheral blood leucocytes[4], in conjunction with fatty acid profiles, should provide further insight into metabolic factors which contribute to the EFA status.

It is recommended that the EFA and LCP in food, tissues and blood components be expressed in absolute amounts per unit weight. This should be done using a suitable standard, preferably heptadecanoic acid together with capillary GLC, so that low levels of biologically important LCP may be identified and quantified. Whilst under some circumstances it may be satisfactory to determine the concentration of the individual fatty acids in the total lipid extract, much more information can be gained by determining the fatty acid concentrations in the phospholipid, unesterified fatty acid, cholesteryl ester and triglyceride fractions[28].

1 Ackman, R.G. (1980): Potential for more efficient methods for lipid analyses. *J. Am. Oil Chem. Soc.* **57**, 821A–829A.

2 Christie, W.W., Nobel, R.C. and Moore, J.H. (1970): Determination of lipid classes by a gas-chromatographic procedure. *Analyst* **95**, 940–944.

3 Cunnane, S.C., Manku, M.S. & Horrobin, D.F. (1984): Accumulation of linoleic and γ-linolenic acids in tissue lipids of pyridoxine deficient rats. *J. Nutr.* **114**, 1754–1761.

4 Cunnane, S.C., Keeling, P.W.N., Thompson, R.P.H. & Crawford, M.A. (1984): Linoleic acid and arachidonic acid metabolism in human peripheral blood leucocytes: comparison with the rat. *Br. J. Nutr.* **51**, 209–217.

5 Cunnane, S.C. & Huang, Y-S. (1985): Species comparisons of the effects of essential fatty acid deficiency on fatty acid composition of total liver phospholipids: implications for the use of 20:3(n-9) to assess EFA deficiency. In *Abstr. 2nd Int. Cong. Essential fatty acids, prostaglandins and leucotrienes*, London, p. 17.

6 Dunbar, L.M. & Bailey, J.M. (1975): Enzyme deletions and essential fatty acid metabolism in cultured cells. *J. Biol. Chem.* **250**, 1152–1153.

7 Faas, F. & Carter, W.J. (1982): Fatty acid desaturation and microsomal lipid fatty acid composition in experimental hypothyroidism. *Biochem. J.* **207**, 29–35.

8 Fiennes, R.N.T-W., Sinclair, A.J. & Crawford, M.A. (1973): Essential fatty acid studies in primates — linolenic acid requirements of capuchins. *J. Med. Primatology* **2**, 155–169.

9 Hassam, A.G., Willis, A.L., Stevens, P. & Crawford, M.A. (1979): The effects of essential fatty acid-deficient diet on the levels of prostaglandins and their fatty acid precursors in the rabbit brain. *Lipids* **14**, 78–80.

10 Holman, R.T. (1960): The ratio of trienoic: tetraenoic acids in tissue lipids as a measure of essential fatty acid requirements. *J. Nutr.* **70**, 405–410.

11 Holman, R.T. (1977): The deficiency of essential fatty acids. In *polyunsaturated fatty acids*, ed W.H. Kanau & R.T. Holman, pp. 163–182. Champaign Il: Am. Oil Chem. Soc.

12 Holman, R.T. (1978): Essential fatty acid deficiency in humans. In *CRC Handbook series in nutrition and food*, ed M. Recheigl, Vol. III, Section E (Nutritional disorders), pp. 335–368. Palm Beach: CRC Press.

13 Holman, R.T., Johnson, S.B. & Hatch, T.F. (1982): A case of human linolenic acid deficiency involving neurological abnormalities. *Amer. J. Clin. Nutr.* **35**, 617–623.

14 Horrobin, D.F. (1985): Do Eskimos and salmon-eating Canadian Indians have a pattern of essential fatty acid (EFA) metabolism different from Europeans. In *Abstr.2nd Int. Cong. Essential fatty acids, prostaglandins and leucotrienes*, London, p. 57.

15 Houstmuller, U.M.T. (1981): Columbinic acid. A new type of essential fatty acid. *Prog. Lipid Res.* **20**, 889–896.

16 Huang, Y.S., Manku, M.S. & Horrobin, D.F. (1984): The effects of dietary cholesterol on blood and liver polyunsaturated fatty acids and on plasma cholesterol in rats fed various types of fatty acid diet. *Lipids* **19**, 664–672.

17 Hwang, D.H. & Kinsella, J.E. (1979): The effects of trans trans methyl linoleate on the concentration of prostaglandins and their precursors in the rat. *Prostaglandins* **27**, 543–559.

18 Kagawa, Y., Nishizawa, M., Suzuki, M., Miyatake, T., Hamamoto, T., Goto, K., Motonaga, E., Izumikawa, H., Hirata, H. & Ebihara, A. (1982): Eicosapolyenoic acids of serum lipids of Japanese islanders with a low incidence of cardiovascular diseases. *J. Nutr. Sci. Vitaminol.* **28**, 441–453.

19 Lagarde, M., Burtin, M., Sprecher, H., Dechavanne, M. & Renaud, S. (1983): Potentiating effect of 5,8,11-eicosatrienoic acid on human platelet aggregation. *Lipids* **18**, 291–294.

20 Lefkowith, J.B. & Needleman, P. (1985): Role and manipulation of eicosanoids in essential fatty acid deficiency. In *Abstr. 2nd Int. Cong. Essential fatty acids, prostaglandins and leucotrienes*, London, p. 154.

21 Maeda, M., Doi, O. & Akamatsu, Y. (1978): Metabolic conversion of polyunsaturated fatty acids in mammalian cultured cells. *Biochim. Biophys. Acta* **530**, 153–164.

22 Mathias, M.M. & Dupont, J. (1979): The relationship of dietary fats to prostaglandin biosynthesis. *Lipids* **14**, 247–252.

23 Maxwell, R.J. & Marmer, W.N. (1983): Systematic protocol for the accumulation of fatty acid data from multiple tissue samples: tissue handling, lipid extraction and class separation, and capillary gas chromatographic analysis. *Lipids* **18**, 453–459.

24 Mohrhauer, H. & Holman, R.T. (1963): The effect of dose level of essential fatty acids upon fatty acid composition of the rat liver. *J. Lipid Res.* **4**, 151–159.

25 Owen, J.M., Andron, J.W., Middleton, C. & Cowey, C.B. (1975): Elongation and desaturation of dietary fatty acid in turbot *Scophthalmus maximus* L., and rainbow trout *Salmo gairdnerii*, Rich. *Lipids* **10**, 528–531.

26 Peluffo, R.O., Nervi, A.M., Gonzales, M.S. & Brenner, R.R. (1984): Effect of different amino acid diets on $\Delta 5$, $\Delta 6$ and $\Delta 9$ desaturases. *Lipids* **19**, 154–157.

27 Pudelkewicz, C., Seufert, J. & Holman, R.T. (1968): Requirements of the female rat for linoleic and linolenic acids. *J. Nutr.* **94**, 138–146.

28 Rajion, M.A., McLean, J.G. and Cahill, R.N.P. (1985): Essential fatty acids in the fetal and newborn lamb. *Aust. J. Biol. Sci.* **38**, 33–40.

29 Rivers, J.P.W., Sinclair, A.J. & Crawford, M.A. (1975): Inability of the cat to desaturate essential fatty acids. *Nature* **258**, 171–173.

30 Rivers, J.P.W. & Frankel, T.L. (1981): Essential fatty acid deficiency. *Br. Med. Bull.* **37**, 59–64.

31 Sherman, A.R., Bartholmey, S.J. & Perkins, E.G. (1982): Fatty acid patterns in iron-deficient maternal and neonatal rats. *Lipids* **17**, 639–643.

32 Sinclair, A.J. & Collins, F.D. (1970): The effect of dietary essential fatty acids on the concentration of serum and liver lipids in the rat. *Br. J. Nutr.* **24**, 971–981.

33 Sinclair, A.J., Slattery, W., McLean, J.G. & Monger, E.A. (1981): Essential fatty acid deficiency and evidence for arachidonate synthesis in the cat. *Br. J. Nutr.* **46**, 93–96.

34 Tinoco, J. (1982): Dietary requirements and functions of α-linolenic acid in animals. *Prog. Lipid Res.* **21**, 1–45.

Dietary essential fatty acids and prostaglandin formation *in vivo*

H.S. HANSEN
Biochemical Laboratory, Royal Danish School of Pharmacy, Universitetsparken 2, DK-2100 Copenhagen Ø, Denmark.

In 1964 it was discovered that arachidonic acid, C20:4(n-6), is a precursor of the diene prostaglandins and since then it has been shown that many other polyunsaturated fatty acids can be transformed by the same enzymatic pathways, Fig. 1. The oxidation products of C20-polyunsaturated fatty acids are called eicosanoids. The physiological significance of most of these eicosanoids are at present unknown, but many different pharmacological effects have been identified. As the discovery of many of the eicosanoids has been made very recently, nutritional studies related to their formation have been related mainly to products of the cyclo-oxygenase pathway, ie prostaglandins, thromboxanes, and prostacylins. Prostaglandins seem to be involved in cardiovascular, renal, and gastro-intestinal physiology as well as in several pathological conditions[2]. Some postulated physiological roles of prostaglandins are summarized in Table 1.

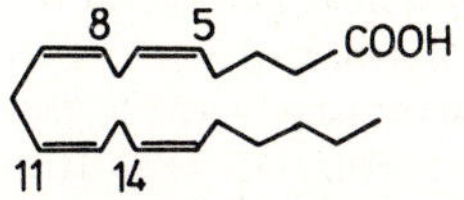

Arachidonic acid — C20:4(n-6)
Formation of eicosanoids

	20:3(n-9)	20:3(n-6)	20:4(n-6)	20:5(n-3)
Prostaglandins and thromboxanes	no	+	+	+
Prostacyclins	no	no	+	+
5-lipoxygenase	+	no	+	+
12-lipoxygenase	+	+	+	+
15-lipoxygenase	no	+	+	+
Cytochrome P_{450}	+	+	+	+

Fig. 1. *The figure shows the ways in which some of the most important of the C20-polyunsaturated fatty acids act as substrates for eicosanoid formation.*

Generally, a cell produces only one or a few eicosanoids. In many cases the prostaglandins can be considered as a defense system (Table 1), which is mobilized during physiological stress, eg normal renal blood flow in the conscious unstressed state is only minimally dependent on renal prostaglandin synthesis, whereas kidney function during extracellular volume depletion and low renal perfusion pressure seems to be dependent on regulatory prostaglandins to some extent[10]. Pathophysiological conditions in which prostaglandin production is increased and in which well-known prostaglandin synthesis inhibitors exert an effect are shown in Table 2.

Precursor pools. In human plasma the concentration of non-esterified arachidonic acid is of the order of 10^{-6} m mol/l[16]. This non-esterified arachidonic acid, the turnover rate of which seems to be closely controlled[15], is probably not available for PG production. The PG-forming cyclo-oxygenase is located in the endoplasmic reticulum in the interior of the cell where the concentration of free arachidonic acid is kept low by esterification by an arachidonyl-CoA synthetase[34]. Arachidonic acid is mainly esterified in the *sn*-2 position of phospholipids. Among the different types of phospholipids phosphatidylinositol may be especially rich in arachidonic

Table 1. *Postulated physiological functions of prostaglandins (TX — thromboxane, PGE & PGF — prostaglandins, PGI — prostacyclin)*

System	PG involved
Cardiovascular	
platelet aggregation	TXA_2, PGI_2
blood flow	PGI_2, PGE_2
closure of ductus arteriosus	PGI_2, PGE_2
Renal	
renin release	PGI_2
water excretion (vasopressin)	PGE_2
blood flow	PGE_2, PGI_2
Gastro-intestinal	
'cytoprotective' effect	PGE_2
blood flow	PGE_2
Reproductive	
uterus contraction	$PGF_{2\alpha}$
luteolysis (non-primate mammals)	$PGF_{2\alpha}$

Table 2. *Conditions of increased eicosanoid formation. (LT — leucotriene, TX — thromboxane, PG — prostaglandin).*

Inflammation (PGE_2, LTs)
Allergic reactions (PGs, TXA_2, LTs)
Mastocytosis (PGD_2)
Hypercalcaemia of cancer (PGE_2)
Bartters syndrome (PGI_2)
Patent ductus arteriosus (PGE_2, PGI_2)
Dysmenorrhoea ($PGF_{2\alpha}$)

acid[32]. The size and types of pool(s) of arachidonate available for eicosanoid production is not known. In platelets arachidonate seems to be derived from both phosphatidylinositol and phosphatidylcholine[30]. It is not clear whether lipoxygenase products and cyclo-oxygenase products originate from the same pool of arachidonic acid, nor is it clear whether different types of stimuli will affect the same pools of arachidonate. Finally it is not clear whether a stimulatory compound in a dose dependent manner will affect the same pool of arachidonate or whether other pools of arachidonate are activated simultaneously. These points are important, especially for an evaluation of the effect of dietary polyunsaturated fatty acids on prostaglandin production. This is because the amount and type of different fatty acids esterified in those phospholipids which serve as storage pools are of great importance for the amount and type of eicosanoids which are formed[18]. Certain polyunsaturated fatty acids are inhibitory or may compete with arachidonate at different enzymatic steps[28]. Figure 2 shows the pathways of free arachidonate in the cell. Release of arachidonate from the phospholipid precursor pool is the triggering step in eicosanoid formation but it is not known to what extent the different metabolic pathways for arachidonate influence the amount of eicosanoid formed.

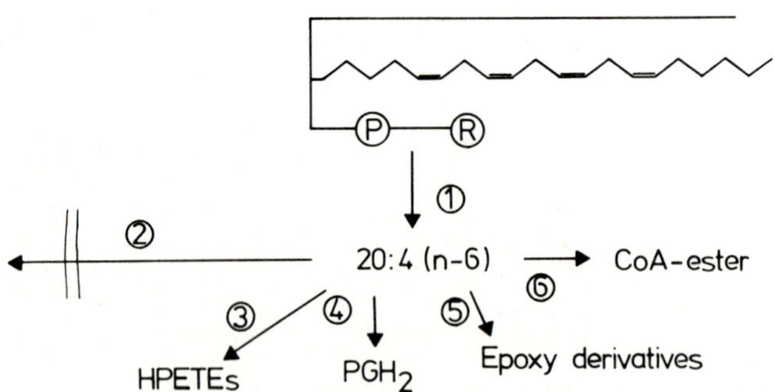

Fig. 2. *Pathways for turnover of intracellular free arachidonic acid.* HPETE: hydroperoxyeicosatretraenoic acid. PGH_2: prostaglandin H_2. (1) release from phospholipid by acylhydrolases; (2) export from the cell; (3) conversion by different lipoxygenases; (4) conversion by cyclo-oxygenase; (5) conversion by cytochrome P_{450}, and (6) esterification by acyl-CoA synthetase.

***In vivo* measurements of eicosanoids in relation to dietary intake of polyunsaturated fatty acid.** From a nutritional point of view there are two aspects of interest in the relationship between essential fatty acids and eicosanoids, ie: (1) is eicosanoid formation decreased during EFA-deficiency and can this explain the description of classical EFA-deficiency symptoms[3,4]; (2) is it possible by dietary means to influence eicosanoid production and thereby influencing physiological or patho-physiological functions?

We have studied urinary PGE_2 excretion in the rat as an example of prostaglandin formation *in vivo*. Prostaglandin E_2 excreted in the urine originates in the kidney where it probably enters the tubule at the level of the loop of Henle[36]. There are several factors besides the biosynthesis of prostaglandins which may influence the level of prostaglandins in urine, eg catabolism both before and after entering the tubular fluid[6,7], pH of tubular fluid[23], urine flow rate[27], but these factors were unlikely to have operated in our experimental rats and we assume therefore, that our measurements of urinary PGE_2 excretion can be used as an index of renal PGE_2 production.

Studies on urinary PGE_2 excretion in the rat in relation to dietary essential fatty acids may be summarized as follows. (1) Urinary PGE_2 excretion can be decreased in EFA-deficient rats, ie young rats fed a fat free diet[17,25], or adult rats starved to nearly half their initial weight and then fed an EFA-deficient diet[8]. However, without the use of severe starvation it takes several weeks before a decreased urinary PGE_2 excretion can be detected[19,31]. (2) The activity of the renal prostaglandin synthetase seems to be increased during EFA-deficiency[26]. (3) Endogenous accumulation of 20:3(n-9) in kidney lipids seems not to affect urinary PGE_2 excretion ([20]Hansen and Jensen, unpublished results). (4) Changing the dietary level of 18:2(n-6) for several weeks in non-EFA-deficient rats seems not to influence urinary PGE_2 excretion[5,7,9,17]. In a study of the effect on urinary PGE_2 excretion by young rats of varying amounts of dietary linoleate (range 0–30 per cent of energy) for 3 months a very good correlation between these two parameters was found[31], but the slope of the correlation curve was rather shallow. Rats raised for three generations on diets containing either 0.3 or 3.0 per cent of energy as linoleate showed a two-fold difference in urinary $PGE_{2\alpha}$ excretion[1]. (5) Feeding (n-3)-fatty acids for several weeks, resulting in the accumulation of 20:5(n-3) in kidney lipids, seems not to affect urinary PGE_2 excretion readily[9,19]. Feeding of 20:3(n-6) to rats seems to increase urinary PGE_1 excretion rather specifically[12,22]. Generally, the formation of PGE_1 is much lower than PGE_2 probably due to the low amounts of 20:3(n-6) in tissue lipids[18].

The overall picture of urinary PGE_2 excretion in the rat indicate that renal PGE_2 formation *in vivo* in non-deficient rats is unaffected by moderate changes over longer periods (weeks) in dietary EFA intake. We have observed that induction of EFA-deficiency in weanling rats results in the appearance of EFA-deficiency symptoms (eg increased evaporative water loss) several weeks before a decrease in urinary PGE_2 excretion can be seen[19]. Our results then seem to show that a decreased production of arachidonic acid metabolites does not explain the appearance of most of the classical EFA-deficiency symptoms. Furthermore, (1) the use of well-known inhibitors of prostaglandin synthesis does not result in the appearance of EFA-deficiency symptoms; (2) columbinic acid (5trans, 9cis, 12cis–18:2) can prevent or reduce some of the EFA-deficiency symptoms, although it is not a prostaglandin precursor[24] and, (3) in the cat, which has a very low capacity for formation of arachidonate from linoleate, dietary linoleate can prevent most of the EFA-deficiency symptoms, eg transepidermal water loss[29]. Linoleic acid apparently has an essential function in the epidermal water premeability barrier of all mammals[21,35]. However, several reports have shown that dietary EFA can affect the formation of other prostaglandins *in vivo* and that this brings about changes in physiological or pathophysiological conditions. Thus, it has been suggested that 20:5(n-3) in the diet of Greenland Eskimos could be the reason for the increased bleeding time[11] and the low risk of coronary heart disease observed in this population and it has been shown that increased intake of 20:5(n-3) by male European volunteers decreased the formation of TXB_2 + TXB_3, and increased the formation of PGI_2 and PGI_3 measured as urinary metabolites[13]. Analyses of urine from Greenland Eskimos living on their traditional diet reveal a similar pattern of metabolites as found in these volunteers[14].

Another example involves the hypercalcaemia of cancer. Some tumours produce large amounts of PGE_2 and it has been postulated that PGE_2 mediates an increase of plasma Ca^{2+} concentrations. In a murine model of hypercalcaemia of cancer, dietary supplementation with menhaden oil for 5–6 weeks resulted in a decrease in plasma Ca^{2+} concentrations as well as plasma levels of 15 keto-13,14-dihydro-PGE_2 as measured by radioimmunoassay[33]. This PGE_2 metabolite in blood can be used as a reliable index of endogenous PG formation[12].

Acknowledgements. E. Aaes-Jørgensen and B. Jensen are thanked for critical reading of the manuscript. The work from this laboratory which is described in this paper has been supported by the Danish Fat Research Foundation and the Danish Medical Research Council (J. No.: 12–4175, 12–4449, 12–4950, and 82–4620).

 1 Alling, C., Becker, W., Jones, A.W. & Änggård, E. (1984): Effects of chronic ethanol treatment on lipid composition and prostaglandins in rats fed essential fatty acid deficient diets. *Alcohol Clin. Exp. Res.* **8**, 238–247.

 2 Änggård, E. (1983): Prostaglandins and related compounds — a general physiological control system. *Scand, J. Urol. Nephrol.* **S75**, 11–18.

 3 Burr, G.O. & Burr, M.M. (1929): A new deficiency disease produced by rigid exclusion of fat from the diet. *J. Biol. Chem.* **82**, 345–367.

 4 Burr, G.O. & Burr, M.M. (1930): On the nature and role of the fatty acids essential in nutrition. *J. Biol. Chem.* **86**, 587–621.

 5 Cachofeiro, V., Lahera, V., Durán, F., Cañizo, F.J., Rodriguez, F.J. & Tresguerres, J.A.F. (1985): Antihypertensive action of dietary linoleic acid. Effects on plasma renin activity, prostaglandins and sodium excretion. *Progr. Lipid Res.* (In press).

 6 Cagen, L.M. & Kauker, M.L. (1983): Metabolism of intratubular prostaglandin E_2 in the rat kidney. *Biochem. Pharmacol.* **32**, 3665–3668.

 7 Cagen, M.L., Killmar, J.T., Warren, W. & Baer, P.G. (1985): Estradiol is responsible for reduced renal prostaglandin dehydrogenase activity in female rats. *Biochim. Biophys. Acta* **833**, 372–378.

 8 Cox, J.W., Rutechi, G.W., Fransisco, L.L. & Ferris, T.F. (1982): Studies of the effects of essential fatty acid-deficiency in the rat. *Circ. Res.* **51**, 694–702.

 9 Croft, K.D., Beilin, L.J., Vandongen, R. & Mathews, E. (1984): Dietary modification of fatty acid and prostaglandin synthesis in the rat. Effect of variations in the level of dietary fat. *Biochim. Biophys. Acta* **795**, 196–207.

10 Dunn, M.J. (1984): Nonsteroidal antiinflammatory drugs and renal function. *Ann. Rev. Med.* **35**, 411–428.

11 Dyerberg, J. & Bang, H.O. (1978): Dietary fat and thrombosis. *Lancet* **1**, 152.

12 Ellis, C.K., Whorton, R., Oelz, O., Sweetman, B.J., Wilkinson, G.R. & Oates, J.A. (1977): Enhanced renal prostaglandin synthesis in renal hypertensive rats fed dihomo-γ-linolenic acid. *Fed. Proc.* **36**, 402.

13 Fischer, S. & Weber, P.C. (1984): Prostaglandin I_3 is formed *in vivo* in man after dietary eicosapentaenoic acid. *Nature* **307**, 165–168.

14 Fischer, S., Weber, P.C. & Dyerberg, J. (1985): The prostacyclin-thromboxane balance is favourably shifted in Greenland Eskimos. *2nd Int. Congr. Essential fatty acids, prostaglandins and leukotrienes*, London, abstract 227.

15 Hagenfeldt, L. (1975): Turnover of individual free fatty acids in man. *Fed. Proc.* **34**, 2246–2249.

16 Hagenfeldt, L., Hagenfeldt, K. & Wennmalm, A. (1975): Turnover of plasma free arachidonic and oleic acid in man and women. *Hormone Metab. Res.* **7**, 467–470.

17 Hansen, H.S. (1981): Essential fatty acid-supplemented diet increases renal excretion of prostaglandin E_2 and water in essential fatty acid-deficient rats. *Lipids* **16**, 849–854.

18 Hansen, H.S. (1983): Dietary essential fatty acids and *in vivo* prostaglandin production in mammals. *Wld Rev. Nutr. Diet.* **42**, 102–134.

19 Hansen, H.S. & Jensen, B. (1983): Urinary prostaglandin E_2 and vasopressin excretion in essential fatty acid-deficient rats: Effect of linolenic acid supplementation. *Lipids* **18**, 682–690.

20 Hansen, H.S. & Jensen, B. (1985): The effect of a single oral dose of ethyl linoleate on urinary prostaglandin E_2 excretion in essential fatty acid-deficient rats. *J. Nutr.* **115**, 39–44.

21 Hansen, H.S. & Jensen, B. (1985): Essential function of linoleic acid esterified in acylglucosylceramide and acylceramide in maintaining the epidermal water permeability barrier. Evidence from feeding studies with oleate, linoleate, arachidonate, columbinate and α-linolenate. *Biochim. Biophys. Acta* **534**, 357–363.

22 Hassall, C.H. & Kirtland, S.J. (1984): Dihomo-γ-linolenic acid reverses hypertension induced in rats by diets rich in saturated fats. *Lipids* **19**, 699–703.

23 Haylor, J., Lote, C.J. & Thewles, A. (1984): Urinary pH as a determinant of prostaglandin E_2 excretion by the conscious rat. *Clin. Sci.* **66**, 675–681.

24 Houtsmüller, U.M.T. (1981): Columbinic acid, a new type of essential fatty acid. *Progr. Lipid Res.* **20**, 889–896.

25 Huang, Y.S., Mitchell, J., Jenkins, K., Manku, M.A. & Horrobin, D.F. (1984): Effect of dietary depletion and repletion of linoleic acid on renal fatty acid composition and urinary prostaglandin excretion. *Prostagland. Leuk. Med.* **15**, 223–228.

26 Kaa, E. (1976): *In vitro* biosynthesis of prostaglandin E_2 by kidney medulla of essential fatty acid-deficient rats. *Lipids* **11**, 693–696.

27 Kirschenbaum, M.A. & Serros, E.R. (1980): Effects of alterations in urine flow rate on prostaglandin E excretion in conscious dogs. *Am. J. Physiol.* **238**, F107–F111.

28 Lands, W.E.M., Hemler, M.E. & Crawford, C.G. (1977): Functions of polyunsaturated fatty acids: biosynthesis of prostaglandins. In *Polyunsaturated fatty acids*, ed W.H. Kunau & R.T. Holman, pp. 193–228, Champaign Il: American Oil Chemist' Society.

29 MacDonald, M.L., Rogers, Q.R. & Morris, J.G. (1984): Nutrition of the domestic cat, a mammalian carnivore. *Ann. Rev. Nutr.* **4**, 521–562.

30 Majerus, P.W., Wilson, D.B., Connolly, T.M., Bross, T.E. & Neufeld, E.J. (1985): Phosphoinositide turnover provides a link in stimulus-response coupling. *Trends Biochem. Sci.* **10**, 168–171.

31 Mathias, M.M. & Mauldin, R.E. (1985): Urinary excretion of prostanoids by rats fed varying amounts of linoleate. *2nd Int. Congr. Essential fatty acids, prostaglandins & leukotrienes*, London, Abstract 124.

32 Michell, R.H. (1975): Inositol phospholipids and cell surface receptor function. *Biochim. Biophys. Acta* **415**, 81–147.

33 Tashijan, A.H., Jr., Voelkel, E.F., Robinson, D.R. & Levine, L. (1984): Dietary menhaden oil lowers plasma prostaglandins and calcium in mice bearing the prostaglandin-producing HSDM$_1$ fibrosarcoma. *J. Clin. Invest.* **74**, 2042–2048.

34 Taylor, A.S., Sprecher, H. & Russell, J.H. (1985): Characterization of an arachidonic acid-selective acyl-CoA synthetase from murine T Lymphocytes. *Biochim. Biophys. Acta* **833**, 229–238.

35 Wertz, P., Cho, E.S. & Downing, D.T. (1983): Effect of essential fatty acid-deficiency on the epidermal sphingolipids of the rat. *Biochim. Biophys. Acta* **753**, 350–355.

36 Williams, W.M., Frölich, J.C., Nies, A.S. & Oates, J.A. (1977): Urinary prostaglandins: Site of entry into renal tubular fluid. *Kidney Int.* **11**, 256–260.

The biochemical basis of relating dietary fatty acids to prostaglandins and leukotrienes

W.E.M. LANDS
Department Biological Chemistry, University of Illinois at Chicago, 1853 W. Polk Street, Chicago, Illinois 60612, USA.

The first committed reaction in the conversion of arachidonic acid to prostaglandins and leukotrienes is catalyzed by fatty acid oxygenases; cyclooxygenase in the case of prostaglandin formation and lipoxygenase in the case of leukotriene formation. These enzymes, which regulate the flow of arachidonate into the eicosanoid pathways, have several striking biochemical characteristics. They exhibit a self-catalyzed inactivation (or 'suicide reaction') which limits the overall amount of eicosanoid that a given enzyme molecule can synthesize[9,14,19,20]. In addition, they exhibit an accelerative self-activated kinetic mode of reaction as a result of the product hydroperoxide serving as an activator for the oxygenation reaction[9,11]. Because of this positive feedback, oxygenases serve as amplifiers of small amounts of lipid hydroperoxides that may be present in tissues. After a small amount of hydroperoxide triggers the oxygenation reaction, the reaction then proceeds to amplify the concentration to much greater levels, enhancing the speed with which eicosanoid biosynthesis can occur. Removal of hydroperoxides from the reaction system suppresses the speed of eicosanoid formation to very low rates[11,13].

These results help emphasize an important regulatory role of lipid peroxides in influencing the speed with which eicosanoid biosynthesis can occur. High amounts of hydroperoxides give high speeds, and low amounts of peroxides tend to give low speeds until the level of hydroperoxide is amplified to an optimal level. Although the combination of the cyclooxygenase with arachidonate is an exquisitely sensitive amplifier of hydroperoxides[8,16], not all polyunsaturated acids react with the cyclooxygenase, and of those that do, not all are very sensitive amplifiers of peroxides. This difference is particularly evident in comparing the eicosatetraenoic acid (20:4n-6) with eicosapentaenoic acid (20:5n-3), the n-6 and the n-3 forms of eicosanoid precursor that are of considerable interest at the present time.

The n-6 acid, arachidonate, is made available by elongation and desaturation of dietary linoleate, and moderate amounts of arachidonate are also available from the meats that we consume in our diet. The eicosapentaenoate is customarily available in our diet through the consumption of seafoods. The eicosapentaenoic acid requires much higher levels of hydroperoxide to sustain the oxygenation reaction than does arachidonate acid[3,10]. As a result, in the presence of small amounts of cellular peroxidases that can scavenge the hydroperoxide activator, we have observed that eicosapentaenoic (20:5n-3) is unable to amplify those small amounts of hydroperoxide to obtain maximum velocity, whereas eicosapentaenoic (20:4n-6) continues to react at near optimum velocities[12]. These results mean that cyclooxygenase-catalysed reactions will tend to be suppressed greatly when eicosapentaenoic is available in the pool of nonesterified fatty acids. Although eicosanoid biosynthesis may proceed in the presence of eicosapentaenoic acid, it seems unlikely that it proceeds at optimum velocity. Therefore the accumulated concentration of eicosanoids at the local site may be insufficient to sustain a physiological response of the sort observed when arachidonate is the substrate. Not only does eicosapentaenoic acid antagonize eicosanoid formation from arachidonate, but the eicosanoids that are formed from eicosapentaenoic acid have been reported to be of much lower biological activity in many situations[4,15,17]. These analogs could antagonize the action of the arachidonate derivatives. As a result, one can predict that modifying the dietary intake of polyunsaturated fatty acids to replace n-6 by n-3 fatty acids, such as are found in diets rich in seafood, could alter appreciably the responses of tissue to stimuli that are mediated by eicosanoids. These alterations may be an underlying basis for the low incidence of certain diseases in the residents of fishing villages that have been reported in epidemiological studies[7]. In particular, the low incidence of atherosclerosis and thrombosis may relate to impaired platelet function by the antagonism of eicosapentaenoic to the formation of arachidonate-derived eicosanoids. Alternatively, the low incidence of breast cancer in Japanese and Eskimo populations[5] may also be related to an antagonism of a cyclooxygenase-mediated[1,2,6] amplifier process that involves n-6 acids in an enhanced tumour proliferation[18].

Finally, one must seriously question whether the relatively low incidence of auto immune diseases, bronchial asthma and psoriasis among Eskimo populations[7] might reflect to some degree a result of the dietary balance in n-3 and n-6 polyunsaturated fatty acid. These questions are now being pursued with increasing vigour by medical researchers around the world. Incorporating the new pharmacological and physiological information in our thinking can help nutritionists modify their assessment of the impact of dietary polyunsaturated fatty acids on the health of humans.

1 Bennet, A. (1982): Prostaglandins, tumor invasiveness and treatment with inhibitors of prostaglandin synthesis. *Progr. in Lipid Res.* **20**, 677–679.
2 Carter, C.A., Milholland, W. & Shea, M.M. (1983): Effect of the prostaglandin synthetase inhibitor indomethacin on 7,12-dimethylbenz(a) anthracene-induced mammary tumorigenesis in rats fed different levels of fat. *Cancer Res.* **43**, 3559–3562.
3 Culp, B.R., Titus, B.G. & Lands, W.E.M. (1979): Inhibition of prostaglandin biosynthesis by eicosapentaenoic acid. *Prostaglandins Med.* **3**, 269–278.
4 Goldman, D.W., Prickett, W.C. & Goetzl, E.J. (1983): Human neutrophil chemotactic and degranulating activities of leukotriene B$_5$ (LTB$_5$) derived from eicosapentaenoic acid. *Biochem. Biophys. Res. Commun.* **117**, 828–288.
5 Karmali, R.A. (1985): Lipid nutrition, prostaglandins and cancer. In *Biochemistry of arachidonic acid metabolism*, ed W.E.M. Lands, pp. 203–212. Boston: Martinus Nijhoff.
6 Kollmorgan, G.M., King, M.M., Kosanke, S.D. & Do, C. (1981): Influence of dietary fat and indomethacin on the growth of transplantable mammary tumors in rats. *Cancer Res.* **43**, 4714–4719.
7 Kromann, N. & Green, A. (1980): Epidemiological studies in the Upernavik District, Greenland. *Acta Med. Scand.* **208**, 401–406.
8 Kulmacz, R.J. & Lands, W.E.M. (1983): Requirements for hydroperoxide by the cyclooxygenase and peroxidase activities of prostaglandin H synthase. *Prostaglandins* **25**, 531–540.
9 Lands, W.E.M. (1979): The biosynthesis and metabolism of prostaglandins. *Ann. Rev. Phyiol.* **41**, 633–652.
10 Lands, W.E.M. & Byrnes, M.J. (1982): The influence of ambient peroxides on the conversion of 5,8,11,14,17-eicosapentaenoic acid to prostaglandins. *Prog. Lip. Res.* **20**, 287–290.
11 Lands, W.E.M., Cook, H.W. & Rome, L.H. (1976): Prostaglandin biosynthesis: consequences of oxygenase mechanism upon *in vitro* assays of drug effectiveness. In *Adv. prostagland. thromb. res. 1* ed B. Samuelsson & R. Paoletti, pp. 7–17. New York: Raven Press.
12 Lands, W.E.M. & Kulmacz, R.J. (1985): The Regulation of the biosynthesis of prostaglandins and leukotrienes. In *Prog. Lipid Res.* ed R.T. Holman. New York: Pergamon Press.

13 Lands, W.E.M., Lee, R.E. & Smith, W.L. (1971): Factors Regulating the Biosynthesis of Various Prostaglandins. *Ann. NY Acad. Sci.* **180**, 107–122.

14 Lands, W.E.M., Letellier, P.E., Rome, R.H. & Vanderhoek, J.Y. (1973): Inhibition of prostaglandin biosynthesis. *Adv. Biosci.* **9**, 15–23.

15 Lee, T.H., Mencia-Huerta, J.-M., Shih, C., Corey, E.J., Lewis, R.A. & Austen, K.F. (1984): Characterization and biologic properties of 5,12-dihydroxy derivatives of eicosapentaenoic acid, including leukotrienes B[5] and the double lipoxygenase product. *J. Biol. Chem.* **259**, 2383–2389.

16 Marshall, P.J., Warso, M.A. & Lands, W.E.M. (1985): Selective microdetermination of lipid hydroperoxides. *Anal Biochem.* **145**, 192–199.

17 Needleman, P., Raz, A., Minkes, N.S., Ferendelli, J.A. & Sprecher, H. (1979): Triene prostaglandins: prostacyclin and thromboxane biosynthesis and unique biological properties. *Proc. Natl. Acad. Sci. USA* **76**, 944–948.

18 Rogers, A.E. (1983): Influence of dietary content of lipids and lipotropic nutrients on chemical carcinogenesis in rats. *Can. Res.* **43**, 2477s–2484s.

19 Smith, W.L. & Lands, W.E.M. (1972): Oxygenation of unsaturated fatty acids by soybean lipoxygenase. *J. Biol. Chem.* **247**, 1038–1047.

20 Smith, W.L. & Lands, W.E.M. (1972): Oxygenation of polyunsaturated fatty acids during prostaglandin biosynthesis by sheep vesicular gland. *Biochem.* **11**, 3276–3285.

Nutrient interactions in fat metabolism

Joyce L. BEARE-ROGERS
Bureau of Nutritional Sciences, Food Directorate, Health Protection Branch, Department of National Health and Welfare, Ottawa, Ontario, Canada K1A OL2.

Interrelationships among dietary lipids involve nutritionally essential and non-essential components. Some of these may be lacking in experimental models which of necessity deviate from usual human practice. One has only to recall that the discovery of the essentiality of linoleic acid occurred with a fat-free diet[8] and that the assessment of the requirement rested on results of adding small increments of linoleate to a basal diet devoid of fat[16]. On the basis of the triene to tetraene ratio, normality appeared when linoleate contributed at least 1 per cent of energy. This situation appeared to be common for mammalian species[17]. Such a criterion for judging adequacy of linoleic acid could not be valid when linolenic acid is fed. Nor would the quantity of linoleic acid converted to arachidonic acid be unaffected by other fatty acids. Linoleic acid as 5.5 per cent of dietary energy has been advocated[20]. Thus, consideration of the fatty acids in the diet of man is changing the early recommendations for essential fatty acids.

Families of essential fatty acids. The (n-6) fatty acids, of which linoleic acid is the prime member, has to compete with the (n-3) fatty acids, of which α-linolenic acids is the prime member, for the 2—positions of glycerylphospholipids in the membranes of many cell types. These fatty acids control the effectiveness of membranes through the conformational changes in the lipid membrane surrounding intrinsic enzymes or transport proteins[30]. That the different essential fatty acids play distinctly different roles is indicated by the concentration of linoleic acid in the acylglycerylceramide of skin[20] and that of docosahexaenoic acid in the photoreceptor membranes of retina[2]. This last fatty acid in the (n-3) series also occurs prominently in the brain[11], in spermatozoa and testes[37]. With its six methylene-interrupted double bonds which cannot rotate, the structure must be rather rigid.

The demonstration of essentiality of (n-3) fatty acids, which have no effect on growth or reproduction, was achieved with deficient rhesus monkeys. They were born of females fed a high linoleic, very-low α-linolenic safflower oil prior to conception, throughout pregnancy and in infant formula while the controls received soybean oil[33]. The visual acuity of the (n-3) fatty-acid-deficient monkeys was significantly lower than the controls at 4 weeks of age and decreased further with time, as did the level of docosapentaenoic acid in the plasma. Upon feeding these monkeys a diet containing fish oil rich in docosahexaenoic acid, the plasma (n-3) fatty acids increased and (n-6) docosahexaenoic acid decreased[15]. This (n-6) fatty acid has been mainly associated with testicular fatty acids[22] but may be altered by (n-3) fatty acids.

Since graduated amounts of (n-3) fatty acids have yet to be used for a sensitive measurement of visual acuity, the dietary requirement based on such an end-point is not established. The relative deposition of (n-6) and (n-3) fatty acids in human fetal tissue during the last trimester of development appeared to be somewhat in excess of six to one[9]. It is not known how closely such a ratio of (n-6) to (n-3) fatty acids in tissue relates to the dietary supply because of the competitive advantage of the (n-3) linolenic acid over linoleic acid for desaturation[3,7].

Female rats deprived of (n-3) fatty acids during pregnancy and lactation produced young with low levels of docosahexaenoic acid and increased (n-6) docosapentaenoic acid in brain tissue, synaptosomal and retinal phospholipids, particularly in phosphatidyl ethanolamine. After a return of the rats to the control diet containing (n-3) fatty acids, the brain acquired a normal fatty acid composition within 9 weeks[33].

The essentiality of the (n-3) fatty acids probably resides with the long-chain derivatives and not with α-linolenic acid itself[18]. That man can synthesize eicosapentaenoic and docosahexaenoic acids from α-linolenic acid is appreciated because strict vegetarians do not have access to the long-chain derivatives in their diets. In the organs of the rat, docosahexaenoic acid can be increased by feeding a source of α-linolenic acid[34]. The effect of chain-length of the dietary (n-3) fatty acids in the rat was studied with a constant level of linoleic acid and a comparison made between α-linolenic acid from linseed oil and the long-chain (n-3) fatty acids from cod liver oil[19]. Both of these sources of (n-3) fatty acids, particularly the latter, decreased the levels of cardiac arachidonic acid and increased the level of docosahexaenoic acid (Figure). The (n-3) polyunsaturated fatty acids from marine oil have been shown to compete with arachidonic acid for the 2—position of cardiac phosphoglycerides[23]. Here it is seen that linolenic acid had less impact on cardiac fatty acids than pre-formed eicosapentaenoic and docosahexaenoic acids from marine oil. Rat heart, unlike human platelets[36] accumulated less eicosapentaenoic acid than docosahexaenoic acid which became the principal replacement of arachidonic acid. The prominence of docosahexaenoic acid in cardiac tissue, as in brain and retinal rods, may indicate a role in neural transmission.

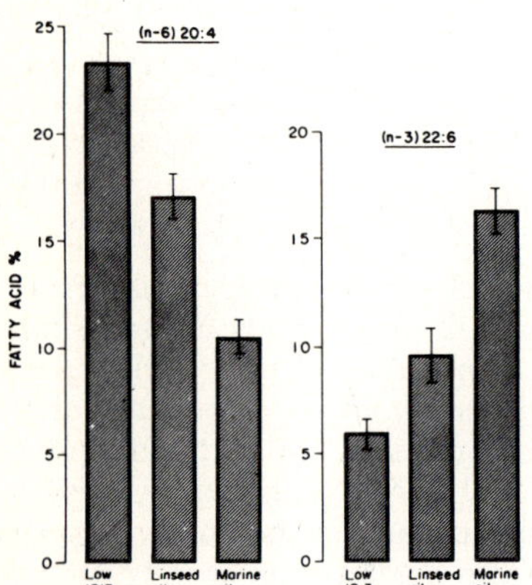

Fig. *Levels of cardiac arachidonic and docosahexaenoic acids in rats fed a diet low in (n-3) fatty acids, with a source of α-linolenic acid from linseed oil, or with a source of marine fatty acids rich in (n-3) acids.* (Holmer & Beare-Rogers, 1985).

A marked accumulation of docosahexaenoic acid in cardiac lipids has been noted when rats were dosed with a marine-oil concentrate rich in eicosapentaenoic and docosahexaenoic acids[34]. No other tissue was as responsive to the ingestion of the (n-3) material and only platelets and erythrocytes accumulated eicosapentaenoic acid. The best indicator of the dietary balance between the (n-6) and (n-3) fatty acids appeared to be the erythrocyte lipids.

The incorporation of essential fatty acids into membranes is related to the selectivity of acyltransferase. Using liver microsomes, it has been observed that the enzyme had a strong preference for arachidonic acid, followed by eicosapentaenoic acid[24]. This might account for the low levels of docosahexaenoic acid found in liver tissue. Consistent with the results of acyltransferase, more arachidonic acid than eicosapentaenoic acid in platelet and liver fatty acids was found after feeding equal quantities of linoleic and linolenic acids[39]. The specificity for activation as well as transacylation may influence the degree of incorporation of an essential fatty acid into a membrane.

Trans unsaturated fatty acids. So long as essential fatty acids are available, other fatty acids, including *trans* isomers of unsaturated fatty acids, are not incorporated into the 2-position of glycerophospholipids. Octadecenoic acids were shown to be incorporated into the 1-position of glyceryl phospholipids, replacing saturated fatty acids[6,21]. The most interesting results that have been attributed to *trans*-unsaturated fatty acids were obtained with diets deficient in essential fatty acids[4,13].

It was shown many years ago that hydrogenated fat increased the need for essential fatty acids[1]. Inhibition of desaturases occurred with various *trans*-unsaturated fatty acids, and indeed with *cis*-isomers as well[28,29]. It should perhaps be noted that the sources of desaturases were liver microsomes obtained from rats that had been maintained for a least 6 months on a diet deficient in essential fatty acids. Wherever other fatty acids are available to compete for active sites on enzymes involved in fatty acid metabolism, the concentration of linoleic acid may be critical.

In an experiment in which linoleic acid was provided, partially hydrogenated vegetable and marine oils in the diet inhibited the Δ6 desaturase, but only the partially hydrogenated marine oil affected the Δ5 desaturase[25]. A partially hydrogenated soybean oil containing isomeric *cis* and *trans* octadecenoic acids (ICTO) was fed with 2 per cent corn oil in the diet to provide a total of 8 per cent linoleic acid, a level which by the usual criteria should have been adequate[26]. In the presence of the high concentration of isomeric fatty acids, (n-9) eicosatrienoic acid increased as a replacement for arachidonic acid, a situation that had been assumed to indicate a deficiency of essential fatty acids. Such findings lead to a questioning of the previously accepted level of adequacy of essential fatty acids when the diet is extraordinarily high in isometric fatty acids. The principal effect of this mixture of dietary fatty acids was a lowering of arachidonic acid in phosphatidyl inositol and phosphatidyl serine. A large increase in docosahexaenoic acid in phosphatidyl serine appeared to have reflected substrate competition for desaturases. The (n-3) fatty acid with one more double bond than the corresponding (n-6) fatty acid in the sequence of desaturations was able to predominate.

Studies on the pattern of fatty acids in membrane constituents indicate that with adequate polyunsaturated fatty acids, *trans*-monounsaturated fatty acids do not occupy the 2-position of glycerylphospholipids nor influence eicosanoid production, but tend to act like saturated fatty acids. The (n-3) fatty acids possess a greater potential than the *trans*-fatty acids to alter the metabolic state of an animal.

Eicosanoids. Compared to a large amount of polyunsaturated fatty acids in membranes where they are esterified in the 2-position of glycerylphospholipids, a small amount of polyunsaturated fatty acids may be used for the synthesis of potent eicosanoids. A balance between the pro-aggregatory thromboxane A_2 in the platelets[14] and the anti-aggregatory prostacyclin in the vessel endothelium[31] was thought to regulate a thrombotic tendency. Unlike thromboxane A_2, thromboxane A_3 lacked similar pro-aggregatory properties in platelets[32].

The low incidence of ischaemic heart disease in the Greenland Eskimos was attributed to their high intake of (n-3) fatty acids from seafood and the inhibition of eicosanoid production from arachidonic acid[12]. This neat theory has been challenged by the failure to find a correspondence between the uptake of eicosapentaenoic into platelet membranes and evidence of a diminished production of thromboxane A_2[32]. The mechanism by which (n-3) fatty acids prolong bleeding times and reduce the thrombotic tendency is still unclear. Studies *in situ* on anti-thrombotic properties of fish oil are limited. Perhaps the most dramatic example of experimental cerebral ischemia was produced in cats by ligation of the left middle cerebral artery[5]. The resulting infarct had a smaller volume with less neurological damage as judged by a gait score and righting reflex in the cats that had received menhaden oil as 8 per cent of energy for 18 to 24 days than in those who had not received such a supplement. The composition of the brain lipids showed no effect of the (n-3) fatty acids which were attributed to inhibiting the synthesis of the series II eicosanoids.

Eicosanoids can also be produced by lipoxygenase for which arachidonic acid and more particularly eicosapentaenoic acid are substrates. The pathway in neutrophils has been described with three possible substrates (arachidonic, eicosapentaenoic and docosahexaenoic acids) which may be acted upon by 5-lipoxygenase[27]. The metabolites of arachidonic acid have been shown to have potent inflammatory actions. In the presence of the long-chain (n-3) fatty acids, there would be curtailment of the production of 5-hydroperoxyeicosatetraenoic acid (5HPETE) from arachidonic acid and the subsequent conversion to leukotriene A_4 and then leukotriene B_4.

There is a complex interrelationship between the metabolites of the cyclo-oxygenase and the lipoxygenase pathways. Prostaglandin E_2 regulates the production of leukotriene B_4. If there is inhibition of the PGE_2 by (n-3) fatty acids, there may actually be an increased generation of the proinflammatory leukotriene B_4. Restriction of the Series II of eicosanoids could conceivably decrease the tendency for thrombosis and increase that of inflammatory disease. For interrelationships of the (n-6) and (n-3) fatty acids in eicosanoid synthesis, both the level and duration of intake are critical variables. Male volunteers who daily swallowed encapsulated preparations containing 3.2 g eicosapentaenoic acid and 2.2 g docosahexaenoic acid produced 58 per cent less leukotriene B_4 after 6 weeks, but 3 weeks was too short a time to produce such an effect[27].

The metabolic fate of polyunsaturated fatty acid depends greatly upon the cellular environment. Tocopherol plays an important role in blocking the oxidation of polyunsaturated fatty acids and inhibiting the formation of lipid hydroperoxides. Selenium as a component of glutathione peroxidase is involved in the degradation of hydroperoxides which could otherwise lead to cellular damage[15]. Thus the relationships between fatty acids and other nutrients are interwoven, and one may affect the requirement of another.

1 Aaes-Jørgensen, E. (1965): Biochemical aspects of hydrogenated oils and isomeric unsaturated fatty acids in nutrition. *Bibl. Nutr. Dieta* **7**, 130–134.

2 Anderson, R.E., Benolken, R.M., Dudley, P.A., Landis, D.J. & Wheeler, T.G. (1974): Polyunsaturated fatty acids of photoreceptor membranes. *Exp. Eye Res.* **18**, 205–213.

3 Arens, M., Könker, S., Werner, G. & Petersen, V. (1984): Ernährungsphysiologische Wirkung unterschiedlicher Gemische von Öl-, Linolund Linolensaüre bei wachsenden Schweinen. *Fette Seifen Anstrichmittel* **86**, 89–92.

4 Beare-Rogers, J.L. (1983): Trans and positional isomers of common fatty acids. In *Advances in nutritional research*, ed H.H. Draper, pp. 171–200. New York: Plenum.

5 Black, K.L., Culp, B., Madison, D., Randall, O.S. & Lands, E.M.W. (1979): The protective effects of dietary fish oil on focal cerebral infarction. *Prostagl. Med.* **3**, 257–268.

6 Blomstrand, R. & Svensson, L. (1983): The effects of partially hydrogenated marine oils on the mitochondrial function and membrane phospholipid fatty acids in rat heart. *Lipids* **18**, 151–170.

7 Brenner, R.R. & Peluffo, R. (1966): Effect of saturated and unsaturated fatty acids on the desaturation *in vitro* of palmitic, stearic, oleic, linoleic and linolenic acids. *J. Biol. Chem.* **241**, 5213–5219.

8 Burr, G.O. & Burr, M. (1929): A new deficiency produced by the rigid exclusion of fat from the diet. *J. Biol. Chem.* **82**, 345–367.

9 Clandinin, J.T., Chappell, J.E., Heim, T., Swyer, P.R. & Chance, G.W. (1981): Fatty acid utilization by high risk low birth weight infants during *de novo* synthesis of tissue. *Early Hum. Devel.* **5**, 355–366.

10 Connor, W.E., Neuringer, M. & Lin, D. (1985): The incorporation of docosahexaenoic acid into the brain on monkeys deficient in ω-3 essential fatty acids. *Am. J. Clin. Nutr.* **41**, 874.

11 Crawford, M.A., Casperd, N.M. & Sinclair, A.J. (1976): Long-chain metabolites of linoleic and linolenic acids in liver and brain in herbivores and carnivores. *Comp. Biochem. Physiol.* **54B**, 395–401.

12 Dyerberg, J., Bang, H.O. & Stoffersen, E. (1978): Eicosapentaenoic acid and prevention of thrombosis and atherosclerosis. *Lancet* **2**, 117–119.

13 Gurr, J.I. (1983): Trans fatty acids: metabolic and nutritional significance. *Int. Dairy Fed.* **166**, 5–18.

14 Hamberg, M., Svenson, J. & Samuelsson, B. (1975): Thromboxanes: a new group of biologically active compounds derived from prostaglandin endoperoxides. *Proc. Nat. Acad. Sci. USA* **72**, 2994–2998.

15 Hoekstra, W.G. (1975): Biochemical functions of selenium and its relation to vitamin E. *Fed. Proc.* **34**, 2083–2089.

16 Holman, R.T. (1960): The ratio of trienoic: tetraenoic acids in tissue lipids as a measure of essential fatty acid requirement. *J. Nutr.* **70**, 405–410.

17 Holman, R.T. (1977): The deficiency of essential fatty acids. In *Polyunsaturated fatty acids*, ed Kunau, W.H. & Holman, R.T. pp. 163–191. Chamgaign, Ill: Am. Oil Chem. Soc.

18 Holman, R.T., Johnson, S.B. & Hatch, T.F. (1982): Reply to letter by Bozian and Moussavien. *Am. J. Clin. Nutr.* **36**, 1254–1255.

19 Hølmer, G. & Beare-Rogers, J.L. (1985): Linseed oil and marine oil as sources of (n-3) fatty acids in rat heart. *Nutr. Res.* (In press).

20 Houtsmuller, V. and Vergroesen, A.J. (1985): Requirements for the (n-6) series of essential fatty acids. In *Proc. 2nd Int. Conf. on Essential fatty acids*, London. (In press).

21 Høy, C.-E. & Hølmer, G. (1981): Incorporation of *cis*-octadecenoic acids into rat liver mitochondrial membrane phospholipids and adipose tissue triglycerides. *Lipids* **16**, 102–108.

22 Høy, C.-E., Hølmer, G., Kaur, N., Byrjalsen, I. & Kirstein, D. (1983): Acyl group distributions in tissue lipids of rats fed evening primrose oil (γ-linolenic acid plus linoleic acid) or soybean oil (α-linolenic acid plus linoleic acid). *Lipids* **18**, 760–771.

23 Iritani, N. & Fujikawa, S. (1982): Competitive incorporation of dietary ω-3 and ω-6 polyunsaturated fatty acids into tissue phospholipids in rats. *J. Nutr. Sci. Vitaminol.* **28**, 621–629.

24 Iritani, N., Ikeda, Y. & Kajitane, H. (1984): Selectivities of l-acylglycerophosphoryl-choline and acyl-CoA synthetase for (n-3) polyunsaturated fatty acids in platelets and liver microsomes. *Biochim. Biophys. Acta* **793**, 416–422.

25 Kirstein, D., Høy, C.-E. & Hølmer, G. (1983): Effect of dietary fats on Δ6- and Δ5-desaturation of fatty acids in rat liver microsomes. *Br. J. Nutr.* **50**, 749–756.

26 Lawson, L.D., Hill, E.G. & Holman, R.T. (1983): Suppression of arachidonic acid in lipids of rat tissues by dietary mixed isomeric *cis* and *trans* octadecenoates. *J. Nutr.* **113**, 1827–1835.

27 Lee, T.H., Drazen, J.M., Lewis, R.A. & Austen, K.F. (1985): Substrate and regulatory functions of eicosapentaenoic and docosahexaenoic acids for the 5-lipoxygenase pathway. *Prog. Biochem. Pharmal.* **20**, 1–17.

28 Mahfouz, M., Johnson, S. & Holman, R.T. (1981): Inhibition of desaturation of palmitic, linoleic and eicosa-8,11,14-trienoic acids *in vitro* by isometric cis-octadecenoic acids. *Biochim. Biophys. Acta* **663**, 58–68.

29 Mahfouz, M.M., Valicenti, A.J. & Holman, R.T. (1980): Desaturation of isomeric *trans*-octadecanoic acids by rat liver microsomes. *Biochim. Biophys. Acta* **618**, 1–12.

30 Mead, J.F. (1984): The non-eicosanoid functions of the essential fatty acids. *J. Lipid Res.* **25**, 1517–1521.

31 Moncada, S., Gryglewski, R., Bunting, S. & Vane, J.R. (1976): An enzyme isolated from arteries transforms prostaglandin endoperoxides to an unstable substance that inhibits platelet aggregation. *Nature* **263**, 663–665.

32 Needleman, P., Raz, A., Minkes, M.S., Ferrendelli, J.A. & Sprecher, H. (1979): Triene prostaglandins: Prostacyclin and thromboxane biosynthesis and unique biological properties. *Proc. Nat. Acad. Sci. USA* **76**, 944–948.

33 Neuringer, M., Connor, W.E., Van Petten, C. & Barstad, L. (1984): Dietary omega-3 fatty acid deficiency and visual loss in infant rhesus monkeys. *J. Clin. Invest.* **73**, 272–276.

34 Roshanai, F. & Sanders, T.A.B. (1985): Influence of different suppplements of n-3 polyunsaturated fatty acids on blood and tissue lipids in rats receiving high intakes of linoleic acid. *Ann. Nutr. metab.* **29**, 189–196.

35 Sanders, T.A.B., Mistry, M. & Naismith, D.J. (1984): The influence of a maternal diet rich in linoleic acid on brain and retinal docosahexaenoic acid in the rat. *Br. J. Nutr.* **51**, 57–66.

36 Sanders, T.A.B. & Younger, K.M. (1981): The effect of dietary supplements of ω-3 polyunsaturated fatty acids on the fatty acid composition of platelets and plasma choline phosphoglycerides. *Br. J. Nutr.* **45**, 501–506.

37 Tinoco, J. (1982): Dietary requirements and function of α-linolenic acid in animals. *Prog. Lipid Res.* **21**, 1–45.

38 Thorngren, M. & Gustafson, A. (1981): Effects of 11-week increase in dietary eicosapentaenoic acid on bleeding time, lipids, and platelet aggregation. *Lancet* **2**, 1190–1193.

39 Weiner, T.W. & Sprecher, H. (1984): Arachidonic acid, 5,8,11-eicosatrienoic acid and 5,8,11,14,17-eicosapentaenoic acid. Dietary manipulation of the levels of these acids in rat liver and platelet lipids. *Biochim. Biophys. Acta* **792**, 293–303.

VII: Protein metabolism

Protein metabolism

Current topics in protein metabolism

PROTEIN METABOLISM

Movement of nitrogenous materials into and out of the gut

J.V. NOLAN

Department of Biochemistry, Microbiology and Nutrition, The University of New England, Armidale, NSW 2351, Australia.

To maintain liveweight, mammals must continually absorb essential amino acids to replace those degraded during protein turnover. To gain weight and produce milk or wool, and for gestation, additional amino acids are required.

Single-stomached animals derive most of their essential amino acid requirements from dietary protein. In humans, customary daily protein intakes vary widely from 0.6 to more than 1.2 g/kg liveweight, ie 50–100 g protein/d. In ruminants and other foregut fermenters such as macropod marsupials, fermentation modifies dietary substances before they undergo gastric digestion, and unfermented dietary and microbial proteins are both sources of amino acids for the host animal. The processes of digestion and absorption and associated N transfers in the small intestine, and fermentation in the large intestine are essentially similar in all mammals (see Figure).

The digestion of protein depends upon enzymes that are secreted into the gut along with other

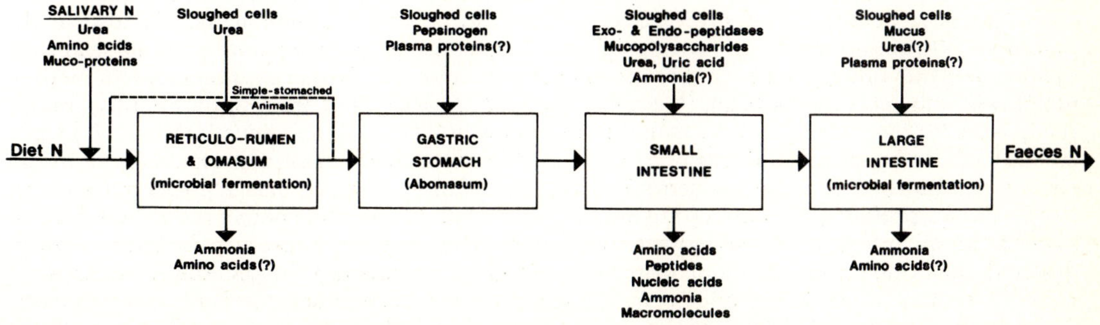

Figure. *Transfers of nitrogenous material into and out of the gut*

proteins from mucous, sloughed epithelial cells and plasma proteins. The amino acids from these endogenous proteins are not totally reabsorbed in the small intestine. After they enter the large intestine, they are not reabsorbed intact; they are either fermented by microorganisms (to amines, ammonia and VFA) or are voided in faeces. Their 'excretion' in this way is one component of 'protein turnover' in the animal[34] and of the animal's minimum protein requirements. Fermentation of endogenous amino acids that enter the foregut of pre-gastric fermenters is likewise an amino acid cost which increases minimum protein requirements. However, amino acids are also synthesized by microbes in the foregut from endogenous as well as dietary N, provided there is a source of fermentable substrate to provide energy for microbial metabolism. Absorption from the small intestine of microbially-synthesized amino acids may thus offset 'excretion' of endogenous amino acids into the foregut. A net gain of N in the foregut is likely to occur only if the ratio of digestible OM: crude protein exceeds 3.5[22]. In ruminants fed higher protein diets, net losses of N occur because absorption of ammonia N is greater than microbial capture of endogenous N.

Entry of endogenous protein into the gut. Endogenous N inputs to the foregut may be considerable relative to N input from the diet. Studies of ^{15}N-ammonia and ^{15}N-urea kinetics in mature 50–60 kg sheep (consuming 1.4 kg DM/d and 15–33 g dietary N/d) indicated that 6–10 g urea-N/d and 8 g/d other organic N (salivary proteins and muco-polysaccharides, sloughed epithelial cells) entered the rumen[25]. It has been estimated that 4–6 g/d of non-urea N entered the rumen of 55 kg sheep consuming 600 g DM/d[40]. Any unfermented portion of these substances would enter the abomasum and augment the 0.5–3.0 g/d of endogenous N of gastric origin[17].

Despite numerous studies, the amounts of endogenous N that normally enter the intestines are still uncertain, but may exceed those of exogenous origin. The amounts entering vary with diet, and notably increase with protein intake (for review, see[13]). Results from a recent study in sheep (P.J. Buttery & J.V. Nolan, unpublished) suggest that amounts of endogenous protein (labelled by intravenous infusion of ^{3}H-leucine) in the duodenum, as well as in the jejunum and ileum, may considerably exceed the amounts of dietary and microbial protein. In contrast, it has been suggested that, in humans, the endogenous entry was 0.30 of that entering from the stomach[33].

Endogenous N also enters the large intestine in plasma proteins, mucous and sloughed cells and the amounts entering can be increased substantially in ruminants infested with gut round-worms[2]. The amino acids in these inputs are not recovered intact and thus add to the minimum protein requirements.

Protein digestion and absorption. Gastric digestion of protein begins with the hydrolytic rupture of peptide bonds by gastric pepsins. The resulting polypeptides are hydrolyzed further in the small intestine to small peptides and amino acids by pancreatic peptidases, secreted in inactive zymogen forms that are activated by enterokinase, and by two distinct groups of oligopeptidases from the brush border and cytosol of mucosal cells (see review[41]). Some workers, eg[20], suggest that intact proteins and other macromolecules are absorbed in normal animals, but probably not in nutritionally-significant amounts. However, these macromolecules may have neural or endocrine activity. The L-forms of free amino acids, and also small peptides (2–6 amino acids) are absorbed, the former by active transport systems that are specific for individual acids or groups of acids[15], and the latter by independent active membrane transport mechanisms[31]. Studies have been cited[29] that show apparent absorption coefficients for mixed feed and microbial amino acids in the small intestine of 0.63–0.77, mean 0.70 ± 0.01, and suggest that essential amino acids, notably methionine, appear to be more efficiently absorbed than non-essential acids; cyst(e)ine, however, has a lower coefficient (0.40 − 0.55), probably because of incomplete reabsorption of endogenous cyst(e)ine secreted into the small intestine in muco-protein. Endogenous proteins appear to be more slowly digested that other proteins and absorption occurs more distally in the small intestine[37], possibly because most endogenous proteins will not have been denatured by gastric pepsins. Absorption coefficients for microbial protein are variable (0.49–0.85) and are often lower than for some vegetable proteins[29,40]. Nucleic acids from food or microorganisms are degraded in the small intestine by a variety of nucleases and associated enzymes and 0.75–0.95 are apparently absorbed[29].

In adult humans the total N flow from the ileum was 0.5–4.0 g N/d, depending on diet, ie 20–160 mg $N/kg^{0.75}/d$ [45]. In ruminants and other foregut fermenters, where undigested microbial debris makes a considerable contribution to N flows, the amounts are greater (3–8 g N/d; 100–370 g $N/kg^{0.75}/d$) and also depend on diet[40]. In the large intestine there is usually a net absorption of N, mainly as ammonia (eg[35]). There is no evidence that peptides or amino acids are absorbed in nutritionally-significant quantities from this part of the gut, although coprophagous animals such as the rabbit benefit from the amino acids synthesized by microbes in the large intestine.

Urea synthesis and transfer to the gut. Urea, synthesized in the liver, is the major end-product of N metabolism in mammals. Urea is not hydrolyzed in germ-free animals[28] and because there are no endogenous mammalian ureases, it is excreted in the urine, or transferred into the gut. Estimates of urea synthesis and degradation in animals have been made by administering ^{14}C-, ^{13}C- or ^{15}N-labelled urea intravenously. Depending on species and physiological state, 0.05–0.90 of the urea synthesized is degraded in the gut (see Table 15 in[45]). Urea is not normally present in ruminal or large intestinal contents because it is rapidly hydrolyzed in the presence of microbial ureases, although it can be present in the small intestine of normal animals and in the large intestine of animals treated with antibiotics[11]. Ammonia from endogenous urea (and other sources) is a major source of N for microorganisms in the intestines of all mammals, and for bacteria (and probably fungi) in the rumen. Amounts of urea degraded in specific regions of the gut can be estimated from the release of $^{14}CO_2$ or ^{15}N-ammonia in these regions after i.v. administration of ^{14}C- or ^{15}N-urea (eg[8]), or from the removal of urea from the blood perfusing various gut segments (eg[19]).

Factors affecting movement of endogenous urea into the gut. Urea enters the gut in saliva and in gastric juice[17,27] and in bile and other secretions. The urea concentrations in these secretions are related to, but are generally lower than, that of blood urea. Urea also enters by diffusion through regions of the gut wall such as the rumen[23] and the human jejunum[12] and ileum[38] although in the dog permeability falls progressively between the duodenum and ileum[30]. Urea concentrations in ileal fluid approach the concurrent concentrations in the blood of humans[16] and of horses and sheep[18]. In rabbits, ileal concentrations may exceed those in plasma[26]. A positive relationship ($P<0.01$; $R^2 = 0.7$) between the concentration (mg N/1) of urea plus ammonia in ileal fluid (Y) and blood urea concentration (X) was found in results from 27 sheep given a variety of diets, viz. $Y = 1.2 + 1.2X$[8]. This implies that blood urea is a major source of ileal ammonia. When ^{15}N-urea was infused intravenously in sheep, the labelling of ammonia-N in the ileum indicated that 0.63 was derived directly from blood urea[7].

The rate of transfer of urea into the rumen varies with protein and readily fermentable carbohydrate content of the diet, time after feeding, stage of growth of the animal, and environmental temperature[36]. In ruminants consuming low N diets, the urea transferred is often insufficient to supplement the dietary N available to meet microbial requirements for N, and both the intake and digestibility of the feed may increase in response to dietary urea supplementation. Whether endogenous urea entry into the rumen is controlled physiologically to the animal's advantage is not clear. Permeability of the rumen wall to urea depends on diet and is reduced in fasted animals, and may be altered by the concentration of rumen metabolites such as VFA[10]. Higher concentrations of VFA, particularly butyrate, and higher partial pressures of CO_2, increase transfer; higher concentrations of ammonia reduce it[36]. It has been argued that bacterial ureases in the cornified layer of the epithelium would enhance the urea concentration gradient across the rumen wall and facilitate urea diffusion[23]. It has been shown that most of the urease in the rumen is produced by bacteria that adhere to the epithelium, and that the rate of production is related inversely to the ammonia concentration in the medium[5]. Thus variations in ureolytic activity could account for variations in the rate of urea diffusion. Differences in urea entry into the rumen both by diffusion, and in saliva, can be accounted for statistically ($R^2 = 0.6$) with knowledge of the extent of OM digestion in the rumen, ruminal ammonia concentration, and blood urea concentration[24]. Why OM digestion accounts for considerably more of the variance than blood urea and ruminal ammonia concentration is not known, although when fermentation rate is increased, CO_2 production is also increased, and increasing the partial pressure of CO_2, through an unidentified indirect effect, increases urea diffusion across the rumen wall[43].

There is uncertainty as to whether urea diffuses across the wall of the large intestine (for review, see[45]), although small amounts do enter the more distal parts of this organ probably in mucin-containing secretions[35]. A number of studies suggest that the large intestine is relatively impermeable to urea (eg[1]) but in some of these studies the normality of the conditions at the epithelium can be questioned, particularly when the lumen was cleaned and perfused. It has been noted that bile acids and fatty-acids present in the digesta of more normal animals may increase the permeability of the wall to small molecules[45]. Cleansing could also affect the microbial populations that adhere to the epithelium. Nevertheless, ^{15}N-urea was infused i.v. in sheep with apparently normal function in the large intestine only negligible amounts of urea were transferred through the wall of the caecum and colon and appeared as ^{15}N-ammonia in the digesta[8]. These result do not, however, exclude the possibility that urea may diffuse through and be degraded close to the epithelium, with the resulting ammonia being absorbed before it has the opportunity to mix in the digesta.

Whether or not endogenous urea diffuses into the large intestine of normal animals, it is arguable that urea diffusion into this organ could disadvantage the animal. Sufficient N enters from the small intestine to supply the microbial requirements for ammonia in this organ; ammonia in excess of these requirements is absorbed, and its resynthesis into urea in the liver is an energy cost to the animal of 4 mol ATP/mol synthesized.

Transfer of other endogenous N into the gut. Other endogenous N-containing materials such as uric acid and creatinine[4] also enter the gut. As with urea, this probably occurs simply because parts of the gut wall are often permeable to relatively small molecules.

Absorption of ammonia from the gut. Ammonia is absorbed from the intestines[14] and the rumen and omasum[35] into the portal blood. It is also actively transported into everted sacs of the ileum of the rat[32].

The dissociation constant for NH_4OH at 37 °C is 10^{-9} ($pK_a = 9$), so at pH values of 7.4 in the blood, or 5.5–7.5 in rumen fluid, more than 0.97 is present in the NH_4^+ form. NH_4^+ being hydrated, charged and having low lipid solubility, penetrates membranes only slowly; NH_3 in contrast is not charged, is lipid-soluble and readily diffuses through membranes. The rate of absorption of ammonia from the gut is governed principally by the trans-epithelial concentration gradient of NH_3 and, to a lesser extent, by the effect, on movement of NH_4^+, of the positive electrical potential of the blood with respect to the mucosa. The electrical gradient is 10–40 mV both for the rumen[39] and large intestine and is dependent on active transport of sodium[6].

The presence of bicarbonate/CO_2 in the gut lumen also affects diffusion of ammonia. In everted sacs of hamster ileum, ammonia absorption was inhibited in the absence of bicarbonate/CO_2[32], and in the isolated colon of the rat the presence of bicarbonate/CO_2 in perfusates increased ammonia absorption[42]. It has been pointed out that diffusion of NH_3 alone would lower H^+ concentration, reduce dissociation of $NH_4^+ \rightarrow NH_3 \pm H^+$, and thus progressively reduce NH_3 absorption[44]. Coupled diffusion of NH_3 and CO_2 would not affect pH or absorption in this way.

Ammonia absorption from rumen contents of anaesthetized sheep at pH 6.5 increased with increasing ammonia concentration, and was enhanced by the concurrent absorption of VFA[21]. Absorption was much reduced at pH 4.5 and was then unaffected by VFA concentration. When ^{15}N-ammonia was used to estimate ammonia absorption in conscious, feeding sheep its values were closely related ($P<0.001; R^2 = 0.85$) to the NH_3 concentration in rumen fluid (calculated according to the Henderson-Hasselbach equation)[40]. These results emphasize the role of nonionic NH_3 as the major form in which ammonia is absorbed from the rumen and other regions of the gut. In humans, the permeability of the large intestine to NH_3 is 4–5 times greater than to NH_4^+[3].

Ammonia absorption from the large intestine is of particular interest to clinicians treating hepatic encephalopathy which is an impairment of brain metabolism believed to occur if ammonia is not removed completely by the liver and enters the systemic blood. One approach to management of this condition in humans is to administer orally a poorly-absorbed, fermentable disaccharide, lactulose. This consistently lowers the pH of colonic digesta and decreases ammonia absorption[9]. Numerous medical researchers have concluded that the success of this treatment results from changes in the bacterial flora present in the colon; none appears to have emphasized the likelihood that the response is to the lactulose acting as a microbial substrate and greatly enhancing fermentative activity of the existing microbial species. Increased microbial utilization of ammonia would reduce ammonia concentration and thus absorption rate; the concomitant increase in VFA production would reduce pH, thereby further reducing nonionic NH_3 concentration and ammonia absorption. Marked increases in colonic gas production and total N excretion in the faeces would be expected under these circumstances.

The so-called hepatic encephalopathy is similar to a condition known as ammonia intoxication that occurs in ruminants given excess urea in the diet. This occurs especially in animals with impaired liver function and is exacerbated by high rumen pH. One treatment is to lower rumen pH, and thus ammonia absorption, by administration of acetic acid.

Concluding comment. A point that emerged whilst surveying the large body of papers and reviews on N transfers between the gut and the body is that medical scientists do not appear to be fully aware of the studies of animal physiologists, and the reverse is also true. It seems therefore pertinent to suggest that scientists from both disciplines would benefit from surveying the literature more widely.

1 Billich, C.O. & Levitan, R. (1969): Effects of sodium concentration and osmolarity on water and electrolyte absorption from the intact human colon. *J. Clin. Invest.* **48**, 1336–1347.

2 Bremner, K.C. (1969): Pathogenic factors in experimental bovine oesophagostomosis. IV. Exudative enteropathy as a cause of hypoproteinemia. *Expl. Parasit.* **25**, 382–394.

3 Castell, D.O. & Moore, E.W. (1971): Ammonia absorption from the human colon. *Gastroenterology* **60**, 33–42.

4 Chadwick, V.S., Jones, J.D., Debongnie, J.-C., Gaginella, T. & Phillips, S.F. (1977): Urea, uric acid and creatinine fluxes through the small intestine of man. *Gut* **18**, A944.

5 Cheng, K.-J. & Wallace, R.J. (1979): The mechanism of passage of endogenous urea through the rumen wall and the role of ureolytic epithelial bacteria in the urea flux. *Br. J. Nutr.* **42**, 553–557.

6 Cooperstein, I.L. & Brockman, S.K. (1959): The electrical potential difference generated by the large intestine: its relation to electrolyte and water transfer. *J. Clin. Invest.* **38**, 435–442.

7 Dixon, R.M. & Nolan J.V. (1983): Nitrogen kinetics in sheep given chopped lucerne (*Medicago sativa*) hay. *Br. J. Nutr.* **50**, 757–768.

8 Dixon, R.M. & Nolan, J.V. (1985): Nitrogen and carbon flows between the caecum, blood and rumen in sheep given chopped lucerne (*Medicago sativa*) hay. *Br. J. Nutr.* (In press).

9 Elkington, S.G., Floch, M.H. & Corn, H.O. (1969): Lactulose in the treatment of chronic portal-systemic encephalopathy. *New Eng. J. Med.* **281**, 408–412.

10 Engelhardt, W.V., Hinderer, S. & Wipper, E. (1978): Factors affecting the endogenous urea-n secretion and utilization in the gastro-intestinal tract. In *Ruminant digestion and feed evaluation*, ed D.F. Osbourn, D.E. Beever & D.J. Thomson, pp. 4.1–4.12. London: Agricultural Research Council.

11 Evans, W.B., Aoyagi, T. & Summerskill, W.H.J. (1966): Gastrointestinal urease in man. II. Urea hydrolysis and ammonia absorption in upper and lower gut lumen and the effect of meomycin. *Gut* **7**, 635–640.

12 Ewe, K. & Summerskill, W.H.T. (1965): Transfer of ammonia in the human jejunum. *J. Lab. Clin. Med.* **65**, 839–847.

13 Fauconneau, G. & Michel, M.C. (1970): In *Mammalian protein metabolism*. ed H.N. Munro, Vol. 4, pp. 481–516. New York: Academic Press.

14 Folin, O. & Denis, W. (1912): Protein metabolism from the standpoint of blood and tissue analysis. 2. The origin and significance of the ammonia in the portal blood. *J. Biol. Chem.* **11**, 161–167.

15 Gardner, M.L.G. (1984): Intestinal assimilation of intact peptides and proteins from the diet — a neglected field? *Biol. Rev.* **59**, 289–331.

16 Gibson, J.A., Sladen, G.E. & Dawson, A.M. (1976): Protein absorption and ammonia production: the effects of dietary protein and removal of the colon. *Br. J. Nutr.* **35**, 61–65.

17 Harrop, C.J.F. (1974): Nitrogen metabolism in the ovine stomach. 4. Nitrogenous components of the abomasal secretions. *J. Agric. Sci., Camb.* **83**, 249–257.

18 Hecker, J.F. (1971): Ammonia and urea in the large intestine of herbivores. *Br. J. Nutr.* **26**, 135–145.

19 Hecker, J.F. & Nolan, J.V. (1971): Arteriovenous differences in concentrations of haemoglobin and urea across the forestomachs of sheep given lucerne chaff. *Aust. J. Biol. Sci.* **24**, 403–405.

20 Hemmings, W.A. (1980): Distributed digestion. *Medical Hypotheses* **6**, 1209–1213.

21 Hogan, J.P. (1961): The absorption of ammonia through the rumen of the sheep. *Aust. J. Biol. Sci.* **14**, 448–460.

22 Hogan, J.P. (1982): Digestion and utilization of proteins. In *Nutritional Limits to animal production from pastures*, ed J.B. Hacker, pp. 245–257, Slough, UK: Commonwealth Agricultural Bureaux.

23 Houpt, T.R. & Houpt, K.A. (1968): Transfer of urea nitrogen across the rumen wall. *Am. J. Physiol.* **214**, 1296–1303.

24 Kennedy, P.M. & Milligan, L.P. (1980): The degradation and utilization of endogenous urea in the gastrointestinal tract of ruminants. A review. *Can. J. Anim. Sci.* **60**, 205–221.

25 Kennedy, P.M. & Milligan, L.P. (1980): Input of endogenous protein into the forestomachs of sheep. *Can. J. Anim. Sci.* **60**, 1029–1032.

26 Knutson, R.S., Francis, R.S., Hall, J.L., Moore, B.H. & Heisinger, J.F. (1977): Ammonia and urea distribution and urease activity in the gastrointestinal tract of rabbits (*Oryctolagus* & *Sylvilagus*). *Comp. Biochem. Physiol.* **58A**, 151–154.

27 Kornberg, H.L., Davies, R.E. & Wood, D.R. (1954): The activity and function of gastric urease in the gut. *Biochem. J.* **56**, 363–372.

28 Levenson, S.M., Crowley, L.V., Horowitz, R.E. & Malm, O.J. (1959): The metabolism of carbon-labeled urea in the germ-free rat. *J. Biol. Chem.* **234**, 2061–2062.

29 Lindsay, D.B. & Armstrong, D.G. (1982): Post-ruminal digestion and the utilization of nitrogen. In *Forage protein in ruminant animal production*, ed D.J. Thomson, D.E. Beever & R.G. Gunn, pp. 13–22. Occasional Publ. No. 6, British Society of Animal Production.

30 Loehry, C.A., Axon, A.T.R., Hilton, P.J., Hider, R.C. & Creamer, B. (1970): Permeability of the small intestine to substances of different molecular weight. *Gut* **11**, 466–470.

31 Matthews, D.M. (1975): Intestinal absorption of peptides. *Phys. Rev.* **55**, 537–608.

32 Mossberg, S.M. & Ross, G. (1967): Ammonia absorption in the small intestine: preferential transport by the ileum. *J. Clin. Invest.* **46**, 490–498.

33 Nixon, S.E. & Mawer, G.E. (1970): The digestion and absorption of protein in man. 1. The site of absorption. *Br. J. Nutr.* **24**, 227.

34 Nolan, J.V. (1983): Minimum requirements for protein in ruminants. *Proc. Nutr. Soc. Aust.* **8**, 107–114.

35 Nolan, J.V., Norton, B.W. & Leng, R.A. (1976): Further studies of the dynamics of nitrogen metabolism in sheep. *Br. J. Nutr.* **35**, 127–147.

36 Norton, B.W., Janes, A.N. & Armstrong, D.G. (1982): The effects of intraruminal infusions of sodium bicarbonate, ammonia chloride and sodium butyrate on urea metabolism in sheep. *Br. J. Nutr.* **48**, 265–274.

37 Ochoa-Solano, A. & Gitler, C. (1968): Digestion and absorption of ingested and secreted proteins labeled with ^{75}Se-selenomethionine and ^{35}S-methionine in gastrointestinal tract of the rat. *J. Nutr.* **94**, 249–255.

38 Pendleton, W.R. & West, F.E. (1932): The passage of urea between the blood and the lumen of the small intestine. *Am. J. Physiol.* **101**, 391–395.

39 Phillipson, A.T. (1955): Sodium transport and its role in the ruminant digestion. *Vet. Record* **67**, 1048–1051.

40 Siddons, R.C., Nolan, J.V. & Beever, D.E. (1985): Nitrogen digestion and metabolism in sheep consuming contrasting forms and levels of dietary nitrogen. *Br. J. Nutr.* (In press).

41 Silk, D.B.A., Grimble, G.K. & Rees, R.G. (1985): Protein digestion and amino acid and peptide absorption. *Proc. Nutr. Soc.* **44**, 63–72.

42 Swales, J.D., Tange, J.D. & Wrong, O.M. (1970): The influence of pH, bicarbonate and hypertonicity on the absorption of ammonia from the rat intestine. *Clin. Sci.* **39**, 769–779.

43 Thorlacius, S.O., Dobson, A. & Sellars, A.F. (1971): Effect of carbon dioxide on urea diffusion through bovine ruminal epithelium. *Am. J. Physiol.* **220**, 162–170.

44 Wrong, O.M. (1971): Intestinal handling of urea and ammonia. *Proc. R. Soc. Med.* **64**, 1025–1026.

45 Wrong, O.M., Edmonds, C.J. & Chadwick, V.S. (1981): *The large intestine: its role in mammalian nutrition and homeostasis*. London: MTP Press.

Interorgan movement of amino acids

E.N. BERGMAN and Jennifer M. PELL
Department of Physiology, New York State College of Veterinary Medicine, Cornell University, Ithaca, New York 14853, USA.

Amino acids simply do not move out from the digestive tract in a general tide to nourish the various tissues. Instead, they have to pass the gut epithelium which is a metabolically-active tissue, and, also, the liver is positioned astride this flow of amino acid traffic to modulate it and interconvert some of the participants. Further, the metabolism of amino acids by the peripheral tissues must be coordinated with gut and liver metabolism and blood concentrations have to be carefully regulated. For these purposes, a number of studies have been made using indwelling catheters in blood vessels to discover what quantities of free amino acids flow from one organ to another. While the total flow of amino acids per unit time is large, studies have shown that only a few amino acids make up the bulk of interorgan movements and that these serve as a means for extensive recycling of nitrogen and carbon. Also, details of these movements reflect physiological adaptations to diet and to stresses such as pregnancy and lactation.

This paper will give an overview of amino acid transport in blood and of metabolism by the liver and specific peripheral tissues. It will deal only with free amino acids and will emphasize work done in the author's laboratory. While most studies have been made on sheep, comparisons will be made, where possible, with cattle, goats and nonruminant animals. Branched-chain amino acids are considered separately in view of their importance and current research interest.

Experimental techinques. Most studies have been performed using multicatheterized adult animals to measure venoarterial (V-A) amino acid concentration differences across various tissues together with measurements of blood flow. Tissues studied have been the portal-drained viscera, liver, kidneys, hindquarters, brain, placenta, fetus and mammary gland. Plasma flow is obtained by subtracting that flow represented by the packed cell volume. Net tissue metabolism thus is calculated by multiplying either the blood or plasma flows by the respective blood or plasma amino acid V-A differences.

The use of plasma, instead of whole blood, previously had been widely accepted and assumed that blood cells make no contribution to amino acids for tissue metabolism. Thus most data available to us today have been obtained by using plasma. More recent work in sheep, dogs and human beings, however, has shown that blood cells can indeed be involved, at least for some amino acids[8–10,13]. Careful consideration of these facts thus become necessary. In sheep[13], the plasma transport rate of all amino acids across four different tissues was less than that of whole blood and thus amino acids, in general, must at least be partially transported by blood cells. In sheep with a packed cell volume of about 25 per cent, most amino acids had a plasma transport rate close to 75 per cent of that of blood, ie the percentage of the blood volume existing as plasma. Glutamine, glutamate, and especially taurine transport in plasma, however, was significantly less that 75 per cent and thus must be transported by blood cells at a greater rate, per unit volume, than by plasma. Measurements of plasma amino acid fluxes thus qualitatively reflect true amino acid transport but do in most cases underestimate total transport to about the same exetent as the packed cell volume. For glutamine and glutamate, however, the underestimation is about 50 per cent of the total and for taurine it is over 95 per cent. Data on humans[10] and dogs[8] corroborate these findings on sheep blood.

Net tissue metabolism of amino acids. *Intestinal disappearance compared with portal blood appearance.* Of all the amino acids present in the lumen of the intestine of sheep, only alanine and serine seem to appear in portal blood in amounts approximately equal to that disappearing from the small intestine[23]. Glutamine, glutamate and aspartate either were not absorbed at all or were actually utilized by the gut tissues. Other amino acids had net rates of portal blood appearance of only 45 to 85 per cent of their intestinal disappearance. Amino acids, of course, can be absorbed as peptides and thus not appear as free amino acids in blood. The data suggest, however, the considerable gut epithelial metabolism must occur for energy production or transaminations[24]. Further, some could be used by the gut mucosae to form protein membranes of chylomicrons or even enzymes that appear in the plasma.

Net metabolism by liver and peripheral tissues. For the sum total of amino acids in adult sheep fed at maintenance levels, the liver removes from the blood approximately the same quantity as that added by the portal-drained viscera[14,25]. At the same time, peripheral tissues such as the kidneys, hindquarters and brain[2,20] remove some amino acids and release others. This, of course, should be expected in that peripheral tissues of adult animals theoretically will be in nitrogen balance and the ultimate fate of most nitrogenous compounds is urea formation in the liver.

In terms of specific or individual amino acids, however, a different picture emerges. The glucogenic amino acids, alanine and glycine, are absorbed in the greatest amounts of all but even more are removed by the liver[14]. The balance is then made up by a large release primarily from the muscles[16,17]. The kidneys also release glycine but, unlike the hindquarters, they remove alanine in significant amounts presumably for renal gluconeogenesis[2]. Other amino acids thus undoubtedly contribute their N or carbon skeletons for this new alanine and glycine formation for transport mainly to the liver.

The three urea-cycle amino acids also are absorbed in significant amounts. The liver, however, removes even more arginine than is absorbed but it releases most of this back into the blood as citrulline and ornithine. Oppositely, both the kidneys and hindquarters release arginine and remove citrulline and ornithine[3]. Urea thus is produced in the liver and arginine, like alanine and glycine, must carry nitrogen away from peripheral tissues. This probably is advantageous to the body in that amino acids can be catabolized in peripheral tissues without the risk of ammonia toxicity.

The metabolism of glutamine and glutamate differs from other amino acids. Glutamine is removed by both gut and liver in large quantities but, again, this is almost exactly balanced by a net movement out of the kidneys, muscles and tissues such as the brain[3,12]. Glutamate, on the other hand, is removed from the blood in only negligible amounts by the gut but is released by liver and removed by peripheral tissues. Glutamine and glutamate thus are interconvertible and the amount of glutamate transported depends upon the quantity of glutamine that is available. Although no glutamate is absorbed, it is present in the diet in greater amounts than any other amino acid. Glutamate thus is metabolized by the gut epithelium during absorption and part of it may be converted to alanine as in other species[19]. The large removal of glutamine from the blood by the gut also is related to this. Studies on the perfused rat intestine[24] show that one-third of the glutamine nitrogen is transaminated for alanine release back into the blood and one-half of the carbon is used for CO_2 production. In normal fed animals, glutamine and glutamate thus share a two-fold relationship. First, they are both used for energy and alanine production in gut tissues and, second, they participate in a cycle for transport of nitrogen out of the peripheral tissues for uptake by the liver for urea formation.

Additionally, the cycling of glutamine and glutamate seems to be of importance in the placenta and fetus. The placenta is capable of producing a large amount of glutamine[15,22], most of which is then transferred to the fetal blood rather than to the maternal blood. After deamination in the fetus, some of the glutamine carbon is then transferred back to the placenta as glutamate, where it is reaminated to glutamine. It thus seems apparent that the placenta is an extremely active tissue, not only synthesizing hormones but also actively metabolizing amino acids and other metabolites. The production of glutamine by the placenta thus permits the metabolism of amino acids without the release of toxic quantities of ammonia into the circulation. It is therefore the fetal liver that produces urea for the eventual disposal of excess ammonia.

Data also are available on total amino acid uptake by the fetus and lactating mammary gland. The subject of metabolism in the fetal lamb has been reviewed[1], and it is now clear that most amino acid concentrations are higher in fetal blood than in maternal blood. The placenta thus must actively transport amino acids to the fetal circulation. While the removal of all individual amino acids has not been clearly worked out, the sum total of amino acid removal by the fetus is definitely greater than that required for fetal protein synthesis. This is especially true for all the essential amino acids, including arginine[15]. The pattern of amino acid uptake by the mammary gland has been investigated in the sheep, cow and goat[5,7,18]. All three species show marked similarities. Essential amino acids, including arginine, are all removed from the blood in amounts equal to or in excess of those needed for milk protein synthesis, while non-essential amino acids seem to be removed in far smaller amounts than are required.

Branched-chain amino acid metabolism. In non-ruminants, muscle tissue classically has been considered to be the major site of catabolism of leucine, isoleucine and valine[11]. In the sheep, however, peripheral catabolism of these essential amino acids seems to be significantly less than in non-ruminants[6,17]. The liver of fed sheep removes roughly 40 per cent of all the branched-chain amino acids absorbed into the blood[4,14] with the remaining 60 per cent removed mainly by the muscles and other tissues such as the brain adiposa and lungs (Fig.). The kidneys actually release some branched-chain amino acids[4]; their source is unknown but they could possibly arise from hydrolysis of plasma proteins in the renal tissues.

The eventual fate of these amino acids in the liver of the sheep (Figure 1) is most probably that of protein (eg albumin) synthesis with subsequent export to the blood[4]. In muscle, however, they are eventually deaminated to their respective ketoacids. A portion of the ketoacids in muscle can then be oxidized to CO_2 but the remainder is returned to the blood for removal by the liver. The amino groups derived from the deaminated amino acids in muscle must then be transferred to form alanine, glycine, glutamine or arginine. In the liver, most of the ketoacids seem to be oxidized to CO_2 and ketone bodies but smaller amounts are reaminated back to the original amino acid. During fasting, hepatic removal is maintained even though portal absorption entirely ceases and the gut actually removes small net amounts from the blood. The major source of these amino acids now is the muscles as clearly shown by their large release from the hindquarters. Also during fasting, ketoacid release from the muscles is maintained or even increased[21].

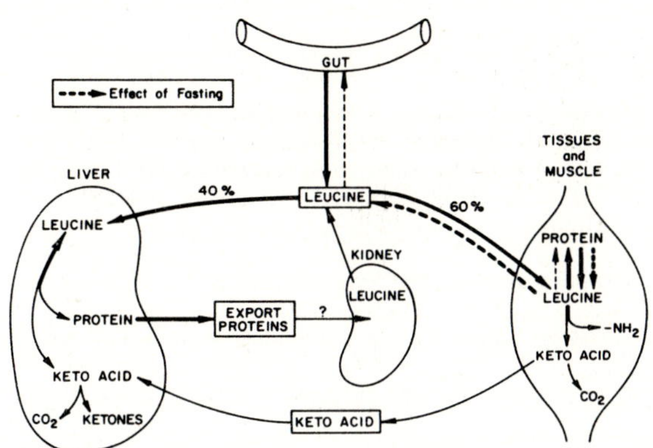

Figure. *Leucine as an example of branched-chain amino acid metabolism in sheep.* During feeding, liver and muscle both remove leucine. Also, muscle releases part of the leucine carbon as the ketoacid for removal by liver; its nitrogen then is transaminated to form other amino acids especially alanine and glutamine. The kidneys release leucine possibly as a result of degradation of plasma proteins. During fasting, muscle releases leucine while liver removal is maintained. Heavy lines indicate major reactions.

In addition to the above individual tissues, the whole-body metabolism of branched-chain amino acids is of interest. Leucine concentrations and turnover in sheep are at least ten-fold greater than that of its ketoacid[4,21]. During fasting, blood concentrations of both compounds increase dramatically. The turnover of the ketoacid also increases somewhat but leucine turnover decreases slightly. The precise reasons for these changes during fasting are unknown but they surely are related to the cessation of leucine absorption, its compensatory increased release by the muscles and probably decreased uptake for protein synthesis by peripheral tissues in general. While the oxidation of leucine is low, more is interconvertible to form the ketoacid during fasting. This probably represents an attempt by the body to conserve an essential amino acid structure during a time of shortage.

1 Bassett, J.M. (1980): Metabolism of the fetus. In *Protein deposition in animals*, ed P.J. Buttery & D.B. Lindsay, pp. 107–123. London: Butterworths.

2 Bergman, E.N., Kaufman, C.F., Wolff, J.E. & Williams, H.H. (1974): Renal metabolism of amino acids and ammonia in fed and fasted pregnant sheep. *Am. J. Physiol.* **226**, 833–837.

3 Bergman, E.N. & Pell, J.M. (1984): Integration of amino acid metabolism in the ruminant. In *Herbivore nutrition in the subtropics and tropics*, ed F.M.C. Gilchrist & R.I. Mackie, pp. 613–628. Craighall: Science Press.

4 Bergman, E.N., Pell, J.M. & Caldarone, E.M. (1984): α-ketoisocaproate (KIC), leucine (LEU) and protein metabolism in fed and starved sheep. *Fed. Proc.* **43**, 463 (Abstr.).

5 Bickerstaff, R., Annison, E.F. & Linzell, J.L. (1974): The metabolism of glucose, acetate, lipids and amino acids in lactating dairy cows. *J. Agric. Sci., Camb.* **82**, 71–85.

6 Buttery, P.J. (1984): Protein turnover and muscle metabolism in the ruminant. In *Herbivore nutrition in the subtropics and tropics*, ed F.M.C. Gilchrist & R.I. Mackie, pp. 597–612. Craighall: Science Press.

7 Davis, S.R., Bickerstaff, R. & Hart, D.S. (1978): Amino acid uptake by the mammary gland of the lactating ewe. *Aust. J. Biol. Sci.* **31**, 123–132.

8 Drewes, L.R., Conway, W.P. & Gilboe, D.D. (1977): Net amino acid transport between plasma and erythrocytes and perfused dog brain. *Am. J. Physiol.* **223**, E320–E325.

9 Elwyn, D.H., Launder, W.J., Parikh, H.C. & Wise, E.M. (1972): Roles of plasma and erythrocytes in interorgan transport of amino acids in dogs. *Am. J. Physiol.* **222**, 1333–1342.

10 Felig, P., Wahren, J. & Räf, L. (1973): Evidence of inter-organ amino-acid transport by blood cells in humans. *Proc. Natl. Acad. Sci. USA* **70**, 1775–1779.

11 Harper, A.E. & Zapalowski, C. (1981): Interorgan relationships in the metabolism of the branched-chain amino and α-ketoacids. In *Metabolism and clinical implications of branched chain amino and ketoacids*, ed M. Walser & J.R. Williamson, pp. 195–203. New York: Elsevier North Holland.

12 Heitmann, R.N. & Bergman, E.N. (1978): Glutamine metabolism, interorgan transport, and glucogenicity in the sheep. *Am. J. Physiol.* **234**, E197–E203.

13 Heitmann, R.N. & Bergman, E.N. (1980): Transport of amino acids in whole blood and plasma of sheep. *Am. J. Physiol.* **239**, E242–E247.

14 Heitmann, R.N. & Bergman, E.N. (1980): Integration of amino acid metabolism in sheep: effects of fasting and acidosis. *Am. J. Physiol.* **239**, E248–E254.

15 Lemons, J.A., Adcock, E.W., Jones, M.D., Naughton, M.A., Meschia, G. & Battaglia, F.C. (1976): Umbilical uptake of amino acids in the unstressed fetal lamb. *J. Clin. Invest.* **58**, 1428–1434.

16 Lindsay, D.B. (1982): Relationships between amino acid catabolism and protein anabolism in the ruminant. *Fed. Proc.* **41**, 2550–2554.

17 Lindsay, D.B. & Buttery, P.J. (1980): Metabolism in muscle. In *Protein deposition in animals*, ed P.J. Buttery & D.B. Lindsay, pp. 125–146. London: Butterworths.

18 Mepham, R.B. & Linzell, J.L. (1966): A quantitative assessment of the contribution of individual plasma amino acids to the synthesis of milk proteins by the goat mammary gland. *Biochem. J.* **101**, 76–83.

19 Neame, K. & Wiseman, G. (1958): The alanine and oxo acid concentrations in mesenteric blood during the absorption of L-glutamic acid by the small intestine of the dog, cat and rabbit *in vivo*. *J. Physiol.* **140**, 148–155.

20 Pell, J.M. & Bergman, E.N. (1983): Cerebral metabolism of amino acids and glucose in fed and fasted sheep. *Am. J. Physiol.* **224**, E282–E289.

21 Pell, J.M., Caldarone, E.M. & Bergman, E.N. (1983): α-ketoisocaproate (KIC) metabolism by tissues of fed and starved sheep. *Fed. Proc.* **42**, 815 (Abstr.).

22 Pell, J.M., Tooley, J., Jeacock, M.K. & Shepherd, D.A.L. (1983): Glutamate and glutamine metabolism by tissues of developing lambs. *J. agric. Sci., Camb.* **101**, 265–273.

23 Tagari, H. & Bergman, E.N. (1978): Intestinal disappearance and portal blood appearance of amino acids in sheep. *J. Nutr.* **108**, 790–803.

24 Windmueller, H.G. & Spaeth, A.E. (1978): Identification of ketone bodies and glutamine as the major respiratory fuels *in vivo* for postabsorptive rat small intestine. *J. Biol. Chem.* **253**, 69–76.

25 Wolff, J.E., Bergman, E.N. & Williams, H.H. (1972): Net metabolism of plasma amino acids by liver and portal-drained viscera of fed sheep. *Am. J. Physiol.* **223**, 438–446.

Protein turnover and food intake

P.J. GARLICK, M.A. McNURLAN, K.C. McHARDY, P.J. REEDS, V.R. PREEDY* and G.A. CLUGSTON†
*Rowett Research Institute, Bucksburn, Aberdeen AB2 9SB, UK; *Cardiothoracic Institute, 2 Beaumont St, London W1N 2DX, UK; †WHO, Indraprastha Estate, Delhi, India.*

Protein metabolism is not only sensitve to nutritional state but also responds to each individual meal. This enables protein to be stored in the tissues during food absorption; an important response, as food intake is never continuous and meals are followed by periods of fasting, which then require the stores to be mobilized. The sensitivity to feeding of rates of whole-body protein synthesis and breakdown and the oxidation of amino acids in man was demonstrated by a study giving continuous i.v. infusion of $(1^{14}C)$ leucine for 24-h periods[2]. Subjects were given regular meals for 12 h and then were fasted for a further 12 h. On changing

Table 1. *Whole-body protein synthesis and amino acid oxidation in men receiving different dietary protein intakes.* Measurements of whole-body protein turnover rate were made by infusion of $[1^{13}C]$leucine in subjects who were either overnight-fasted or receiving regular small meals. Calculated from data of Yang *et al.* quoted in Young *et al.* (1983).

Protein intake (g/kg B.Wt. per day)	Fed		Fasted	
	Synthesis	*Oxidation*	*Synthesis*	*Oxidation*
0	2.2	0.4	2.6	0.3
0.3	2.3	0.3	2.4	0.4
0.6	3.3	0.3	2.8	0.3
1.5	4.2	0.9	3.5	0.4

from feeding to fasting protein synthesis fell by 27 per cent and protein breakdown rose by 36 per cent: amino acid oxidation was particularly sensitive and fell to less than a half of the rate in the fed state. The net result of these changes was a switch from net anabolism of protein in the fed state to net catabolism in the fasted state.

Similar acute responses of protein turnover to food intake have been observed in a number of other laboratories (eg[1,8,11]). The magnitude of the effect is related to the nutritional state and to the protein content of the meals given. When obese subjects were given a protein-free, low-energy diet for 3 weeks, protein synthesis was depressed and no longer responded to the intake of food, either as the protein free diet or when meals containing protein were reintroduced[3]. Table 1 shows data from V.R. Young's group, who measured rates of protein metabolism in the fed and fasted state in young men given meals containing different amounts of protein. As the dietary protein intake increased the rate of body protein synthesis increased also, particularly during feeding. Only at the very highest intake of protein (1.5 g/kg B.Wt. per day) was amino and oxidation increased, and then only in the fed state. This suggests that the priority is for storage of protein by an increase in protein synthesis: oxidation increases only when this process is saturated. Although the subjects in Table 1 were adapted to their diets for one week before measurements were made, very similar effects of meals containing different amounts of protein have been observed[1], without prior adaptation to the diet.

Measurement of amino acid oxidation in parallel with indirect calorimetry also allows the disposition of carbohydrate and fat from the meals to be determined. Table 2 shows an example in which 8 per cent of energy expenditure in the fasted state was derived from protein, 24 per cent from carbohydrate and 68 per cent from fat. On feeding, the protein contribution rose to 20 per cent, and carbohydrate to 62 per cent, but fat fell to only 19 per cent, demonstrating a switch from predominantly fat oxidation in fasting to predominantly carbohydrate in feeding. During feeding, energy intake greatly exceeded utilization, and the excess was stored, the largest component of storage being as carbohydrate.

Table 2. *Disposition of the energy of protein, carbohydrate and fat in fed and fasted human subjects.* Rates are expressed as kJ (kcal)/h per 70 kg B.Wt. ($n = 3$). Subjects were either fasted overnight or were given small meals hourly after an overnight fast. Protein oxidation was measured by infusion of $[1^{13}C]$leucine and carbohydrate and fat oxidation by indirect calorimetry. Unpublished data of McHardy, McNurlan & Garlick.

	Fasted	Fed		
	Oxidized	*Oxidized*	*Intake*	*Stored*
Protein	25 (6)	59(14)	109 (26)	50(12)
Carbohydrate	67(16)	180(43)	506(121)	326(78)
Fat	188(45)	54(13)	301 (72)	247(59)

Although the hormonal mechanisms controlling storage of carbohydrate and fat following meals have been extensively investigated, less is known about the control of protein storage. It has been shown that in man, a high proportion of the increase in whole-body protein synthesis on feeding can be attributed to a stimulation in muscle protein synthesis[11]. Measurements of rates of protein synthesis in rat tissues have also shown that muscle is particularly sensitive to food deprivation[12]. It is therefore important to understand which hormones and metabolite concentrations control the increase in muscle protein synthesis after feeding. Many studies have been made with isolated or perfused muscles, showing that insulin, amino acids and glucose can all stimulate protein synthesis (eg[5,7]). However, although the plasma concentrations of these substances rise after feeding, their role in the response to feeding in the whole animal is not yet clear.

Table 3. *Muscle protein synthesis in fasted rats after refeeding or i.v. infusion of glucose, amino acids or insulin.* Young male rats were fasted overnight before refeeding for 1 h or infusion of glucose, an amino acid mixture (1 h) or insulin (0.5 h). Muscle protein synthesis was measured during the last 10 min and rates are expressed as percentages of the rate obtained in fasted animals. Indomethacin or anti-insulin serum were injected i.v. just before refeeding or infusion. Data from Garlick *et al.*, 1983; Reeds *et al.*, 1985 and unpublished data of Garlick, Preedy and Reeds.

Treatment	Protein synthesis (per cent of fasted)	Plasma insulin ($\mu U/ml$)
Refed	128	40
Glucose	98	41
Amino acids	97	11
Glucose + amino acids	122	26
Insulin	107	38
Insulin	126	>140
Refed + anti-insulin serum	97	0
Insulin + indomethacin	109	>140
Refed + indomethacin	100	–

Table 3 shows the effects of a range of treatments on muscle protein synthesis in post-absorptive rats. There was an increase in protein synthesis when food was given, but 1-h infusions of neither amino acids nor glucose had any effect. However, when amino acids and glucose were given together there was an increase in protein synthesis, illustrating the more potent response when amino acids act in combination with glucose, or possibly with the insulin secreted in response to glucose.

Table 3 also shows the result of insulin infusion on muscle protein synthesis in post-absorptive rats. When low rates of infusion were employed, so that plasma insulin concentrations were similar to those in refed rats, there was no increase in protein synthesis. However, when higher concentrations of insulin were achieved, there was an increase in protein synthesis, almost as great as that induced by feeding. This suggests that insulin is involved in the food intake response, but as with amino acids, at the concentrations found in refed animals it acts in combination with some other factor. Insulin is, however, an essential component of the response to food, as the normal increase in muscle protein synthesis when post-absorptive rats are refed does not occur when anti-insulin serum is given i.v. before feeding.

Insulin has recently been shown to act on protein synthesis in incubated rabbit muscles *in vitro* by a mechanism requiring the synthesis of prostaglandins[9]. The data in Table 3 show that indomethacin, a drug that inhibits the synthesis of prostaglandins, also prevents the stimulation by insulin of protein synthesis in rat muscle *in vivo*. Furthermore, since indomethacin inhibits the action of insulin, and insulin is essential for the stimulation of muscle protein synthesis by food intake, it seemed likely that the drug would inhibit the response to food. This is indeed the case, as i.v. injection of indomethacin immediately prior to feeding completely abolished the normal increase in protein synthesis (Table 3). Potentially this interference with the response to food by an inhibitor of prostaglandin synthesis could have important consequences for the vast numbers of patients treated with indomethacin or similar non-steroidal anti-inflammatory drugs for conditions such as arthritis. However, our preliminary attempts to demonstrate a similar effect in volunteers taking indomethacin immediately before commencing measurement of whole-body protein turnover with (^{15}N) glycine have failed to detect an effect of the drug (Table 4). In conclusion, the ability to regulate protein turnover rates when food is given is an important response that allows the body to store protein, as well as carbohydrate and fat, in the face of a fluctuating dietary supply. The control factors are not yet completely understood, but insulin and amino acid concentrations in the plasma appear to have an important role.

Table 4. *Effect of indomethacin on the response of whole-body protein turnover to feeding in man.* Measurements of nitrogen flux (g N/9 h) were made by single dose of [^{15}N]glycine with measurements of the excretion of label in urinary urea and ammonia (Fern *et al.*, 1981). Indomethacin (100 mg) was given 2 h before the isotope. Unpublished data of McNurlan, McHardy, Reeds and Garlick.

Subject	Fasted	Fed	Fed + indomethacin
1	12.6	21.6	24.2
2	11.1	22.5	20.4
3	14.0	19.3	19.1
Mean	12.6	21.1	21.2

Acknowledgements. The authors are grateful to the Medical Research Council for financial support and to the Scottish Hospitals Endowment Research Trust for the award of the Cruden Scholarship to KMcH.

1 Clague, M.B., Keir, M.J., Wright, P.D. & Johnston, I.D.A. (1983): The effects of nutrition and trauma on whole-body protein metabolism in man. *Clin. Sci.* **65**, 165–175.

2 Clugston, G.A. & Garlick, P.J. (1982): The response of protein and energy metabolism to food intake in lean and obese man. *Hum. Nutr.: Clin. Nutr.* **36C**, 57–70.

3 Clugston, G.A. & Garlick, P.J. (1982): The response of whole-body protein turnover to feeding in obese subjects given a protein-free, low-energy diet for three weeks. *Hum. Nutr.: Clin. Nutr.* **36C**, 391–397.

4 Fern, E.B., Garlick, P.J., McNurlan, M.A. & Waterlow, J.C. (1981): The excretion of isotope in urea and ammonia for estimating protein turnover in man with [^{15}N] glycine. *Clin. Sci.* **61**, 217–228.

5 Fulks, R.M., Li, J.B. & Goldberg, A.L. (1975): Effects of insulin, glucose and amino acids on protein turnover in rat diaphragm. *J. Biol. Chem.* **250**, 290–298.

6 Garlick, P.J., Fern, M. & Preedy, V.R. (1983): The effect of insulin infusion and food intake on muscle protein synthesis in postabsorptive rats. *Biochem. J.* **210**, 669–676.

7 Li, J.B., Higgins, J.E. & Jefferson, L.S. (1979): Changes in protein turnover in skeletal muscle in response to fasting. *Am. J. Physiol.* **236**, E222–E228.

8 Motil, K.J., Mathews, D.E., Bier, D.M., Burke, J.F., Munro, H.N. & Young, V.R. (1981): Whole-body leucine and lysine metabolism: response to dietary protein intake in young men. *Am. J. Physiol.* **240**, E712–E721.

9 Reeds, P.J. & Palmer, R.M. (1983): The possible involvement of prostaglandin $F_{2\alpha}$ in the stimulation of muscle protein synthesis by insulin. *Biochem. Biophys. Res. Commun.* **116**, 1084–1090.

10 Reeds, P.J., Hay, S.M., Glennie, R.T., Mackie, W.S. & Garlick, P.J. (1985): The effect of indomethacin on the stimulation of protein synthesis by insulin in young post-absorptive rats. *Biochem. J.* **227**, 255–261.

11 Rennie, M.J., Edwards, R.H.T., Halliday, D., Matthews, D.E., Wolman, S.L. & Milward, D.J. (1982): Muscle protein synthesis measured by stable isotope techniques in man: the effects of feeding and fasting. *Clin. Sci.* **63**, 519–523.

12 Waterlow, J.C., Garlick, P.J. & Millward, D.J. (1978): *Protein turnover in mammalian tissues and in the whole body.* Amsterdam: North Holland.

13 Young, V.R., Munro, H.N., Mathers, D.E. & Bier, D.M. (1983): Relationship of energy metabolism to protein metabolism. In *New aspects of clinical nutrition*, ed G. Kleinberger & E. Deutsch, pp. 43–73. Basel: Karger.

Nutritional aspect of amino acid oxidation

A. YOSHIDA
Department of Agricultural Chemistry, Nagoya University, Nagoya 464, Japan.

Nitrogen balance has been used very often for the measurement of both protein requirement and the nutritional quality of food proteins. Since amino acids containing labelled carbon became available, many studies have been carried out showing the metabolism of the carbon skeleton of amino acids. The nitrogen balance method is simple and convenient but takes several days for the urine collection and one cannot specify the specific amino acid source of excreted nitrogen. When a ^{14}C-labelled amino acid is used, ^{14}CO$_2$ can be collected immediately after the dose of ^{14}C-amino acid and the oxidation of specific labelled amino acid can be observed.

The rate of amino acid oxidation can be modified by the composition of diet and the feeding regimen. Oxidation of amino acids has been employed for the estimation of the requirement and the utilization of amino acids.

Effect of dietary level of protein on amino acid oxidation. The metabolic changes occurring in animals due to dietary protein deficiency are significant, but animals can survive for a considerable period on a protein-free diet. Assuming the existence of an adaptive mechanism, the overall metabolism of some amino acids *in vivo* was tested by measurement of their CO$_2$ production in animals fed on low-protein diets[9]. The results indicated that the oxidative degradation of leucine and phenylalanine, measured *in vivo* in rats fed a 2 per cent casein diet for eight weeks, was markedly decreased as compared with the control rats which were fed the Purina Lab Chow diet, whereas that of glutamate and alanine was apparently unaffected. This phenomenon was accompanied by increased incorporation of ^{14}C-leucine into liver proteins. The existence of an adaptive mechanism that functions to conserve an indispensable carbon skelton was suggested. Similar results were obtained using [1-^{14}C]-leucine and [1-^{14}C]-valine[17]. The dehydrogenase activity of the respective ketoacids in muscle was significantly reduced when animals were fed the protein-free diet, whereas amino transferase activities in liver and muscle were not significantly altered. It was suggested that the ketoacid dehydrogenases are responsible for regulating the amino acid oxidation.

The effect of the dietary level of protein on the oxidation of lysine *in vivo* and *in vitro* was investigated in rats[18]. The rate of oxidation increased with each increase in the concentration of dietary protein. The lysine-degrading activity of liver homogenates from rats fed 10 or 20 per cent casein diets remained essentially constant but the activity in homogenates from rats fed 40 or 60 per cent casein diets was much increased. The authors suggested that the changes in the activity of lysine-ketoglutarate reductase would be involved in this metabolic adaptation.

On the other hand the decreased oxidation of ^{14}C-amino acid mixture, lysine, valine or leucine by protein-deficient rats when animals were not previously fasted, was not demonstrated in another study[11]. However, when animals were fasted for 16 h, the catabolism of mixed amino acids and of lysine given intragastrically was decreased. Neither the catabolism of valine nor that of leucine decreased in protein-deficient rats even after fasting.

Neale & Waterlow[13] further investigated the metabolism of ^{14}C-labelled essential amino acids given by intragastric or i.v. infusions to rats fed normal and protein-free diets. Uniformly labelled amino acids (leucine, lysine, valine or phenylalanine) were continuously infused by intragastric or i.v. routes for 4 h, after overnight fast into rats which had been fed a normal or a protein-free diet for 20 d. They showed no difference between the protein-depleted and normal rats in the proportion of labelled amino acid oxidized. The results are therefore in conflict with others in which the tracer was given by single injection. As pointed out by these authors[12], the distribution a single injection of ^{14}C-labelled amino acid in tissues may be different from that resulting from continuous infusion of the labelled amino acid. Initially after a single injection there is a preferential uptake of radioactivity by the liver and viscera and later by the peripheral tissues. Therefore, the initial output of $^{14}CO_2$ after single injection of ^{14}C-amino acid may predominantly reflect the rate of oxidation in the liver and viscera. With a continuous infusion, ^{14}C-amino acid distributes fairly uniformly in the body, and the changes in the rate of oxidation in liver and viscera might be masked by the large contribution of muscle and other extrahepatic tissues where the rate of oxidation may not be affected significantly by the dietary level of protein.

Effect of dietary level of a single amino acid on amino acid oxidation. Not only the depletion of protein but the deficiency or excess of a single amino acid can also affect the oxidation of amino acids. Animals lose more body weight when fed a threonine-deficient diet than do animals fed a lysine-free diet[16,22]. There was speculation that a certain homoeostatic mechanism may operate in animals fed the lysine-deficient diet[19]. The breakdown of ^{14}C-lysine to respiratory $^{14}CO_2$ within 1 h after intraperitoneal injection into rats fed a lysine-free diet for 5 d, decreased to about one-half of the control value. In the case of ^{14}C-threonine, however, there was no significant difference in the recovery of respiratory $^{14}CO_2$ between rats fed the threonine-free diet and those fed the control diet. These results may indicate that the lysine catabolism of rats fed the lysine-free diet is depressed, whereas the threonine catabolism in rats fed the threonine-free diet is not greatly affected.

The first step of lysine degradation is considered to be catalized by lysine ketoglutarate reductase. The effect of dietary lysine on the activity of the reductase in rats was examined[5]. The reductase activity was clearly induced by the high lysine diet, but no difference in the activities was found between the group fed the protein-free diet and that fed the basal diet (0.42 per cent lysine). The induction of lysine ketoglutarate reductase activity by a high-lysine diet was demonstrated by others[10]; but the activity of this enzyme in rats fed the lysine-free diet was not especially low as compred with that of the basal diet group. Lysine may be conserved well in the body of animals fed the usual quantity of lysine and only when dietary concentrations of lysine are excessively high is the oxidation of lysine stimulated with the induction of lysine ketoglutarate reductase. In an investigation of the effect of the dietary level of threonine on oxidation of threonine and threonine dehydratase activity *in vivo*; the rate of oxidation of threonine was low when intake was in the range of the requirement for maximum growth, but increased thereafter as threonine intake increased. (Other workers have shown that liver threonine activity was not affected by the dietary level of threonine). The effect of dietary histidine on histidine oxidation was also studied by the same authors[6]. During *ad-libitum* consumption of experimental diets containing [U-^{14}C]-histidine, $^{14}CO_2$ production in rats remained low until dietary histidine content exceed 0.25 per cent then it increased linearly. Liver histidase responded to the dietary level of protein but not to the dietary level of histidine. Liver histidine concentration is usually below the K_m value of histidase, and this can account for the rate of oxidation of histidine increasing with increased intake of histidine, as the authors suggested[6].

Use of amino acid oxidation for the determination of amino acid requirement. When amino acid is present in the diet in suboptimal amounts, a large proportion of this amino acid will be used for protein synthesis. As the dietary supply exceeds the animal's needs for protein synthesis, excess amino acid would be mainly oxidized to CO_2 except for lipogenesis and gluconeogenesis. Accordingly, the increased oxidation of an amino acid could be used as an indicator of amino acid requirement. The relationship in rats between the dietary concentration of lysine and *in vivo* oxidation of lysine was investigated using [U-^{14}C]-lysine[3]. The oxidation of lysine did not increase markedly until the dietary lysine intake was increased above that concentration at which average daily gain was maximal, and it was concluded that the oxidation technique provides a means for estimating the dietary amino acid requirement. Similarly, histidine and threonine requirements were estimated from the inflection point of the oxidation curve[6,7].

When compared with growth assay, the oxidation method needs only a short time and may also be applicable to the maintenance requirement of adult animals or slowly growing large animals. This method has been employed for the estimation of the amino acid requirement of piglets. Monitoring the oxidation of either [1-^{14}C]-phenylalanine or [1-^{14}C]-histidine was used to determine histidine requirement[8]. In diets containing more than 4 g histidine/kg, oxidation of [^{14}C]-phenylalanine was minimal. But when the diet contained less than 4 g histidine/kg, phenylalanine oxidation increased. In contrast, when there was over 4 g histidine/kg diet, the oxidation of histidine was increased and thus confirmed the good agreement of the results of direct and indirect oxidation methods.

Endogenous loss of amino acids and the maintenance requirement of amino acids. For the basis of the estimation of protein requirements for maintenance obligatory nitrogen loss is determined. On a similar basis, an attempt was made to estimate the maintenance requirement of leucine or methionine from the endogenous loss of leucine and methionine using [1-^{14}C]-leucine and [1-^{14}C]-methionine in young adult rats[12,13]. Rats were given the labelled amino acid by stomach tube and were maintained on the low protein basal diet for 17 d and then transferred to a lower-protein diet or a cystine and methionine-free diet. They determined the expired ^{14}CO$_2$ after a fairly long time of feeding the low-protein diet or the S-amino-acids-deficient diet to ensure the uniform distribution of the ^{14}C-labelled amino acid in the various organs. From these experiments, they calculated the absolute loss of endogenous amino acids. The rate of endogenous oxidation of leucine was higher than the maintenance requirement determined in an earlier study, while that of endogenous methionine oxidation was in good agreement with it[15] and with another study[2]. The fractional loss of ^{14}CO$_2$ was constant regardless of the methionine intake[14].

Catabolic specificity of endogenous amino acids. If a specific amino acid in the amino acid pool is catabolized faster than the other amino acids, this amino acid would become limiting in animals fed a protein-free diet. Or, when some tissue proteins containing a large amount of a specific amino acid turn over rapidly, the amino acid would become limiting when animals to not consume a protein-containing diet. The limiting amino acid in the dietary proteins is often calculated and discussed. The nitrogen-sparing effect of whole egg protein was demonstrated and the suggestion made that it was mainly due to its methionine content[4]. On the other hand, the addition of 0.3 per cent of methionine together with 0.3 per cent of threonine to a protein-free diet markedly alleviated the body-weight loss and reduced the urinary nitrogen excretion in rats[22]. The effect was much greater than that of methionine alone. Urinary excretion of urea in rats fed the protein-free diet was 82 mg for 3 d. But the rats of the group supplemented with methionine and threonine excreted only 23 mg of urea. Addition of methionine alone also reduced the urinary excretion of urea, but not so significantly as seen in the methionine-plus-threonine supplemented group. Urinary excretion of allantoin and creatinine was not affected by the supplementation of methionine or methionine-plus-threonine. Thus the nitrogen-sparing effect of methionine and threonine is mainly due to the reduced excretion of urea.

The supplementation of methionine and threonine to the protein-free diet did not decrease the activities of amino-acid-catabolizing enzymes and urea cycle enzymes[23]. The plasma concentration of most of the free amino acids except threonine was reduced by the supplementation with methionine and threonine suggesting the increased utilization of the endogenous amino acids following supplementation with these two essential amino acids.

When ^{14}C-lysine or ^{14}C-histidine was injected into rats receiving the methionine and threonine-supplemented diet, the expiration of ^{14}CO$_2$ was significantly reduced as compared with that of the protein-free control diet group. These observations also indicate the improved reutilization of endogenous free amino acids following the addition of methionine and threonine to the protein-free diet.

Tissue polyribosomal profiles are considered to reflect the state of protein synthesis. When methionine and threonine were added to the protein-free diet, the ratio of liver monosomes and disomes to total ribosomes was significantly reduced suggesting stimulated liver protein synthesis[20]. In addition to methionine and threonine, small amounts of valine, isoleucine and tryptophan together with a nonspecific nitrogen source (glutamic acid) were added to the protein-free diet and resulted in a further reduction in the body weight loss and increase nitrogen balance[21]. The further addition of all the remaining essential amino acids (phenylalanine, leucine, histidine and lysine) maintained the body weight and the nitrogen equilibrium.

From these results, it may be postulated that when rats were fed the protein-free diet, the extent of deficiency of each essential amino acid is not equal but methionine would be the first limiting, and threonine, the second. These differences in the extent of deficiency in endogenous amino acids would be due to the differences in the catabolic rate of endogenous amino acids.

The high rate of oxidation of methionine, as compared with the other essential amino acids, has been reported[1] and may relate to our observation on the specific endogenous nitrogen-sparing effect of methionine and threonine. When rats were fed a diet deficient in one essential amino acid, nitrogen balance was naturally negative. However, the extent of negative nitrogen balance depended on the kinds of essential amino acid deficient[24]. When the deficient amino acid was methionine or threonine, rats showed severe negative nitrogen balance. But when lysine or histidine was deficient in the diet, rats showed only slightly negative nitrogen balance. This nutritional specificity of amino acid would be explainable by the specificity of each amino acid catabolism. The nutritional specificity of amino acids would be especially significant for estimating the limiting amino acid of dietary protein in low protein intake.

As stated above, the oxidation of amino acids is affected by dietary protein, amino acid composition, and by other dietary conditions, and may be an useful tool for monitoring the nutritional status of the animal insofar as it is limited by supply of protein and amino acids.

1 Aguilar, T.S., Harper, A.E. & Benevenga, N.J. (1972): Efficiency of utilization of indispensable amino acids for growth by the rat. *J. Nutr.* **102**, 1199–1208.
2 Ashida, K. & Yoshida, A. (1975): Nutritional specificities of essential amino acids and their relationships to evaluation of the nutritional quality of dietary proteins. *Proc. IX Int. Cong. Nutr., Mexico* 1972. **3**, 321–331.
3 Brookes, I.M., Owens, F.N. & Garrigus, U.S. (1972): Influence of amino acid level in the diet upon amino acid oxidation by the rat. *J. Nutr.* **102**, 27–36.
4 Brush, M., Willman, W. & Swanson, P.P. (1947): Amino acids in nitrogen metabolism with particular reference to the role of methionine. *J. Nutr.* **33**, 389–410.
5 Funahashi, K. (1973): Regulation of lysine metabolism. MS Thesis. Nagoya University.
6 Kang-Lee, Y. AE. & Harper, A.E. (1977): Effect of histidine intake and hepatic histidase activity on the metabolism of histidine *in vivo*. *J. Nutr.* **107**, 1427–1443.
7 Kang-Lee, Y. AE. & Harper, A.E. (1978): Threonine metabolism *in vivo*: effect of threonine intake and prior induction of threonine. *J. Nutr.* **108**, 163–175.
8 Kim, K.I., McMillan, I. & Bayley, H. (1983): Determination of amino acid requirement of young pigs using an indicator amino acid. *Br. J. Nutr.* **50**, 369–382.
9 McFarlane, I.G. & von Holt, C. (1969): Metabolism of amino acids in protein-calorie-deficient rats. *Biochem. J.* **111**, 557–563.
10 Muramatsu, K. Takada, R. (1978): Adaptive response of liver and kidney lysine-ketoglutarate reductase in rats fed dietary lysine and protein. *Rep. Res. Committee of Essential Amino Acids (Japan)*, No. 78, 23–26.
11 Neale, R.J. (1971): Adaptation of amino-acid metabolism in protein-depleted rats. *Nature New Biology* **231**, 117–118.
12 Neale, R.J. & Waterlow, J.C. (1974): The metabolism of ^{14}C-labelled essential amino acids given by intragastric or intravenous infusion to rats on normal end protein-free diets. *Br. J. Nutr.* **32**, 11–25.
13 Neale, R.J. & Waterlow, J.C. (1977): Endogenous loss of leucine and methionine in adult male rats. *Br. J. Nutr.* **37**, 259–268.
14 Neale, R.J. & Waterlow, J.C. (1983): Rate of endogenous methionine oxidation in rats at different levels of methionine intake. *Br. J. Nutr.* **50**, 157–162.
15 Said, A.K. & Hegsted, D.M. (1970): Response of adult rats to low dietary levels of essential amino acids. *J. Nutr.* **100**, 1363–1376.
16 Sidransky, H. & Baba, T. (1960): Chemnical pathology of acute amino acid deficiencies III. Morphologic and biochemical changes in young rats fed valine- or lysine- devoid diets. *J. Nutr.* **70**, 463–471.
17 Sketcher, R.D. & James, W.P.T. (1974): Branched-chain amino acid oxidation in relation to catabolic enzyme activities in rats given a protein-free diet at different stages of development. *Br. J. Nutr.* **32**, 615–623.
18 Soliman, A-G.M. & Harper, A.E. (1971): Effect of protein content of diet on lysine oxidation by the rat. *Biochim. Biophys. Acta.* **244**, 146–154.
19 Yamashita, K. & Ashida, K. (1969): Lysine metabolism in rats fed lysine-free diet. *J. Nutr.* **99**, 267–273.
20 Yokogoshi, H. & Yoshida, A. (1979): Effect of supplementation of methionine and threonine on hepatic polyribosome profile in rats interval-fed a protein free diet. *J. Nutr.* **109**, 148–154.
21 Yokogoshi, H. & Yoshida, A. (1981): Sequence of limiting amino acids for the utlization of endogenous amino acids in rats fed a protein free diet. *Nutr. Rep. Int.* **23**, 517–523.

22 Yoshida, A., Leung, P.M.B., Rogers, Q.R. & Harper, A.E. (1966): Effect of amino acid imbalance on the fate of the limiting amino acid. *J. Nutr.* **89**, 80–90.

23 Yoshida, A. & Moritoki, K. (1974): Nitrogen sparing action of methionine and threonine in rats receiving a protein free diet. *Nutr. Rep. Int.* **9**, 159–169.

24 Yoshida, A. (1978): Nutritional evaluation of protein and scoring method. *Rep. Res. Committee of Essential Amino Acids (Japan)*, No. 79, 12–15.

★   ★   ★

CURRENT TOPICS IN PROTEIN METABOLISM

Basal protein metabolism and protein requirements

P.J. REEDS and M.F. FULLER
Rowett Research Institute, Bucksburn, Aberdeen, Scotland AB2 9SB.

There are three main routes of loss of body protein. (1) integumental losses — largely due to desquamation of the skin, some loss of hair (this being a significant component in animals) and some small losses in sweat; (2) losses due to the continuing catabolism of amino acids, and (3) losses into the intestine, either as enterocytes, as hepatic, intestinal and pancreatic enzyme secretion or as mucous. We wish, in this paper, to concentrate on the second and third of these components.

Amino acid catabolism. Although the phenomenon of protein turnover is now well-established it is important to recognise that the turnover of tissue proteins does not directly lead to a loss of amino acids. Because of the quantitative relationship between protein turnover (in adult man approximately 300 g per day under basal conditions) and protein intake (approximately 70 g per day) a high proportion of the amino acids released by tissue protein breakdown must be recycled, often within the cell in which they have originated[7]. On the other hand the catabolism of the essential amino acids represents a true loss from the body.

It is clear that, even in individuals that are receiving no dietary protein, amino acid catabolism, although suppressed, continues. Typically in man the equivalent of 20 g of protein are lost in amino acid catabolism each day[3,8]. The immediate question is: why do these losses continue under circumstances in which the conservation of body protein would seem to be of great importance?

Part of the answer may be that complete loss of amino acid catabolic enzymes cannot occur because the retention of this metabolic activity confers the adaptive advantage of maintaining the ability of the organism to dispose of an abrupt increase in dietary protein. A second factor may be the role of amino acids as substrates for the production of ATP. It is rare for naturally-occurring diets to be specifically deficient in protein. Generally a combined energy and protein deficit exists. Undoubtedly reducing the energy intake of subjects that are receiving no protein (eg progression to the fasted state) leads to an increase in body protein loss of about 16 g per day. Conversely the ingestion of carbohydrate by fasting individuals lowers urinary nitrogen excretion. It is unknown whether the interaction between dietary energy and nitrogen excretion is indicative of some specific role for amino acids in energy metabolism. It seems unlikely that their use as substrates for glucose synthesis is of critical importance.

The third potential influence on basal amino acid catabolism does, however, relate to a specific pathway of amino acid utilization that is not directly related to protein metabolism. If under basal conditions proteins of a constant composition are degraded and resynthesised then it is important to maintain an appropriate pattern of amino acids within the cell. This is analogous to the need to provide an optimum pattern of dietary amino acids for growth. In the absence of dietary amino acids the disproportionate loss of a single essential amino acid will disturb the cellular free-amino-acid pattern and limit the resynthesis of cellular proteins. The result of this will be a relative excess of the other amino acids and this in its turn will lead to their catabolism.

Under basal conditions methionine seems to occupy a pivotal position in the overall amino acid economy. It behaves as the 'first limiting' amino acid under fasting and protein-free conditions and perhaps at body nitrogen equilibrium. Thus the provision of methionine to animals receiving no dietary protein reduces the rate of body protein loss[10]. Recent work with chicks suggests also that the addition of methionine to protein-free diets stimulates muscle protein synthesis.

There may be two reasons that underlie this specific requirement for methionine. First, integumental losses of protein, especially hair and wool, appear to continue under conditions where body protein loss occurs and these proteins are relatively rich in the sulphur amino acids. Second, methionine has an important role as a source of methyl groups. These groups, derived from the catabolism of methionine among other precursors, are involved in the synthesis of choline, a significant component of the membrane phospholipids. Furthermore, a number of proteins, most notably the contractile proteins actin and myosin, are modified after translation by the methylation of specific histidine and lysine residues. Because these methylated amino acids are not reutilized for protein synthesis their loss after degradation places a permanent drain on methyl group donors.

Nitrogen losses in the intestine. A further and potentially large loss of nitrogen from the body is via the intestinal tract and this has important practical and nutritional consequences. The most immediate consequence lies in the effect that endogenous intestinal nitrogen loss has on the assessment of the digestibility of dietary proteins and hence the prediction of safe levels of intake of given diets. Until recently the large majority of the available estimates of protein digestibilities were 'apparent', ie calculated as the net disappearance of nitrogen or amino acids between the diet and the faeces. Yet it has been known for many years that the largest component of faecal nitrogen in hind-gut bacterial protein[5]. These grow by fermenting undigested dietary constituents, especially carbohydrate, and by transforming and assimilating a variety of nitrogen sources. The amino acid composition of faeces is relatively fixed and bears little relationship to the amino acid digestibilities measured from faecal samples give little or no information about the true digestibility of the dietary amino acids.

In animals, at the practical level of dietary assessment, this problem has been solved by the measurement of amino acid digestibility at the terminal ileum. There appears to be little absorption of amino acids (as opposed to nitrogen) in the hind-gut so that the pre-caecal disappearance of dietary amino acids represents the amount of amino acids that is potentially available for the maintenance of body protein and for production processes.

Nevertheless, the fact remains that faecal nitrogen represents the transformation and sequestration of at least three sources of nitrogen: undigested dietary protein, undigested endogenous protein losses and urea.

Contribution of urea to faecal nitrogen. There is much circumstantial and some direct evidence that a portion of faecal nitrogen output is derived from urea nitrogen. The provision of additional energy, either by carbohydrate infusion into the hind-gut[11] or by addition of indigestible but fermentable carbohydrate to the diet[5], increases the output of faecal nitrogen and at the same time reduces urinary nitrogen and urea excretion. Similarly there is a general relationship between the rate of urea recycling (ie the difference between urea excretion and synthesis) and the output of faecal nitrogen. Urea recycling (measured with carbon-labelled urea) is also increased by the presence of indigestible carbohydrate in the diet. Finally, when monogastric animals received ^{15}N-labelled ammonium salts, label appeared in faecal nitrogen[1]. As it appeared that the labelled essential amino acids in faecal protein had similar isotope abundances they seemed to have a common precursor and the presence of additional fermentable carbohydrate in the hind-gut increases the loss of ^{15}N in the faeces when the animals received ^{15}N-ammonium salts.

Surprisingly there is relatively little formal quantitative information on this subject. Recent work in both rabbits[2] and in man[9] has suggested that only a small proportion (15–25 per cent) of caecal ammonia is derived from plasma urea. In man the degree to which urea ^{15}N contributed to faecal nitrogen was very low (6–7 per cent) and it was concluded[9] that the hind-gut was not the main site for urea hydrolysis and recycling. Clearly this is an important area of ignorance.

Contribution of endogenous protein to faecal nitrogen output. As with urea there is much qualitative evidence to show that endogenous proteins, secreted into the gut, contribute to faecal nitrogen loss. Comparison of the amino acid composition of the digesta in the terminal ileum suggests that part has been derived from endogenous sources[12]. Experiments in which the labelling of terminal ileal contents have been measured in animals receiving either labelled dietary proteins or i.v.-infused labelled amino acids also have demonstrated a contribution of host proteins to the digesta[1,6]. Given that little or no amino acid (as opposed to ammonia N) is absorbed from the hind-gut, these losses at the terminal ileum are a true loss of protein from the body. This is of importance as it represents a loss of essential amino acids and also represents a loss of the energy that has been expended in synthesising the protein that is lost by this route.

Measurements in pigs receiving protein-free diets suggest that up to 0.6 g protein per kg B.Wt. can be lost each day at the terminal ileum. This represents 60 per cent of the losses of protein by amino acid catabolism. Moreover the value may be an underestimate of the scale of protein loss in the intestine as the nature of the diet (particularly its fibre content) can influence endogenous nitrogen loss are also rich in dietary fibre, the effect of this component on nitrogen loss may have important nutritional consequences.

Exact quantification of these losses has not been made. Work carried out in the DDR, in which animals were infused intravenously with nitrogen labelled glycine and leucine, suggests that a very high proportion of the terminal ileal digesta proteins are derived from endogenous sources. In these experiments the prolonged intravenous infusion of labelled amino acids labelled the ileal protein to an isotope abundance that approached that of the free amino acids in plasma and this confirmed the conclusions drawn from earlier work with ^{14}C labelled dietary protein[6]. Recent work with chemically modified proteins[4] represents a new approach to formal quantitative studies carried out in animals that are receiving commonly available diets, and may allow the nutritional significance of these findings to be established.

1 Bergner, H., Bergner, U. & Simon, O. (1983): Measurement of ^{15}N-amino acid excretion and endogenous N-secretion in [15]N- and ^{14}C-labelled pigs. In *Proc. 4th EAAP Symposium on Protein metabolism and nutrition*, INRA Publication 16, pp. 339–342. Paris: INRA.

2 Forsythe, S.J. & Parker, D.S. (1985): Urea turnover and transfer to the digestive tract in the rabbit. *Br. J. Nutr.* **53**, 183–190.

3 Garlick, P.J., Clugston, G.A. & Waterlow, J.C. (1980): Influence of low-energy diets on whole-body protein turnover in obese subjects. *Am. J. Physiol.* **238**, E235–E244.

4 Hagemeister, H. & Erbersdobler, H. (1985): Chemical labelling of dietary protein by transformation of lysine to homoarginine: A new technique to follow intestinal digestion and absorption. *Proc. Nutr. Soc.* (In press).

5 Mason, V.C. & Palmer, R. (1973): The influence of bacterial activity in the alimentary canal of rats on faecal nitrogen excretion. *Acta Agric. Scand.* **23**, 141–150.

6 Nasset, E.S. (1965): Role of the digestive system in protein metabolism. *Fed. Proc.* **24**, 953–958.

7 Waterlow, J.C., Garlick, P.J. & Millward, D.J. (1978): *Protein turnover in mammalian tissues and in the whole body*, Amsterdam: North Holland.

8 Winterer, J., Bistrian, B.R., Bilmazer, C., Blackburn, G.L. & Young, V.R. (1980): Whole body protein turnover, studied with ^{15}N-glycine, and muscle protein breakdown in mildly obese subjects during a protein-sparing diet and a brief total fast. *Metabolism* **29**, 575–581.

9 Wrong, O.M., Vinci, A.J. & Waterlow, J.C. (1985): The contribution of endogenous urea to faecal ammonia in man, determined by ^{15}N labelling of plasma urea. *Clin. Sci.* **68**, 193–199.

10 Yoshida, A. & Moritoki, K. (1974): Nitrogen sparing action of methionine and threonine in rats receiving a protein-free diet. *Nutr. Rep. Int.* **9**, 159–168.

11 Zebrowska, T., Zebrowska, H. & Buraczewska, L. (1980): The relationship between amount and type of carbohydrates entering the large intestine and nitrogen excretion in faeces and urine of pigs. In *Proc. 3rd EAAP Symposium on Protein metabolism and nutrition*, EAAP Publication No. 27, pp. 222–226.

12 Zebrowska, T., Simon, O., Munchmeyer, R., Wolf, E., Bergner, H. & Zebrowska, H. (1982): Flow of endogenous and exogenous amino acids along the gut of pigs. *Arch. Tier.* **32**, 431–444.

The influence of infection on protein metabolism in skeletal muscle

Vickie E. BARACOS
Department of Animal Science, University of Alberta, Edmonton, Canada T6G 2P5.

Metabolic response to infection. Generalized body wasting and muscle protein depletion are common clinical signs associated with febrile infection, sepsis and trauma. Even infections which are brief, mild or highly localized cause detectable losses of body protein[2,13,17]. In the adult, there is an abrupt transition into negative N balance[2,7,30]. In rapidly growing young, there is typically an impairment of growth[17]. Body protein loss is proportional to the severity and to the duration of the insult, and is greater than would be expected on the basis of reduced food intake alone. When infections are chronic or complicated by injuries, surgery or burns, up to one-third of total body protein can be lost[30]. This condition is, in itself, considered life-threatening.

The atrophy of skeletal muscle results from increased protein degradation, decreased protein synthesis, or both. Several studies on patients with sepsis or trauma have suggested that the negative N balance results from an accelerated degradation of cellular protein, particularly in skeletal muscle[5,6,8,9,13,19,23]. For example, measurements of arteriovenous differences in amino acids show that muscle is in considerable negative amino acid balance[7,9]. The reported effects of fever, infection and trauma on protein synthesis in muscle and in the whole body are conflicting[9,13,18,22,25]. Protein synthesis is likely to be suppressed by the lack of amino acid precursors, when food intake is reduced.

The catabolism of muscle would appear to be coupled to a number of anabolic processes related to host defence[2], including activation and proliferation of phagocytes and lymphocytes and antibody synthesis. In addition to a general increase in hepatic protein synthesis, a variety of proteins which are not ordinarily produced in large quantities are synthesized within the liver. These include the acute phase reactants (fibrinogen, haptoglobin, serum amyloid A, C-reactive protein, α_2-macrofetoprotein), the metallothioneins and proteins involved in the function of the kinin, complement and coagulation systems. The synthesis of these proteins, whose functions are related to immunocompetance, maintenance of organ function and healing, could utilize amino acids derived from muscle protein.

The rise in muscle protein breakdown following infection is also associated with an increase in the *de-novo* synthesis of alanine by muscle, and an increased rate of oxidation of amino acids in the whole body[24,29,31]. As in fasting[14], the net breakdown of protein in muscle and the release of amino acids, especially alanine, provides substrates for hepatic gluconeogenesis or for direct oxidation. Thus muscle is used as a source of metabolizable energy, apparently to satisfy increased overall metabolic energy expenditure. Metabolic rate may rise 10 to 20 per cent in mild infection, and up to 50 per cent in severe infection[21,30]. In extreme cases where infection is complicated by multiple trauma or burns, metabolic rates may be up to double the predicted normal value[30]. Since this elevated metabolism is generally accompanied by anorexia, muscle serves as an important store of nutrients.

The role of interleukin-1 in coordination of host response to infection. Purposeful signals coordinate host response to infection at the level of many tissues. Endocrine responses include participation by the anterior and posterior pituitary glands, the adrenal cortex, the thyroid and the endocrine pancreas (in recent review[2]). In addition, Interleukin-1 has emerged as a factor signalling diverse aspects of host responses to antigens, infection, inflammation and injury. This product of mononuclear phagocytes is a protein of approximately 15 kd MW, and is similar or highly related to 'endogenous pyrogen', 'leukocyte endogenous mediator', 'lymphocyte activating factor' and 'mononuclear cell factor'[10]. Its actions include the initiation of fever at the level of the hypothalamus, induction of acute phase protein synthesis in the liver and lymphocyte activation (Figure). Interleukin-1 also signals systemic metabolic responses such as the net breakdown of protein in skeletal muscle and the release of amino acids from this tissue[1]. When rat muscles were incubated with purified human Interleukin-1, net protein degradation increased, while protein synthesis was not affected. Interleukin-1 stimulated the production of a prostaglandin (PG) namely PGE_2 by the muscles by 2.5 to 10 – fold. The addition of indomethacin, an inhibitor of PG synthesis, prevented the enhancement of PGE_2 synthesis and of protein breakdown by Interleukin-1[1]. The stimulation of proteolysis by Interleukin-1 was also markedly decreased by Ep-475, an inhibitor of lysosomal thiol proteases. These observations suggested that Interleukin-1 signals the muscle protein catabolism which accompanies fever and infection, an effect involving local production of PGE_2 and an activation of lysosomal proteolysis.

Evidence supporting a role for Interleukin-1 in muscle protein catabolism *in vivo* has been obtained by Clowes and coworkers[8,9]. These investigators isolated a peptide from the plasma of septic patients which stimulated protein degradation in rat muscle *in vitro*. This 'proteolysis-inducing factor' or 'PIF', like Interleukin-1, also induces a variety of 'acute phase' reactions including lymphocyte activation and hepatic protein synthesis, but does not induce fever (Figure)[1,20]. PIF has a molecular weight of approximately 4 kd, which may be a circulating fragment of Interleukin-1, since a 4 kd peptide with the same activities appears spontaneously in purified preparations of 15 kd Interleukin-1[11]. The relative amounts of circulating 15 kd Interleukin-1 and of the 4 kd fragment are not known. Factors influencing the rate of appearance of the 4 kd piece and its subsequent clearance or breakdown remain to be defined.

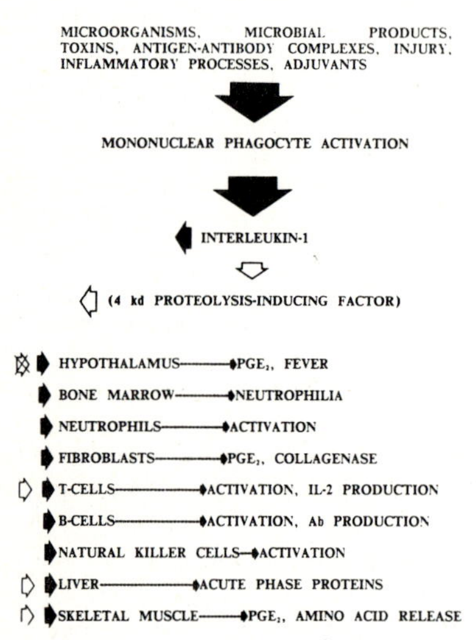

Figure. *Schematic representation of the actions of Interleukin-1 and of its 4 kd fragment (proteolysis-inducing factor) on different cell types.* Dark arrows indicate the activities of Interleukin-1. Open arrows indicate the known activities of the proteolysis-inducing factor.

Two recent studies have implicated PG and lysosomal thiol proteases in the muscle protein catabolism which accompanies infection: that *Eschericia coli* sepsis in the rat was shown to be accompanied by increased muscle protein degradation and PGE_2 release, these effects being inhibited by the administration of indomethacin *in vivo*[12], while muscle atrophy and loss of muscle contractile function were shown to accompany *Streptococcus pneumoniae* sepsis in the rat[27]. These effects were abolished when animals were treated systemically with inhibitors of prostaglandin synthesis or leupeptin, an inhibitor of lysosomal thiol proteases. It is not yet known if the muscle protein loss accompanying surgery, trauma or burn injury occurs by a similar mechanism.

Implications for nutritional support of the infected patient. Host response to infection thus comprises a complex cascade, including a mixture of anabolic and catabolic processes, involving many different tissues and interorgan relationships. The adaptive value of metabolic alterations accompanying infection needs to be more clearly defined. Muscle protein stores are utilized during a generalized increase in metabolic rate, accompanied by reduced food intake. The catabolism of muscle proteins would appear to represent the mobilization of a relatively expendible and labile store to satisfy requirements for amino acids and metabolizable energy. It is possible that this ability to mobilize peripheral protein stores has important survival value. Clowes & coworkers[4,26] studied the peripheral production rates of amino acids, and their central clearance rates in patients receiving no parenteral amino acid infusions. Both of these processes were elevated three to five-fold in survivors of sepsis. By contrast, patients who failed to survive had on average less than half the peripheral production and central clearance rates of amino acids. These results suggest that an adequate supply of amino acids may be essential to survival in the critically ill, and provides a rationale for the vigorous nutritional support of the infected patient.

We must determine to what extent undesirable changes can be altered by exogenous nutritional support. For example, oral protein intake or parenteral feeding tend to reduce the peripheral release of amino acids from muscle, to accelerate their visceral uptake, and improve N balance[4,19,24,28]. Prior malnutrition or protein deficiency results in reduced production of Interleukin-1 in humans and rabbits[3,15,16], as well as depleted whole-body protein reserves. This situation may result in an inability to increase muscle protein degradation, and reduce the supply of amino acids available for synthetic processes essential to immunocompetance and healing, including Interleukin-1 synthesis.

It is possible that in certain circumstances the catabolism of skeletal muscle during infection could be actively suppressed. The initiation of this process by Interleukin-1, although apparently of value to the host, ultimately results in a cumulative protein loss which threatens survival. If the nutritional status of the patient can be maintained, then inhibition of muscle protein breakdown may not affect survival or recovery rates. If this is the case, then inhibitors of PG synthesis which are effective at the level of skeletal muscle may prove useful in maintaining muscle mass and function, and prevent a potentially catastrophic protein loss.

Acknowledgements. The author is grateful to Drs C.A. Dinarello, A.L. Goldberg and G.H.A. Clowes Jr. for their support, enthusiasm and many useful discussions.

1 Baracos, V.E., Rodemann, H.P., Dinarello, C.A. & Goldberg, A.L. (1983): Stimulation of muscle protein degradation and prostaglandin E$_2$ release by leukocytic pyrogen (Interleukin-1). *New Engl. J. Med.* **308**, 553–558.

2 Beisel, W.R. (1984): Metabolic effects of infection. *Prog. Fd Nutr. Sci.* **8**, 43–75.

3 Bell, R. & Hoffman-Goetz, L. (1983): Effect of protein deficiency on endogenous-pyrogen mediated acute phase protein responses. *Can. J. Physiol. Pharmacol.* **61**, 376–380.

4 Bigatello, L.M., Clowes, G.H.A. Jr & Loda, M. (1985): The effects of amino acid parenteral alimentation on central plasma clearance rates, differentiating survivors and deaths in trauma, sepsis and gangrene. *Surg. Forum* (In press).

5 Birkhahn, R., Long, C., Fitkin, D., Geiger, J. & Blakemore, W. (1980): Whole body protein metabolism due to trauma in man measured with L-[1-^{14}C]-leucine. *Surgery* **88**, 294–300.

6 Clague, M., Keir, J., Wright, P. & Johnson, I. (1983): The effects of nutrition and trauma on whole body protein metabolism in man. *Clin. Sci.* **65**, 165–175.

7 Clowes, G.H.A. Jr, Randall, H. & Cha, C.J. (1980): Amino acid and energy metabolism in septic and traumatized patients. *J. Parenteral & Enterol Nutr.* **4**, 195–205.

8 Clowes, G.H.A. Jr, George, B. & Ryan, N. (1982): Induction of accelerated proteolysis and amino acid release from skeletal muscle by a potent nonprotein factor in the plasma of septic patients; in *The role of chemical mediators in the pathophysiology of acute illness and injury*, ed R. McConn pp. 327–341 New York: Raven Press.

9 Clowes, G.H.A. Jr, George, B.C., Villee, C.A. Jr, & Saravis, C.A. (1983): Muscle proteolysis induced by a circulating peptide in patients with sepsis or trauma. *New Engl. J. Med.* **308**, 545–552.

10 Dinarello, C.A. (1984): Interleukin-1. *Rev. Infect. Dis.* **6**, 51–95.

11 Dinarello, C.A., Clowes, G.H.A. Jr, Gordon, H.A., Saravis, C.A. & Wolff, S.M. (1984): Cleavage of human Interleukin-1: Isolation of a peptide fragment from plasma of febrile humans and activated monocytes. *J. Immunol.* **133**, 1332–1338.

12 Fagan, J. & Goldberg, A.L. (1985): Muscle protein breakdown, PGE$_2$ and fever, upon bacterial infection, in *'The physiologic, metabolic and immunologic actions of Interleukin-1'*, ed M. Kluger, Ann Arbor, Michigan, June, 1985 New York: Alan R. Liss (In press).

13 Garlick, P., McNurlan, M., Fern, E., Tomkins, A. & Waterlow, J.L. (1980): Stimulation of protein synthesis and breakdown by vaccination. *Br. Med. J.* **281**, 263–265.

14 Goldberg, A.L. & Chang, T.W. (1978): Regulation and significance of amino acid metabolism in muscle. *Fed. Proc.* **37**, 2301–2307.

15 Hoffman-Goetz, L., McFarlane, D., Bistrian, B.R. & Blackburn, G.L. (1981): Febrile and plasma iron responses of rabbits injected with endogenous pyrogen from malnourished patients. *Am. J. Clin. Nutr.* **32**, 1423–1427.
16 Keenan, R.A., Moldawer, L.L., Yang, R.D., Kawamura, I., Blackburn, G.L. & Bistrian, B.R. (1982): An altered response by peripheral leukocytes to synthesize or release luekocyte endogenous mediator in critically ill, protein malnourished patients. *J. Lab. Clin. Med.* **100**, 844–857.
17 Keilman, A. (1977): Weight fluctuations after immunization in a rural preschool child community. *Am. J. Clin. Nutr.* **30**, 592–598.
18 Kien, C., Young, V.R., Rothbough, D. & Burke, J. (1978): Increased rates of whole body protein synthesis and breakdown in children recovering from burns. *Ann Surg* **187**, 383–391.
19 Leverve, X., Guignier, M., Carpentier, F., Serre, J.C. & Caravel, J.P. (1984): Effect of parenteral nutrition on muscle amino acid output and 3-methylhistidine excretion in septic patients. *Metabolism* **33**, 471–477.
20 Loda, M., Clowes, G.H.A. Jr, Dinarello, C.A., George, B.C., Lane, B. & Richardson, W. (1984): Induction of hepatic protein synthesis by a peptide in blood plasma of patients with sepsis and trauma. *Surgery* **96**, 204–213.
21 Long, C.L. (1977): Energy balance and carbohydrate metabolism in infection and sepsis. *Am. J. Clin. Nutr.* **30**, 1301–1310.
22 Long, C.L., Jeevanadam, M., Kim, B.M. & Kinney, J.M. (1977): Whole body protein synthesis and catabolism in septic man. *Am. J. Clin. Nutr.* **30**, 1340–1344.
23 Long, C.L., Birkhahan, R., Geiger, J., Betts, J., Schiller, W. & Blakemore, W. (1981): Urinary excretion of 3-methylhistidine: an assessment of muscle protein catabolism in adult normal subjects and during malnutrition, sepsis and skeletal trauma. *Metabolism* **30**, 765–776.
24 Pittiruti, M., Seigel, J.H., Sganga, G., Coleman, B., Wiles, C.E. III., Belzberg, H., Wedel, S. & Placko, R. (1985): Increased dependence of leucine in posttraumatic sepsis: leucine/tyrosine clearance ratio as an indicator of hepatic impairment in septic multiple organ failure syndrome. *Surgery* (In press).
25 Rennie, M.J. & Harrison, R. (1984): The effects of injury, disease and malnutrition on protein metabolism in man. *Lancet* **1**, 323–325.
26 Rosenblatt, S., Clowes, G.H.A. Jr, George, B.C., Hirsch, E. & Lindberg, B. (1983): Exchange of amino acids by muscle and liver in sepsis. *Archs. Surg.* **118**, 167–175.
27 Ruff, R.L. & Secrist, D. (1984): Inhibitors of prostaglandin synthesis or Cathepsin B prevent muscle wasting due to sepsis in the rat. *J. Clin. Invest.* **73**, 1483–1486.
28 Shaw, S.N., Elwyn, D.H., Askanazi, J., Iles, M., Schwarz, Y. & Kinney, J.M. (1983): Effects of increasing nitrogen intake on nitrogen balance and energy expenditure in nutritionally depleted adult patients receiving parenteral nutrition. *Am. J. Clin. Nutr.* **37** , 930–940.
29 Wannemacher, R.W. (1977): Key roles of various individual amino acids in host response to infection. *Am. J. Clin. Nutr.* **30**, 1340–1344.
30 Wilmore, D.W. & Kinney, J.M. (1981): Panel report on the nutritional support of patients with trauma or infection. *Am. J. Clin. Nutr.* **34**, 1213–1222.
31 Yang, R.D., Moldawer, L.L., Sakamoto, A., Keenan, R.A., Matthews, D.E., Wolfe, R.R., Young, V.R., Wannemacher, R.W. & Blackburn, G.L. (1983): Leukocyte endogenous mediator alters protein dynamics in the rat. *Metabolism* **32**, 654–60.

Regulation of protein turnover in primary cultured hepatocytes

A. ICHIHARA and K. TANAKA
Institute for Enzyme Research, School of Medicine, University of Tokushima, Tokushima 770, Japan.

Liver has diverse functions and its regulation of synthesis and degradation are unique. Primary cultures of adult rat hepatocytes are a very good experimental system for use in studies on complex liver functions[1]. In this paper we report the features of protein turnover in the liver shown with this system.

Isolation and culture of hepatocytes. Parenchymal hepatocytes were isolated from adult rats by perfusion of the liver with collagenase, and were cultured as monolayers for several days in Williams' medium E supplemented with 10 per cent calf serum and various hormones[10].

Nitrogen balance of hepatocytes. Protein turnover of hepatocytes can be calculated from changes in the concentrations of urea, ammonia and amino acids in the culture medium. In a medium containing low concentrations of amino acids, the cells release amino acids by protein degradation, with little formation of urea or ammonia, showing that their protein metabolism is in a catabolic state[9]. On the other hand, in a medium containing high concentrations of amino acids, they show marked uptake of amino acids, with formation of much urea, but little ammonia, indicating anabolic protein metabolism. Thus, the nitrogen balance of the hepatocytes increase with increase in the amino acid concentration in the medium, due to increased protein synthesis and decreased protein degradation. Their nitrogen balance changes from negative to positive on increase in the amino acid concentration from 0.5 to 1.0 mM. Insulin enhances the positive nitrogen balance, while glucagon depresses it.

Hormonal regulation of protein synthesis. Overall protein synthesis in hepatocytes is stimulated by insulin and glucocorticoid, but repressed by glucagon[10]. These hormones have similar effects on the synthesis of plasma proteins. However, the synthesis of intracellular enzymes related to amino acid degradation is increased by glucocorticoid, isoproterenol and glucagon and inhibited by insulin and catecholamine (alpha$_1$)[5]. The effects of these hormones appear to be exerted at the transcriptional level.

Two pools of amino acids for protein synthesis. In hepatocyte culture, depletion of amino acids in the medium causes a rapid decrease in synthesis of proteins to be secreted with no change in proteins in the cells for 40 h and then their gradual decrease[6]. In these conditions, polysomes on the rough endoplasmic reticulum are degraded specifically with the appearance of many autophagic vacuoles, suggesting increasing degradation of intracellular proteins. Addition of leupeptin to the medium inhibits synthesis of intracellular proteins only when the amino acid concentration of the medium is low. These facts suggest that when the amino acid supply from the medium is sufficient, the amino acids are used for syntheses of both intra- and extracellular proteins and the breakdown of intracellular proteins is low, but that when the supply of extracellular amino acids is low, synthesis of serum proteins is reduced, while that of intracellular proteins still continues, because protein degradation increases and the amino acids derived from this degradation are reutilized for synthesis of intracellular proteins only. It is very interesting that the amino acid supply regulates the synthesis of intra- and extracellular proteins in different ways, and also regulates protein degradation, possibly in lysosomes. This is interpreted to imply that in these conditions liver tends to sacrifice synthesis of extracellular proteins which are not essential for survival of the cells, but to maintain synthesis of housekeeping proteins.

Mechanism of degradation of hepatic proteins. Lysosomal protease inhibitors, such as leupeptin and E-64, cause only 20–30 per cent inhibition of long-lived proteins and have no effect on degradation of those with short half-lives[8]. However, in conditions of amino acid deprivation, lysosomal activity increases and the degradation of proteins with long half-lives doubles. This accelerated rate is decreased by addition of leupeptin or EGTA. On the other hand, these lysosomal inhibitors have no effect on the degradation of abnormal proteins containing amino acid analogues. Thus there seem to be two distinct pathways of protein degradation in hepatocytes. One is the lysosomal route, which plays a major role in nutritional regulation and is related to the formation of autophagic vacuoles, while the other is the non-lysosomal route, which is unaffected by the above conditions, but regulated by the energy supply. The latter mechanism may be important in disposal of defective proteins, which may be formed even in normal cells and are hazardous to the cells. Although the mechanism of the non-lysosomal system is unknown, we recently found a latent endoprotease in the liver cytosol. This enzyme is unusually large (Mr = 750 000) and has multiple active sites with different specificities for various substrates and it could be the protease involved in the non-lysosomal system[7].

Growth of hepatocytes and protein metabolism. Mature hepatocytes in cultures at low cell density can be induced to proliferate by insulin, epidermal growth factor and a factor secreted from platelets (not PDGF)[2]. Under these conditions amino acid transport and protein synthesis increase (synthesis of serum proteins does not change), while liver specific functions including amino acid degradation decrease. In cultures at high cell density, activities related to growth decreases and liver specific functions increase[4]. Therefore, regulation of the metabolism of proteins and amino acids in hepatocytes is different in growing and quiescent states.

Recently we found that in hepatocytes, collagen synthesis is required for DNA synthesis. If proline in omitted from the medium, or inhibitors of collagen synthesis are added, then DNA synthesis is markedly inhibited. The collagen synthesized may be a component of the intercellular matrix, which gives a favourable environment for hepatocyte growth[3].

Conclusion. In the body, liver synthesizes a variety of proteins, not only for housekeeping, but also for secretion as serum proteins. Their turnovers are in dynamic states, and they have long and short half-lives. Their levels are controlled not only by dietary proteins, but also by various hormones, which affect the rates of their synthesis and degradation. Protein synthesis is controlled at two sites, membrane bound and free polysomes. Protein degradation occurs by lysosomal and non-lysosomal pathways. Two states of the cell cycle must also be considered in protein turnover: the quiescent (differentiated) and growing (undifferentiated) states. The latter should be divided into the normal regenerating and abnormal tumorigenic states. Moreover, recent studies have shown that the architecture of liver tissue is important for functions including protein metabolism and thus the findings obtained in experiments should be interpreted taking into account all the variables described above.

Acknowledgement. This work was supported by Research Grants from the Ministry of Education, Science and Culture of Japan.

1　Ichihara, A., Nakamura, T. & Tanaka, K. (1982): Use of hepatocytes in primary cultures for biochemical studies on liver functions. *Mol. Cell. Biochem.* **43**, 145–160.

2　Nakamura, T. & Ichihara, A. (1985): Control of growth and expression of differentiated functions of mature hepatocytes in primary culture. *Cell Struct. Funct.* **10**, 1–16.

3　Nakamura, T., Teramoto, H., Tomita, Y. & Ichihara, A. (1984): L-proline is an essential amino acid for hepatocytes growth in culture. *Biochem. Biophys, Res. Commun.* **122**, 884–891.

4　Nakamura, T., Yoshimoto, K., Nakayama, Y., Tomita, Y. & Ichihara, A. (1983): Reciprocal modulation of growth and differentiated functions of mature rat hepatocytes in primary culture by cell-cell contact and cell membranes. *Proc. Natl. Acad. Sci. USA* **80**, 7229–7233.

5　Noda, C., Nakamura, T. & Ichihara, A. (1983): Alpha-adrenergic control of enzymes of amino acid metabolism in primary cultures of adult rat hepatocytes. *J. Biol. Chem.* **258**, 1520–1525.

6　Tanaka, K. & Ichihara, A. (1983): Different effects of amino acid deprivation on syntheses of intra- and extracellular proteins in rat hepatocytes in primary culture. *J. Biochem. (Tokyo)* **94**, 1339–1348.

7　Tanaka, K. & Ichihara, A. (In prep): Purification and characterization of high molecular weight and multifunctional protease from liver cytosol.

8　Tanaka, K., Ikegaki, N. & Ichihara, A. (1981): Effect of leupeptin and pepstatin on protein turnover in adult rat hepatocytes in primary culture. *Arch. Biochem. Biophys.* **208**, 296–304.

9　Tanaka, K., Kishi, K. & Ichihara, A. (1979): Biochemical studies on liver functions in primary cultured hepatocytes of adult rats II. Regulation of protein and amino acid metabolism. *J. Biochem. (Tokyo)* **86**, 863–870.

10　Tanaka, K., Sato, M., Tomita, Y. & Ichihara, A. (1978): Biochemical studies on liver functions in primary cultured hepatocytes of adult rats I. Hormonal effects on cell viability and protein synthesis. *J. Biochem. (Tokyo)* **84**, 937–946.

VIII: Protein energy interrelationships

METABOLIC ADAPTATION TO LOW INTAKES

Adaptation and regulation — general concepts

J.C. WATERLOW
London School of Hygiene & Tropical Medicine, Keppel Street, London WC1E 7HT, UK.

Fifteen years ago P.P. Cohen and I organised a one-day symposium on nutritional adaptation at a meeting of the Pan-American Health Organization[6]. I had been working in Jamaica on severely malnourished children, and my main interest was to identify, explain and if possible reverse the metabolic changes and the pathological disturbances that often led to death. However, I gradually realized that this was a one-sided approach. Clearly these children had been adapted for some time to a state of malnutrition and then the adaptation broke down. It was perhaps more important to understand the mechanisms that enable children to survive and function in an adverse environment as well as they do, and to find out why, in the majority of cases, the mechanisms of adaptation do not break down.

Since then a great deal more has been found out about protein and energy metabolism in mammalian organisms under different conditions and it is the aim of this Symposium to pull some of this knowledge together and see what kind of a picture we can build up of adaptive processes in malnutrition.

I do not think it is useful to try to define precisely what is meant by words such as adaptation, homoeostasis, regulation. This subject has been discussed in more detail elsewhere[7]. I would like, however, to begin with some remarks about the general concept of adaptation and its characteristics. First, we have to distinguish between genetic, metabolic and social or behavioural adaptation, although they often overlap. For example, ethnic groups who have lived for thousands of years by keeping animals and in whose diet milk plays an important part retain their intestinal lactase in adult life, whereas most of us lose it. This appears to be a genetically determined metabolic adaptation (eg[4]). At the other end of the scale, many of us believe that behavioural changes, ie economies in physical activity, may play an important part in adaptation to low energy intakes. Such adaptations are clearly not without cost.

Secondly, an adapted state is one that is capable of being maintained. Sometimes the concept of a set point, as with a thermostat, may be useful. Adaptation would represent a change in set point; regulation summarizes the mechanisms by which conditions are maintained at the set point. Examples of an altered set point would be the increase in red cell mass at high altitude or in plasma volume on prolonged exposure to heat. I wonder whether the somewhat lower obligatory nitrogen losses found in orientals compared with other ethnic groups[3] could be regarded as an altered set point in nitrogen metabolism. The same might apply to the lower BMRs that have been recorded in Indians compared with Caucasians[5]. Both these important phenomena need to be more widely studied; nor do we know the extent to which they are genetically determined.

Thirdly, any realistic discussion of adaptation must tackle the question: adaptation in respect to what? It is necessary to define the characteristics or functions that adaptation, in teleological terms, is trying to preserve. In the case of high altitude the key function is oxygen transport; in adaptation to hot climates it is the maintenance of heat transfer and relatively constant body temperature. In these well worked out physiological examples, adaptation is related to functions for which there is a recognized range of normality. To paraphrase Claude Bernard's dictum that the fixity of the internal environment is the condition of a free life, one might say that adaptation is the condition of normal function. Unfortunately, in most nutritional contexts there is no clear definition of the range of normality. We generally rely either on statistical limits, eg the so-called normal range of plasma albumin, or on subjective judgements about the quality of life, eg that voluntary activity should never be restricted by an inadequate energy intake.

There is one characteristic that cannot be omitted from any discussion of adaptation: that is the question of body size and body weight or lean body mass (LBM). In adaptations to low intakes of energy and protein, must a 'successful' adaptation in principle maintain a fixed body weight for any given person? Or can the weight be allowed to vary, and if so, within what range? If, after maintaining a constant weight for 10 years I consistently eat a little more or a little less, my weight will rise or fall to a new steady state. We know something about the upper limit of acceptable body weight, in terms of body mass index (BMI) from the data that have been accumulated on the morbidity and mortality associated with obesity. We know much less about the lower limit although it is of far greater importance in the context of this symposium. The conventional range of 'acceptable' BMI is currently given as 18–25[1]. However, I believe that this value for the lower limit is an artefact of Western societies. The poor Indian labourers described by Shetty[5] were active and performed well in standard physiological tests although their BMI was only 15–16. Anorexic subjects, as described, for example, by Forbes and co-workers[2] are typically hyperactive physically, with a BMI of about 14. We need much more sensitive tests of function to assess the lower limit of BMI that could be regarded as an acceptable adaptation.

The question of body size is particularly important in children. I refer to the hotly debated issue of whether stunting in linear growth should be regarded as an acceptable adaptation. If one takes the moral point of view that children have a right to develop their innate growth potential, then stunting is an acceptable adaptation only to the extent that it helps children to survive. That is certainly one criterion, but hardly an adequate one, since one may then ask: Survive in what condition? It would not be profitable to pursue this point further. I only make it to emphasize that in any general discussion of adaptation it is impossible to avoid concepts such as 'adequate', 'acceptable', 'normal' range, 'normal' function, etc. This is a philosophical problem that has to be recognized even though it cannot be solved. Many of the arguments, such as the one about stunted children, simply represent differences in value judgements.

I think it is more profitable to concentrate on particular mechanisms of adaptation or response, such as changes under various conditions in enzyme activities or metabolic fluxes. These can be described and analysed without the need for value judgements. The papers in this Symposium represent a variety of contributions to this approach. I believe that the nature and extent of metabolic adaptation to low intakes of energy and protein is one of the most important subjects in nutritional science at the present time.

1 Bray, G.A. ed (1979): *Obesity in America*. Proceedings of the 2nd Fogarty International Center Conference on Obesity, Washington, DC. US Department of Health, Education & Welfare. NIH Pubn. No. 79.
2 Forbes, G.B., Kreipe, R.E., Lipinski, B.A. & Hodgman, C.H. (1984): Body composition changes during recovery from anorexia nervosa: comparison of two dietary regimes. *Am. J. Clin. Nutr.* **40**, 1137–1145.

3 Huang, P.C., Chong, H.E. & Rand, W.M. (1972): Obligatory urinary and fecal nitrogen losses in young Chinese men. *J. Nutr.* **102**, 1605–1614.

4 Kretchmer, N. (1981): Food: a selective agent in evolution. In *Food, nutrition and evolution*, ed D.N. Walcher & N. Kretchmer, pp. 37–48. New York: Masson.

5 Shetty, P.S. (1984): Adaptive changes in basal metabolic rate and lean body mass in chronic undernutrition. *Hum. Nutr. Clin. Nutr.* **38C**, 443–452.

6 Waterlow, J.C. (1971): The concept of "normal" in nutrition. In *Metabolic adaptation and nutrition*, pp. 76–80. Scientific Publication No. 222, Pan American Health Organization, Washington, DC.

7 Waterlow, J.C. (1985): Postscript. In *Nutritional adaptation in man*, ed K. Blaxter & J.C. Waterlow, pp. 233–235. London: John Libbey.

Range of variation in energy expenditure and scope for regulation

Anna FERRO-LUZZI
National Institute of Nutrition, Via Ardeatina, 546, Rome, Italy.

Energy spent in daily life varies between and also within individuals. This is not surprising because people have a variety of jobs and leisure activities, and operate under different constraints. To show the extent of this variability I selected field studies on energy expenditure published in such a way as to permit individual values to be retrieved (Table 1) and encompassing a wide variety of habitats, occupations and ethnic groups. Less developed countries (LDC) feature in 15 of the 21 studies, but there were roughly equal numbers of

Table 1. *Study groups (males) of energy expenditure under real life conditions, selected on the basis of criteria suggested by Durnin & Ferro-Luzzi, 1982, carried out by direct assessment of time-use and energy costs, and whose results had been reported in such a way as to allow retrieval of individual values.*

Study No.	Group	Sample Size (n)	Length of Survey (d)	Ref.
	LDC Rural habitat			
1	Lowland subsistence horticulture (New Guinea)	42	5	27
2	Highland subsistence horticulture (New Guinea)	40	5	27
3	Peasants (Upper Volta)	11	6	6
4	Agricultural labourers (Guatemala)	18	7	30
5	Rice farmers (Philippines)	9	7	18
6	Agricultural labourers (Philippines)	32	7	22
7	Fishermen (Philippines)	33	7	22
8	Agricultural labourers: Spring (Iran)	10	1	7
9	Agricultural labourers: Summer (Iran)	14	1	7
10	Agricultural labourers: Autumn (Iran)	10	1	7
11	Agricultural labourers: Winter (Iran)	12	1	7
	LDC Urban habitat			
12	Shoemakers (Philippines)	10	7	19
13	Clerk typists (Philippines)	10	7	17
14	Jeepney drivers (Philippines)	10	7	20
15	Textile mill workers (Philippines)	25	7	2
	Western world			
16	University students (UK)	6	14	25
17	Cadets (UK)	12	14	11
18	Infantry recruits (UK)	35	21	10
19	Antarctic study team	12	82	1
20	Shipyard workers (Italy)	149	7	26
21	Aged, retired homes (Italy)	67	7	28
	Total	567	5067 (subject days)	

Table 2. *Interindividual variability expressed as coefficient of variation (CV): of 567 subjects. This sample was obtained by pooling the study groups listed in Table 1.*

Sample size (n)	Mean length of survey (d)	Mean Body wt (kg)	Energy expenditure (kcal (MJ)/d)			CV (%)
			Mean	−2sd	+2sd	
567	9	64.1	2843 (11.9)	1512 (6.3)	4088 (17.1)	23.2

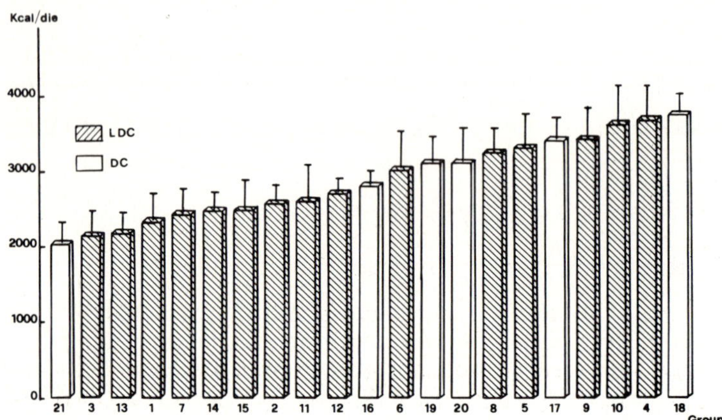

Fig. 1. *Mean interindividual variability (within groups and between groups) of 24-h energy expenditure of study groups from developed (DC) and less developed (LDC) countries. Mean intragroup CV = 12%; mean intergroup CV = 19%. For identification of groups, refer to Table 1. Error bars represent s.ds.*

subjects from LDC and developed countries (DC). Pooling all the subjects from the studies, a sample was obtained of 567 healthy active adult males whose habitual energy expenditure has been assessed, by time and motion coupled with direct measure of energy cost, for an average of 9 days per subject (Table 2). This admittedly very heterogeneous group had a mean daily energy expenditure of 2843 kcal (11.9 MJ), 44 kcal (184 kJ)/kg body weight, with a coefficient of variation (CV) of 23 per cent indicating that about one-third of the subjects spent less than 2200 kcal (9.2 MJ) and more than 3500 kcal (14.6 MJ)/d. Some 3 per cent had expenditures exceeding 4000 kcal (16.7 MJ)/d or below 1500 kcal (6.3 MJ)/d. Such remarkable variability might have been anticipated on the basis of the wide variety of life-styles and occupations represented.

However, Fig. 1 shows that, while noticeably reduced, an average 12 per cent variability still persisted when the 567 individuals were regrouped according to their original categories based on their jobs. The argument in this case might be that job denominations are poor descriptors of energy expenditure[26] and that the observed variability may be justified by this rather imprecise categorization and grouping. It would be legitimate, nevertheless, to ask whether this range of variability reflects a capacity of the human organism to regulate its energy output. The fact that intraindividual variance of total energy expenditure has been found to account for the largest part of the observed interindividual variance lends support to this hypothesis[24]. My own analysis on 478 subjects of the large pooled sample confirms that CV intra—is almost as large as CV inter—individuals (Table 3). According to Margen[24] CV intra reflects the capacity to adapt (regulate) intake and expenditure in such a way that the expected value of daily energy balance is zero and the co-variance between daily energy balance K days apart is constant over time'. As 'metabolic mechanisms which may lead to variation in energy utilization are known', Margen draws the conclusion that 'it seems more likely that the body regulates its energy balance by varying the efficiency of energy utilization'.

Table 3. *Mean group intraindividual variability expressed as coefficient of variation (CV) of 24-h energy expenditure observed on 478 subjects, each studied for an average of 7 days.*

Study No. (reference)	Group	Sex	Sample size (n)	Length of survey (d)	CV (%)
1[27]	New Guinea lowlands	m	42	6	15.7 ± 6.9
2[27]	New Guinea highlands	m	40	5	10.3 ± 4.4
22[27]	New Guinea lowlands	f	40	6	13.1 ± 5.8
23[27]	New Guinea highlands	f	42	5	9.5 ± 4.3
20[26]	Shipyard workers	m	149	7	11.5 ± 5.0
24[13]	University staff	f	4	29	5.5 ± 1.6
21[28]	Old men in retirement homes	m	67	7	4.5 ± 2.8
25[28]	Old women in retirement homes	f	57	7	5.0 ± 4.2
17[11]	British cadets	m	12	14	12.4 ± 3.2
3[6]	Upper Volta farmers	m	11	6	6.3 ± 3.1
26[6]	Upper Volta farmers	f	14	6	6.3 ± 2.7
	Total		478	3247	9.7 ± 5.8

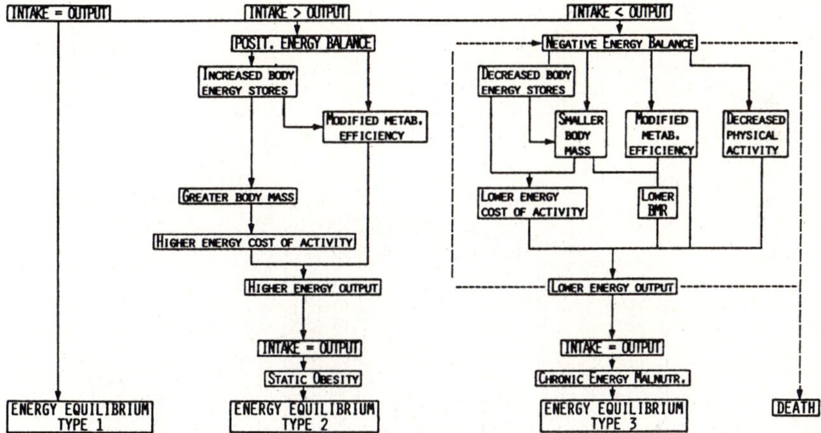

Fig. 2. *Postulated mechanisms to achieve energy equilibrium under different energy balance conditions (modified from[13]).*

While this might indeed be invoked to explain dynamic changes within the individual, the extent to which metabolic variations in energy utilization can contribute to counter the challenge of chronic energy malnutrition, is unknown.

Current hypotheses on adaptation to negative energy balance. The current thinking about the ways in which an organism is supposed to respond to energy unbalance are summarized in Fig. 2, where it can be seen that adaptation represents the outcome of complex integration of several different processes. Very little is known about the timing and the sequence with which the three mechanisms are called into action, the nature of their complex interactions and the respective contributions to total energy sparing. Furthermore, it is conceivable that long-term exposure may elicit mechanisms that may differ from those evoked by acute, severe short-term energy deprivation, and there is no guarantee that well-fed or obese subjects will react in the same way as subjects with lower energy stores.

Two phases can be distinguished in normal individuals subjected to negative energy balance. Initially there is a dynamic phase during which body stores are called upon to fill the energy gap. Within a brief lapse of time, other compensatory mechanisms come into operation, behavioural, metabolic and morphological.

In the second, static phase, a new equilibrium is achieved at a lower level; at this stage the individual who has gone through this postulated adaptive process is expected to exhibit the more or less permanent sequelae of adaptation, ie a smaller body size, a lower BMR, a diminished level of habitual physical activity and possibly a modified metabolic efficiency of energy handling.

Epidemiological evidence. Obviously the best way to explore the existence and modes of action of these putative adaptive mechanisms would be to study the dynamic phase of the process. On the other hand, considering that a large proportion of humanity is presumed or suspected to have experienced life-long exposure to energy deprivation, it would be legitimate to expect that the above mentioned sequelae would be largely represented among LDC populations and thus easily accessible for investigation.

Referring back to the studies mentioned previously LDC male subjects were lighter (56.5 kg) than DC ones (73.4 kg) and this by itself would cause energy sparing, independently of whether or not the smaller body size is the outcome of a process of adaptation to energy deprivation. What is interesting, however, is that, controlling for body weight, LDC subjects do *not* appear to spend less energy than the priviledged DC subjects (Fig. 3). Two conclusions are possible. Either that these LDC study groups had not experienced the challenge of chronic energy malnutrition, or, if they had, they had not made adjustments to their physical activity in order to spare energy.

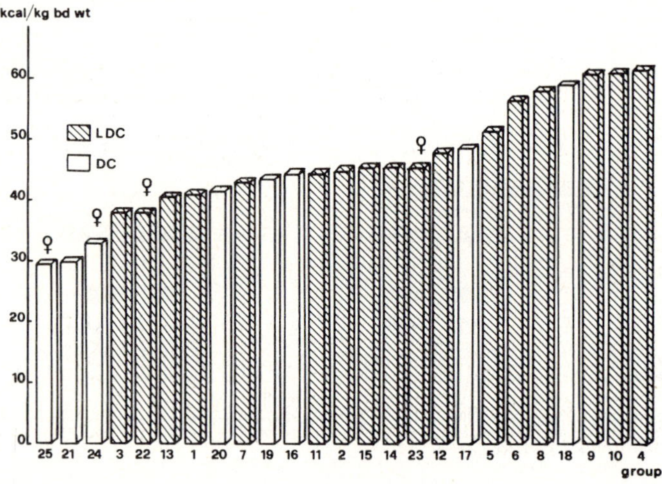

Fig. 3. *Mean interindividual variability (within groups and between groups) of energy expenditure standardized for body weight (kcal/kg body weight) of various study groups from developed (DC) and less developed (LDC) countries. Mean intragroup CV = 14%; mean intergroup CV = 20%.* To identify groups, refer to Table 1 and Table 3.

Total energy expenditure can be broken down into two main components: BMR, that usually represents two-thirds to three quarters of total energy output, and physical activity making up almost all the rest.

Concerning physical activity, it has been possible to verify on a small number of the selected study groups (Nos. 1, 20 and 24, Table 1), that net energy expenditure, even after standardization for body size, makes the greatest contribution to the observed interindividual differences in energy expenditure within an homogeneous group of subjects (14 to 41 per cent). The reason why people nominally engaged in the same type of activity spend so widely differing amounts of energy is not clear, but might reasonably be interpreted to reflect: (1) the fact that the same activity might have a different energy cost for different people; (2) the fact that people do in reality slightly different things.

With regard to BMR, differences in metabolic rate have been reported in the literature in association with ethnicity[2,3,29]. Interpretation of these data is not straightforward as the ethnic groups for which a lower BMR has consistently been reported are likely to have experienced, at some stage in their life, some degree of nutritional stress. However, there is evidence that metabolic rate has a genetic component[14,16].

Differences in the energy cost of lying, sitting and standing has also been recently reported[15] for normal, well-nourished individuals belonging to different ethnic groups. The differences were in the range of 10–17 per cent even after standardization for fat-free mass (FFM) and careful matching of the subjects. As the subjects had been selected in such a way as to exclude past or present exposure to poor nutrition, the authors suggest the possibility of an overestimation of FFM for the non-European groups, due to the use of prediction equations developed for Caucasians[9].

That the nutritional background can play a role in the level of metabolic rate, superimposing its effect on the genetic component, is beyond doubt. Several well-controlled experiments[4,5,23] have shown that previously well-fed subjects exhibit a drop in BMR which occurs mostly during the first few weeks of exposure to severe energy deprivation. Some 16 per cent of it has been attributed to a true, possibly hormone — mediated change in the metabolic efficiency of energy utlization. Besides the classical semistarvation and fasting experiments, some recent Indian data have contributed a further element of great interest to this issue. Shetty[29] was able to show that, within an ethnically homogeneous group, significant interindividual differences in BMR existed in association with past (and current?) exposure to malnutrition and persisted even after standardization for FFM. The differences ranged between 5 per cent (when results were standardized for body weight) and 14 per cent (when standardized for FFM). In the 60s, Banerjee[2,3] obtained similar results, but reported that BMRs were normalized when O_2 uptake was expressed on the basis of cell mass, thus implying that abnormal hydration of malnourished subjects could fully account for the apparent drop in BMR.

Two alternative mechanisms, not mutually exclusive, can be postulated to explain low BMR and may be of relevance to the issue of adaptation to energy deprivation. One relates to the morphological argument, the other attempts to explain the difference on the basis of systematic modifications in the efficiency of energy metabolism. The first approach is based on the observation that various organs and tissues have highly different respiratory rates per unit weight. Visceral organs such as liver, brain and kidneys contribute about 56 per cent of total basal heat production, while muscle only 18 per cent. It is obvious that if the proportion contributed by the different organs to FFM varies, this will inevitably be reflected in the energy spent per unit FFM. I have calculated that if one's liver, brain and kidneys were to represent 3.5 per cent of total body weight instead of the normal 4.7 per cent, this by itself would cause a 14 per cent drop in total BMR, about 251 kcal (1050 kJ). There is evidence that, besides being the expression of a genetic, biological variability, organ sizes may be altered also by environmental stressors.

Speculations on impact of adaptive changes. Let us consider a typical adult male from a LDC, presumed to have been exposed, since early life, to chronic energy malnutrition resulting in shorter stature, but appropriate body mass index (kg/m^2) — Table 4. Because of smaller body size, his BMR as well as the cost of his physical activity, especially that involving body displacements, will be lower. For the sake of simplicity, we shall assume that the decrease is linearly related to body weight. Weighing 60 kg instead of 70 kg would save 153 kcal (640 kJ)/d on BMR. Total energy expenditure at a physical activity level (PAL, total energy expenditure/BMR) of 1.86, a fairly average level[12], would be 2970 kcal (12.4 MJ)/d, representing a saving of 285 kcal (1.2 MJ)/d compared to a well-fed and fully grown counterpart with a similar PAL. The stunted individual would spend a net 23 kcal/kg body weight for physical work, a value indistinguishable from the 21 kcal/kg of the normal individual.

A 16 per cent drop in the BMR of the metabolically adapted individual would cause a net energy saving of 521 kcal (2.18 MJ)/d (for a PAL of 1.86). The integrated response (morphological and metabolic) would spare 761 kcal (3.18 MJ)/d. In other words, while

Table 4. *Postulated effects of adaptation to low energy intakes in adult males (adapted from Ferro-Luzzi, 1985).*

		Normal	'Adapted'		
			For BMR	For size	For size & BMR
Height	cm	175	175	165	165
Weight	kg	70	70	60	60
Body mass index	kg/m^2	23	23	22	22
BMR	kcal(MJ)/d	1750(7.32)	—	1597(6.68)	—
Adapted BMR	kcal(MJ)/d	—	1470(6.15)	—	1341(5.61)
Expenditure at 1.86 PAL*	kcal(MJ)/d	3255(13.6)	2734(11.4)	2970(12.4)	2494(10.4)
Net energy saving over 'normal'	kcal(MJ)/d	—	521(2.18)	285(1.19)	761(3.18)
Net energy for work	kcal(MJ)/d	1505(6.30)	1264(5.29)	1373(5.74)	1153(4.82)
	kcal(kJ)/kg	21(88)	12(50)	23(96)	19(79)

*Physical activity level

maintaining his PAL of 1.86, the stunted subject would be spending 2494 kcal (10.4 MJ)/d (or 42 kcal (176 kJ)/d per kg body weight) instead of the 3255 kcal (13.62 MJ)/d (or 47 kcal (197 kJ)/d per kg). This represents quite a remarkable saving in energy expenditure (23 per cent) and an extremely convenient survival strategy, inasmuch the adapted individual would have avoided being trapped in the notorious vicious circle of decreased physical activity[12,13]. Adjustments in physical activity are, in fact, the third postulated mechanism of adaptation and indeed, while being the least desirable, is the one that might be potentially the most powerful one. A net energy saving of about 1000 kcal (4.18 MJ)/d would be theoretically possible by dropping from an activity level of 1.86 down to a survival value of 1.20. Such a level however, is incompatible with almost any motor activity, other than a bare minimum of personal care. A PAL of 1.50 would probably permit survival at an acceptable maintenance level. At this level the adapted individual would spend some 2000 kcal (8.37 MJ)/d and would still be able to perform a reasonable amount of physical work.

Conclusions. We have seen that: (1) the energy spent by LDC subjects is no less than that spent by the well-nourished DC counterparts, when body weight is corrected for; and their PAL is quite comparable, if not actually higher, suggesting no curtailment of physical activity (Table 4); (2) their body size is significantly smaller; (3) their BMR might be lower, and (4) very little, if any, documentation exists on whether the efficiency of their metabolic handling of energy is modified.

The evidence provided by the studies reviewed above suggests but does not prove that body size changes may be the pivotal response of the average man to chronic exposure to marginal energy deprivation under real life conditions.

Acknowledgements. The research work reported here was supported by CNR (National Research Council), Italy, special grant IPRA, subproject 3, paper no. 728.

1 Acheson, K.J., Campbell, I.T., Edholm, O.G., Miller, D.S. & Stock, M.J. (1980): The measurement of daily energy expenditure — an evaluation of some techniques. *Am. J. Clin. Nutr.* **33**, 1155–1164.

2 Banerjee, S. & Bhattacharya, A.K. (1964): Basal metabolic rates of boys and young adults of Rajasthan. *Indian J. Med. Res.* **52**, 1167–1172.

3 Banerjee, S. & Sen, R. (1958): Body composition of Indians and its relation to basal metabolic rate. *J. Appl. Physiol.* **12**, 29–33.

4 Benedict, F.G., Miles, W.R., Roth, P. & Smith, H.M. (1919): Human vitality and efficiency under prolonged restricted diet. *Carnegie Inst. Wash. Publ.* No. 280.

5 Benedict, F.G. (1915): A study of prolonged fasting. *Carnegie Inst. Wash. Publ.* No. 203.

6 Bleiberg, F., Brun, T.A., Goihman, S. & Lippman, D. (1981): Food intake and energy expenditure of male and female farmers from Upper-Volta. *Br. J. Nutr.* **45**, 505–515.

7 Brun, T.A., Geissler, C.A., Mirbagheri, I., Hormozdiary, H., Bastani, J. & Hedayat, H. (1979): The energy expenditure of Iranian agricultural workers. *Am. J. Clin. Nutr.* **32**, 2154–2161.

8 Durnin, J.V.G.A. & Ferro-Luzzi, A. (1982): Conducting and reporting studies on human energy intake and output: suggested standards. *Am. J. Clin. Nutr.* **35**, 624–626.

9 Durnin, J.V.G.A. & Womersley (1974): Body fat assessed from total body density and its estimation from skinfold thicknesses: measurements on 481 men and women aged from 16–72 years. *Br. J. Nutr.* **33**, 77–97.

10 Edholm, O.G., Adam, J.M., Heavy, M.J.R., Wolff, K.S., Goldsmith, R. & Best, T.W. (1970): Food intake and energy expenditure of army recruits. *Br. J. Nutr.* **24**, 1091–1107.

11 Edholm, O.G., Fletcher, J.G., Widdowson, E.M. & McCance, E.A. (1955): The energy expenditure and food intake of individual men. *Br. J. Nutr.* **2**, 286–300.

12 Ferro-Luzzi, A. (1984): Energy intakes as predictors of energy balances in free-living populations. In *Energy intake and activity*, ed E. Pollitt & P. Amante, pp. 79–99. New York: Alan R. Liss.

13 Ferro-Luzzi, A. (1985): Marginal energy malnutrition: some speculations on preeminent energy sparing mechanisms. *Proc. IUBS Symp. on Working capacity in tropical populations*, (in press).

14 Fontaine, E., Savard, R., Tremblay, A., Després, J.P., Poehlman, E. & Bouchard, C. :1985): Resting metabolic rate in monozygotic and dizygotic twins. *Acta Genet. Med. Gemellol.* **34**, (in press).

15 Geissler, C.A. & Aldouri, M.S.H. (1985): Racial differences in the energy cost of standardized activities. *Ann. Nutr. Metab.* **29**, 40–47.

16 Griffiths, M. & Payne, P.R. (1976): Energy expenditure in small children of obese and non obese parents. *Nature* **260**, 698–700.

17 Guzman de, M.P.E., Cabrera, J.P., Basconcillo, R.O., Gaurano, A.L., Yuchingtat, G.P., Tan, R.M., Kalaw, J.M. & Recto, R.C. (1978): A study of the energy expenditure, dietary intake and pattern of daily activity among various occupational groups. 5. Clerk-typists. *Philippine J. Nutr.* **31**, 147–156.

18 Guzman de, M.P.E., Dominguez, S.R., Kalaw, J.M., Basconcillo, R.O. & Santos, V.F. (1974): A study of the energy expenditure, dietary intake and pattern of daily activity among various occupational groups. Laguna rice farmers. *Philippine J. Nutr.* **27**, 53–65.

19 Guzman de, M.P.E., Dominguez, S.R., Kalaw, J.M., Buning, M.N., Basconcillo, R.O. & Santos, V.F. (1974): A study of the energy expenditure, dietary intake and pattern of daily activity among various occupational groups. 2. Marikina shoemakers and housewives. *Philippine J. Nutr.* **27**, 21–30.

20 Guzman de, M.P.E., Kalaw, J.M., Tan, R.H., Recto, R.C., Basconcillo, R.O., Ferrer, V.T., Tombokon, M.S., Yuchingtat, G.P. & Gaurano, A.L. (1974): A study of the energy expenditure, dietary intake and pattern of daily activity among various occupational groups. 3. Urban jeepney drivers. *Philippine J. Nutr.* **27**, 182–188.

21 Guzman de, M.P.E., Recto, R.C., Cabrera, J.P., Basconcillo, R.O., Gaurano, A.L., Yuchingtat, G.P. & Abanto, Z.U. (1979): A study of the energy expenditure, dietary intake and pattern of daily activity among various occupational groups. 6. Textile-mill workers. *Philippine J. Nutr.* **32**, 134–148.

22 Guzman de, M.P.E., Yuchingtat, G.P., Abanto, Z.U., Cabrera, J.P. & Agustin, C.P. (1981): A study of the energy expenditure, dietary intake and pattern of daily activity among various occupational groups. 8. Fishermen. *Philippine J. Nutr.* **34**, 168–182.

23 Keys, A., Brozek, K., Henshel, A., Mickelson, O. & Taylor, K.L. (1950): *The biology of human starvation*. Minneapolis: University of Minnesota Press.

24 Margen, S. (1984): Auto-regulatory processes to maintain energy balance in the individual. In *Energy intake and activity*, ed E. Pollitt & P. Amante, pp. 57–76. New York: Alan R. Liss.

25 Norgan, N.G. & Durnin, J.V.G.A. (1980): The effects of 6 weeks of overfeeding on the body weight, body composition and energy metabolism of young men. *Am. J. Clin. Nutr.* **33**, 978–988.

26 Norgan, N.G. & Ferro-Luzzi, A. (1978): Nutrition, physical activity and physical fitness in contrasting environments. In *Nutrition, physical fitness, and health; Int. Series on Sport Sciences*, ed J. Parizkova & V.A. Rogozkin, pp. 167–193. Baltimore: University Park Press.

27 Norgan, N.G., Ferro-Luzzi, A. & Durnin, J.V.G.A. (1974): The energy and nutrient intake and the energy expenditure of 204 New Guineas adults. *Phil. Trans. R. Soc. B.* **268**, 309–348.

28 Scaccini, C., Borgioni, G., D'Amicis, A. & Ferro-Luzzi, A. (1985): Age related physical activity in old people. *XIII Int. Congress of Nutrition*, Abstr.

29 Shetty, P.S. (1984): Adaptive changes in basal metabolic rate and lean body mass in chronic undernutrition. *Hum. Nutr.: Clin. Nutr.* **38C**, 443–451.

30 Viteri, F.E., Torun, B., Galicia, J.C. & Herrera, E. (1971): Determining energy costs of agricultural activities by respirometer and energy balance techniques. *Am. J. Clin. Nutr.* **24**, 1418–1430.

The roles of substrate cycles in provision of precision in metabolic control and in expenditure of energy

E.A. NEWSHOLME
Department of Biochemistry, University of Oxford, South Parks Road, Oxford, OX1 3QU, UK.

Energy expenditure is increased under a variety of conditions when the body carries out either physical or chemical work. The efficiency with which this energy is expended in relation to the work done has been investigated in depth and it is usually considered to be about 25 per cent[12]. The implicit assumption is that all the energy not transformed into work can be classified as wasted. However, this must represent a myopic view of energy consumption since it does not take into account the energy that is expended to provide for control and regulation of *all* the processes involved in the expenditure of energy. Regulation occurs at many different levels and the preoccupation of biologists and physiologists with nervous and endocrine control may explain a prevalent viewpoint that the amount of energy expended in regulation is quantitatively trivial. A recent quantitative approach to the subject of metabolic regulation provides at least the basis not only for testing model systems of regulation but also for investigating the energy cost of metabolic regulation[8]. The magnitude of the problem that faces the body is illustrated by consideration of just three everyday situations.

—(1) A normal Western diet contains a high proportion of carbohydrate, approximately 300 g of carbohydrate being ingested everyday. If this is consumed equally during three meals/day this means that more than 100 g are consumed at each meal, which is sufficient to increase the blood glucose level more than 30-fold. That this does not happen is due to the precision of the mechanisms that control the blood glucose level. Some of the extra glucose absorbed will be converted to glycogen in muscle and liver which have the capacity to store over 400 g of glucose[15]. However, the *total* capacity for the synthesis of glycogen in man is probably more than 1 g of glucose per min so that, if feeding caused complete activation of glycogen synthase, it could rapidly result in hypoglycaemia, coma and possibly death. Indeed eating is a dangerous activity; it is made safe by the precision of control mechanisms.

—(2) In order to complete the 100 metre sprint in a respectable time the rate of conversion of glycogen to lactate must be increased more than 1000-fold: in other words, from resting to maximum acceleration the activities of all the enzymes of glycolysis must increase by more than 1000-fold[15]. Similarly, for the average individual walking rapidly upstairs or running to catch the last bus or train probably requires an increase in glycolysis of several hundredfold in any individual. However, the control must be precise not only for increasing the rate of anaerobic glycolysis to a sufficient level to provide the ATP for the physical activity, but also for decreasing it! It can be calculated that the capacity for maximum glycolysis in human muscle is such that if the glycolytic enzymes were fully activated, enough protons would be produced in about four min to lower the pH of the body to 2.0! Indeed walking upstairs is a dangerous activity; it is made safe by the precision of control mechanisms.

—(3) During endurance exercise (eg marathon running) the fat store in the adipose tissue is made available in the blood-stream as fatty acid. The hydrolysis of triacylglycerol occurs in the adipose tissue and fatty acids are transported to the muscle via the blood-stream. This provides an extremely important source of energy for muscle during endurance exercise[15]. It can be calculated that, if the rate of mobilisation of fatty acid was overstimulated by just 1 per cent, in about 60 min the concentration of plasma fatty acid could double to reach a concentration of perhaps 4 mmol/l, which would be highly dangerous. Endurance exercise is a dangerous activity; it is made safe by the precision of control mechanisms.

Sensitivity in metabolic regulation. Sensitivity in metabolic regulation can be defined as the quantitative relationship between the relative change in enzyme activity and the relative change in concentration of the regulator. (If the concentration of a regulator (x) changes by Δx, the relative change is $\Delta x/x$; similarly if the flux (J) changes by ΔJ, the relative change is $\Delta J/J$. The sensitivity of J to the change in concentration of (x) is given by the ratio $(\Delta J/J):(\Delta x/x)$ and this sensitivity is indicated by the symbol s[8,9]. For example, if the concentration of a regulator increases two-fold, the question arises, how large an increase in enzyme activity will this produce? The greater the response of enzyme activity to a given increase in regulator concentration, the greater is the sensitivity.

There are several important mechanisms for increasing sensitivity which include multiplicity of regulators, cooperativity (ie sigmoid response of enzyme activity to regulator concentration) interconversion cycles and substrate cycles. These have been discussed in detail in several reviews[8,9,14,15]. However, attention will be focused in this discussion on substrate cycles which have the capacity to expend a considerable amount of energy[8].

Substrate cycle. It is possible for a reaction that is non-equilibrium in the forward direction of a pathway ($A \rightarrow B$) to be opposed by a reaction that is non-equilibrium in the reverse direction of the pathway ($B \rightarrow A$). Both reactions must be chemically distinct so that they will be catalysed by separate enzymes. Then, a substrate cycle between A and B occurs if the two enzymes are simultaneously catalytically active. For every molecule of A converted to B and back again to A, chemical energy must be converted to heat, which is lost to the environment. An example of a substrate cycle is the fructose 6-phosphate (F6P)/fructose bisphosphate (FBP) cycle.

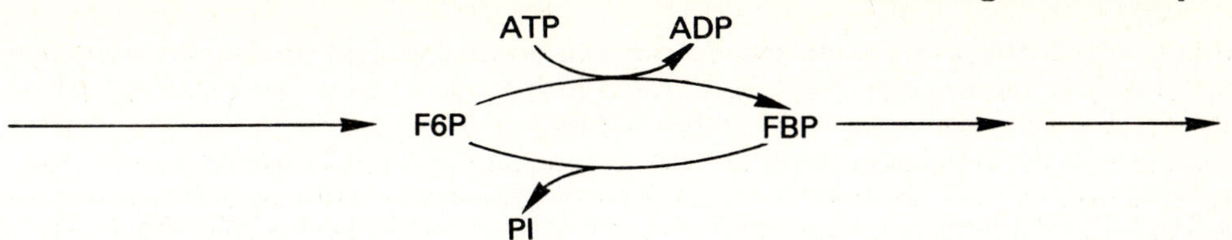

The role of a cycle can best be understood when it is appreciated that, in some conditions, an enzyme activity may have to be reduced to values closely approaching *zero*. Even with a sigmoid response this would require that the concentration of an activator be reduced to almost zero or that of an inhibitor to an almost infinite level. Such enormous changes in concentration probably never occur in living organisms, since they would cause osmotic and ionic problems and unwanted side reactions. However, the net flux through a reaction can be reduced to very low values (approaching zero) via a substrate cycle. Thus as the concentration of the product of the forward enzyme (ie FBP in the above example) reaches a low level it is converted back to substrate by the reverse enzyme (fructose bisphosphatase). This ensures that the net forward flux is very low despite a finite activity of the forward enzyme and a moderate concentration of an activator of 6-phosphofructokinase. If the concentration of this activator is increased by only a small amount, above that at which the activities of the two enzymes are almost identical (and the flux is almost zero), the activity of 6-phosphofructokinase will increase so that the net flux through the reaction will increase from almost zero to a moderate rate. Such a cycle therefore provides a large improvement in sensitivity; indeed, it can be seen as a means of producing a threshold (or almost threshold) response with a simple metabolic system. Indeed the cycle provides an improvement in sensitivity without changing the properties or characteristics of the enzyme catalysing the forward reaction in the pathway and for this reason can be seen to be different from the other mechanisms for improving sensitivity: this has also been shown to be the case when the precise quantitative role of substrate cycles in metabolic control is considered[9]. One advantage of the substrate-cycling mechanism for increasing sensitivity is that the extent of this increase varies according to the rate of cycling, in other words sensitivity is proportional to the ratio, cycling rate: flux[8].

Considerable evidence has now been obtained to demonstrate this variability in cycling rate. (1) The precise rate of the triacylglycerol/fatty acid cycle can be measured by comparing the rates of fatty acid and glycerol production by adipose tissue, or by following the rates of incorporation of $[^3H]$ from $[^3H]_2O$ into the glycerol and fatty acid moieties of triacylglycerol. In isolated adipose tissue of the rat the cycling rate is increased markedly by β-adrenergic agents and the effect is abolished by the β-blocker propranolol[1]. Furthermore, the rate of this cycle in white adipose tissue of the mouse *in vivo* is doubled by feeding and increases five-fold by a β-adrenoreceptor agonist and, in brown adipose tissue, it is increased three-fold by such an agonist and doubled by exposure to the cold for 4 h [2]. (2) The precise rate of the fructose 6-phosphate/fructose bisphosphate cycle can be measured from the changes in the $[^3H]/[^{14}C]$ radioactivity ratio in hexose-monophosphates and fructose bisphosphate after isolation and separation from a tissue that has been utilizing $[5-^3H, 6-^{14}C]$ glucose. The hormone adrenaline, or other β-adrenoreceptor agonists, increases the cycling rate up to ten-fold in the isolated epitrochlearis muscle of the rat. This stimulation occurs at physiological concentrations of the hormone and is abolished by propanolol[4,5].

There are several conditions in which the concentrations of catecholamines are known to be raised in which increased sensitivity in metabolic control would be very advantageous, in which the rate of some substrate cycles is also known to be increased and in which thermogenesis is known to be increased. These conditions include stress, the absorptive period after a meal (thermic response to food) and in the period after exercise. These conditions are discussed below.

Stress. Both anxiety-related and aggression-related stress increase the plasma levels of catecholamines. The nor-adrenaline level is raised more in anxiety-stress whereas that of adrenaline is raised more in aggression stress. However, stress conditions in modern society are not always related to primitive 'fight or flight' situations. Driving a car in crowded traffic conditions or debating at a committee meeting can be stressful and can lead to an increase in plasma catecholamines[3]; and Beryl Bainbridge in her novel *Injury time* has emphasised the energy loss in anxiety stress caused by simple family problems.

'Keep your lid on' said Lucy. She began to comb her hair at the mirror. Strands of hair and crumbs of bread fell to the hearth. Binney could feel a pulse beating in her throat. She burned with fury. No wonder she never put on an ounce of weight. The daily aggravation the children caused her was probably comparable to a five-mile run or an hour with a skipping rope.

Measurements of the precise rates of cycling between fructose 6-phosphate and fructose 1,6-bisphosphate in muscle and between triacylglycerol and fatty acid in both brown and white adipose tissue have demonstrated that catecholalmines increase the rate of these cycles[1,2,4,5]. Increased cycling rates would be advantageous in providing sensitivity for metabolic regulation during stress conditions in preparation of the animal for increased fuel supply and increased fuel utilisation that would occur in 'fight or flight'. They would also cause conversion of chemical energy into heat, that is 'burning off' of excess energy and prevent weight gain (as was so clearly described by Beryl Bainbridge) or help in the loss of excess fat from the adipose tissue stores. Such a mechanism would be consistent not only with the accepted anticipatory role of catecholamines but also with their well-established thermogenic action[16].

Postexercise oxygen consumption. It is well established that, in the period after exercise, more oxygen is consumed than is required to support resting metabolism; this phenomenon is known as oxygen debt, recovery oxygen or, more recently, extra post-exercise oxygen consumption (EPOC). The latter can be divided into three phases: the rapid phase, the slow phase, and the ultraslow phase. The rapid phase may be explained by replenishment of creatine phosphate stores and reoxygenation of myoglobin and haemoglobin; the slow phase may be partly explained by reconversion of lactate to glucose and glycogen, but the amount of extra oxygen consumed in this phase is usually considerably larger than can be explained by carbohydrate synthesis. The consumption of oxygen in the slow component that cannot be explained by lactate conversion to glycogen, and all the oxygen consumption in the ultraslow phase, may be due to stimulation of the rates of substrate cycles. Indeed it has now been shown that the fructose 6-phosphate/fructose bisphosphate cycle in the isolated incubated muscle is stimulated after a single bout of exercise in the rat[6]. Prolonged stimulation of cycles after exercise could be caused by a prolonged elevation in the level of catecholamines: there is evidence that the plasma level of adrenaline is elevated after endurance exercise, for example, it is elevated for at least 48 h after a marathon race[13]. Of course, rates of other cycles (eg triacylglycerol fatty acid cycle, protein/amino acid cycle) could also be elevated for long periods after exercise. In this case, exercise would be beneficial in control of body weight, not only for the energy losses incurred during the exercise, but also because a considerable amount of energy may be lost *after* the exercise has finished.

Recently, in very carefully controlled studies, it has been shown that after 60–90 min of exercise (at about 60 per cent of VO_2 max) in human volunteers, oxygen consumption was elevated for at least 24 h after cessation of exercise[10,11]. Of considerable importance is the fact that the respiratory exchange ratio was found to be lowered for most of this 24 h period indicating a greater rate of fat oxidation after exercise[11]. Since these subjects were allowed to eat only simple carbohydrate meals after exercise, and since the plasma glycerol and fatty acid levels were elevated, these findings suggest that triacylglycerol is being mobilised from the adipose tissue depots and utilised by muscle and perhaps other tissues and that the rate of the triacylglycerol/fatty acid cycle is enhanced.

The significance of increased rates of cycling would be to increase the sensitivity of metabolic control so that the increased rates of metabolism during exercise can return *gradually* and *smoothly* to the normal resting level during the recovery period.

Thermic response to food. The increase in heat production that occurs after a meal (the thermic response to food) has many properties that are consistent with stimulation of cycling rates[14] which provide indirect support for the hypothesis that increased rate of substrate cycling can explain the thermic response to food. More direct evidence is now available: it has been shown[7] that the rate of the fructose 6-phosphate/fructose bisphosphate cycle in isolated muscle is decreased by 24 h starvation and it has been shown, in rats and mice, that the rate of the triacylglycerol/fatty acid cycle is increased by feeding in white and brown adipose tissue *in vivo*[2]. Furthermore, these effects are removed by administration of a β-adrenoreceptor blocker. This suggests that the stimulation of cycling rates during feeding is due to increased level of catecholamines. Since fasting decreases and eating or overeating increases the activity of the sympathetic nervous system[17] it would be expected that the level of nor-adrenaline would be increased in these tissues after feeding but would be decreased by 24 h starvation. The author suggests that the role of the increased sympathetic activity after a meal is *primarily* to provide higher rates of substrate cycling which would increase the sensitivity of processes that control the rates of degradation and synthesis of fuel stores. It means that a significant proportion of the energy ingested in the meal *must* be lost as heat during assimilation to provide for sensitivity in metabolic control.

1 Brooks, B.J., Arch, J.R.S. & Newsholme, E.A. (1982): Effects of hormones on the rate of the triacylglycerol/fatty acid substrate cycle in adipocytes and epididymic fat pads. *FEBS Lett.* **146**, 327–330.
2 Brooks, B.J., Arch, J.R.S. & Newsholme, E.A. (1983): Effect of some hormones on the rate of the triacylglycerol/fatty acid substrate cycle in adipose tissue of the mouse *in vivo*. *Biosci. Rep.* **3**, 263–267.
3 Carruthers, M.E. (1977): The chemical anatomy of stress. In *Beta-blockers and the Central Nervous System*, ed P. Kielholz, pp. 53–58, Stuttgart: Hans Huber.
4 Challiss, R.A.J., Arch, J.R.S. & Newsholme, E.A. (1984): The rate of substrate cycling between fructose 6-phosphate and fructose 1,6-bisphosphate in skeletal muscle. *Biochem. J.* **221**, 153–161.
5 Challiss, R.A.J., Arch, J.R.S., Crabtree, B. & Newsholme, E.A. (1984): Measurement of the rate of substrate cycling between fructose 6-phosphate and fructose bisphosphate in skeletal muscle by using a single isotope technique. *Biochem. J.* **223**, 849–853.
6 Challiss, R.A.J., Arch, J.R.S. & Newsholme, E.A. (1985): The rate of substrate cycling between fructose 6-phosphate and fructose bisphosphate in skeletal muscle from cold-exposed, hyperthyroid or acutely exercised animals. *Biochem. J.* (In press).
7 Challiss, R.A.J., Arch, J.R.S. & Newsholme, E.A. (1985): Starvation for 24 h decreases fructose 6-phosphate/fructose bisphosphate substrate cycling in skeletal muscle. *Biochem. Soc. Trans.* **13**, 269–270.
8 Crabtree, B. & Newsholme, E.A. (1978): Sensitivity of a near-equilibrium reaction in a metabolic pathway to changes in substrate concentration. *Eur. J. Biochem.* **89**, 19–22.
9 Crabtree, B. & Newsholme, E.A. (1985): A quantitative approach to metabolic control. *Curr. Topics Cellul. Regul.* **25**, 21–76.
10 Hermansen, L., Grandmontagne, M., Maehlum, S. & Ingnes, I. (1984): Post-exercise elevation of resting oxygen uptake: possible mechanisms and physiological significance. In *Physiological chemistry of training and detraining*, pp. 119–129. Basel: Karger.
11 Maehlum, S., Grandmontagne, M., Newsholme, E.A. & Sejersted, O.M. (1985): Magnitude and duration of excess post-exercise oxygen consumption in healthy subjects. *Metabolism* (in press).
12 Margaria, R. (1976): *Biomechanisms and energetics of muscular exercise*, Oxford: Clarendon Press.
13 Maron, M.B., Horvath, S.M. & Wilkerson, J.E. (1977): Blood biochemical alterations during a recovery from competitive marathon running. *Eur. J. Appl. Physiol.* **36**, 231–238.
14 Newsholme, E.A. & Crabtree, B. (1976): Substrate cycles in metabolic regulation and heat generation. *Biochem. Soc. Symp.* **41**, 61–110.
15 Newsholme, E.A. & Leech, A.R. (1983): *Biochemistry for the medical sciences*. Chichester: John Wiley.
16 Steinberg, D. (1963): Fatty acid mobilization — mechanisms of regulation and metabolic consequences. *Biochem. Soc. Symp.* **24**, 111–144.
17 Young, J.B. & Landsberg, L. (1977): Stimulation of the sympathetic nervous system during sucrose feeding. *Nature* **269**, 615–617.

Dynamics of protein metabolism and their relation to adaptation

A.A. JACKSON
Tropical Metabolism Research Unit, University of the West Indies, Mona, Kingston 7, Jamaica. (Present address: Department of Nutrition, University of Southampton, UK).

Over the past decade or so an increasing interest in the dynamics of whole-body protein metabolism has served to enrich our understanding of the way in which protein synthesis and breakdown change in response to a range of environmental and pathological stimuli[30,32,33]. The picture that emerges is one of great complexity, and we are beginning to gain an appreciation of the intricacy of the various control mechanisms. For any given individual the state of protein metabolism at a point in time will be determined by a number of interrelated factors: the previous dietary intake, and the current intake especially in relation to both the absolute and relative intake of energy and protein. Further changes can be identified in association with the habitual level of activity or the relative metabolic demands. There is a vast expanding literature dealing with every facet from the molecular level to the highest levels of integration. My paper considers protein metabolism at the level of the whole body and attempts to delineate the basic pattern in the normal before considering some of the adaptive changes that might be expected in different physiological or pathological states. The term adaptive is used here in the sense outlined by Waterlow[31] that the adaptive state is a response to a particular environment and is maintained as long as the environmental factors which brought it about continue to operate; it is a state which is of benefit to the organism because it makes it possible to maintain the integrity of function.

General consideration. *Oral vs intravenous (i.v.) feeding.* The methods used for the measurement of protein turnover in the whole body utilize isotopically-labelled amino acids, which are administered either orally or i.v. for varying periods of time and attention has been drawn to the important difference that the route of presentation of the isotope has on the answer obtained[6]. Using the single dose approach the point was made, the importance of which can only be fully appreciated with a constant or intermittent infusion: it now seems clear that when the isotope is given orally, a higher value for amino acid flux, and hence turnover, is usually obtained, compared to i.v. isotope, for leucine[12] or glycine[23,38] (Fig. 1). The difference may be quite large, with oral isotope giving results 30 to 100 per cent higher than i.v. The magnitude of the difference is more obvious in studies of shorter duration. The observation is not altogether new[34,37] and has been attributed to a difference in the handling of amino acids in the gut and liver. The important, but little understood, role that the red cell performs in the interorgan transport of amino acids has been demonstrated[5], raising the important question of the extent to which measurements made on plasma samples give values for flux that are representative. The point is illustrated in Fig. 2 which shows the relative enrichment of alanine in plasma, red cells, urinary urea and ammonia following the oral or i.v. presentation of ^{15}N alanine over 18 h in normal males[22]. This difference in the handling of amino acids may represent a specific example of a more general phenomenon whereby flux is reduced by 20 per cent (100 mgN/kg per d) in subjects receiving i.v. nutrition compared to an oral intake[28]. The difference has been attributed to the digestive and absorptive activity of the gastrointestinal tract. However, given the extent to which the gastrointestinal tract is involved in modulation the dietary pattern of amino acids before presentation to the liver[5], this could have important implications for specific complications of parenteral feeding such as the development of hepatic steatosis[9,10,15].

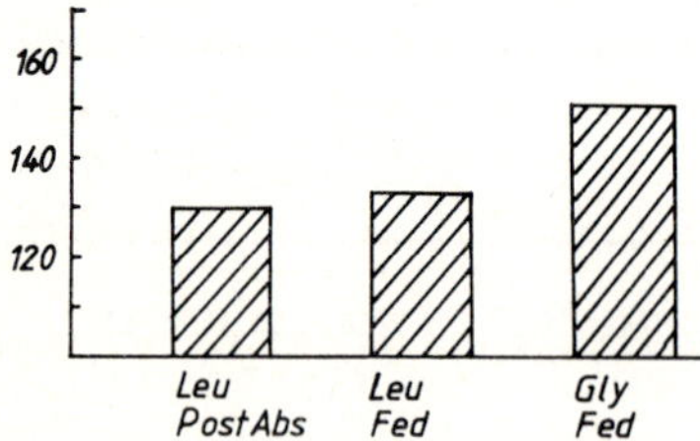

Fig. 1. *A comparison of the flux measured with either leucine, or glycine, in the fed or post-absorptive state, between the oral or i.v. presentation of isotope (oral flux expressed as a percentage of the i.v. flux).*

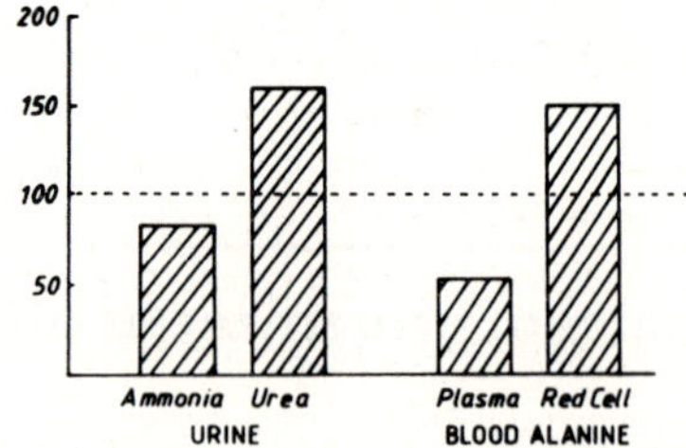

Fig. 2. *The relative enrichments in urinary urea, and ammonia and alanine in plasma and red cells following oral or i.v. prime, intermittent infusion of ^{15}N-alanine over 18 hours (oral value expressed as a percentage of the i.v.)*

Duration of study. The second consideration is the time over which the measurements are made. In general, to date, the i.v. methods have been preferred as they are of much shorter duration than the oral methods, although recently we have developed the oral end-product method to give reliable measurements in 2 to 3 h [23]. As one would expect, with time, there is a return of label from protein to the amino acid pool[27] so that the longer it takes to make the measurements, the lower the values obtained for turnover. Garlick's group have shown[19] that when flooding doses of labelled amino acid were used to measure turnover in rats over a period of minutes, there was a far greater contribution to the total turnover than had been appreciated of proteins which turnover rapidly. This particularly applies to the activity of the gut and liver, and may serve to increase the value for total turnover by more than 50 per cent. It is likely that we have a similar situation in man which would mean that the longer oral methods in particular have tended to give values for turnover which are significant underestimates.

Enterohepatic nitrogen pool. It might be concluded that both the oral and i.v. methods have tended to underestimate the contribution to total turnover of the enterohepatic nitrogen pool. In normal man, 30 per cent of the urea produced is hydrolysed in the body. By measuring the kinetics of urea in the body it is possible to measure the flux through the pool of nitrogen to which hydrolysed urea contributes[16]. The values obtained, about 210 mgN/kg per d, closely approximates the estimated endogenous production of nitrogen from proteins and amino acids in the gastrointestinal tract[5], an amount that exceeds the dietary intake, and may represent as much as 30 per cent of total body flux. Urea nitrogen only contributes about one-fifth to this pool, which accounts for the relatively low contribution of urea to faecal nitrogen[36]. The flow through this pool is greatly reduced in the postprandial state[5], in association with a virtual absence of urea hydrolysis[18]. It may be of significance that the enterohepatic flux of nitrogen measured in this way, is of similar magnitude to the difference in total body flux measured with the oral against the i.v. method. The metabolic function of the gastrointestinal tract and its contents may be of far greater importance, both quantitatively and qualitatively than previously recognised[14], and may help to put in perspective the suggestion that muscle accounted for more than 50 per cent of whole-body protein turnover[25].

Energy cost of protein turnover. The two approaches that have been used to assess the energy cost of protein turnover give disparate results. In the biochemical approach the factorial cost of the energy required for synthesizing peptide bonds for a measured value of protein turnover, have been summated to account for about 15 to 20 per cent of basal energy expenditure[30]. The physiological approach, in which protein turnover and energy expenditure are regressed against each other, gives a much higher value, of about 30 per cent for animals and man[15,20,24]. If the measurements of protein turnover had consistently given an underestimate of one-third to one-half, as discussed above, this would go a long way to bringing the two estimates into line by increasing the assessment made with the biochemical approach. The clinical importance of what might appear at first sight to be a relatively small difference is perhaps demonstrated in a study we recently carried out on children with sickle-cell disease before and after splenectomy for hypersplenism (V. Badaloo & A.A. Jackson, unpublished observations). Nitrogen flux was reduced from 1.15 g N/kg per d to 0.75 g N/kg per d by splenectomy, resulting in a theoretical saving of 18 kJ/kg per d (4.3 kcal/kg per d) an amount sufficient to allow for the deposition of balanced new tissue of about 1 g/kg per d. Emond (unpublished observations) has shown that this same group of children all experienced a significant height spurt following splenectomy, possibly associated with the saving in energy expenditure.

Functional demand. The extent to which the pattern of amino acids taken in the diet matches the body's requirement is expressed as protein quality, but is only understood at the most superficial level and is worthy of much greater detailed investigation. Thus it has been shown[8] that proteins differed in their relative efficiency according to the method by which their value was assessed; the regeneration of liver protein, haemoglobin or granulocytes, or the maintenance of nitrogen balance. Likewise, the metal moiety of metalloproteins can exert a similar effect on the pattern of protein being synthesized, iron in regenerating haemoglobin[2] or zinc for synthesizing metallothionein[3]. The extent to which various, and on a marginal intake, conflicting, demands can be satisifed will be modulated by the relative functional demands of the organism at that point in time[15]. This consideration is especially important in relation to the role that non-essential nitrogen, the first limiting 'nutrient' when protein intake is reduced, plays in metabolism and the extent to which both dispensable and non-dispensable amino acids can be synthesized in the body in quantitatively significant amounts[10,14,38].

During growth there is net synthesis of new tissue, with a consequent demand for energy and nutrients in excess of maintenance requirements. In both experimental animals[17,24] and man[4,7] this is brought about by an increase in protein synthesis, with an associated increase in protein breakdown, hence net accretion has a measurable inefficiency. Of great interest is the protein intake required to maintain adequate growth and the efficiency with which it is utilised. Although it has been shown[29] that the rate of catch up weight gain during recovery from malnutrition is proportional to the energy intake, there have been a number of suggestions that the weight gained may not represent balanced tissue, but rather demonstrates a limitation of lean tissue deposition with a preponderance of fat[15]. One marker for the effective demand for nitrogen in relation to the dietary intake is the extent to which the body adapts to minimize the loss in the form of urinary urea. Where the demand for nitrogen is not fully satisfied by the diet the relative rate of urea nitrogen recycling through the bowel increases[11]. Thus during recovery from malnutrition the rate at which urea nitrogen is recycled and made available for synthetic reactions is determined by the demand, as measured by the rate of weight gain.

Normal pregnancy and lactation represents one of the most fascinating physiological problems in nitrogen metabolism, about which very little is known. Over the 9 months of gestation there are large shifts in the pattern of metabolic demands to satisfy the needs of the products of conception, and subsequently during lactation for the production of export milk protein. Even our knowledge of the net accretion of nitrogen over the course of a pregnancy is incomplete. We have recently measured protein turnover in a group of women, during the first, second and third trimester of pregnancy[4] (Fig. 3). We were surprised to find that the most

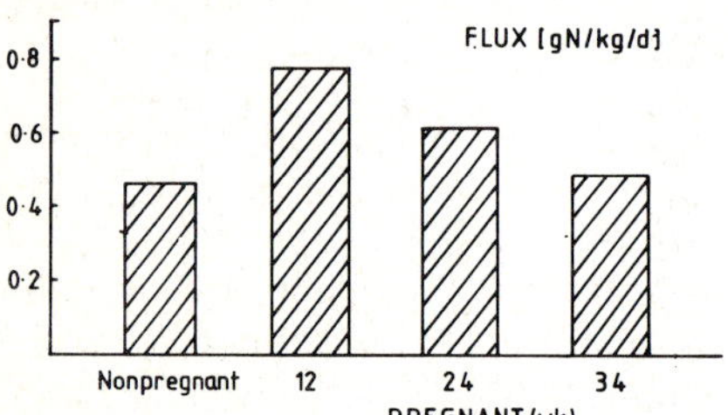

Fig. 3. *Whole-body protein turnover in normal and pregnant Jamaican women, measured with a prime, intermittent infusion of ^{15}N-glycine and urinary ammonia over 18 h.*

intense increase in protein turnover was already taking place by the time of our first measurement at 12 weeks, well before there was any marked development in fetal or placental mass, or maternal weight gain. By the third, trimester, at the time of most rapid fetal growth, the rate of turnover was decreasing to the range of non pregnant women, expressed per unit of body weight, although there was obviously an absolute increase. It is not possible to say the relative contribution made by maternal or fetal tissues to the intense changes seen in the first trimester, but clearly these were associated with a shift, or reordering of the relative demands rather than net accumulation. These data suggest that the marked increase in both synthesis and breakdown observed during growth, that has been ascribed to the inherent inefficiency of tissue deposition, may in fact represent in part a much more structured process of 'remodelling' of the protein mass.

Pathological states. It is particularly difficult to obtain clear insights into the changes in nitrogen metabolism in pathological states, not only because there are intense changes taking place over short periods of time, but also because in any one individual a number of factors are likely to be operative at the same time, each of which will exert its own effect on protein turnover, not necessarily in the same direction (Table 1). Thus, for example in cystic fibrosis, once there is adequate control of the dietary intake, there is no evidence of a change in turnover associated

Table 1. *The main factors likely to modify whole-body protein turnover in disease states.*

Duration and intensity of insult
Nutritional state — general/specific
Appetite — anorexia
Activity — immobility
Infection — local/general response
   fever
   acute phase proteins
   immune response
Tissue destruction
Tissue repair

Table 2. *Comparison of nitrogen dynamics between normal adults and sickle-cell patients (HbSS) in a stable state (mgN/kg per d).*

	Normal	*HbSS*
Dietary intake	200	200
Urea production	139	238
Urea hydrolysed	41	110
Flux through N pool	210	295
Total body N flux	780	1280

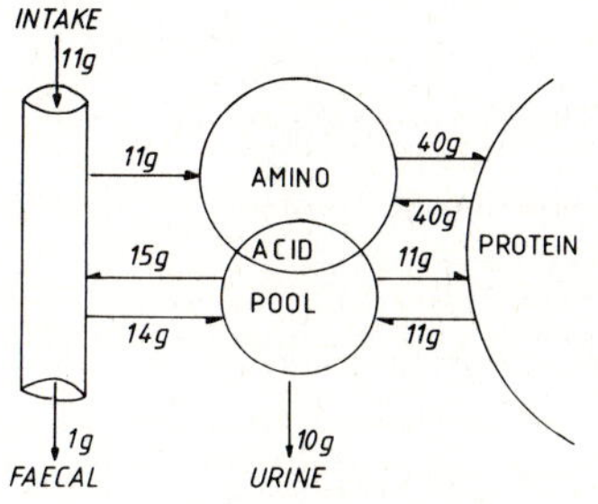

Fig. 4. *Outline of the dynamics of nitrogen metabolism in the whole body, assuming that virtually all dietary nitrogen is absorbed and that the metabolic activity in the lower bowel represents endogenous sources of nitrogen (gN/d).*

with the chronic disease[21] except in the presence of an acute infection[13]. It was demonstrated[35] that the plane of protein nutrition at the time of trauma had a more important determinant effect on the outcome than the quality of care or nutritional management given after the trauma[38]. We have used patients with sickle cell disease (HbSS) as a model to study the effect of a persistent drain on the nitrogen economy of the body provoked by increased breakdown of red cells. Table 2, shows that in HbSS an increase in protein turnover[1] is associated with an increase in urea production. A greater proportion of the urea produced is hydrolysed, and the nitrogen made available for metabolic interaction[11]. Hence, at a normal protein intake, the sickler responds to conserve nitrogen in the same way as seen in normal individuals on a low protein intake. In other words the stimulus to retain nitrogen is related to the imbalance between demand and dietary availability. It is likely that with a higher demand the proteins being synthesized are specific and thus the individual will be more susceptible to an imbalanced dietary pattern of amino acids. The gastrointestinal tract may play an important role in either setting or offsetting an appropriate pattern[5,14]. The exact control and function of urea hydrolysis in intermediary nitrogen metabolism is unclear, but in this regard the demonstration that urea recycling is reduced to almost insignificant levels on a very low dietary intake[18], and that it is abolished[26] on a very high protein intake, have special relevance.

Conclusion. The progressive development of the techniques for measuring nitrogen kinetics in the whole body, and the application of these techniques to the study of an increasing range of clinical and metabolic states, has served to confirm the value of this approach for developing an understanding of the control and regulation of this fundamental process. For the future, there is the need to develop methods which adequately quantify the relative contribution of proteins that turn over rapidly, with special emphasis on the activity of the gastrointestinal tract (Fig. 4). It is necessary to identify the extent to which changes in gastrointestinal metabolism reflect the contribution of the gut itself as distinct from the activity of the luminal contents. The gut has the characteristics of not only being the most flexible in terms of its potential for adaptation, but also most susceptible to modulation by dietary manipulation.

Acknowledgements. I should like to acknowledge the support of the Wellcome Trust and thank V. Badaloo, B. de Benoist, E. Forrest, J. Hibbert and C. Persaud for assisting in the preparation of this manuscript.

1 Badaloo, V. (1985): Measurement of protein turnover and metabolic rate in sickle cell anaemia. MSc thesis, University of the West Indies.

2 Beard, J.L., Huebers, H.A. & Finch, C.A. (1984): Protein depletion and iron deficiency in rats. *J. Nutr.* **114**, 1396–1401.

3 Brady, F.O. & Helvig, B. (1984): Effect of epinephrine and norepinephrine on zinc thionein levels and induction in rat liver. *Am. J. Physiol.* **247**, E318–E322.

4 de Benoist, B., Jackson, A.A., Hall, J. St. E. & Persaud, C. (1985): Whole body protein turnover in Jamaican women during normal pregnancy. *Hum. Nutr.: Clin. Nutr.* **39C**, 167–179.

5 Elwyn, D.H. (1970): The role of the liver in regulation of amino acid and protein metabolism. In *Mammalian protein metabolism IV*, ed H.N. Munro, pp. 523–557 Academic Press, New York.

6 Fern, E.B., Garlick, P.J. & Waterlow, J.C. (1985): Apparent compartmentation of body nitrogen in one human subject: its consequences in measuring the rate of whole-body protein synthesis with ^{15}N. *Clin. Sci.* **68**, 271–282.

7 Golden, M.H.N., Waterlow, J.C. & Picou, D. (1977): Protein turnover, synthesis and breakdown before and after recovery from protein-energy malnutrition. *Clin. Sci. Molec. Med.* **53**, 473–477.

8 Guggenheim, K. & Buechler-Czaczkes, E. (1950): The effect of quantity and quality of food proteins on the regeneration of liver protein in protein depleted rats. *Br. J. Nutr.* **4**, 161–165.

9 Hall, R..I., Grant, J.P., Ross, L.H., Coleman, R.A., Bozovic, M.G. & Quarfordt (1984): Pathogenesis of hepatic steatosis in the parenterally fed rat. *J. Clin. Invest.* **74**, 1658–1668.

10 Harper, A.E. & Elvehjem, C.A. (1957): A review of the effects of different carbohydrates on vitamin and amino acid requirements. *Agric. Fd Chem.* **5**, 754–758.

11 Hibbert, J.M. & Jackson, A.A. (1985): Increased urea metabolism in sickle cell disease. *W. Indian Med. J.* **34**, (Suppl)., 38.

12 Hoerr, R.A., Matthew, B.E., Bier, D.M., Blackburn, G.L. & Young, V.R. (1984): Splanchnic bed metabolism of leucine in man measured by simultaneous intravenous and intragastric infusion of stable isotope tracers of leucine. *Am. J. Clin. Nutr.* **39**, 687.

13 Holt, T.L., Ward, L.C., Francis, P.J., Isles, A., Cooksley, W.G.E., & Shepherd, R.W. (1985): Whole body protein turnover in malnourished cystic fibrosis patients and its relationship to pulmonary disease. *Am. J. Clin. Nutr.* **41**, 1061–1066.

14 Jackson, A.A. (1983): Amino acids: essential and non essential? *Lancet* **1**, 1034–1037.

15 Jackson, A.A. (1985): Nutritional adaptation in disease and recovery. In *Nutritional adaptation in man*, ed K. Blaxter & J.C. Waterlow, pp. 111–126. London: John Libbey.

16 Jackson, A.A., Picou, D. & Landman, J. (1984): The non-invasive measurement of urea kinetics in normal man by a constant infusion of ^{15}N-urea. *Hum. Nutr.: Clin. Nutr.* **38C**, 339–354.

17 Laurent, G.J., Sparrow, M.P. & Millward, D.J. (1978): Changes in rates of protein synthesis and breakdown during hypertrophy of the anterior and posterior latissimus dorsi muscles. *Biochem. J.* **176**, 407–417.

18 Long, C.L., Jeevanandam, M. & Kinney, J.M. (1978): Metabolism and recycling of urea in man. *Am. J. Clin. Nutr.* **31**, 1367–1382.

19 McNurlan, M.A., Tomkins, A.M. & Garlick, P.J. (1979): The effect of starvation on the rate of protein synthesis in rat liver and small intestine. *Biochem. J.* **178**, 373–379.

20 Nuramatsu, T. & Okumura, J-I (1985): Whole-body protein turnover in chicks at early stages of growth. *J. Nutr.* **115**, 483–490.

21 Parsons, H.G., Beaudry, P. & Pencharz, P. (1985): The effect of nutritional rehabilitation on whole body protein metabolism of children with cystic fibrosis. *Pediatr. Res.* **19**, 189–192.

22 Persaud, C. (1983): Studies of ^{15}N-alanine metabolism in man. MSc thesis, University of the West Indies.

23 Persaud, C., Jackson, A., Badaloo, V. & de Benoist, B. (1985): Protein turnover measured in 3 hours with ^{15}N-glycine and urinary ammonia. XIII International Congress of Nutrition, Abstract.

24 Reeds, P.J., Cadenhead, A., Fuller, M.F., Lobley, G.E. & McDonald, J.D. (1980): Protein turnover in growing pigs. Effects of age and food intake. *Br. J. Nutr.* **43**, 445–455.

25 Rennie, M.J., Edwards, R.H.T., Halliday, D., Matthews, D.E., Wolman, S.L. & Millward, D.J. (1982): Muscle protein synthesis measured by stable isotope techniques in man: the effects of feeding and fasting. *Clin. Sci.* **63**, 519–523.

26 Richards, P. & Brown, C.L. (1975): Urea metabolism in an azotaemic women with normal renal function. *Lancet* **2**, 207–209.

27 Schwenk, W.F., Tsalikian, E., Beaufree, B. & Haymond, M.W. (1985): Recycling of an amino acid label with prolonged isotope infusion: implications for kinetic studies. *Am. J. Physiol.* **248**, E482–E487.

28 Sim, A.J.M., Wolfe, B.M., Young, V.R., Clarke, D. & Moore, F.D. (1979): Glucose promotes whole-body protein synthesis from infused amino acids in fasting man. *Lancet* **1**, 68–72.

29 Waterlow, J.C. (1961): The rate of recovery of malnourished infants in relation to the protein and calorie levels of the diet. *J. Trop. Pediat.* **7**, 16–22.

30 Waterlow, J.C. (1984): Protein turnover with special reference to man. *Q. J. exp. Physiol.* **69**, 409–438.

31 Waterlow, J.C. (1985): What do we mean by adaptation. In *Nutritional adaptation in man*, ed K.Z. Blaxter & J.C. Waterlow, pp. 1–11. London: John Libbey.

32 Waterlow, J.C., Garlick, P.J. & Millward, D.J. (1978): Protein turnover in mammalian tissues and in the whole body. Amsterdam: North Holland.

33 Waterlow, J.C. & Stephen, J.M.L. (1981): *Nitrogen metabolism in man.* Applied Science Publishers, London.

34 Watts, R.W.E. & Crawhall, J.C. (1959): The first glycine metabolic pool in man. *Biochem. J.* **73**, 277–286.

35 Whipple, A.O. (1940): The critical latent or lag period in the healing of wounds. *Ann. Surg.* **112**, 481–488.

36 Wrong, O.M., Vince, A.J. & Waterlow, J.C. (1985): The contribution of endogenous urea to faecal ammonia in man, determined by ^{15}N labelling of plasma urea. *Clin. Sci.* **68**, 193–199.

37 Wu, H. & Bishop, C.W. (1959): Pattern of N[15]-excretion in man following administration of N[15]-labeled glycine. *J. Appl. Physiol.* **14**, 1–5.

38 Yu, Y.M., Yong, R.D., Matthews, D.E., Wen, Z.M., Burke, J.F., Bier, D.M. & Young, V.R. (1985): Quantitative aspects of glycine and alanine nitrogen metabolism in postabsorptive young men: effects of level of nitrogen and dispensable amino acid intake. *J. Nutr.* **115**, 399–410.

Enzymatic basis for adaptive changes in amino acid metabolism

A.E. HARPER

Departments of Nutritional Sciences and Biochemistry, College of Agricultural and Life Sciences, University of Wisconsin-Madison, 420 Henry Mall, Madison, Wisconsin 53706, USA.

Higher animals tolerate a wide range of nutritional conditions and are able to restore the concentrations of solutes in body fluids toward standard steady-state conditions after a perturbation. This ability to adapt to changes in the supply of nutrients requires coordination of metabolic responses. Cannon (1929) coined the term 'homoeostasis'[4] to describe this attribute of living systems. For the survival of organisms during periods when intakes of food or specific nutrients are marginal to inadequate, metabolic systems that contribute to maintenance of homoeostasis must respond appropriately. During periods when the protein intake of an organism is low, survival depends upon highly efficient conservation of the nutritionally-indispensable amino acids. Although the ability of homoeothermic organisms to adjust to a low intake is characterized as adaptation, the metabolic responses that contribute to such adjustments are both regulatory and adaptive. The major systems for regulation of amino acid metabolism and for maintaining homoeostasis of blood and body fluid amino acid concentrations are those for protein synthesis and degradation, and those for catabolism of amino acids. Adaptation to low intakes of protein is associated mainly with changes in the rates of various reactions in these systems.

Channelling of amino acids into systems for protein synthesis. Efficient utilization of amino acids for synthesis of tissue proteins during periods when protein intake is low depends upon channelling the limited amounts of amino acids in the food consumed preferentially into systems for protein synthesis and away from those for amino acid degradation. Evidence that this occurs comes from studies *in vivo* of the oxidation of [^{14}C]-labelled amino acids by animals consuming diets in which the concentration of a labelled indispensable amino acid ranged from well below to well above that required for maximal growth[16,20,21]. When histidine intake was below the estimated requirement of about 40 mg/day, the amount of histidine oxidized did not exceed 10 per cent of the amount absorbed. As the dietary content of histidine was increased above the requirement, the rate of histidine oxidation increased directly with increasing histidine intake without any change occurring in the activity of histidase, the initial and limiting enzyme in the degradative pathway. Similar patterns of oxidation, with only 5 to 10 per cent of the absorbed amino acid being oxidized when intake was low, have been observed in similar studies with other amino acids. Recovery of radioactivity from the carcasses of the rats used in studies of this type[2,20,21] indicated that 85–90 per cent of the label from the amino acid absorbed when intake was not excessive was retained in the carcass. These observations reveal how efficiently amino acids are conserved by higher animals when protein intake is low.

Protein intake, tissue amino acid concentrations and protein synthesis. Amino acids are channelled into pathways for protein synthesis through reactions by which they are combined with transfer-RNA (tRNA) to form aminoacyl-tRNAs. The Michaelis constants (Km) of many of the aminoacyl-tRNA synthetases, the catalysts for these reactions, are of the order of 1–50 μM for amino acids; liver concentrations of amino acids of rats fed a low protein diet (60 g lactalbumin/kg) range from 30 to 500 μM; the Km of the amino acid-degrading enzymes of liver are generally in the millimolar range[15,30]. Thus, even when liver amino acid concentrations are as low as they are in rats consuming a low-protein diet, aminoacyl-tRNA synthetases should be functioning at high rates and tRNAs should be highly charged. Also, the activities of the synthetases are elevated in liver, but not in muscle, of protein-depleted rats[37]. These responses should increase the efficiency of channelling of whatever amino acids are available into pathways for protein synthesis in the liver. Amino acid-degrading enzymes, in contrast, will be far from saturated with substrate under these conditions, so rates of amino acid degradation should be low.

Rates of synthesis of protein by cell-free systems prepared from livers of rats with widely different protein intakes have recently been measured[6]. The system[8] incorporated methionine at a rate approaching 10 per cent of that reported for liver *in vivo* [40]. When protein synthesis was not limited by amino acid supply in the medium, the highest rates of protein synthesis were observed with preparations from rats that had been fed either protein-free or low protein diets (6 g casein/kg). This adaptive response should contribute to the efficient capture of amino acids by liver of protein-depleted rats[40], and to the rapid recovery noted when protein-depleted rats are fed a diet containing an adequate amount of protein[24].

As the capacity of protein-depleted rats for synthesis of liver proteins is elevated, a disproportionately high rate of incorporation of amino acids into liver proteins might be expected, with the result that the supply of amino acids for other tissues would be inordinately depleted. This occurs to only a limited extent, and mainly when malnutrition is severe[41], presumably in part because the system for protein synthesis in liver is highly responsive to changes in amino acid supply. In a study of relationships between circulating amino acid concentrations and protein synthesis by the isolated perfused liver, it was noted[11] that the rate of protein synthesis increased as perfusate amino acid concentrations were increased from fasting blood concentrations to about 5-fold the fasting values. In a further study[6] with the soluble system prepared from liver of protein-depleted rats—the system that was highly active when amino acid supply was not limiting—protein synthesis was depressed (from 177 to 76 pmoles of methionine incorporated in 160 min/mg protein) if amino acid concentrations in the incubation medium were as low as those of blood from rats fed a low-protein diet.

With the perfused liver system the quantity of tRNA-bound amino acids was not depressed when amino acid supply was low, but binding of initiation factors by 40S ribosomal subunits was[11]. These and other similar observations[27] suggest that reduced ability to initiate protein synthesis is an adaptive response of mammals to an inadequate supply of amino acids. Such a response should reduce the possibility that a disproportionate amount of the available amino acids will be incorporated into liver when the protein intake of an animal is low.

Protein intake and amino acid transport. Hepatic amino acid transport is stimulated in animals consuming high-protein diets[39], but effects of low protein intakes on amino acid transport have received only limited attention. Uptake of the non-metabolizable amino acid, α-aminoisobutyric acid (AIB), by liver slices prepared from rats at various times after they have been fed a single meal, is greatly elevated within one hour if the meal is rich in protein. The stimulation of AIB transport declines steadily after one hour, indicating that this is a short-lived adaptation to an influx of amino acids. AIB uptake by liver cells from rats fed a low-protein diet (130 g casein/kg) was about half that of cells from rats fed an excessively high-protein diet (900 g casein/kg)[9].

A high protein intake stimulates glucagon release[7]; both glucagon administration and a high protein intake increase cyclic-AMP concentration and AIB uptake by liver[38]. By following the rate of decay of the stimulation of AIB transport in liver slices from rats given a single subcutaneous injection of glucagon, the induced transport system was shown to have a half-life of only 0.8 h. Although the patterns of response of AIB transport after glucagon administration and after a high-protein meal are similar, whether the basis for the responses to these two stimuli are the same has not been established.

In a study of AIB uptake by liver slices from rats fed a low-protein diet (60 g casein/kg) it was observed[39] that the responsiveness of the AIB transport system after the rats were intubated with an amino acid load (1 g casein hydrolyzate), declined within 4 d to about half of that observed for those consuming a higher-protein diet. Reduced stimulation of hepatic uptake of amino acids from a meal containing protein in rats that have become adjusted to a low protein intake should make more amino acids available for protein synthesis in peripheral tissues. As responsiveness of this transport system in liver is restored within a short period of time when such animals begin to consume a high-protein diet, there would appear to be coordination among adaptive responses of transport systems and those of systems for amino acid conservation and catabolism under these conditions.

Protein intake and amino acid catabolism. Changes that occur in the rate of amino acid catabolism when the protein intake of an animal is altered depend upon the properties of enzymes and may represent either regulatory or adaptive responses. With a fixed amount of enzyme, the rate of an enzymatic reaction increases, usually in hyperbolic fashion, with increasing substrate concentration until the enzyme becomes saturated with substrate. This occurs also with tissue preparations and *in vivo*. In a study with the isolated perfused rat hindquarter[19] as leucine concentration in the perfusate was increased from 0.1 to 0.5 mM, the rate of leucine oxidation increased from about 0.5 to 5.5 nmol/g muscle per min.

The amount of active enzyme present in a tissue is the other major variable that determines the rate of an enzymatic reaction, with the rate increasing directly with increasing content of active enzyme in a tissue. The activities of most of the amino-acid-degrading enzymes in liver change in parallel with changes in the protein intake of an animal[12,32]. When rats that have been consuming a diet containing 180 g casein/kg are subsequently fed 800 g casein/kg diet, histidase activity increases seven-fold within 10 d. When protein is deleted from the diet of rats that have been consuming a diet containing 800 g casein/kg, histidase activity falls within another 10 d to one-ninth of the value for animals fed the high protein diet[34].

Measurements of this type made *in vitro* may not always represent measurements of enzyme that is functional *in vivo*. However, when the effect of protein intake on the rate of clearance of a load of histidine (50 mg/100 g body weight i.p.) from the blood of rats was examined, rate constants for clearance were 0.5, 0.25, and 0.15, respectively, for rats consuming diets containing 400 g, 120 g and 40 g casein/kg. Thus, in rats with low protein intakes, low histidase activity was associated with a slow rate of removal of histidine from body fluids.

Some enzymes exist in both active and inactive forms. Phenylalanine hydroxylase, the catalyst for the conversion of phenylalanine to tyrosine, the initial and rate-limiting step in the degradation of phenylalanine, is such an enzyme. It can be activated several-fold in a number of ways[18], among them by its substrate[35]. The activity also increases in animals treated with glucagon. Glucagon stimulates both phosphorylation of the enzyme by a cyclic-AMP-dependent protein kinase[18] and phenylalanine metabolism in rats *in vivo*[14].

Allosteric activation of phenylalanine hydroxylase by its substrate should also occur *in vivo* as activation is about half-maximal in the presence of 0.06 mM phenylalanine, about the concentration in livers of rats fed a low-protein diet. Also, as the Km of the enzyme is 0.2 to 0.3 mM, but appears to increase when the enzyme is fully activated[22], the rate of phenylalanine degradation by rats with low intakes of protein should be low. This should contribute to conservation of phenylalanine, but in malnourished subjects can lead to depletion of tyrosine[3].

Tryptophan oxygenase, the initial enzyme in the pathway for degradation of tryptophan, is only partially in the active form in liver. It also is activated by its substrate. This activation is associated with increased binding of the haematin cofactor to the inactive apoenzyme to form active holoenzyme[10]. Also, the rate of intracellular degradation of tryptophan oxygenase is reduced by tryptophan[33]. Thus, with low tryptophan concentration in the liver of animals consuming a low-protein diet (only about 0.03 mM), tryptophan oxygenase activity will be low, an adaptive response that should contribute to conservation of this amino acid.

A direct relationship is observed between the protein intake of animals and the activities of many enzymes of amino acid metabolism in liver that do not appear to be regulated by specific mechanisms. Among these are arginase and ornithine aminotransferase (OT)[32]. Rates of both synthesis and degradation of liver arginase in rats adjusting from a high (700 g/kg) to a low (80 g/kg) protein diet were measured by immunological and isotopic techniques[31]; when the protein content of the diet was reduced, arginase content decreased by almost 75 per cent within 6 d as the result of a steady decrease in the rate of enzyme synthesis and a marked increase in the rate of degradation. Similarly, when the protein content of the diet of rats was reduced from 600 g to 120 g/kg, OT activity decreased to 25 per cent of the original value as the result of increased enzyme degradation and decreased synthesis[5]. Thus, reduced enzyme capacity when protein intake is inadequate, can occur through regulation of the rates of both synthesis and degradation.

In a study of the mechanism of induction of ornithine aminotransferase (OAT), antibody to the enzyme and cloned DNA complementary to mRNA for OAT was prepared[26] enabling OAT mRNA and OAT levels to be quantified in hepatocytes from rats fed a 600 g protein/kg or a protein-free diet. Enzyme activities and rates of enzyme synthesis differed by 100-fold between the two groups, whereas the quantity of mRNA differed by only about two-fold. Further, the amount of radioactivity in OAT released from polysomes after initiation of protein synthesis had been inhibited allowed estimation of the rate of initiation of synthesis of OAT which was 23-fold greater in hepatocytes from rats fed the high-protein than in those from rats fed the protein-free diet[26]. Thus, levels of some amino-acid-degrading enzymes can be modified as the result of changes in efficiency of translation of mRNA in response to changes in amino acid supply.

The enzyme system for branched-chain amino acid (BCAA) catabolism differs from those for degradation of other indispensable amino acids in that it is distributed throughout all of the tissues of the body and the activity of the initial enzyme in the pathway, branched-chain amino acid aminotransferase (BCAAT), is much higher in tissues other than liver than that of the second enzyme, branched-chain ketoacid dehydrogenase (BCKAD), the catalyst for oxidation of the product of the transamination reaction[17].

BCKAD is present in most tissues in active and inactive states. The enzyme is inactivated by phosphorylation and is activated by removal of the phosphate group[29]. The proportion of BCKAD in the active state *in vivo* can be estimated by measuring the activity in tissues prepared in the presence and absence of fluoride, which inhibits activation of BCKAD by phosphatase. The enzyme is less than 40 per cent, and may be as little as 20 per cent, in the active form in liver from rats fed a low-protein diet, but is almost fully active in liver from rats fed a high-protein diet. In muscle, the degree of activation is less than 15 per cent and is little influenced by protein intake of animals[13,28].

As the activity of BCAAT is high in most tissues and that of BCKAD, except in liver, changes little when protein intake is low, rapid degradation of BCAA would be anticipated. Despite this, the rate of degradation of leucine by the rat *in vivo* is low when protein intake is low, as it is for other amino acids. How then is this conservation of BCAA accomplished? BCAA transamination is a highly reversible reaction. As the concentration of glutamate, one of the products of the BCAAT reaction, is high in most cells, ranging from 2 to above 5 mM, this should favour conversion of BCKA to BCAA and result in low concentrations of BCKA in tissues[23]. Concentrations of BCKA measured in tissues are on the order of 10 to 20 µM. Thus, it would appear that the relative concentrations of substrates and products of the BCAAT reaction in tissues tend to keep BCKA concentrations and hence the rate of BCAA oxidation low when intake of protein is low[25]. Measurements of the fate of the BCAA carbon-skeleton using doubly-labelled amino acids indicate that up to 80 per cent of BCKA formed may be reaminated to BCAA[36]. Whether these mechanisms should be considered regulatory, adaptive, or both, is an open question, but the end result is conservation of BCAA when protein intake is low.

1 Aguilar, T.S., Benevenga, N.J. & Harper, A.E. (1974): Effect of dietary methionine level on its metabolism in rats. *J. Nutr.* **104**, 761–771.

2 Aguilar, T.S., Harper, A.E. & Benevenga, N.J. (1972): Efficiency of utilization of indispensable amino acids for growth by the rat. *J. Nutr.* **102**, 1199–1208.

3 Antener, I., Verwilghen, A.M., van Geert, C. & Mauron, J. (1981): Biochemical study of malnutrition. Part V. Metabolism of phenylalanine and tyrosine. *Internat. J. Vit. Res.* **51**, 297–306.

4 Cannon, W.B. (1929): Organization for physiological homeostasis. *Physiol. Rev.* **9**, 399–431.

5 Chee, P.Y. & Swick, R.W. (1976): Effect of dietary protein and tryptophan on the turnover of rat liver ornithine aminotransferase. *J. Biol. Chem.* **251**, 1029–1034.

6 Eisenstein, R.S. (1984): Characterization and applications of a protein synthesis system from rat liver. Ph. D. Thesis, University of Wisconsin-Madison. Madison, Winconsin.

7 Eisenstein, A.B. & Strack, I. (1971): Effect of high protein feeding on gluconeogenesis in rat liver. *Diabetes* **20**, 577–585.

8 Eisenstein, R.S. & Harper, A.E. (1984): Characterization of a protein synthesis system from rat liver: Translation of endogenous and exogenous messenger RNA. *J. Biol. Chem.* **259**, 9922–9928.

9 Fafournoux, P., Remesy, C. & Demigne, C. (1982): Stimulation of amino acid transport into liver cells from rats adapted to a high-protein diet. *Biochem. J.* **206**, 13–18.

10 Feigelson, P. & Greengard, O. (1962): Regulation of liver tryptophan pyrrolase activity. *J. Biol. Chem.* **237**, 1908–1913.

11 Flaim, K.E., Peavy, D.E., Everson, W.V. & Jefferson, L.S. (1982): The role of amino acids in the regulation of protein synthesis in perfused rat liver. I. Reduction in rates of synthesis resulting from amino acid deprivation and recovery during flow-through perfusion. *J. Biol. Chem.* **257**, 2932–2938.

12 Freedland, R.A. & Szepesi, B. (1971): Control of enzyme activity: Nutritional factors. In *Enzyme synthesis and degradation in mammalian systems*, ed M. Rechcigl, pp. 103–140. Basel: Karger.

13 Gillim, S.E., Paxton, R., Cook, G.A. & Harris, R. (1983): Activity state of the branched chain α-ketoacid dehydrogenase complex in heart, liver, and kidney of normal, fasted, diabetic, and protein-starved rats. *Biochem. Biophys. Res. Commun.* **111**, 74–81.

14 Haley, C.J. & Harper, A.E. (1982): Glucagon stimulation of phenylalanine metabolism. The effects of acute and chronic glucagon treatment. *Metabolism* **31**, 524–532.

15 Harper, A.E. (1974): Control mechanisms in amino acid metabolism. In *The control of metabolism*, ed J.D. Sink, pp. 49–74. University Park and London: Pennsylvania State University Press.

16 Harper, A.E. & Benjamin, E. (1984): Relationship between intake and rate of oxidation of leucine and α-ketoisocaproate in vivo in the rat. *J. Nutr.* **114**, 431–440.

17 Harper, A.E., Miller, R.H. & Block, K.P. (1984): Branched-chain amino acid metabolism. *Ann. Rev. Nutr.* **4**, 409–454.

18 Hasegawa, H. & Kaufman, S. (1982): Spontaneous activation of phenylalanine hydroxylase in rat liver extracts. *J. Biol. Chem.* **257**, 3084–3089.

19 Hutson, S.M., Cree, T.C. & Harper, A.E. (1978): Regulation of leucine and α-ketoisocaproate metabolism in skeletal muscle. *J. Biol. Chem.* **253**, 8126–8133.

20 Kang-Lee, Y.A. & Harper, A.E. (1977): Effect of histidine intake and hepatic histidase activity on the metabolism of histidase activity on the metabolism of histidine in vivo. *J. Nutr.* **107**, 1427–1443.

21 Kang-Lee, Y.A. & Harper, A.E. (1978): Threonine metabolism in vivo: Effect of threonine intake and prior induction to threonine dehydratase in rats. *J. Nutr.* **108**, 163–175.

22 Kaufman, S. & Mason, K. (1982): Specificity of amino acids as activators and substrates for phenylalanine hydroxylase. *J. Biol. Chem.* **257**, 14667–14678.

23 Krebs, H.A. & Lund, P. (1977): Aspects of the regulation of the metabolism of branched-chain amino acids. *Adv. Enz. Regul.* **15**, 375–394.

24 Mendes, C.B. & Waterlow, J.C. (1958): The effect of a low-protein diet, and of refeeding, on the composition of liver and muscle in the weanling rat. *Br. J. Nutr.* **12**, 74–88.

25 Miller, R.H. & Harper, A.E. (1984): Metabolism of valine and 3-methyl-2-oxobutanoate by the isolated perfused kidney. *Biochem. J.* **224**, 109–116.

26 Mueckler, M.M., Merrill, M.J. & Pitot, H.C. (1983): Translational and pretranslational control of ornithine aminotransferase synthesis in rat liver. *J. Biol. Chem.* **258**, 6109–6114.

27 Pain, V.M., Lewis, J.A., Huvos, P., Henshaw, E.C. & Clemens, M.J. (1980): The effects of amino acid starvation on regulation of polypeptide chain initiation in Ehrlich ascites tumor cells. *J. Biol. Chem.* **255**, 1486–1491.

28 Patston, P.A., Espinal, J. & Randle, P.J. (1984): Effects of diet and of alloxan-diabetes on the activity of branched-chain 2-oxo acid dehydrogenase complex and of activator protein in rat tissues. *Biochem. J.* **222**, 711–719.

29 Randle, P.J., Fatania, H.R. and Lau, K.S. (1984): Regulation of the mitochondrial branched-chain 2-oxoacid dehydrogenase complex of animal tissues by reversible phosphorylation. In *Enzyme regulation by reversible phosphorylation, further advances*, ed P. Cohen, pp. 1–26. Amsterdam: Elsevier.

30 Rogers, Q.R. (1976): The nutritional and metabolic effects of amino acid imbalances. In *Protein metabolism and nutrition*, ed K.N. Boorman, P.J. Buttery, D. Lewis, R.J. Neale & H. Swan, pp. 279–301. London: Butterworth.

31 Schimke, R.T. (1964): The importance of both synthesis and degradation in the control of arginase levels in rat liver. *J. Biol. Chem.* **239**, 3808–3817.

32 Schimke, R.T. & Doyle, D. (1970): Control of enzyme levels in animal tissues. *Ann. Rev. Biochem.* **39**, 929–976.

33 Schimke, R.T., Sweeney, E.W. & Berlin, C.M. (1965): The roles of synthesis and degradation in the control of rat liver tryptophan pyrrolase. *J. Biol. Chem.* **240**, 322–331.

34 Schirmer, M.D. & Harper, A.E. (1970): Adaptive responses of mammalian histidine-degrading enzymes. *J. Biol. Chem.* **245**, 1204–1211.

35 Shiman, R. & Gray, D.W. (1980): Substrate activation of phenylalanine hydroxylase. A kinetic characterization. *J. Biol. Chem.* **255**, 4793–4800.

36 Staten, M.A., Bier, D.M. & Matthews, D.E. (1984): Regulation of valine metabolism in man: a stable isotope study. *Am. J. Clin. Nutr.* **40**, 1224–1234.

37 Stephen, J.M.L. & Waterlow, J.C. (1968): Effect of malnutrition on activity of two enzymes concerned with amino acid metabolism in human liver. *Lancet* **2**, 118–119.

38 Tews, J.K., Colosi, N.W. & Harper, A.E. (1975): Amino acid transport and turnover of a transport system in liver slices from rats treated with glucagon and antibiotics. *Life Sci.* **16**, 739–750.

39 Tews, J.K. & Harper, A.E. (1976): α-Aminoisobutyric acid transport in liver slices from rats fed low protein meals. *J. Nutr.* **106**, 1497–1506.

40 Waterlow, J.C. & Garlick, P.J. (1975): Metabolic adaptations to protein deficiency. In *Alcohol and abnormal protein biosynthesis*, ed M.A. Rothschild, M. Oratz & S.S. Schreiber, pp. 67–94, New York: Pergamon.

41 Waterlow, J.C., Garlick, P.J. & Millward, D.J. (1977): Amino acid supply and protein turnover. In *Clinical nutrition updates: amino acids*, ed H.L. Greene, M.A. Holliday & H.N. Munro, pp. 1–9. Chicago, IL: American Medical Association.

Role of energy metabolism in regulation of protein requirements

B. TORUN
Division of Nutrition and Health, Institute of Nutrition of Central America and Panama (INCAP), Apartado Postal 1188, Guatemala City, Guatemala.

Energy intake and protein metabolism. An increase in energy intake with constant dietary protein can reduce nitrogen excretion and increase nitrogen balance[16]. This is more marked with protein intakes below or near the requirement level and it has also been demonstrated when energy in excess of expenditure is fed[1,2,6,8]. But there is a limit to the effect of dietary energy: when the diet does not provide adequate amounts of protein, additional intakes of energy beyond a given amount will not further improve nitrogen balance.

It is to be expected that, when energy intake cannot satisfy energy demands, more protein is oxidized, thus increasing urinary nitrogen excretion and decreasing nitrogen balance, but this is not always the case. In a study of the energy requirements of preschool children with a constant intake of vegetable proteins equivalent to 1.2 g milk protein/kg per d, two consecutive reductions of 10 per cent in dietary energy at 40 d intervals did not affect nitrogen retention measured 17–20 and 37–40 d after each dietary change[25]. Energy expenditure diminished with the first reduction in energy intake and weight gain decreased after the second reduction; growth in height was not affected and there were no consistent changes in urinary creatinine excretion related to the levels of energy intake. It may be that the compensatory decrease in energy expenditure, the protein ingestion at a safe level of intake, the good nutritional status of the children and their hygienic living conditions prevented a nitrogen loss with the reduction in energy intake. It is possible that if the low energy intake had continued longer, if the children had become ill with the frequency that is customary in developing countries or if their dietary protein had been marginal (ie, closer to the average requirement for their age), they might have gone into negative nitrogen balance.

Studies in India also failed to show an association between energy intake and nitrogen balance. In one study[10], children 4 years old ate diets that provided 1, 1.3, 1.6 and 2 g protein, and 80 or 100 kcal (334 or 418 kJ)/kg per d. With three of those levels of protein intake, nitrogen balance fell with the lower energy intake in only two of three children. In another study with adults[9], an increase in dietary energy from 44–56 kcal (184–234 kJ)/kg per d improved nitrogen retention when the men ate 1.0 but not 1.2 g protein/kg per d.

These findings indicate that nitrogen balance is more sensitive to changes in dietary energy when protein intake is relatively low. They also suggest that when protein intake is adequate, the body is better protected in terms of nitrogen metabolism against a moderate decrease in energy intake.

The protein-sparing effect of dietary energy has been demonstrated by means other than nitrogen balance. For example, amino acids labelled with stable isotopes showed that, in men with a protein intake of 0.6 g/kg per d, an energy intake 25 per cent in excess of maintenance requirements reduced the rate of leucine oxidation from (mean ± s.d.) 18.0 ± 8.3 to 12.4 ± 8.7 μmol/kg per h, and increased net protein retention[15].

The experimental evidence of the effects of energy intake on protein metabolism has raised the question whether protein requirements have been underestimated for populations prone to have marginal or deficient energy intakes. On the other hand, have such populations adapted to use more efficiently their low energy intakes and preserve body protein? Although a decrease in energy expenditure in response to low energy intake may diminish the risk of body protein loss, it is not known how long such a response can be effectively sustained. Furthermore, this should be regarded as a transient compensation of low intakes and not as a desirable adaptation in view of the physical, emotional and social costs of diminished energy expenditure, which usually is achieved through a reduction in physical activity.

Another important related question is whether protein requirements are higher for individuals with low bodily store of energy and whose dietary intakes are sometimes marginal and sometimes adequate, as occurs in groups of migrant workers or persons subject to seasonal changes in food availability.

The most logical answer to these questions would be to raise the dietary protein recommendations. However, this is more expensive and often more difficult than increasing the availability of dietary energy sources. The question, then, that also needs to be answered is whether increasing the recommendations for energy intake in populations with constraints to eat more protein will reduce their protein requirements.

Dietary energy substrates. The effects of dietary energy on protein metabolism vary with the source of energy. Both carbohydrates and lipids enhance nitrogen and amino acid metabolism, but carbohydrates have specific actions that make them more effective than fats in promoting the utilization of dietary protein, at least transiently. The administration of carbohydrates at a given protein intake or while fasting, reduces the urinary excretion of nitrogen more than fat does and results in better nitrogen retention[17]. With isocaloric, isonitrogenous diets having carbohydrate: fat ratios of 1:1 and 2:1, the higher nitrogen-sparing effect of carbohydrate relative to fat was more pronounced at lower levels of energy and protein intakes[20] and it made no difference whether sucrose or dextrins and maltose were the principal dietary carbohydrates[19].

The effects of carbohydrates on protein metabolism have also been shown in relation to specific amino acids. The oral or i.v. administration of glucose produces a transient decrease in plasma amino acid concentration, specially the branched-chain amino acids and other large neutral amino acids, such as methionine, phenylalanine, tyrosine and tryptophan[13]. This is accompanied by an increase in synthesis or a reduction in catabolism of muscle protein. Conversely, dietary carbohydrate restriction, as in high-protein, low-carbohydrate diets, leads to increased accumulation of plasma branched-chain amino acids after protein feeding or after intravenous infusion of leucine[7]. This is probably due to reduced utilization of those amino acids, which are the major substrates for restoration of muscle tissue after protein feeding.

The effects of giving 25 per cent excess of dietary energy either as sucrose plus a glucose polymer, butter fat, or combination of both, on the metabolism of whole body leucine and lysine have been explored.[15]. The former is metabolized mainly in peripheral tissues and the latter in liver. Net leucine retention in the fed state increased more with the carbohydrate or mixed supplementations than with fat alone. Whole body flux of both amino acids did not change, but leucine flux was greater than lysine with the various energy sources and two levels of energy intake. This suggests that identical dietary conditions may elicit different responses from different essential amino acids.

Glucose administration also influences the metabolism of the non-essential amino acid alanine, increasing its *de novo* synthesis, its release to the circulating plasma and its whole body flux[4,21].

In addition to its influence on the metabolism of circulating amino acids, dietary carbohydrate also interacts with amino acids from the same meal. Giving protein and carbohydrates as separate meals can lead to nitrogen loss from the body, which is reversed by giving these two nutrients in the same meal[3].

The mechanisms by which carbohydrate exerts these effects on protein metabolism are not fully understood. They are partly mediated by the insulin released in response to carbohydrate absorption or infusion[17]. The simultaneous infusion of insulin and glucose produces a decrease in plasma urea concentration and urinary nitrogen excretion several times greater than the decrease observed when glucose is infused alone[5]. Another possible mechanism of the effects of glucose may be through its suppression of glucagon release. Glucagon infusion increases the synthesis of urea at the expense of the free amino acid pool and probably also by hydrolysis of visceral protein, and it increases urinary nitrogen excretion[29]. A small increase in plasma glucagon concentration was observed when carbohydrates were restricted in the diet[7].

The evidence that carbohydrates spare protein more efficiently than fat raises important practical questions, such as: Is there a more efficient use of dietary proteins among populations whose dietary energy is derived 70–80 per cent from carbohydrates? If so, will their protein requirements be affected by the dietary changes induced by migrations, cultural changes and access to processed foods?

But there may also be adaptive changes in protein metabolism with the long-term ingestion of diets rich in fat. Although the stimulation of muscle protein synthesis and reduction of catabolism observed with carbohydrate are not the same when fat is fed as a single meal, the studies with patients on long-term parenteral feeding[11] indicate that the administration of fat as a major energy source on a regular basis over long periods of time may be as effective as carbohydrate in promoting nitrogen retention and net protein synthesis.

Physical activity and energy expenditure. Physical activity and its resultant energy expenditure influence protein metabolism. That influence appears to be transient during periods of physical training, but some effects may be long-lasting. However, their importance in terms of adaptation to chronically low dietary intakes by persons who are continuously active has not been clearly defined.

Weanling rats with dietary intakes retricted by 25 or 50 per cent grew better when they were forced to exercise daily in a revolving drum, than pair-fed animals forced to remain inactive in small metabolic cages that restricted their movements[26]. In spite of their higher energy expenditure with identical dietary intakes, the active rats gained more weight, retained more body protein as determined by carcass analysis and grew more in length than the inactive animals. These results were replicated in an experiment with a cross-over design, where on day 14 one half of the active animals were forced to remain inactive for two more weeks, and *vice versa*[27]. Further evidence of the beneficial effect of energy expenditure on protein metabolism and overall growth was provided by studies in preschool-aged children recovering from PEM[24]. When a programme of moderate systematic exercise was added to the dietary therapy, children with an increase of approximately 25 per cent in total daily energy expenditure compared with that of pair-fed control patients, grew more in height and although weight gains were similar in both groups, the more active children gained more lean body mass based on their urinary creatinine excretion, basal oxygen consumption and anthropometric measurements.

Investigators from Berkeley[1,23] studied the effects on nitrogen retention in young men of changes in energy balance, induced by modifying either energy intake or expenditure. In three separate experiments, energy balance was made positive by increasing intake relative to expenditure, or negative by either decreasing intake or increasing physical work. Protein intake was maintained constant at 0.57 or 0.8 g/kg per d. In every instance, mean nitrogen balance fell with the decrease in energy balance, but it fell less when the reduction in energy balance was due to increased work than to a lower energy intake. When energy balance was achieved through equivalent changes in energy intake and expenditure, nitrogen balance was more positive —or less negative— as physical activity and energy expenditure increased. On the average, the men were in negative nitrogen balance with 0.57 g dietary protein/kg per d, and in positive nitrogen balance when they were more active and ate 0.8 g protein/kg per d. These results indicate that physical activity has an anabolic effect on protein metabolism, even under conditions of marginal protein intakes, but the effect is more pronounced when energy balance is maintained and dietary protein is not a limiting factor.

This protein-sparing effect of exercise was also reported in middle-aged men on a weight reducing diet, who lost less lean body mass when the restricted energy intake was accompanied by an increase in physcial activity[28]. In contrast with the beneficial effects of exercise, inactivity reduces the rate of protein synthesis and produces a marked negative nitrogen balance, eg in men who had been immobilized for several days in a plaster cast[22]. Post-mortem tissue analysis of active and inactive rats confirmed that muscle mass is lost with physical inactivity[26], and hypokinetic rats had increased muscle protein catabolism, as suggested by marked increments in urinary excretion of urea and 3-methylhistidine[18], contrary to the effects of exercise which depresses the degradation of 3-methylhistidine-containing proteins and reduces the urinary excretion of that amino acid[14].

Physical activity also influences the metabolism of specific amino acids. This has been reviewed by several authors[12,14,31,32]. In general, exercise increases the oxidation of branched-chain amino acids and the release of alanine from muscle. The significance of these changes in amino acid metabolism is not yet clear for persons who have a chronic marginal dietary protein intake or who regularly engage in heavy physical work and it is not known whether exercise induces a greater need for branched-chain amino acids among such persons.

In summary, most of the evidence indicates that increased energy expenditure has a beneficial effect on protein metabolism, particularly when the diet supplies enough energy to satisfy the demands of physical activity. These observations may be of major importance for persons in developing countries who have relatively low protein and energy intakes and whose occupations demand constant or seasonal heavy energy expenditures. It is conceivable that when energy balance is sustained, the protein requirement to maintain existing lean body mass may be less for a chronically active individual than for one who is inactive. Conversely, marked inactivity, as in immobilized patients, produces a loss of muscle mass. Whether greater protein intakes will help to counteract this negative effect, remains to be proven.

Conclusions. This review of the effects of energy intake and metabolism on amino acid protein metabolism raises important questions related to protein requirements, such as: Since protein recommendations are based on research done with adequate or surfeit dietary energy, have protein requirements been underestimated for populations prone to have marginal or deficient energy intakes? On the other hand, since exercise has an anabolic effect, are protein requirements lower for persons who are almost always physically active? Should dietary protein recommendations be higher for individuals with low body stores of energy and whose energy intakes fluctuate between adequate and deficient, or who engage in seasonal activities with different levels of energy expenditure? Will an increase in physical activity help to protect children from the deleterious effects of mild or moderate protein malnutrition? Since carbohydrates enhance protein metabolism more than fats, will protein requirements increase in persons who change the proportion of those energy sources in their diets? If that were the case, is this a transient effect that will disappear with metabolic adaptations to the higher fat intakes? The answer to these questions and others that may arise will shed further light on the interactions of energy and proteins, and allow us to make better dietary recommendations.

1 Butterfield, G.E. & Calloway, D.H. (1984): Physical activity improves protein utilization in young men. *Br. J. Nutr.* **51**, 171–184.
2 Calloway, D. (1975): Nitrogen balance of men with marginal intakes of protein and energy. *J. Nutr.* **105**, 914–923.
3 Cuthbertson, D.P. & Munro, H.N. (1939): The relationship of carbohydrate metabolism to protein metabolism: I. The roles of total dietary carbohydrate and of surfeit carbohydrate in protein metabolism. *Biochem. J.* **33**, 128–142.
4 Felig, P. (1973): The glucose–alanine cycle. *Metabolism* **22**, 179–207.
5 Fuller, M.F., Weekes, T.E.C., Cadenhead, A. & Bruce, J.B. (1977): The protein-sparing effect of carbohydrate. 2. The role of insulin. *Br. J. Nutr.* **38**, 489–496.
6 Garza, C., Scrimshaw, N.S. & Young, V.R. (1976): Human protein requirements: the effect of variations in energy intake within the maintenance range. *Am. J. Clin. Nutr.* **29**, 280–287.
7 Gelfand, R.A., Hendler, R.G. & Sherwin, R.S. (1979): Dietary carbohydrate and metabolism of ingested protein. *Lancet* **2**, 65–68.

8 Inoue, G., Fujita, Y., Niiyama, Y. (1973): Studies on protein requirements of young men fed egg protein and rice protein with excess and maintenance energy intakes. *J. Nutr.* **103**, 1673–1687.

9 Iyengar, A. & Narasinga Rao, B.S. (1979): Effect of varying energy and protein intake on nitrogen balance in adults engaged in heavy manual labour. *Br. J. Nutr.* **41**, 19–25.

10 Iyengar, A.K., Narasinga Rao, B.S. & Reddy, V. (1979): Effect of varying protein and energy intakes on nitrogen balance in Indian preschool children. *Br. J. Nutr.* **42**, 417–423.

11 Jeejeebhoy, K.N., Anderson, G.H., Nakhooda, A.F., Greenberg, G.R., Sanderson, I. & Marliss, E.B. (1975): Metabolic studies in total parenteral nutrition with lipid in man: comparison with glucose. *J. Clin. Invest.* **57**, 125–136.

12 Lemon, P.W.R. & Nagle, F.F. (1981): Effects of exercise on protein and amino acid metabolism. *Med. Sci. Sports Exercise* **13**, 141–149.

13 Martin-DuPan, R., Mauron, C., Glaeser, B., Wurtman, R.J. (1982): Effect of various oral glucose doses on plasma neutral amino acid levels. *Metabolism* **31**, 937–943.

14 Millward, D.J., Davies, C.T.M., Holliday, D., Wolmen, S.L., Matthews, D. & Rennie, M. (1982): Effect of exercise on protein metabolism in humans as explored with stable isotopes. *Fed. Proc.* **41**, 2686–2691.

15 Motil, K.J., Bier, D.M., Matthews, D.E., Burke, J.F., Young, V.R. (1981): Whole body leucine and lysine metabolism studied with (1-13C)-leucine and (α-15N)-lysine. Response in healthy young men given excess energy intakes. *Metabolism* **30**, 783–791.

16 Munro, H.N. (1951): Carbohydrate and fat as factors in protein utilization and metabolism. *Physiol. Rev.* **31**, 449–488.

17 Munro, H.N. (1964): General aspects of the regulation of protein metabolism by diet and by hormones. In *Mammalian protein metabolism*, ed H.N. Munro & J.B. Allison, vol. 1, p. 381–481. New York: Academic Press.

18 Musacchia, A.J., Deavers, D.R., Meininger, G.A. & Davies, T.P. (1980): A model for hypokinesia; effects on muscle atrophy in the rats. *J. Appl. Physiol. Environ. Exercise Physiol.* **48**, 479–486.

19 Richardson, D.P., Scrimshaw, N.S. & Young, V.R. (1980): The effect of dietary sucrose on protein utilization in healthy young men. *Am. J.. Clin. Nutr.* **33**, 264–272.

20 Richardson, D.P., Wayler, A.H., Scrimshaw, N.S. & Young, V.R. (1979): Quantitative effect of an isoenergetic exchange of fat for carbohydrate on dietary protein utilization in healthy young men. *Am. J. Clin. Nutr.* **32**, 2217–2226.

21 Robert, JJ., Bier, D.M., Zhao, X.H., Matthews, D.E. & Young, V.R. (1982): Glucose and insulin effects on de novo amino acid synthesis in young men: studies with stable isotope labeled alanine, glycine, leucine and lysine. *Metabolism* **31**, 1210–1218.

22 Schoenheyder, F., Heilskov, N.C.S., Olesen, K. (1954): Isotopic studies and mechanism of negative nitrogen balance produced by immobilization. *Scand. J. Clin. Lab. Invest.* **6**, 178–188.

23 Todd, K.S., Butterfield, G.E., Calloway, D.H. (1984): Nitrogen balance in men with adequate and deficient energy intake at three levels of work. *J. Nutr.* **114**, 2107–2118.

24 Torun, B., Schutz, Y., Bradfield, R., Viteri, F.E. (1976): Effect of physical activity upon growth of children recovering from protein–calorie malnutrition. *Proc. 10 Int. Congr. Nutr.* pp. 247–29. Kyoto: Victory-sha Press.

25 Torun, B. & Viteri, F.E. (1981): Energy requirements of pre-school children and effects of varying energy intakes on protein metabolism. In *Protein–energy requirements of developing countries: evaluation of new data*, ed B. Torun, V.R. Young & W.M. Rand, pp. 229–241. Tokyo: United Nations University.

26 Viteri, F.E. (1973): Efecto de la inactividad sobre el crecimiento de ratas alimentadas con una dieta adecuada, a niveles de ingestión calórica normal, y restringidos. In *Nuevos Conceptos sobre Viejos Aspectos de la Desnutrición*, pp. 207–229. México: Academia Mexicana Pediatria.

27 Viteria, F.E. & Torun. B. (1981): Nutrition, physical activity, and growth. In *The biology of normal human growth*, ed M. Ritzen *et al.*, pp. 265–273. New York: Raven Press.

28 Weltman, A., Matter, S. & Stamford, B.A. (1980): Caloric restriction and/or mild exercise effects on serum lipids and body composition. *Am. J. Clin. Nutr.* **33**, 1002–1009.

29 Wolfe, B.M., Culebras, J.M., Aoki, T.T., O'Connor, N.E., Finley, R.J., Kaczowka, A. & Moore, F.D. (1979): The effects of glucagon on protein metabolism in normal man. *Surgery* **86**, 248–257.

30 Young, V.R., Munro, H.N., Matthews, D.E. & Bier, D.M. (1983): Relationship of energy metabolism to protein metabolism. In *New aspects of clinical nutrition*, ed G. Kleinberg & E. Deutsch, pp. 43–73. Basel: Karger.

31 Young, V.R., Robert, J.J., Motil, K.J., Matthews, D.E., Bier, D.M. (1981): Protein and energy intake in relation to protein turnover in man. In *Nitrogen metabolism in man*, ed J.C. Waterlow, pp. 419–447. London: Applied Science Publishers.

32 Young, V.R. & Torun, B. (1981): Physical activity: impact on protein and amino acid metabolism and implications for nutritional requirements. In *Nutrition in health and disease and international development*, ed A.E. Harper & G.K. Davis, pp. 57–85. New York: Alan R. Liss.

Hormonal responses to low intakes in relation to adaptation

D.J. MILLWARD
Nutrition Research Unit, Department of Human Nutrition, London School of Hygiene & Tropical Medicine, St Pancras Hospital, London NW1 2PE, UK.

Whilst the importance of the link between the hormonal and metabolic responses to undernutrition is beyond argument, it remains exceedingly difficult to judge the causal significance of hormonal changes when they are known. The systemic responses reflect not only the circulating levels which are measureable but also the tissue sensitivity which is seldom assessed, and in any case there are few targets which are not subject to multiple hormonal regulation[36]. In this paper I intend to focus on the likely consequences of changes in two hormones, somatomedin C and the principal thyroid hormone, T_3, since marked changes in their concentrations occur in malnourished individuals and might be expected to occur in populations on low food intakes, and there is evidence to indicate that they may mediate important changes which might be considered to be adaptive.

Somatomedin C (SMC). This is one of the two insulin-like growth hormone-dependent peptide growth factors involved in the regulation of somatic growth. Somatomedin C (insulin-like growth factor I), mediates postnatal growth with bone as a primary target, the other, insulin-like growth factor II, mediating fetal growth[28,29]. Plasma concentrations are highest in the 2nd and 3rd decades of life[12] and there are particular changes during the pubertal growth spurt[30]. In young adults its concentration falls on fasting with restoration on refeeding, dependent on intakes of both dietary energy and protein[12]. In growing rats reductions in growth associated with protein or energy-deficiency involve reduced SMC levels[31], and in *ad-lib*-fed very young rats there is a striking relationship with dietary protein concentration and SMC, the highest hormone concentrations occurring with diets containing 15 per cent of their energy as protein, the optimum protein : energy ratio for growth.

Reduced SMC levels are found in children with severe PEM[34]. Plasma concentrations of growth hormone and cortisol are both elevated and there are low levels of insulin and SMC. The SMC and free cortisol are negatively correlated which is particularly significant since cortisol is known to inhibit both SMC synthesis from growth hormone and its action on chondrocytes (see[34]). Thus in these studies the elevated cortisol is seen as an inhibitory response, in marked contrast to prior interpretations of the increases in PEM (eg[35]) which associated the increase in cortisol with an 'adaptive' response mediating the muscle wasting in the marasmic child and preserving albumin synthesis[3].

These changes raise the obvious question as to whether reduced SMC levels could be responsible for stunting in children, an important response whether adaptive or not. Although stunting reflects reduced energy and protein intakes there is evidence that it is particularly related to protein-deficiency (see[9]). This is indicated by increased growth in height in protein-supplementation studies in infants[7,18] and in school children of which the best example is the studies of Malcolm and coworkers on the Bundi boarding school children in New Guinea[16,17]. These children were fed a low-protein diet (exclusively taro and sweet potato), which did not allow optimal growth in height even when fed at a 60 per cent higher level.

While no hormone concentrations have been measured in any of these supplementation studies, it seems likely that reduced SMC concentrations could not only be responsible for the growth inhibition in undernutrition in general, but could specifically mediate stunting in response to very-low-protein diets. However, this emphasis on SMC as the regulator of growth in height is not to ignore the importance of the other hormones involved, particularly insulin, corticosteroids and thyroid hormone[19]. It is the case, however, that SMC does appear to be much more a single function hormone than any others involved in growth regulation, and it may well play the primary role in growth regulation. Its plasma concentration may prove to be a sensitive and much less ambiguous index of nutritional status.

Thyroid hormones. Relatively small imbalances in energy intake and expenditure are associated with measurable changes in thyroid hormones[8], and there are marked changes in response to undernutrition. In adults with PEM, low levels of T_3 have been reported[32]. In severe malnutrition in children the changes are particularly marked[11,25]. Although the extent to which T_4 is reduced is variable (in some cases increases have been reported[25]) the invarient finding of low levels of T_3 coupled with the report of low levels of free T_3[27], means that there can be no doubt that there is an actual hypothyoid state, in contrast to the confusing literature on the response to protein-energy deficiency in rat models[4,5].

Thyroid hormone action at the cellular level involves two types of processes, ie the metabolic rate and consequent energy balance, and growth and development through its influence on gene expression, protein synthesis and turnover.

Metabolic rate. There is no doubt that severe energy deficiency and associated reduced thyroid hormones is associated with a reduced resting metabolic rate (RMR), and given the fact that such reductions are also observed when the RMR is related to lean body mass[14] or total body K^2, it can be assumed that actual metabolic changes have occurred in individual tissues. Little is known of the mechanism of these changes although there is some indication of a reduced ion pumping in severely malnourished children, since the Na-K ATPase activity in leucocytes is reduced[26].

Protein metabolism in children. Malnourished children can conserve N when energy intakes fall[13] and rates of whole-body protein turnover are depressed[10], so it might be thought that the reduced protein degradation, which is one known response to reduced thyroid status[24], is an adaptive response. However, this ignores the possibility that the reduced T_3 is a major factor in mediating the reduced protein synthesis since this is an equally important target for the hormone[22]. Thus the relative importance of these two effects of T_3 will determine on whether the responses are adaptive or detrimental in the growing child.

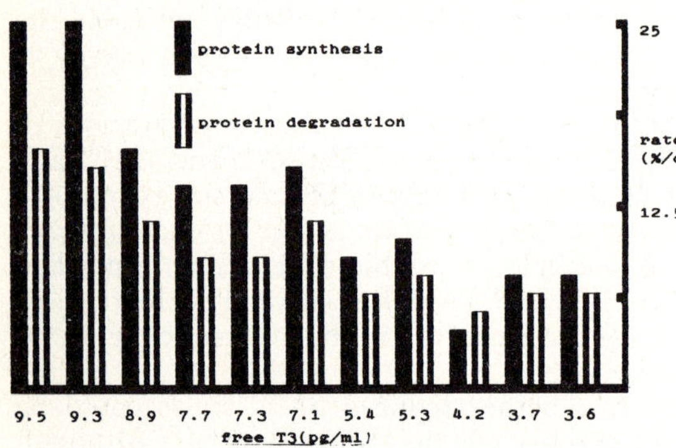

Fig. 1. *Relationship between thyroid hormone status and muscle protein turnover in rat skeletal muscle.* The rates were measured *in vivo* in young rats fed diets of varying protein content ranging from 20 to 0.5 per cent protein for two weeks. The protein-deficient diets induced reductions in growth rates (shown as the difference between the rate of protein synthesis and degradation), and in free T_3 in proportion to the degree of deficiency so the results represent increasing protein deficiency from left to right (Jepson & Millward, unpublished).

Although it is probably not possible to answer this point completely we can go some way by examining the responses of muscle protein synthesis and degradation to malnutrition and T_3 in growing rats. Our results (Fig. 1) show that both processes superficially appear to be related to T_3 with the highest rates of growth, protein synthesis and degradation occurring in the well fed rats with highest levels of free T_3. When these data are analysed in terms of the relationship between protein turnover and growth, protein synthesis is more steeply related to growth than degradation. Thus a fixed change in synthesis will effect growth more than the same change in degradation. Furthermore, analysis of the relationship between T_3 and muscle protein synthesis and degradation indicates that once again synthesis is more steeply related to T_3 than degradation implying that reduced T_3 will be detrimental for growth.

We have to be cautious with this type of analysis since there are other hormonal factors which influence both synthesis and degradation which are to some extent covariants with T_3. Thus, insulin is an important determinant of muscle protein synthesis[22] and in these experiments falls in parallel with T_3. However, we believe that insulin is only active on muscle protein synthesis at relatively low concentrations[23]. Furthermore, as discussed elsewhere[19], apart from the very low rates of protein synthesis associated with the most severe undernutrition where the reduced protein synthesis does reflect a reduced rate of translation (the site of insulin action), the major reason for the reduced protein synthesis in these experiments is a reduced muscle RNA, and ribosomal RNA synthesis is a primary target for T_3[21].

What this means is that during growth a fall in T_3 may well be inhibitory because of its greater effect on synthesis than degradation, rather than being adaptive which would be the case if it enabled conservation of body protein or allowed growth at the reduced synthesis rate by further reducing degradation.

Protein metabolism in the adult. In the adult the situation is different since the main objective of any adaptive change in undernutrition would be conservation, rather than growth of body protein. Without the need for an excess of protein synthesis over degradation, it is more likely that the reduced T_3 can mediate the adaptation by reducing protein degradation. Indications that this happens are typified by the report of Koppeschaar *et al*[15] who showed in obese adults that the reduction in N loss and achievement of near balance over the first few weeks of a low-protein low-calorie diet was reversed when T_3 was administered and N excretion was doubled.

Whether such adaptations associated with reduced T_3 would enable N-balance to be achieved at low intakes is particularly relevant to the thesis[33] that protein requirements in adults are not fixed, but rather defined by values which are the upper and lower limits of a range of intakes which allow balance to be achieved.

In the adult there are continuous diurnal changes in body protein reflecting the meal-eating pattern, so that overall N-balance is achieved by depositing sufficient protein after a meal to balance losses in the post-absorptive state. As recently reviewed[20], because the extent of protein deposition following a meal is a function of the protein intake it follows that if balance is to be achieved at low intakes then the losses in the post-absorptive phase must be reduced to balance the low rate of deposition during feeding. In other words (Fig. 2*a*) the amplitude of the diurnal cycling of body N must be low.

Is there any evidence that reduced T_3 can allow such an adaptation? The crucial change is the reduction in post-absorptive losses. This does occur as indicated above in the weight-reducing obese adult. Also, in sheep, the reduced T_3 level associated with reduced food intake is accompanied by reduced fasting N-loss[1]. A possible metchanism is shown in the scheme in Fig. 2*b*. This is an extension of the idea recently described[20]. It shows the predicted changes in whole body protein synthesis and degradation in the fed and fasted state which would allow N-balance to be achieved at different levels of intake and thyroid hormone status. The crucial points are that protein degradation increases with dietary intake and T_3 status, and the magnitude of the gains in the fed state and fasting losses increase with intake because of increasing diurnal swings in protein synthesis. There is a range of intakes over which losses balance gain but a lower limit determined by the fact that N losses do not fall to zero but to some minimum value and so the intake must allow this value of gain in the fed state. The upper limit is less important but is the intake at which the diurnal expansion of body protein is maximum.

For this to occur, what is needed is not only a fall in degradation with intake and T_3 status but also a reduction in the sensitivity of protein synthesis and degradation to fasting and feeding so that the diurnal swings in the two processes are minimised. As yet, the extent to which thyroid hormone does regulate the sensitivity of tissue protein synthesis and degradation to factors such as insulin, and the acute hormonal mediators of the response to food intake, is poorly understood, although it is known that reduced thyroid hormone status reduces the responsiveness of glucose metabolism in muscle and adipocytes to insulin[6].

The consequence of such changes, if the model is valid, is that reduced thyroid status would enable diurnal cycling of body N, which would result in decreased requirements for N balance and also have the added important consequence of allowing balance to be achieved on lower

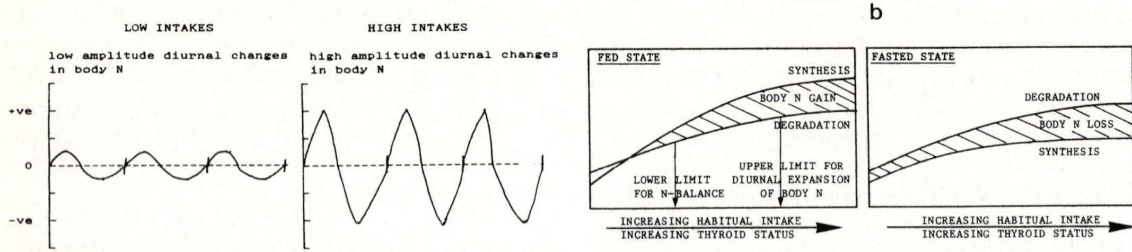

Fig. 2. *Mechanisms for the maintenance of nitrogen balance in the adult on low and high intakes. (a) Diurnal cycling of N-balance at low and high intakes.* Because there is net deposition after a meal and post-absorptive losses, body nitrogen content exhibits diurnal cycling. Furthermore since the magnitude of the deposition varies with the intake the amplitude of the cycling varies with intake, and balance on low intakes can only be achieved with low-amplitude cycling. *(b) Relationship between whole body protein synthesis and degradation in the fed and fasted state, habitual intake and thyroid status.* These are hypothetical curves (constructed from literature values[20]) showing the changes in protein synthesis and degradation necessary to mediate the cyclical changes in body protein — shown in (a) — and allow balance to be achieved over a range of intakes. Degradation increases with intake and thyroid status and there are increasingly large swings in protein synthesis with feeding and fasting. The lower limit for balance is the intake necessary to allow sufficient net synthesis to replace the fasting losses which cannot fall below a minimum value. It is argued that thyroid hormones play a key role by not only regulating protein degradation but also by controlling the sensitivity of protein synthesis to the acute regulatory influences of feeding.

quality dietary protein. This is because the requirement for essential amino acids would be much less if there was little net protein deposition after a meal[20].

1 Blum, J.W., Gingins, M., Vitins, P. & Bickel, H. (1980): Thyroid hormone levels related to energy and nitrogen balance during weight loss and regain in adult sheep. *Acta Endocrinol.* **93**, 440–447.

2 Brooke, O.G. & Cocks, T. (1974): Resting metabolic rate in malnourished babies in relation to total body potassium. *Acta Paediatr. Scand.* **63**, 817–825.

3 Coward, W.A. & Lunn, P.G. (1981): Biochemistry and physiology of kwashiorkor and marasmus. *Br. Med. Bull.* **37**, 19–24.

4 Cox, M.D., Dalal, S.S., Heard, C.R.C. & Millward, D.J. (1984): Metabolic rate and thyroid status in rats fed diets of different protein-energy values; importance of free T3. *J. Nutr.* **114**, 1609–1616.

5 Cox, M.D. & Millward, D.J. (1985): Thyroid status and metabolic rate in protein-deficient rats. *Br. J. Nutr.* **54**, 321.

6 Czech, M.P., Malbon, C.C., Kerman, K. & Gitomer, W. (1980): Effect of thyroid status on insulin action in rat adipocytes and skeletal muscle. *J. Clin. Invest.* **66**, 574–582.

7 Fomon, S.J., Filer, L.J., Ziegler, E.E., Bergmann, K.E. & Bergmann, R.L. (1977): Skim milk in infant feeding. *Acta Paediatr. Scand.* **66**, 17–30.

8 Garrel, D.R., Todd, K.S., Pugeat, M.M. & Calloway, D.H. (1984): Hormonal changes in normal men under marginally negative energy balance. *Am. J. Clin. Nutr.* **39**, 930–936.

9 Golden, M. (1985): The consequences of protein deficiency in man and its relationship to the features of kwashiorkor. In *Nutritional adaptation in man*, ed K. Blaxter & J.C. Waterlow, pp. 169–188. London: John Libbey.

10 Golden, M.H.N., Waterlow, J.C. & Picou, D. (1977): Protein turnover, synthesis and breakdown before and after recovery from malnutrition. *Clin. Sci. Mol. Biol.* **53**, 473–477.

11 Ingenbleek, Y. & Beckers, C. (1975): Triiodothyronine and thyroid-stimulating hormone in protein calorie malnutrition in infants. *Lancet* **2**, 845–846.

12 Isley, W.L., Underwood, L.E. & Clemmons, D.R. (1983): Dietary components that regulate serum somatomedin-c concentrations in humans. *J. Clin. Invest.* **71**, 175–182.

13 Jackson, A. (1985): Nutritional adaptation in disease and recovery. In *Nutritional adaptation in man*, ed K. Blaxter & J.C. Waterlow, pp. 111–126. London: John Libbey.

14 Keys, A., Brozek. J., Henschel, A. & Mickelsen, O. (1950): *The biology of human starvation*. Minneapolis Press: Minneapolis.

15 Koppeschaar, H.P.F., Meinders, A.E. & Schwarz, F. (1983): Metabolic responses in grossly obese subjects treated with a low calorie diet with and without T3 treatment. *Int. J. Obesity* **7**, 133–141.

16 Lampl, M., Johnston, F.E. & Malcolm, L.A. (1978): The effect of protein suplementation on the growth and skeletal maturation of New Guinea school children. *Ann. Hum. Biol.* **5**, 219–227.

17 Malcolm, L.A. (1970): Growth retardation in a New Guinea boarding school and its response to supplementary feeding. *Br. J. Nutr.* **24**, 297–305.

18 McIntosh, N., Shaw, J.C.L. & Taghizadeh, A. (1977): Accumulation of nitrogen and collagen in the femur of the human fetus and the effects of premature birth. *Ped. Res.* **11**, 1023–1025.

19 Millward, D.J. (1985): The effect of dietary energy and protein on growth as studied in animal models. In *Energy and protein needs of infancy* ed S.J. Foman & W. Heird. London: Academic Press.

20 Millward, D.J. (1985): Human protein requirements: the physiological significance of changes in the rate of whole body protein turnover. In *Energy and substrate metabolism in man*, ed J.S. Garrow & D. Halliday, pp. 135–144. London: John Libbey.

21 Millward, D.J. (1985): Physiological regulation of proteolysis in muscle. *Biochem. Soc. Trans.* **13**. (In press)

22 Millward, D.J., Bates, P.C., De Benoist, B., Brown, J.G., Cox, M.C., Halliday, D., Odedra, N. & Rennie, M.J. (1983): Protein Turnover: the nature of the phenomenon and its physiological regulation. In *Protein metabolism and nutrition*. Les Colloques de l'INRA 16, EAPP Publ. **31**, 69–96.

23 Millward, D.J., Odedra, B. & Bates, P.C. (1983): Role of insulin, corticosterone and other factors in the acute recovery of muscle protein synthesis on refeeding food-deprived rats. *Biochem. J.* **216**, 583–587.

24 Millward, D.J., Bates, P.C., Brown, J.G., Cox, M.C., Giugliano, R., Jepson, M. & Pell, J. (1985): Role of thyroid, insulin and corticosteroid hormones in the physiological regulation of proteolysis in muscle. In *Intracellular protein catabolism*. Prog. Clin. Biol. Res. **180**, 531–542. New York: Alan R. Liss.

25 Onuora, C., Ajitsingh, G.M. & Etta, K.M. (1983): Thyroid status in various degrees of protein calorie malnutrition in children. *Clin. Endocrinol.* **19**, 87–93.

26 Patrick, J. & Golden, M.H.N. (1977): Leucocyte electrolytes and sodium transport in protein energy malnutrition. *Am. J. Clin. Nutr.* **30**, 1478–1481.

27 Payne-Robinson, H.M., Betton, H. & Jackson, A.A. (1984): Free and total T3 and T4 in malnourished Jamaican infants. *Biochem. Soc. Trans.* **12**, 511–512.

28 Perdue, J.F. (1984): Chemistry, structure, and function of the insulin-like growth factors and their receptors: a review. *Can. J. Biochem. Cell. Biol.* **62**, 1237–1245.

29 Phillips, L.S. & Vassilopoulou-Sellin, R. (1980): Somatomedins. *New Engl. J. Med.* **302**, 371–380; 438–446.

30 Preece, L.S., Cameron, N., Donmall, M.C., Dunger, D.B., Holder, A.T., Preece, J-B., Seth, J., Sharp, G. & Taylor, A.M. (1984): *The endocrinology of male puberty*. In *Human growth & development* ed J. Borms *et al.*, pp. 23–38. London: Plenum Press.

31 Prewett, T.E.A., D'Ercole, A.J., Switzer, B.R. & Van Wyk, J.J. (1982): Relationship of serum immunoreactive somatomedin—c to dietary protein and energy in growing rats. *J. Nutr.* **112**, 144–150.

32 Rastogi, G.K., Sawnhey, R.C., Panda, N.C. & Tripathy, B.B. (1974): Thyroid hormone levels in adult protein calorie malnutrition (PCM). *Horm. Metab. Res.* **6**, 528–529.

33 Sukhatme, P.V. & Margen, S. (1978): Models for protein deficiency. *Am. J. Clin. Nutr.* **31**, 1237–1248.

34 Smith, I.F., Latham, M.C., Azubuike, J.A., Butler, W.R., Phillips, L.S., Pond, W.G. & Enwonwu, C.O. (1981): Blood levels of cortisol, insulin, growth hormone and somatomedin in children with marasmus, kwashiorkor, and intermediate forms of protein energy malnutrition. *Proc. Soc. Exp. Biol. Med.* **167**, 607–611.

35 Whitehead, R.G. & Alleyne, G.A.O. (1972): Pathophysiological features of importance in protein calorie malnutrition. *Br. Med. Bull.* **28**, 72–78.

36 Young, V.R. (1985): Mechanisms of adaptation to protein malnutrition. In *Nutritional adaptation in man*, ed K. Blaxter & J.C. Waterlow, pp. 189–218. London: John Libbey.

$\star\quad\star\quad\star$

NUTRIENT SUPPLY AND RESPONSE

Absorbed nutrients and gastro-entero-pancreatic hormonal production in relation to the composition of the food

A.A. RERAT
Laboratoire de Physiologie de la Nutrition, INRA — CNRZ, 78350 Jouy-en-Josas, France.

During the last 10 years two opposite concepts have been used to study intestinal transport and absorption of nutrients. First, the disappearance of nutrients from the intestine has been measured by a quantitative *in vivo*[9], or a non-quantitative *in vitro*[36], method of analysis to describe their hydrolysis and transport and to explain the mechanisms involved. Secondly, post-prandial appearance of nutrients in the body fluids (blood or lymph) have been measured by draining the digestive tract by a systematic quantitative analysis in the pig based on a simultaneous measurement of the porto-arterial differences in the concentration of nutrients and of the portal blood flow rate[35]. This method has two advantages as it permits accurate description of the absorption steps and demonstration of how nutrients are modified in the digestive lumen as affected by the microflora and in the gut wall due to the metabolism of the cells, but it requires long observation periods (18 h) for the establishment of full balances. This method may contribute to understanding the factors responsible for the metabolism of nutrients and to the establishment of whether the synchronized supply of nutrients to the tissues, whether they be amino acids[6] or energy and protein[11], is really necessary for protein synthesis. Because of lack of space, I will concentrate here on the absorption of carbohydrates and protein end-products measured by the latter method and the production of gastro-entero-pancreatic regulatory peptides, with the pig as an experimental animal.

Absorption kinetics and balance of carbohydrates of various dietary origins. *Influence of the nature and quantity of carbohydrates with a constant load of proteins.* In 3-month-old animals with an adult enzyme capacity, fed with carbohydrate containing meals[33,34] and a constant load of protein (about 100 g per meal), the amounts of reducing sugars appearing in the portal vein were variable according to the sugar ingested and, except for lactose, increased simultaneously with the level of ingestion. For example, after intake of 800 g, the amounts of reducing sugars absorbed were the greatest when glucose and sucrose were fed and exceeded those recorded with maize starch and, even more, with lactose. With the smallest levels of intake, digestion was nearly finished within 8 h after the meal as the porto-arterial differences almost returned to zero. According to the absorption balance, utilisation of glucose by the gut cell-wall ranged from 14 to 21 g/h[34].

How can these differences between carbohydrates be explained? In the case of lactose, the rather low absorption coefficient was almost reduced by half when the level of intake doubled: accordingly, there is a limiting factor in non-conditioned animals, probably involving the hydrolysis of lactose. This was well shown on the contrary when lactose was hydrolysed prior to its ingestion, the absorption rate thus achieved being more than two-fold higher[32]. In the case of starch, the digestion rate seemed to be limited more by the speed of degradation and absorption, than by gastric emptying which was quick enough to induce a large accumulation of starch in the proximal intestine during the first hours after the meal[4].

Influence of the load of protein[22]. When pigs received the same amount (800 g) of starch-based diets with increasing fish protein levels, the absorption rate of reducing sugars 8 h after the meal decreased with increasing dietary protein level (86.5, 72.0 and 56.2 per cent for 0, 14 and 28 per cent protein respectively), much more than what could be expected by the rather constant uptake by the cell wall. Thus, the addition of protein to protein-free diets might cause either a slowing down of gastric emptying — but this does not seem to be the case[28] — or a slowing down of the absorption probably depending on a competition between glucose and amino acids[12].

Nature of the hydrolysis products appearing in the blood circulation. With respect to fed-sucrose and lactose, the proportion of glucose in the reducing sugars absorbed was greater than that which might be expected (50 per cent) from their chemical composition[33]. Thus, the absorption of the fructose or galactose moieties of these carbohydrates was slower than that of glucose, or a fraction of them was transformed into glucose during digestion and absorption. The latter hypothesis was confirmed for galactose by the fact that within 5 h after the meal the amount of absorbed glucose exceeded that ingested when hydrolysed lactose was used[32].

Absorption of organic acids. The microbial degradation of complex carbohydrates or more simple ones in the gut lumen leads to formation of organic acids and carbonic acid as well as methane and

Table 1. *Production of volatile fatty acids (mmol ± s.e.m.) according to time elapsed after the meal in conscious pigs[25].*

| | Time after meal (h) | | | |
	0–8	8–16	16–24	0–24
Acetic acid	472.1 ± 103.9	469.1 ± 231.9	349.1 ± 97.4	1290.3 ± 341.8
Propionic acid	219.1 ± 37.0	250.0 ± 69.3	196.7 ± 40.7	665.8 ± 141.4
Butyric acid	73.0 ± 22.5	74.9 ± 21.6	64.5 ± 26.2	212.4 ± 46.8
Isovaleric acid	16.2 ± 2.8	14.1 ± 0.8	16.0 ± 0.5	46.3 ± 2.0
Valeric acid	9.3 ± 2.5	10.9 ± 0.9	9.4 ± 0.8	29.6 ± 3.7
Total	789.7 ± 153.2	819.0 ± 316.6	635.7 ± 151.6	2244.3 ± 526.2

hydrogen[16]. The transport of volatile fatty acids (VFA) through the mucosa of the pig caecum and colon is very efficient[1], as shown by the appearance of VFA in the efferent blood from the gut during digestion[3,5].

The amounts of VFA appearing in the portal vein of animals fed a diet containing 6 per cent crude fibre[25] (Table) represented about 600 gross kcal (2.5 MJ)/24 h and could vary with the meal frequency[24] and type of diet (Rérat *et al.*, unpublished). When passing the intestinal barrier the absorbed mixture was enriched with acetic acid at the expense of butyric acid[25]. Rather large amounts of VFA were retained during their passage through the mucosa[7,10].

The quantity of lactic acid appearing in the portal blood circulation during digestion of various carbohydrates[34] was rather large (2.5–3.5 g/h) and corresponded to 30–40 per cent of the difference between the amounts of sugars disappearing from the gut lumen and the amounts of reducing sugars appearing in the portal vein.

Absorption of protein hydrolysis products. During the last few years, exchanges of nitrogenous compounds between the portal blood and the gut have been quantified in the pig using meals containing proteins or mixtures of peptides or amino acids (AA).

Variations according to the nature of ingested proteins[15,18,26,31]. Comparison of the absorption of protein nutrients from two feeds of rather similar composition (barley and wheat) and a different one (fish meal) showed that the chronology of digestion of these three feedstuffs was different. The greatest digestion rate was obtained with wheat proteins and seemed to be almost as fast as that with fish protein in a semi-synthetic diet. The digestion rate of wheat carbohydrates was definitely less than that of wheat protein, but this was not the case for barley. This possibility of a differential digestion of proteins and carbohydrates may have important nutritional consequences especially for the improvement of nitrogen retention by manipulation of the energy.

After a large increase in the blood concentration of nutrients in the first hours after the meal and before the following meal, the portal blood levels reached again the systemic blood levels[17], indicating that exogenous nutrients were no longer supplied to the portal blood. The overall absorption balance could then be established. Digestion of wheat proteins was sooner and lasted a little less long (15 h) than that of barley proteins (17 h). Digestion of wheat (22 h) and barley (20 h) carbohydrates lasted longer than that of their proteins. The large difference between the amounts disappearing from the digestive tract (about 89 per cent for wheat, and 80 per cent for barley[8]) and the amounts appearing in the portal blood (70 and 60 per cent, respectively) could only be explained by the appearance of dietary components in a different chemical form resulting from their metabolism by the microflora of the large intestine or by the intestinal cell wall. The activity of this tissue corresponded to a large uptake of dietary components as shown by its very high turnover rate[2].

With the experimental level of intake of these three proteins (wheat, barley, fish) the pattern of the mixture of essential amino acids (EAA) absorbed within 8 h closely depended on the profile of the EAA ingested without fully resembling it. Thus, whatever the protein ingested, the overall absorption rate of branched EAA and threonine was similar to that of the mixture; the absorption rate of histidine and aromatic AA was much faster; contrary to that, the total cumulative absorption of lysine, sulphur AA and especially arginine was slower. In this example, it seemed that the chronology of degradation of proteins and absorption of their EAA was the same whatever their intake pattern.

In the mixture of non-essential amino acids (NEAA) absorbed within 8 h, a large excess of alanine and glycine and marked deficiencies of aspartic and glutamic acid were observed. This corresponded with transaminations in the gastro-intestinal cell wall[13,14]. Furthermore, fairly high amounts of ornithine (1.8–2.3 g/8 h) and citrulline (0.8–1.1 g/8 h) appeared in the portal blood[31].

Variations according to molecular weight. Solutions containing peptides of low molecular weight introduced into the duodenum[24] led to an early occurrence of much larger amounts of amino acids in the portal vein than solutions containing only free amino acids in the same proportions as those of the hydrolysate. During the short post-prandial period of observation (5 h) the amounts appearing exceeded those introduced into the duodenum except when large amounts of amino acids were used. This emphasizes the importance of endogenous nitrogen turnover during enteral nutrition based on such components.

Endogenous nitrogen recycling. The endogenous contribution to the supply of AA in the portal vein was measured by means of protein-free diets offered in the middle of sequences of meals with a normal protein level[23,30]. The amounts absorbed corresponded to about 2 g mixture per hour. For some essential AA such as lysine, the quantities absorbed during a post-prandial period of 7 h could represent 1/4 or 1/5 of that which was absorbed from cereal proteins after feeding of a normal meal.

Furthermore, the intestinal efferent blood was more ammonia-rich during digestion than the systemic blood[19]. Thus, absorption of this substance was generally steady (15–19 mmol/h) and tended to increase with time after the meal, which would support a proposal that deamination of the ileal dietary residues occurred. This ammonia may also be derived from urea secreted into the gut (9–13 mmol/h), but the total amount of absorbed ammonia nitrogen corresponded only to a maximum of 80 per cent of the urea nitrogen taken up[20,31]; on the other hand, 20 per cent at least of the urea secreted into the digestive tract under the usual feeding conditions seemed to be used for synthesis of microbial proteins.

In conclusion, digestion is a more or less rapid process depending on dietary proteins. Furthermore, together with other phenomena such as the competition of simple compounds (saccharoses, amino acids) for sites of transport and addition of endogenous substances, metabolism by the microflora and the intestinal cell wall may affect the amount of nutrients appearing in the portal vein and contribute to changes in the composition of nutrient mixtures absorbed.

Production of gastro- entero-pancreatic regulatory peptides in relation to the composition of the diet. When pigs were fed the same amount (800 g) of a semi-synthetic diet with different levels of fish meal proteins 0, 14 and 28 per cent), variations in the quantities and composition of absorbed nutrients caused large variations in the kinetics of secretion of some regulatory peptides[21,22]. Each regulatory peptide behaved differently according to the composition of the diet. *Insulin*: the amount released during the total post-prandial period (1080 μg/8 h) after the 14 per cent protein meal was significantly higher than that released after the protein-free diet (691 μg/8 h). This was also the case for the amount released during the 3rd hour. Most insulin was released soon after meal ingestion, as evidenced by the fact that 40–47 per cent of the total 8 h insulin release was completed within 2 h. *Glucagon*: although the total amount released increased from 48.5 to 93.6 μg/h when the protein content increased from 0 to 28 per cent, the differences between the 8 h responses were not significant. The amount released in the 2nd hour after the 28 per cent protein meal was significantly higher than that following the protein-free diet. *Gastrin*: the total 8 h release was 2.2 times higher after the 28 per cent protein than after the protein-free meal. About 30 per cent of the release occurred within 2 h. From 2 to 8 h, the response to the 28 per cent protein meal (2.1–2.9 μg/h) was consistently greater than the responses to the 14 per cent (1.0–2.1 μg/h) or the protein-free meal (0.8–1.4 μg/h). *Somatostatin*: the 28 per cent protein diet gave the greatest response both in terms of hourly production (7–11 μg/h) and total release. However, large inter-individual variations made the differences between meals non significant.

Interrelationships between hourly amounts of nutrients and regulatory peptides appearing in the portal blood. There were very close relationships between the hourly α-aminonitrogen absorption and glucagon (r = 0.72, n = 24) and gastrin (r = 0.78, n = 24) secretion in the same time interval. The hourly pancreatic polypeptide production was closely correlated with insulin production (r = 0.80, n = 24).

Conclusions. Quantitative nutrient absorption kinetics, and production of regulatory gastro-entero-pancreatic peptides, may be described by means of a technique based on differences in the porto-arterial concentration combined with the portal blood flow rate. The following results were obtained. (1) Digestion of carbohydrates and appearance of their degradation products in the body are more or less rapid according to the nature of these sugars. Digestion of lactose is particularly long whereas absorption of glucose and digestion of sucrose are rather quick. The length of time of starch digestion is intermediate. Hydrolysed lactose components are absorbed much more rapidly than non-hydrolysed lactose. (2) Digestion of various proteins (such as wheat, barley and fish meal) does not take place at the same rate, barley amino acids being available for the body later than wheat amino acids. (3) Mixtures of nutrients are liable to be modified during digestion and cell transport because of the differential hydrolysis, as well as the competition for absorption and metabolism by the intestinal cell wall. Some essential amino acids are absorbed more rapidly (aromatic AA), others more slowly (sulphur AA, arginine). Glutamic acid nitrogen is transaminated to alanine. A rather large fraction of fructose and galactose is transformed into glucose. (4) During digestion, volatile fatty acids supplying a rather large amount of energy (about 600 kcal [2.5 MJ]/24 h) and lactic acid (2.5 to 3.5 g/h) appear in the body. (5) There is a close relationship between the quantities of α-amino nitrogen absorbed and the secretion of glucagon and gastrin as well as between the secretion of insulin and pancreatic polypeptide.

1 Argenzio, R.A. & Southworth, M. (1975): Sites of organic acid production and absorption in gastrointestinal tract of the pig. *Am. J. Physiol.* **228**, 454–460.

2 Arnal, M., Obled, C. & Attaix, D. (1983): Renouvellement des protéines et flux d'acides aminés au cours du développement. IVème Symp. Int. Métabolisme et Nutrition Azotés, Clermont-Ferrand (France) 5–9 Sept. 1983. In *Les Colloques de l'INRA, No. 16*, **I**, pp. 117–136. Paris: INRA.

3 Barcroft, J.R., McAnally, R.A. & Phillipson, A.T. (1944): Absorption of volatile acids from the alimentary tract of the sheep and other animals. *J. Exp. Biol.* **20**, 120–129.

4 Cuber, J.C. & Laplace, J.P. (1979): Evacuation gastrique de la matière sèche d'un régime semi-purifié à base d'amidon de maïs chez le porc. *Annls Biol. Anim. Biochim. Biophys.* **19**, 899–905.

5 Friend, D.W., Nicholson, J.W.G. & Cunningham, H.M. (1964): Volatile fatty acid and lactic acid content of pig blood. *Can. J. Anim. Sci.* **44**, 303–308.

6 Geiger, E. (1950): The role of time factor in protein synthesis. *Science* **111**, 594–599.

7 Imoto, S. & Namioka, S. (1978): VFA production in the pig large intestine. *J. Anim. Sci.* **47**, 467–478.

8 Keys, J.E. & De Barthe, J.V. (1974): Site and extent of carbohydrate, dry matter, energy and protein digestion and the rate of passage of grain diets in swine. *J. Anim. Sci.* **39**, 57–62.

9 Laplace, J.P., Darcy-Vrillon, B. & Picard, M. (1985): Evaluation de la disponibilité des acides aminés: choix raisonné d'une méthode. *J. Rech. Porcine en France* **17**, 353–370.

10 Ly, J. (1974): Caecal function in the pig: VFA content and utilization by the caecal wall. *Cuban J. Agric. Sci.* **8**, 247–254.

11 Munro, H.N. (1949): The relationship of carbohydrate metabolism to protein metabolism. III. Further observations of time of carbohydrate ingestion as a factor in protein utilization by the adult rat. *J. Nutr.* **39**, 375–391.

12 Murer, H., Sigrist Nelson, K. & Hopler, U. (1975): On the mechanism of sugar and aminoacid interaction in intestinal transport. *J. Biol. Chem.* **250**, 7392–7396.

13 Neame, K.D. & Wiseman, G. (1958): The alanine and oxo acid concentration in mesenteric blood during the absorption of L-glutamic acid by the small intestine of the dog, cat and rabbit in vivo. *J. Physiol. London* **140**, 148–155.

14 Pion, R., Fauconneau, G. & Rérat, A. (1963): Etude cinétique de la composition en acides aminés du sang porte chez le porc. *Annls Biol. Anim. Biochem. Biophys.* **3**, 31–37.

15 Rérat, A. (1977): Mesure quantitative *in vivo* de l'absorption chez le porc. Application aux sucres et aux acides aminés. In *1er Coll. sur la réanimation entérale à faible débit continue*, pp. 47–62. Paris: Inserm.

16 Rérat, A. (1978): Digestion and absorption of carbohydrates and nitrogenous matters in the hindgut of the omnivorous non-ruminant animal. *J. Anim. Sci.* **46**, 1808–1837.

17 Rérat, A. (1981): Chronologie et bilans de l'absorption des sucres réducteurs et de l'azote α-aminé chez le porc selon la nature des aliments. *Bull. Acad. Nat. Med.* **165**, 1131–1137.

18 Rérat, A. (1982): Absorption des sucres et des acides aminés chez le porc. In *Digestive physiology in the pig.* ed J.P. Laplace, T. Corring & A Rérat, pp. 63–87. Paris: INRA.

19 Rérat, A. & Aumaitre, A.A. (1971): Absorption de l'azote uréique et ammoniacal chez le porc. Résultats préliminaires. *Annls Bioch. Anim. Biophys.* **11**, 348–350.

20 Rérat, A & Buraczewska, L. (1985): Postprandial quantitative kinetics of urea and ammonia nitrogen exchanges between the digestive tract and the portal blood in conscious pigs receiving a diet with or without urea. *Arch. Tierernähr.* (In press)

21 Rérat, A., Chayvialle, A., Kandé, J., Vaissade, P. & Vaugelade, P. (1984): Cinétique de la production de quelques hormones de l'aire splanchnique (insuline, glucagon, gastrine, somatostatine) après ingestion de rapas à taux variables de protéines chez le porc éveillé. *Reprod. Nutr. Dévelop.* **24**, 773.

22 Rérat, A., Chayvialle, J.A., Kandé, J., Vaissade, P., Vaugelade, P. & Bourrier, Ph. (1985): Metabolic and hormonal effects of test meals with various protein contents in pigs. *Cand. J. Physiol. Pharmacol.* (In press).

23 Rérat, A., Corring, T. & Laplace, J.P. (1976): Protein digestion and absorption. In *Protein metabolism and nutrition*, EAAP publ. No. 16, ed D.J.A. Cole, K.N. Boorman, P.J. Buttery, D. Lewis, R.J. Neale & M. Swan. pp. 97–138. London: Butterworth.

24 Rérat, A., Fiszlewicz, M., Giusi, A. & Vaugelade, P. (1985): Variations postprandiales de la production et de

l'absorption des acides gras volatils dans le tube digestif du porc éveillé selon la fréquence des repas antérieurs. *36th Annual Meeting. EAAP*. Kallithea-Kassandra-Ilalkidiki, Grece, 30 Sept.–3 Oct. (In press).

25 Rérat, A., Fiszlewicz, M., Herpin, P., Vaugelade, P. & Durand, M. (1985): Mesure de l'apparition dans la veine porte des acides gras volatils formés au cours de la digestion chez le porc éveillé. *C.R. Acad. Sci. Paris* **300**, série III, 467–470.

26 Rérat, A., Kandé, J., Jung, J., Vaissade, P. & Vaugelade, P. (1980): Absorption of aminoacids of different dietary origin in the pig. *3rd EAAP Symposium on protein metabolism and nutrition*, Braunschweig, May 1980, (E.A.A. publ. 27) **1**, 243–251.

27 Rérat, A., Lisoprawski, C., Vaissade, P. & Vaugelade, P. (1979): Métabolisme de l'urée dans le tube digestif du porc; données préliminaires qualitatives et quantitatives. *Bull. Acad. Vét. Fr.* **52**, 333–346.

28 Rérat, A. & Lougnon, J. (1963): Etude sur le transit digestif chez le porc. *Annls Biol. Anim. Biochim. Biophys.* **3**, 21–30.

29 Rérat, A., Simoes-Nunés, C., Lacroix, M., Vaugelade, P. & Vaissade, P. (1985): Cinétique comparée d'apparition dans la veine porte de l'azote α-aminé provenant de mélanges de petits peptides ou d'acides aminés libres de même composition introduits dans le duodénum chez le porc éveillé. *C.R. Acad. Sci. Paris.* **300**, série III, 293–296.

30 Rérat, A., Vaissade, P., Vaugelade, P., Robin, D., Robin, P. & Jung, J. (1977): Determination of nature and quantity of endogenous nitrogen absorbed during the digestion a protein-free meal in the pig. *Vth Int. Symp. on Amino Acids*, D₃, Budapest, pp. 1–8.

31 Rérat, A., Vaissade, P. & Vaugelade, P. (1979): Absorption kinetics of amino acids and reducing sugars during digestion of barley or wheat in pig: preliminary data. *Annls Biol. Anim. Biochim. Biophys.* **19**, 739–747.

32 Rérat, A., Vaissade, P. & Vaugelade, P. (1983): Cinétique d'absorption du glucose et du galactose après ingestion de lactose ou de lactose hydrolysé chez le porc. *Bull. Acad. Nat. Med.* **167**, 297–303.

33 Rérat, A.A., Vaissade, P. & Vaugelade, P. (1984): Absorption kinetics of some carbohydrates in conscious pigs. 1. Qualitative aspects. *Br. J. Nutr.* **51**, 505–515.

34 Rérat, A.A., Vaissade, P. & Vaugelade, P. (1984): Absorption kinetics of some carbohydrates in conscious pigs. 2. Quantitative aspects. *Br. J. Nutr.* **51**, 517–529.

35 Rérat, A., Vaugelade, P. & Villiers, P.A. (1980): A new method for measuring the absorption of nutrients in the pig: critical examination In *Current concepts of digestion and absorption in pigs*, ed A.G. Low & I.G. Partridge, pp. 177–216. Reading, England: NIRD.

36 Smith, M.W. (1980): In vitro measurements of intestinal function. In *Current concepts of digestion and absorption in pigs*, ed A.G. Low & I.G. Partridge, pp. 157–172. Reading, England: NIRD.

Gut hormones and the disposition of food

V. MARKS
Division of Clinical Biochemistry, Department of Biochemistry, University of Surrey, Guildford, Surrey, UK.

Sixty years were to elapse after the first use of the term 'hormone' before the gut itself was widely appreciated to be, not only the largest endocrine gland in the body, but also the source of the greatest number and variety of different hormones, many of which have only been discovered in the past 10 years or so[2].

One of the main reasons for the re-awakened interest in the gut as an endocrine organ was a number of contemporaneous discoveries, amongst which that of the role of humoral factors released from the gut in response to the ingestion of glucose in the secretion of insulin[16], was amongst the most important. From this study it became apparent that nutrients were not only concerned with the regulation of gut function itself, but also with the disposition, within the body, of the absorbed nutrients themselves.

Improvements in peptide hormone isolation, purification and characterisation, coupled with the discovery of how to measure them by immunoassay at the very low concentrations at which they occur in blood[35] led to an explosive growth of interest in the gut as an endocrine organ. In spite of this, precise knowledge of the physiological role of the by now more than 20 gastrointestinal hormones that have been isolated and characterised and even synthesized is still remarkably meagre[2,17].

Gastrointestinal hormones. All of the 20 or so gastrointestinal hormones — excluding serotonin, but including those of the pancreatic islets — so far identified are polypeptides, varying in molecular size from roughly 1000–10 000 daltons. Many occur in more than one molecular form — both in the gut and in the blood — and are characterized by possession of a C—terminal amide group. This is so characteristic a feature of this group of compounds that it has been used as a method of isolating and identifying new and previously uncharacterized hormonally active compounds from gut extracts[30].

Sequence analysis of the various hormones has revealed analogies which have led to some of them being grouped together as 'families' with what is thought to be a common phylogenetic background. Nevertheless, small, to quite large, differences in molecular structure do occur in the 'same' hormone isolated from different species as a result of one or more amino acid deletions or substitutions. This seems often to have remarkably little effect upon their pharmacological and/or immunological properties but can sometimes cause subtle changes which, unless, recognised, can lead to grossly erroneous conclusions.

Each of the gastrointestinal hormones is associated with a unique and microscopically identifiable cell type and appears to have a normal pattern of distribution which may be distorted by, or in, disease.

Classification. One classification of the gastrointestinal hormones based on current beliefs about their functional significances is into (a) those predominantly concerned with regulation of gastrointestinal function itself and (b) those with a predominantly or exclusively metabolic role. Amongst hormones in the latter category whose production is confined to the intestinal tract and not to have 'migrated' during evolution into the pancreatic islets, GIP is both the best known and the best studied. The acronym GIP was originally used to describe its mode of discovery as a gastric (acid) inhibitory polypeptide but GIP is now considered more appropriately to stand for glucose (dependent) insulinotropic hormone or probably, best of all, for nothing in particular and to be merely the name of a hormone whose importance, in health and disease, can still only be surmized from clinical and experimental observations in man and animals[3]. It is mainly with GIP, as probably the most important — though almost certainly not the sole representative — of the group of hormones whose production and secretion is influenced by the constituents and nature of the diet, and which themselves are concerned with disposition of those constituents within the body[17,19] that the rest of this paper will deal.

Entero-insular axis. The term 'Entero-insular axis' was used[33] to embrace all of those gut factors which contribute to the enhanced secretion of insulin following ingestion of foods over and above that which could be accounted for by the increase in nutrient concentration in the arterial blood perfusing the endocrine pancreas[16]. GIP has emerged as the main contender for the role of mediator of intestinal augmentation of insulin release.

GIP. The hormone occurs in blood in two major molecular forms; one, GIP 5000, is well characterized and has been sequenced and synthesized; the other, GIP 8000, is still largely uninvestigated and is recognised mainly by virtue of its ability to cross-react with many, but not all, GIP—specific antisera[14]. GIP 5000 — hereafter referred to simply as GIP — is a linear polypeptide of 42 amino acids and the human form — which has been sequenced and synthesized — differs by only two amino acids from the porcine variety[21]. Earlier descriptions of GIP as a 43 amino acid polypeptide led to futile synthesis of biologically relatively inert compounds and confusion in the literature. The small but importance differences between human and porcine GIP are reflected in their behaviour towards certain GIP antisera used for the measurement of GIP in plasma and tissues and this too has caused confusion[13].

GIP is produced by the K-cells of the intestinal mucosa which are found mostly in the duodenum and jejunum but also, in smaller numbers, in the ileum, especially in genetic obesity[9,25].

GIP was isolated by Brown and co-workers from the side fractions of what had hitherto been the purest preparations of cholecystokinin/pancreozymin (CCK/PZ) available in the quest for enterogastrone, the hypothetical inhibitor of gastric acid secretion. As purification of the CCK/PZ proceeded and it became more potent as a stimulant of pancreatic exocrine function its effectiveness in blocking gastric acid secretion diminished. The side fraction on the other hand increased in gastric inhibitory activity and led to the isolation of a hitherto unrecognised hormone, namely GIP. Following demonstration of its insulin-stimulatory properties[6,31] GIP was rapidly installed as a likely candidate for the role of the intestinal mediator of the augmented insulin secretory response observed when glucose was taken orally instead of administered intravenously.

The first contender for this role was the hormone secretin[16], but, although it does possess insulin-stimulatory properties, other considerations made its continued candidacy, at least as a major factor, improbable. The same applies to CCK/PZ, gastrin and the glucagon cross-reacting materials[26] which are present in the gut and released in response to appropriate stimulation.

An insulin-releasing polypeptide extracted from porcine intestinal mucosa[31] was later proved (unpublished observations) to be contaminated with GIP which the same group[32] confirmed was an extremely potent insulin secretagogue — but only in the presence of mild to moderate hyperglycaemia[1,6].

Pharmacological actions. It is controversial whether the ability of GIP to stimulate insulin release represents a genuine physiological function of GIP or merely a pharmacological action[27]. The bulk of evidence supports the concept of a physiological role since much of the contra-evidence[27] was based on misconceptions of identity between human and porcine GIP[13]. Even so, the most ardent supporters of a physiological role for GIP as mediator of alimentary augmentation of insulin secretion concede that it is unlikely to be the only factor involved. Indeed it is now recognised that there is participation by the autonomic nervous system — with afferent impulses arising from glucoreceptors in the intestinal mucosa[20] — as well as by other, as yet poorly identified, hormones. Amongst the latter, consideration must be given to peptide histidine-isoleucine (PHI) and at least some of the glucagon-like immunoreactants found in the gut and which are released in a specific and well-defined pattern in response to nutrient ingestion.

Other ways — in addition to its direct action through modulation of insulin secretion — by which GIP can participate in the disposition of absorbed nutrients is by a direct effect upon disposal of chylomicrons by activation of lipoprotein lipase in adipocytes thereby promoting clearance from the plasma[8,34]. GIP appears also to have an effect upon the interraction between insulin and glucagon upon isolated adipocytes and possibly hepatocytes *in vitro*[5].

Control of GIP secretion. GIP secretion is stimulated by the presence, in the small bowel, of fat, carbohydrate and protein in descending order of potency[3]. Under certain circumstances GIP may be released in response to the presence of acid in the duodenum — but the evidence is conflicting.

There was some question whether the type of GIP secreted in response to fat and carbohydrate in the gut might be different but this now seems unlikely[3,14]. Nevertheless the regulatory processes for secretion of GIP by the two kinds of nutrient appear to be different and independent of each other.

Only the actively absorbed sugars, glucose and galactose, and the complex carbohydrates giving rise to them in the course of digestion stimulate the release of GIP[29]. If for any reasons, such as lack of the appropriate pancreatic and/or mucosal enzymes, hydrolysis does not occur in the upper intestine, there is little or no GIP secretion even in response to a nutrient that normally produces it. Thus lactose, which is a potent stimulus to GIP secretion in normal adult Caucasians, does not stimulate GIP secretion in apparently healthy Africans and Asiatics with minimal lactose intolerance even though glucose does[18]. Similarly the normal stimulatory effect of sucrose is inhibited by the sucrase inhibitor acabose[10] and even that of glucose itself is blocked by phloridzin which interferes with active transport of glucose across cell membranes[29]. Further evidence that it is active transport rather than molecular configuration of the sugar that is involved in stimulation of GIP secretion comes from experiments in animals using sugar analogues[29].

Amongst the major human nutrient carbohydrates only fructose and the polyols xylitol and sorbitol are non-stimulatory to GIP secretion in the absence of disease causing digestive or absorptive disturbances. The pathophysiological relevance of this fact is unknown.

The role of fibre. The presence in the gut of some types of dietary fibre, of which guar is the best studied example, markedly impairs the stimulatory effect upon GIP secretion of carbohydrates and to a lesser extent of mixed meals[22]. It has no affect upon stimulation of GIP secretion by fat[24], suggesting that interference has more to do with the chemical than with the physical nature of the fibre. The latter is, however, also clearly important[4]. It might be supposed that delayed digestion of food in the upper intestinal tract — where the majority of K-cells occur — might lead to reduced total, but more prolonged, GIP release as digestion proceeds in the lower jejunum and ileum.

Stimulation of GIP secretion by fat is confined to fatty acids that are actively converted into chylomicrons in the intestinal mucosa[7]. Neither short nor medium-chain fatty acids or triglycerides stimulate GIP release,[7,15] nor do long-chain triglycerides until and unless they are hydrolysed by pancreatic lipases. Preliminary evidence suggests that unsaturated are more potent than saturated long-chain fatty acids in stimulating GIP release[15], but the degree of unsaturation seems not to be important. Fat, but not glucose, stimulated GIP secretion is reduced by insulin providing the basis for a negative feedback control system.

In species such as the rat, which normally consumes a low-fat diet, provocation of GIP secretion by fat loading is enhanced by prior high-fat feeding[12]. This does not appear to happen in human beings who do, however, show a significant reduction in the ability of exogenous and probably endogenous, insulin to inhibit fat-induced GIP secretion after a prolonged period of high-fat feeding[23]. This observation is consistent with reports that feedback control of GIP secretion by insulin is lost in obese subjects and suggests that ingestion of an habitually high-fat diet can interfere with the normal feedback control of GIP and possibly the whole of the entero-insular axis. This would, in turn, lead to hyperinsulinism and insulin resistance, with or without hyperglycaemia, and the possible production, or at least perpetuation, of obesity. There is indeed evidence that not only is the number and distribution of K-cells increased in the gut in human and animal obesity[9,25] but that excessive amounts of GIP, which are not inhibited by the exaggerated insulinaemia provoked

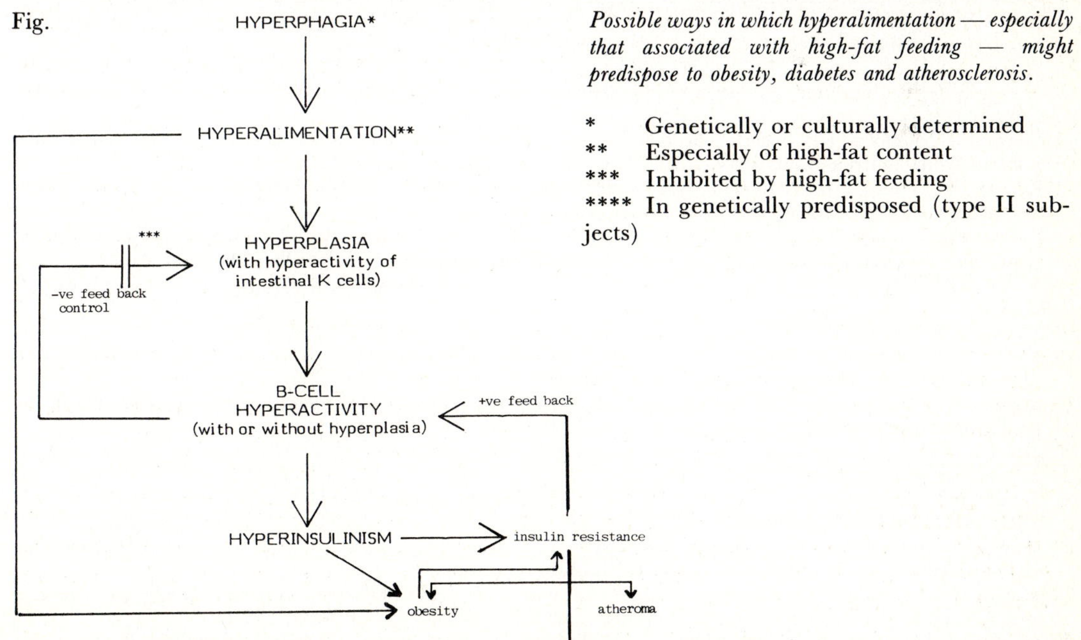

Fig.   *Possible ways in which hyperalimentation — especially that associated with high-fat feeding — might predispose to obesity, diabetes and atherosclerosis.*

*   Genetically or culturally determined
**   Especially of high-fat content
***   Inhibited by high-fat feeding
**** In genetically predisposed (type II subjects)

simultaneously, are released into the blood in response to stimulation by food. Since insulin[28] and hyperinsulinism — or at least insulin-resistance[11] is atherogenic the induction of hyperlipaemia or at least interference with its feedback control by high-fat feeding suggests a mechanism whereby high dietary-fat intake might predispose to development of atheroma without involving the cholesterol hypothesis.

The Figure summarizes our preliminary thoughts on the possible role of gut hormones, in particular GIP, in the pathogenesis of some types of obesity and atherosclerosis. Though based largely upon the genetically-obese animal model it is consistent with many observations on obese human subjects and healthy human volunteers undergoing short-term feeding experiments.

Clearly the gut should no longer be looked upon, as it has been for so long, as involved only in the digestion and absorption of nutrients from the food but also with their disposition within the body.

1 Andersen, D.K., Elahi, D., Brown, J.C., Tobin, J.D. & Andres, R. (1978): Oral glucose augmentation of insulin secretion: interactions of gastric inhibitory polypeptide with ambient glucose and insulin levels. *J. Clin. Invest.* 62, 152–168.

2 Bloom, S.R. & Polak, J.M. (editors) (1981): *Gut hormones*. Edinburgh: Churchill Livingstone.

3 Brown, J.C. (1982): *Gastric inhibitory polypeptide*. Berlin: Springer-Verlag.

4 Collier, G. & O'Dea, K. (1982): Effect of physical form of carbohydrate on the postprandial glucose, insulin, and gastric inhibitory polypeptide responses in type 2 diabetes. *Am. J. Clin. Nutr.* **36**, 10–14.

5 Dupre, J., Greenidge, N., McDonald, T.J., Ross, S.A. & Rubinstein, D. (1976): Inhibition of actions of glucagon in adipocytes by gastric inhibitory polypeptide. *Metabolism* **25**, 1197–1199.

6 Dupre, J., Ross, S.A., Watson, D. & Brown, J.C. (1973): Stimulation of insulin secretion by gastric inhibitory polypeptide in man. *J. Clin. Endocrinol. Metab.* **37**, 826–828.

7 Ebert, R. & Creutzfeldt, W. (1985): Fat-induced secretion of gastric inhibitory polypeptide is coupled to chylomicron formation. *Acta Endocrinol.* **108**, 42.

8 Eckel, R.H., Fujimoto, W.Y. & Brunzell, J.D. (1979): Gastric inhibitory polypeptide enhanced lipoprotein lipase activity in cultured preadipocytes. *Diabetes* **28**, 1141–1142.

9 Flatt, P.R., Bailey, C.J., Kwasowski, P., Page, T. & Marks, V. (1984): Plasma immunoreactive gastric inhibitory polypeptide in obese hyperglycaemia (ob/ob) mice. *J. Endocr.* **104**, 249–256.

10 Folsch, U.R., Ebert, R. & Creutzfeldt, W. (1981): Response of serum levels of gastric inhibitory polypeptide and insulin to sucrose ingestion during long-term application of acarbose. *Scand. J. Gastroenterol.* **16**, 629–632.

11 Garcia-Webb, P., Bonser, A.M., Whiting, D. & Masarei, J.R.L. (1983): Insulin resistance — a risk factor for coronary heart disease? *Scand. J. Clin. Lab. Invest.* **43**, 677–685.

12 Hampton, S.M., Kwasowski, P., Tan, K., Morgan, L.M. & Marks, V. (1983): Effect of pretreatment with a high fat diet on the gastric inhibitory polypeptide and insulin responses to oral triolein and glucose in rats. *Diabetologia* **24**, 278–281.

13 Krarup, T. & Holst, J.J. (1984): The heterogeneity of gastric inhibitory polypeptide in porcine and human gastrointestinal mucosa evaluated with 5 different antisera. *Regulatory Peptides* **9**, 35–46.

14 Krarup, T., Holst, J.J. & Larsen, K.L. (1985): Responses and molecular heterogeneity of IR-GIP after intraduodenal glucose and fat. *Regulatory Peptides* (In press)

15 Kwasowski, P., Flatt, P.R., Bailey, C.J. & Marks, V. (1985): Effects of fatty acid chain length and saturation on gastri-inhibitory polypeptide release in obese hyperglycaemia (ob/ob) mice. *Biosci. Rep.* (In press)

16 McIntyre, N., Holdsworth, C.D. & Turner, D.S. (1964): New interpretation of oral glucose tolerance. *Lancet* **2**, 20–21.

17 Marks, V. & Morgan, L. (1982): Gastrointestinal hormones. *Molec. Aspects Med.* **5**, 225–292.

18 Marks, V. & Morgan, L. (1984): The entero-insular axis. In *Recent advances in diabetes*, ed M. Nattrass & J.V. Santiago, pp. 55–71. Edinburgh: Churchill Livingstone.

19 Marks, V. & Turner, D. (1977): The gastrointestinal hormones with particular reference to their role in the regulation of insulin secretion. *Essays Med. Biochem.* **3**, 109–152.

20 Mei, N., Arlhac, A. & Boyer, A. (1981): Nervous regulation of insulin release by the intestinal vagal glucoreceptors. *J. Auton. Ner. Syst.* **4**, 351–363.

21 Moody, A.J., Thim, L. & Valverde, I. (1984): The isolation and sequencing of human gastric inhibitory peptide (GIP). *FEBS Letters* **172**, 142–148.

22 Morgan, L.M., Goulder, T.J., Tsiolakis, D., Marks, V. & Alberti, K.G.M.M. (1979): The effect of unabsorbable carbohydrate on gut hormones. *Diabetologia* **17**, 85–89.

23 Morgan, L.M., Tredger, J.A., Hampton, S.M. & Kwasowski, P. (1983): Effect of diet upon response to oral fat and glucose in man; modification in control of the enteroinsular axis. *Scand. J. Gastroenterol.* **18**, 99–101.

24 Morgan, L.M., Tredger, J.A., Madden, A., Kwasowski, P. & Marks, V. (1985): The effect of guar gum on carbohydrate-, fat- and protein-stimulated gut hormone secretion: modification of postprandial gastric inhibitory polypeptide and gastrin responses. *Br. J. Nut.* **53**, 467–475.

25 Polak, J.M., Pearse, A.G.E., Grimelius, L. & Marks, V. (1975): Gastrointestinal apudosis in obese hyperglycaemic mice. *Virchows Arch. B Cell Path.* **19**, 135–150.

26 Samols, E. & Marks, V. (1967): Nouvelles conceptions sur la signification functionelle du glucagon pancreatique et extra pancreatique. *J. Annu. Diabetol. Hotel Dieu* **7**, 43–56.

27 Sarson, D.L., Wood, S.M., Kansal, P.C. & Bloom, S.R. (1984): Glucose-dependent insulinotropic polypeptide augmentation of insulin: physiology or pharmacology? *Diabetes* **33**, 389–393.

28 Stout, R.W. (1981): The role of insulin in atherosclerosis in diabetics and non-diabetics. *Diabetes* **30**, Suppl. 2, 55–57.

29 Sykes, S., Morgan, L.M., English, J. & Marks, V. (1980): Evidence for preferential stimulation of gastric inhibitory polypeptide in the rat by actively transported carbohydrates and their analogues. *J. Endocr.* **85**, 201–207.

30 Tatemoto, K. & Mutt, V. (1980): Isolation of two novel candidate hormones using a chemical method for finding naturally occurring polypeptides. *Nature* **285**, 417–418.

31 Turner, D.S., Shabaan, A., Etheridge, L. & Marks, V. (1973): The effect of an intestinal polypeptide fraction on insulin release in the rat *in vitro* and *in vivo*. *Endocrinology* **93**, 1323–1328.

32 Turner, D.S. Etheridge, L., Jones, J., Marks, V., Meldrum, B., Bloom, S.R. & Brown, J.C. (1974): The effect of the intestinal polypeptide, IRP and GIP on insulin release and glucose tolerance in the baboon. *Clin. Endocr.* **3**, 489–493.

33 Unger, R.H. & Eisentraut, A.M. (1969): Entero-insular axis. *Archs. Intern. Med.* **123**, 261–266.

34 Wasada, T., McCorkle, K., Harris, V., Kawai, K., Howard, B. & Unger, R.H. (1981): Effect of gastric inhibitory polypeptide on plasma levels of chylomicron triglycerides in dogs. *J. Clin. Invest.* **68**, 1106–1107.

35 Yalow, R.S. & Berson, S.A. (1960): Immunoassay of endogenous plasma insulin. *J. Clin. Invest.* **39**, 1157–1175.

Integration of nutrient intake, nutrient utilization and physiological state

D.B. LINDSAY and V.H. ODDY
AFRC Institute of Animal Physiology, Babraham, Cambridge CB2 4AT, UK.

Nutrition would perhaps be simpler if we had only to consider mature subjects, in energy and nitrogen balance. In animal nutrition we are predominantly interested in production, when animals are depositing nutrients either as new tissue or as some secreted product. In this paper we consider two states — pregnancy and lactation — in which animals adapt to meet their increased nutrient demands. We discuss only changes in sheep, because we are not aware of comparable studies in other animals. This means that our results cannot strictly be generalized but some of the findings may apply more widely.

Most of the work has been done with sheep fitted with catheters in portal, hepatic, mesenteric and recurrent tarsal veins and the carotid artery. From nutrient concentrations in blood samples drawn from them, and relevant blood flow measurement we could quantify nutrient exchange across the gastrointestinal tract, liver and hindlimb muscle. The general technique was as described by Pethick *et al.*[10]. For pregnant or lactating sheep, catheters were implanted at 60–70 days of pregnancy, and maintained until lactation and beyond if possible. Experiments were done at about 120–130 d pregnancy and about 20–30 d of lactation, lambs being allowed to remain with the ewe.

Nutrient intake. We allowed food intake to increase in pregnancy and lactation to follow the pattern of energy requirement. In terms of metabolizable energy (ME) food intake was about 30 per cent greater in pregnancy, and nearly doubled in lactation compared with dry sheep. Intake was estimated only approximately since in addition to a pelleted concentrate offered morning and night, long hay was freely available, the intake of which was estimated after substracting scattered residues.

In sheep, as a consequence of ruminant fermentation, the form of absorbed nutrients is quite different from that in the diet. The major energy-yielding nutrients produced in ruminants are the volatile fatty acids (acetate, propionate and butyrate) (VFA). Of these there is good evidence for extensive catabolism of butyrate to ketones in the rumen wall. The sum of the VFA plus ketones entering the portal circulation, expressed as ME (MJ/day) varied from 2.8 (dry) to 5.4 (lactating) and accounted for only 30–40 per cent of ingested ME. The proportion was similar in dry and lactating sheep, but may have been slightly more in pregnant animals. In most of the animals glucose was used by the gut and glycolysis could have accounted for some of the lactate produced. On some diets, rich in concentrates, some glucose may be absorbed (see, eg[5]); catabolism of propionate is also possible in the rumen wall, so that some may be absorbed as lactate and/or pyruvate. We therefore estimated the sum of glucose, lactate and pyruvate appearing, and used only values where this sum was positive. On this basis, the maximum additional contribution to absorbed ME was about 7–8 per cent in dry sheep; and in pregnant and lactating animals 4–5 per cent — not appreciably different. There was a slight increase in the proportion of potentially glucogenic precursors to about 36–39 per cent in pregnancy and lactation, compared with 34 per cent in dry sheep, due, presumably, to increased concentrate intake. The proportion of ME attributable to VFA is substantially less than is commonly assumed. Absorption of isobutyrate, isovalerates or valerate was not estimated; but these in sum would contribute less than 5 per cent to ME (eg[10]); technical factors may also lead to some underestimation. However, our estimate (33–41 per cent) is not greatly different from an estimate (43 per cent) in studies in cattle[4]. One reason for these rather low estimates is suggested from our measurements of oxygen consumption by the gastrointestinal tract, which ranged from 16–29 per cent of that of the whole animal, with higher values in lactating animals, especially those suckling twins. Much nutrient oxidized at this site is derived from within the gastrointestinal tract, and thus never enters the portal vein. About 30 per cent of acetate is oxidized in this way[4,10].

It seems that there is an increased proportion of the food ME available in pregnancy and lactation, although in lactation (and perhaps in twin-pregnant sheep) this increase is partly offset by the increased metabolic activity of the gastrointestinal tract.

Oxygen consumption by the liver increased in pregnancy and even more so during lactation, but only in proportion to whole body oxygen use. In dry and pregnant animals the total of gut and hepatic oxygen consumption accounted for about 40 per cent of the total by the animal, in lactation the sum was just over 50 per cent.

The nitrogen intake of the pregnant animals (26 g/d) was only slightly greater than that of the dry animals (23 g/d); but there was a large increase in the lactating group (51 g/d). There was a moderate increase in NH_3-N absorbed (7–9–12 g/d from dry to pregnant to lactating) and more so in total α-amino-N (2–6–11 g/d). Thus the fraction of dietary nitrogen absorbed was from 40–60 per cent; less than the expected nitrogen digestibility of 60–70 per cent. There was only a modest improvement in efficiency in pregnancy and lactation. However the fraction absorbed as α-amino-N was substantially increased (25 per cent in dry, 41 per cent in pregnant and 47 per cent in lactating animals).

We are unable at present to explain the rather small amount of dietary nitrogen apparently absorbed, although we suspect that a number of factors may be involved (eg, absorption of peptides and of lymph protein). It is clear nevertheless that there is a substantial increase in the direct absorption of α-amino-N in pregnancy and lactation; and that this is more than might be expected on the basis of the increase in nitrogen intake. A change in pattern is also seen in respect of the liver. The NH_3 absorbed from the gut is removed by the liver (102 per cent in dry and pregnant animals, that is, some removal of peripherally produced as well as gut ammonia; and 89 per cent in lactating sheep). The fraction of α-amino-N removed by the liver, however, is decreased — from 169 per cent in dry, to 41 per cent in pregnant and 29 per cent in lactating animals.

Ruminants are known to be dependent on gluconeogenesis to meet their glucose needs, and this is increased in pregnancy and lactation (in these studies, glucose output by the liver was about 48 mg/min in dry, and 112 mg/min in pregnant and lactating sheep). The question is sometimes raised, therefore, whether there may be competition for amino acids between the needs of gluconeogenesis and protein requirements. In this study, propionate taken up by the liver was sufficient for about 70 per cent of glucose released. However, glycerol taken up brought the amount of carbon available for gluconeogenesis to about 85 per cent; and lactating uptake increased it to well over 100 per cent — in pregnant and lactating as well as dry sheep. There is thus no requirement at all for amino acid use for gluconeogenesis. If all the α-amino-N taken up by the liver were used for gluconeogenesis, amino acids could contribute 11–13 per cent of glucose put out by the liver. Of individual amino acids, alanine uptake by the liver could contribute less than 1 per cent to glucose in pregnancy, and about 6 per cent in lactation. In studies with ^{14}C-alanine in pregnant sheep, about 4 per cent of glucose was apparently derived from alanine. This may perhaps indicate a significant use of alanine for gluconeogenesis in the kidney, which contributes to about 15 per cent of glucose production[1]. Even so, there may be no net transfer of alanine to glucose because of peripheral production of alanine from glucose. The other major gluconeogenic amino acid is glutamine[3]. In pregnant and lactating ewes hepatic uptake of glutamine was actually less than glutamic output, suggesting no net usage for gluconeogenesis. Studies with ^{14}C-threonine also suggest little use of this for gluconeogenesis in pregnant or lactating sheep[2]. Thus in adequately fed sheep there is no shortage of carbon precursors for gluconeogenesis; and no likely amino acid limitation due to this need.

Adaptation by peripheral tissues. Although the liver appears to have ample precursor supply to meet glucose needs in pregnancy and lactation, other strategies may be used to ensure adequate availability of glucose from the pregnant uterus or the mammary gland. A similar technique has been used to assess net glucose utilization (ie corrected for lactate production) by muscle, and uterus or mammary gland, in dry, pregnant or lactating sheep[7]. Diets of differing energy content were also used. The rate of glucose production at any given stage of pregnancy or lactation was substantially less in sheep eating a low-energy oaten hay than those eating lucerne. This confirms findings reported earlier[12]. It was also observed that glucose uptake by the uterus was similar across different diets[7]. This was achieved through a fall in maternal glucose utilization, partly by muscle, but more strikingly in maternal non-muscle ('remainder') tissues. In late pregnancy, there was also a marked fall in 'remainder' glucose, so that uterine and muscle uptake accounted for almost all glucose used. In lactation there was no reduction in glucose utilization by 'remainder' tissues, due chiefly to enhanced feed intake. Although muscle glucose was reduced on the low-energy diet there were no specific changes in pregnancy and lactation, except perhaps some increase in muscle lactate output in late pregnancy and early lactation.

'Remainder' glucose utilization is partly that of the brain. This is unchanged in pregnancy[6] and probably in lactation. Another important site is the gut. We found net glucose utilization (corrected for lactate and pyruvate output) was greatly reduced in pregnancy and lactation (equivalent to 'late' pregnancy and 'early' lactation of Oddy *et al.*[7]). One mechanism by which lactate production in muscle may be increased (and thus net glucose utilization reduced) is through mobilisation of depot fat, with an increase in circulating free fatty acids (FFA). Oddy and co-workers[9] have shown that a rising FFA concentration is significantly related to increased lactate output, and hence decreasing net utilization of glucose by muscle. Whether this mechanism is also effective in the gastrointestinal tract is not known.

In addition to a reduced net glucose utilization (through elevated lactate production), there is also reduced acetate utilization (at a given arterial acetate concentration) by muscle in lactation[11]. It seems likely that this is of significance in making more acetate available for the mammary gland, for when a diet containing a high proportion of concentrates is eaten, there is no longer reduced acetate utilization by muscle. This condition usually results in a fall in the proportion of fat in milk.

There are also peripheral adaptations to protein metabolism. It is found that wool growth (per unit of feed intake) is depressed in both pregnant and lactating sheep and this seems not to be determined by sulphur or probably energy availability[9]. The rate of muscle protein synthesis seems to be actually increased in pregnant and lactating sheep; however the rate of protein degradation may be increased even more, so that there is a net loss of muscle protein, particularly in late pregnancy[15]. Probably net gain or loss of protein is determined by a dietary interaction, as is seen for wool protein, since it has been shown that in the muscle of pregnant and lactating sheep the net exchange of tyrosine (which, we believe, reflects loss or gain of protein) is significantly correlated with loss or gain of body weight[14]. The increased turnover of muscle protein in pregnancy and lactation may increase the sensitivity of response to nutrient availability.

Hormonal influences. It is certain that the adaptations occurring in pregnancy and lactation are determined by hormonal factors. A fairly full survey of such hormonal changes have been reported[13]. In particular, there is some reduction of plasma insulin and a marked increase in plasma growth hormone. However, in pregnancy, there are also increases of progesterone and ovine placental lactogen (OPL), and in lactation of prolactin. We cannot assess their relative importance in inducing metabolic changes. Nevertheless, we have emphasized the interaction of diet with metabolic changes in pregnancy and lactation, and it is perhaps pertinent to note that diet will alter hormonal responses. This is shown elegantly in a study of plasma ovine placental lactogen[8] — a hormone thought to redirect glucose from maternal to uterine use. Increasing metabolizable energy intake resulted in a progressive lowering of OPL. At a given energy intake, however, the presence of two fetuses compared with one elevated the plasma OPL.

In conclusion, it seems that changes occurring in pregnancy and lactation are of two types. One sort is inevitable — such as an increase in food intake in lactation; and consequent increased metabolism of the liver and gastrointestinal tract. The other may be regarded as dependent on the extent of nutrient intake. If it is ample to meet increased productive demands, then readjustment is minimal; but if intake is not sufficient, then adjustments may be made to direct nutrients where they are most needed.

1 Bergman, E.N., Brockman, R.P. & Kaufman, C.P. (1974): Glucose metabolism in ruminants: comparison of whole-body turnover with production by gut, liver, and kidneys. *Fed. Proc.* **33**, 1849–1854.

2 Egan, A.R. & Macrae, J.C. (1979): Amino acid catabolism and gluconeogenesis in sheep. *Ann. Rech. Vet.* **10**, 376–378.

3 Heitmann, R.N. & Bergman, E.N. (1978): Glutamine metabolism, interorgan transport, and glucogenicity in the sheep. *Am. J. Physiol.* **234**, E197–E203.

4 Huntington, G.B., Reynolds, P.J. & Tyrrell, H.F. (1983): Net absorption and ruminal concentrations of metabolites in nonpregnant dry Holstein cows before and after intraruminal acetic acid infusion. *J. Dairy Sci.* **66**, 1901–1908.

5 Janes, A.N., Parker, D.S., Weekes, T.E.C. & Armstrong, D.G. (1984): Mesenteric venous blood flow and the net absorption of glucose in sheep fed dried grass or ground maize based diets. *J. agric. Sci., Camb.* **103**, 549–553.

6 Lindsay, D.B. & Setchell, B.P. (1976): The oxidation of glucose, ketone bodies and acetate by the brain of normal and ketonaemic sheep. *J. Physiol. (Lond.)* **259**, 801–823.

7 Oddy, V.H., Gooden, J.M., Hough, G.M., Teleni, E. & Annison, E.F. (1985): Partitioning of nutrients in Merino ewes 2. Glucose utilization by skeletal muscle, the pregnant uterus and the lactating mammary gland in relation to whole body glucose utilization. *Aust. J. Biol. Sci.* **38**, 95–108.

8 Oddy, V.H. & Jenkin, G. (1981): Diet and fetal number influence ovine placental lactogen concentration. *Proc. Nutr. Soc. Aust.* **6**, 151.

9 Oddy. V.H. & Lindsay, D.B. (1986): Metabolic and hormonal interactions and their potential effects of growth. In *Control and manipulation of animal growth*, ed P.J. Buttery, N.B. Haynes & D.B. Lindsay. London & Boston: Butterworths (In press).

10 Pethick, D.W., Lindsay, D.B., Barker, P.J. & Northrop, A.J. (1981): Acetate supply and utilization by the tissues of the sheep in-vivo. *Br. J. Nutr.* **46**, 97–110.

11 Pethick, D.W. & Lindsay, D.B. (1982): Acetate metabolism in lactating sheep. *Br. J. Nutr.* **48**, 319–328.

12 Steel, J.W. & Leng, R.A. (1973): Effects of plane of nutrition and pregnancy on gluconeogenesis in sheep 1. The kinetics of glucose metabolism. *Br. J. Nutr.* **30**, 451–473.

13 Vernon, R.G., Clegg, R.A. & Flint, D.J. (1981): Metabolism of sheep adipose tissue during pregnancy and lactation; adaptation and regulation. *Biochem. J.* **200**, 307–314.

14 Vincent, R. (1984): Protein metabolism in sheep. Ph D Thesis, University of Cambridge.

15 Vincent, R. & Lindsay, D.B. (1985): Effect of pregnancy and lactation on muscle protein metabolism in sheep. *Proc. Nutr. Soc.* **44**, 77A.

The prediction of responses to nutrients

C. FISHER
Agricultural and Food Research Council, Poultry Research Centre, Roslin, Midlothian EH25 9PS, Scotland.

A classical purpose of nutritional research has been to define nutrient requirements. Tables of requirements, which are an end point of this research, are widely used, but in animal nutrition at least, this approach can be criticized on two grounds. First, it must be recognized that objective criteria for determining requirements are economic and not biological. The selection of economic optima requires a statement of rate of response to nutrients and this replaces the idea of a fixed requirement applicable under all conditions. Secondly, requirements and rates of response, will vary in different circumstances. Tables of requirements are now being replaced by methods of calculation which more accurately reflect the circumstances in which nutrition is being practised.

In poultry nutrition it has been argued elsewhere[14] that the failure to incorporate the theoretical principles of prediction into the scientific development of the topic has both limited progress and led to poorly designed, repetitive experimental work.

Prediction implies extrapolation. Extrapolation, that is, of observations from experimental subjects to subjects both in general and in the future. Prediction depends on theory. An adequate theory is essential if the relationship between experimental and future subjects is to be explored. Even if the theory is the rather unimaginative one, 'all subjects are the same', it is a theory and should be explicitly acknowledged. Finally prediction is quantitative. Quantitative or mathematical theories of response are required and this leads to consideration of simulation and modelling and their role in nutrition.

These ideas are not new. They were first promulgated formally by econometricians[9] but this group failed to find a satisfactory solution to the problem of predicting biological response. However, it is still true that research in this area is mainly aimed at empirical description of biological mechanisms and that compartmentalism (eg between types of animal) and reductionism, as opposed to integration, dominates the experimental approaches that are used. By introducing nutritional theory as a topic for debate and argument, a framework would be provided within which knowledge can accumulate in a more systematic and useful way.

Prediction: problems and approaches. Nutritional prediction raises several problems which require formal treatments. The discussion of mathematical modelling in agriculture by France & Thornley[17] probably provides the best general review of the topic whilst two books merit close study[9,33]. Here, a few selected topics only can be discussed.

Mathematical modelling. The application of mathematical modelling to nutrition has been discussed[17] and also in relation to ruminant nutrition[19], defining a model as 'a set of mathematical equations that represent the behaviour of a system' and suggesting a three-way classification into dynamic or static, deterministic or stochastic and mechanistic or empirical models. This is useful — although the classes are not always mutually exclusive and many existing models contain elements of both types. Ideal theories for the prediction of nutritional response would be dynamic, stochastic and mechanistic; that is they would explicitly consider time as a variable, they would take account of variation and they would reflect current understanding of the causation of the mechanism of response. To the writer's knowledge no such model has yet been produced, but in some areas considerable progress has been made by models which incorporate two out of these three.

Bounds and levels. It is accepted that nutrient response and requirements depend on many factors concerned with the animal, the feed and the environment, and some of these must be included as explicit variables in the prediction theory. However, if all possible interactions are considered the system will rapidly become too complex and some pragmatic guide-lines must be adopted. In agricultural practice the type of animal (genotype), major dietary variables, environmental temperature and economic conditions are probably the minimum requirements. Some factors may have to be ignored because they are too complex or difficult to describe; the effects of sub-clinical disease and 'level of husbandry' are examples.

Theories for predicting nutrient response can be elaborated at many levels; the population, herd or flock, the individual animal, organs, tissues, cells and so on. Some of the properties of this organisational hierarchy have been discussed[17]. There is virtue in using the highest level possible consistent with the overall objectives or the work. One unavoidable feature seems to be that mechanistic descriptions of the relationship between nutrient supply and response can only be defined for the individual animal. Prediction for populations must be derived by averaging the results for a known population of individuals and it is important that the average differs from the response of the average animal[8]. Recognition of this distinction allows very simple biological models to acquire elegant formal and valuable utilitarian properties[7,15].

For animal feeding in general the description of whole animals by simple factorial statements representing the major components of metabolism have been successful[10,23,39]. Schemes for rationing dairy cows have largely been elaborated at this level[1]. The description of transformations and exchanges in the rumen, however, requires representation of the major biochemical pathways[3,18]. The simulation of metabolism at the whole animal level[21] seems to be more appropriate for evaluating concepts and hypotheses for research purposes than for the prediction of nutrient responses in practice. The view that metabolic modelling will be required to achieve practical objectives has widespread support, however.

Elements of prediction. A static and simple statement of nutrient requirement allows most of the elements of a satisfactory prediction theory to be identified. Thus:

$$cR_i = (dR_i/dt)/(dF/dt)$$

$$\text{and} \quad dR_i/dt = \frac{a_i}{e_i} (dO/dt) \text{------------} + b_i W^n$$

$$\begin{aligned}
\text{where} \quad cR_i &= \text{desired concentration of resource i in feed} \\
(dR_i/dt) &= \text{desired rate of intake of resource i} \\
(dF/dt) &= \text{rate of food intake} \\
a_i &= \text{concentration of resource i in output (O)} \\
e_i &= \text{efficiency of utilization of feed resource i} \\
dO/dt &= \text{rate of output} \\
b_1 W^n &= \text{maintenance requirement for bodyweight, W.}
\end{aligned}$$

Six elements of general theory can then be recognised[11]: (1) a sufficient description of the animal, (2) scales for resources, (3) nutrient requirements, (4) food intake and diet selection, (5) allocation of deficient resources and recovery from deficiency, and (6) Stochastic elements; individuals and populations.

A *sufficient description of the animal* is required since resources are either stored untransformed in the body (eg essential amino acids) or used in metabolism. Therefore animal characteristics (dO/dt and W in the example) are major determinants of requirements. The concept of *potential output* is central since the limits to response must be defined. Very small increments of response are of economic importance and therefore the limit must be estimated precisely. The estimation of potential output presents a problem since observed production levels are invariably lower. Mathematical models which may fairly be assumed to describe potential output may fit actual observations less well, especially in growing animals, thus creating problems in parameter estimation. This topic is of great importance[38] but cannot be explored here.

A sufficient description will be applicable to animals differing in age, sex and genotype. It has been proposed[10] that potential growth can be described in terms of a Gompertz function, relating protein growth to time and, by allometric relationships amongst body components, scaled to mature protein mass. Pigs have been characterized in terms of protein growth[39]. Standardized growth equations have been discussed[29] and a theory encompassing both growth and food intake[33]. Recent work[34] raises the possibility that potential growth in the pig is limited by food intake, a concept which adds a new, and important, dimension to growth analysis. Descriptions of lactation curves are mainly empirical[22] but a mechanistic model of milk production has been presented[28]. Egg production has been considered less. Attempts to quantify the deposition and utilization of nutrients in pregnancy, in this case in the sow, have recently been exemplified[31].

Maintenance, represented here as a simple function of body weight, is a concept of great value in quantitative nutrition, although it is difficult to define on theoretical grounds. Body-weight is the most readily available predictor although body protein mass may be more appropriate. The effects of body composition and of great technical difficulties in measuring maintenance probably exacerbate the confusion over scaling rules. It has been proposed that maintenance should be scaled to $W_A^{-0.27}$ where W_A is mature body size[36]. This proposal leads to some interesting and unexpected results and there is no doubt that maintenance, both the concept and the problems of measurement, is a topic that merits more attention. Whether attempts to do this in mechanistic terms, by considering metabolic functions, will be useful, remains to be seen.

Most existing theories of animal performance assume predetermined feeding levels (input). To predict *ad-libitum* intake it appears that some objective must be attributed to the animal. Without this it is logically impossible to predict a voluntary activity such as food intake. Only Emmans[10] has explicitly incorporated such ideas into his theory; he attributes to growing animals the two objectives of achieving maximum protein growth and attaining a desired body composition. Similar ideas, but based on energy needs, are implicit in other theories of food intake[5,10].

Scales for resources are required suitable for describing feed resources and relating them to animal functions. Scales for energy, nitrogen, amino acids, mineral elements and vitamins are required. Except for energy, and the N-supply to ruminants, the problems of definition are largely solved, though great practical difficulties remain. Scales for describing the energy contributions of feeds are still evolving and, in ruminant animals, at least, may eventually require consideration of a wide range of chemical substrates to predict animal response[3]. The same is true of the N-supply to ruminants[4].

Nutrient requirement is now given a more limited meaning as the amount of each resource needed for a unit of each function. That it is a listing of the coefficients e_i for each resource and output function (O). In some cases, eg amino acid utilization for egg production, and probably growth, it appears that constant values can be used in practical schemes of prediction. However, more biological theories of nutrient utilization are required and this remains a major challenge for research.

A variety of approaches can be used to complete the table of efficiencies. Economic pressures will determine that most emphasis is placed on protein, amino acid and energy utilization. It has been shown[13] how the analysis of response data can be used to assess amino acid utilization and this is probably the simplest case. For exchanges in ruminant animals complex function will probably be required to represent the coefficient e_i at the whole animal level, although post-ruminal utilization may be found to be similar to single-stomached animals. In some circumstances, eg trace mineral requirements, reasonable 'guess-timates' may prove to be adequate.

Prediction of food intake is clearly essential if nutrient supply is to be controlled in animals fed *ad-libitum*. Even in well-defined situations, such as laying hens in cages, this remains a significant problem. Earlier approaches were mainly based on empirical regression equations relating intake to observable variables such as yield, bodyweight and temperature for laying hens[6] for dairy cows[39] as examples). More mechanistic approaches[5] and in particular the work of Forbes[16] on ruminants seek to explain how an animal eats to meet its requirements, basically for energy, by a balance of positive stimuli and negative feed-back controls of hunger and satiety. In contrast a more general biological theory has been proposed[10]; that an animal has a 'desired' food intake which will provide enough of the first-limiting feed resources to achieve its objectives. An empirical theory of growth and food intake has been proposed[33].

The allocation of deficient resources and the recovery from a state of deficiency are important in some systems of animal production and short-periods of deficiency and recovery are frequently a source of variation even in simple and short-term experiments. On controlled feeding animals are, by definition, short of the first-limiting resource. Under *ad-libitum* feeding, deficiencies may also occur because of short-term limitations on intake eg familiarisation to a change of diet. In both cases information is required to describe how priorities between different functions are allocated. The development and use of nutritional reserves is an important component of both natural and agricultural strategies.

Similarly the metabolic consequences of deficiency during a subsequent recovery period must be quantified. The concepts of compensatory growth or production are important components of agricultural systems which reflect or exploit seasonal variations in food supply.

Finally in any response theory consideration must be given to *stochastic elements* and to the distinction between *individuals and populations*. As noted above, prediction of animal response can only logically be at the level of the individual animal. Consideration of populations raises two issues; variability and covariability of model elements and the extension of prediction to populations.

The second of these is easily dealt with provided the population structure can be defined. Fisher *et al.*[15] show how statements of the variance and covariance in dO/dt and W can be used to generate a diminishing-response population curve from a linear model describing the response of an individual. These principles were formalized by Curnow[7].

Response curves. Many experiments done to determine nutrient requirements for a specific response are interpreted by examination, by some sort of interval or range test or by fitting two intersecting straight lines ('broken-line' model,[35]). All of these are readily shown to be formally unsatisfactory[26] and, more importantly, to lead to erroneous conclusions. Two dimensional response models are, in general, rather limited descriptions of the system of nutritional response, but because they form a widely used, but little considered methodology, they are briefly mentioned here.

Table. *Some non-linear models for describing nutrient-response relationships.*

Type	*Reference*	*Type*	*Reference*
1. Log-log, with plateau	Almquist (1953)	4. Logistic	Ware *et al.* (1980)
2. Exponential curves		5. Mitscherlich	Gibney *et al.* (1977)
— sigmoidal	Robbins *et al.* (1979)	6. Equation based on saturation kinetics	Morgan *et al.* (1975)
— diet space and	Parks (1973)		Curnow (1973)
response	Nelder (1966)	7. 'Broken-line' for individuals yielding diminishing response for populations	
3. Inverse polynomials	Curnow (1986)		
	Morris & Blackburn (1982)		

Discontinuity of response, as in the 'broken-line' model seems unlikely[35] and continuous, curvilinear response models are widely accepted. Some recently suggested models are summarized in the Table. Inverse polynominals[39] seem to offer a class of equations, the application of which to nutrition remains to be worked out[8].

Most writers in this field attribute the curvilinearity of response as a general characteristic of living organisms and deriving from widely accepted kinetic principles. The model described by Fisher *et al.*[15] however shows that all of the observed curvilinearity can be explained by the variability of individuals in output characteristics, the individuals themselves showing 'broken-line' responses. This very simple theory leads to useful formal properties for interpreting experimental data[7] and calculating economically optimum requirements[12]. Consideration of growing animals[13] suggests that the 'broken-line' model can reasonably be assumed to apply to one animal at one time. Curvature of response is then attributable both to variations in output of one individual over time and to variations between individuals.

Discussion. It is essential that more rigorous and formal theory should be introduced into the study of nutrient requirements and response. The challenge of developing theories and models to describe whole animals at the metabolic level will require the resources of many closely collaborating research groups. This type of collaboration is appearing in ruminant nutrition and is to be applauded.

1 Agricultural Research Council (1980): *Nutrient requirements of ruminant livestock*. Slough: Commonwealth Agricultural Bureaux.

2 Almquist, H.J. (1953): Interpretation of amino acid requirement data according to the Law of Diminishing Returns. *Archs. Biochem. Biophys.* **44**, 245–247.

3 Baldwin, R.L., Koong, L.J. & Ulyatt, M.J. (1977): A dynamic model of ruminant digestion for evaluation of factors affecting nutritive value. *Agric. Systems* **2**, 255–288.

4 Black, J.L., Beever, D.E., Faichney, G.J., Howart, B.R. & Graham, N.McC. (1981): Simulation of the effects of rumen function on the flow of nutrients from the stomach of sheep: part 1 — description of a computer programme. *Agric. Systems* **6**, 195–219.

5 Booth, D.A. (editor) (1978): *Hunger models: comparative theory of feeding control*. London: Academic Press.

6 Byerly, T.C. (1979): Prediction of the food intake of laying hens. In *Food intake regulation in poultry*, ed K.N. Boorman & B.M. Freeman, pp. 327–363. Edinburgh: British Poultry Science.

7 Curnow, R.N. (1973): A smooth population response curve based on an abrupt threshold and plateau model for individuals. *Biometrics* **29**, 1–10.

8 Curnow, R.N. (1986): The statistical approach to nutrient requirements. In *Nutrient requirements of poultry and nutritional research*, ed C. Fisher & K.N. Boorman. London: Butterworths. (In press).

9 Dent, J.B. & Casey, H. (1967): *Linear programming and animal nutrition*. London: Crosby Lockwood.

10 Emmans, G.C. (1981): A model of the growth and feed intake of ad libitum fed animals particularly poultry. In *Computers in animal production*, ed G.M. Hillyer, C.T. Whittemore & R.G. Gunn, pp. 103–110. Occ. Pubn No 5 British Society of Animal Production.

11 Emmans, G.C. & Fisher, C. (1986): Problems in nutritional theory. In *Nutrient requirements of poultry and nutritional research*, ed C. Fisher & K.N. Boorman. London: Butterworths. (In press)

12 Fisher, C. (1976): Protein in the diets of the pullet and laying bird. In *Protein metabolism and nutrition. EAAP Publ. No 16*, ed D.J.A. Cole, K.N. Boorman, P.J. Buttery, D. Lewis, R.J. Neale & H. Swan, pp. 323–351. London: Butterworths.

13 Fisher, C. (1983): The physiological basis of the amino acid requirements of poultry. In *Protein metabolism and nutrition. Les Colloques de l'INRA No 16*, ed M. Arnal, R. Pion & D. Bouin, pp. 385–404.

14 Fisher, C. (1983): Nutrition and growth: experimental methods. *Proc. IV Europ. Poult. Nutr. Symp.*, pp. 1–16. Tours, France.

15 Fisher, C., Morris, T.R. & Jennings, R.C. (1973): A model for the description and prediction of the response of laying hens to amino acid intake. *Br. Poult. Sci.* **14**, 469–484.

16 Forbes, J.M. (1980): A model of the short-term control of feeding in the ruminant: effects of changing animal or feed characteristics. *Appetite* **1**, 21–41.

17 France, J. & Thornley, J.H.M. (1984): *Mathematical models in agriculture*. London: Butterworths.

18 France, J., Thornley, J.H.M. & Beever, D.E. (1982): A mathematical model of the rumen. *J. Agric. Sci. Camb.* **99**, 343–353.

19 France, J., Thornley, J.H.M. & Beever, D.E. (1984): Opinion: mechanistic modelling in ruminant nutrition and production. *Res. Devel. Agric.* **1**, 65–71.

20 Gibney, M.J., Dunne, A. & Kinsella, I.A. (1977): The use of the Mitscherlich equation in describe amino acid response curves in the growing chick. *Nutr. Rep. Int.* **20**, 501–510.

21 Gill, M., Thornley, J.H.M., Black, J.L., Oldham, J.D. & Beever, D.E. (1984): Simulation of the metabolism of absorbed energy-yielding nutrients in young sheep. *Br. J. Nutr.* **52**, 621–649.

22 Goodall, E.A. & Sprevak, D. (1985): A Bayesian estimation of the lactation curve of a dairy cow. *Anim. Prod.* **40**, 189–193.

23 Graham, N. McC., Black, J.L., Faichney, G.J. & Arnold, G.L. (1976): Simulation of growth and production in sheep. *Agric. Syst.* **1**, 113–138.

24 Moore, A.J. (1985): A mathematical equation for animal growth from embryo to adult. *Anim. Prod.* **40**, 441–453.

25 Morgan, P.H., Mercer, L.P. & Flodin, N.W. (1975): General model for nutritional responses of higher organisms. *Proc. Nat. Acad. Sci. USA.* **72**, 4327–4331.

26 Morris, T.R. (1983): The interpretation of response data from animal feeding trials. In *Recent advances in animal nutrition — 1983*, ed W. Haresign, pp. 13–23. London: Butterworths.

27 Morris, T.R. & Blackburn, H.A. (1982): The shape of the response curve relating protein intake to egg output for flocks of laying hens. *Br. Poult. Sci.* **23**, 405–424.

28 Neal, H.D.StC. & Thornley, J.H.M. (1983): The lactation curve in cattle: a mathematical model of the mammary gland. *J. Agric. Sci., Camb.* **101**, 389–400.

29 Neal, H.D.StC., Thomas, C. & Cobby, J.M. (1984): Comparison of equations for predicting voluntary intake by dairy cows. *J. Agric. Sci., Camb.* **103**, 1–10.

30 Nelder, J.A. (1966): Inverse polynomials, a useful group of multi-factor response functions. *Biometrics* **22**, 303–315.

31 Noblet, J., Close, W.H., Heavens, R.P. & Brown, D. (1985): Studies on the energy metabolism of the pregnant sow. 1. Uterus and mammary tissue development. *Br. J. Nutr.* **53**, 251–265.

32 Parks, J.R. (1973): Diet space and response surfaces. *J. Theor. Biol.* **42**, 349–358.

33 Parks, J.R. (1982): *A theory of feeding and growth of animals*. Berlin: Springer Verlag.

34 Pekas, J.C. (1985): Animal growth during liberation from appetite suppression. *Growth* **49**, 19–27.

35 Robbins, K.R., Norton, H.W. & Baker, D.H. (1979): Estimation of requirements from growth data. *J. Nutr.* **109**, 1710–1714.

36 Taylor, StC.S. (1980): Genetic size — scaling rules in animal growth. *Anim. Prod.* **30**, 161–165.

37 Ware, G.O., Phillips, R.D., Parrish, R.S. & Moon, L.C. (1980): A comparison of two non-linear models for describing intake-response relationships in higher organisms. *J. Nutr.* **110**, 765–770.

38 Whittemore, C.T. (1981): Animal production response prediction. In *Computers in animal production*, ed G.M. Hillyer, C.T. Whittemore & R.G. Gunn, pp. 47–63. Occ. Pubn No 5, British Society of Animal Production.

39 Whittemore, C.T. & Fawcett, R.H. (1976): Theoretical aspects of a flexible model to simulate protein and lipid growth in pigs. *Anim. Prod.* **22**, 87–96.

IX: Vitamins

Research developments in folate and vitamin B$_{12}$ nutrition

Research developments in vitamin A nutrition

Workshop

RESEARCH DEVELOPMENTS IN FOLATE AND VITAMIN B$_{12}$ NUTRITION

Folate status and folate requirements

V. HERBERT

Hematology & Nutrition Research Laboratory, Veterans Administration Medical Center, Bronx, New York 10468 and State University of New York Downstate Medical Center, Brooklyn, New York 11203, USA.

Assessing folate status. Going from normality to folate deficiency, megaloblastic anaemia is a continuum starting with negative folate balance and proceeding through three sequential stages, or degrees of folate depletion, each defined by the appearance of specific biochemical and/or haematologic markers (Table and Figure).

The first evidence of negative folate balance is a folate level below 3 ng folate/ml serum. Serum folate stabilizes below 3 ng/ml after only 2 to 3 weeks of negative folate balance[7,21,22,28]. A single observation of low serum folate does not mean that treatment with folate is indicated, but serial low folates over more than a month mean that stores are low[33].

Folate depletion is a state of reduced folate stores characterized by a fall in the red-cell folate level to below 160 ng folate/ml erythrocytes[7,21,22,24,28], a level at which there is little reserve to be called on in times of increased demand but no biochemical or functional deficit. Red-cell and liver-folate stores fall together as folate deficiency progresses[21,49].

Folate depletion may be primary, or secondary to vitamin B$_{12}$ deficiency. Due to lack of B$_{12}$, folate is trapped as methylfolate[29,30,41], which is a poor substrate for polyglutamate synthesis[46]. This results in decreased production of tissue-folate stores, which are mainly polyglutamates, and leakage of short-chain-length folates from cells, with resultant tissue-folate depletion[46].

In addition to primary and secondary folate deficiency, there is also selective folate deficiency in one cell line but not another[21,26,28,37].

The second stage of folate depletion is folate deficient erythropoiesis (Figure) characterized first by an abnormal diagnostic deoxyuridine (dU) suppression test on bone marrow cells—ie, inadequate DNA synthesis corrected by methylfolate[6,28,39] — and then on peripheral blood lympho-

443

Table. *Sequential events in the development of folate deficiency megaloblastic anaemia in persons consuming an experimental diet containing almost no folate (< 5 µg of folate daily)*[21,28,31].

Sequential changes	Time of appearance[a]
Low serum folate (< 3 ng/ml); slight increase in size of average bone marrow normoblast	3 weeks
Hypersegmentation in neutrophils in bone marrow (lobe average > 3.5); dU suppression test abnormal in bone marrow	5 weeks
Hypersegmentation in peripheral blood; bone marrow shows increased and abnormal mitoses and basophilic intermediate megaloblasts; dU suppression test abnormal in peripheral blood lymphocytes	7 weeks
Bone marrow shows some large metamyelocytes and a number of polychromatophilic intermediate megaloblasts	10 weeks
High urine formiminoglutamate (FIGLU)	13 weeks
Orthochromatic intermediate megaloblasts in bone marrow	14 weeks
Low red blood cell folate	17 weeks
Macro-ovalocytosis; many large metamyelocytes in bone marrow	18 weeks
Overtly megaloblastic marrow	19 weeks
Anaemia	20 weeks

[a]After initiation of diet

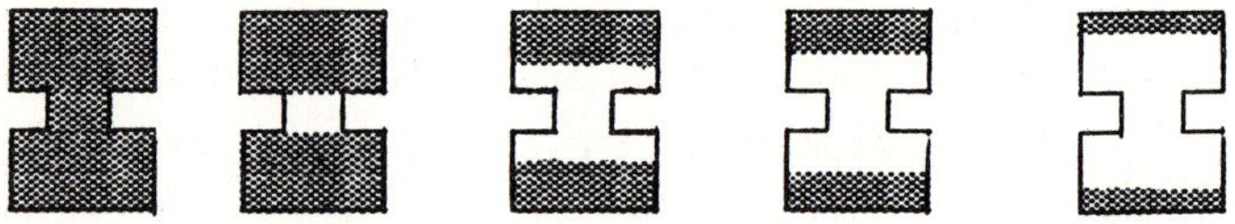

	Normal	Negative folate balance	Folate depletion	Folate-deficient erythropoiesis	Folate deficiency anaemia
Liver folate					
Plasma folate					
Erythron folate					
Serum folate, ng/ml	> 5	< 3	< 3	< 3	< 3
RBC folate, ng/ml	> 200	> 200	< 160	< 120	< 100
Diagnostic dU suppression	Normal	Normal	Normal	Abnormal	Abnormal
Hypersegmentation[a], lobes per nucleus	Absent		Absent	Present	Present
Liver folate, µg/g	> 3	> 3	< 1.6	< 1.2	< 1
Erythrocytes	Normal		Normal	Normal	Macro-ovalocytic
MCV	Normal		Normal	Normal	Elevated
Haemoglobin, g/dl	> 12		> 12	> 12	< 12
Plasma clearance of i.v. folate	Normal		Normal	Increased	Increased

[a]Normal lobe average = 3.2 ± 0.15 lobes per nucleus[14,37]

Figure. *Sequential stages in the development of folate deficiency*. In the first three lines, the area of the shaded boxes in the normal individual shows the relative quantities of folate in each compartment and the sequentially increasingly unshaded areas its proportional disappearance during successive stages of folate deficiency development. In our laboratory, in 100 normal adults, arithmetic mean serum folate = 8.125 ± 5.06 ng/ml, and geometric mean serum folate = 6.92 with range (± 2 s.d.) = 1.89 to 21.8. In the same 100, arithmetic mean red cell folate = 359.5 ± 158.2 ng/ml and geometric mean red cell folate = 329.7 with range (± 2 s.d.) = 129.8 to 773.3. Boxes enclose laboratory abnormalities which characterize onset of the stage indicated in the column heading.

cytes[13,15,28]. This second stage has been referred to as 'subclinical deficiency' or 'subtle megaloblastic anaemia[6,28]. The diagnostic dU suppression test becomes clearly abnormal when intracellular folate levels fall to <200 ng folate/10^9 cells, in normal cells[9] and malignant cells[47].

The third stage of folate depletion, folate deficiency anaemia (Figure), is characterized by the appearance of macro-ovalocytic erythrocytes and a low haemoglobin level. Folate deficiency without anaemia (ie, folate depletion and folate deficient erythropoiesis) is more prevalent than with anaemia.

Hidden folate deficiency is common in patients with defects in haemoglobin synthesis, such as iron deficiency and thalassaemia[28]. In these situations, for unknown reasons, serum and red-cell folate are artificially elevated despite lymphocyte and bone-marrow folate depletion, demonstrable by dU suppression tests diagnostic for folate deficiency[14,15,20]. The diagnosis is confirmed by giving low-dose (100–200 μg/d) folate therapy and observing the ensuing reticulocytosis and rise in haemoglobin. Larger doses can produce haematologic response in patients who just have vitamin B_{12} deficiency[23].

Folate requirements. The minimal daily input folate requirement to sustain normality (ie, to sustain normal DNA synthesis) in the absence of increased metabolic need is in the range of 50 μg for adults (about 1 μg/kg b.wt)[21,25,31,52]. Complicated cases may fail to respond to such doses[34,38]. Hyperthyroidism, pregnancy, haemolytic anaemia[7,28,36], need for intensive care[1,2], or any other sustained metabolic drain, may increase folate need up to six- to eight-fold. Loss of folate from the liver, on an intake of essentially no folate (ie, 2 μg folate daily), as assessed by liver biopsies, varies from 35 to 47 μg daily[19]. Obvious folate deficiency in bone marrow and peripheral blood does not appear until liver folate falls below 1 μg/g[19].

In Canada, the mean national daily folate intake at ages 12 to 65 is approximately 3 μg/kg b.wt[5], which permits maintenance of normal and similar liver-folate levels in both sexes[35]. Of 560 assayed livers from children and adults, only two had folate content below 3μg/g of liver[35]. From this, one can conclude that North American daily dietary intake of approximately 1 μg folate/kg b.wt keeps liver folate >1 μg/g liver in more than 99 per cent of cases, and approximates the minimal daily requirement to sustain DNA normality but low stores. Daily dietary folate intake correlates significantly with red-cell folate[4], and red-cell folate reflects liver folate fairly closely[7,26,51].

On the United Kingdom diet, which contains about 190 μg folate/d[4,40,48], a daily oral supplement of 100 μg pteroylglutamic acid (PGA) prevented any fall in mean red-cell folate during pregnancy[8]. In women with poor folate stores, folate deficiency was as effectively prevented by 300 μg PGA daily in a food that impaired folate availability by 44 per cent (thereby reducing the effective dose to 168 μg PGA daily) as it was by higher doses or more efficient vehicles[10]. Maternal milk folate content may be as high as 50 to 60 μg/l[50], suggesting a need for a daily supplement in that range for lactating women with minimal stores. However, supplementation may be unnecessary in lactating women in the socio-economic middle class[16].

In a premature infant, 50 μg to 100 μg/d is adequate to prevent the folate deficiency that commonly accompanies childhood haemolytic anaemias[2]. In 20 infants aged 2 to 11 months, the nutritional adequacy of diets providing 3.6 μg of folate/kg body weight per d over 6 to 9-month periods has been demonstrated[3]. In full-term infants, liver stores are about 224 μg[45]. The needs of infants are adequately met by human or cow's milk, which contains 50 to 60 μg folate/liter[18,50], but not by goat milk, which has a much lower folate content[27]. Milk from humans, cows, and goats contains a factor essentially unaffected by pasteurization which facilitates folate uptake by gut cells[11,12].

Folate needs of the elderly are similar to those of younger adults[43]. On diets estimated to contain 135 μg folate/d, 21 elderly men and women living at home sustained red-cell folate greater than 100 ng/ml and were haematologically normal; but nine had red-cell folate below 150 ng/ml[4]. Red-cell folate was not lower in achlorhydrics[44], suggesting that their reduced *percentage* absorption may be compensated for by the increased *quantities* of folate supplied by the increased colonies of enteric bacteria[32].

A higher serum folate:erythrocyte folate ratio has been found in the elderly than the young in the USA and in China[17,42].

1 Amos, R.J., Amess, J.A.L., Hind, C.J. & Mollin, D.L. (1982): Incidence and pathogenesis of acute megaloblastic bone marrow change in patients receiving intensive care. *Lancet* **2**, 835–839.

2 Amos, R.J., Amess, J.A.L., Nancekievill, D.G. & Rees, G.M. (1984): Prevention of nitrous oxide-induced megaloblastic changes in bone marrow using folinic acid. *Br. J. Anaesthesiol.* **56**, 103–107.

3 Asfour, R., Wahbea, N., Waslien, C., Guindi, S. & Darby, W.J. (1977): Folacin requirements of children. III. Normal infants. *Am. J. Clin. Nutr.* **30**, 1098–1105.

4 Bates, C.J., Fleming, M., Paul, A.A., Black, A.E. & Mandal, A.R. (1980): Folate status and its relation to vitamin C in healthy elderly men and women. *Age and Ageing* **9**, 241–248.

5 Canada Bureau of Nutritional Sciences, Dept. of Health & Welfare (1977): *Nutrition Canada: Food consumption report.* (Ottawa).

6 Carmel, R. & Karnaze, D.S. (1985): The deoxyuridine suppression test identifies subtle cobalamin deficiency in patients without typical megaloblastic anaemia. *J. Am. Med. Ass.* **253**, 1284–1287.

7 Chanarin, I. (1979): *The megaloblastic anaemias*, 2nd edn. Oxford: Blackwell Scientific Publications.

8 Chanarin, I., Rothman, D., Ward, A. & Perry, J. (1968): Folate status and requirement in pregnancy. *Br. Med. J.* **2**, 390–394.

9 Colman, N. & Herbert, V. (1980): Abnormal lymphocyte deoxyuridine suppression test: A reliable indicator of decreased lymphocyte folate levels. *Am. J. Haemat.* **8**, 169–174.

10 Colman, N., Green, R. & Metz, J. (1975): Prevention of folate deficiency by food fortification. II. Absorption of folic acid from fortified staple foods. *Am. J. Clin. Nutr.* **28**, 459–464.

11 Colman, N., Hettiarachchy, N. & Herbert, V. (1981): Detection of a milk factor that facilities folate uptake by intestinal cells. *Science* **211**, 1427–1429.

12 Colman, N., Chen, J.-F., Gavin, W. & Herbert, V. (1981): Factors affecting enhancement by milk of folate uptake into intestinal cells. *Blood* **58** (Suppl. 1), 26A.

13 Das, K.C. & Herbert, V. (1978): The lymphocyte as a marker of past nutritional status: Persistence of abnormal lymphocyte deoxyuridine (dU) suppression test and chromosomes in patients with past deficiency of folate and vitamin B_{12}. *Br. J. Haemat.* **38**, 219–233.

14 Das, K.C., Herbert, V., Colman, N. & Longo, D. (1978): Unmasking covert folate deficiency in iron-deficient subjects with neutrophil hypersegmentation: dU suppression tests on lymphocytes and bone marrow. *Br. J. Haemat.* **39**, 357–375.

15 Das, K.C., Manusselis, C. & Herbert, V. (1980): Simplifying lymphocyte culture and the deoxyuridine suppression test by using whole blood (0.1 ml) instead of separated lymphocytes. *Clin. Chem.* **26**, 72.

16 Ek, J. (1983): Plasma, red cell, and breast milk folacin concentrations in lactating women. *Am. J. Clin. Nutr.* **38**, 929–935.

17 Ettinger, S. & Colman, N. (1985): Altered relationship between red cell and serum folate in the aged, suggesting impaired erythrocyte folate transport. *Fed. Proc.* **44**, 1283.

18 FAO/WHO Expert Group (1970): *Requirements of ascorbic acid, vitamin D, vitamin B_{12}, folate and iron.* WHO Tech. Rep. Ser. No. 452. Geneva: World Health Organization.

19 Gailani, S.D., Carey, R.W., Holland, J.F. & O'Malley, J.A. (1970): Studies of folate deficiency in patients with neoplastic diseases. *Cancer Res.* **30**, 327–333.

20 Green, R., Kuhl, W., Jacobson, R., Johnson, C., Carmel, R. & Beutler, R. (1982): Masking of macrocytosis by α-thalassemia in blacks with pernicious anemia. *New. Engl. J. Med.* **307**, 1322.

21 Herbert, V. (1962): Experimental nutritional folate deficiency in man. *Trans Ass. Am. Physns.* **75**, 307–320.

22 Herbert, V. (1962): Minimal daily adult folate requirement. *Archs. Int. Med.* **110**, 649–652.

23 Herbert, V. (1963): Current concepts in therapy: megaloblastic anemia. *New Engl. J. Med.* **268**, 201–203; 368–371.

24 Herbert, V. (1964): Studies of folate deficiency in man. *Proc. Roy. Soc. Med.* **57**, 377–384.

25 Herbert, V. (1968): Nutritional requirements for vitamin B_{12} and folic acid. *Am. J. Clin. Nutr.* **21**, 743–752.

26 Herbert, V. (1977): Folic acid requirement in adults (including pregnant and lactating females) (pp. 247–255); Summary of the workshop (pp. 277–293). In *Folic acid: biochemistry and physiology in relation to the human nutrition requirement*. National Research Council. Washington DC: Food and Nutritional Board, National Academy of Sciences.

27 Herbert, V. (1981): Nutritional anaemias of childhood — folate, B_{12}: The megaloblastic anemias. In *Textbook of pediatric nutrition* pp. 133–144. ed R.M. Suskind New York: Raven Press.

28 Herbert, V. (1985): Biology of disease: megaloblastic anaemia. *Lab. Invest.* **52**, 3–19.

29 Herbert, V. & Das, K.C. (1976): The role of vitamin B_{12} and folic acid in hemato- and other cell-poiesis. *Vit. Hormones* **34**, 1–30.

30 Herbert, V & Zalusky, R. (1962): Interrelations of vitamin B_{12} and folic acid metabolism: folic acid clearance studies. *J. Clin. Invest.* **41**, 1263–1276.

31 Herbert, V., Colman, N. & Jacob, E. (1980): Folic acid and vitamin B_{12}. In *Modern nutrition in health and disease*, ed R.S. Goodhart & M.E. Shils, pp. 229–259. Philadelphia: Lea & Febiger.

32 Herbert, V., Drivas, G., Manusselis, C., Mackler, B., Eng, J. & Schwartz, E. (1984): Are colon bacteria a major source of cobalamin analogues in human tissues? 24-hour human stool contains only abot 5 µg cobalamin but about 100 µg apparent analogue (and 200 µg folate). *Trans Ass. Am. Physns.* **97**, 161–171.

33 Herbert, V., Colman, N. & Drivas, G. (1985): A proposed model of sequential stages in the development of folate deficiency anemia. *Blood* **66**, (Suppl. 1). (In press)

34 Hoogstraten, B., Cuttner, J. & Natovitz, B. (1964): Sequence of recovery from multiple manifestations of folic acid deficiency. *J. Mt. Sinai Hosp.* **31**, 10–16.

35 Hoppner, K. & Lampi, B. (1980): Folate levels in human liver from autopsies in Canada. *Am. J. Clin. Nutr.* **33**, 862–864.

36 Lindenbaum, J. (1977): Folic acid requirement in situations of increased need. In *Folic acid: Biochemistry and physiology in relation to the human nutrition requirement*, pp. 256–276. National Research Council. Washington, DC: Food and Nutrition Board, National Academy of Sciences.

37 Lindenbaum, J. & Nath, B. (1980): Megaloblastic anaemia and neutrophil hypersegmentation. *Br. J. Haemat.* **44**, 551.

38 Marshall, R.A. & Jandl, J.H. (1960): Response to 'physiologic' doses of folic acid on megaloblastic anemia. *Archs. Int. Med.* **105**, 352.

39 Metz, J., Kelly, A., Swett, V.C., Waxman, S. & Herbert, V. (1968): Deranged DNA synthesis by bone marrow from vitamin B_{12} deficient humans. *Br. J. Haemat.* **14**, 575.

40 National Research Council (1977): *Folic acid: biochemistry and physiology in relation to the human nutrition requirement.* Washington, DC: Food and Nutrition Board, National Academy of Sciences.

41 Noronha, J.M. & Silverman, M. (1962): On folic acid, vitamin B_{12}, methionine, and formiminnoglutamate metabolism. In *Vitamin B_{12} and intrinsic factor*, 2nd Eur. Symp. pp. 728–736. ed H.C. Heinrich. Stuttgart: Ferdinand Enke.

42 Ran, J.-Y., Colman, N., Wang, Y.L., Drivas, G. & Herbert, V. (1985): Folate and B_{12} status in young and elderly without/with carcinoma in China. *Clin. Res.* **33**, 760A.

43 Rosenberg, I.H., Bowman, B.B., Cooper, B.A., Halsted, C.H. & Lindenbaum, J. (1982): Folate nutrition in the elderly. In 'Symposium on the evidence relating selected vitamins and minerals to health and disease in the elderly population in the United States'. *Am. J. Clin. Nutr.* **36** (Suppl), 1060–1066.

44 Russell, R.M., Krasinski, S.D. & Samloff, I.M. (1984): Correction of impaired folic acid (PteGlu) absorption by orally administered HCl in subjects with gastric atrophy. *Clin. Res.* **32**, 633A.

45 Salmi, H.A. (1963): Comparative studies on vitamin B_{12} in developing organism and placenta. *Ann. Acad. Sci. Fenn.* **103** (Suppl.).

46 Shane, B. & Stoksted, E.L.R. (1985): Vitamin B_{12}-folate interrelations. *Ann. Rev. Nutr.* **5**, 115–141.

47 Steinberg, S.E., Fonda, S., Campbell, C.L. & Hillman, R.S. (1983): Cellular abnormalities of folate deficiency. *Br. J. Haemat.* **54**, 605–612.

48 Spring, J.A., Robertson, J. & Buss, D.H. (1979): Trace nutrients. 3. Magnesium, copper, zinc, vitamin B_6, vitamin B_{12}, and folic acid in the British national household food supply. *Br. J. Nutr.* **41**, 487–493.

49 Weir, D.G., McGing, P.G. & Scott, J.M. (1985): Commentary: folate metabolism, the enterohepatic circulation and alcohol. *Biochem. Pharmacol.* **34**, 1–7.

50 WHO (1968): *Nutritional anemias: report of a WHO scientific group.* WHO Tech. Rep. Ser. No. 405. Geneva: World Health Organization.

51 Wu, A.I., Chanarin, I., Slavin, G. & Levi, A.J. (1975): Folate deficiency in the alcoholic — its relationship to clinical and haematological abnormalities, liver disease, and folate stores. *Br. J. Haemat.* **29**, 469–478.

52 Zalusky, R. & Herbert, V. (1961): Megaloblastic anaemia in scurvy with response to 50 μg folic acid daily. *New Engl. J. Med.* **265**, 1033–1038.

Update on folate-binding proteins

Madeleine A. KANE*, J.F. KOLHOUSE and S. WAXMAN
Chemotherapy Foundation Laboratory, Departments of Neoplastic Diseases and Medicine, Mount Sinai Medical Center, 1 Gustave L. Levy Place, New York, New York 10029 and (JFK) Division of Hematology, Department of Medicine, University of Colorado Health Sciences Center, 4200 E. Ninth Avenue, Denver, Colorado 80262, USA.

The essential role of folates in cellular biochemistry is well-established, but the nature of the participation by folate binding proteins has been disputed. The term folate binding protein should be reserved for the high-affinity folate binding proteins which have affinity constants (K_a) for folic acid (PteGlu) in the range 10^{-9}–10^{-10}M. Folate binding proteins are a family of immunologically cross-reactive glycoproteins which exist in particulate and soluble forms.

Folate binding protein: a saturable membrane carrier? The mechanisms of folate uptake by cells has been controversial. This may be the result of transport studies using cells grown in tissue culture media which contain $2 - 4 \times 10^{-6}$M folic acid, 100-fold higher than the normal plasma folate concentration. A folate uptake with specificity for reduced folates and K_a about

*Dr Kane is the recipient of a Charles Revson Foundation Fellowship and a National Research Service Award

10^{-6}M has been proposed as the relevant physiologic folate transport system[4,5,7,13]. That these affinity constants are two to three orders of magnitude lower than those reported for other recognized membrane receptors has been largely ignored, as has the fact that the observed uptake occurs in a concentration range 100-times higher than the folate concentration in human plasma (10–50 nM).

In contrast the membrane-associated folate binding protein possesses properties which make it a logical candidate for the physiologic folate transport protein. Not only is the affinity of folate binding proteins for PteGlu in the range of other receptors for their ligands, but it is also high for $CH_3H_4PteGlu$, and is the ligand of choice for future studies of folate binding proteins.

At normal plasma folate concentrations, unlike the putative reduced folate transport system, folate binding proteins would be saturated with endogenous ligand. In fact, endogenous folate must be removed in order to expose folate binding sites in milk. Folate binding proteins appear to be integral membrane proteins which have been identified on the surfaces of cells, eg human erythrocytes[3], human nasopharyngeal epidermoid carcinoma cells[2], myeloblasts[14]. Thus membrane-associated folate binding proteins have physiological ligand affinity in the proper range, exist saturated with endogenous ligand under physiological conditions, and are in the proper location to function as folate transport proteins. Examples of experimental data that support a transport function follow.

Studies of human nasopharyngeal epidermoid carcinoma (KB) cells in culture. KB cells contain large amounts of membrane-associated folate binding protein compared with other human cells[11]. They can be maintained in medium containing near physiological folate levels (> 10 nM)[10]. After five or six passes through this low folate medium, the folate content of KB cells fell to 4 pmol per 10^6 cells, their doubling time increased, the cells became megaloblastic; however, after 12–15 passes in this medium, their growth rate and their morphology returned to normal compared with cells maintained in the usual high folate medium[10]. Specific folate uptake by intact KB cells which were adapted to physiological folate levels increased ten-fold for (^{3}H)PteGlu, and more than 40-fold for (^{14}C)$CH_3H_4PteGlu$; the K_a for uptake was 5 nM and 6 nM (if only the 1-diastereomer of $CH_3H_4PteGlu$ is considered), respectively. Folate uptake was inhibited in a dose-dependent manner by anti-human placental folate receptor anti-serum, but not control serum (both sera were exhaustively dialysed to remove free folate), suggesting that an immunologically cross-reactive folate binding protein was involved in the uptake[2].

Two folate binding proteins were found in KB cells: a soluble folate binding protein, which they released into their growth medium, but which was not present in the cells, and a cellular folate binding protein with the characteristics of an integral membrane protein[8–10]. This compartmentation provided a convenient model for studying the biochemical interrelationship of the two folate binding proteins (See next Section).

In the KB cells adapted to near physiological folate concentrations, the levels of both the membrane-associated and soluble folate binding proteins were elevated four-to-five-fold as measured either by (^{3}H)PteGlu binding after endogenous folate removal or by radioimmunoassay, indicating regulation by extracellular folate concentration[8]. $CH_3H_4PteGlu$ exhibited high-affinity binding to the purified membrane-associated folate binding protein[9]. The KB cell membrane-associated folate binding protein bound large amounts of Triton X-100, consistent with the hydrophobicity of its membrane location[1,9]. While 40 per cent of the total cell-associated folate binding protein was released intact from the cell surface by trypsin treatment of intact KB cells, the remainder was associated with intracellular membranes[2]. The intracellular portion may, in part, be due to folate receptor recycling and may function in controlling the availability of intracellular folate coenzymes.

The biochemical interrelationship of the soluble and membrane-associated folate binding proteins. The immunologic cross-reactivity of the two forms of folate binding proteins demonstrates a close structural homology between them. This has led to the speculation that soluble folate binding proteins arise by specific proteolytic cleavage of the membrane-associated folate binding protein precursor[12] or that the particulate folate binding proteins may consist of subunits of the soluble folate binding proteins. The subunit relationship was initially supported by the observations that a large and a small folate binding protein could be identified in many tissues, eg milk, serum, placenta. In the presence of Triton X-100, the large folate binding protein had an $M_r = 160\,000$, and the small folate binding protein, an $M_r = 40\,000$[1,8]; however on sodium dodecyl sulfate (SDS) polyacrylamide gel electrophoresis (PAGE), both had $M_r = 40\,000$[1,8]. However, when the degree of detergent binding was determined based on sedimentation by sucrose density gradient ultracentrifugation in water and in deuterium oxide, 75 per cent of the M_r of the large folate binding protein was due to bound Triton X-100. In addition, detergent has been observed to enhance folate binding. The folate binding protein purified from cow's whey exhibited a five-to-ten-fold increase in (^{3}H)PteGlu binding in the presence of the detergents Triton X-100 (0.8–1 per cent) or cetyltrimethylammonium bromide (5–10·mM) or in serum[6]. Although this folate binding protein was purified without detergent being present and had an $M_r = 29\,800$ by sedimentation equilibrium, this activation by detergent suggests that it may be predominantly the particulate form.

The calculated molecular weights for the purified soluble milk proteins are all very similar (30 000) and consistently slightly lower than the calculated molecular weights for the purified particulate proteins (except for rat kidney). This supports the hypothesis that the particulate folate binding protein is anchored in the cell membrane by a tail of hydrophobic amino acids, and that the extracellular portion is cleaved, with the folate binding site intact, to release the soluble folate binding protein. For example, the soluble serum folate binding protein in adult serum may arise from a hepatic membrane-associated folate binder; fetal serum folate binding protein may arise primarily from the placental folate receptor; urine folate binding protein may arise from that in the renal tubule brush border membrane, and soluble folate binder in cerebrospinal fluid may arise from the choroid plexus.

The observation that KB cells grown in tissue culture release soluble folate binding protein into their medium, but the membrane-associated folate binding protein is the only cell-associated one, provides a convenient model system for studying the biochemical relationship of the two proteins. Pulse-chase studies in which KB-cell folate binding proteins were endogenously labelled with (^{35}S)methionine, purified, and their specific activities determined at various times after the pulse, produced results consistent with a precursor-product relationship[8].

Conclusions. Folate binding proteins, which possess high affinity for PteGlu and CH_3H_4PteGlu, the major extracellular physiologic folate, exist in two immunologically related forms: (1) soluble extracellular, cytosolic and vesicular proteins, and (2) particulate integral membrane proteins. The membrane-associated folate binding proteins are probably involved in folate translocation across cell membranes, and may control the availability of folate coenzymes inside the cell as well. The soluble folate binding proteins appear to be a heterogeneous group with diverse functions. Current evidence suggests that the two folate binding proteins in human KB cells and human milk are related in the precursor-product manner. Extracellular folate concentration regulates the levels of both the soluble and membrane-associated folate binding proteins in human KB cells, but the metabolic level at which this regulation occurs requires further study.

1 Antony, A.C., Utley, C.S., Marcell, P.D. & Kolhouse, J.F. (1982): Isolation, characterization and comparison of the solubilized particulate and soluble folate binding proteins from human milk. *J. Biol. Chem.* **257**, 10081–10089.
2 Antony, A.C., Kane, M.A. & Kolhouse, J.F. (1983): Characterization of a membrane protein involved in folate transport by malignant human cells. *Blood* **62**, 35a.
3 Antony, A.C., Kane, M.A. & Kolhouse, J.F. (1985): Identification and characterization of a human erythrocyte membrane folate receptor. *Clin. Res.* **33**, 333A.
4 Chabner, B.A. (1982): Methotrexate. In *Pharmacologic principles of cancer treatment*, ed B. Chabner, pp. 229–255. Philadelphia: W.B. Saunders.
5 Goldman, I.D. (1971): The characteristics of membrane transport of amethopterin and the naturally occurring folates. *Ann. NY Acad. Sci.* **186**, 400–422.
6 Hansen, S.I., Holm, J. & Lyngbye, J. (1982): Detergent activation of the binding protein in the folate radioassay. *Clin. Chem.* **28**, 117–118.
7 Henderson, G.B., Grzelakowska-Sztabert, B., Zevely, E.M. & Huennekens, F.M. (1980): Binding properties of the 5-methyl-tetrahydrofolate-methotrexate transport system in L1210 cells. *Archs. Biochem. Biophys.* **202**, 144–149.
8 Kane, M.A., Antony, A.C. & Kolhouse, J.F. (1984): The inter-relationship of the two folate binding proteins of human head and neck cancer cells. *Clin. Res.* **32**, 310a.

9 Kane, M.A., Antony, A.C. & Kolhouse, J.F. (1984): Folic acid and N[5]methyltetrahydrofolate share a common membrane-associated binding protein in KB cells. *Blood* **64**, 40a.

10 Kane, M.A., Kolhouse, J.F. Schreiber, C. & Waxman, S. (1985): Human cancer cells with an extremely low folate requirement. *Clin. Res.* **33**, 577A.

11 McHugh, M. & Cheng, Y.C. (1979): Demonstration of a high affinity folate binder in human cell membranes and its characterization in cultured human KB cells. *J. Biol. Chem.* **254**, 11312–11318.

12 Rothenberg, S.P., Fischer, C.D. & da Costa, M. (1978): Binding of N^5,N^{10}-methylene tetrahydrofolate and the inhibition of thymidylate synthesis by a folate binding protein. *Biochim. Biophys. Acta* **543**, 340–348.

13 Sirotnak, F.M. (1980): Correlates of folate analog transport, pharmacokinetics and selective antitumor action. *Pharmacol. Ther.* 71–101.

14 Waxman, S. (1979): Studies on the origin of serum folate binding protein. In *Chemistry and biology of pteridines*, ed R.L. Kisliuk & G.M. Brown, pp. 619–624. North Holland: Elsevier.

Vitamin B$_{12}$ (cobalamin, Cbl)-binding proteins

Sally P. STABLER and R.H. ALLEN
Division of Hematology, Department of Medicine, University of Colorado Health Sciences Center, 4200 E. 9th Avenue, Denver, CO 80262, USA.

As indicated in Table 1 the cobalamin (Cbl)-binding proteins can be divided into three groups based on their localization and functional properties. These groups consist of the three well-characterized extracellular Cbl-transport proteins, the two intracellular Cbl-dependent enzymes, and an uncertain number of intracellular Cbl-transport proteins which must exist, although that have neither been identified nor characterized.

Table 1. *Mammalian Cbl-binding proteins*

I. Extracellular Cbl-transport proteins
  (1) R protein
  (2) Intrinsic factor
  (3) Transcobalamin II
II. Intracellular Cbl-dependent enzymes
  (1) L-methylmalonyl-CoA mutase
  (2) Methionine synthetase

III. Intracellular Cbl-transport proteins
  (1) Lyososomal export?
  (2) Mitochondrial import?
  (3) Mitochondrial export?
  (4) Cellular export?
    (a) General?
    (b) Ileal?
    (c) Hepatic?
      (i) Plasma?
      (ii) Biliary?

Table 2. *Quantitative daily cellular uptake of endogenous Cbl from normal human plasma*[3]

Cbl-transport proteins	Endogenous plasma Cbl (total µg)	Half-life for Cbl clearance (h)	Cbl clearance (µg/24 h)	Site of clearance
Transcobalamin I	0.6–0.8	240	< 0.1	Unknown
Transcobalamin II	0.1–0.2	0.1	15–30	Many cell types
Transcobalamin III	0.0–0.1	0.05	0–30	Hepatocytes
Total	0.90		15–60	

Extracellular Cbl-transport proteins. Three classes of extracellular Cbl-transport proteins exist, ie 'R' protein, intrinsic factor and transcobalamin II. The amino acid portion of each of these proteins has a molecular weight of approximately 40 000 and consists of a single polypeptide chain with a single Cbl-binding site. Despite these similarities, each of the three classes is coded for by a separate structural gene, and these proteins differ structurally, immunologically, and in their functional characteristics[1,11].

R protein and intrinsic factor are both involved in the gastrointestinal transport of Cbl. Once liberated from food protein by HCl and pepsin in the stomach, dietary CBl is bound by R protein which has a much higher affinity for Cbl at acid pH than does intrinsic factor. In the jejunum, pancreatic proteases partially degrade the R protein moiety, and the Cbl is then transferred to intrinsic factor. The formation of the intrinsic factor-Cbl complex is essential for Cbl absorption, since ileal receptors bind intrinsic factor-Cbl with high affinity while failing to bind R protein-Cbl or free Cbl. The functional advantage in having Cbl bound to R protein in gastric juice in unknown, but could involve protection of Cbl or the destruction of Cbl analogues[2,9].

A number of uncertainties exist concerning the ileal phase of Cbl absorption including such critical areas as to how Cbl enters ileal mucosal cells, how Cbl exits from ileal mucosal cells, and the nature of the role and fate of intrinsic factor during these processes[4].

Cbl in plasma is bound to one of the three transcobalamins (transCbl) known as transcobalamin I, transcobalamin II, and transcobalamin III. transCbl I and transCbl III are R proteins. How and at what point Cbl becomes bound to these three proteins is unknown. It is possible that Cbl becomes bound to transCbl II within ileal mucosal cells, but this is far from established. Even if Cbl does bind to transCbl II within ileal mucosal cells, it is unclear whether ileal mucosal cells actually synthesize significant amounts of transCbl II, since it is possible that transCbl II might be taken up and utilized from plasma[1,4,11].

As Table 2 shows, transCbl II is the most important Cbl-transport protein based both on the amount of Cbl actually transported from plasma to cells and on the fact that only transCbl II facilitates the uptake of Cbl by many and probably all cells within the body. transCbl III may transport a significant amount of Cbl, but delivers Cbl only to hepatocytes. transCbl I contains the majority of Cbl present in plasma, but is probably unimportant since its prolonged plasma survival results in an insignificant amount of Cbl-transport, and since it does not appear to facilitate Cbl uptake by any cell[1,3,11].

The mechanism by which transCbl II facilitates the uptake of Cbl by cells involves the sequential binding of transCbl II to cell surface receptors, internalization, formation of secondary lysosomes, and finally degradation of transCbl II with the subsequent release of Cbl. The initial binding to cell surface receptors is mediated by the transCbl II moiety and occurs irrespective of whether the Cbl-binding site is empty, occupied by Cbl, or occupied by a wide variety of Cbl analogues that bind to transCbl II with high affinity[1,3,11].

The mechanism by which transCbl III mediates the uptake of Cbl by hepatocytes is very similar to that utilized by transCbl II, although the receptors for transCbl III are clearly different. They consist of the well-characterized receptors for asialoglycoproteins and bind to oligosaccharide side chains that contain terminal galactose residues. The initial binding to cell surface receptors is mediated by the transCbl III moiety and occurs regardless of whether the Cbl-binding site is empty, occupied by Cbl, or occupied by a wide variety of Cbl analogues that bind to transCbl III with high affinity[1,3,11].

Intracellular Cbl-dependent enzymes. The vast majority of intracellular Cbl is bound to the two mammalian Cbl-dependent enzymes, L-methylmalonyl-CoA mutase and methionine synthetase. The mutase is located within mitochondria, utilizes adenosyl-Cbl as an essential cofactor, and catalyses the conversion of L-methylmalonyl-CoA to succinyl-CoA. The synthetase is located in the cytoplasm, utilizes methyl-Cbl as an essential cofactor, and catalyses the conversion of N^5-methyltetrahydrofolate and homocysteine to tetrahydrofolate and methionine, respectively[5,6,13].

At least 80 per cent of intracellular Cbl is tightly bound to the two Cbl-dependent enzymes with the remainder being present in unbound form. A storage form of Cbl does not exist. The proportion of Cbl bound to the mutase and the proportion bound to the synthetase varies greatly among different tissues (Table 3). What factors regulate the marked differences in distribution of Cbl between these two enzymes is not known[7,8,10,13].

The amount of intracellular Cbl is much less than that required to saturate both

Table 3. *Distribution of intracellular Cbl between the two mammalian Cbl-dependent enzymes in various tissues.* (Values represent the percentage of Cbl bound to the enzyme).

Tissue	L-methylmalonyl-CoA mutase	Methionine synthetase
Rabbit liver[7]	95	5
Rat liver[8]	60	40
Human placenta[13]	20	80
Human fibroblasts[10]	5	95

Table 4. *Effects on rats of subcutaneous injections of 500 μg of OH-Cbl every other day for 14 d. Eight control and eight experimental animals were studied.* (Values represent concentrations as % of the control).

Serum Cbl: 5200* *Liver Cbl:* 490* *Liver methylmalonyl-CoA mutase:* 170*

Liver methionine synthetase: 270* *Serum methylmalonic acid:* 41* *Serum succinic acid:* 130

Serum homocysteine: 63* *Serum methionine:* 100 *Serum cysteine:* 93

*$P < 0.01$ (significantly different from the control).

Cbl-dependent enzymes. Mutase is only 5–10 per cent saturated with Cbl and it appears likely that the synthetase is also only partially saturated with Cbl[6–8,10,13]. These observations suggest that there may be some advantage in limiting the amount of intracellular Cbl and that this limitation might be utilized to regulate the activities of the two Cbl-dependent enzymes. Recent studies, which are summarized in Table 4, indicate that the amount of intracellular Cbl is, in fact, rate-limiting for both of the mammalian Cbl-dependent enzymes. This conclusion is based on the fact that the levels of both enzymes increase following the administration of Cbl to laboratory animals. More importantly, these changes are not *in vitro* artifacts, since serum levels of methylmalonic acid and homocysteine both decrease significantly following such Cbl administration. The rationale or advantage in limiting and regulating the activities of both Cbl-dependent enzymes is unknown.

Intracellular Cbl-transport proteins. The extracellular Cbl-transport proteins described above are required for the cellular uptake of Cbl, since Cbl is a relatively large, water soluble vitamin that diffuses poorly across cell membranes. This property also makes it extremely likely that intracellular Cbl-binding proteins exit to facilitate the transport of Cbl across membranes of intracellular organelles, and across plasma membranes during the process by which Cbl exits from cells, although such proteins have not been identified, much less characterized. It appears likely, for example, that some type of Cbl-binding protein exists to facilitate the exit of Cbl from lysosomes which occurs following the lysosomal degradation of transCbl II and transCbl III. Cbl-binding proteins would also appear to exist for the poorly understood processes by which Cbl is taken up by mitochondria and released from this intracellular organelle.

Finally, Cbl-binding proteins would appear to be required for the mechanisms by which Cbl exits from cells following the uptake of transCbl II-Cbl and transCbl III-Cbl. The situation with respect to hepatocytes is particularly interesting, since Cbl can exit from these cells either into bile or by returning to plasma. Studies performed with a number of Cbl analogues indicate that these two exit processes are saturable, and that they have structural specificities that differ from each other and from the structural specificities of each of the extracellular Cbl-transport proteins, R protein, intrinsic factor, and transCbl II. These studies indicate that different Cbl-transport proteins exist for biliary release and for plasma release of Cbl[7].

The case for the existence of unidentified intracellular Cbl-transport proteins has recently been strengthened by the description of a patient with the phenotype of Cbl deficiency, but in whom the defect was actually localized to an inability of Cbl to be released from lysosomes. It is likely, although not proven, that this defect involves an abnormality or the lack of an intracellular Cbl-binding protein required for the export of Cbl from lysosomes[12].

1 Allen, R.H. (1975): Human vitamin B$_{12}$ transport proteins. *Prog. Hematol.* **9**, 57–84.
2 Allen, R.H., Seetharam, B., Podell, E.R. & Alpers, D.H. (1978): Effect of proteolytic enzymes on the binding of cobalamin to R protein and intrinsic factor. *In vitro* evidence that a failure to partially degrade R protein is responsible for cobalamin malabsorption in pancreatic insufficiency. *J. Clin. Invest.* **61**, 47–54.

3 Allen, R.H. (1976): Annotation: The plasma transport of vitamin B_{12}. *Br. J. Haematol.* **33**, 161–171.

4 Donaldson, R.M., Jr. (1985): Editorial: How does cobalamin (vitamin B_{12}) enter and traverse the ileal cell? *Gastroenterology* **88**, 1069–1076.

5 Kolhouse, J.F. & Allen, R.H. (1977): Recognition of two intracellular cobalamin-binding proteins and their identification as methylmalonyl-CoA mutase and methionine synthetase. *Proc. Natl. Acad. Sci. USA* **74**, 921–925.

6 Kolhouse, J.F., Utley, C.S. & Allen, R.H. (1980): Isolation and characterization of methylmalonyl-CoA mutase from human placenta. *J. Biol. Chem.* **255**, 2708–2712.

7 Kolhouse, J.F. & Allen, R.H. (1977): Absorption, plasma transport and cellular retention of cobalamin analogues in the rabbit. Evidence for the existence of multiple mechanisms that prevent the absorption and tissue dissemination of naturally occurring cobalamin analogues. *J. Clin. Invest.* **60**, 1381–1392.

8 Kondo, H., Osborne, M., Kolhouse, J.F., Binder, M.J., Podell, E.R. & Allen, R.H. (1981): Nitrous oxide has multiple deleterious effects on cobalamin-dependent enzymes in rats. *J. Clin. Invest.* **67**, 1270–1283.

9 Marcoullis, G., Parmentier, Y., Nicolas, J.P., Jimenez, M. & Gerard, P. (1980): Cobalamin malabsorption due to nondegradation of R proteins in the human intestine. *J. Clin. Invest.* **66**, 430–440.

10 Mellman, I., Willard, H.F. & Rosenberg, L.E. (1978): Cobalamin binding and cobalamin-dependent enzyme activity in normal and mutant human fibroblasts. *J. Clin. Invest.* **62**, 952–960.

11 Nexo, E. & Olesen, H. (1982): Intrinsic factor, transcobalamin and haptocorrin. In *B_{12}*, ed D. Dolphin, vol. 2, pp. 57–85. New York: John Wiley.

12 Rosenblatt, D.S., Hosack, A., Matiaszuk, N.V., Cooper, B.A. & Laframboise, R. (1985): Defect in vitamin B_{12} release from lysosomes: Newly described inborn error of vitamin B_{12} metabolism. *Science* **228**, 1319–1320.

13 Utley, C.S., Marcell, P.D., Allen, R.H., Antony, A.C. & Kolhouse, J.F. (1985): Isolation and characterization of methionine synthetase from human placenta. *J. Biol. Chem* (In press)

Role of the vitamin B_{12} and folate-binding proteins in milk

N.M.F. TRUGO and D.N. SALTER
Instituto de Nutricao, Universidade Federal de Rio de Janeiro, 21910 Rio de Janeiro — Brazil; Animal and Grassland Research Institute, Shinfield, Reading, Berkshire, RG2 9AQ, UK.

Both vitamin B_{12} and folate in milk are strongly attached to specific 'binder' proteins which, as in human milk and sow's milk, may be present in considerable excess. These vitamin-binding proteins may have an important physiological role. It has been suggested[4,5] that they may strongly influence the vitamin economy of the sucking mammal and the ecology of its intestinal microflora. The uptake *in vitro* of folic acid and vitamin B_{12} by a selection of bacteria commonly found in the small intestine is inhibited by unsaturated milk folate and B_{12} binders[4] and growth is prevented[2]. They may also act as a trapping mechanism to accumulate the vitamins from the maternal blood into milk. In addition, they may fulfil a protective role in the mammary gland, by inhibiting the growth of vitamin-dependent mastitis pathogens.

To postulate a role for these binders in the gut is to presuppose that they are not readily degraded by the gut proteases. In a study with 6-day-old kids a high proportion of the folate binding protein in goat's milk was resistant to digestion[8]. Experiments with piglets up to a month old similarly showed that about 80 per cent of the saturated and 50 per cent of the unsaturated vitamin B_{12} binder was resistant to proteolysis *in vivo*[15].

Influence of vitamin B_{12}-binding protein from milk on the absorption of vitamin B_{12}.
Intrinsic factor promotes the intestinal absorption of vitamin B_{12} in all the mammalian species that have so far been studied[1]. However, the absorption process has been investigated mainly in adult animals and the situation in the neonatal period may be different. It has been shown that sucking piglets absorbed and retained the vitamin efficiently in the first 2 weeks of life, despite the virtual absence of intrinsic factor, which becomes fully established by about 2 to 3 weeks after birth. The influence of the vitamin B_{12} binders from milk on absorption of vitamin B_{12} has been investigated more recently both *in vivo* and *in vitro*, using piglets as models and sow's milk as the source of binder[13,14].

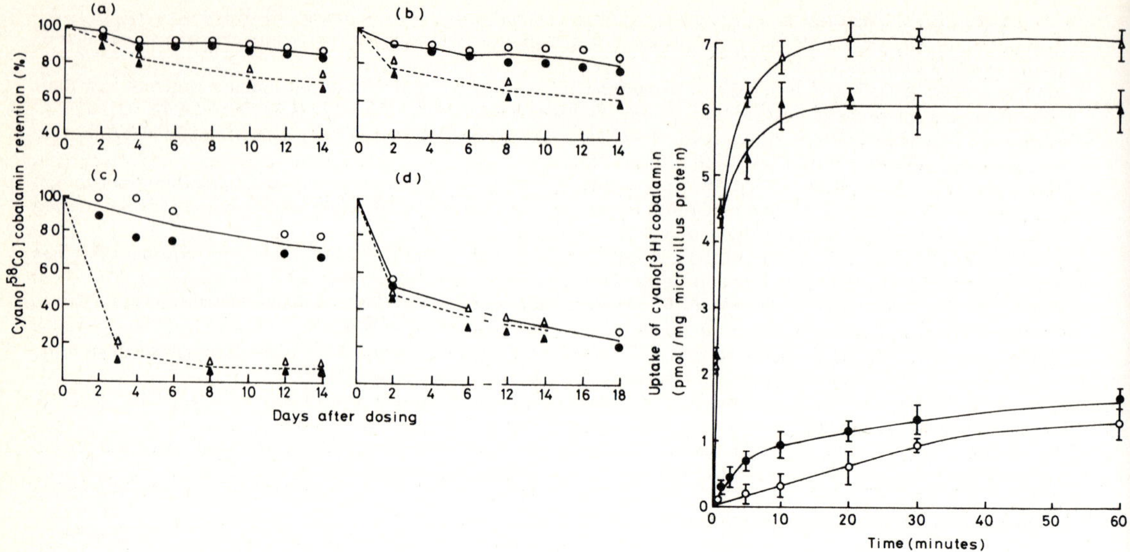

Fig. 1 (above, left). *Percentage retention over a period of 14 d (or 18 d) of a test dose of cyano [^{58}Co]-cobalamin given orally to suckled and weaned piglets at birth (a) and at 3 (b), 7 (c) and 14 (d) days post partum.* Suckled piglets: (○, ●), individual values; (———), mean. weaned piglets: (△, ▲), individual values; (-----), mean. The two piglets dosed at birth in the weaned group were kept with the sow for 2 d after dosing. At day 2 *post partum* they were then weaned with the remaining six piglets from the same litter[14].

Fig. 2 (above, right). *Time course of uptake of cyano [^{3}H]-cobalamin by microvillus membrane vesicles.* Membrane vesicles (0.05 mg protein) were incubated in buffer solution (50 mM HEPES/50 mM MES/50 mM NaCl/2 mM MgSO$_4$) at pH 7.0. The incubation mixtures contained 3 nmol cyano [^{3}H]-cobalamin/mg microvillus protein, without (○, ●) and with (△, ▲) an equivalent amount of vitamin B$_{12}$-binder. Vesicles were prepared from the lower small intestine of 7-d-old (○, △) and 28-d-old (●, ▲) piglets. Values are means ± sem of triplicate determinations[13].

Studies in vivo. From birth to 7 d of age suckled piglets consistently absorbed and retained a higher proportion of a single oral dose of cyano [^{58}Co]-cobalamin than did piglets receiving a diet containing no vitamin B$_{12}$-binder (Fig. 1)[13]. But by day 14 the efficiency of uptake by the suckled animals was similar to that in the early-weaned piglets, suggesting that by this stage intrinsic factor was regulating uptake in both groups. Since the milk binder might have facilitated uptake indirectly, by preventing uptake of vitamin B$_{12}$-binder by intestinal bacteria, the results obtained could not be interpreted unequivocally to demonstrate that the vitamin B$_{12}$-binder exerted a specific and direct effect on vitamin B$_{12}$ absorption.

Studies in vitro. Uptake of cyano [G^{3}H]-cobalamin or cyano [^{57}Co]-cobalamin by microvillus membrane vesicles prepared from the small intestine of piglets aged 7 and 28 d was strongly promoted by the vitamin B$_{12}$-binding protein isolated from sow's milk (Fig. 2)[13]. Uptake of bound vitamin B$_{12}$ was saturable, dependent on pH, the maximum uptake at around pH 7.0, and Mg^{2+} or Ca^{2+} were required for maximum uptake. Uptake of free vitamin B$_{12}$ was much less dependent on pH and was independent of Mg^{2+} and Ca^{2+}.

Kinetic analysis showed that the uptake of vitamin B$_{12}$ by the vesicles was a saturable process, and the Scatchard plot of equilibrium binding data revealed a single class of binding sites and a maximum binding capacity of 25–30 pmol/mg microvillus protein. The dissociation constant, K$_d$, was 0.53 and 0.57 μM for the bound vitamin, for vesicles isolated respectively from 7- and 28-d-old piglets. Attachment of the vitamin B$_{12}$-binder from sow's milk to the brush border membrane of intestinal epithelial cells was demonstrated in another experiment[12]. It occurred independently of the presence of the vitamin, as was evident from examination of the ileal mucosa of piglets, using an immunoflourescence technique, after incubation of the binder *in vivo* in ligated intestinal segments, in the presence and absence of vitamin B_{12}.

Using the preparations of microvillus membrane vesicles and radioiodinated binder, it was found that the binding sites were specific for the milk binder and that intrinsic factor did not compete for the same binding sites[13]. Intrinsic factor promoted uptake of vitamin B_{12} only in vesicles prepared from the lower third of the small intestine, as was expected, since intrinsic factor-mediated uptake of vitamin B_{12} is restricted to the ileum, in the pig as in other animal species[10]. Comparing the effects of intrinsic factor and the milk binder, the former was more effective in promoting vitamin B_{12} uptake in membrane vesicles from 28-d-old piglets whereas the milk binder had a greater effect in those from 7-d-old piglets. Thus, the milk binder may play only a transitory role in vitamin B_{12} absorption; the intrinsic-factor mechanism clearly becomes the predominant mode of uptake in the older animals. In the adult pig, as in man and in the guinea-pig, R-proteins from milk, saliva, gastric juice and blood plasma had no effect on vitamin B_{12} uptake by ileal mucosal homogenates[6].

The influence of folate binding protein in milk on the absorption of the folates. It has been shown[3] that uptake of folic acid by rat enterocytes was enhanced two- to three-fold when it was given in a bound form in skimmed goat's milk, but it was not shown unequivocally that the enhancement was caused by the specific folate binding protein.

Recently, it was shown[7] that the uptake of pteroylmonoglutamate and 5-methyltetrahydrofolate by brush border membrane vesicles and enterocytes isolated from the small intestine of 6 to 10-d-old kids was strongly promoted by folate binding protein isolated from goat's milk. With the membrane vesicles, uptake of 5-methyltetrahydrofolate was increased more than 100-fold, the degree of the increase being dependent on the molar ratio of binding protein to folate with an optimal effect at 1.0 to 2.5 (Table 1). Competitive binding tests

Table 1. *The effect of folate binding protein (FBP) on folate uptake by microvilli.* Microvilli were incubated with (^{14}C)–MTHF (0.5, 1 or 2 μM) together with various concentrations of FBP for 30 min. Microvilli were separated by filtration and assayed for radioactivity. Results are the means of six determinations. MTHF: 5-methyltetrahydrofolate.

	Folate uptake by microvilli (pmol MTHF/mg membrane protein)		
Initial MTHF concentration (μM):	0.5	1.0	2.0
Molar ratio FBP:MTHF			
0	0.4	1.2	2.0
0.25	12.5	11.1	42.9
0.50	22.0	25.5	80.3
1.0	50.2	76.8	276.0
2.5	71.9	149.0	294.0
5.0	77.8	119.0	49.7

with various milk proteins, albumins and binding proteins in 5-fold excess indicated that binding was specific for milk folate binding proteins, competition with bound ^{125}I-labelled goat's milk folate binding protein being observed only with goat's or cow's milk binders (Table 2). Kinetic studies and equilibrium binding data indicated that uptake of the binding protein and of bound folate were saturable processes. However, the Scatchard plot of the equilibrium binding data for the ^{125}I-labelled binding protein uptake by brush border membrane vesicles was non-linear, presumably in consequence of the microheterogeneity of the protein previously reported[9]. The observation that uptake of free folates by intestinal microvilli in the absence of the milk folate binding protein was very inefficient[11], amounting to only about 0.1 per cent of the dose at physiological concentrations, was confirmed. In the presence of the purified-milk folate binding protein folate uptake increased to 15 per cent of the added dose.

Table 2. *The competitive effect of other proteins on folate binding protein (FBP) binding.* Microvilli were incubated for 15 min with $10\,\mu g$ $(0.57\,\mu M)$ (^{125}I)-FBP and a five-fold (a–h) or 20-fold (i) molar excess of competing protein. Microvilli were separated by filtration and assayed for radioactivity. Results are the means of six determinations (except for (i)-3 determination), with s.e.m. in parentheses.

Competing protein	(^{125}I)-FBP uptake (μg-mg membrane protein)	[a]
(a) None	10.57 (0.85)	
(b) Bovine serum albumin	12.84 (3.1)	> 0.7
(c) α-Lactalbumin	12.31 (2.69)	0.7
(d) β-Lactoglobulin	7.64 (0.87)	0.2
(e) Ovalbumin	8.2 (0.89)	0.2
(f) Lactoferrin	8.56 (2.81)	0.6
(g) Cow's milk FBP	6.67 (2.05)	0.1
(h) Goat's milk FBP (5 ×)	6.41 (1.12)	0.05
(i) Goat's milk FBP (20 ×)·	1.4	< 0.01

[a]Student's t-test was applied to the values (compared with values in the absence of competing protein) and the results are shown as probabilities (P).

Acknowledgements. The authors thank Dr J.E. Ford for his suggestions and valued discussions.

1 Chanarin, I. (1979): *The megaloblastic anaemias*, 2nd edn, Oxford: Blackwell.

2 Cole, C.B., Scott, K.J., Henschel, M.J., Coates, M.E., Ford, J.E. & Fuller, R. (1983): Trace-nutrient-binding proteins in milk and the growth of bacteria in the gut of infant rabbits. *Br. J. Nutr.* **49**, 231–240.

3 Colman, N., Hettiarachy, N. & Herbert, V. (1981): Detection of a milk factor that facilitates folate uptake by intestinal cells. *Science* **211**, 1427–1429.

4 Ford, J.E. (1974): Some observations on the possible nutritional significance of vitamin B_{12}- and folate binding proteins in milk. *Br. J. Nutr.* **31**, 243–257.

5 Ford, J.E., Scott, K.J., Sansom, B.F. & Taylor, P.J. (1975): Some observations on the possible nutritional significance of vitamin B_{12}- and folate binding proteins in milk. Absorption of $[^{58}Co]$ cyano cobalamin by suckling piglets. *Br. J. Nutr.* **34**, 469–492.

6 Hooper, D., Alpers, D.H., Burger, D.H., Mehlman, C.S. & Allen, R.H. (1973): Characterization of ileal vitamin B_{12} binding using homogeneous human and hog intransic factors. *J. Clin. Invest.* **52**, 3074–3083.

7 Salter, D.N. & Blakeborough, P. (1985): Folate transport in the small intestine of the neonatal kid: the influence of milk folate binder on uptake by isolated enterocytes and microvilli. *National Institute for Research in Dairying, Report 1984–5.* University of Reading, 1985.

8 Salter, D.N. & Mowlem, A. (1983): Neonatal role of milk folate binding protein: studies on the course of digestion of goat's milk folate binder in the 6-day-old kid. *Br. J. Nutr.* **50**, 589–596.

9 Salter, D.N., Scott, K.J., Slade, H. & Andrews, P. (1981): The preparation and properties of folate binding protein from cow's milk. *Biochem. J.* **193**, 469–476.

10 Seetharam, B. & Alpers, D.H. (1982): Absorption and transport of cobalamin (vitamin B_{12}). *Abstr. Rev. Nutr.* **2**, 343–370.

11 Selhub, J. & Rosenberg, I.H. (1981): Folate transport in isolated brush border membrane vesicles from rat intestine. *J. Biol. Chem.* **256**, 4489–4493.

12 Trugo, N.M.F. (1984): Vitamin B_{12} absorption in the neonatal piglet. Studies on the physiological role of vitamin B_{12}-binding protein in milk. PhD Thesis, University of Reading.

13 Trugo, N.M.F., Ford, J.E. & Salter, D.N. (1985): Vitamin B_{12} absorption in the neonatal piglet. 3. Influence of vitamin B_{12}-binding protein from sow's milk on uptake of vitamin B_{12} by microvillus membrane vesicles prepared from small intestine of the piglet. *Br. J. Nutr.* **54**, 269–284.

14 Trugo, N.M.F., Ford, J.E. & Sansom, B.F. (1985): Vitamin B_{12} absorption in the neonatal piglet. 1. Studies in vivo on the influence of the vitamin B_{12}-binding protein from sow's milk on the absorption of vitamin B_{12} and related compounds. *Br. J. Nutr.* **54**, 245–256.

15 Trugo, N.M.F. & Newport, M.J.. (1985): Vitamin B_{12} absorption in the neonatal piglet. 2. Resistance of the vitamin B_{12}-binding protein in sow's milk to proteolysis in vivo. *Br. J. Nutr.* **54**, 257–268.

Folates in embryonic development and old age

C.J. SCHORAH and N. HABIBZADEH
Departments of Paediatrics and Chemical Pathology, University of Leeds, Leeds LS2 9JT, UK.

Folic acid itself, pteroylmonoglutamate, comprises only about 1 per cent of the folate of the average diet. Other biologically active derivates found in the diet of man are produced from folic acid by reduction, further conjugation with glutamic acid and combination with 1C components in various oxidation states. For our purposes here, however, the terms folic acid and folate will be applied generally to folic acid and its metabolites with biological activity in man.

The metabolism of folic acid is complex. Our knowledge of this process is incomplete, and this causes uncertainty when we consider the role of, and requirements for, folic acid in man. We may find that folate requirements are no more than those which are needed to prevent overt macrocytic anaemia. The current evidence, however, particularly during pregnancy and old age suggests that this is not the case.

It is these two population groups that we wish to examine in more detail. For simplicity we will largely be considering folate alone but this is artificial. It is unusual in man to find a single nutrient depletion in the presence of an adequate supply of others. In addition, the metabolism of folic acid itself involves other essential micronutrients[17]. It is therefore important to remember that if folate supplies are insufficient for optimum health the body will also probably lack other nutrients.

Folate requirements during embryonic development. In industrialized societies individuals are arguably closer to the threshold of overt deficiency of folic acid than they are for almost any other organic micronutrient. This is illustrated by the number of pregnant women who develop folate deficiency and become anaemic unless they receive folate supplements[2,3,7]. There is little evidence to suggest that this folate deficiency produces serious effects on the fetus in late pregnancy[15], although there may be some reduction in fetal weight[8]. However, it has been observed that some fetal malformations, especially neural tube defects (NTD), which arise early in pregnancy, occur most frequently in those populations with the poorest diet[10]. Low average levels of folic acid along with some decrease in vitamin C have also been found in early pregnancy in women who subsequently gave birth to an NTD-affected infant[21].

An unrandomized trial of multivitamin supplements has recently suggested that a considerable reduction in the prevalence of the condition can be affected by appropriate periconceptional multivitamin supplementation[20]. Whilst a multivitamin supplement was given in these studies, the most likely effective agent is folic acid. This is because of its known role in cell division and because a smaller randomized study has suggested that folic acid alone was effective in reducing the prevalence of NTD[9].

Folate in general embryonic development. If adequate folate provision is important for rapidly dividing neural tissue, one might expect it to be equally essential for general embryonic development. Severe lack of an essential micronutrient will often have disastrous effects on the development of the fetus[5]. We have attempted to study the effect of less severe nutrient depletion by examining maternal depletion of folic acid in the pregnant guinea-pig.

Folic acid intakes in the guinea-pigs were adjusted during early pregnancy (3rd to 17th day) so that no effects of deficiency were observed in maternal white or red cell morphology, weight gain, food intake, or general health and activity. These intakes of folic acid ($106 \pm 8\,\mu g/d$), which we have called intermediate, were similar to those that had been recommended by some workers for the adult guinea-pig[14].

Maternal blood levels of folic acid and outcome of pregnancy in these guinea-pigs were compared with those that had been supplied with folic acid at approximately four times this intake (Tables 1, 2). Blood levels are considerably lower in the intermediate group and are not

Table 1. *Average folic acid intakes during days 3–17 of pregnancy with blood levels measured on day 17 in two groups of guinea-pigs given different folic acid intakes.*

		Folic acid (mean values ± s.d.)		
Folate intake	*No. of animals*	*Intake (μg/d)*	*Serum (μg/l)*	*Erythrocyte (μg/l)*
Intermediate	41	106 ± 8	1.1 ± 1.7	83 ± 35
Supplemented	29	465 ± 61	8.0 ± 3.3	211 ± 77

Table 2. *Reproductive outcome in terms of number of live and dead fetuses on the 36–37 day of gestation (mean numbers ± s.d.) in two groups of guinea-pigs given different intakes of folic acid.* These results and those in Table 1 are the pooled values for two separate experiments, details of these and other experimental groups are reported in full elsewhere[6].

		Live		Resorbed or aborted		
Folate intake	*No. of pregnancies*	*Number*	*Mean per conception*	*Number*	*Mean per conception*	*Live as % of implantations*
Intermediate	41	74	1.8 ± 2.1	118	2.9 ± 2.2	38
Supplemented	29	113	3.9 ± 1.8	27	0.9 ± 1.6	81

dissimilar from the lowest levels seen in the maternal blood of some women during early pregnancy[21]. In terms and number of live fetsues and abortions the supplemented group does significantly better than the group receiving the intermediate intake. Indeed, the number of live fetuses in the supplemented group is rather better than the average outcome of pregnancy reported for this strain[4]. One other animal species, the rat, has been reported to be affected by marginal folate deficiency during early pregnancy[13].

It is always dangerous to extrapolate from animal models to the human, but an increase nutrient recommendation is only made in women in the second and third trimesters. The guinea pig results might suggest that folate intakes ought also to be increased during the periconceptional period.

Folate in the elderly. In the United Kingdom the elderly appear to be at particular risk of undernutrition[19]. The cause of this would appear primarily to be reduced intake, with metabolic factors further compromising nutrition in acute disease[19]. Whilst the undernutrition tends to be non-specific, folate deficiency is a common finding. Folate deficiency occurs in patients presenting with acute psychiatric problems[16]. In a number of elderly subjects with mental illness and peripheral neuropathy, folate deficiency has been found to be the direct cause of their condition[1,11,12,22] and not all these patients had overt signs of folate deficiency such as macrocytic anaemia.

It is probable that folate deficiency is the cause of only a small proportion of diseases of the central nervous system, but folate deficiency, may lead to a less severe impairment of mental performance in a larger number of elderly subjects.

Low folate levels are also present in other elderly patients who are sick. We have examined the nutritional status of patients with fracture of the femur; their general nutritional status was poor, but in many the folic acid values were especially low compared with long-stay hospital patients of similar age (Table 3). Of those with low folates 50 per cent had a macrocytosis (mean cell volume > 96 fl) compared with only 10 per cent who had normal folates. The assessment of these patients was made within 24 h of the fracture and the trauma itself might have affected their serum folate concentrations. However, some of those who survived still had a low folate 6 months later (Table 3).

Increases in folate reserves following therapy. Whilst it remains speculative that improved folate intake in the two age groups that we have examined will lead to improvement in health, the indications are that some improvement can be expected. It is therefore necessary to enquire how we can increase the folate reserves of these populations.

Table 3. *Mean concentrations (± s.d.) of folic acid in the serum and red blood cells (RBC) of elderly female patients with fracture of the femur and of long-stay hospital patients of similar age, together with percentages of subjects showing folate deficiency.*

Patient group	No. subjects	Serum folate (μg/l)	% Subjects with low serum folate[a]	RBC folate (μg/l)	% Subjects with: Low RBC folate[b]	Macrocytosis[c]
Fracture						
On admission	24	2.3 ± 1.6	42	197 ± 87	30	29
6 months after fracture	8	2.7 ± 1.6	38	166 ± 59	25	38
Long-stay	15	4.9 ± 3.2	7	250 ± 117	14	7

[a] < 1.5 μg/l; [b] < 150 μg/l; [c] Mean corpuscular volume > 96 fl

Table 4. *Mean changes (± s.d.: range in parentheses) in blood folic acid concentration in five elderly women supplemented with 400 μg of folate/d and in six controls given a placebo.*

	Folic acid (μg/l) in			
	Serum		Erythrocyte	
	Placebo	Supplemented	Placebo	Supplemented
Before supplementation	4.2 ± 2.4 (1.9 − 7.3)	2.8 ± 2.7 (1.1 − .6.8)	224 ± 56 (127 − 267)	173 ± 80 (79 − 275)
After 40d supplementation	4.9 ± 2.8 (1.2 − 7.1)	15.6 ± 10.0 (3.7 − 32)	208 ± 65 (108 − 273)	302 ± 108 (199 − 462)

We have studied the effect on blood folate levels of physiological doses of pteroylmonoglutamate (at about the UK recommended daily allowance for pregnancy) in both pregnant women[18] and in the elderly (Table 4). The results show that considerable increases in the blood vitamin concentrations were achieved by these supplements. It is probable, therefore, that in most of these subjects improved folate status could be achieved by improved diet and that increases in intakes smaller than we used would also be effective.

1 Botez, M.I., Peyronnard, J.M., Bachevalier, J. & Charron, L. (1978): Polyneuropathy and folate deficiency. *Archs. Neurol.* **35**, 581–584.

2 Chanarin, I. (1979): Distribution of folate deficiency. In *Folic acid in neurology, psychiatry and internal medicine*, ed M.I. Botez & G.H. Reynolds, pp. 7–28. New York: Raven Press.

3 Cooper, B.A., Cantile, G.S.D. & Brunton, L. (1970): The case of folic acid supplement during pregnancy. *Am. J. Clin. Nutr.* **23**, 848–854.

4 Dunkin, G.W., Hartley, P., Lewis-Faning, E. & Russell, W.T. (1930): A comparative biometric study of the albino and coloured guinea-pigs. *J. Hyg.* **30**, 311–330.

5 Habibzadeh, N. (1983): The effects of folic acid and vitamin C on the fertility and reproduction of the guinea-pig. PhD thesis, University of Leeds.

6 Habibzadeh, N., Schorah, C.J. & Smithells, R.W. (1986): The effects of maternal folic acid and vitamin C nutrition in early pregnancy on pregnancy outcome in the guinea-pig. *Br. J. Nutr.* **55**, 23–35.

7 Herbert, V. (1970): Folic acid deficiency. *Am. J. Clin. Nutr.* **23**, 841—842.

8 Iyengar, L. & Rajalakshmi, K. (1975): Effect of folic acid supplement on birth weight of infants. *Am. J. Obstet. Gynecol.* **122**, 332–336.

9 Lawrence, K.M., James, N., Miller, M.H., Tennant, G.B. & Campbell, H. (1981): Trial of folate treatment to prevent recurrence of neural tube defect. *Br. Med. J.* **282**, 1509–1511.

10 Leck, I. (1974): Causation of neural tube defects: clues from epidemiology. *Br. Med. Bull.* **30**, 158–163.

11 Manzoor, M. & Runcie, J. (1976): Folate-responsive neuropathy: report of 10 cases. *Br. Med. J.* **1**, 1176–1178.

12 Melamed, E., Reches, A. & Hershko, C. (1975): Reversible central nervous system dysfunction in folate deficiency. *J. Neurol. Sci.* **25**, 93–98.

13 Morgan, B.L.G. & Winick, M. (1978): Effects of folic acid supplementation during pregnancy in the rat. *Br. J. Nutr.* **40**, 529–533.

14 Navia, J.M. & Hunt, C.E. (1976): Nutrition, nutritional disease and nutrition research applications. In *The biology of the guinea-pig*, ed J.E. Wagner & P.J. Manning, p. 238. New York: Academic Press.

15 Pritchard, J.A., Scott, D.E., Whalley, P.J. & Haling, R.F. (1970): Infants of mothers with megaloblastic anaemia due to folate deficiency. *J. Am. Med. Ass.* **211**, 1982–1984.

16 Reynolds, E.H. (1976): Neurological aspects of folate and vitamin B$_{12}$ metabolism. *Clin. Haematol* **5**, 661–696.

17 Schorah, C.J. (1983): Commentaries. In *Prevention of spina bifida and other neural tube defects*, ed J. Dobbing, pp. 63–66; 110–112. London: Academic Press.

18 Schorah, C.J., Wild, J., Hartley, R., Sheppard, S. & Smithells, R.W. (1983): The effect of periconceptional supplementation on blood vitamin concentrations in women at recurrent risk for neural tube defect. *Br. J. Nutr.* **49**, 203–211.

19 Schorah, C.J. & Margan, D.B. (1985): Nutritional deficiencies in the elderly. *Hospital Update* **11**, 353–360.

20 Smithells, R.W., Nevin, N.C., Seller, M.J., Sheppard, S., Harris, R., Read, A.P., Fielding, D.W., Walker, S., Schorah, C.J. & Wild, J. (1983): Further experience of vitamin supplementation for prevention of neural tube defect recurrences. *Lancet* **1**, 1027–1031.

21 Smithells, R.W., Sheppard, S. & Schorah, C.J. (1976): Vitamin deficiencies and neural tube defects. *Archs. Dis. Childh.* **51**, 944–950.

22 Strachan, R.W. & Henderson, J.G. (1967): Dementia and folate deficiency. *Quart. J. Med.* **36**, 189–204.

Cobalamins in clinical medicine

J.C. LINNELL and H.R. BHATT
Departments of Chemical Pathology and Child Health, Vincent Square Laboratories of Westminster Children's Hospital, Charing Cross & Westminster Medical School, London SW1V 2RH, UK.

One hundred and thirty years ago, Thomas Addison provided the world with a proper description of the 'progressive and crippling disease' which, thanks to Biermer, later became known as pernicious anaemia. Others before this time, including Combe (1822)[3] and Andral (1823)[1] had been aware of the curious, recurring and invariably fatal effects of this *idiopathic anaemia*, though it now seems likely that the first account of the disease was given almost 100 years before Addison, by Christophorus Godofredus Pichler in his treatise entitled *Anaemia: theory and practice illustrated*, published in 1756[17].

It is remarkable that today, though the great nutritional value of vitamin B$_{12}$ is universally recognised, the involvement of cobalamins in metabolic processes is still incompletely understood. To many, vitamin B$_{12}$ is of interest only because of its haematological effects, but recent research has highlighted the ever widening importance of cobalamins in clinical medicine, in conditions ranging from malnutrition to mental retardation, diabetes to leukaemia and optic atrophy to alcoholism. The cobalamin coenzymes, methylcobalamin (MeCbl) and adenosylcobalamin (AdoCbl) are needed by every cell in the body and the ability to estimate these directly should increase our understanding of various diseases[11]. In man, MeCbl is involved in the transmethylation of homocysteine to methionine, while AdoCbl is required for the isomerisation of methylmalonyl CoA to succinyl CoA and of *alpha*-to *beta*-leucine. MeCbl is important since a block in the methylation of homocysteine to methionine leads to failure of DNA synthesis and megaloblastic changes which can be life-threatening. AdoCbl deficiency causes a build-up of methylmalonic acid and consequent metabolic acidosis which if undiagnosed likewise threatens life, especially in neonates. Methylmalonic acidaemia also interferes with fatty acid and myelin synthesis[10].

Estimation of cobalamins. Until recently, the only practical method for estimating cobalamins individually in small biological samples has been the chromato-bioautographic technique using thin-layer chromatography[14,15]. The method is sufficiently sensitive to detect the very low (picogram) levels of cobalamins in blood and other tissues, and can identify a deficiency or imbalance in any of the forms of the vitamin even when the total Cbl is normal[7,11].

Recently, cobalamins have been separated by high-performance liquid chromatography[5,9] but detection remains a serious problem.

Distribution in the body. MeCbl, the major circulating form of the vitamin in plasma, accounts for some 55–85 per cent of the total Cbl, but is reduced disproportionately in pernicious anaemia and dietary cobalamin deficiency[6,15]. In genetic errors of metabolism where synthesis of both coenzymes is defective, the plasma MeCbl is disproportionately low despite a normal or raised plasma total Cbl[11]. Conversely, in acquired myeloproliferative diseases both MeCbl and total Cbl in plasma are raised[15] and synthesis of MeCbl from labelled cyanocobalamin *in vivo* is increased[8].

AdoCbl is the predominant form of the vitamin in all cells, including cells undergoing maturation in the bone marrow and peripheral blood cells. Its proportion and concentration vary widely in different tissues, however, from some 50 per cent in the spleen, for example, to over 80 per cent in the liver[14]. Alcohol-induced cirrhosis can lead to release of AdoCbl into the blood, with a corresponding rise in plasma AdoCbl, which may be of diagnostic value. In experimental diabetes there appears to be a disturbance in cobalamin metabolism, since methylmalonic acid excretion is abnormally increased despite raised cobalamin levels in plasma and tissues[2]. Similar findings have recently been made in human diabetes suggesting a link between insulin-dependent glucose homoeostasis and cobalamin metabolism.

In leukaemia patients treated by bone marrow grafting, chemotherapy ablates transcobalamin II, the key carrier protein required for cell-uptake of cobalamins. Successful engraftment is indicated by the reappearance of transcobalamin II in the circulation, which precedes other markers[16].

Rapid growth, both pre- and postnatal, is associated with an increased rate of DNA turnover, which depends on cobalamin-mediated transmethylation of homocysteine to methionine. Unlike liver and other tissues, which contain two enzymes able to synthesize and recycle methionine from homocysteine, viz betaine-homocysteine methyltransferase (EC 2.1.1.5) and methionine synthetase (EC 2.1.1.13), brain contains only the cobalamin-dependent methionine synthetase[4]. This appears to be the route by which methionine is recycled in the brain[19]. In fetal brain, MeCbl accounts for a much higher percentage of the total cobalamin than in adult brain[13], underlining the key part this coenzyme plays in normal brain development. In fetal alcohol syndrome the most prominent features are growth retardation, microcephaly, abnormal neuronal migration and malformations of the face and cardiovascular system. A number of these features are also prevalent in genetic disorders of cobalamin metabolism. We have recently found high levels of methylmalonic acid and acetaldehyde in the liver and brain of a 'fetal alcohol' baby who died at 3 months of age.

Diagnostic probes. Information about possible disturbances of cobalamin metabolism in various clinical conditions may be assessed by studies in cultured cells, eg skin fibroblasts or phytohaemagglutinin-stimulated lymphocytes. In human lymphocytes *in vitro*, synthesis of MeCbl and AdoCbl may readily be estimated. MeCbl synthesis is stimulated by added folate compounds and depressed by folate antagonists such as methotrexate (MTX) or 5-fluorouracil. The MTX-induced depression of MeCbl synthesis in these cells can be overcome by added folinic acid[18]. Such studies indicate, for example, the importance of MeCbl and an intact methionine synthase pathway for effective operation of the 'folinic acid rescue' procedure used during cancer chemotherapy with folate antagonists.

Inherited diseases of cobalamin metabolism can be life-threatening. Following diagnosis by blood and urine analysis, and institution of appropriate treatment, the patient can be monitored by simple tests recently developed for sulphur-containing amino acids (Bhatt & Linnell, unpublished) and organic acids[12]. Characterization of the genetic defect requires estimation of the relevant enzymes and cobalamin coenzymes in suitable cells such as cultured fibroblasts[11].

Current world problems of nutrition underline the importance of vitamins. Despite the many advances made in the cobalamin field in recent years, much still remains to be done if the full involvement of cobalamins in clinical medicine is to be understood and the nutritional consequences realised.

Acknowledgements. We are indebted to the Children's Medical Charity for their financial support and to Professor A. Fleck for Departmental facilities.

1 Andral, G. (1823): Cited in Chanarin I. (1969): The megaloblastic anaemias. Oxford: Blackwell.

2 Bhatt, H.R., Linnell, J.C. & Matthews, D.M. (1983): Can faulty vitamin B_{12} metabolism produce diabetic neuropathy? *Lancet* **2**, 572.

3 Combe, J.S. (1822): Cited in Chanarin I. (1969): The megaloblastic anaemias. Oxford: Blackwell.

4 Finkelstein, J.D., Kyle, W.E. & Harris, B.J. (1971): Methionine metabolism in mammals: regulation of homocysteine methyltransferase in rat tissue. *Archs. Biochem. Biophys.* **146**, 84–92.

5 Frenkel, E.P., Kitchens, R.C.L. & Prough, R. (1979): High-performance liquid chromatographic separation of cobalamins. *J. Chromatog.* **174**, 393–400.

6 Gimsing, P., Hippe, E. & Nexo, E. (1979): Determination of the plasma cobalamins by one-dimensional thin-layer chromatography. In *Vitamin B_{12}* ed B. Zagalak & W. Friedrich, pp. 665–669. Berlin: De Gruyter.

7 Gimsing, P. & Nexo, E. (1983): The forms of cobalamin in biological materials. In *The Cobalamins* ed C.A. Hall, pp. 8–29. Edinburgh: Churchill Livingstone.

8 Hall, C.A., Horch, C. & Begley, J.A. (1979): The forms and transport of plasma cobalamins in normal man and in myeloproliferative states. *J. Lab. Clin. Med.* **94**, 772–780.

9 Jacobsen, D.W., Green, R., Quadros, E.V. & Montejano, Y.D. (1982): Rapid analysis of cobalamin and related corrinoid analogs by high-performance liquid chromatography. *Analyt. Biochem.* **120**, 394–403.

10 Linnell, J.C. (1986): The role of cobalamins in cyanide detoxication. In *Clinical and experimental toxicology of cyanides*, ed T.C. Marrs & B. Ballantyne, Bristol: John Wright & Sons (In press).

11 Linnell, J.C. & Matthews, D.M. (1984): Cobalamin metabolism and its clinical aspects. *Clin. Sci.* **66**, 113–121.

12 Linnell, J.C., Miranda, B., Bhatt, H.R., Dowton, S.B. & Levy, H.L. (1983): Abnormal cobalamin metabolism in a megaloblastic child with homocystinuria, cystathioninuria and methylmalonic aciduria. *J. Inher. Metab. Dis.* **6** (Suppl. 2), 137–139.

13 Linnell, J.C. (1975): The fate of cobalamin *in vivo.* In *Cobalamin: biochemistry and pathophysiology,* ed B.M. Babior, pp. 287–333. New York: Wiley-Interscience.

14 Linnell, J.C., Hoffbrand, A.V., Hussein, H.A-A., Wise, I.J. & Matthews, D.M. (1974): Tissue distribution of coenzyme and other forms of vitamin B_{12} in control subjects and patients with pernicious anaemia. *Clin. Sci. Mol. Med.* **46**, 163–172.

15 Linnell, J.C., Hoffbrand, A.V., Peters, T.J. & Matthews, D.M. (1971): Chromatographic and bioautographic estimation of plasma cobalamins in various disturbances of vitamin B_{12} metabolism. *Clin. Sci.* **40**, 1–16.

16 Naparstek, E., Rachmilewitz, B., Rachmilewitz, M., Fuks, Z. & Slavin, S. (1983): Serum transcobalamin levels as an early indicator of engraftment following bone marrow transplantation. *Br. J. Haematol.* **55**, 229–234.

17 Pichler, C.G. (1756): Anaemia: theory and practice illustrated, MD thesis, University of Tubingen.

18 Quadros, E.V., Matthews, D.M., Hoffbrand, A.V. & Linnell, J.C. (1976): Synthesis of cobalamin coenzymes by human lymphocytes *in vitro* and the effects of folates and metabolic inhibitors. *Blood* **48**, 609–619.

19 Spector, R., Coakley, G. & Blakely, R. (1980): Methionine recycling in brain: a role for folates and vitamin B_{12}. *J. Neurochem.* **34**, 132–137.

★　★　★

RESEARCH DEVELOPMENTS IN VITAMIN A NUTRITION

Recent developments in the biochemistry of vitamin A

J.A. OLSON
Department of Biochemistry and Biophysics, Iowa State University, Ames, Iowa 50011, USA.

Here I will consider the following topics: current methodology for the measurement of retinoids and carotenoids[2,6,11,12,18,24,26], digestion, absorption and storage[3,13,17,21,22,27,28], plasma transport and uptake by target cells[9,14,15,19,23], metabolism[7,10,20] and function[1,4,5,8,16,25,29,30].

Methodology. During the last decade, high pressure liquid chromatography (HPLC) has been used increasingly for the separation of vitamin A and carotenoids. Different metabolites of vitamin A, various retinoids, isomeric mixtures, various retinyl esters and carotenoids have all been separated by the proper selection of suitable columns and solvents. HPLC has the advantage of maintaining the stability of the retinoid or carotenoid during isolation, short analysis time, high sensitivity and good resolution. Usually detection is by UV visible absorption spectrophotometry. Recently, retinol has also been isolated in good yield with little isomerization during analysis by gas liquid chromatography coupled with mass spectrometry.

Digestion, absorption and storage. Vitamin A and carotenoids in food aggregate into lipid globules that are emulsified by bile in the small intestine. After ester hydrolysis by pancreatic lipases, lipids in mixed micelles are absorbed by intestinal cells. Within the mucosa provitamin A carotenoids are cleaved to retinal. The latter is reduced, then esterified and incorporated into chylomicrons. The latter enter the general circulation through the lymph.

In the liver, the stellate cells and the parenchymal cells (hepatocytes) are primarily involved in the storage and release of vitamin A. The stellate cells, which comprise 2 to 5 per cent of the total cells in the liver, are small perisinusoidal cells, whereas the parenchymal cells, which comprise 60 to 75 per cent of total liver cells, are by far the largest liver cells. Within parenchymal cells, the retinyl ester associated with the chylomicron remnant is hydrolysed to retinol, which might then be bound by retinol-binding protein (RBP), esterified to retinyl ester, transferred to the stellate cell, or metabolized largely to oxidized and conjugated products. In the mobilization of vitamin A from the liver, the reverse process obviously takes place. Possibly, a specific interstitial retinol-binding protein (IRBP) might ferry retinol back and forth between these two cells in the liver as it does in the retina.

The two enzymes predominantly involved in the storage and release of vitamin A, and possibly in its control, are retinyl ester synthase (or acyl coenzyme A:retinol acyl transferase) and retinyl ester hydrolase. Indeed, retinyl ester synthase is increased in activity when high doses of vitamin A are given, but does not seem to be depressed in vitamin-A-deficiency. The hydrolase activity is also the same in deficiency as in adequate vitamin A status. Furthermore, the hydrolase is not inhibited by retinoic acid, which has been implicated as a possible control factor for vitamin A release. Interestingly, the crude hydrolase is more active on 13-*cis* retinyl ester than on the all-*trans* form. Possibly, more than one type of synthase and hydrolase exist in the liver.

Plasma transport and uptake by target cells. Vitamin A, in the form of all-*trans* retinol, combines with apo-retinol binding protein in parenchymal cells. Holo-RBP is then released through the Golgi apparatus into the plasma. Retinoic acid, on the other hand, in the form of its beta-glucuronide, is released into the bile and then is recycled back to the liver. Both retinoic acid and retinoyl beta-glucuronide have now been identified as endogenous plasma components in healthy humans.

Target tissues, which consist primarily of epithelial cells, seem to contain cell-surface receptors for holo-RBP. Vitamin A might be transported into cells by two different processes: (1) by transfer of vitamin A alone into the cell, to the exclusion of its carrier, retinol-binding protein or (2) by receptor-mediated endocytosis of holo-RBP. Within cells, retinol can be oxidized to retinoic acid, and both retinoids can combine with specific cellular retinoid-binding proteins.

Metabolism. Quite apart from the metabolic transformations already indicated, a large variety of other metabolic processes take place, such as the isomerization from all-*trans* to 11-*cis* vitamin A and the interconversion of the 13-*cis* and all-*trans* isomers. Vitamin A is also converted, particularly in the liver but also in other tissues, to a wide spectrum of oxidized and chain-shortened products. These oxidized metabolites, because of their very low biological activity, are generally considered to be inactive excretion products.

β-Carotene, the most active provitamin A carotenoid, is cleaved by 15,15′ beta-carotenoid dioxygenase into retinal. Some provitamin A carotenoids may also be converted to vitamin A by stepwise cleavage of the conjugated chain. In man carotenoids are found primarily in the adipose tissue but also in other tissues. Little is known of the subsequent metabolism of carotenoids in mammalian species.

Function. The best defined function of vitamin A is in vision. In response to a photon of light, 11-*cis* retinaldehyde in rhodopsin is converted to an all-transoid form, which triggers a series of conformational changes. One of these conformers, and probably metarhodopsin, interacts with G protein (transducin), which ultimately leads to the activation of a phosphodiesterase which cleaves cyclic GMP to GMP. These changes in cytosolic concentrations of cGMP and GMP lead to the closing of the sodium channel of the rod outer segment. The resultant membrane hyperpolarization is then transmitted as an electrical signal to other cells of the retina. Calcium may well play a role in this sequence, but apparently not by direct release from the disc membrane into the cytosol.

The second major function of vitamin A is in cellular differentiation. Perhaps the strongest current hypothesis is that retinol and retinoic acid bind in the cytosol to specific cellular retinoid-binding proteins, which then interact at discrete sites on chromatin in the nucleus. This interaction in turn gives rise to a stimulation or inhibition of gene transcription. On the other hand, in some cell lines, such as the HL60 cell, retinoic acid can induce a rapid induction of transglutaminase, even though the cell does not contain the appropriate retinoid-binding protein. Thus, the possibility exists that the action of retinoids may be at the level of the cellular membrane rather than directly in the nucleus.

Retinoids also cause marked changes in cell surface glycoproteins, which have been associated with the ability of cells to bind to each other and to an appropriate surface. Such actions of vitamin A could also have profound effects on cellular differentiation.

Carotenoids may show physiological actions, such as the enhanced fertility of cows that are seemingly independent of their conversion into vitamin A. Although subsequent studies have not always agreed with the original finding, carotenoids are known to concentrate in the corpus luteum of the cow, and carotenoid cleavage activity has been detected in that organ.

Some carotenoids, including those that are not converted into vitamin A, might also be protective against cancer induced by UV radiation and possibly by other carcinogenic and prooxidant molecules. As very effective quenchers of singlet oxygen, carotenoids may serve a protective role against neoplasm independent of their nutritional importance.

Acknowledgement. Many of the studies cited in this paper were supported by grants from the National Institutes of Health (AM-32793 and EY-03677) and from the Competitive Research Grants Office, US Department of Agriculture (84-CRCR-1-1418).

1 Ahlswede, L. & Lotthammer, K.H. (1978): Investigation of a specific vitamin A-independent action of β-carotene on bovine fertility. *Dtsch. Tierarztl. Wochenschr.* **85**, 7–12.

2 Arroyave, G., Chichester, C.O., Flores, H., Glover, J., Mejia, L.A., Olson, J.A., Simpson, K.L. & Underwood, B.A. (1982): Biochemical methodology for the assessment of vitamin A status. Int. Vitamin A Consult, Gp. Washington DC: The Nutrition Foundation.

3 Blomhoff, R., Holte, K., Naess, L. & Berg, T. (1984): Newly administered [³H] retinol is transferred from hepatocytes to stellate cells in liver for storage. *Exp. Cell Res.* **150**, 186–193.

4 Burton, G.W. & Ingold, K.U. (1984): β-Carotene: an unusual kind of lipid antioxidant. *Science* **224**, 569–573.

5 Chytil, F. & Ong, D.E. (1984): Cellular retinol and retinoic acid-binding proteins. In *The retinoids*, ed M.B. Sporn, A.B. Robert & D.S. Goodman. Vol. 2, pp. 89–123. New York: Academic Press.

6 Clifford, A.J., Tondeur, Y., Lautamo, R., Jennings, W., Jones, A.D., Furr, H.C., Olson, J.A. & DeLuca, L.M. (1985): An improved GC/MS technique for analysis of vitamin A. *Fed. Proc.* **44**, 771.

7 DeLuca, H.F. (1979): Retinoic acid metabolism. *Fed. Proc.* **38**, 2519–2523.

8 DeLuca, L.M. (1977): Direct involvement of vitamin A in glycosyl transfer reactions of mammalian membrane. *Vitam. Horm.* **35**, 1–57.

9 Fong, S.-L., Liou, G.I., Alvarez, R.A. & Bridges, C.D. (1984): Purification and characterization of a retinol-binding glycoprotein synthesized and secreted by bovine neural retina. *J. Biol. Chem.* **259**, 6534–6542.

10 Frolik, C. (1984): Metabolism of retinoids. In *The retinoids*, Vol. 2., ed M.B. Sporn, A.B. Roberts & D.S. Goodman. pp. 177–208. New York: Academic Press.

11 Frolik, C.A. & Olson, J.A. (1984): Extraction, separation and chemical analysis of retinoids. In *The retinoids*, Vol. 1, ed M.B. Sporn, A.B. Roberts & D.S. Goodman. pp. 181–233. New York: Academic Press.

12 Furr, H.C., Amedee-Manesme, O. & Olson, J.A. (1984): Gradient reversed-phase high pressure liquid chromatographic separation of naturally occurring retinoids. *J. Chromatog.* **309**, 299–307.

13 Goodman, D.S. (1984): Biosynthesis, absorption and hepatic metabolism of retinol. In *The retinoids*, Vol. 2, ed M.B. Sporn, A.B. Roberts & D.S. Goodman, pp. 1–39. New York: Academic Press.

14 Goodman, D.S. (1984): Plasma retinol-binding protein. In *The retinoids*, Vol. 2, ed M.B. Sporn, A.B. Roberts & D.S. Goodman, pp. 41–88. New York: Academic Press.

15 Heller, J. (1975): Interactions of plasma retinol-binding protein with its receptor. Specific binding of bovine and human retinol-binding protein to pigment epithelial cells from bovine eyes. *J. Biol. Chem.* **250**, 3613–3619.

16 Johnson, J.D. & Davies, P.J.A. (1985): Retinoic acid induction of transglutaminase in cells lacking cellular retinoic acid binding protein (CRABP). *Fed. Proc.* **44**, 544.

17 Knook, D.L., Seffelaar, A.M. & deLeeuw, A.M. (1982): Fat-storing cells in the rat liver: their isolation and purification. *Exp. Cell Res.* **139**, 468–471.
18 Landers, G. & Olson, J.A. (1984): Statistical solvent optimization for the separation of geometric isomers of retinol by HPLC. *J. Chromatog.* **291**, 51–57.
19 Newcomer, M.E., Jones, T.A., Aqvist, J., Sundelin, J., Eriksson, U., Rask, L. & Peterson, P.A. (1984): The 3-dimensional structure of retinol-binding protein. *EMBO J.* **3**, 1451–1454.
20 Olson, J.A. (1983): Formation and function of vitamin A. In *Biosynthesis of isoprenoid compounds*, Vol. 2, ed J.W. Porter and S.L. Spurgeon, pp. 371–412. New York: Wiley-Interscience.
21 Olson, J.A. (1984): Vitamin A. In *Handbook of vitamins*, ed L.J. Machlin. pp. 1–43. New York: M. Dekker.
22 Olson, J.A. & Gunning, D. (1983): The storage form of vitamin A in rat liver cells. *J. Nutr.* **113**, 2184–2191.
23 Peterson, P.A., Nillsen, S.F., Ostberg, L., Rask, L. & Vahlquist, A. (1974): Aspects of the metabolism of retinol-binding protein and retinol. *Vitam. Horm.* **32**, 181–214.
24 Simpson, K.L. (1983): Relative value of carotenoids as precursors of vitamin A. *Proc. Nutr. Soc.* **42**, 7–17.
25 Sporn, M.B. & Roberts, A.B. (1983): Role of retinoids in differentiation and carcinogenesis. *Cancer Res.* **43**, 3034–3040.
26 Taylor, R.F. (1983): Chromatography of carotenoids and retinoids. *Adv. Chromatog.* **22**, 157–213.
27 Underwood, B.A. (1984): Vitamin A in animal and human nutrition. In *The retinoids*, ed M.B. Sporn, A.B. Roberts & D.S. Goodman, pp. 281–392. New York: Academic Press.
28 Wake, K. (1980): Perisinusoidal stellate cells (fat-storing cells, interstitial cells, lipocytes), their related structure in and around the liver sinusoids, and vitamin A-storing cells in extrahepatic organs. *Int. Rev. Cytol.* **66**, 303–353.
29 Wolf, G. (1984): Multiple functions of vitamin A. *Physiol. Rev.* **64**, 873–937.
30 Zile, M.H. & Cullum, M.E. (1983): The function of vitamin A: current concepts. *Proc. Soc. Exp. Biol. Med.* **172**, 139–152.

Structural analysis of some retinoid-binding proteins

U. ERIKSSON, C.O. BÅVIK, Eva HANSSON, B.C. LAURENT, J. LUNDVALL, H. MELHUS, M.H.L. NILSSON, J. SUNDELIN and P.A. PETERSON
Department of Cell Research, The Wallenberg Laboratory, University of Uppsala, Box 562, S-751 22 Uppsala, Sweden.

A common property of the fat-soluble vitamins is their insolubility in aqueous media. Based on this consideration, few would contest that the fat-soluble vitamins exert their molecular functions either dissolved in the lipid bilayers of membranes or in association with membrane-embedded or water-soluble proteins. While vitamin E may perform its biological role according to the former principle, vitamins A, D and K seem to accomplish their actions according to the latter. The binding between fat-soluble vitamins and specific proteins may also be a prerequisite for the appropriate transport and metabolism of the vitamin. This is exemplified by vitamin A, whose transport and function seem to be intimately associated with a number of proteins[19,21]. These proteins sequentially transfer the vitamin to the site of action. Thus, following absorption of vitamin A alcohol (retinol) and its dietary precursors in the small intestine, and storage of the vitamin in the liver, further mobilization of retinol requires transport by the plasma retinol-binding protein (RBP)[8]. This protein carries retinol to the target cells, which display a cell surface receptor recognizing the transport protein[9,18]. Two intracellular proteins with a ubiquitous tissue distribution display affinity for retinol and retinoic acid, respectively. It is conceivable that these proteins, the cellular retinol-binding protein (CRBP) and the cellular retinoic-acid-binding protein (CRABP), ascertain that the metabolically active form of the vitamin reaches its ultimate destination. This may vary in different types of cells inasmuch as the retinoids seem to fulfil at least two discrete functions. While the general function of the vitamin in organs outside of the eye is undefined its role in the visual process is known in great detail. Thus, in the eye vitamin A aldehyde (retinaldehyde) associates with opsin to form the visual pigments[5]; a process that involves at least two other, tissue-specific retinoid-binding proteins[14,20]. It would not be surprising if, in the process of unravelling the general function(s) of vitamin A, other tissue-specific retinoid-binding proteins were identified. However, the three retinoid-binding proteins RBP, CRBP and CRABP appear to have functional roles that are common to all vitamin-A-requiring tissues. In this brief review some recent information will be summarized as regards the structures and the tissue distribution of the three proteins.

The plasma retinol-binding protein. In plasma vitamin A mainly occurs as retinol bound to RBP. This protein is synthesized in the liver and consists of a single polypeptide chain with a molecular weight of 21 000[8,19]. The RBP-retinol complex is noncovalently associated with a tetrameric thyroxine-binding protein, prealbumin[10,17]. Upon delivery of retinol to target cells, RBP becomes modified and loses its affinity for prealbumin[18]. Due to the low molecular weight of the non-complexed form of RBP it is removed from plasma by glomerular filtration and finally catabolised in the kidney tubules[26].

Apart from binding retinol and prealbumin, RBP is recognized by a cell surface receptor. All these interactions would tend to conserve the structure of RBP during evolution. This view is supported by the primary structures of human, rabbit and rat RBP inasmuch as more than 90 per cent of the residues are identical[22]. The three-dimensional structure of RBP[15] shows that the highly conserved aminoterminal two-thirds of the molecule forms a coil and a barrel-like structure of two sheets with anti-parallel β-strands. The β-sheet core is followed by an α-helix while the most carboxyterminal part does not form any obvious structural domain. The species specific residues are mainly present in the carboxyterminal part of RBP. The retinol-binding site lies inside the barrel and constitutes a hydrophobic cleft, which is closed at one end. The β-ionone ring of retinol is buried innermost in this cleft. The residues in contact with retinol are recruited from several of the β-strands and are mainly hydrophobic in nature.

Recently, we have isolated and sequenced the rat RBP gene which spans over 6.9 kilobases. The gene is divided into 6 exons with the introns varying in size from 81 basepairs to 4.4 kilobase pairs[13]. Interestingly, several of the discrete structural domains present in RBP seem to be encoded in separate exons.

Detailed knowledge of the RBP structure will allow studies of how retinol is delivered to target cells. Such analyses, now under way, should clarify whether the receptor structure for RBP on the surface of target cells will induce release of retinol by the general scheme of adsorptive endocytosis or whether other mechanisms may be operative.

Intracellular vitamin-A-binding proteins. Despite the fact that CRBP and CRABP appear to be highly selective as regards the binding of their ligands[3], the two 16 000-dalton proteins are highly homologous in primary structure[23,24]. The amino acid sequence of human CRBP, as deduced from the nucleotide sequence of a cDNA clone[4], bears striking similarities to rat CRBP. In fact, out of the 135 residues only five differ between the two proteins. This may indicate that CRBP, similar to RBP, is involved in several molecular interactions in addition to the binding of retinol.

The two intracellular retinoid-binding proteins belong to a protein family encompassing several other members. Thus, myelin protein P2[12], the hepatic and the intestinal fatty acid-binding proteins (L-FABP and I-FABP)[1,25] and mouse protein 422[2] display statistically significant homologies to CRBP and CRABP. Proteins P2 and 422 seem to be as related to the retinoid-binding proteins as are the latter to each other.

Early studies[27] clearly demonstrated that some cells and tissues are adversely affected by the lack of vitamin A. Several epithelia, the trachea and the urogenital tract, the germinal epithelium of the testis and the eye show abnormalities in vitamin A deficiency. In contrast, the liver, the gastrointestinal tract and the kidney, apart from the urothelium, appear normal or only mildly affected by deficiency of the vitamin. It is interesting to correlate this information with the tissue and cellular distribution of the two retinoic-binding proteins. The abundance of CRBP in tissues and cells through which retinol may pass transitorily[7,11,16] suggests that CRBP participates in the intracellular transport of retinol in cells involved in the resorption, storage and mobilization of retinol[6]. However, CRBP may have dual functions since it also occurs in several tissues and cells with no known involvement in the transport of retinol. CRBP may act as an intracellular acceptor for retinol in these tissues.

The tissues and cellular distribution of CRABP is clearly different from that of CRBP inasmuch as it seems to be more closely restricted to tissues that are known targets for vitamin A[7]. In several of the tissues exhibiting the most overt signs of retinol-deficiency both CRABP and CRBP are present. Most cells under normal nutritional conditions obtain vitamin A as retinol. This raises the interesting possibility that retinol is converted to retinoic acid in the target tissues. Retinoic acid or metabolites thereof may consequently be the active forms of the vitamin.

Conclusion. The molecular modes of operation of CRBP and CRABP are most likely similar in view of their structural homology. The information cited above may be interpreted to mean that both proteins exhibit intracellular transport functions. If so, it remains to be established to what acceptor structures they deliver their ligands. Such putative acceptors for the retinoids may well define the elusive general function(s) of vitamin A.

1 Alpers, D.H., Strauss, A.W., Ockner, R.K., Bass, N.M. & Gordon, J.I. (1984): Cloning of a cDNA encoding rat intestinal fatty acid binding protein. *Proc. Natl. Acad. Sci. USA* **81**, 313–317.
2 Bernlohr, D.A., Angus, C.W., Lane, M.D., Bolanowski, M.A. & Kelly, Jr, T.J. (1984): Expression of specific mRNAs during adipose differentiation: identification of an mRNA encoding a homologue of myelin P2 protein. *Proc. Natl. Acad. Sci. USA* **81**, 5468–5472.
3 Chytil, F. & Ong, D.E. (1983): Cellular retinoid-binding proteins. In *The retinoids*, ed M.B. Sporn, A. Roberts & D.S. Goodman, Vol. 2, pp. 90–125. New York: Academic Press.
4 Colantuoni, V., Cortese, R., Nilsson, M., Lundvall, J., Båvik, C.-O., Eriksson, U., Peterson, P.A. & Sundelin, J. (1985): Cloning and sequencing of a full length cDNA corresponding to human cellular retinol-binding protein. *Biochem. Biophys. Res. Com.* **130**, 431–439.
5 Dratz, E.A. & Hargrave, P.A. (1983): The structure of rhodospin and the rod outer segment disk membrane. *Trends Biol. Sci.* **8**, 128–131.
6 Eriksson, U., Das, K., Busch, C., Nordlinder, J., Sällstrom, J., Sundelin, J. & Peterson, P.A. (1984): Cellular retinol-binding protein: quantitation and distribution. *J. Biol. Chem.* **259**, 13464–13470.
7 Eriksson, U., Hansson, E., Nordlinder, H., Busch, C., Sundelin, J. & Peterson, P.A. (In prep): Quantitation and tissue localization of the cellular retinoic acid-binding protein.
8 Goodman, D.S. (1983): Plasma retinol-binding protein. In *The retinoids*, ed M.B. Sporn, A. Roberts & D.S. Goodman, Vol. 2, pp. 42–89. New York: Academic Press.
9 Heller, J. (1975): Interactions of plasma retinol-binding protein with its receptor. Specific binding of bovine and human retinol-binding protein to pigment epithelium cells from bovine eyes. *J. Biol. Chem.* **250**, 3613–3619.
10 Kanai, M., Raz, A. & Goodman, D.S. (1968): Retinol-binding protein: the transport protein for vitamin A in plasma. *J. Clin. Invest.* **47**, 2025–2044.
11 Kato, M., Kato, K. & Goodman, D.S. (1984): Immunocytochemical studies on the localization of plasma and of cellular retinol-binding proteins and of transthyerin (prealbumin) in rat liver and kidney. *J. Cell Biol.* **98**, 1696–1704.
12 Kitamura, K., Suzuki, M., Suzuki, A. & Uyemura, K. (1980): The complete amino acid sequence of the P2 protein in bovine peripheral nerve myelin. *FEBS Lett.* **115**, 27–30.
13 Laurent, B.C., Nilsson, M.H.L., Båvik, C.-O., Jones, T.A., Sundelin, J. & Peterson, P.A. (1985): Characterization of the rat retinol-binding protein gene and its comparison to the three dimensional structure of the protein. *J. Biol. Chem.* (In press).
14 Liou, G.I., Bridges, C.D.B., Fong, S.-L., Alvarez, R.A. & Gonzales-Fernandez, F. (1982): Vitamin A transport between retina and pigment epithelium — an interstitial protein carrying endogenous retinol (interstitial retinol-binding protein). *Vision Res.* **22**, 1457–1468.
15 Newcomer, M., Jones, T.A., Åqvist, J., Sundelin, J., Eriksson, U., Rask, L. & Peterson, P.A. (1984): The three-dimensional structure of retinol-binding protein. *EMBO J.* **3**, 1451–1454.
16 Ong, D.E., Crow, J.A. & Chytil, F. (1983): Radioimmunochemical determination of cellular retinol- and cellular retinoic acid-binding proteins in cytosols of rat tissues. *J. Biol. Chem.* **257**, 13385–13389.
17 Peterson, P.A. & Berggård, I. (1971): Isolation and properties of a human retinol-binding protein. *J. Biol. Chem.* **246**, 25–33.
18 Rask, L. & Peterson, P.A. (1976): In vitro uptake of vitamin A from the retinol-binding plasma protein to mucosal epithelial cells of the monkey's small intestine. *J. Biol. Chem.* **251**, 6360–6366.
19 Rask, L., Anundi, H., Böhme, J., Eriksson, U., Fredriksson, Å., Nilsson, S.F., Vahlquist, A. & Peterson, P.A. (1980): The retinol-binding proteins. *Scand. J. Lab. Clin. Invest.* **40** Suppl. **154**, 45–61.
20 Stubbs, G.W., Saari, J. & Futterman, S. (1979): 11-cis retinal-binding protein from bovine retina. Purification and partial characterization. *J. Biol. Chem.* **259**, 8529–8533.
21 Sundelin, J., Eriksson, U., Melhus, H., Nilsson, M., Lundvall, J., Båvik, C.-O., Hansson, E., Laurent, E. & Peterson, P.A. (1985): Cellular retinoid binding proteins. In *Chemistry and physics of lipids*. Elsevier Scientific Publishers Ireland Ltd. (In press).

22 Sundelin, J., Laurent, B.C., Anundi, H., Trägårdh, L., Larhammar, D., Björk, L., Eriksson, U., Åkerström, B., Jones, T.A., Peterson, P.A. & Rask, L. (1985): Amino acid sequence homologies between rabbit, rat and human serum retinol-binding proteins. *J. Biol. Chem.* **260**, 6472–6480.
23 Sundelin, J., Anundi, H., Trägårdh, L., Eriksson, U., Lind, P., Ronne, H., Peterson, P.A. & Rask, L. (1985): The primary structure of rat liver cellular retinol-binding protein. *J. Biol. Chem.* **260**, 6488–6493.
24 Sundelin, J., Das, S., Eriksson, U., Rask, L. & Peterson, P.A. (1985): The primary structure of bovine cellular retinoic acid-binding protein. *J. Biol. Chem.* **260**, 6494–6499.
25 Takahashi, K., Odani, S. & Ono, T. (1982): Primary structure of rat liver Z-protein. *FEBS Lett.* **140**, 63–66.
26 Vahlquist, A., Peterson, P.A. & Wibell, L. (1973): Metabolism of the vitamin A transporting protein complex. I. Turnover studies in normal persons and in patients with chronic renal failure. *Eur. J. Clin. Invest.* **3**, 352–362.
27 Wolbach, S.B. & Howe, P.R. (1925): Tissue changes following deprivation of fat soluble A vitamin. *J. Exp. Med.* **42**, 753–778.

Physiological effects of vitamin-A-deficiency

Vinodini REDDY
National Institute of Nutrition, Hyderabad-500 007, India.

Vitamin A is essential for normal vision, for maintaining integrity of the epithelial cells and for a wide variety of metabolic functions. Acute vitamin-A-deficiency, although affecting many tissues of the body, is clinically and socially most significant in its disruption of the cornea resulting in permanent blindness. In the world today, 200 000 to 500 000 children become blind every year as a result of this deficiency. A more precise figure is unavailable since mortaility is extremely high in those who lose sight. Much of the information available today on the molecular changes involved has come from experimentation in animals. In recent times, however, there has been a spurt of interest in human studies.

Ocular manifestations. Mild deficiency of vitamin A in man leads to night-blindness and conjunctival lesions, while more severe deficiency results in corneal damage. The term 'xerophthalmia' is used to indicate all eye lesions that result from vitamin-A-deficiency.

Night-blindness. Deficiency of vitamin A leads to delayed synthesis of rhodopsin and impaired dark-adaptation resulting in night-blindness. Testing dark-adaptation in young children is difficult especially in the field. In a study carried out in Indonesia, the symptoms of night-blindness were found to be far more sensitive, and easier to diagnose, than dark-adaptation tests[26]. Twice as many children had a history of night-blindness compared with those in whom conjunctival lesions were detected. The value of this method, however, will depend upon the care with which the case history is elicited and the extent to which the phenomenon is recognized by the community.

Colour vision. Although vitamin-A-deficiency is known to cause disturbance of rod function, there is little information regarding its effect on the cone function. In adult patients with biliary cirrhosis who had impaired dark-adaptation and defective colour-vision, vitamin-A-treatment produced a significant improvement[2]. This may be related to hepatic function rather than vitamin A status, since other workers have reported that the defects in colour-vision disappeared after the patients recovered from the acute stage of liver disease[5]. Studies in Indian children with night-blindness and conjunctival lesions revealed no abnormality in colour-vision[22].

Conjunctival lesions. Loss of transparency, dryness and wrinkling of bulbar conjunctiva are characteristic of conjunctival xerosis. Early stages, are, however, not easy to identify clinically. Staining with rose bengal or lissamine green has been suggested, but subsequent studies have indicated that it is not a reliable method[8].

Bitot spot is more readily recognized and, therefore, a more useful sign in a field survey. In some adults and older children, Bitot spots are firmly adherent and do not respond to vitamin-A-therapy. In view of this, their relationship to vitamin-A-deficiency has been questioned. In pre-schoolchildren, however, Bitot spots are generally accompanied by xerosis of conjunctiva and/or night-blindness and indicate acute vitamin-A-deficiency[23].

Corneal lesions. Severe vitamin-A-deficiency resulting in corneal damage is almost always seen in children below 5 years, and is frequently associated with PEM and infection. Even before the clinical lesions become evident, changes occur in the corneal epithelium which can be detected by slit lamp examination after fluoroscein staining. Punctate keratopathy has been observed in many children with night-blindness and conjunctival xerosis whose cornea appear normal on clinical examination[25].

Loss of lustre, haziness and dryness are characteristic of corneal xerosis. This can be completely reversed with vitamin-A-therapy but in untreated cases it progresses rapidly to keratomalacia and blindness. The precise pathophysiology of keratomalacia is still unknown. There is some experimental evidence to suggest that corneal ulceration may be mediated through the enzyme collagenase, synthesised by the corneal epithelium[20]. Serum is known to contain powerful collagenase inhibitors — $\alpha 2$ macroglobulin and $\alpha 1$ antitrypsin, and such natural inhibitors may possibly diffuse into the stroma and normally protect it from autodigestion. In severe protein deficiency, which is invariably associated with keratomalacia, the levels may go down altering the defence mechanism. The epithelial changes can also invite secondary infection which can produce corneal damage by direct invasion as well as by activation of the enzyme collagenase. Higher isolation rate of pathogenic organisms from keratomalacia cases support this hypothesis[19].

Systemic effects. Extra-ocular effects of vitamin-A-deficiency reported in animal modes include reduced food intake, impaired growth, epithelial changes, altered immune response and disturbance of reproductive process. These effects have not been confirmed in man.

Follicular hyperkeratosis has been observed in depletion studies on adults[24], but it is a nonspecific sign and is rare in young children. In this study, abnormalities were also observed in taste and smell.

Lysosomal instability. Regulation of membrane stability is one of the physiological functions of Vitamin A. The release of acid hydrolases from lysosomes of liver cells has been shown to be greatly enhanced in vitamin-A-deficient rats. There have been few studies to determine whether in human vitamin-A-deficiency, lysosomal stability is altered. In Indian children with clinical signs of vitamin-A-deficiency, urinary excretion of two lysosomal enzymes — aryl sulphatase and acid phosphatase — was increased and the levels were restored to normal after treatment with vitamin A[21]. Children with kwashiorkor have also been found to excrete higher levels of lysosomal enzymes. This may be due to associated vitamin-A-deficiency as the enzyme levels showed a substantial fall after administration of the vitamin[7].

Sulphate metabolism. Impaired synthesis of sulphated mucopolysaccharide has been reported in vitamin-A-deficient rats. Recently studies were conducted in human subjects to investigate this aspect. It was observed that children suffering from vitamin-A-deficiency not only excreted low amounts of mucopolysaccharide but that the sulphated fraction constituted only 30 per cent as against 70 per cent in normal subjects[13]. Homogenates of colonic mucosa obtained from vitamin-A-deficient children were found to incorporate ^{35}S less effectively into mucopolysaccharides than did colonic homogenates from normal children, and treatment with vitamin A corrected this defect[14]. These studies suggest that sulphate metabolism is altered in human vitamin-A-deficiency.

Anaemia. Studies in experimental animals as well as in human volunteers have shown that iron metabolism is altered in vitamin-A-deficiency. Adult men receiving vitamin-A-deficient diet developed a moderate degree of anaemia despite adequate intake of iron[6]. The anaemia did not respond to iron therapy until vitamin supplements were started. These results support the concept that vitamin A is essential for normal haematopoiesis.

Xerophthalmia and nutritional anaemia coexist in many poor communities. A study was carried out in Indian children to investigate the possible relationship between the two deficiency diseases. Haemoglobin levels were found to be significantly lower in children with plasma vitamin A below 20 μg/dl than in those with normal levels[16]. Supplementation with vitamin A resulted in a significant increase in the levels of haemoglobin and serum iron. Since the absorption of iron is not altered in vitamin-A-deficiency[18], hypoferraemia may be explained on the basis of impaired mobilization of iron from the stores. This is supported by the results of animal studies which show that vitamin-A-deficiency is associated with increased amounts of iron in the liver[11].

These observations suggest that, apart from iron deficiency, hypovitaminosis A may also contribute to the prevalence of anaemia in poor communities. In Indonesia, vitamin-A-supplementation increased blood values of both vitamin A and haemoglobin[17]. In Guatemala, the national programme of vitamin-A-fortification of sugar not only improved vitamin A status of the population but also had a favourable effect on iron metabolism[12].

Resistance to infection. Vitamin A has been called the 'anti-infective' vitamin. Although the epithelial changes and reduced mucous production are primary factors, altered immune mechanisms also contribute to lowered resistance to infection. Both the humoral and the cell-mediated immune responses have been shown to be altered in vitamin-A-deficient rats. There is, however, little information on immunocompetence in human vitamin-A-deficiency.

In Indian children who had clinical signs of vitamin-A-deficiency, the lysosomal content of leucocytes was found to be significantly reduced[15]. Studies on cell-mediated immunity showed that the number of circulating T lymphocytes is reduced, but their response to phytohaemagglutinin is not altered[1]. Antibody titres following diphtheria and tetanus toxoids were similar in vitamin-A-deficient and normal children[9]. Administration of vitamin A did not enhance the immune response[4]. These observations are contrary to those made in laboratory animals and indicate that the humoral immune response is not altered in human vitamin-A-deficiency.

In poor communities where vitamin-A-deficiency is widespread, infection rates are also high. However, it is difficult to establish the causal relationship because there are a number of concommitant variables that influence the morbidity rates. A study carried out in Indonesian children showed that xerophthalmia was associated with increased risk of respiratory disease and diarrhoea[28]. It has also been found[3] that infection rates were similar in malnourished children with and without xerophthalmia but that the former showed significant bacteruria.

In children with severe PEM, mortality was found to be four-fold higher when they had xerophthalmia as well[10]. The effect of vitamin-A-deficiency is difficult to assess in such children since they suffer from severe degrees of PEM that could have independently contributed to the high mortality. Recently a study was carried out in Indonesia to see whether mild xerophthalmia, which is much more common in children, is associated with increased mortality[27]. Ocular signs of vitamin-A-deficiency like night-blindness and/or Bitot spots were seen in about 5 per cent of the children. The mortality rate among these children was four times higher than in those without eye lesions. These observations suggest that inadequate vitamin-A-nutrition, apart from causing eye lesions, may contribute to other health risks in young children.

1 Bhaskaram, C. & Reddy, V. (1975): Cell mediated immunity in iron and vitamin deficient children. *Br. Med. J.* **3**, 522–523.

2 Bronte-Stewart, J.M. & Foulds, W.S. (1975): Acquired dyschromatopsia in vitamin A deficiency. *Mod. Probl. Ophthal.* **10**, 133–136.

3 Brown, K.H., Gaffar, A. & Alamgir, S.M. (1979): Xerophthalmia, protein calorie malnutrition and infections in children. *J. Pediat.* **95**, 651–656.

4 Brown, K.H., Rajan, M.M., Chakraborty, J. & Aziz, K.M.A. (1980): Failure of a large dose of vitamin A to enhance the antibody response to tetanus toxoid in children. *Am. J. Clin. Nutr.* **33**, 212–217.

5 Fialkow, P.J., Thuline, H.C. & Fenster, L.F. (1966): Lack of association between cirrhosis and the common types of colour blindness. *New Engl. J. Med.* **275**, 584–587.

6 Hodges, R.E., Sauberlich, H.E., Canham, J.E., Wallace, D.L., Bucker, R.B., Mejia, L.A. & Mohanram, M. (1978): Hematopoietic studies in vitamin A deficiency. *Am. J. Clin. Nutr.* **31**, 876–885.

7 Ittyerah, T.R., Dumm, M.E. & Bachawat, B.K. (1967): Urinary excretion of lysosomal aryl sulphatases in kwashiorkor. *Clin. Chim. Acta* **17**, 405–414.

8 Kusin, J.A., Soewondo, W. & Parlindungan Dinaga, H.S.R. (1979): Rose bengal and lissamine green vital stains; useful diagnostic aids for early stages of xerophthalmia. *Am. J. Clin. Nutr.* **32**, 1559–1564.

9 Kutty, P.M., Mohanram, M. & Reddy, V. (1981): Humoral immune response in vitamin A deficient children. *Acta Vitaminol. Enzymol.* **4**, 231–235.

10 McLaren, D.S., Shirajian, E., Tehalian, M. & Khoury, G. (1965): Xerophthalmia in Jordan. *Am. J. Clin. Nutr.* **17**, 117–130.

11 Mejia, L.A., Hodges, R.E., Mohanram, M., Rucker, R.B., Arroyave, G. & Viteri, F. (1976): Anemia in vitamin A deficiency. *Clin. Res.* **24**, 315–319.

12 Mejia, L.A. & Arroyave, G. (1982): The effect of vitamin A fortification of sugar on iron metabolism in pre-school children in Guatemala. *Am. J. Clin. Nutr.* **36**, 87–93.

13 Mohanram, M. & Reddy, V. (1971): Urinary excretion of acid mucopolysaccharide in kwashiorkor and vitamin A deficient children. *Clin. Chim. Acta* **34**, 93–96.

14 Mohanram, M. & Reddy, V. (1973): Incorporation of ^{35}S sulphate into acid mucopolysaccharide of colon in vitamin A deficient children. *Int. J. Vit. Nutr. Res.* **43**, 56–60.

15 Mohanram, M., Reddy, V. & Mishra, S. (1974): Lysozyme activity in plasma and leukocytes of malnourished children. *Br. J. Nutr.* **32**, 313–316.

16 Mohanram, M., Kulkarni, K.A. & Reddy, V. (1977): Hematological studies in vitamin A deficient children. *Int. J. Vit. Nutr. Res.* **47**, 389–393.

17 Muhilal & Karyadi, D. (1984): Highlight of current studies; considerations for programme intervention. In *Human nutrition, better nutrition, better life*, ed V. Tanphaichitr, W. Dahlan, V. Suphakarn and A. Valyasevi, pp. 191–195. *Proc. IV Asian Congr. Nutr.* Bangkok: Aksornsmai.

18 National Institute of Nutrition (1977): *Annual report.* p. 60. Hyderabad: National Institute of Nutrition.

19 National Institute of Nutrition (1981): *Annual report*, pp. 48–49. Hyderabad: National Institute of Nutrition.

20 Pirie, A., Webb, Z. & Burleigh, M.C. (1975): Collagenase and other proteinases in the cornea of retinol deficient rat. *Br. J. Nutr.* **34**, 297–309.

21 Reddy, V. & Mohanram, M. (1971): Urinary excretion of lysozomal enzymes in hypovitaminosis and hypervitaminosis A in children. *Int. J. Vit. Nutr. Res.* **41**, 321–326.

22 Reddy, V. & Vijayalakshmi (1977): Colour vision in vitamin A deficiency. *Br. Med. J.* **1**, 81.

23 Reddy, V. (1978): Vitamin A deficiency and blindness in Indian children. *Ind. J. Med. Res.* **68** (Suppl), 26–37.

24 Sauberlich, H.E., Hodges, R.E. & Wallace, D.L. (1974): Vitamin A metabolism and requirements in humans studied with the use of labelled retinol. *Vit. Horm.* **32**, 251–275.

25 Sommer, A., Emram, M. & Tamba, T. (1979): Vitamin A responsive punctate keratopathy in xerophthalmia. *Am. J. Ophthal.* **87**, 330–333.

26 Sommer, A., Hussaini, G., Muhilal, Tarwotjo, I., Susanto, D. & Saroso, J.S. (1980): History of night blindness; a simple tool for xerophthalmia screening. *Am. J. Clin. Nutr.* **33**, 887–891.

27 Sommer, A., Hussaini, G., Tarwotjo, I. & Susanto, D. (1983): Increased mortality in children with mild vitamin A deficiency. *Lancet* **1**, 585–588.

28 Sommer, A., Katz, J. & Tarwotjo, I. (1984): Increased risk of respiratory disease and diarrhoea in children with preexisting mild vitamin A deficiency. *Am. J. Clin. Nutr.* **40**, 1090–1095.

Vitamin A and mechanisms of immunity

R. LOTAN
Department of Tumor Biology (Box 108), The University of Texas, M.D. Anderson Hospital and Tumor Institute at Houston, Texas 77030, USA.

The immune response is affected by changes in the hormonal and nutritional status of the organism. Nutrient deficiency or excess may affect immune functions by altering differentiation of immunocompetent cells or cells that regulate the development of immune responses. Various studies have demonstrated that vitamin A and certain retinoids increase resistance to microbial infections, stimulate skin-graft rejection, reverse immunodepression and augment host anti-tumour responses (for recent reviews see[13,14,19,23,26,39]).

Effects of retinoids on humoral immune responses. Vitamin A has been shown to increase the number of antibody-forming cells in the spleen of mice immunized with sheep red blood cells[11] or with proteins[6,18]. It has been reported[37] that vitamin A markedly enhanced production of antibodies to a T-independent antigen. A study of IgG$_1$ and IgE responses to ovalbumin revealed that retinoids act as adjuvants to augment a secondary response[6,7,10].

These results were consistent with a direct effect of retinoids on B cells. Indeed, recent studies, using human tonsillar lymphocytes sensitized to sheep erythrocytes, have clearly demonstrated that retinoic acid can enhance antibody response by acting directly on B cells[32].

Effects of retinoids on cell-mediated immune responses. *T-lymphocytes.* It has been observed[1] that retinoic acid enhances phytohaemagglutinin (PHA) response of human peripheral blood lymphocytes, whereas high doses of retinol inhibited mitogenic response of human lymphocytes[35]. In contrast, an enhancement of the blastogenic response of human thymocytes to PHA has been observed[34]. The PHA response *in vitro* of lymphocytes from cancer patients treated systemically with retinyl palmitate or 13-cis retinoic acid was also stimulated[28].

An improvement in response of immunosuppressed cancer patients to cutaneous delayed hypersensitivity antigens has been observed[28,31]. In a mouse model we found no stimulatory effect of retinoic acid on delayed type hypersensitivity (DHT). High retinoic acid doses actually suppressed DTH[16]. In contrast another study, under different conditions[4], found a stimulation of DHT to sheep erythrocytes in mice. It has been observed[36] that the TMMP analogue of ethyl retinoate augmented PHA-induced suppressor-cell activity while retinoic acid was ineffective.

Several lines of evidence support the conclusion that retinoids enhance anti-tumour cell-mediated cytotoxicity: (1) immunogenic tumours were inhibited whereas nonimmunogenic tumours were not affected by retinoids; (2) abrogation of host immune system by whole-body irradiation, by thymectomy, by injection of anti-lymphocyte serum, by cyclosporin A treatment or by transplantation in nu/nu mice abolished the anti-tumour effects of the retinoids, and (3) there was no correlation between sensitivity to growth inhibition by retinoids in culture and *in vivo*[19,20,29]. Our studies[15,16,21,24] demonstrated that retinoic acid as well as other retinoids can stimulate the induction of cytotoxic T cells both *in vivo* and *in vitro*. The cytotoxic cells were induced only in the presence of an immunogen, and they were specific for H-2 antigens in allogeneic immunization and for tumour antigens in syngeneic systems. Essentially similar results were reported by others[9,25]. Enhancement of natural killer (NK) activity by retinoic acid has been observed[22]; however, it has also been found that retinoic acid inhibits the spontaneous activity of human NK cells[2]. Others[9,25,33] found that retinoic acid had little, if any, influence on the development, cytotoxic potential, or activity of NK cells.

Macrophages. Retinoids have been shown to affect the growth and differentiation of normal myeloid progenitor cells and the function of mature macrophages. There are conflicting reports regarding the effect of retinoids on clonal growth of stem cells committed to the granulocyte-macrophage lineage (CFU-GM). Some studies have found that retinoic acid can enhance colony stimulating factor-induced clonal growth of human CFU-GM[3,17]. In contrast, others reported suppression of growth of CFU-GM by retinoids[5,8].

Retinoids can also modulate the function of mature, differentiated macrophages *in vivo* and in culture. Thus, the ability of vitamin A to increase resistance to *Listeria monocytogenes* suggests that the vitamin enhances the functional capacities of phagocytic cells[12]. Treatment of aging mice with retinoic acid increased the activity of peritoneal macrophages[9]. It has been observed[30] that whereas the expression Fc receptors and the subsequent phagocytosis of opsonized cells was suppressed by retinoids, the production of the tumoricidal enzyme arginase was augmented. Treatment of rats with vitamin A rendered their alveolar macrophages tumoricidal and increased their phagocytic activity[38].

Effects of retinoids on lymphokines. Although absence of effect of retinoic acid on interleukin-2 (IL-2) production by human thymocytes has been reported[33], there has been a recent report that dietary supplementation with retinyl acetate increases in mice the proportion of T cells that produce IL-2[27]. Similarly, it has been reported[14] that spleen cells from retinoic acid-injected mice have an increased ability to produce IL-2 in mixed lymphocyte cultures. These findings suggest that one way by which retinoids may enhance cell-mediated cytotoxity is by stimulating T-helper-cell proliferation or IL-2 production, or both.

Conclusions. In spite of some conflicting results, the majority of studies indicate that retinoids can modulate various immunological responses both *in vivo* and in culture. In many cases the effect of vitamin A and retinoids is beneficial as they augment cellular and humoural immune responses to pathogens and cancer. Although retinoids exert direct effect on the growth and differentiation of different tumour cells, the augmentation of immune responses *in vivo* plays an important role in their anti-tumour activity.

1 Abb, J. & Deinhardt, F. (1980): Effects of retinoic acid on the human lymphocyte response to mitogens. *Exp. Cell Biol.* **48**, 169–179.
2 Abb, J., Abb, H. & Deinhardt, F. (1982): Effect of retinoic acid on the spontaneous and interferon-induced activity of human natural killer cells. *Int. J. Cancer* **30**, 307–310.
3 Aglietta, M., Piacibello, W., Sanavio, F., Visconti, A. & Gavosto, F. (1982): Retinoic acid enhances the growth of only one subpopulation of granulomonocyte precursors. *Acta Haematol.* **71**, 97–99.
4 Athanassiades, T.J. (1981): Adjuvant effect of vitamin A palmitate and analogs on cell-mediated immunity. *J. Natl. Cancer Inst.* **67**, 1153–1156.
5 Bailey-Wood, R., May, S. & Jacobs, A. (1985): The effect of retinoids on CFU-GM from normal subjects and patients with myelodysplastic syndrome. *Br. J. Haematol.* **59**, 15–20.
6 Barnett, J.B. (1983): Immunomodulating effects of 13-cis-retinoic acid on the IgG and IgM response of Balb/C mice. *Int. Archs. Allergy Appl. Immunol.* **72**, 227–233.
7 Barnett, J.B. & Bryant, R.L. (1980): Adjuvant and immunosuppressive effects of retinol and tween 80 on IgG production in mice. *Int. Archs Allerg. Appl. Immunol.* **63**, 145–152.
8 Bradley, E.C., Ruscetti, F.W., Steinberg, H., Paradise, C. & Blaine, K. (1983): Inhibition of differentiation and proliferation of colony-stimulating factor-induced clonal growth of normal human marrow cells *in vitro* by retinoic acid. *J. Natl. Cancer Inst.* **71**, 1189–1192.
9 Bruley-Rosset, M., Hercend, T., Martinez, J., Rappaport, H. & Mathe, G. (1981): Prevention of spontaneous tumours of aged mice by immunopharmacologic manipulation: study of immune antitumor mechanisms. *J. Natl. Cancer Inst.* **67**, 1113–1119.
10 Bryant, R.L. & Barnett, J.B. (1979): Adjuvant properties of retinol on IgE production in mice. *Int. Archs Allergy. Appl. Immunol.* **59**, 69–74.
11 Cohen, B.E. & Cohen, I.K. (1973): Vitamin A: adjuvant and steroid antagonist in the immune response. *J. Immunol.* **111**, 1376–1380.
12 Cohen, B.E. & Elin, R.J. (1974): Vitamin A-induced nonspecific resistance to infection. *J. Infect. Dis.* **129**, 597–600.
13 Dennert, G. (1984): Retinoids and the immune system: immunostimulation by vitamin A. In *The retinoids*, Vol. 2, ed M.B. Sporn, A.B. Roberts & D.S. Goodman, pp. 373–390. New York: Academic Press.
14 Dennert, G. (1985): Immunostimulation by retinoic acid. In *Retinoids, differentiation and disease*, Ciba Foundation Symposium No 113, pp. 117–131. London: Pitman.
15 Dennert, G., Crowley, C., Kouba, J. & Lotan, R. (1979): Retinoic acid stimulation of the induction of mouse killer T cells in allogeneic and syngeneic systems. *J. Natl. Cancer Inst.* **62**, 89–94.
16 Dennert, G. & Lotan, R. (1978): Effects of retinoic acid on the immune system: Stimulation of T-killer cell induction. *Eur. J. Immunol.* **8**, 23–29.
17 Douer, D. & Koeffler, H.P. (1982): Retinoic acid enhances colony stimulating factor-induced clonal growth of normal human myeloid progenitor cells *in vitro*. *Exp. Cell Res.* **138**, 193–198.
18 Dresser, D.W. (1968): Adjuvanticity of vitamin A. *Nature* **217**, 527–529.
19 Eccles, S.A. (1985): Effects of retinoids on growth and dissemination of malignant tumours: Immunological considerations. *Biochem. Pharmacol.* **34**, 1599–1610.
20 Felix, E.L., Loyd, B. & Cohen, M.H. (1975): Inhibition of the growth and development of a transplantable murine melanoma by vitamin A. *Science* **189**, 886–888.
21 Glaser, M. & Lotan, R. (1979): Augmentation of specific tumor immunity against a syngeneic SV40-induced sarcoma in mice by retinoic acid. *Cell. Immunol.* **45**, 175–181.
22 Goldfarb, R.H. & Herberman, R.B. (1981): Natural killer cell reactivity: regulatory interactions among phorbolester, interferon, cholera toxin, and retinoic acid. *J. Immunol.* **126**, 2129–2135.
23 Lotan, R. (1980): Effects of vitamin A and its analogs (retinoids) on normal and neoplastic cells. *Biochim. Biophys. Acta* **605**, 33–91.
24 Lotan, R. & Dennert, G. (1979): Stimulatory effects of vitamin A analogs on induction of cell-mediated cytotoxity *in vivo*. *Cancer Res.* **39**, 55–58.
25 Malkovsky, M., Dore, C., Hunt, R., Palmer, L., Chandler, P. & Medawar, P.B. (1983): Enhancement of specific antitumor immunity in mice fed a diet enriched in vitamin A acetate. *Proc. Natl. Acad. Sci. USA* **80**, 6322–6326.
26 Malkovsky, M. & Medawar, P.B. (1984): Retinoids and *in vivo* immunity to transplantable tumors: a terra relatively incognita. *Immunol. Today* **5**, 178–180.
27 Malkovsky, M., Medawar, P., Thatcher, D.R., Toy, J., Hunt, R., Rayfield, L.S. & Dore, C. (1985): Acquired immunological tolerance of foreign cells is impaired by recombinant interleukin 2 or vitamin A acetate. *Proc. Natl. Acad. Sci. USA* **82**, 536–538.
28 Micksche, M., Cerni, C., Kokron, O., Titscher, R. & Wrba, H. (1977): Stimulation of immune response in lung cancer patients by vitamin A therapy. *Oncology* **34**, 234–238.
29 Patek, P.Q., Collins, J.L., Yogeeswaran, G. & Dennert, G. (1979): Anti-tumor potential of retinoic acid stimulation of immune mediated effectors. *Int. J. Cancer* **24**, 624–628.

30 Rhodes, J. & Oliver, S. (1980): Retinoids as regulators of macrophage function. *Immunology* **40**, 467–472.

31 Serrou, B., Cupissol, D. & Rosenfeld, C. (1982): Immune imbalance and immune modulation in solid tumor patients: new insights. *Rec. Res. in Cancer Res.* **80**, 9–16.

32 Sidell, N., Famatiga, E. & Golub, S.H. (1984): Immunological aspects of retinoids in humans. II. Retinoic acid enhances induction of hemolytic plaque-forming cells. *Cell. Immunol.* **88**, 374–381.

33 Sidell, N., Famatiga, E., Shau, H. & Golub, S.H. (1985): Immunological aspects of retinoids in humans. III. Effects of retinoic acid on the natural killing of tumor cells. *J. Biol. Res. Mod.* **4**, 1–11.

34 Sidell, N., Rieber, P. & Golub, S.H. (1984): Immunological aspects of retinoids in humans. I. Analysis of retinoic acid enhancement of thymocyte response to PHA. *Cell. Immunol.* **87**, 118–125.

35 Skinnider, L.F. & Giesbrecht, K. (1979): Inhibition of phorbol myristate acetate and phytohemagglutinin stimulation of human lymphocytes by retinol. *Cancer Res.* **39**, 3332–3334.

36 Soppi,. E., Tertti, R., Soppi, A., Toivanen, A. & Jansen, C.T. (1982): Differential *in vitro* effects of retinate and retinoic acid on the PHA and ConA induced lymphocyte transformation, suppressor cell induction and leukocyte migration inhibitory factor (LMIF) production. *Int. J. Immunopharmacol.* **4**, 437–443.

37 Sugimura, K., Azuma, I., Yamamura, Y., Imada, I. & Morimoto, H. (1976): The effect of Ubiquinone-7 and its metabolites on the immune response. *Int. J. Vit. Nutr. Res.* **46**, 464–471.

38 Tachibana, K., Sone, S., Tsubura, E. & Kishino, Y. (1984): Stimulatory effect of vitamin A on tumoricidal activity of rat alveolar macrophages. *Br. J. Cancer* **49**, 343–348.

39 Watson, R.R. & Moriguchi, S. (1985): Cancer prevention by retinoids: role of immunological modifications. *Nutr. Res.* **5**, 663–675.

Vitamin A status, carotene and cancer prevention

Barbara A. UNDERWOOD
*National Eye Institute, National Institutes of Health Building 31, Room 6A-08, 9000 Rockville Pike
Bethesda, Maryland 20205, USA.*

Vitamin-A-deficiency, much like some cancers, results in the loss of cellular differentiation. It is quite reasonable, therefore, to postulate that vitamin A has a role in cancer prevention. This hypothesis has received much attention in recent years particularly because *in vitro* studies have shown that the addition of naturally-occurring retinoids to culture systems inhibits proliferation of undifferentiated cells. Because vitamin A itself is a fat-soluble substance that accumulates in mammals, particularly in hepatic tissue, and can lead to toxicity, derivatives that are not stored but are anticarcinogenic have been sought for preventive and therapeutic usage in man. Some promising synthetic retinoids have been found that are effective in culture and in some animal models[12,18]. Some of these may, on further testing, prove effective against some kinds of human cancers. It is difficult to extrapolate, however, from the Petri dish or controlled animal models to living conditions of man where many unknown factors may alter how substances interact with cells. Evidence in man for an association between vitamin A status and cancer is derived from two kinds of epidemiologic studies, observational studies and case-control studies. Because of methodological limitations inherent in epidemiological studies of either kind, risk factors can be identified but not definitive cause-effect relationships. A clinical trial in man is the best methodological approach toward establishing causation and studies of this kind are now in progress. The available evidence for an association between vitamin A status and cancer from observational and case-control epidemiological studies and some clinical trials now in progress are reviewed below.

Epidemiological evidence. *Dietary intake studies.* Several observational studies among varied populations are reported that have suggested an association between vitamin A status and some cancer prevalence. These studies, most of which have measured 'status' by the dietary intake of vitamin A, have not definitely established the nature of this association. One reason for the variability in findings is that different parameters have been used for assessing vitamin A intake. For example, some have assessed the total dietary intake of vitamin A activity as retinol equivalents, while others have evaluated dietary preformed and precursor vitamin A separately. Still others have created a vitamin A index or vegetable index based on food groups. In general, observational studies indicate that an association with preformed vitamin A (retinol) intake is not consistently found, a weak relationship to total vitamin A intake occurs and the most consistent association is with the intake of a green and yellow fruit and/or vegetable index. These latter food groups, of course, contain precursor carotenoids rather than preformed forms of vitamin A. A variable portion of the total carotenoids in these food groups, depending upon the particular foods included, is β-carotene.

The case-control approach can provide a somewhat more reliable methodology than descriptive studies for identifying risk factors associating diet and disease. A number of such studies, some retrospective and others prospective, are reported and recently have been evaluated[15]. They tend to confirm that the consumption of green and yellow fruits and vegetables is negatively correlated with the risk of some, but not all, types of cancers[8]. Squamous or small cell carcinomas are most consistently reported to be negatively associated with carotenoid intake. However, serum levels of total carotenoids are not consistently reported to be significantly correlated with cancer risk[20].

Until now there is no established metabolic role in man for carotenoids other than as precursors of retinol. Currently the most widely endorsed hypothesis for a mode of action of carotenoids in cancer prevention is their ability to quench singlet oxygen and, in the absence of the latter, as an antioxidant[2]. Hence, carotenoids may act in a way complementary to tocopherols in certain tissues of species such as man that deposit yellow fat. However, the fruits and vegetables that contain carotenoids also contain other substances, such as plant sterols, phenols and other micro-nutrients, some of which also are antioxidants (eg, vitamin C and selenium). These substances as yet have not been ruled out as possible anticancer constituents[3]. As Ames[1] has pointed out, just as foods contain anticancer agents, they also contain naturally-occurring mutagens and carcinogens. It is likely, therefore, that several substances in the food supply, and in the particular food groups of interest, are involved and that it is the relative balance of these in the diets of individuals and populations that determines outcomes.

Serum vitamin A levels. Serum vitamin A values have been used as a measure of vitamin A status in both retrospective and prospective case-control studies. The results have been variable[15]. One of the first studies that reported a positive protective association with higher blood levels of vitamin A was not confirmed in subsequent follow-up studies in the same population[16]. Recently, all the data from three large studies from which serum vitamin A values were available on cancer cases and matched controls have been pooled for statistical analysis; no evidence of a relationship between serum retinol levels and the risk of cancer in all sites combined or of lung cancer was found[17].

Serum values of vitamin A and carotenoids are known to be poor reflectors of vitamin A status and therefore this lack of an association with cancer prevalence cannot exclude the possibility that there is an association at the tissue level. To determine this will require a more definitive means of establishing relative levels of vitamin A status in target tissues than provided by the gross measures of dietary or serum parameters now used[19].

Evidence from clinical trials. As noted, epidemiological studies are limited to establishing associated factors in disease risk, but it is prospectively designed, randomized, double-blind clinical trials that offer the greatest potential for assigning causation to specific nutrient-disease relationships. Such studies are expensive to conduct. They must be carefully designed to be both cost-effective and provide reliable evidence about a positive, inverse, or null effect of an intervention. Several clinical trials are now in progress or anticipated[5,7,10]. Their outcome over the next several years should provide the evidence needed before considering intervention programmes for the public. While waiting for definitive answers, prudent practice is to follow the principles in the guide-lines published by the special committee assembled for the National Research Council that pertains particularly to the US diet[4]. The committee takes special caution, based on currently available evidence, in avoiding suggesting that dietary supplements of individual nutrients (including retinoids) convey any benefit in preventing cancer.

Assessment of vitamin A status. As noted before, neither dietary intake nor serum values of vitamin A or carotenoids alone are an adequate measure of relative vitamin A status except at the extremes of deficiency or excess. Newer measures are being sought. Some are still at the laboratory stage in development and others are being applied under various clinical and natural conditions to check their applicability and reliability[14].

One new functional approach, referred to as the relative dose response (RDR), appears to be promising for identifying humans whose liver reserves are depleted to a level that places them at risk[6]. The test is based on newer knowledge of factors that control the levels of retinol-binding protein (RBP) in the liver, the release of vitamin A from hepatic tissue and the pathway through the liver of newly ingested vitamin A under conditions of vitamin A deficit or adequacy[11]. However, this approach as well as some newer clinical approaches that use filter paper conjunctival impressions to determine the relative presence of goblet and keratinized cells[9], only detect individuals whose status is below a threshold level of deficiency. Above this threshold they are not linearly related to the vitamin A found in liver tissue. Further, there is little information as to how any of these parameters of vitamin A status relate to the levels found in nonhepatic tissue, both those that are healthy and those are are diseased, such as cancerous tissue[13]. Until better methods for determining relative levels of vitamin A status are found, even if associations with cancer prevention are established, it will be difficult to determine critical tissue threshold levels for cancer prevention.

Conclusion. In summary, the evidence for an association between vitamin A status and cancer is not clearly documented. This lack is due in part to the unavailability of a good indicator of relative levels of vitamin A in tissues, hence a reliable means of determining true vitamin A status. Clinical trials now in progress may provide more definitive evidence in the near future. Clearly there is need for additional research to determine the true nature of the association between vitamin A status and cancer prevention before public policy can be reliably made and advice to the public confidently given[19].

1 Ames, B.N. (1983): Dietary carcinogens and anticarcinogens. *Science* **221**, 1256–1264.

2 Burton, G.W. & Ingold, K.U. (1984): Beta-carotene: an unusual type of lipid antioxidant. *Science* **224**, 569–573.

3 Colditz, G.A., Branch, L.G., Lipnick, R.J., Willett, W.C., Rosner, B., Posner, B.M. & Hennekens, C.H. (1985): Increased green and yellow vegetable intake and lowered cancer deaths in an elderly population. *Am. J. Clin. Nutr.* **41**, 32–36.

4 Committee on Diet, Nutrition and Cancer (1982): *Diet, nutrition and cancer.* National Research Council, Washington DC: National Academy of Science.

5 Ershow, A.G., Zheng, S-F., Li, G., Li, J., Yang, C.S. & Blot, W.J. (1984): Compliance and nutritional status during feasibility study for an intervention trial in China. *J. Natl Cancer Inst.* **73**, 1477–1481.

6 Flores, H., Campos, F., Araujo, C.R.C. & Underwood, B.A. (1984): Assessment of marginal vitamin A deficiency in Brazilian children using the relative dose response procedure. *Am. J. Clin. Nutr.* **40**, 1281–1289.

7 Goodman, G.E., Alberts, D.S., Earnst, D.L. & Meyskens, F.L. (1983): Phase I trials of retinol in cancer patients. *J. Clin. Oncology* **1**, 394–399.

8 Graham, S. (1984): Epidemiology of retinoids and cancer. *J. Natl Cancer Inst.* **73**, 1423–1428.

9 Hatchell, D.L. & Sommer, A. (1984): Detection of ocular surface abnormalities in experimental vitamin A deficiency. *Archs Ophthalmol.* **102**, 1389–1393.

10 Hennekens, C.H. (1984): Issues in the design and conduct of clinical trials. *J. Natl Cancer Inst.* **73**, 1473–1476.

11 Loerch, J.D., Underwood, B.A. & Lewis, K.C. (1979): Response of plasma levels of vitamin A to a dose of vitamin A as an indicator of hepatic vitamin A reserves in rats. *J. Nutr.* **109**, 778–786.

12 Moon, R.C., McCormick, D.L. & Metha, R.G. (1983): Inhibition of carcinogenesis by retinoids. *Cancer Research (Suppl.)* **43**, 2469s–2475s.

13 Muto, Y. & Moriwaki, H. (1984): Antitumor activity of vitamin A and its derivatives. *J. Natl Cancer Inst.* **73**, 1389–1393.

14 Olson, J. (1984): Serum levels of vitamin A and carotenoids as reflectors of nutritional status. *J. Natl Cancer Inst.* **73**, 1439–1444.

15 Palgi, A. (1984): Vitamin A and lung cancer: a perspective. *Nutr. & Cancer* **6**, 105–120.

16 Peleg, I., Heyden, S., Knowles, M. & Hames, C.G. (1984): Serum retinol and risk of subsequent cancer: extension of the Evans County, Georgia, study. *J. Natl Cancer Inst.* **73**, 1455–1458.

17 Seigel, D. (1984): Discussion of case-control studies of Peleg, Stahelin, and Willett. *J. Natl Cancer Inst.* **73**, 1469–1470.

18 Sporn, M.R. & Roberts, A.B. (1983): Role of retinoids in differentiation and carcinogenesis. *Cancer Res.* **43**, 3034–3040.

19 Underwood, B.A. (1984): Summary of research needs. *J. Natl Cancer Inst.* **73**, 1489.

20 Willett, W.C., Polk, B.F., Underwood, B.A., Stampfer, M.J., Pressel, S., Rosner, B., Taylor, J.O., Schneider, K. & Hames, C.G. (1984): Relation of serum vitamins A and E and carotenoids to the risk of cancer. *New Engl. J. Med.* **310**, 430–434.

Operational research to combat vitamin-A-deficiency: the case of Indonesia

Ignatius TARWOTJO
Directorate of Nutrition, Ministry of Health, Jakarta, Indonesia

Vitamin-A-deficiency has been recognized as a major public health problem in Indonesia for well over 10 years and this paper describes a vitamin A programme implemented by the Ministry of Health as a series of 'generations', punctuated with specific, targeted and well-thought out 'operational research' activities. The results of each generation have influenced the next in a very direct sense.

Phase 1: Initiation of Indonesia's vitamin A programme. In 1973, the problem of xerophthalmia had already been recognized and efforts were underway to design and test a pilot study in 20 sub-districts in Java in which vitamin A (200 000 IU) capsules were distributed to all children between 1 and 4 years of age. These children were chosen because they were the most likely to suffer a high mortaility from malnutrition and disease. Collaboration between WHO, UNICEF, HKI, and the Ministry of Health was necessary to implement the project.

The operational research design consisted of two components. The first was a clinical study designed to determine the biological effectiveness of vitamin A capsules in preventing xerophthalmia. It was a double-blind propsective experimental/placebo study with the determination of eye signs of xerophthalmia by examination teams at 6-monthly intervals, following a baseline examination. The second aspect was to test the effectiveness and efficiency of the capsule distribution system.

The major clinical findings of the study were: (1) administration of 200 000 IU vitamin A led to a significant decrease of xerophthalmia in the experimental group; (2) xerophthalmia was deemed to be easily reversible, and (3) it could not be determined if vitamin A could effectively reduce blindness.

Operationally, effectiveness was defined in terms of coverage of the target population, and efficiency was measured in terms of capsules per worker per day administered and cost per capsule distributed. The major findings were: (1) vitamin A capsules were accepted by the population and appropriate under field conditions; (2) coverage of the target population was feasible by the method used; (3) administrative support was critical to capsule distribution; (4) average cost per capsule distributed was US$ 0.19.

As a result of this study, operational guide-lines were established which proved useful for Indonesia. On the basis of this information, the government decided to expand the vitamin A capsules programme to include 7 million preschool-age children during 1974–1979.

Phase II: Planning and implementation of a comprehensive epidemiologic research study. Based on the premise that operational research was a sound method for prevention planning, a meeting was held in Indonesia in November 1974 called by both WHO and USAID, to address the control of vitamin-A-deficiency, including priorities for research and action.

The first study was a longitudinal, prospective study of 5000 pre-school children, who were to be reexamined every three to four months for 2 years.

The second study was also prospective and was a detailed clinical, biochemical, bacteriological and histopathological study of children with corneal and non-corneal xerophthalmia. The last study was a national survey of the prevalence of xerophthalmia conducted in 24 provinces of

Indonesia. The findings of the project included the following: (1) vitamin-A-deficiency is a public health problem in Indonesia; (2) dark green leafy vegetables are available in the family diet but consumed less frequently by children; (3) consumption of edible fat is low in xerophthalmic children; (4) a majority of xerophthalmic children eat three potentially fortifiable items: mono-sodium glutamate (MSG), wheat and refined sugar; (5) measles precipitates nutritional blindness in many instances; (6) vitamin A can reduce the incidence of nutritional blindness; (7) cases of xerophthalmia tend to cluster about a small geographical area; (8) cases of mild xerophthalmia tend to have a higher relative risk of mortality than matched controls; (9) night blindness is a sensitive and specific indicator of xerophthalmia.

From these results, which were obtained in 1980, the national vitamin A programme became even more focused. The nature of the problem was clearly defined, the solutions identified, and momentum established to test these interventions. The question now was how to implement programmes to address the problem given limited available resources. The next round of operational research was to help answer these questions.

Phase III: Consolidation of the national vitamin A programme. By the end of 1980 the problem and its solutions were identified. In the short run, vitamin A capsules supplied by UNICEF could be distributed either as a special programme or as part of a larger nutrition and primary health care effort. The effort was to improve the effectiveness and efficiency of capsule distribution and to explore long-term solutions which would eventually eliminate the need to outside aid in the form of capsules. This second strategy would require changes in the feeding behaviour of the population and the need to devise mechanisms whereby vitamin A could get to the target population through the fortification of foodstuffs.

Improvement of capsule coverage. By 1982 vitamin A capsule distribution had become a routine part of the Family Nutrition Improvement Programme (FNIP). Coverage of the target population was low and the programme was not run efficiently. An operational research project was designed to test the effectiveness and efficiency on the island of Lombok in the province of Nusa Tenggara Barat, one of the 15 high-risk provinces.

The operational research project tested the effectiveness and efficiency of vitamin A capsule delivery on a 6-month cycle in the form of mini campaigns, compared to routine administration of capsules. Operationally, the 6-month effort, when combined with health education, could result in increased vitamin A coverage of the target population. The result of this effort coloured the decision to plan capsule distribution as part of the national FNIP but on 6-month cycles.

Evaluation of different capsule distribution systems and their impact on vitamin-A-deficiency. In previous studies coverage estimates were most often based on *capsules provided* rather than on *children receiving capsules*, and no information of those not receiving capsules was available. Furthermore, questions remained on the efficacy of periodic massive dosing of vitamin A as a nutritional 'topping up' strategy in the presence of a basal diet low in the vitamin, systemic infections etc. To investigate these issues, a study was proposed for Aceh (another of the high-risk provinces) to: (1) assess the coverage and reasons why children did or not receive capsules; (2) assess the impact of periodic massive dosing of vitamin A on children under 5 years of age on the incidence of xerophthalmia; (3) demonstrate the difference in mortality rates between those areas with different capsule distribution systems.

The method used consisted of an assessment of the effectiveness of two capsule programmes: the on-going vitamin A distribution as part of the national FNIP to specific target groups, and the distribution of vitamin A to any child with signs of xerophthalmia. Project villages were censused, families interviewed and children examined for xerophthalmia and capsules distributed on 6-month cycles with a follow-up for examination. This was a prospective 2-year study and the preliminary results indicate: (1) high risk villages tend to be near the main roads and market towns which are generally the larger villages in the area; (2) the same high-risk villages also tend to be the least well covered, while rural villages have less of a vitamin-A-deficiency problem and higher coverage; (3) providing vitamin A capsules to parents or guardians of the children is not an effective means of treating children, for they often do not receive the capsules; (4) the length of training of the distributor and his/her age and education all influence distribution but do not affect coverage; (5) villages with low-coverage with vitamin A had a higher prevalence of xerophthalmia and coverage was inversely proportional to the prevalence of xerophthalmia, and (6) children in villages with low coverage of vitamin A had a relative risk of mortality 30 per cent higher than high-coverage villages.

Use of communication strategies to encourage nutrition status changes. Health education/communication was deemed needed to change the behaviour of mothers with regard to feeding dark green leafy vegetables to children. Two operational research projects were carried out to assess the viability of this method of intervention. In the first, conceptual testing was done to assess the types of education methods needed and a workshop was held to prepare the strategy and the project carried out. In a pretest-posttest non-equivalent control group design, areas with communication/education programmes were compared to areas without this intervention in terms of the nutritional status of the children.

Although measuring the impact of education is difficult, results indicated that in areas where nutrition education was implemented, there were large and significant differences in nutritional status of children as compared to areas with no nutrition education. Based on these results, which were not vitamin-A-specific, the Ministry of Health has decided to place greater emphasis on improving the nutrition education component of the FNIP with the help of HKI.

Another operational research project was established to test whether or not, in areas where radios are prevalent, radio messages could influence mothers' purchasing, preparation and feeding of children low-cost dark green leafy vegetables. A baseline survey was conducted, messages developed and aired and a follow-up made to households and mothers indicated that radio is a good medium for this purpose and a phase II project proposal is being developed to assess actual knowledge and behaviour change.

Fortification. Subsequent to the national xerophthalmia survey which identified potentially fortifiable foodstuffs, a feasibility study was carried out which identified MSG as the most easily fortifiable product. The project is again a pretest-posttest non-equivalent control group design implemented in West Java. One area is getting fortified MSG, the other area not. The initial surveys collected information on MSG consumption, blood and breast-milk samples, and on the results of examination of the children's eyes. Information on household and village characteristics was also collected.

Although analysis is still being done on the data, the results indicate that in those target areas where the fortified product was consumed, xerophthalmia was significantly lower than in areas with the non-fortified product but overriding social and political consequences of using MSG as the vehicle may prevent the national expansion of the project.

Phase IV: Planning for the future. The operational studies which have been carried out have influenced the development, planning and expansion of the vitamin A programme in Indonesia.

This trend will continue with studies now in the planning stages. The Directorate of Nutrition, together with the Directorate of Epidemiology and Immunization of the Ministry of Health, is planning to carry out a 2-year prospective study measuring the impact on child mortality of a combined vitamin-A-immunization campaign in Aceh province. Again, this will be a study, totally operational in nature, to assess the effectiveness of combining these two interventions and their impact.

In addition to the above, and based on results of earlier studies, the Directorate will be defining a model of vitamin-A-deficiency surveillance and containment based on the clustering phenomenon. In addition, a cost analysis study will be undertaken to determine whether liquid vitamin A distribution, as part of the FNIP can significantly reduce the unit cost of vitamin A distribution, anticipating reductions in the availability of donated vitamin A capsules.

Biological interactions and nutrition: a workshop report

J.C. SOMOGYI, D. HÖTZEL and M. FUJIWARA (Organizers)
Universities of Zurich, Bonn and Kyoto.

The organizers and participants in this workshop had as their goal a state-of-the-art presentation of the positive and negative effects of biological interactions in nutrition, pharmacology and clinical medicine.

In his introductory remarks *J.C. Somogyi* discussed classifications within this complex field and the need to modify classifications with the expansion of knowledge. In this context, he cited the example of his classification of antimetabolites and antivitamins into two groups which included: (1) structurally similar compounds which compete with the physiological analogue and (2) structure-modifying compounds that destroy or decrease the effect of vitamins either by modifying the molecular structure or by forming complexes with the vitamin. He pointed out that it would be impossible to fit calcium-channel blockers into either of these categories.

In a paper on the interactions between thiamin and some food components by *S. Vimokesant, B. Panijpan and P. Reunwongsa*, (Department of Biochemistry Mahidol University, Bangkok, Thailand) *B. Panijpan* described the thiamin-deficiency occurring in elderly Thai women, who are heavy tea-drinkers and who also chew tea leaves. If these women could be induced to stop chewing or drinking tea at meal times, their thiamin status could be improved. The thiamin antagonists in tea had been identified as polyphenolic compounds and it had been shown that ascorbic acid could reduce the severity of this chemically induced thiamin deficiency in the rat. In a discussion of this paper, *J.C. Somogyi* commented that in his own earlier experiments, he had found that among dihydrophenols, the number and position of the OH groups are of primary significance in determining the anti-thiamin effect.

Y. Itokawa, (University of Kyoto) discussed the interrelations between thiamin, magnesium and calcium. In the rat, thiamin deficiency reduces the severity of magnesium depletion induced by dietary restriction. In cases of human thiamin-deficiency, associated with inadequate magnesium status, both thiamin and magnesium should be given.

D. Hotzel, (University of Bonn) discussed sulphite toxicity in relation to B vitamin status.

Vitamin K antagonists were discussed by *R. Olson*, (State University of New York) who grouped these antagonists into those, such as broad-spectrum antibiotics which inhibit the gut biosynthesis of menaquinone, vitamin A and other retinoids which inhibit the absorption of vitamin K, vitamin E and also the cephalosporin antibiotics which block the carboxylation reaction, coumarin anticoagulants which block the interconversion of K vitamers and a further drug group which included phenytoin, which block the effects of vitamin K by unknown mechanisms.

A further contribution to advances in the field of fat-soluble vitamins was offered by *S. Berger*, (Warsaw Agricultural University). He paid special attention to the effect of changing the levels of vitamin A and vitamin E in animal and human diets and showed that by changing the ratios of these nutrients in the diet, their levels in the blood and tissues could be altered. He also suggested that we should reconsider optimal levels of vitamins A and E in human diets in the light of their anticancer potential.

H. Weiser, (Hoffmann-La Roche, Basel) presented a paper on the interrelations between polyunsaturated fatty acids and vitamin E co-authored by *A.W. Kormann* in which the hypothesis was supported that vitamin E not only has potent antioxidant effects but also that it influences the metabolism of arachidonic acid. The role of vitamin E in reducing the toxicity of anticancer drugs was also discussed. *W. Hopff*, (Pharmacology Institute University of Zurich) described the modes of action of calcium-channel blockers. They may either bind to the surface of the calcium-channels and so modify membrane excitability or they may compete with coordinating sites for calcium or they may enter into cells thus substituting for calcium. This latter effect was characteristic of inorganic lanthanum compounds and not of the calcium-channel blockers in current use as cardiovascular agents.

D.R. Fraser, (Dunn Nutritional Laboratory, Cambridge) described interactions between calcium and other components of food. He stressed that while most of the interactions of calcium with other nutrients or non-nutrient food compounds, resulted in complex formation which decrease calcium absorption, lactose and casein both promote calcium absorption.

D.A. Roe, (Division of Nutritional Sciences, Cornell University) reviewed the established risks of drug-induced nutritional deficiencies and then described risks that have arisen recently not only because of the availability of new drugs, but also because certain drugs, such as cholestyramine, were being prescribed for use in children and for very prolonged periods of time, even for a lifetime. She emphasized that there was a particular risk of drug-induced malnutrition when drugs having this potential were given to very malnourished patients. Further, she indicated that drug-induced malnutrition could usually be prevented if the risk was recognized and that such risk assessment could now be achieved using computerized knowledge base management systems. The individual papers were followed by general discussion and the workshop was summarized by *R. Olson*.

X: Trace elements

The epidemiology of iodine deficiency disorders in China, India and Africa

The effects of iodine deficiency on development

Research developments in zinc nutrition

Research developments in iron nutrition

Workshop

THE EPIDEMIOLOGY OF IODINE DEFICIENCY DISORDERS IN CHINA, INDIA AND AFRICA

Neurological disorders in cretins of different types in China

T. MA and T.Z. LU
Institute of Clinical Endocrinology, Tianjin Medical College, Tianjin, China.

Iodine-deficiency disorders are still a significant problem in China. More than a quarter of our one billion population lives in the original iodine-deficient area; however 90 per cent of them are under treatment by an iodisation programme at present but still there are 11 million goitre patients. The real disaster of the iodine-deficiency is the retardation of brain development in children. There are more than 200 000 typical cretins in various endemic areas of China and the subclinical cases number many times more than the above figure. After the iodisation programme, the typical cretin was very rarely found but the subclinical cretins (we prefer to use the term sub-cretins) could still be found. The real cause of this persistency of sub-cretins is still being studied. Inadequate and irregular iodisation should be considered as a cause.

We have two types of cretinism in China. The major type is neurological cretinism which is found in most of the areas in which cretinism is endemic. Myxoedematous cretinism is the minor type which is found chiefly in the north-west part of China and these patients are nearly always found together with neurological cretins.

The clinical features of neurological cretinism in China are similar to those of the neurological cretinism found in other areas of the world, such as in the mountainous areas of the Alps and the Andes and in New Guinea. The neurological triad, ie mental retardation, deaf-mutism, and spastic paralysis are the principal symptoms.

The neurological cretins of Guizhou Province may be the most typical neurological cretins in China. Besides the mental retardation and deaf-mutism, the neuromuscular defects are particularly remarkable. Although subclinical hypothyroidism with slight lowering of T_4 and a slightly increased T_3 and TSH have been detected among the cretins, no single case of frank myxoedema has been found there.

Examination of 247 cases of endemic cretinism in the South-eastern part of Guizhou revealed that mental retardation is the most significant neurological manifestation and is present in all of the cretins there, but that its severity varies[3]. Hearing defects have been detected in almost all cretins there and its severity varies. Speech defects have been found in 94.8 per cent of the cretins there. Neuromuscular defects could be seen in the branches of the spinal as well as the cranial nerves. Spinal nerve defects could be demonstrated in almost all the cretins. These symptoms occurred in different combinations. Cranial nerve defects have been found in 58 cretins there.

Chengde is another typical endemic area of neurological cretinism in China and 80 cases have been examined there[1]. All of the cases have marked neurological defects. Two cases exhibited frank myxoedema in addition to the neurological symptoms. Mental defects have been found in all of the cretins in this area. Hearing and speech defects are common. The defect in hearing is correlated with the defect in vestibular response in this group of patients. As we know, the centre of hearing and the centre of balance lie quite remote from each other in the brain. Therefore we suspect that this lesion might be located in the inner ear rather than in the brain. Recently an Australian neurologist Dr. J.G. Morris (personal communication) examined a group of neurological cretins in Xin-Zhou county of Shanxi Province and found that there is no auditory first wave, that means the cochlea cannot respond to a sound stimulus to produce an electrical potential. This finding also supports the hypothesis that the lesion causing deafness might be located in the inner ear. However some lesion in another part of the auditory tract or the temporal lobes of brain cound not be excluded. No retardation of conductivity of peripheral nerve trunks could be demonstrated. No particular sign of cerebellar lesion could be demonstrated yet the special gait and the impaired performance of fine skilled manipulations might be the sum result of some disturbances in the pyramidal tract, the extrapyramidal tract and cerebellum. There is no evidence of involvement of vegetative functions dependent on hypothalamus and autonomic system. Temperature regulation, fluid balance, sleep and appetite are quite normal in neurological cretins. Functions of limbic and cingulate system seem to be intact.

Xinin is a region where a mixed type of certinism is endemic. Most of the cretin patients there have some signs of hypothyroidism, including myxoedema. Even for the patients having frank myxoedema, typical upper motor neurone paralysis could be demonstrated. The feeblemindedness and deaf-mutism of those patients are also quite similar to the neurological cretins in Chengde. Dr. J.G. Morris examined some patients with myxoedema in Xinin and found that most patients show no auditory first wave. No delay of conductivity of peripheral nerve trunks was demonstrated. From these findings we can say the neurological symptoms of the mixed type cretin are quite similar to those of the neurological cretin.

There are both neurological and myxoedematous types of cretins in Hetan[2]. The neurological cretins there have upper motor neurone symptoms with hypothyroidism signs, including myxoedema (similar to the mixed type cretin in Xinin); but the myxoedematous cretins in Hetan have very few upper motor neurone signs, feeblemindedness or deaf-mutism, and the coordinative movements are quite well preserved. Some typical myxoedematous cretins in Hetan could undertake an interpreter job between Uyghur and Han languages and some can dance in a coordinated way to the tempo of their folk music.

The cretin patients in Liang-cheng county[2] are considered to be myxoedematous. However the myxoedema is not so severe as in the myxoedematous type cretins in Hetan; but most of them have no upper motor neurone lesion signs prior to the thyroxine treatment. The upper motor neurone signs became gradually obvious during the disappearance of the myxoedema.

From the various features of neurological manifestations in the different areas of endemic hypothyroidism known in China, we may conclude that every cretin patient has congenital brain lesions, however their severity is various, and only a proportion of cretin patients have postnatal hypothyroidism.

1 Lu, T.Z., Zhang, J. & Ma. T. *et al.* (1965): Clinical observation on endemic cretinism of Chengde Region. *Tianjin Med. Pharm. J.* **7** (1), 1. (In Chinese).
2 Ma, T. *et al.* (1982): The present status of endemic goiter and endemic cretinism in China. 4 (4), **13**.
3 Zeng, K.H. *et al.* (1982): Neuropsychiatrical changes of 247 cases of endemic cretin in south-eastern part of Gui-zhou. *Chin. J. Neuropsychiat.* **15**, 154. (In Chinese).

Iodine-deficiency and neonatal hypothyroidism in India

N. KOCHUPILLAI, M.M. GODBOLE, C.S. PANDAV*, M.G. KARMARKAR, MANJU MEHTA† and M.M.S. AHUJA
*Departments of Endocrinology and Metabolism, *Centre for Community Medicine and †Department of Psychiatry, All-India Institute of Medical Sciences, New Delhi-110 029, India.*

The reported incidence of neonatal hypothyroidism (NH) in developed countries without iodine-deficiency or endemic goitre varies from 1 in 2500 to 1 in 8000 births[1,2]. NH screening is not adopted as a measure to prevent mental retardation in any of the developing countries. Recently, we reported 4 per cent incidence of NH in the Gonda district of Uttar Pradesh (UP) belonging to the sub-Himalayan endemic goitre belt[4-6]. We also reported significantly lower mean thyroxine (T_4) values and elevated mean TSH values in the 'normal' new-born from Gonda[4]. We have now extended these studies to several other areas of India with varying degress of iodine-deficiency and goitre prevalence. In two severely iodine-deficient villages belonging to areas with very high incidence of NH, we also studied the intelligence quotient (IQ) of school children and prevalence of nerve deafness in the village population.

Results. The overall prevalence of goitre in the district of Deoria was 80 per cent; 3 to 5 per cent cretinism was observed in the seriously goitrous flood-prone villages of the district. The survey of the incidence of goitre and of I.Q. and audiometry measurements clearly show that significant neurological damage occurs in the population living in villages which are seriously iodine-deficient with a high incidence of NH.

The results (see Tables 1–3) permit the following conclusions: (a) The incidence of NH as reflected in blood T_4 and TSH levels is significantly higher in regions of India with iodine-deficiency and endemic goitre. (b) The incidence of NH varies from 0.6 per cent to 13 per cent, depending on the severity of iodine-deficiency as assessed by the pattern of urinary iodide excretion, as well as the prevalence of goitre and cretinism in the affected population. (c) In populations with very high incidence of NH due to iodine-deficiency, besides overt cretinism, sub-cretinous neurological damage occurs in a substantial proportion of the population.

High incidence of NH in iodine-deficient areas with endemic goitre and or cretinism have been reported from Zaire and Sicily[8,9]. From Zaire 10 per cent of NH was reported as reflected in cord blood hormone levels at birth[9] — the authors have also shown that a good proportion of these children remain hypothyroid in the post-weaning period to end up as typical myxoedematous cretins. According to these authors, the continued hypothyroidism through childhood and adolescence in these patients is because of cassava consumption which aggravates the iodine-deficient state.

Table 1. *Iodine-deficiency and incidence of neonatal hypothyroidism (NH) in different geographical areas.*

Area	Goitre prevalence (%)	Cretinism (%)	Urinary Iodine Excretion[a]	Incidence of NH (%)
Deoria	80	3–5	V	13. 3
Gorakhpur	60–70	0–4	V	8. 5
Gonda	60	0–4	V	7. 5
Delhi	29	Nil	II & III	0. 6
Kerala	1.3	Nil	NA	0.12

[a]Follis, 1964[3].

Table 2. *Distribution of intelligence quotient[a] in survey and in the normal population.*

Age (yrs)	No Subjects	Intelligence quotient				
		≤ 69	70–79	80–89	90–109	110–119
Survey population						
6 to 10	10	2	3	4	1	–
11 to 16	50	12	17	11	9	1
Total	60	14	20	15	10	1
	100%	23.3%	33.3%	25%	16.7%	1.7%
Normal population		–	–	–	–	–
	100%	2.2%	6.7%	16.1%	50.0%	16.1%

[a]Bhatia's Battery of Performance Tests, Malin's Intelligence Scale, Bender Visual Motor Gestalt Tests[7].

Table 3. *Audiometry results in Ramdham village, Deoria District of U.P., India.*

Goitre prevalence	No. of subjects studied	Sensorineuronal loss	Conductive loss
95%	93	18	1

A study of blood from 180 new-born children from a severe endemic region of Sicily with goitre and cretinism revealed 9.3 per cent incidence of NH at birth[8]. On following-up these children for a period of from 6 weeks to 10 months transient hypothyroidism was found which lasted more than 12 weeks in a significant proportion of the detected neonatal hypothyroids.

A variety of factors seem to make it safe to conclude that a good proportion of the detected new-born with hypothyroidism may remain so, long enough postnatally to end up with significant neurological damage. These facts include: (a) the severe degree of hypothyroxinemia observed in the present set of new-born, (b) the severity of iodine-deficiency in the areas of study and the demonstrated low-iodine content in the breast-milk of the mothers belonging to these areas (N. Kochupillai, unpublished) and (c) the evidence of significant sub-cretinous brain damage occurring in a striking proportion of children at the Primary Health Centres with high incidence of NH. The above facts, when taken together, can be interpreted to mean that environmental iodine-deficiency is causing much more brain damage than is evidenced by overt cretinism in the millions of people living in the sub-Himalayan endemic goitre belt.

Overt cretinism may indeed be the mere tip of an iceberg of neurological damage occurring due to environmental iodine-deficiency in the indigent populations. The findings of the present study demonstrate that nutritional iodine-deficiency is a far more serious health problem than it appears in the guise of goitre or cretinism and that it is a potentially serious threat to health in regions inhabitated by hundreds of millions of people in the developing world.

1 Illig, R. & Gitzelmann, R. (1977): Screening for congenital hypothyroidism. *J. Pediat.* **91**. 348–349.
2 Irie, M. & Naruse, H. (1979): Mass screening of neonatal hypothyroidism. In *Neonatal screening for inborn errors of metabolism*, ed H. Bickel, R. Guthrie & G. Hammerser. Berlin: Springer Verlag.

3 Follis, R.H. (1964): Recent studies on iodine malnutrition and endemic goitre. *Med. Clins. North Am.* **48**, 1919.
4 Kochupillai, N. (1984): Neonatal thyroid status in Iodine deficient environments of the sub-Himalayan region. *Indian J. Med. Res.* **80**, 293.
  5 Kochupillai, N. *et al.* (1984): Thyroid status among new-borns from iodine-deficient environments in India. *Proc. 4th Asian Congr. Nutr.*, Bangkok.
6 Kochupillai, N., Godbole, M.M., Pandav, C.S., Karmarkar, M.G., Mithal, A. & Ahuja, M.M.S. (1985): Iodine deficiency and neonatal hypothyroidism. In *Iodine nutrition, thyroxine and brain development*, ed V. Ramalingaswami. New Delhi: Tata-McGraw Hill. (In press).
7 Murthy, H.N. (1965): Short scale of Bhatia Battery performance test of intelligence. Trans All-India Institute of Mental Health, Bangalore.
8 Sava, L., Delange, F., Belfiore, A., Purrello, F. & Vigneri, R. (1984): *J. Clin. Endocrinol. Metab.* **59**, 90–95.
9 Thilly, C.H., Delange, F., Lagasse, R., Bourdoux, P., Ramioul, I., Berquist, H. & Ermans, A.M. (1978): Fetal hypothyroidism and maternal thyroid status in severe endemic goiter. *J. Clin. Endocrinol. Metab.* **47**, 354–360.

Endemic goitre and cretinism in Africa

F.P. KAVISHE
Tanzania Food and Nutrition Centre, PO Box 977, Dar es Salaam, Tanzania.

Iodine-deficiency disorders (IDD), manifesting mainly as endemic goitre and cretinism, are no longer a world-wide problem. Technical advances in mass iodine supplementation since the Ohio trials in 1920[8], coupled with a massive socio-economic development in the advanced countries have now relegated the disease to the long list of problems 'peculiar' to the developing countries. Since the health effects of iodine-deficiency go far beyond those of endemic goitre and cretinism and include conditions like still births, abortions, congenital anomalies and various forms of physical and mental retardation, a control programme is not only socially but economically desirable.

This paper examines, albeit not exhaustively, the problem of endemic goitre and cretinism in Africa according to available data. It recommends further data collection, inter-regional African cooperation in control/eradication programmes and calls for more support for Africa by international organizations as stipulated in the 1978 World Food Council's (WFC) declaration, which adopted a global target for goitre eradication in the next decade. This will also be consistent with WHO/UNICEF's global declaration of health for all by year 2000 (HFA/2000).

The epidemiology of endemic goitre and cretinism in Africa. For various technical, economic and administrative reasons, the epidemiologic data available on the problem of IDD in Africa is almost completely confined to endemic goitre alone, and the extent of other disorders caused by iodine-deficiency remains completely unexplored, with the exception of endemic cretinism which has been mentioned in a few reports. Assuming a continental average prevalence rate of 10 per cent for endemic goitre and 0.1 per cent for cretinism, an estimated 50 million people and 5 million people may be afflicted with endemic goitre and cretinism respectively in Africa.

Endemic goitre. Although the information from the various countries is not always representative of the actual situation, due to poor sampling techniques and too few observations, nevertheless it gives an idea of the extent of the problem and may motivate concerned authorities to establish control programmes. The Table summarizes the situation regarding endemic goitre in a few African countries. It can be seen that with only a few exceptions endemic goitre is of public health significance according to WHO criteria in almost all the countries shown in the Table. The Figure shows the assumed distribution of goitre in Africa, ie it remains essentially that compiled by Kelly & Snedden in 1960[6] and updated by Demaeyer *et al.* in 1979[2], with only a few

Table. *The prevalence of endemic goitre and cretinism in some African countries.*

Name of country	Year of survey	Age groups surveyed (years)	Number examined	Goitre prevalence (%)	Cretinism prevalence (%)
Cameroon	1969	All	39 980	58.0	?
Central African Republic	1971	All	?	<1.0	?
Chad	1941	All	?	100.0	?
Ethiopia	1965	1–12	1115	29.5	?
Ivory Coast	1966–69	All	14 798	18.5	?
Ghana	1961–62	Adults	826	13.5	?
Kenya	1962–64	Children	28 250	30.2	?
Kenya	1969	All	?	64.0	?
Kenya	1972	Children	?	62.0	?
Libya Arab Jamahiriya	1974	11–20	741	46.0	?
Mali	1968	Children	?	48.5	?
Niger	1968	Children	1300	12.5	?
Senegal	1970	All	12 000	39.5	?
Senegal	1976	All	2424	39.5	?
Sudan	1975	< 20	2919	9.4	?
Tunisia	1973–75	All	10 789	2.6	?
Tanzania	1953–70	All	?	73.0	?
Tanzania	1980–81	6–19	55 573	47.8	?
Zaire (Ubangi)	1982	All	4407	76.8	4.7
Zambia	1971	All	54 830	50.5	?
Zimbabwe	1968	All	550	45.0	?

additions particularly in East and Central Africa. The largest addition is a national goitre survey done in Tanzania in 1980–1981 where more than 55 000 primary school children were examined. It appears that the situation regarding endemic goitre in Africa has remained fairly stable within the past 20 years or so, because there have been no sustained endemic goitre control programmes in any country.

Endemic cretinism. The situation regarding endemic cretinism in Africa has not been documented to the extent of that of endemic goitre, possibly due to the shortage of medical skills needed in the diagnosis and the large samples required when doing community surveys. Overt clinical cretinism of 3 per cent was found in one village (Magoye in Njombe district) in the Southern highlands of mainland Tanzania where the visible goitre rate was above 60 per cent[9] and in a National Goitre Survey (Kavishe *et al.*[5]) several cretins were observed in areas where the gross goitre prevalance was above 60 per cent.

Endemic goitre studies in Idjwi island, Lake Kivu, Democratic Republic of the Congo found a prevalence of cretinism of 1.1 per cent in the northern area where the goitre prevalence was 54.4 per cent but found no cretins in the south-west and south-east where the goitre prevalences were 5.3 per cent and 17.5 per cent, respectively[3]. In the Kungu zone, in Zaire, a progressive increase of myxoedematous cretinism was found when the prevalence of goitre reached a critical threshold of 50 per cent of the population[1]. It has been recognized generally that when the iodine intake of a population is below 20 µg per person per day, up to 10 per cent of the children may be affected by endemic cretinism.

Deaf-mutism and endemic goitre. An epidemiologic association between deaf-mutism and endemic goitre has been observed in some parts of the world. There are other causes of deaf-mutism in areas when endemic goitre is prevalent, and these must be excluded if an epidemiological correlation with goitre is contemplated. This was evident in a national goitre survey done in Tanzania in 1980–1981[5]. In this survey the correlation between the prevalence (viz number of population affected/number of total population) of visible goitre rate and that of crude deaf-mutism was poor (r = 0.3; n = 23) probably because other causes of deaf-mutism were not properly eliminated and the number of the total population was under-estimated. When other causes are excluded, the presence of high rates of deaf-mutism in a high goitre-endemic area would reflect subclinical endemic cretinism.

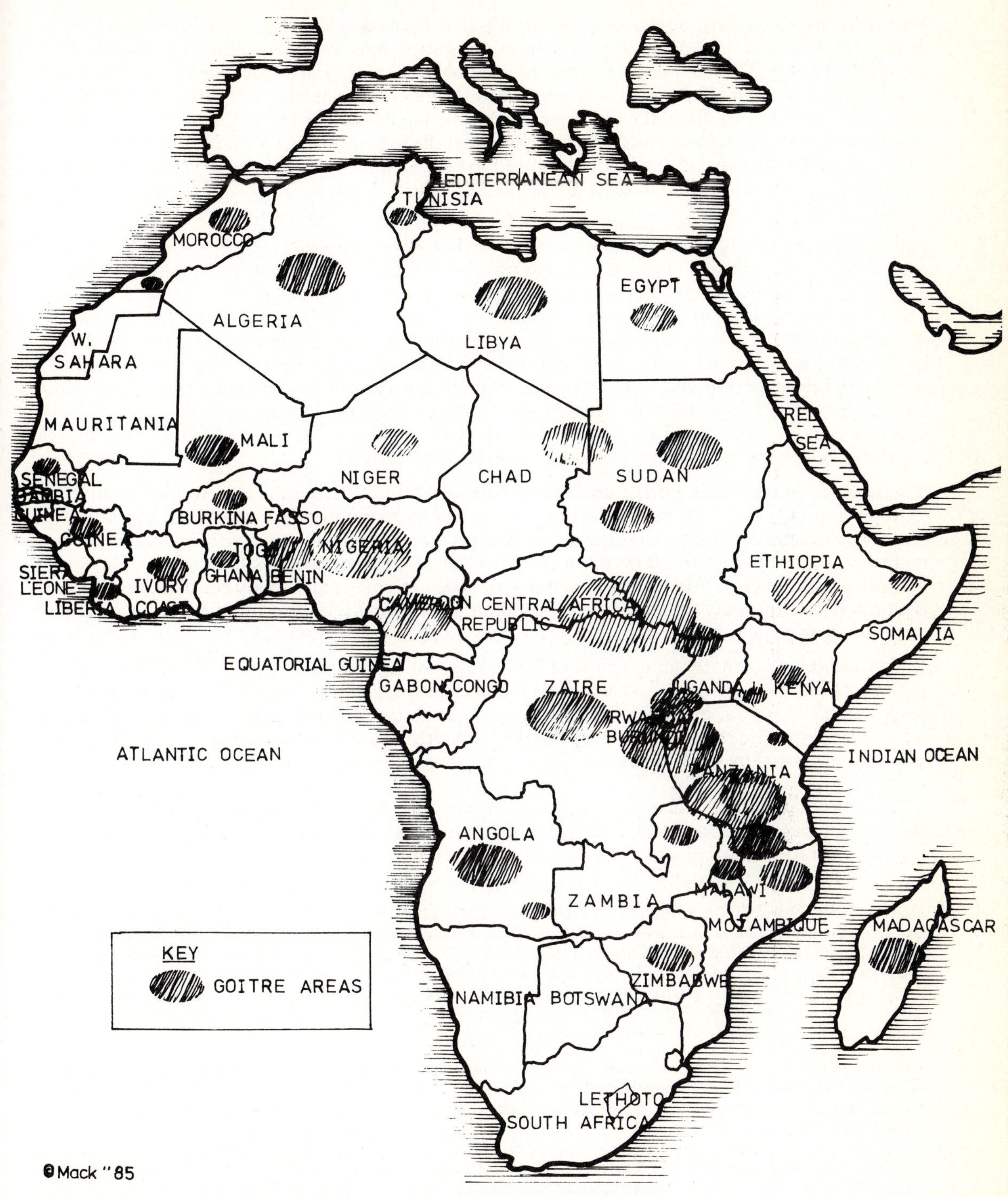

Figure. *The geographical distribution of endemic goitre in Africa (1939–1985)*

The aetiology of goitre and cretinism in Africa. *Iodine-deficiency.* As in other continents the central aetiological factor in the endemics of goitre and cretinism in Africa is dietary iodine-deficiency. This is reflected in the geographical distribution of the disease, which seems to clearly follow geological features suspected to be deficient in iodine. In these endemic areas, food and water arising from the soils contain iodine far below the levels found in areas where goitre and cretinism are not endemic. In Tanzania, the iodine level in water in the Ukinga area where goitre prevalence is high has been found to be less than 1 μg per litre, as compared to Dar es Salaam (coast) tap water which is 4.7 μg per litre and 47 μg per litre of water from the Indian Ocean.

Goitrogenic factors. Only one goitrogen has been fairly well implicated as a cause of endemic goitre and cretinism in Africa. This is cassava in Zaire[1]. Although cabbage is known to have goitrogenic activity, no association was found between the prevalence of goitre in Ukinga Tanzania and the level of cabbage consumption[7]. Millet has also been implicated as a factor in the goitre endemics of Sudan. On the basis of epidemiologic data in goitrogenous patients living in the southern part of Senegal, it was observed that the thyroid swelling was negatively correlated with the patients' retinol status, implicating vitamin-A-deficiency as a goitrogenic factor[4]. However, it has been stressed in all cases that the goitrogenic activity of these substances is superimposed on a primary iodine-deficiency. This makes iodine-deficiency a necessary factor for the goitre and cretinism endemics in Africa.

The control of endemic goitre and cretinism in Africa. During the last decade or so, some African countries have attempted rather unsuccessfully to institute goitre control programmes mainly by iodination of salt. In some areas pilot projects have tested the use of iodinated oil as a means of controlling goitre. The main drawback in these programmes has been the lack of a definite national policy and its implementation. IDD are potentially easily controllable diseases if national governments are convinced as to their public health importance and are willing and capable of taking action.

Conclusions. As seen, the magnitude of the problem of endemic goitre and cretinism in various regions of Africa is of public health significance, although in certain areas, it has not been well-defined. National mapping using simple, cheap and yet rapid epidemiological methods is recommended. The surveys can use low level health and education cadres, and the survey methods proposed by DeMaeyer *et al.*[2] are easily reproducible. School children would make an easily reachable population.

It is recommended that control programmes be done on an inter-country regional cooperation basis. International and regional organizations and concerned governments should actively take the initiative and start regional programmes for the control of endemic goitre and cretinism. For example salt iodination could be a regional project.

Acknowledgements. I would like to thank J.C. Waterlow of London School of Hygiene and Tropical Medicine and B. Hetzel of the Commonwealth Scientific and Industrial Research Organization, Australia, for encouraging my participation in this conference. F. Delange of the University of Brussels Belgium provided me with copies of their work concerning goitre and cretinism in Zaire, and Dr Ingenbleek of Nestlé Products Technical Assistance Research Department, Switzerland, provided me with copies of his work about vitamin-A-deficiency and goitre. I thank them all. Last but not least, I would like to thank the ODA for sponsoring my attendance and the Tanzania Food and Nutrition Centre for allowing my participation in this Congress.

1 Delange, F., Iteke, F.B. & Ermans, A.M. (1982): *Nutritional factors involved in the goitrogenic action of cassava.* Ottawa, Canada: International Development Research Centre.

2 DeMaeyer, E.M., Loweinstein, F.W. & Thilly, C.H. (1979): *The control of endemic goitre.* Geneva: World Health Organization.

3 Ermans, A.M., Thilley, C., Vis, H.L. & Delange, F. (1969): Studies on Idjiwi Island Lake Kiru Democratic Republic of the Congo: permissive nature of iodine deficiency in the development of endemic goitre. In *Endemic goitre* ed J.B. Stanbury. Report of the PAHO Scientific group on Research on Endemic Goitre, Puebla, Mexico. 27–29 June 1968, pp. 101–117. Scientific Publication 193. Washington: PAHO.

4 Ingenbleek, Y. & De Visscher, M. (1979): Hormonal and nutritional status: critical conditions for endemic goitre epidemiology? *Metabolism* **28**, 9–19.

5 Kavishe, F.P., Kalinga, L., Ljungqvist, B.G., Mlingi, N.L. & Bunga, B.E. (1983): The prevalence and control of endemic goitre in Tanzania. Tanzania Food and Nutrition Centre Report No. 818.

6 Kelly, F.C. & Snedden, W.W. (1960): *Endemic goitre*. WHO Monograph Series No. 44. Geneva: WHO.
7 Latham, M.C. (1965): The aetiology, prophylaxis and treatment of endemic goitre in Ukinga, Tanzania. *East Afr. Med. J.* **42**, 489.
8 Marine, D. & Kimball, O.P. (1921): The prevention of simple goitre in man. *J. Am. Med. Ass.* **77**, 1068–1070.
9 Wachter, W., Mvungi, M.G., Triebel, E., Van Thiel, D., Marschner, I., Wood, W.G., Habermann, J., Pickardt, C.R. & Scriba, P.C. (1985): Iodine deficiency, hypothyroidism and endemic goitre in Southern Tanzania. *J. Epidem. Community Hlth.* **39**, 263–270.

Juvenile hypothyroidism and thiocyanate overload after weaning

C.H. THILLY, P. BOURDOUX, P. NGO BEBE, B. SWENNEN and J. VANDERPAS
IRS-CEMUBAC, Kinshasa, Zaïre, and Brussels University, Belgium; School of Public Health CP1 590/7, route de Lennik 808, B-1070 Bruxelles, Belgium.

In Ubangi, Zaire, a very severe endemic goitre occurs and it has been customary to consider its main hazard to public health to be the concomitant occurrence of 2 to 6 per cent of cretin and cretinoid subjects. However we have clearly demonstrated that, in addition to cretinism, low-birthweight, high perinatal and infantile mortality and low psychomotor development in larger groups of infants also occurs[3,4].

Apart from severe iodine-deficiency, the presence of a supplementary endemic goitrogenic factor, namely excess thiocyanate (SCN), resulting from the consumption of large quantities of poorly detoxified cassava has also been well-demonstrated[1], so that it is not clear whether the range of abnormalities observed are linked to the iodine-deficiency alone or also to thiocyanate overload.

Mothers eating cassava have high thiocyanate levels in the serum which readily crosses the placenta[2] and cassava consumption by children starts early in life, as complementary foods during the long breast-feeding period and also after weaning. Therefore the aim of the present work was to study the thyroid function of children at risk together with the incidence of both goitrogenic factors and to relate them to the feeding pattern.

Results. Figure 1 presents the mean serum TSH, T4, free T4 (FT4), T3 and T3/T4 ratio at birth and between 0 to 3, 3 to 6, 6 to 9 and 9 to 12 months of age. Values at birth in the new-born of iodine-treated mothers are also given for comparison. At birth, subnormal T4 is accompanied by a high TSH (18.0 µU/ml), significantly higher than the value (7.2 µU/ml) observed in the new-born from treated mothers ($P < 0.001$). Compared with the values obtained at birth, the usual increase in T3 and thus in the T3/T4 ratio were observed in the 0–3 months untreated group. From the 2nd to the 3rd and 4th trimesters, none of the parameters studied present any significant variation so that during the 1st year of life there is certainly no degradation of the thyroid function but rather a stabilization or even a very slight improvement. The means for the same parameters in the age groups < 1, 1 to 4, 4 to 7 years old and in young adults are shown in the Table. Control values in 0 to 7 years old Belgians are also given. Compared with the first year of life, one observes in the next two age groups, further degradation of the thyroid function, characterized by an important and significant decrease of T4 and FT4 and significant increase of serum TSH. T3 is unchanged. Some further but quite small degradation of the thyroid function is then observed in young adults.

From the same data, it has been calculated that, in the 4 to 7 compared with the < 1 year age group, the percentage of children with T4 < 4 µg/dl is 65 per cent compared with 32 per cent ($P < 0.001$), those with TSH > 50 µU/ml: 42 per cent compared with 24 per cent ($P < 0.05$) and those with both T4 less than 4 µg/dl and T3 less than 110 ng/dl are 15 per cent compared with 6 per cent ($P > 0.05$).

Figure 2 shows the incidence of goitre, serum SCN concentration and urinary iodine (I)

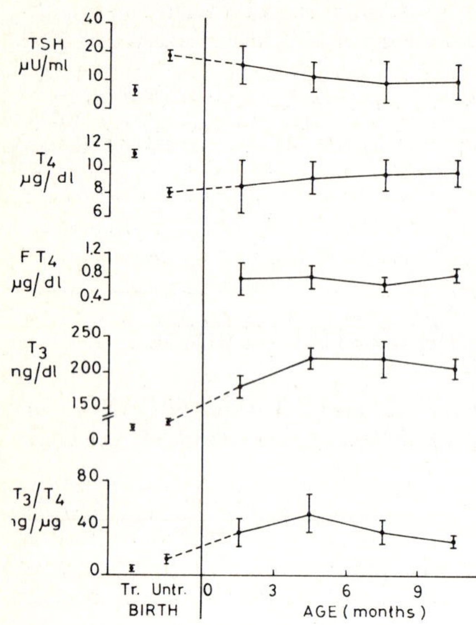

Table. *Comparison of the mean serum T4, Free T4 (FT4), T3, TSH and T3/T4 ratio in different age groups of Ubangi and in Belgian controls.*

	Belgian Controls (0–7 years)	Age (Years)			
		< 1	*1 to 4*	*4 to 7*	*15 to 30*
Serum T4 (µg/dl)	9.8 (174)	9.6 (79)	5.8*** (53)	4.8*** (66)	4.1*** (775)
Serum FT4 (µg/dl)	1.51	0.81	0.64ns	0.60*	0.48***
Serum T3 (ng/dl)	193	210	207ns	189ns	181ns
Serum TSH (µU/ml)	2.9	10.4	10.1ns	24.3*	24.1**
Serum T3/T4	22	38	60*	64**	–

Significance levels compared with < 1 year age group; number of subjects in parentheses. *$P < 0.05$, **$P < 0.01$, ***$P < 0.001$.

Fig. 1 (left). *Mean ± s.e.m. of serum TSH, T4, free T4 (FT4), T3 and T3/T4 ratio at birth (Untr.) and between 0 to 3, 3 to 6, 6 to 9 and 9 to 12 months of age in children from Ubangi. For comparison mean of the same parameters at birth in new-born from iodine-treated mothers (Tr).*

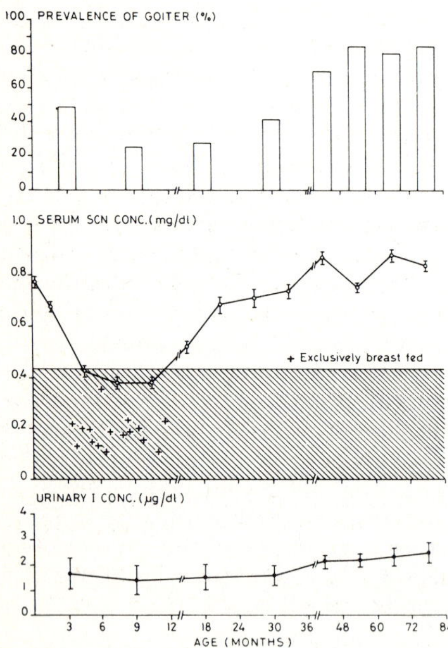

Fig. 2. *Prevalence of goitre (upper section) serum thiocyanate (SCN) concentration (middle section) and urinary iodine (I) concentration (lower section) against age. For SCN, the shaded area represents the normal range.*

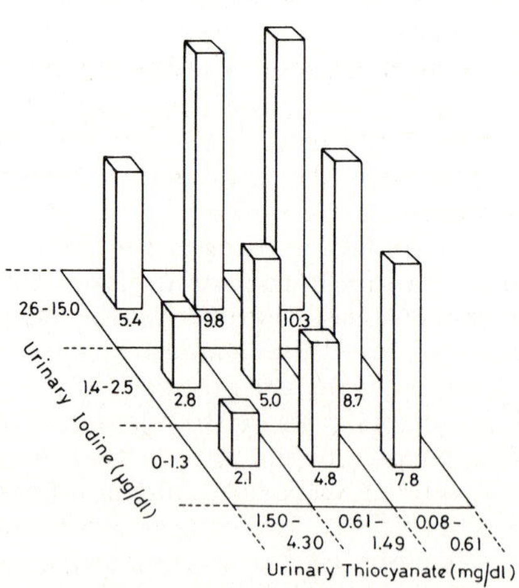

Fig. 3. *Mean serum T4 (µg/dl), shown under each block, as a function of urinary iodine (µg/dl) and thiocyanate (mg/dl) concentrations.*

concentration from 0 to 7 years of age. The incidence of goitre is 49 per cent at 3 months, reaches a minimum of 25 per cent during the 2nd semester and then progressively increases to reach a plateau of 75 per cent from the age of 3 years. The urinary I concentration is low and does not show any significant changes, indicating severe I-deficiency throughout the age period studied. In contrast, serum SCN concentration varied markedly and the shape of the curve is parallel to that of the incidence of goitre. At birth the mean is 0.75 mg/dl and correlated closely with the maternal values suggesting its placental transfer. During the first 3 months of life, the concentration decreases quickly to the upper limit of the normal range. It stays at this level between 3 and 12 months of age and then increases again to its maximum adult value at 3 years of age. The decrease of serum SCN corresponds to breast-feeding and the increase after 1 year of age corresponds to the progressive supplementation and weaning with foods consisting mainly of cassava. Between 3 and 12 months of age, a few individual SCN values of children still exclusively breast-fed have also been represented. They are in the normal range. Compared with a high serum SCN concentration in Ubangi mothers at delivery (0.77 mg/dl), its mean concentration in their milk is 0.33 mg/dl and is not significantly different from that obtained in the milk from Belgian mothers.

Figure 3 presents in a stereogram the mean value of serum T4 in nine subgroups of these children classified in tertiles by their urinary I and SCN concentrations. The mean serum T4 values are spread from the very low value of 2.1 µg/dl for the children with the more severe iodine-deficiency and thiocyanate overload to a normal 10.3 µg/dl for those without such exposure to either goitrogenic factor.

Conclusion. In the area of endemic goitre incidence in Ubangi there are two separate periods of risk during which a supplementary goitrogenic factor, excess dietary SCN, is present, The first period is at the end of fetal life and during the perinatal period during which we have demonstrated that 12 per cent of the new-born suffer neonatal hypothyroidism responsible for the impairment of brain maturation and also low birthweight, high perinatal mortality and low developmental quotient[4]. Prolonged breast-feeding exerts an important protective effect, because SCN it is not present in human milk, so that during the 1st year of life there is no further degradation of the thyroid function.

The second period of risk is after weaning when a late thyroid failure appears as a consequence of the recurrence of SCN overload. It explains the high proportion of cretinoids observed in Ubangi, characterized by less severe mental retardation and no neurologic defects but by stunted growth and florid hypothyroidism. The number of children affected with juvenile hypothyroidism is much larger than that of those affected with perinatal hypothyroidism. It may thus constitute the main public health complication in that area of deficiency.

While there is no question that it is the occurrence of the SCN overload which explains the extreme severity and the nature of the complication of this disease, it has to be remembered that iodine prophylaxis during pregnancy, lactation and weaning, entirely prevents the occurrence of all symptoms.

1 Bourdoux, P., Delange, F., Gérard, M., Mafuta, M., Hanson, A. & Ermans, A.M. (1978): Evidence that cassava ingestion increases thiocyanate formation: a possible etiologic factor in endemic goiter. *J. Clin. Endocr. Metab.* **46**, 613–621.

2 Delange, F., Bourdoux, P., Lagasse, R., Hanson, A., Mafuta, M., Courtois, P., Seghers, P. & Thilly, C. (1980): Effects of thiocyanate during pregnancy and lactation on thyroid function in infants. In *Role of cassava in the etiology of endemic goitre and cretinism*, ed A.M. Ermans, N.M. Mbulamoko, F. Delange & R. Ahluwalia, pp. 121–126. Ottawa: International Development Research Centre.

3 Ermans, A.M., Bourdoux, P., Lagasse, R., Delange, F. & Thilly, C. (1980): Congenital hypothyroidism in developing countries. In *Neonatal thyroid screening*, ed G.N. Burrow & J.H. Dussault, pp. 61–73. New York: Raven Press.

4 Thilly, C., Lagasse, R., Roger, G., Bourdoux, P. & Ermans, A.M. (1980): Impaired fetal and postnatal development and high perinatal death-rate in a severe iodine deficient area. In *Thyroid research VII*, ed J.R. Stockigt & S. Nagataki, pp. 20–23. Canberra: Australian Academy of Sciences.

THE EFFECTS OF IODINE DEFICIENCY ON DEVELOPMENT

The effects of iodine-deficiency on fetal development in the sheep and the marmoset

B.S. HETZEL and B.J. POTTER
CSIRO Division of Human Nutrition, Kintore Avenue, Adelaide, 5000 South Australia, Australia.

The relation between dietary iodine-deficiency in man and endemic cretinism has now been well established by epidemiological studies[4]. These include descriptive studies dating from the Sardinian Commission (1848), analytic studies and finally the results of a controlled trial with iodised oil injection in the New Guinea Highlands[10]. The prevention of cretinism by correction of iodine-deficiency in the mother was demonstrated in this trial and in another controlled trial in Zaire. This finding has been confirmed subsequently with uncontrolled observations following iodization programmes in Indonesia and other countries[2,4].

These observations raise questions about the mechanism involved — particularly as to whether the iodine-deficiency is acting through the maternal and/or fetal thyroid or possibly directly on brain development[6,10].

To this end animal models have been investigated. Earlier studies include the guinea-pig and the rat, but the Australian merino sheep and the marmoset (*Callithrix jacchus jacchus*) have provided the most successful models. The sheep offers the advantage that surgical procedures can be carried out readily in both mother and fetus while the marmoset offers the advantage of a nonhuman primate much more closely related to man.

It is well-known that the timing of brain development varies between species. In the human, the maximum growth occurs around the time of parturition which is also the maximum growth time of the pig brain (termed 'perinatal brain developer'). In the rat (and rabbit) the maximum growth is postnatal (termed 'postnatal brain developer'). In the sheep and the monkey the maximum growth is prenatal, termed 'prenatal brain developers'[1,6]. As has been pointed out[1], comparisons can be made between species if the stages rather than the ages of brain development are taken into account.

Iodine-deficiency in sheep. Severe iodine-deficiency has been produced in sheep[14] with a low-iodine diet of crushed maize and pelleted pea pollard (8–15 µg iodine/kg) which provided 5–8 µg iodine per day. After a period of 5 months, although body weights were maintained, iodine-deficiency was evident with the appearance of goitre, low plasma values for thyroxine (T_4) and triiodothyronine (T_3) values, elevated TSH levels and low daily urinary excretion of iodine. Control animals received the same diet, but were supplemented with 2 mg sodium iodide administered by subcutaneous injections each week, or by an iodised oil injection (1 ml = 400 mg iodine). The ewes were mated with normal fertile rams, dates of conception established, and fetuses delivered at 56, 70, 98 and 140 d gestation by hysterotomy[14].

Goitre was evident from 70 d in the iodine-deficient fetuses and, thyroid histology revealed evidence of hyperplasia from 56 d gestation. The increase in thyroid weight was associated with a reduction in fetal thyroid iodine content, reduced plasma T_4 values and increased plasma TSH (Table 1).

The iodine-deficient fetuses at 140 d were grossly different in physical appearance from the control fetuses[4]. They exhibited reduced weight, absence of wool growth, goitre, varying degrees of subluxation of the foot joints and deformation of the skull. There was also delayed bone maturation as indicated by delayed appearance of epiphyses in the limbs[4,14].

There was a lowered brain weight and brain DNA as early as 70 d, indicating a reduction in cell number probably due to reduction in the speed of neuroblast multiplication which normally occurs from 40–80 d in the sheep[8]. Although brain protein was reduced in the deficient fetuses the ratio protein: DNA and protein content were reduced to less than normal in the 98 d and 140 d fetal brains (Table 2).

Table 1. *Effect of severe dietary iodine-deficiency on maternal and fetal thyroid function in sheep.* Potter et al., (1982)[14].

Gestational age (d)		56	70	98	140
Maternal plasma	I-defic.	(5) 37^a	(6) 17^a	(5) 15^a	(7) 19^a
T$_4$(nmol/l)	Control	(3)126	(4)134	(5)141	(3)137
Maternal plasma	I-defic.	(5) 54	(6)120^a	(5)125^b	(7)109^a
TSH(ng/ml)	Control	(3) 6	(4) 7	(5) 5	(3) 11
Fetal plasma	I-defic.	(5) 3^b	(6) 4^a	(5) 4^a	(7) 6^a
T$_4$(nmol/l)	Control	(2) 10	(4) 25	(5)125	(3)216
Fetal plasma	I-defic.	(5) 56	(6)165^a	(5)170^a	(7)211^a
TSH(ng/ml)	Control	(2) 12	(4) 11	(5) 13	(3) 12
Fetal thyroid	I-defic.	(5)0.01	(6)0.37^b	(5)4.30^a	(7)12.69^a
weight (g)	Control	(3)0.05	(4)0.08	(5)0.28	(3) 0.99
Fetal thyroid	I-defic.	(5)0.06	(6)1.15^c	(5)8.7^c	(7) 29^b
iodine(μg/ whole gland)	Control	(3)0.24	(4)8.79	(5)146.9	(3)2636

[a]$P<0.001$, [b]$P<0.01$, [c]$P<0.05$ (two-tailed 't' test) comparing the iodine-deficient value and the corresponding control figure in the same column and row. (Number of observations shown in parentheses).

Table 2. *Effect of severe dietary iodine-deficiency on fetal brain development in sheep.* Potter et al., (1982)[14].

Gestational age (d)		56	70	98	140
Brain wt (g)	I-defic.	(5) 1.79	(7) 4.20^c	(5)19.0	(7)46.4^b
	Control	(3) 1.68	(4) 5.01	(5)22.1	(6)53.8
Cell number	I-defic.	8.86	14.2^c	27.8^b	62.6^a
(mg DNA)	Control	8.37	16.2	32.5	74.5
Cell size	I-defic.	9.31	12.4	25.2	40.3
(protein:DNA)	Control	8.95	12.8	26.6	44.1
Body wt (g)	I-defic.	31.7	101^c	662	2930^b
	Control	32.2	129	753	3820

[a]$P<0.001$, [b]$P<0.01$, [c]$P<0.05$ (two-tailed 't' test). Number of observations shown in parentheses.

Retardation of fetal brain development in severe dietary iodine-deficiency was revealed also by histological studies at 140 d gestation[14]. Delayed maturation of the cerebellum was shown by reduced migration of cells from the external granular layer to the internal granular layer and increased density of Purkinje cells. The greater density of Purkinje cells indicates a reduction in Purkinje cell arborisation with the molecular layer. In the cerebral hemispheres the cells were more densely packed in the motor and visual areas while the pyramidal neurons in the hippocampus were denser in some areas indicating severe retardation in neuropil growth in both subfields.

Evidence of retarded myelination in the cerebral hemispheres and brainstem was provided by lowered cholesterol: DNA ratios, and an increased water content in the brain at 140 d was further confirmation of brain retardation in iodine-deficiency[14].

The effect of iodine on this retarded fetal brain development due to iodine-deficiency has been investigated with a single intramuscular injection of iodised oil containing 500 mg iodine given at 100 d gestation[13]. In injected animals, the difference between iodine-deficient and control fetal brain weights was reduced from 10.8 per cent to 6 per cent by the iodised oil injection. The difference in body weight was also reduced and maternal and fetal plasma T$_4$ values were restored to normal[13].

The effects of iodine-deficiency and the iodised oil administration on cerebellum and cerebral hemispheres are summarized in the Figure.

The effects of severe iodine-deficiency on fetal brain development in the sheep were more severe but similar to those of fetal thyroidectomy carried out at 50–60 d or at 98 d[7]. Maternal thyroidectomy carried out some 6 weeks before pregnancy had a significant effect of fetal brain development in mid-gestation[11]. The combination of maternal thyroidectomy and fetal thyroidectomy at 98 d produces more severe effects than that of iodine-deficiency (Figure)[5].

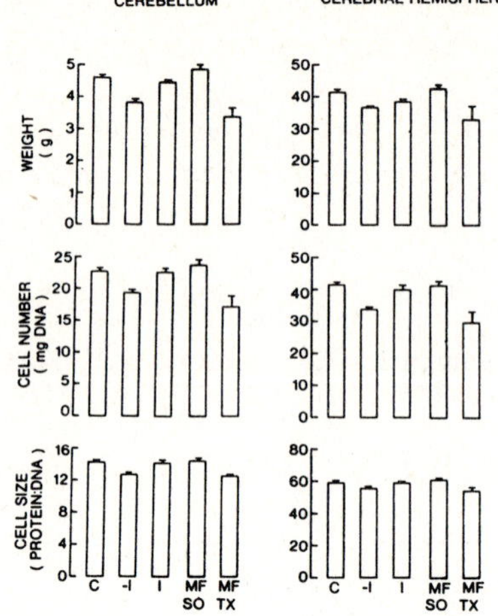

Figure. *Comparison of brains of sheep fetuses at 140 d gestation.* C = Control; −I = iodine-deficient; I = iodine at 100 d; MFSO = mother+fetus sham-operated; MFTX = mother+fetus thyroidectomised. From Hetzel (1983)[2] with permission.

The findings following maternal, fetal and combined thyroidectomy suggest that the effect of iodine-deficiency on fetal brain development is mediated by the combination of reduced maternal and fetal thyroid secretion and not by a direct effect of iodine[4,5,10]. The effect of reduced maternal secretion occurs in the 1st half of pregnancy and the effect of reduced fetal secretion in the latter half of pregnancy. The conclusion is consistent with recent evidence in the rat of the passage of maternal thyroxine across the placental barrier early in pregnancy[3,9,15].

Iodine-deficiency in the marmoset. Severe iodine-deficiency has been produced in the marmoset (*Callithrix jacchus jacchus*) with a mixed diet of maize (60 per cent), peas (15 per cent), torula yeast (10 per cent) and dried iodine-deficient mutton (10 per cent) derived from the iodine-deficient sheep produced in the study already described[14]. There was a gross reduction in maternal T_4 levels (Table 3) with grossly reduced thyroid iodine. After a year on the diet the animals were allowed to become pregnant and the new-born animals were studied following the 1st pregnancy and then again following the 2nd pregnancy. The effects on brain development are summarized in Table 3. Significant effects were apparent in the 2nd pregnancy.

Table 3. *Effect of iodine-deficiency on fetal brain development in the marmoset. Values at birth.* Modified from Potter *et al.*[12].

		Plasma T4 (nmol/l)		Brain		
		Maternal	*Fetal*	*Weight (g)*	*DNA mg in whole brain ('cell number')*	*Cell size (Protein: DNA)*
Control	Mean	182[aaa,bb]	>400[aaa,bbb]	3.4[bb]	7.90[ab]	31.3[bb]
(n = 6)	s.e.m.	± 15	–	± 0.08	± 0.10	± 0.7
Iodine-deficiency	Mean	16[aaa]	75[aaa]	3.50[ccc]	7.40[a]	30.9[c]
(1st pregnancy)	s.e.m.	± 3	± 17	± 0.06	± 0.15	± 0.9
(n = 8)						
Iodine-deficiency	Mean	11[bb]	40[bbb]	2.97[bb,ccc]	7.17[b]	27.8[bb,c]
(2nd pregnancy)	s.e.m.	± 3	± 8	± 0.11	± 0.28	± 0.7
(n = 4)						

[a,b,c]$P < 0.05$, [aa,bb,cc]$P < 0.01$, [aaa,bbb,ccc]$P < 0.001$: Values within a column with the same superscript differ significantly.

There was other evidence of hypothyroidism in the form of impaired hair growth and some skull deformity but there were no striking effects on epiphyseal development. In general the findings in this primate resemble those in the sheep.

Conclusions. The findings from these two animal models confirm the necessity of iodine for normal brain development. The effects in the sheep are apparent early in pregnancy (70 d) indicating a slowing of neuroblastic multiplication before the fetal thyroid is secreting. There is now good evidence of the passage of maternal thyroxine across the placental barrier in the rat[9,15]. Other effects observed in the iodine-deficient sheep include a high rate of still births (10 per cent) compared with less than 1 per cent in the control animals receiving the iodine supplement. The findings indicate general effects on growth and development which justify the term iodine-deficiency disorders (IDD) rather than 'goitre' to denote the effects of iodine-deficiency.

The findings in the marmoset indicate fetal hypothyroidism as the main effect of severe iodine-deficiency during pregnancy in a nonhuman primate. This corresponds to the condition of myxoedematous cretinism in man[7]. So far in both species, the classical features of human neurological cretinism — deaf-mutism and spastic diplegia[2,6] have not been observed, but only limited observations have so far been made in the postnatal period. The marmoset model is very appropriate for longer-term behavioural observations. These need to be made in order to further elucidate the effects of iodine-deficiency on development.

1 Dobbing, J. (1974): The later development of the brain and its vulnerability. In *Scientific foundations of paediatrics*, ed J.A. Davis & J. Dobbing. pp. 565–577. London: Heinemann Medical.

2 Hetzel, B.S. (1983): Iodine deficiency disorders (IDD) and their eradication. *Lancet* **2**, 1126–1129.

3 Hetzel, B.S., Potter, B.J., Mano, M.T., Belling, G.B., McIntosh, G.I. & Cragg, B.G. (1984): Brain development in the iodine deficient ovine fetus. In *Endocrinology*, ed F. Labrie & L. Proulx, pp. 731–734. *Proc. 7th Int. Cong. Endocrinol.*, Quebec. Amsterdam: Excerpta Medica.

4 Hetzel, B.S. & Potter, B.J. (1983): Iodine Deficiency and the Role of Thyroid Hormones in Brain Development. In *Neurobiology of the trace elements*, ed I.E. Dreosti & R.M. Smith, pp. 83–133, New Jersey: Humana Press.

5 Hetzel, B.S., Potter, B.J., McIntosh, G.H., Mano, M.T., Belling, G.B., Martin, D.M., Hua, C. & Cragg, B.G. (1983): A comparison of the effect of maternal and fetal thyroidectomy with that of severe iodine deficiency on fetal brain development at 140 days gestation in the sheep. In *Current problems in thyroid research*, ed N. Ui, K. Torizuka, S. Nagataki & K. Miyai, pp. 345–348. Proc. 2nd Asia and Oceania Thyroid Association, Tokyo. Amsterdam: Excerpta Medica.

6 Hetzel, B.S. & Hay, I.D. (1979): Thyroid function, iodine nutrition and fetal brain development. *Clin. Endocrinol.* **11**, 445–460.

7 McIntosh, G.H., Potter, B.J., Hetzel, B.S., Hua, C.H. & Cragg, B.G. (1982): A quantitative morphological and biochemical study comparing 60 and 98 day fetal thyroidectomy on brain development in the newborn lamb. *J. Comp. Path.* **92**, 599–607.

8 McIntosh, G.H., Baghurst, K.I., Potter, B.J. & Hetzel, B.S. (1979): Fetal brain development in the sheep. *Neuropathol. Appl Neurobiol.* **5**, 103–114.

9 Obregon, M.J., Mallol, J., Pastor, R., Morreale de Escobar, G. & Escobar del Ray, F. (1984): L-thyroxine and 3,5,3'-triiodo-L-thyronine in rat embryos before onset of fetal thyroid function. *Endocrinology*, **114**, 305–307.

10 Pharoah, P.O.D., Buttfield, I.H. & Hetzel, B.S. (1971): Neurological damage to the fetus resulting from severe iodine deficiency during pregnancy. *Lancet* **1**, 308–310.

11 Potter, B.J., McIntosh, G.H., Mano, M.T., Chavedej, J., Hua, C.H., Cragg, B.G. & Hetzel, B.S. (1985): The effect of maternal thyroidectomy prior to conception on fetal brain development in sheep. *Acta Endocrinologica* **112**, 93–99.

12 Potter, B.J., Mano, M.T., Belling, G.B. & Hetzel, B.S. (1984): Iodine deficiency and fetal development in the marmoset. *Proc. Endocrin. Soc. Aust.* **27**, p. 26.

13 Potter, B.J., Mano, M.T., Belling, G.B., Martin, D.M., Cragg, B.G., Chavedej, J. & Hetzel, B.S. (1984): Restoration of brain growth in fetal sheep after iodised oil administration to pregnant iodine-deficient ewes. *J. Neurol. Sci.* **66**, 15–26.

14 Potter, B.J., Mano, M.T., Belling, G.B., McIntosh, G.H., Hua, C., Cragg, B.G., Marshall, J., Wellby, M.L. & Hetzel, B.S. (1982): Retarded fetal brain development resulting from severe dietary iodine deficiency in sheep. *Neuropathol. Appl. Neurobiol.* **8**, 303–313.

15 Woods, R.J., Sinha, A.K. & Ekins, R.P. (1984): Uptake and metabolism of thyroid hormones by the rat fetus in early pregnancy. *Clin. Sci.* **67**, 359–363.

Effects of iodine-deficiency on the motor performance of children in Papua New Guinea

K.J. CONNOLLY and P.O.D. PHAROAH
Department of Psychology, University of Sheffield, Sheffield, S10 2TN; and Department of Community Health, University of Liverpool, Liverpool, L69 3BX, UK.

Contact was first made with the people of the Jimi valley in the Western Highlands Province of Papua New Guinea in 1953. By 1956 a patrol post was established in the valley and medical patrols began. It was later noticed that the incidence of cretinism in several villages in the middle Jimi was high. Although it was widely believed that cretinism was associated with iodine-deficiency a clear demonstration had not been made. A correlation was reported between iodine prophylaxis and a decline in cretinism[13] but this was criticized on methodological grounds[6].

A census was undertaken in the middle Jimi in 1966 and 16 500 people were enrolled in a trial, alternate families receiving either an injection of iodinated oil or a saline placebo. The results of the trial have been reported in full[11]; follow-up over a period of 6 years found six cretins out of 687 children born to women given the iodine supplement, of these five were conceived prior to injection. In the control group 31 cretins were found among a total of 688 children, five of whom were conceived before the placebo was given. Further evidence about the importance of iodine came from the observation that the disease was of recent onset in the Jimi valley. Following first contact with Europeans in 1953 there was a sharp rise in the prevalence of cretinism; from about 0.1 per cent before 1953 rising in the late 1950s and early 1960s to a peak of 15 per cent in 1965 (Figure). The increase in prevalence was found to be due to an increased incidence attributed to a change in the source of salt used by the people; their original source of salt was found to have a very high iodine content[10].

Whether iodine-deficiency had an all-or-none effect was not evident from the early follow-up examination of the two groups of children: it was argued[5] that deaf-mute cretins in an Ecuadorian Andean population were not a discontinuous group of physically and neurologically retarded individuals. The alternative hypothesis is that cretins represent the most severely affected end of a continuum of physical, neurological and behavioural development. The hypothesis of a continuum of effect was examined in the Jimi population by comparing the performance of the ostensibly normal children, that is excluding the cretins, born to mothers in the iodine and saline groups.

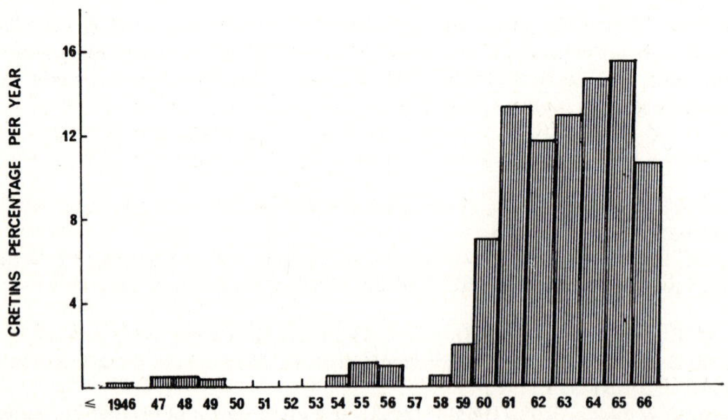

Figure. *Annual prevalence of cretinism in the Jimi valley of Papua New Guinea.* Reproduced by kind permission of the Editor of *The Lancet*.

The motor performance of children born to mothers given either an iodine supplement or saline placebo was examined[2]. The evaluation of motor skills (and of course intellectual performance) in such a population is extremely difficult and tests had to be selected with several constraints in mind; materials and equipment had to be carried into remote mountain areas, few if any facilities (such as a power source) were available, time for testing was limited, tests must be sensitive over an age range, they must be valid and reliable. And most difficult of all the requirements of the tests must be explained to the children non-verbally; the language barrier is formidable. A number of tests were employed[2] which measured grip strength, speed of movement, and speed/accuracy in one- and two-handed tasks. A screening test for motor impairment developed for use in a Western developed country was also used. Over five of the villages involved in the original trial 208 children were found and tested; 115 from the iodine group and 79 from the control. The difference in numbers is largely a reflection of differential mortality in the two groups. The investigation was conducted under double-blind conditions, that is to say neither the persons administering the tests nor the children knew whether their mothers had been given an iodine or a saline injection.

The data obtained from the investigation of these two groups of clinically normal children showed that they differed in terms of skilled motor ability. The difference is apparent in tasks requiring both speed and accuracy in performance though not on grosser measures of strength or simple speed of movement. The findings, which are clear and statistically significant, give support to the hypothesis that dietary iodine-deficiency during development can lead to sub-clinical deficits. Support for this conclusion is provided from data collected in central Java[1].

One reason why iodine is important functionally is because it is a component of the two thyroid hormones thyroxine (T_4) and triiodothyronine (T_3). In conditions of iodine deficiency the concentration of serum T_4 falls, but T_3 remains in the normal range or even rises[9], so maintaining clinical euthyroidism. The compensating mechanism for iodine-deficiency involves a rise in TSH which produces an enlargement of the gland — a goitre. Thus, although people in an iodine-deficient region may be clinically euthyroid and indistinguishable from normal, biochemical analysis will reveal abnormalities.

In 1970 and 1971 blood samples were taken from women of childbearing age, several of whom were pregnant at the time, and T_3 and T_4 were measured. The offspring from some of these women were amongst the sample subsequently reported on[2] and the data on these children were examined in relation to maternal hormone levels during pregnancy. Significant correlations were found for the 22 cases between tests involving speed and accuracy (pegboard and bead-threading, r = 0.48, $P < 0.05$ and r = 0.54, $P < 0.01$ respectively) and maternal T_4 level[11]. Correlations between the child's performance and maternal T_3 were low and non-significant.

Subsequently measures of motor performance were again made on those children for whom data on maternal hormone status were available. Measures of height were also obtained. A further 20 cases were collected (there was partial overlap with the 22 cases referred to above). The effect of maternal T_4 on motor performance was again significant at $P < 0.05$ level but maternal T_4 level had no effect on the child's height. No association was found between maternal T_3 and motor performance or height[12].

A further patrol undertaken in the spring of 1985 set out to find all the children born to mothers who were pregnant when blood samples were taken in 1970 and 1971, and again make measurements of motor performance. From the 65 cases where maternal hormone status was measured 44 children were found, 18 had died and three were not located. Satisfactory measurements were obtained on 41 cases. The analysis of the data is not yet completed but preliminary findings indicate that the effect is still present in the larger sample. Again no relationship with height was found.

Although the number of cases is relatively small and the circumstances under which measurements were made less than ideal the relationship between maternal T_4 in pregnancy and the child's subsequent motor performance is clear and strong. There is evidence of a spectrum of sub-clinical deficits associated with depletion of maternal T_4. It is possible that maternal hormone levels were proxy measures for the child's hormonal status, but this seems to us unlikely because no relationship was found with the child's height. Also there is evidence that the damage occurs early in pregnancy before the fetal thyroid is itself functional[8].

It is possible that elemental iodine *per se* is vital to the neurological development of the fetus by some process not involving the synthesis of thyroid hormones, but a more plausible explanation of the effect is that maternal thyroxine crosses the placenta and is used by the fetus. Early in gestation and before the fetal thyroid becomes functional at around 12 weeks the only source of thyroxine available to the fetus is from the mother. Attempts to establish the extent of hormone transport across the placenta have led to a consensus that transfer of T_3 and T_4 is negligible[7]. However, much of the evidence relates to a period following the functional development of the fetal thyroid, by which time T_4 of maternal origin may no longer be required. Preliminary experiments on rats during the first 2 weeks of pregnancy[3] indicate a rapid accumulation of T_4 of maternal origin in fetal tissue. Another related factor may be the circulating thyroid-binding proteins which may play a specific role in the redistribution of hormone delivery through the body during pregnancy. The maintenance of an adequate supply of T_4 to the placenta and hence to the fetus is a function that thyroxine-binding globulin is well suited to fulfil (a detailed hypothesis along these lines has been developed[4]).

The findings summarized here support the view that the consequences of iodine-deficiency on the early development of the nervous system range from severe pathology of the motor system to sub-clinical deficits in performance which can be detected by careful quantitative procedures. The findings underline the importance of public health measures directed at iodine supplementation and suggest that they should be given a higher priority in those areas where endemic goitre and cretinism are present.

1 Bleichrodt, N., Dreuth, P.J.D. & Querido, A. (1980): Effects of iodine deficiency on mental and psychomotor abilities. *Am. J. Phys. Anthrop*, **53**, 55–67.
2 Connolly, K.J., Pharoah, P.O.D. & Hetzel, B.S. (1979): Fetal iodine deficiency and motor performance during childhood. *Lancet* **2**, 1149–1151.
3 Ekins, R.P., Sinha, A.K., Woods, R.J., Connolly, K.J. & Pharoah, P.O.D. (1983): Placental transfer of thyroxine in early pregnancy. Abst. presented at 13th Scientific Meeting of the Thyroid Club, London.
4 Ekins, R.P. (1985): Roles of serum thyroxine-binding proteins and maternal thyroid hormones in fetal development. *Lancet* **1**, 1129–1132.
5 Greene, L.S. (1973): Physical growth and development, neurological maturation and behavioural functioning in two Ecuadorian Andean communities in which goitre is endemic. *Am. J. Phys. Anthrop.* **38**, 119–134.
6 Koenig, P. & Veraguth, P. (1961): Studies on thyroid function in endemic cretins. In *Advances in thyroid function*. ed R. Pitt-Rivers. London: Pergamon Press.
7 Larsen, P.R. (1982): The thyroid. In *Cecil's textbook of medicine*. ed J.B. Wyngaarden & L.H. Smith. Philadelphia: Saunders.
8 Pharoah, P.O.D., Buttfield, I.H. & Hetzel, B.S. (1971): Neurological damage to the fetus resulting from severe iodine deficiency during pregnancy. *Lancet* **1**, 308–310.
9 Pharoah, P.O.D., Lawton, N.F., Ellis, S.M., Williams, E.S. & Ekins, R.P. (1973): The role of triiodothyronine (T_3) in the maintenance of euthyroidism in endemic goitre. *Clin. Endocrinol.* **2**, 193–199.
10 Pharoah, P.O.D. & Hornabrook, R.W. (1974): Endemic cretinism of recent onset in New Guinea. *Lancet* **2**, 1038–1040.
11 Pharoah, P.O.D., Connolly, K.J., Hetzel, B.S. & Ekins, R.P. (1981): Maternal thyroid function and motor competence in the child. *Develop. Med. Child Neurol.* **23**, 76–82.
12 Pharoah, P.O.D., Connolly, K.J., Ekins, R.P. & Harding, A.G. (1984): Maternal thyroid hormone levels in pregnancy and the subsequent cognitive and motor performance of the children. *Clin. Endocrinol.* **21**, 265–270.
13 Wespi, H.J. (1945): Abnahme der traubstummheit in der Schweiz als volge der Kropfprophylaxe mit jodiertem Kochsalz. *Schweiz med. Wschr.* **28**, 625–630.

★ ★ ★

RESEARCH DEVELOPMENTS IN ZINC NUTRITION

Zinc metabolism — coordinate regulation as related to cellular function

R.J. COUSINS
Food Science and Human Nutrition Department, Institute of Food and Agricultural Sciences, Gainesville, Florida 32611, USA.

There is a large volume of quantitative data suggesting that in tissues of both animals and humans the zinc concentration is maintained within a very narrow range. In contrast, there is an evolving body of kinetic data which suggests zinc turnover is rapid in many tissues. Acute disease and stress alter these processes by coordinately regulated mechanisms involving pancreatic, adrenal and pituitary hormones and leukocytic factors. In addition to responding to these hormonal stimuli, the amount of zinc absorbed from the dietary supply may also have a homoeostatic regulatory effect. In this brief review, the biochemical mechanisms related to the absorption and metabolism of zinc as it relates to the function of this essential nutrient will be discussed.

Absorption. Once zinc is sufficiently separated from the bulk of the dietary components to which it can bind, it is transported across the brush border membrane surface, probably in a chelated form, and absorbed into the cell. Experiments with isolated brush border membrane vesicles suggest that this transport process has both saturable and diffusive (non-mediated) components[12]. Kinetic analysis of transport suggested the velocity is increased when rats from which the vesicles were obtained were fed a zinc-deficient diet. Under these conditions, the Km was not influenced. When the kinetics of absorption were measured using an isolated, vascularly-perfused rat intestine, the transfer of zinc to the portal effluent provided evidence of a non-mediated and mediated component[17]. The Km for the mediated component was 55 μM and the Vmax was 3.3 nmol/min. The fact that the mediated component was responsible for a greater proportion of the total zinc absorbed when the luminal zinc concentration was low, may have particular relevance to zinc absorption in humans. Although zinc deficiency has been clearly demonstrated in humans an adaptation to a fairly low level of zinc intake must occur since a very low intake is necessary to show manifestations of deficiency. This adaptation may occur through the increased activity of a mediated transport system.

Transfer of zinc from enterocytes to the plasma compartment is not well understood. Recent evidence suggests that there is no influence of dietary zinc on transport across the basolateral membrane surface, however, there does appear to be a requirement for ATP[13]. Albumin is the protein that transports zinc between the intestine and liver[15,16]. Data suggest that the concentration of albumin presented to the serosal surface receptors of the intestine may be a help to control the rate of zinc absorption. Thus, the plasma albumin concentration may be a factor in zinc malabsorption which frequently accompanies diseases resulting in hypoalbuminaemia.

Metabolism. Kinetics studies have revealed newly ingested zinc is rapidly transferred from the plasma compartment to other tissues, particularly the liver[10]. For this reason, a considerable amount of attention has been given to the relationship between plasma and liver zinc levels. Kinetic studies with isolated rat liver parenchymal cells have shown that zinc uptake is biphasic[14]. This describes the summation of two uptake processes; a slow uptake process which represents primarily exchange with existing hepatocyte zinc and a rapidly taken up zinc pool which is a precursor of the more slowly exchangeable zinc. Kinetics of the slow uptake phase showed a Km of 9.5 μM when albumin was present in the incubation medium. This value is close to the normal plasma zinc concentration in animals and man. When the magnitude of ^{65}Zn uptake by hepatocytes, over a period of 20 h, is compared with the total cellular zinc concentration approximately 67 per cent of the total cellular zinc concentration can be accounted for as zinc that has been exchanged with the medium within that time period. This indicates zinc turnover by hepatocytes is particularly rapid and that acute physiological changes could rapidly alter uptake kinetics.

In order to define more closely the hormonal regulation of hepatic zinc metabolism, we studied the effect of glucocorticoids (viz dexamethasone), Bt$_2$cAMP, epinephrine and glucagon in experiments with both intact animals and isolated hepatocytes. It was clear from studies with intact rats that the induction of liver metallothionein was inversely related to the serum zinc concentration. This exponential function can be accentuated by using actinomycin D treatment to elevate serum zinc concentration and concomitantly suppress liver metallothionein to below basal levels. To define which of the hormones were acting by a primary effect at the level of hepatocytes, companion experiments were carried out with isolated liver hepatocytes that were incubated with these hormones, at concentrations known to regulate other metabolic processes. Each hormone was shown individually to stimulate zinc uptake/exchange rates and when two or more hormones were added to the culture medium there was an additive effect. Moreover, addition of insulin to the culture medium abolished the effect of glucagon on zinc uptake/exchange rates. Metallothionein mRNA levels in hormone-stimulated hepatocytes and intact rats were increased by each hormone and the extent of induction was comparable to the cellular total metallothionein content. Although the effects of the individual hormones varied with concentration and time, it is clear that each of the hormones is a direct inducer of metallothionein gene expression.

Coordinate regulation of metallothionein gene expression and the concomitant changes in zinc metabolism that occur as a result of this induction process, ie the ability of hepatocytes to produce more binding sites for zinc exchange is relevant to clinical findings. A rapid depression of serum zinc levels was observed in patients during corticosteroid therapy[9]. When steroid therapy was eliminated, serum zinc concentrations returned to normal. A decrease in plasma zinc concentrations by 12 h after administration of either methylprednisolone or dexamethasone was observed[22]. The extent of the depression appeared to be related to the dose of corticosteroid administered. Chronic changes in corticosteroid secretion has also been related to changes in the serum zinc concentration in a fashion that would be anticipated based upon experimental evidence with intact animals and isolated cells as well as from clinical studies. In particular, it was shown[10] that patients with Addison's disease (adrenalcortical insufficiency) had abnormally elevated concentrations, whereas patients with Cushing's syndrome (associated with corticosteroid excess), had serum zinc concentrations significantly below normal levels. Streptozotocin-induced hyperglucagonaemia and diabetes is associated with hepatic zinc accumulation and metallothionein induction[7]. ACTH infusion, it was shown[8], lowered the serum zinc concentration in patients with normal serum zinc concentrations, but not in those subjects that had depressed serum zinc levels at the time of infusion. When the serum was fractionated by gel filtration chromatography, it was shown that the reduction was accounted for only by a low molecular weight zinc-binding protein, presumably albumin. It was proposed that the depression of serum zinc levels associated with acute disease is related to a hormonal cycle initiated by ACTH secretion.

Considering that the plasma zinc concentration accounts for an extremely small amount of zinc deposited in various tissues, particularly liver and muscle, it is clear that relatively small shifts in cellular uptake will not be noticed when total tissue zinc levels are used as a measurement. Lack of an effect of prednisolone on liver zinc concentrations[19] could be explained on that basis. Experiments with isolated hepatocytes showed that the phenomenon of zinc transfer between the external medium (plasma) and these cells can be hormonally regulated in a way that would be expected based upon clinical findings. Nevertheless, the possibility that zinc excretion contributes in some way to the serum zinc depression associated with stress cannot be ruled out. It was showed that glucagon infusion increases zinc excretion by the perfused dog kidney[21]. Intact animal studies have also shown that infusion of amino acids can increase urinary zinc excretion[20,22]. These would accompany muscle protein catabolism caused by stress, infection and acute disease. The major aspects of the hormonal control of mammalian zinc metabolism are shown in the Figure.

The teleological explanation for the reduction in plasma zinc associated with acute disease and hormonal imbalance remains enigmatic. It has been suggested that hypozincaemia is necessary for the increase of phagocytic activity of inflammatory cells since this is normally inhibited by Zn^{2+} [2]. An alternative explanation for the response is that this depression is a consequence of the need for enhanced zinc uptake into cells. During the acute phase response increased metabolic activity of certain cells including the liver, is such that there may be an increased production of zinc- containing proteins as well as an increase in the activity of zinc metalloenzymes. The role of zinc in gene expression has been well established[11] and growth and development of a variety of cells including leukocytes may require zinc at a number of stages of differentiation. A leukocytic factor has been demonstrated[5,6], similar to interleukin 1, which causes increased metallothionein mRNA levels, metallothionein synthesis and hypozincaemia. Since these leukocytic factors control many phases of the acute phase response[4], these zinc-related phenomena may have important functions in host defense. It is also possible that zinc is able to stabilize cellular membranes[1] and in this way contributes to the overall host

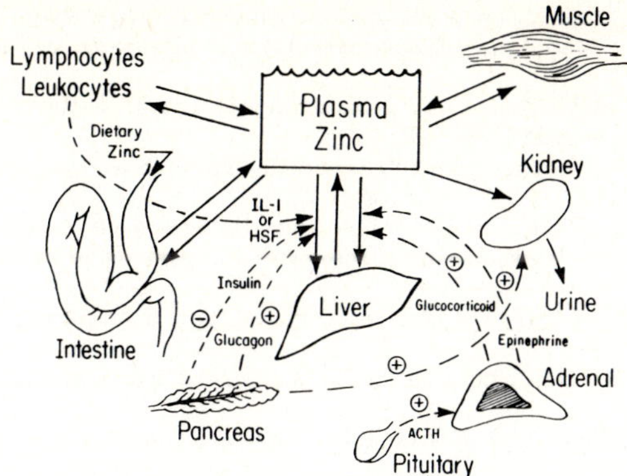

Figure. *Principal points of the hormonal control of zinc metabolism.* Solid lines indicate a metabolic pathway for zinc. Broken lines indicate hormonal or other stimulus. Indicated: ⊕ positive or ⊖ negative influence.

defense response. In this regard, it is of interest that we have been able to show a zinc-related decrease in chemically induced peroxidation in isolated hepatocytes[3]. Moreover, zinc appears to cause a reduction of free radical production by hepatocytes. Since the phenomenon is responsive to zinc, it is possible that induction of metallothionein in hepatocytes contributes to the free radical suppressing effect of zinc. This later suggestion is supported by *in vitro* evidence[18] which shows that metallothionein is a potent suppressor of hydroxyl radicals, but not superoxide radicals.

Conclusion. There is an increasing body of evidence suggesting that zinc metabolism is under definitive coordinate regulation involving adrenaline, glucocorticoids and glucagon. The demonstration that interleukin-1-like factors derived from leukocytes also exert potent influences over zinc metabolism suggests the metal has important functions in one or more phases of the acute phase response.

1 Bettger, W.J. & O'Dell, B.L. (1981): A critical physiological role of zinc in the structure and function of biomembranes. *Life Sci.* **28**, 1425–1438.

2 Chvapil, M. (1977): The role of zinc in the function of some inflammatory cells. In *Progress in clinical and biological research*, ed G.J. Brewer, pp. 103–122. New York: Alan R. Liss.

3 Coppen, D.E., Cousins, R.J. & Richardson, D.E. (1985): Effect of zinc on chemically induced peroxidation in rat liver parenchymal cells in primary culture. *Fed. Proc.* **44**, 6404 Abst.

4 Dinarello, C.A. (1984): Interleukin-1 and the pathogenesis of the acute-phase response. *New Engl. J. Med.* **311**, 1413–1418.

5 DiSilvestro, R.A. & Cousins, R.J. (1984): Translational regulation of rat liver metallothionein levels by glucagon. *Fed. Proc.* **43**, 3310 Abst.

6 DiSilvestro, R.A. & Cousins, R.J. (1984): Mediation of endotoxin-induced changes in zinc metabolism in rats. *Am. J. Physiol.* **247**, E436-E441.

7 Failla, M.L. & Kiser, R.A. (1983): Hepatic and renal metabolism of copper and zinc in the diabetic rat. *Am. J. Physiol.* **244**, E115–E121.

8 Falchuk, K.H. (1977): Effect of acute disease and ACTH on serum zinc proteins. *New Engl. J. Med.* **296**, 1129–1133.

9 Flynn, A., Pories, W., Strain, W.H., Hill, O.A. Jr. & Fratianne, R.B. (1971): Rapid serum-zinc depletion associated with corticosteroid therapy. *Lancet* **2**, 1169–1171.

10 Henkin, R.I. (1974): On the role of adrenocorticosteroids in the control of zinc and copper metabolism. In *Trace element metabolism in animals*, 2nd edn W.G. Hoekstra, J.W. Suttie, H.E. Ganther & W. Mertz, pp. 647–641. Baltimore MD: University Park Press.

11 Mazus, B., Falchuk, K.H. & Vallee, B.L. (1984): Histone formation, gene expression and zinc deficiency in *Euglena gracilis*. *Biochemistry*. **23**, 42–47.

12 Menard, M.P. & Cousins, R.J. (1983): Zinc transport by brush border membrane vesicles from rat intestine. *J. Nutr.* **113**, 1434–1442.

13 Oestreicher, P. & Cousins, R.J. (1984): Zinc transport by basolateral membrane vesicles from rat small intestine. *Fed. Proc.* **43**, 4646 Abst.

14 Pattison, S.E. & Cousins, R.J. (1985): Zinc uptake and metabolism by hepatocytes. *Fed Proc.* (In press).

15 Smith, K.T. & Cousins, R.J. (1980): Quantitative aspects of zinc absorption by isolated, vascularly perfused rat intestine. *J. Nutr.* **110**, 316–323.

16 Smith, K.T., Failla, M.L. & Cousins, R.J. (1979): Identification of albumin as the plasma carrier for zinc absorption by perfused rat intestine. *Biochem. J.* **184**, 627–633.

17 Steel, L. & Cousins, R.J. (1985): Kinetics of zinc absorption by luminally and vascularly perfused rat intestine. *Am. J. Physiol.* **248**, G46-G53.

18 Thornalley, P.J. & Vasak, M. (1985): Possible role for metallothionein in protection against radiation-induced oxidative stress. Kinetics and mechanism of its reaction with superoxide and hydroxyl radicals. *Biochim. Biophys. Acta.* **827**, 36–44.

19 Turnlund, J. & Margen, S. (1979): Effect of glucocorticoids and zinc deficiency on femur and liver zinc in rats. *J. Nutr.* **109**, 467–472.

20 Van Rij, A.M., Godfrey, P.J. & McKenzie, J.M. (1979): Amino acid infusions and urinary zinc excretion. *J. Surg. Res.* **26**, 293–299.

21 Victery, W., Levenson, R. & Vander, A.J. (1981): Effect of glucagon on zinc excretion in anesthetized dogs. *Am. J. Physiol.* **240**, F299–F305.

22 Yunice, A.A., Czerwinski, A.W. & Lindeman, R.D. (1981): Influence of synthetic corticosteroids on plasma zinc and copper levels in humans. *Am. J. Med. Sci.* **181**, 68–74.

Zinc bioavailability to humans*

N.W. SOLOMONS
Division of Nutrition and Health, Institute of Nutrition of Central America and Panama, Guatemala City, Guatemala; and Center for Studies in Sensory Impairment, Aging and Metabolism of the National Committee of the Blind and Deaf of Guatemala, Guatemala City, Guatemala.

The theme of zinc bioavailability in humans has become topical, given the demonstration of human zinc-deficiency[26]. There are a number of extensive reviews of the topic[2,20,31,32]. This review treats issues of zinc's biological availability as related to *humans* and *human dietetics*.

Intestinal absorption of zinc. The intestinal absorption of zinc is homoeostatically regulated and subject to influence by intraluminal factors. Figure 1 illustrates the routes of transport and mechanisms of regulation for zinc's absorption by intestinal cells. In the lumen, zinc is separated from the matrices of foods by mechanical and digestive processes, then possibly bound by a low-molecular-weight binding-species of pancreatic origin[1,11]. The cellular uptake of zinc is a carrier-mediated, saturable process[9,30]. The induction of metallothionein, an intracellular sulfhydryl-rich metal-binding protein is the basis for intestinal regulation of zinc movement. Elevation of metallothionein levels leads to sequestration of zinc within the intestinal cell[19]. Transfer of zinc from the enterocyte to the plasma is the rate limiting process in zinc absorption[9], and probably an energy-dependent process. The major route for excretion of endogenous zinc is pancreatic secretion[22].

In isotopic studies in human experiments, fractional absorption of zinc has ranged for 43 to 69 per cent while it ranges for 14 to 41 per cent for meals[32], providing evidence that dietary factors condition absorptive efficiency from the human diet.

Definition and concept of nutrient biological availability. The use of the term 'biological availability' with respect to zinc in human diets was introduced in 1973, in conjunction with calculations of adequate dietary intakes from distinct regional cuisines[29,35]. For most purposes, bioavailability has been synonymous with fractional absorption by the intestine[3,31]. However, a strong case has been made for a more ample definition[20]: 'Bioavailability is the proportion of a nutrient in food which is absorbed and utilized'; by utilization is meant, 'the process of transport, cellular assimilation and conversion to a biologically active form(s)'. In experimental

*INCAP Publication — I-1425.

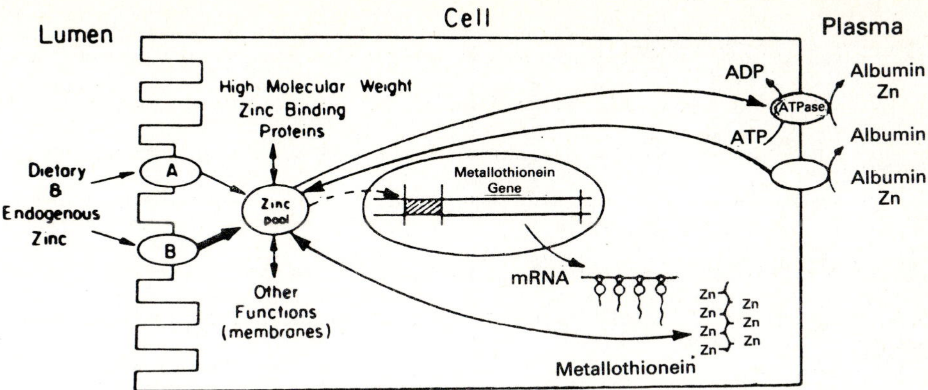

Fig. 1. *Schematic representation of zinc absorption by intestinal cells.* Carrier-mediated zinc transport at the brush border membrane is shown as A and B. Transport when an adequate amount of zinc is in the diet is shown as A, while the apparent increase in transport observed when the dietary supply is low is shown as B. Interactions of zinc with intracellular macromolecules are indicated as is the regulation of the metallothionein gene by dietary and plasma zinc. The active transport step is shown at the basolateral membrane. Transfer of cellular zinc to and from plasma albumin is also shown. After Solomons & Cousins, 1984[32]. Reproduced with permission.

animals, haemoglobin repletion in anaemic rats[23] or reversal of pancreatic degeneration in selenium-deficient chicks[4] have served as indices of iron and selenium bioavailability with *utilization* as the definitive index. In studying repletion of platelet glutathione peroxidase in Finnish men fed selenium of various dietary sources a conscious transfer was made of this paradigm to human bioavailability studies[12]. In surveying the literature on human zinc biology, several studies are found in which an index of transport, tissue incorporation or growth have been measured in the context of long-term feeding of one or another diets contrasting in chemical characteristics.

Dietary factors and zinc bioavailability to humans. Our discussion here concerns observations in human subjects in which some index of zinc storage, transport or function has been evaluated over time in response to a specific dietary treatment. Many substances have been classified as enhancers or inhibitors of zinc bioavailability in experimental animal studies or human metabolic balance experiments[12,20,31,32]. Of these dietary factors, suitable observations have been made in people with human milk, unrefined cereals, soya-based diets, and inorganic iron.

Human breast-milk. In studies from Japan[21] and Denver, Colorado[15] comparing plasma zinc levels of breast- and bottle-fed infants at 3 or 6 months of life, circulating zinc concentrations were found to be significantly higher in breast-fed cohorts, despite a lesser net content of zinc in the breast-milk diets.

Dietary fibre and phytate. There is sufficient evidence from animal experiments that phytic acid and dietary fibre components are the major inhibitory factors that influence zinc availability in unrefined cereal grains[5,10]. When fed to volunteers in metabolic studies, whole-wheat flatbreads produced negative zinc balance[28]. Growth failure and altered zinc kinetics were shown in adolescent boys in rural Egypt consuming an unleavened flatbread[25]; evidence for a detrimental effect of this high-fibre, high-phytate food on zinc bioavailability was the dramatic growth spurt seen when a zinc-rich hospital diet was fed to these subjects.

Soyabean protein foods. When soya, a phytic acid-rich food, is fed to humans as a sole source of dietary protein, zinc appears to be less available than from non-soya-based foods. This has

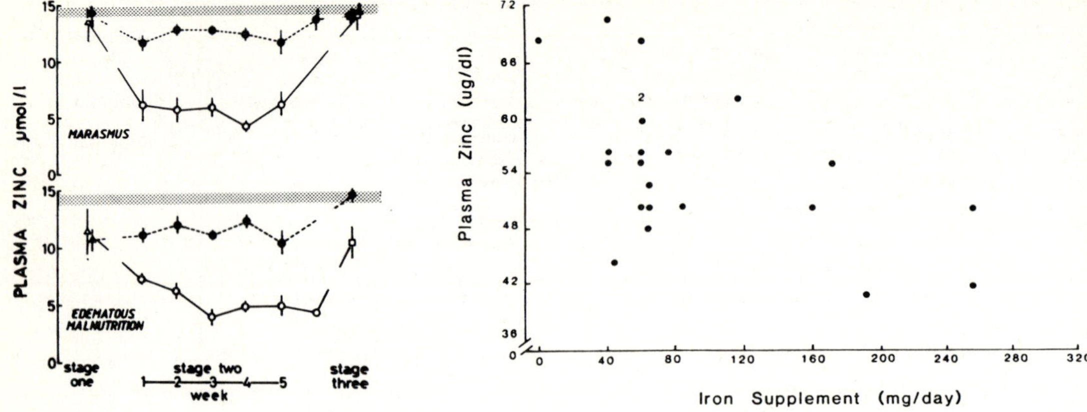

Fig. 2 (Above, left). *Plasma zinc concentration during recovery from severe malnutrition.* The upper graphs are for children with an admission diagnosis of marasmus and the lower graphs for children with edematous malnutrition. $\triangle$ and $\blacktriangle$, maintenance diet; $\bullet$, cow's milk based formula; $\bigcirc$, soya protein based formula; $\square$ and $\blacksquare$, mixed diet. The open symbols are for children given the soya diet and the closed symbols for those given the cow's milk diet. The shaded horizontal bars represent the mean ± SEM for the control children. Vertical bars show SEMs. From Golden & Golden (1981)[13]; reproduced with permission.

Fig. 3 (Above, right). *Plot of plasma zinc concentration at 9 months of gestation versus the level of prenatal supplementation.* From Hambidge *et al.*, 1983[14]; reproduced with permission.

been proven true for malnourished Jamaican children fed soya- and milk-based recovery diets[13] (Fig. 2), and healthy American infants fed milk or soya formulas[7,8]. Circulating zinc levels were lower in soya-fed subjects in all studies, and growth rates lagged in the Jamaican children's recoveries.

Progressive reduction was found in plasma and neutrophil (but not erythrocyte) zinc levels in adult men who were switched from their usual mixed animal-protein diets to soya diets for 3 months[6].

Inorganic iron. In 1970, a competitive interaction of chemically-similar ions was described[17]. Iron and zinc are two such metals[16,24]. Several long-term experiences in humans suggest an effect of high Fe/Zn ratios on circulating zinc transport. When marginal zinc intakes (< 3.5 mg daily) were fed to adult volunteers, 20-mg daily intakes of iron (Fe/Zn ratios = 5.7:1) allowed plasma zinc levels to be maintained about 70 μg/dl, whereas with iron intakes of 130 mg (Fe/Zn ration = 48:1) plasma zinc concentration was reduced to below 70 μg/dl[27].

Cow-milk-based infant formulas, with and without added iron, were compared as to their effects on plasma zinc levels after 1 or 2 months of feeding; the Fe/Zn rations of 0.4:1 and 2.2:1 produced significantly different mean plasma zinc levels, with mean concentrations being lower in the group fed the high-iron diet[7,8]. High iron contents of milk-based formula may also accentuate the effect of a low zinc content, as suggested by the poorer growth of infants fed an iron-fortified diet without supplementary zinc[34].

In two recent studies of pregnant women, inverse associations between circulating levels of zinc and the amount of iron consumed as part of the prenatal vitamin-mineral supplementation regimen were encountered. In Denver, Colorado in the 3rd trimester, higher iron intakes were clearly correlated with lower plasma zinc (Fig. 3)[14]. Throughout the course of pregnancy, consistently lower mean serum zinc concentrations were found in the cohort of women taking more than 30 mg of iron supplement daily[2]. It has been noted that many over-the-counter nutrient supplement preparations on the market have Fe/Zn ratios well over 3:1 and sometimes as high as 25:1[33]. Thus, in situations in which the tendency is to prescribe abundant iron in the diet, infancy and pregnancy, longitudinal studies suggest that depression in zinc transport in the blood can be the consequence due to poor bioavailability of the zinc.

Conclusions. The extent of our knowledge related to human zinc biology from experiments or observations conducted directly in man is limited, specifically if the more ample definition of nutrient bioavailability[18,20] incorporating a concept of nutrient *utilization* is applied. In the present survey, in which effects of dietary factors were evaluated in terms of either zinc transport or tissue incorporation *in vivo*, or growth, enhanced zinc biological availability from breast-milk and reduced bioavailability of zinc of high-fibre diets, soyabean protein diets and non-haem iron can be demonstrated. Further studies using a definition of availability that goes beyond simple intestinal uptake are needed to refine further our knowledge for human diets.

1 Boosalis, M.G., Evans, G.M. & McClain, C.J. (1983): Impaired handling of orally administered zinc in pancreatic insufficiency. *Am. J. Clin. Nutr.* **37**, 268–271.
2 Breskin, M.W., Worthington-Roberts, B.S., Knopp, R.H., Brown, Z., Mottet, N.K. & Mills, J.L. (1983): First trimester serum zinc concentration in human pregnancy. *Am. J. Clin. Nutr.* **38**, 943–953.
3 Burk, R.F. & Solomons, N.W. (1985): Trace elements and vitamins and bioavailability as related to wheat and wheat foods. *Am. J. Clin. Nutr.* **41**, 1091–1102.
4 Cantor, A.H., Langevin, M.L., Noguchi, T. & Scott, M.L. (1975): Efficacy of selenium in selenium compounds and feedstuffs for prevention of pancreatic fibrosis in chicks. *J. Nutr.* **105**, 106–111.
5 Caprez, A. & Fairweather-Tait, S.J. (1982): The effect of heat treatment and particle size of bran on mineral absorption in rats. *Br. J. Nutr.* **48**, 467–475.
6 Cossack, Z.T. & Prasad, A.S. (1983): Effect of protein source on the bioavailability of zinc in human subjects. *Nutr. Res.* **3**, 23–31.
7 Craig, W.J., Balbach, L., Harris, S. & Vyhmeister, N. (1984): Plasma zinc and copper levels of infants fed different milk formulas. *J. Am. Coll. Nutr.* **3**, 183–186.
8 Craig, W.J., Balbach, L. & Vyhmeister, N. (1984): Zinc bioavailability and infant formulas. *Am. J. Clin. Nutr.* **39**, 981–983.
9 Davies, N.T. (1980): Studies on the absorption of zinc by rat intestine. *Br. J. Nutr.* **43**, 189–203.
10 Davies, N.T. & Nightingale, R. (1975): The effects of phytate on intestinal absorption and secretion of zinc and whole-body retention of Zn, copper, iron and manganese in rat. *Br. J. Nutr.* **34**, 243–258.
11 Evans, G.W., Grace, C.I. & Votava, H.J. (1975): A proposed mechanism for zinc absorption in the rat. *Am. J. Physiol.* **228**, 501–505.
12 Forbes, R.M. & Erdman, J.W. Jr. (1983): Bioavailability of trace mineral elements. *Ann. Rev. Nutr.* **3**, 213–231.
13 Golden, B.E. & Golden, M.H.N. (1981): Plasma zinc, rate of weight gain and energy cost of tissue deposition in children recovering from severe malnutrition on a cow's milk or soya protein based diet. *Am. J. Clin. Nutr.* **34**, 892–899.
14 Hambidge, K.M., Krebs, N.F., Jacobs, M.A., Favier, A. Guyette, L. & Ikle, D.M. (1983): Zinc nutritional status during pregnancy: a longitudinal study. *Am. J. Clin. Nutr.* **37**, 429–442.
15 Hambidge, K.M., Walravens, P.A., Casey, C.E., Brown, R.M. & Bender, C. (1979): Plasma zinc concentration of breast-fed infants. *J. Pediatr.* **94**, 607–608.
16 Hamilton, D.L., Bellamy, J.E.C., Valberg, J.D. & Valberg, L.S. (1978): Zinc, cadmium and iron interaction during intestinal absorption in iron-deficient mice. *Can. J. Physiol. Pharmacol.* **56**, 384–388.
17 Hill, C.H. & Matrone, G. (1970): Chemical parameters in the study of *in vivo* and *in vitro* interactions of transition elements. *Fed. Proc.* **29**, 1474–1481.
18 Levander, O.A., Alfthan, G., Arvilommi, H., Gref, C.G., Huttunen, J.K., Kataje, M., Koivistoinen, P. & Pikkarainen, J. (1983): Bioavailability of selenium to Finnish men as assessed by platelet glutathione peroxidase activity and other blood parameters. *Am. J. Clin. Nutr.* **37**, 887–897.
19 Menard, M.P., McCormick, C.C. & Cousins, R.J. (1981): Regulation of intestinal metallothionein biosynthesis in rats by dietary zinc. *J. Nutr.* **111**, 1353–1361.
20 O'Dell, B.L. (1984): Bioavailability of trace elements. *Nutr. Rev.* **43**, 301–308.
21 Ohtake, M. (1977): Serum zinc and copper levels in healthy Japanese infants. *Tohoku J. Exp. Med.* **123**, 265–270.
22 Pekas, J.C. (1966): Zinc-65 metabolism: Gastrointestinal secretion by the pig. *Am. J. Physiol.* **211**, 407–413.
23 Pla, G.W. & Fritz, J.C. (1970): Availability of iron. *J. Assoc. Off. Anal. Chem.* **53**, 791–800.
24 Pollack, S., George, J.N., Reba, R.C., Kaufman, R.M. & Crosby, W.A. (1965): The absorption of nonferrous metals in iron deficiency. *J. Clin. Invest.* **44**, 1470–1473.
25 Prasad, A.S. (1966): Metabolism of zinc and its deficiency in human subjects. In *Zinc metabolism*, ed A.S. Prasad, pp. 250–301, Springfield: Charles C. Thomas.
26 Prasad, A.S. (1982): Clinical and biochemical spectrum of zinc deficiency in human subjects. In *Clinical, biochemical, and nutritional aspects of trace elements*, ed A.S. Prasad, pp. 3–62. New York: Alan R. Liss.
27 Prasad, A.S., Rabbani, P., Abbasii, A., Bowersox, E. & Spivey Fox, M.R. (1978): Experimental zinc deficiency in humans. *Ann. Intern. Med.* **89**, 483–490.

28 Reinhold, J., Faradji, B., Abadi, P. & Ismail-Beigi, F. (1976): Decreased absorption of calcium, magnesium, zinc and phosphorus by humans due to increased fiber and phosphorus consumption as wheat bread. *J. Nutr.* **106**, 493–503.
29 Sandstead, H.H. (1973): Zinc nutrition in the United States. *Am. J. Clin. Nutr,* **26**, 1251–1260.
30 Smith, K.T. & Cousins, R.J. (1980): Quantitative aspects of zinc absorption by isolated, vascularly perfused rat intestine. *J. Nutr.* **110**, 316–323.
31 Solomons, N.W. (1981): Biological availability of zinc in humans. *Am. J. Clin. Nutr.* **35**, 1048–1075.
32 Solomons, N.W. & Cousins, R.J. (1984): Zinc. In *Absorption and malabsorption of mineral nutrients,* ed N.W. Solomons & I.H. Rosenberg, pp. 125–197. New York: Alan R. Liss.
33 Solomons, N.W. & Jacob, R.A. (1981): Studies on the bioavailability of zinc in humans: Effects of heme and nonheme iron on the absorption of zinc. *Am. J. Clin. Nutr.* **34**, 475–482.
34 Walravens, P.A. & Hambidge, K.M. (1976): Growth of infants fed a zinc-supplemented formula. *Am. J. Clin. Nutr.* **29**, 1114–1121.
35 World Health Organization. (1973): *Trace elements in human nutrition.* Tech. Report Series 532, p. 9. Geneva: WHO.

Zinc in pregnancy

M. KIRCHGESSNER and Anna M. REICHLMAYR-LAIS
Institut für Ernährungsphysiologie, Technische Universität München, D-8050 Freising-Weihenstephan, FRG.

Animal reproduction involves modifications in the metabolism of macro and micro-nutrients, because there is a need to meet the demands of production as well as those of maintenance. In this paper phenomena of Zn (zinc) supply and metabolism during gestation are presented.

The element zinc fulfils essential functions in reproduction in the main as a constituent or activator of enzymes and hormones. Functions of Zn in connection with the onset and efficient completion of parturition[3] and with the antibacterial activity of the amniotic fluid[20] have been unrecognized until recently. To meet the requirement resulting from these functions not only the quantity of dietary Zn plays a role, but also its utilization which may be influenced by numerous factors such as absorption, intermediate metabolism, excretion and interactions with other dietary constituents.

Zn absorption in pregnancy. The elevated requirement for Zn in the case of reproduction is met not only by higher feed intake, which is not so marked as during lactation, but also by an increased absorbability of dietary Zn which results at least partially from hypertrophy of the intestine especially in the late stages of pregnancy[2]. When the Zn supply was adequate, using *in vitro* experiments with everted intestinal sacs an increased Zn adsorption at the intestinal wall and a greater Zn absorption into serosal solution of pregnant rats in comparison with non-pregnant was demonstrated[22]. There was a sharp increase in absorption as pregnancy advanced in parallel with the growing accumulation of Zn in reproductive products[24]. A short time before parturition the absorption decreased. The decline in Zn absorption continued during lactation. Similarly, in pregnant sows, an increased apparent Zn absorption (intake minus faecal excretion) was found, which was again reduced shortly before parturition, perhaps caused by hormonal changes leading to parturition[13].

Super-retention and tissue distribution during pregnancy. In an experiment with sows a positive Zn retention in pregnant animals appeared only in the case of sufficient supply with Zn[13]. In this case the pregnant sows retained a greater quantity of zinc in reproductive organs and fetuses. The quantity retained by the reproducing organism exceeding the accumulation in conception products is defined as super-retention or as gravidity anabolism. This phenomenon is already known for nitrogen[15] and other trace elements, especially copper[14]. In experiments with pregnant rats such an anabolic effect could be demonstrated only in liver[21]. In comparison with nongravid control animals the Zn content in liver of gravid rats was elevated in parallel with the increased liver mass in pregnancy. The increase in liver Zn content was also dependent on dietary Zn supply. After lactation the Zn content of the liver was not different from that of the control animals indicating that the reserves are mobilized during lactation. The Zn concentration in serum, in contrast to the liver, of these gravid rats declined even in the case of a supply exceeding the requirement[21]. This fact which has been reported in several experiments with different species including human (eg[23]) may result from the hormonal balance during pregnancy. In other soft tissues, muscle and femur only negligible changes of Zn content occurred if Zn supply was adequate[12,18,24]. In amniotic fluid, Zn concentration increases during pregnancy[19]. Further studies are necessary to clarify super-retention during gravidity.

Placental transfer of Zn. As well as the maternal absorption, the placental transfer is important for supply of Zn to fetuses. The Zn content of the placenta increases in the course of pregnancy and approaches an asymptotic value[24]. The placental permeability to Zn increases at the same time as that during which fetuses accumulate most of their Zn[1].

Suboptimal and deficient Zn supply during pregnancy. An insufficient Zn supply affects the Zn status of the mother as well as the fetus. In addition to a reduced feed intake and even a loss of body weight[17] rats receiving insufficient Zn during pregnancy had reduced Zn concentration in serum, uterus and placenta, whereas the Zn concentration in liver and kidneys was not affected[16]. Zinc binding capacity of serum and the activity of alkaline phosphatase in serum connected with a so called response technique are suggested for diagnosis of maternal Zn deficiency[10]. The diagnostic value of Zn concentration in serum is however of very limited use because it is affected by numerous factors.

Maternal dietary zinc deprivation during pregnancy affects embryonic and fetal development as Hurley and coworkers repeatedly demonstrated with rats. Resorption of implantation sites, congenital malformations involving all organ systems and reduced birth weights were recorded as abnormalities. Even transitory periods of zinc-deficiency were teratogenic indicating that maternal stores could not adequately be mobilized[8]. Therefore, an adequate Zn supply during the whole pregnancy is indispensable. Biochemical abnormalities in fetuses are also apparent[7]. In the lung, synthesis of the pulmonary surfactant phospholipids is depressed. The biochemical development and enzymatic differentiation of the pancreas is abnormal. A reduced synthesis of nucleic acids connected with chromosomal aberrations may be decisive for the congenital malformations. In this connection a decrease in uptake of tritiated thymidine into the whole body and into DNA itself as well as of activity of thymidine kinase and DNA polymerase has been demonstrated.

In experiments with rats as well as with pigs the fetal Zn content was reduced resulting from insufficient maternal Zn supply (eg[11,16]). In new-born pigs the Zn content of the 'storage organ' liver and femur was impaired, whereas the spleen and kidney showed no changes. Even in massive Zn-deficiency the fetal brain of rats was not depleted although the brain weight of Zn-deficient fetuses was less than that of control animals[17]. Additionally the total cell number was reduced while the cytoplasmic nuclear ratio was increased indicating an impairment of cell division in the brain.

There is some evidence that deficiency of Zn may be also related to abnormal development in man[5,9].

Excessive Zn supply during pregnancy. Especially high Zn concentrations in maternal and fetal tissues result from increased maternal Zn supply during pregnancy, whereas copper content was reduced not only in maternal, but also in fetal tissues[4]. Because of the interactions between copper and zinc the ratio zinc/copper in the diet should generally be taken into consideration. If a diet is deficient in one of these elements, a deficiency or an excess of the other may alleviate the deficiency effects[6].

Conclusion. For the normal progress of gestation and parturition as well as fetal development the element Zn plays an essential role. The increased requirement especially in the last third of gestation resulting from accumulation in conception products and from super-retention induces an increased Zn absorption. In spite of the increased absorption dietary Zn intake should be sufficient. To meet the requirements not only the dietary content is relevant but also factors which influence the utilization of Zn. To clarify the roles of Zn in reproduction further model studies are necessary. Because of limitations of human experimentations, precisely controlled experiments with animals are unavoidable.

1 Anon (1976): Zinc deficiency in pregnant, fetal and young rats. *Nutr. Rev.* **34**, 84–86.
2 Boyne, R., Fell, B.F. & Robb, I. (1966): Surface area of the intestinal mucosa in the lactating rat. *J. Physiol.* **183**, 570–575.
3 Bunce, G.E., Wilson, G.R., Mills, C.F. & Klopper, A. (1983): Studies on the role of zinc in parturition in the rat. *Biochem. J.* **210**, 761–767.
4 Cox, D.H., Schlicker, S.A. & Chu, R.C. (1969): Excess dietary zinc for the maternal rat and zinc, iron, copper, calcium and magnesium content and enzyme activity in maternal and fetal tissues. *J. Nutr.* **98**, 459–466.
5 Hambidge, K.M., Neldner, K.H. & Walravens, P.A. (1975): Zinc, acrodermatitis enteropatica, and congenital malformations. *Lancet* **1**, 577–578.
6 Hurley, L.S., Keen, C.L. & Lönnerdal, B. (1983): Aspects of trace element interactions during development. *Fed. Proc.* **42**, 1735–1739.
7 Hurley, L.S. (1981): The roles of trace elements in foetal and neonatal development. *Phil. Trans. R. Soc. Lond. B* **294**, 145–152.
8 Hurley, L.S. & Mutch, P.B. (1973): Prenatal and postnatal development after transitory gestational zinc deficiency in rats. *J. Nutr.* **103**, 649–656.
9 Jameson, S. (1976): Effects of zinc deficiency in human reproduction. *Acta Med. Scand.* Supp **593**, 1–89.
10 Kirchgeßner, M., Reichlmayr-Lais, A.M. & Roth, H.-P. (1983): Possibilities for the diagnosis of trace element deficiency. In *Trace elements — analytical chemistry in medicine and biology*, Vol. 2, ed P. Brätter, P. Schramel. Berlin, New York: Walter de Gruyter.
11 Kirchgeßner, M., Roth-Maier, D.A., Reithmayer, F. & Spörl, R. (1985): Zum Zinkstatus neugeborener Ferkel bei suboptimaler Zinkversorgung der Sauen während der Trächtigkeit. *Z. Tierphysiol., Tierernährg. u. Futtermittelkde.* **54**, 20–25.
12 Kirchgeßner, M. & Schneider, U.A. (1978): Zum Trächtigkeitsanabolismus von Zink. *Arch. Tierernährg.* **28**, 211–220.
13 Kirchgeßner, M., Spörl, R. & Roth-Maier, D.A. (1980): Exkretion im Kot und scheinbare Absorption von Kupfer, Zink, Nickel und Mangan bei nichtgraviden und graviden Sauen nach unterschiedlicher Spurenelement-versorgung. *Z. Tierphysiol., Tierernährg. u. Futtermittelkde.* **44**, 98–111.
14 Kirchgeßner, M. & Spörl, R. (1975): Zum Trächtigkeitsanabolismus an Kupfer in Abhängigkeit von der Cu-Versorgung. *Z. Tierphysiol., Tierernährg. u. Futtermittelkde.* **36**, 75–86.
15 Lenkeit, W. (1972): Der mütterliche Stoffwechsel während der Gravidität. In *Handbuch der tierernährung Bd. 2 Leistung und Ernährung* ed W. Lenkeit & K. Breirem, p. 115, Hamburg, Berlin: P. Parey.
16 Masters, D.G., Keen, C.L., Lönnerdal, B. & Hurley, L.S. (1983): Comparative aspects of dietary copper and zinc deficiencies in pregnant rats. *J. Nutr.* **113**, 1448–1451.
17 McKenzie, J.M., Fosmire, G.J. & Sandstead, H.H. (1975): Zinc deficiency during the latter third of pregnancy; effects on fetal rat brain, liver and placenta. *J. Nutr.* **105**, 1466–1475.
18 Mutch, P.B. & Hurley, L.S. (1974): Effect of zinc deficiency during lactation on postnatal growth and development. *J. Nutr.* **104**, 828–842.
19 Rösick, U., Rösick, E. & Brätter, P. (1983): Determination of zinc in amniotic fluid in normal and high risk pregnancies. *J. Clin. Chem. Clin. Biochem.* **21**, 363–372.
20 Schlievert, P., Johnson, W. & Galask, R.P. (1976): Bacterial growth inhibition by amniotic fluid. V. Phosphate/zinc ratio as predictor of bacterial growth-inhibitory activity. *Am. J. Obstet. Gynecol.* **125**, 899–905.
21 Schneider, U.A. & Kirchgeßner, M. (1979): Veränderungen der Retention von Zink im Organismus während der Gravidität. *Nutr. Metab.* **23**, 241–249.
22 Schwarz, F.J., Kirchgeßner, M. & Sherif, S.Y. (1981): Zur intestinalen Absorption von Zink während der Gravidität und Laktation. *Res. Exp. Med. Berl.* **179**, 35–42.
23 Swanson, Ch. A. & King, J.C. (1982): Zinc utilization in pregnant and non pregnant woman fed controlled diets providing the zinc RDA. *J. Nutr.* **112**, 697–707.
24 Williams, R.B., Davies, N.T. & McDonald, I. (1978): The effect of pregnancy and lactation on copper and zinc retention in the rat. *Br. J. Nutr.* **38**, 407–416.

Zinc and the neonate

P.J. AGGETT, T. STACK and D.J. LLOYD
Department of Child Health, University Medical Buildings, Aberdeen AB9 2ZD, UK.

Circumstantial evidence suggests that the metabolism of zinc in the human neonate differs from that in the adult and that it adapts to meet the demands of extrauterine life. The overall concentration of zinc (20 mg Zn/kg B.Wt.) in the new-born is less than that in the adult (25–30 mg Zn/kg B.Wt.), and its distribution is different also. It has been calculated that in the neonate the liver contains approximately 25 per cent of the total body zinc and the skeleton about 40 per cent compared with about 10 per cent and 25 per cent in those respective tissues in adulthood[16]. Additionally, studies in pigs indicate that the pale unexercised muscles of piglets contain less zinc than their mature counterparts[6]. Whether these altered relative distributions of zinc involve endogenous or exogenous sources of the metal has not been elucidated.

Changing concentrations and intracellular distributions of zinc in the neonatal liver have been noted in a number of mammals[3]. This involves the association of zinc (and copper) with the low molecular weight protein metallothionein. Although there is some interspecies variation in the time, ie late gestation or early infancy, at which hepatic metallothionein concentrations are maximal, they fall subsequently and reach adult-like levels around the age of weaning[3]. Immunohistochemical localisation of metallothionein in the livers of rat pups shows that there is a dimunition of intranuclear metallothionein between birth and 14 d *post partum* at which time the protein reaction was localized predominantly in the cytoplasmic pattern typical of adult animals. The physiological significance of this altered pattern is unknown but there has been speculation that in these circumstances metallothionein may be acting as a reservoir for zinc[14]. Indeed, at the same time as these events occur, the hepatic concentrations of zinc fall, and less of the metal is associated with metallothionein[3,14], even though, because of hepatic growth, the total amount of zinc in the liver increases.

The intestinal absorption and secretion of zinc may also change with maturation. In the first week of life, human neonates fed a synthetic formula had a net intestinal loss of zinc[7], however older infants have a net intestinal uptake of zinc as evidenced by balance studies[19]. In contrast preterm infants fed pasteurized human breast-milk can be in gross negative zinc balance, in some cases for up to 60 d of age[9]. Even though another study has found net intestinal absorption of zinc in preterm infants fed their own mothers' milk or a preterm formula[11] their net retention of zinc did not match calculated intrauterine accretion rates of the element. Hence it is not surprising that symptomatic zinc-deficiency has been described in pretern infants. Eleven such cases have been reported[1,2,4,8,12,15,17,18,20]. The gestations of these infants varied between 26 and 34 weeks, and their birth-weights between 0.71 and 2.2 kg. Boys predominate, and the histories of three of the four reported girls included extensive periods of parenteral feeding[5,17]. All these cases were breast-fed infants presenting at about three months of age. One report describes a similar experience in seven infants fed a formula derived from cow's milk[5], but the account is not extensive enought to assess all the cases reliably.

The development of zinc-deficiency in such cases has been attributed to a low intake of zinc from their mother's breast-milk, to increased faecal losses, and to a low body content of zinc at birth; all of which leave the baby unable to meet the post-natal anabolic requirements. It has been suggested that the adventitious release of zinc during remodelling of the skeleton may provide enough metal to maintain growth and other essential processes such as protein synthesis[16]. However, it has been shown, in weanling rats, that the release of zinc from bone is susceptible to the dietary supply of calcium[13]. In animals fed a diet with a low calcium and zinc content, $4.5 \pm 0.4\,\mu g$ (mean $\pm$ s.d.) of zinc was released from the humerus over a 4-week experimental period in contrast to animals supplied with a low zinc but adequate calcium diet who released only $0.3 \pm 0.4\,\mu g$ of zinc. Thus the skeleton may not be a reliable source of zinc in the ex-preterm neonate. Additionally there can be speculation that the stresses experienced during their clinical management may derange the normal regulation of zinc metabolism in preterm infants. For example many factors which induce the synthesis of metallothionein could interfere with the physiological redistribution of zinc in the liver; additionally, starvation and infection may cause net catabolism of tissues, such as muscle, and reduce what little zinc these tissues may contain.

Metabolic balance studies in one zinc-deficient preterm neonate demonstrated a marked intestinal loss of the element (8.4 µmol/kg per 24 h) with an intake of zinc of 1.24 µmol/kg per 24 h[1]. The child was losing endogenous zinc in the stools and was unable to reabsorb it adequately but a jejunal mucosal biopsy from that same child showed, relative to biopsies from older children, an enhanced ability *in vitro* to take up radiozinc from an incubation medium. Apart from the studies of Mendelson *et al.*[11] another recent investigation, using the stable isotope ^{70}Zn, has demonstrated that preterm neonates born with weights appropriate for their gestational age are able to absorb quite efficiently zinc given as a single bolus dose of 2 µmol/kg B.Wt.: babies being fed their own mothers milk or a preterm formula absorbed (mean ±s.d.) 68.4 ± 4.6 per cent and 66.4 ± 3.8 per cent of the dose respectively[10]. The design of the study was not wholly physiological, but it would seem that if such infants are at risk of developing zinc-deficiency one has to seek other possible causes apart from immature intestinal absorptive mechanisms. This is further evidenced by our unpublished experiences with another preterm boy who, at 3 months of age, developed zinc-deficiency with a plasma zinc of 4 µmol/l and a plasma alkaline phosphatase activity of 104 units/l. His oral intake of zinc was low at 2.0 µmol/kg per 24 h, even so he had a net intestinal absorption and maximal whole body retention of zinc of 1.13 and 0.66 µmol/kg per 24 h respectively. The response to zinc supplements of this baby's clinical and biochemical features left little doubt that, in spite of the intestinal absorption of zinc, he was zinc-deficient.

The requirements for zinc, their dependence on gestational maturity, and their fluctuation with growth rates, have not been delineated. For this to be achieved considerably more insight is needed into the neonatal homoeostasis of zinc, the mechanisms and regulation of its post natal changes, and into the influence of other nutrients and systemic stress on zinc metabolism. This may be asking a lot, but this is a singularly important challenge.

1 Aggett, P.J., Atherton, D.J., More, J., Davey, J., Delves, H.T. & Harries, J.T. (1980): Symptomatic zinc deficiency in a breast-fed preterm infant. *Archs Dis. Child.* **58**, 547–550.

2 Ahmed, S. & Blair, A.W. (1981): Symptomatic zinc deficiency in a breast-fed infant. *Archs Dis. Child.* **56**, 315.

3 Bakka, A. & Webb, M. (1981): Metabolism of zinc and copper in the neonate: changes in the concentration and contents of thionein-bound Zn and Cu with age in the livers of the new born of various mammalian species. *Biochem. Pharmacol.* **30**, 721–725.

4 Blom, I., Jameson, S., Krook, F., Larsson-Stymne, B. & Wranne, L. (1980): Zinc deficiency with transitory acrodermatitis enteropathica in a boy of low birth weight. *Br. J. Dermatol.* **104**, 459–464.

5 Bonifazi, E., Rigillo, N., De Simone, B. & Meneghini, C.L. (1980): Acquired dermatitis due to zinc deficiency in a premature infant. *Acta Derm. Venerol.* **60**, 449–451.

6 Cassens, R.G., Hoekstra, W.G., Faltin, E.C. & Briskey, E.J. (1967): Zinc content and subcellular distribution in red versus white porcine skeletal muscle. *Am. J. Physiol.* **221**, 688–692.

7 Cavell, P.A. & Widdowson, E.M. (1964): Intakes and excretions of iron, copper and zinc in the neonatal period. *Archs Dis. Child.* **139**, 496–501.

8 Connors, T.J., Czarnecki, D.B. & Haskett, M.I. (1983): Acquired zinc deficiency in a breast-fed premature infant. *Archs Dermatol.* **119**, 319–321.

9 Dauncey, M.J., Shaw, J.C.L. & Urman, J. (1977): The absorption and retention of magnesium, zinc and copper by low birth weight infants fed pasteurised human breast milk. *Pediatr. Res.* **11**, 991–997.

10 Ehrenkranz, R.A., Ackerman, B.A., Nelli, C.M. & Jangorbhani, M. (1984): Determination with stable isotopes of the dietary bioavailability of zinc in premature infants. *Am. J. Clin. Nutr.* **40**, 72–81.

11 Mendelson, R.A., Bryan, M.H. & Anderson, G.H. (1983): Trace mineral balances in preterm infants fed their own mothers milk. *J. Pediatr. Gastro. Nutr.* **2**, 256–261.

12 Murphy, J.F., Gray, O.P., Rendall, J.R. & Hann, S. (1985): Zinc deficiency: a problem with preterm breast milk. *Early Hum. Devl.* **10**, 303–307.

13 Murray, E.J. & Messer, H.H. (1981): Turnover of bone zinc during normal and accelerated bone loss in rats. *J. Nutr.* **111**, 1641–1647.

14 Panemangalore, M., Banerjee, D., Onosaka, S. & Cherian, M.G. (1983): Changes in the intracellular accumulation and distribution of metallothionein in rat liver and kidney during postnatal development. *Devl. Biol.* **97**, 95–102.

15 Parker, P.H., Helinek, G.L., Meneely, R.L., Stroop, S., Ghishan, F.K. & Green, H.L. (1982): Zinc deficiency in a premature infant fed exclusively human milk. *Am. J. Dis. Child.* **136**, 77–78.

16 Shaw, J.C.L. (1979): Trace elements in the fetus and young infant. *Am. J. Dis. Child.* **133**, 1260–1268.

17 Sivasubramanian, K.N. & Henkin, R.I. (1978): Behavioural and dermatologic changes and low serum zinc and copper concentrations in two premature infants after parenteral alimentation. *J. Pediatr.* **93**, 847–851.

18 Weymouth, R.D., Kelly, R. & Landsdell, B.J. (1982): Symptomatic zinc deficiency in a premature infant. *Aust. Paediatr. J.* **1B**, 208–210.

19 Ziegler, E.E., Edwards, B.B., Jensen, R.L., Filer, L.J. & Foman, S.J. (1978): Zinc balances studies in normal infants. In *Trace element metabolism in man and animals — 3.* ed M. Kirchgessner, pp. 292–295. Freising-Weihenstephan: Arbeitskieis fur Tierernährungsforschung.

20 Zimmerman, A.W., Hambidge, K.M., Lepow, M.L., Greenberg, R.D., Stover, M.L. & Casey, C.E. (1982): Acrodermatitis in breast–fed premature infants: evidence for a defect of mammary zinc secretion. *Pediatrics* **59**, 176–183.

Zinc-deficiency

K.M. HAMBIDGE, Nancy F. KREBS and P.A. WALRAVENS
University of Colorado, Health Sciences Center, 4200 East Ninth Avenue, Denver, Colorado 80262, USA.

The aim of this paper is to provide a selective review of the evidence derived from our studies in North America in support of the hypothesis that chronic, mild, or marginal zinc-deficiency occurs in some sections of the population. Attention will be focused on the infant, young child, and lactating woman. A second aim is to speculate as to why zinc-deficiency may occur despite the evidence that the human may have a significant ability to adapt to restricted zinc intake.

Evidence for zinc-deficiency in infants and young children. Though the laboratory assays may be useful in group comparisonsof zinc nutrition[4], the sensitivity and reliability of the assays that are currently available are inadequate for the detection or confirmation of mild human zinc-deficiency. Hence confirmation has been and is still dependent on the demonstration of improvement in an impaired zinc-dependent physiological function with appropriate levels of dietary zinc supplementation in studies that are randomized and adequately controlled. This approach also indicates the benefits that accrue from partial or complete correction of the putative deficiency state. Three randomized, double-blind controlled zinc supplementation studies have been completed in this centre[7] and a fourth is in progress[15]. The primary biological function that has been examined in each of these investigations is physical growth. In the animal model, the extent to which growth velocity is improved depends on the severity of the dietary zinc restriction, and some diminution of growth rate occurs even with very mild dietary zinc restriction[16]. Excess zinc may actually impair growth[2] and there is no evidence for a pharmacological growth-promoting effect of zinc. Moreover, the quantities of supplemental zinc that have been used in these studies were very modest such that the total daily zinc intake has been maintained within an acceptable dietary range. Hence, any increase in growth velocity associated with the zinc supplement under these circumstances can be interpreted to indicate the correction or prevention of a growth-limiting zinc-deficiency state.

Two of our supplementation studies have involved young Denver children with height-for-age percentiles ≤ 10th[5,14]. The subjects were aged 2 to 6 years and were primarily Mexican-American children from low-income families. The zinc supplement or placebo was administered for 6 months in the first study, and for 1 year in the second. A total of 29 male pairs and 20 female pairs completed one of the two studies. In both of these studies the mean increment in height and height-for-age Z score for the zinc supplemented children (combined sexes and boys) was significantly greater than the corresponding increments for the children who had received the placebo. (Z scores are standard deviations around the mean, which in these studies is the 50th percentile of the National Center for Health Statistics growth curves). No significant differences occurred between test and control girls, but only seven female pairs were included in the most recent study and more extensive research is warranted. The difference in height increments between zinc supplemented boys and paired controls were also significant when the changes were expressed as percentages of initial height. Linear regression analysis on each individual's longitudinal height data at 0, 3, 6, 9 and 12 months was performed. The average difference in slopes of the zinc supplemented versus the paired control boys was significant ($P < 0.05$, one-tailed t-test). These differences, though statistically significant, were quite small (12–14 per cent or < 1 cm/year). However, the very small quantities of supplemental zinc consumed and the lack of any change in biochemical indices of zinc status of the zinc supplemented children relative to the controls, both suggest that a maximal effect may not have been achieved.

Increases in food intake between the beginning and the end of the more recent study were also found to be significantly greater for the zinc supplemented than for the control children[9]. Mean calculated intakes for energy increased from levels below most reported intakes for this age group, and below levels recommended by WHO/FAO, up to a mean level that was comparable with that of other groups of children who have been investigated. The mean energy intake of the placebo group of children remained relatively low.

The aetiology of this growth-limiting zinc-deficiency syndrome, which is probably not limited to any one ethnic or socio-economic group[3], has not been completely elucidated. Calculated dietary zinc intakes averaged about 5 mg/day or about half the RDA. This was only about 15–20 per cent lower than calculated intakes from middle-income Denver children of the same age[6]. However, if the intake for the middle-income children had been borderline, it is quite possible that this difference could be of considerable practical significance. The growth percentiles of these children started to decline in infancy, with a typical pattern of failure to thrive due to malnutrition. Hence, if zinc-deficiency is one aetiological factor in the poor growth of these children, the onset of this deficiency must also have occurred in early post-natal life. Currently, a study is in progress to determine the effects of dietary intervention with zinc supplements at an early stage after the commencement of declining growth percentiles. Initial results of this randomized, double-blind, controlled study have demonstrated a significant improvement in weight-for-age Z scores of the zinc supplemented infants compared with the controls receiving a placebo over a 6-month period[15]. Quantitative data on weaning practices are not yet available to determine what effect these are likely to have on the zinc status of this population. However, it is worth noting that only a very small percentage of the children in these studies were breast-fed for more than a few weeks.

Zinc in human milk and maternal zinc intake during lactation. Our studies of zinc supplementation in lactation[10] are of more recent origin and have not yet included randomized, blind-controlled studies. However, the results of initial studies indicate that lactating women are at risk from sub-optimal zinc nutrition, especially with prolonged lactation, and that sub-optimal maternal zinc intake is associated with lower milk zinc concentrations. This observation has a parallel in cows, which have a decline in milk zinc concentration with mild zinc-deficiency under 'field' conditions[11]. The administration of a daily zinc supplement, sufficient to raise the total daily zinc intake to the level of the RDA of 25 mg[12], was associated with a mean rate of decline in milk zinc concentrations over the first 9 months of lactation that was significantly less than for a similar group of lactating women who did not receive a zinc supplement. It has been calculated[10] that the zinc intake of fully-breast fed infants after the age of 7 months would be insufficient to meet minimal requirements even assuming 100 per cent net absorption of zinc from breast-milk in the case of mothers who did not receive a zinc supplement. By this stage of lactation milk zinc concentrations were 50 per cent lower than in the zinc supplemented group. These observations could have nutritional implications for those infants who continue to depend on mother's milk for most of their nutrients during the second half of infancy and beyond. The importance of adequate zinc uptake for optimal growth of formula-fed infants has been documented in an earlier study[13].

Plausibility of mild chronic zinc-deficiency syndromes. Are there valid reasons for rejecting the hypothesis that nutritional zinc-deficiency as an isolated phenomenon can occur in the free-living population in a relatively affluent country? In addressing this question, two factors merit special consideration. First, it has been shown experimentally that zinc balance in normal adults is altered relatively little by severe dietary zinc restriction due to a notable adaptation that leads to increased absorption of dietary zinc and decreased excretion of endogenous zinc[8]. However, it has not been shown whether this degree of adaptation is possible on all mixed diets. In the young, 'adaptive' mechanisms may conceivably include a diminution of growth velocity and during lactation adaptation may include decreased zinc secretion by the mammary gland. Neither of these possibilities are necessarily acceptable. Second is the argument that diets cannot be deficient in zinc if they are commonly used and, as a corollary, that the current RDAs must be set too high, especially during pregnancy and lactation, as they are at a level which is not reached by the great majority of subjects. This argument is, at best, very tenuous. For example, paleolithic diets that were commonly consumed 40 000 years ago[1] may have typically provided more than 160 g of protein per day to lactating women with a daily energy intake of 8.37 MJ (2000 kcal). Calculations based on the mean dietary zinc:protein ratio for lactating women in Denver[10] indicate that these diets would have provided more than 20 mg of zinc per day. There is very little evidence to support the occurrence of significant genetic changed over this time interval and it is unlikely that human zinc homoeostatic mechanisms have changed significantly. Hence, current diets that are influenced extensively by food processing and fortification and that reflect relatively recent changes in agricultural and feeding practices should not be accepted as providing optimal quantities of zinc without careful evaluation.

Conclusion. Evidence has been presented, based on the results of randomized, blind-controlled studies of dietary zinc supplementation, that mild chronic zinc-deficiency occurs in some otherwise normal infants and growing children in North America. Documented sequelae are growth retardation and decreased food consumption. There is evidence to suggest that nutritional zinc-deficiency occurs in lactation, especially with prolonged lactation, leading to decreased zinc concentrations in breast-milk. Based on the circumstances in which these individuals were identified it is suggested that mild nutritional zinc-deficiency may occur quite commonly as a single nutrient deficiency in North America.

Acknowledgements. Supported by grant AM 12432 from the National Institutes of Health, National Institue of Arthritis, Diabetes, Digestive and Kidney Diseases, and by grant RR-69 from National Institutes of Health, General Clinical Research Centers.

1 Eaton, S.B. & Konner, M. (1985): Paleolithic nutrition. *New Engl. J. Med.* **312**, 283–289.
2 Golden, M. (discussant in): Hambidge, K.M. (1985): Clinical deficiencies: when to suspect there is a problem. In *Trace elements in nutrition of children*, ed R.K. Chandra, p. 12. New York: Nestlé Nutrition, Vevey/Raven Press.
3 Hambidge, K.M., Hambidge, C., Jacobs, M.A. & Baum, J.D. (1972): Low levels of zinc in hair, anorexia, poor growth and hypogeusia in children. *Ped. Res.* **6**, 868–874.
4 Hambidge, K.M., Walravens, P.A., Brown, R.M., Webster, J., White, S., Anthony, M. & Roth, M.L. (1976): Zinc nutrition of preschool children in the Denver Head Start Program. *Am. J. Clin. Nutr.* **29**, 734–738.
5 Hambidge, K.M. & Walravens, P.A. (1978): Zinc supplementation of low income preschool children. In *Trace element metabolism in man and animals-3*, ed M. Kirchgessner, pp. 296–299. Weihenstephan Arbeitskreis für Tierernährungsforschung.
6 Hambidge, K.M., Chavez, M.N., Brown, R.M. & Walravens, P.A. (1979): Zinc nutritional status of young middle-income children and the effects of consuming zinc-fortified breakfast cereals. *Am. J. Clin. Nutr.* **32**, 2532–2539.
7 Hambidge, K.M., Krebs, N.F. & Walravens, P.A. (1985): Growth velocity of young children receiving a dietary zinc supplement. *Nutr. Res.* (In press).
8 King, J.C. (1985): Assessment of human zinc requirements. *J. Am. Dietet. Assoc.* (In press).
9 Krebs, N.F., Hambidge, K.M. & Walravens, P.A. (1984): Increased food intake of young children receiving a zinc supplement. *Am. J. Dis. Child.* **138**, 270–273.
10 Krebs, N.F., Hambidge, K.M., Jacobs, M.A. & Oliva-Rasbach, J. (1985): The effects of a dietary zinc supplement during lactation on longitudinal changes in maternal zinc status and milk zinc concentrations. *Am. J. Clin. Nutr.* **41**, 560–570.
11 Miller, W.J., Neathery, M.W., Gentry, R.P., Blackmon, D.M. & Stake, P.E. (1974): Adaptations in zinc metabolism by lactating cows fed a low-zinc practical-type diet. In *Trace element metabolism in animals-II*, ed W.G. Hoekstra, J.W. Suttie, W.E. Ganther, W. Mertz, pp. 550–552. New York: University Park Press.
12 Recommended Dietary Allowances (1980): Food and Nutrition Board, National Academy of Sciences, Washington, DC.
13 Walravens, P.A. & Hambidge, K.M. (1976): Growth of infants fed a zinc supplemented formula. *Am. J. Clin. Nutr.* **29**, 1114–1121.

14 Walravens, P.A., Krebs, N.F. & Hambidge, K.M. (1983): Linear growth of low income preschool children receiving a zinc supplement. *Am. J. Clin. Nutr.* **38**, 195–201.
15 Walravens, P.A., Koepfer, D.M., Hambidge, K.M. & Casey, C.E. (1985): Zinc supplementation in infants with failure to thrive: effects on weight gains. *Clin. Res.* **33**, 134A.
16 Williams, R.B. & Mills, C.F. (1970): The experimental production of zinc deficiency in the rat. *Br. J. Nutr.* **24**, 989–1003.

Assessment of zinc status and requirements

Ananda S. PRASAD
Department of Medicine, Wayne State University School of Medicine, Harper-Grace Hospitals, 3990 John R, Detroit, Michigan 48201 and Veterans Administration Medical Center, Allen Park, Michigan, USA.

In 1961, for the first time, deficiency of zinc was suspected to occur in human subjects[14]. Its occurrence was documented first from the Middle East in 1963[15]. During the last two decades, it has become obvious that the nutritional deficiency of zinc in humans is fairly prevalent throughout the world. In addition to Iran and Egypt, zinc-deficiency in humans has now been reported from Turkey, Portugal, Morocco, Yugoslavia and other developing countries.

Nutritional deficiency of zinc occurring in children and infants has also been recognized in the United States. A study from Denver in 1972 identified several children from middle and upper income families who had significantly decreased zinc levels in the hair and retarded growth[3]. Nutritional problems related to zinc have now been encountered in certain population segments of other developed countries as well. Old age, pregnancy, lactation and alcoholism are also associated with higher incidence of poor zinc nutrition. Predominant use of cereal proteins by the majority of the world population is an important predisposing factor for zinc-deficiency. The availability of zinc in such diets is poor because of high phosphate and phytate content. Zinc deficiency is likely to occur in conditions requiring an increased zinc intake. These conditions include the rapid growth age period in infants and children and pregnancy and lactation.

Zinc-deficiency has been reported in patients with malabsorption syndrome, chronic renal disease following total parenteral nutrition for 6 to 10 weeks without zinc supplementation, and following penicillamine therapy to a patient with Wilson's disease[5].

Hyperzincuria over an extended period may lead to zinc depletion. Conditions associated with hypercatabolic states such as surgery, burns, multiple injuries, major fractures, diabetes mellitus, protein deprivation and starvation usually exhibit hyperzincuria. Use of chelating agents such as penicillamine may also result in excessive zinc loss in the urine. Patients with cirrhosis of the liver, nephrotic syndrome and sickle cell disease have hyperzincuria[12,13]. Several of their clinical manifestations are due to zinc-deficiency and are corrected by zinc supplementation.

At present, two genetic disorders, acrodermatitis enteropathica (AE) and sickle cell disease, are known to be associated with zinc-deficiency[2]. The clinical manifestations of AE seem to be completely reversible with zinc supplementation. In this review, clinical manifestations and laboratory diagnosis of zinc-deficiency will be presented. A brief discussion of bioavailability of zinc will also be provided.

Clinical manifestations of zinc-deficiency. Growth retardation, hypogonadism in males, poor appetite, mental lethargy and skin changes were the typical clinical features of chronically zinc-deficient subjects from the Middle East as reported by the author in the early sixties[10,11]. These features were corrected by zinc supplementation.

Recently, abnormal dark adaptation in alcoholic cirrhotics has been related to a deficiency of zinc[8]. Zinc administration to these patients corrected the abnormal dark adaptation. Similar clinical observations have been made in some zinc-deficient, sickle cell anaemia patients[19]. It has been proposed that the effect of zinc on the retina may be mediated by an enzyme, retinene reductase, which is known to be zinc-dependent.

The conclusion that zinc can promote the healing of cutaneous sores and wounds has been controversial for several years. Most studies now provide evidence that zinc supplementation promotes wound healing in zinc-deficient patients and that zinc therapy in zinc-sufficient subjects is not effective for wound healing.

Abnormalities of taste have been related to a deficiency of zinc in many clinical conditions by some investigators[4,6]. Decreased taste acuity (hypogeusia) has been observed in zinc-deficient subjects with liver disease, malabsorption syndrome, thermal burns or chronic uraemia and in subjects following administration of penicillamine or histidine. It appears that depletion of zinc may lead to decreased taste acuity, but not all cases of hypogeusia are due to zinc-deficiency. The role of zinc in hypogeusia needs to be delineated further.

The dermatological manifestations of severe zinc-deficiency include progressive bullous-pustular dermatitis of the extremities and the oral, anal, and genital areas, combined with paronychia and generalized alopecia such as seen in AE. Infection with *Candida albicans* is a frequent complication. These manifestations are seen in cases with severe deficiency of zinc.

Neuropsychiatric signs include irritability, emotional disorders, tremors and occasional cerebellar ataxia. The patients generally have retarded growth and males exhibit hypogonadism. Zinc therapy has been shown to produce remarkable improvements and is considered to be a life-saving measure in these subjects.

In adults, a mild deficiency of zinc as induced by an experimental diet resulted in weight loss, decreased plasma testosterone concentration, and decreased sperm count. Following supplementation with zinc all the above mentioned manifestations were reversed[1,16].

Laboratory diagnosis of zinc-deficiency. Measurement of zinc level in plasma is useful provided the sample is not haemolyzed or contaminated. In conditions of acute stress, following myocardial infarction or acute infections, zinc from the plasma compartment may redistribute to other tissues, thus making an assessment of zinc status in the body a difficult task[12]. Intravascular haemolysis would also increase the plasma zinc level inasmuch as the content of red cell zinc is much higher than the plasma.

Many investigators have utilized plasma copper:zinc ratio for clinical assessment in certain diseases. It has been suggested that an increase in this ratio in patients with malignancy may indicate activity of the disease and poor prognosis.

Zinc in the red cells and hair also may be used for assessment of body zinc status. Because these tissues turn over slowly, the zinc levels do not reflect recent changes with respect to body zinc stores. Zinc determination, in cells such as neutrophils, lymphocytes, and platelets on the other hand, appear to reflect the body zinc status more accurately and therefore are very useful parameters.

Urinary excretion of zinc is decreased as a result of zinc-deficiency. Thus, determination of zinc in 24 h urine may be of additional help in diagnosing zinc-deficiency, provided cirrhosis of the liver, sickle cell disease, chronic renal disease, and other conditions known to cause hyperzincuria are ruled out. Hyperzincuria may be associated with zinc-deficiency in the above mentioned disorders.

A metabolic balance study may clearly distinguish zinc-deficient from zinc-sufficient subjects[16]. Recently, an oral zinc tolerance test has been utilized for diagnostic purposes[9,18].

The activities of many zinc-dependent enzymes have been shown to be affected adversely in zinc-deficient tissues. Three enzymes, alkaline phosphatase, carboxypeptidase and thymidine kinase, appear to be most sensitive to zinc restriction in that their activities are affected adversely within 3 to 6 days of institution of a zinc-deficient diet to experimental animals. In human studies, the activities of deoxythymidine kinase in proliferating skin collagen and alkaline phosphatase activity in neutrophils were shown to be sensitive to dietary zinc intake. As a practical test, quantitative measurement of alkaline phosphatase activity in neutrophils may be a useful adjunct to neutrophil zinc level determination in order to assess body zinc status in man. Following supplementation with zinc to deficient subjects, a prompt response in the activities of sensitive enzymes is observed.

Cell-mediated immune functions are affected adversely as a result of zinc-deficiency. Skin tests for anergy, natural killer cell activity, proliferative responses of peripheral blood lymphocytes, T-helper and suppressor functions, serum thymic hormone (Facteur Thymique Serique) assay, chemotaxis and a correlation of the above tests with zinc concentration of lymphocytes and neutrophils may provide valuable tools for the diagnosis of zinc-deficiency in humans in the future. Obviously much more scientific work is needed in this area.

Metabolic requirements and bioavailability of zinc. Most data in the literature suggest that the metabolic requirement of zinc for a 50 to 80-kg subject is approximately 4–6 mg per day. If these values represent amount which must be absorbed and delivered to the blood daily, then dietary zinc must equal 9 to 15 mg/day presuming that absorption of zinc is approximately 40 per cent. The majority of studies for developed countries have reported daily zinc intake to be in that range. The recommended daily dietary allowance of zinc for an adult according to National Research Council, National Academy of Sciences, USA should be 15 mg.

Several factors such as phytate and fibre are known to affect the bioavailability of zinc. The overall effect of food fibre on zinc balance remains controversial and it is probable that different sources of food fibre may have different effects on zinc bioavailability. Composition of the meals, including level and source of protein, calcium and iron content and presence of natural chelators such as phytates and oxalates are variables that affect bioavailability and thus dietary requirement of zinc[17]. The significance and quantitative relationship of each of these in human diets remains to be established. Other factors which may affect dietary zinc requirement include zinc status of the body, genetic background, geographic location, energy expenditure and amount of exercise, medications, stress (physical and mental), dietary additives (such as EDTA), alcohol consumption and diseases such as malignancy, malabsorption syndrome, renal disease, sickle cell anaemia and myocardial infarction.

In general, the animal studies have shown that dietary phytate:zinc molar ratios exceeding 15 results in decreased bioavailability of dietary zinc. In limited human studies, phytate:zinc molar ratio of 8 to 12 did not appear to affect the bioavailability of zinc[7]. However, when this ratio exceeded 20 in another study[16], it was reported to be unfavourable to the bioavailability of zinc in human subjects.

Thus the phytate:zinc molar ratio is very important in cases where daily dietary zinc intake is well below RDA, in cases where the metabolic requirement of zinc is increased such as growing infants, children, pregnant and lactating women and in those who consume large quantities of grain and legumes with little or no meat or seafood.

Conclusion. Zinc-deficiency in human subjects is fairly prevalent throughout the world. Many dietary factors are known to affect the bioavailability of zinc and therefore requirement of zinc may vary from one part of the world to another depending upon the nature of the diet. Measurement of zinc in cells such as lymphocytes and platelets and assay of lymphocyte functions may provide good assessment of zinc status in humans.

Acknowledgements. Supported in part by grants from the National Heart, Lung, and Blood Institute, Sickle Cell Center grant, a grant from the National Institute of Arthritis, Metabolic, and Digestive Diseases, NIH, and a grant from Veterans Administration Research Service.

1 Abbasi, A.A., Prasad, A.S., Rabbani, P. & DuMouchelle, E. (1980): Experimental zinc deficiency in man. Effect on testicular function. *J. Lab. Clin. Med.* **96**, (3), 544–550.

2 Barnes, P.M. & Moynahan, E.J. (1973): Zinc deficiency in acrodermatitis enteropathica. Multiple dietary intolerance treated with synthetic diet. *Proc. R. Soc. Med.* **66**, 327–329.

3 Hambidge, K.M. & Walravens, P.A. (1976): Zinc deficiency in infants and preadolescent children. In *Trace elements in human health and disease*, ed A.S. Prasad, Vol. 1, pp. 21–31. New York: Academic Press.

4 Henkin, R.I. & Bradley, D.F. (1969): Regulation of taste acuity by thiols and metal ions. *Proc. Natl. Acad. Sci. USA.* **62**, 30–37.

5 Klingberg, W.G., Prasad, A.S. & Oberleas, D. (1976): *Trace elements in human health and disease*, ed A.S. Prasad, pp. 51–65. New York: Academic Press.

6 Mahajan, S.K., Abbasi, A.A., Prasad, A.S., Rabbani, P., Briggs, W.A. & McDonald, F.D. (1982): Effect of oral zinc therapy on gonadal function in hemodialysis patients. *Ann. Int. Med.* **97**, 357–361.

7 Morris, E.R. & Ellis, R. (1982): Dietary phytate/zinc molar ratio and zinc balance in humans. In *Nutritional*

bioavailability of zinc, ed G.E. Inglett, pp. 159–172. American Chemical Society Symposium Series, Washington DC: Am. Chem. Soc.

8 Morrison, S.A., Russel, R.M., Carney, E.A. & Oaks, E.V. (1978): Zinc deficiency. A cause of abnormal dark adaptation in cirrhotics. *Am. J. Clin. Nutr.* **31**, 276–281.

9 Oelshlegel, F.J. & Brewer, G.J. (1977): Absorption of pharmacologic doses of zinc. In *Zinc metabolism: in current aspects in Health and Disease*, ed G.J. Brewer & A.S. Prasad, pp. 299–311. New York: Alan R. Liss.

10 Prasad, A.S. (1966): Metabolism of zinc and its deficiency in human subjects. In *Zinc metabolism*, ed A.S. Prasad, pp. 250–303, Springfield, Illinois: Charles C Thomas.

11 Prasad, A.S. (1978): *Trace elements and iron in human metabolism*, pp. 251–329. New York: Plenum.

12 Prasad, A.S. (1982): Clinical and biochemical spectrum of zinc deficiency in human subjects. In *Clinical, biochemical and nutritional aspects of trace elements*, ed A.S. Prasad, Vol. 6, pp. 3–62. New York: Alan R. Liss.

13 Prasad, A.S. (1982): Clinical disorders of zinc deficiency. In *Clinical applications of recent advances in zinc metabolism*, pp. 89–119, New York: Alan R. Liss, Inc.

14 Prasad, A.S., Halsted, J.A. & Nadimi, M. (1961): Syndrome of iron deficiency anemia hepatosplenomegaly, hypogonadism, dwarfism and geophagia. *Am. J. Med.* **31**, 532–546.

15 Prasad, A.S., Miale, A., Farid, Z., Schulert, A. & Sandsted, H.H. (1963): Zinc metabolism in patients with syndrome of iron deficiency anemia, hypogonadism and dwarfism. *J. Lab. Clin. Med.* **61**, 537–549.

16 Prasad, A.S., Rabbani, P., Abbasi, A., Bowersox, E. & Fox, M.R.S. (1978): Experimental zinc deficiency in humans. *Ann. Intern. Med.* **89**, 483–490.

17 Smith, J.C. Jr., Morris, E.R. & Ellis, R. (1983): Zinc requirements, bioavailabilities and recommended dietary allowances. In *Zinc deficiency in human subjects*, ed A.S. Prasad, A.O. Cavdar, G.J. Brewer & P.J. Aggett, pp. 147–169. New York: Alan R. Liss.

18 Sullivan, J.F., Jetton, M.M. & Burch, R.E. (1979): A zinc tolerance test. *J. Lab. Clin. Med.* **93**, 485–492.

19 Warth, J.A., Prasad, A.S., Zwas, F. & Frank, R.N. (1981): Abnormal dark adaptation in sickle cell anemia. *J. Lab. Clin. Med.* **98**, 189–194.

★ ★ ★

RESEARCH DEVELOPMENTS IN IRON NUTRITION

Bioavailability of iron in food

M. LAYRISSE
Instituto Venezolano de Investigaciones Científicas (IVIC), Laboratorio de Medicina Experimental, Apartado 1827, Caracas, Venezuela.

The introduction of the extrinsic label method for the measurement of iron absorption from food enabled a distinction to be made between two forms of iron haem and non-haem, in terms of iron absorption[10,19,23]. The first group is comprised of haemoglobin and myoglobin. The second group, non-haem, is comprised of a variety of iron compounds present in animal and vegetable foods, ferric and ferrous iron salts. In the muscle and viscera of animals non-haem iron is found principally in the form of the two major iron storage compounds, ferritin and haemosiderin[13,21,28].

In the lumen of the gastro-intestinal tract the absorption of iron from the haem present in haemoglobin and myoglobin behaves as a single pool, in terms of absorption, and can be measured by mixing small amounts of labelled rabbit haemoglobin with the meat to be tested for iron absorption[19,23]. The iron from vegetables, eggs, ferric and ferrous salts and possibly milk form another pool (non-haem) which shows a completely different absorption pattern from the haem pool. This pool can be measured by mixing small amounts (traces or 0.1 mg of iron) of ferric chloride or other soluble iron salt with one of the vegetable foods of the meal[6,10,19,23].

Ferritin and haemosiderin may be considered as a subgroup of the non-haem iron pool. When purified, their iron is less well absorbed than vegetable foods because of its tendency to polymerize, but the absorption is high when they are integrated into meat or viscera[35].

A small amount of labelled purified rabbit ferritin may be used to measure the absorption from ferritin and haemosiderin present in animal foods. It is known that the iron absorption from either iron oxide or iron hydroxide alone is poor but less is known about the behaviour of these compounds when introduced into the gut as iron contamination of foods[14,20].

It may be stated as a general rule that the iron from the haem pool is very well absorbed, about 15–20 per cent in normal subjects and about 25–35 per cent in iron deficient subjects, and its absorption is not affected by inhibiting substances present in vegetable and some animal foods. On the other hand, iron from the non-haem pool is less well absorbed than haem iron, only about 2–5 per cent in normal and 5–10 per cent in iron deficient subjects. Its absorption is reduced by the inhibitors mentioned above and is increased by the presence of ascorbic acid and meat in the meal tested (Fig. 1).

	Food of vegetable origin							Food of animal origin				
	Spinach	Black beans	Maize	Milled rice	Soybean	Lettuce	Wheat	Eggs	Fish	Hemoglobin	Veal liver	Veal Muscle
Dose of foods Fe mg	2	3–4	2–4	2–4	3–4	1–1.7	2–4	3	1–2	3–4	2–4	2–3
Nº Cases normals Iron deficients	9 7 2	61 44 17	260 120 140	54 30 24	59 32 27	13 10 3	34 19 15	27 11 16	63 40 23	50 29 21	74 51 23	89 49 40

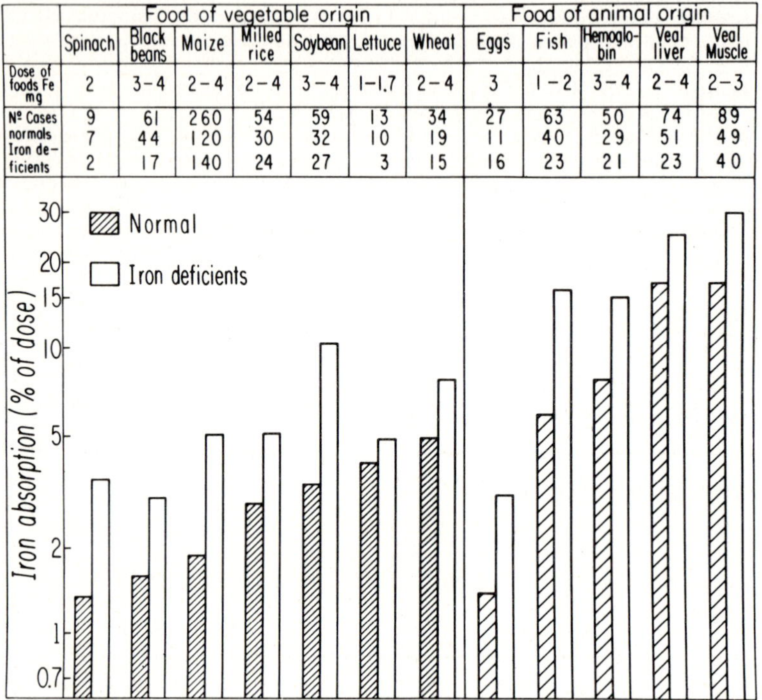

Fig. 1. *Iron absorption from vegetable and animal foods in normal and iron deficient subjects.* The data from rice were taken from Aung-Than-Batu *et al.*, 1976[2] and Hallberg, L., personal communication; data from eggs iron-absorption from Callender *et al.*, 1970[8]; and Bjorn-Rasmussen *et al.*, 1972[7] and the other data were taken from various studies by Layrisse *et al.*, 1969[22]; Layrisse & Martinez-Torres, 1983[24].

Inhibitors and enhancers of iron absorption. Early studies of iron absorption from a single food, into which radioactive iron was biosynthetically incorporated, indicated that the great difference in absorption between vegetable and animal foods was not entirely due to the chemical characteristics of the iron and these foods most probably contain substances that inhibit or enhance the iron absorption. Later studies demonstrated that these substances, called ligands, not only affect the iron absorption from the food in which they are present but also the iron absorption from other foods in the same meal[23]. There is only sparse information on the nature and mechanism by which these ligands govern the absorption of the dietary iron.

The inhibiting ligands for iron absorption are in excess in the majority of vegetable foods, affecting not only the absorption of the intrinsic iron of the food but also that of a large amount of extrinsic iron. This was clearly demonstrated when 100 g of maize was able to reduce the absorption of 60 mg of iron in the form of ferric iron[25]. It is possible that the low absorption of iron observed from cereals and legumes is due to their high content of phytate and polyphenols[12,39]. The strong inhibiting effect of tea, coffee and also of legumes is probably due to a polyphenol, tannin[1,15,16,29,38,40]. The mechanism of the inhibitory effect of soya protein is still undefined[12]. Apparently, the fibre content of a diet has little effect on non-haem iron

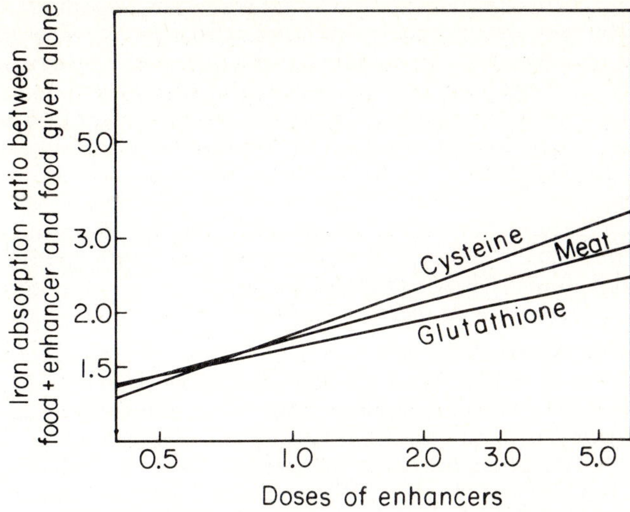

Fig. 2. *Geometrical regression line calculated from the mean iron absorption between that obtained from maize administered with increasing doses of cysteine, glutathione and beef meat and that obtained from maize given alone.* The correlation coefficient was 0.99, 0.94 and 0.98 and the standard error was 0.08, 0.09 and 0.05 for cysteine, glutathione and beef meat, respectively (Layrisse *et al.*, 1984[2]).

absorption[17]. It has been suggested that the phosphoproteins contained in eggs are the ligands that depress the absorption of non-haem iron taken in the same meal. The measurement of iron absorption from milk to which traces of labelled iron were added, indicated that while the absorption from breast-milk averages 49 per cent, for cow's milk it is only 10–12 per cent[37,41,42]. It is not known if the iron label added to the milk truly reflects the absorption of the intrinsic iron.

Amongst enhancing substances are organic acids in the vegetables that facilitate iron absorption, the most effective being ascorbic acid, but others such as lactic, citric and malic acids also show a positive effect on the absorption of non-haem iron. Thus, besides the fruits, especially tropical fruits such as papaya, guava and orange, with a high content of ascorbic acid, other vegetable foods including turnip, cabbage, cauliflower, broccoli, tomato, pumpkin and beetroot, also enhance iron absorption[4,18,43].

Meat, liver and probably other viscera increase the absorption of haem and non-haem iron. Purified haem is poorly absorbed but its absorption is increased three to four times when it is integrated into the haemoglobin molecule and experiences a further increase when integrated as haemoglobin and myoglobin into meat[9,32]. Many studies in the last 15 years have demonstrated the enhancing effect of various kinds of meat and liver on iron absorption from vegetable foods[5,11,30,32–34]. Studies in humans showed that cysteine is the only amino acid that mimics the enhancing effect of meat on the absorption of non-haem iron[31,36]. Recent studies suggest that the effect of meat on non-haem iron absorption occurs at the stage in which cysteine is in the peptide form, rather than as the free amino acid[27,45] (Fig. 2). The effect of meat on the absorption of haem iron is less well understood. It has been suggested that products of protein digestion prevent the polymerization of haem and thus facilitate its absorption[9].

Effect of iron dose. A significant difference may not be expected in iron absorption from the administration of a single food or a meal when the amount of non-haem iron varies between 1 and 4 mg. However, statistical differences are found when the amount of non-haem iron varies more than 10-fold. The only one iron compound that defies this rule is ferritin. It seems that the intestinal mucosal barrier does not discriminate the iron liberated from ferritin, to the same extent that it does with other forms of iron (Layrisse — unpublished observation).

The amount of enhancers in the meal is the main determinant of the increase in non-haem iron absorption. It has been observed that a dose of 5–10 mg of ascorbic acid administered in a purified form or contained in the vegetables, is sufficient to promote the absorption of 1 mg of vegetable iron, and the absorption shows a greater increase when the dose of the vitamin is also increased[4,26]. Similar results have been found with varying doses of meat, cysteine and cysteine-containing peptides[26]. Since the inhibitors of iron absorption are in excess in vegetables and some animal foods, it may be expected that an increased consumption of foods containing these inhibitors does not result in an increase in the absorption of non-haem iron.

Culinary preparation of foods. An excess of heat in culinary preparations produces adverse effects on both non-haem and haem iron absorption. It is known that heat denatures ascorbic acid and in consequence reduces its enhancing effect on the absorption on non-haem iron. Intense and prolonged heat also transforms the haem into other forms of iron which are less available for absorption[44]. The iron absorption from the Venezuelan maize bread called 'arepa', is about twice the absorption from the Mexican 'tortilla'. Differences in absorption are found between brown and white flour[3], and between polished and unpolished rice[7].

Acknowledgement. The information presented here was supported in part by the Consejo Nacional de Investigaciones Científicas of Venezuela and by the United Nations University.

1 Acosta, A., Amar, M., Cornbluth-Szarfac, S., Dillman, E., Fosi, M., Gongora-Biachi, R., Grebe, G., Hertrampf, E., Kremenchuzky, S., Layrisse, M., Martínez-Torres, C., Morón, C., Pizarro, T.M., Reynafarje, C., Stekel, A., Villavicencio, D. & Zuniga, H. (1984): Iron absorption from typical Latin American Diets. *Am. J. Clin. Nutr.* **39**, 953–962.

2 Aung-Than-Batu, Then-Than & Thane-Toe. (1976): Iron absorption from Southeast Asian rice-based meals. *Am. J. Clin. Nutr.* **29**, 219–225.

3 Bjorn-Rasmussen, E. (1973): Food iron absorption in man. III. Effect of iron salt, ascorbic acid and desferrioxamine on the isotopic exchange between native food iron and extrinsic inorganic iron tracer. *Scand. J. Haematol.* **11**, 391–397.

4 Bjorn-Rasmussen, E. & Hallberg, L. (1974): Iron absorption from maize. Effect of ascorbic acid on iron absorption from maize supplemented with ferrous sulfate. *Nutr. Metab.* **16**, 94–100.

5 Bjorn-Rasmussen, E. & Hallberg, L. (1979): Effect of animal proteins on the absorption of food iron in man. *Nutr. Metab.* **23**, 192–202.

6 Bjorn-Rasmussen, E., Hallberg, L. & Walker, R.B. (1972): Food iron absorption in man. I. Isotopic exchange between food iron and inorganic iron salt added to food: Studies on maize, wheat and eggs. *Am. J. Clin. Nutr.* **25**, 317–323.

7 Bjorn-Rasmussen, E., Hallberg, L. & Walker, R.B. (1973): Food iron absorption in man. II. Isotopic exchange of iron between labelled foods and between a food and iron salt. *Am. J. Clin. Nutr.* **26**, 1311–1319.

8 Callender, S.T., Marney, S.R. & Warner, G.T. (1970): Eggs and iron absorption. *Br. J. Haemat.* **19**, 657–665.

9 Conrad, M.E., Cortell, S., Williams, H.L. & Foy, A.L. (1968): Polymerization and intraluminal factors in the absorption of haemoglobin-iron. *J. Lab. Clin. Med.* **68**, 659–668.

10 Cook, J.D., Layrisse, M., Martínez-Torres, C., Walker, R.B., Monsen, E.R. & Finch, C.A. (1972): Food iron absorption measured by an extrinsic tag. *J. Clin. Invest.* **51**, 805–815.

11 Cook, J.D. & Monsen, E.R. (1976): Food iron absorption in human subjects. III. Comparison of the effect of animal proteins on nonheme iron absorption. *Am. J. Clin. Nutr.* **29**, 859–867.

12 Cook, J.D., Morck, T.A. & Lynch, S.R. (1981): The inhibitory effect of soy products on non-heme iron absorption in man. *Am. J. Clin. Nutr.* **34**, 2622–2629.

13 Derman, D.P., Bothwell, T.H., Torrance, J.D., Macphail, A.P., Bezwoda, W.R., Charlton, R.W. & Mayet, F.G.H. (1982): Iron absorption from ferritin and ferric hydroxide. *Scand. J. Haematol.* **29**, 18–24.

14 Derman, D.P., Sayers, M.H., Lynch, S.R., Charlton, R.W., Bothwell, T.H. & Mayet, F.G.H. (1977): Iron absorption from a cereal diet containing cane sugar fortified with ascorbic acid. *Br. J. Nutr.* **38**, 261–269.

15 Disler, P.B., Lynch, S.R., Charlton, R.W. & Bothwell, T.H. (1975): The effect of tea on iron absorption. *Gut.* **16**, 193–200.

16 Disler, P.B., Lynch, S.R., Torrance, J.D., Sayers, M.H., Bothwell, T.H. & Charlton, R.W. (1975): The mechanisms of the inhibition of iron absorption by tea. *S. Afr. J. Med. Sci.* **40**, 109–116.

17 Gillody, M., Bothwell, T.H., Charlton, R.W., Torrance, J.D., Bezwoda, W.R., Macphail, A.P., Derman, D.P., Novelli, L., Morall, P. & Mayet, F.G.H. (1984): Factor affecting the absorption of iron from cereals. *Br. J. Nutr.* **51**, 37–46.

18 Gillody, M., Bothwell, T.H., Charlton, R.W., Torrance, J.D., Bezwoda, W.R., Mills, W. & Mayet, F.G.H. (1983): The effect of organic acids, phytates and polyphenols on the absorption of iron from vegetables. *Br. J. Nutr.* **49**, 331–342.

19 Hallberg, L. & Bjorn-Rasmussen, E. (1972): Determination of iron absorption from whole diet. A new two-pool model using two radioiron isotopes given as haem and non-haem iron. *Scand. J. Haematol.* **9**, 193–197.

20 Hallberg, L., Bjorn-Rasmussen, E., Rossander, L., Suwanik, R., Pleehachinda, R. & Tuntawiroon, M. (1983): Iron absorption from some Asian meals containing contamination iron. *Am. J. Clin. Nutr.* **37**, 272–277.

21 Layrisse, M. (1985): Iron absorption from ferritin. In *Sideropenic conditions and physiotherapeutic role of an iron containing protein*, ed M. Layrisse, G. Ceccarelli & M. Ciampini, pp. 71–76. Rome: Antonio Delfino Edit.

22 Layrisse, M., Cook, J.D., Martínez-Torres, C., Roche, M., Kuhn, I.N. & Finch, C.A. (1969): Food iron absorption: A comparison of vegetable and animal foods. *Blood.* **33**, 430–443.

23 Layrisse, M. & Martínez-Torres, C. (1972): Model for measuring dietary absorption of heme iron: test with a complete meal. *Am. J. Clin. Nutr.* **25**, 401–411.

24 Layrisse, M. & Martínez-Torres, C. (1983): *Absorción del hierro a partir de los alimentos*, p. 32. Caracas: Editorial Arte.

25 Layrisse, M., Martínez-Torres, C., Cook, J.D., Walker, R.B. & Finch, C.A. (1973): Iron fortification of food. Its measurement by the extrinsic tag method. *Blood* **41**, 333–352.

26 Layrisse, M., Martínez-Torres, C. & Gonzalez, M. (1974): Measurement of the total daily dietary absorption by the extrinsic tag model. *Am. J. Clin. Nutr.* **27**, 152–162.

27 Layrisse, M., Martínez-Torres, C., Leets, I., Taylor, P. & Ramírez, J. (1984): Effect of histidine, cysteine, glutathione and beef meat on iron absorption in man. *J. Nutr.* **114**, 217–223.

28 Layrisse, M., Martínez-Torres, C., Renzi, M. & Leets, I. (1975): Ferritin iron absorption in man. *Blood* **45**, 689–698.

29 Layrisse, M., Martínez-Torres, C., Renzi, M., Velez, F. & Gonzalez, M. (1976): Sugar as a vehicle for iron fortification. *Am. J. Clin. Nutr.* **29**, 8–18.

30 Layrisse, M., Martínez-Torres, C. & Roche, M. (1968): The effect of interaction of various foods on iron absorption. *Am. J. Clin. Nutr.* **21**, 1175–1183.

31 Martínez-Torres, C. & Layrisse, M. (1970): Effect of amino acids on iron absorption from a staple vegetable food. *Blood* **35**, 669–682.

32 Martínez-Torres, C. & Layrisse, M. (1971): Iron absorption from veal muscle. *Am. J. Clin. Nutr.* **24**, 521–540.

33 Martínez-Torres, C., Leets, I. & Layrisse, M. (1975): Iron absorption from fish. *Archs Latin. Nutr.* **25**, 199–210.

34 Martínez-Torres, C., Leets, I., Renzi, M. & Layrisse, M. (1974): Iron absorption from veal liver. *J. Nutr.* **104**, 983–993.

35 Martínez-Torres, C., Renzi, M. & Layrisse, M. (1976): Iron absorption by humans from ferritin and hemosiderin. *J. Nutr.* **106**, 128–135.

36 Martínez-Torres, C., Romano, E. & Layrisse, M. (1981): Effect of cysteine on iron absorption in man. *Am. J. Clin. Nutr.* **34**, 322–328.

37 McMillan, J.A., Oski, F.A., Lourie, R.M., Tomarelli, R.M. & Landaw, S.A. (1977): Iron absorption from human milk. Simulated human milk and proprietary formulas. *Pediatrics* **60**, 896–900.

38 Morck, T.A., Lynch, S.R.. & Cook, J.D. (1983): Inhibition of food iron absorption by coffee. *Am. J. Clin. Nutr.* **37**, 416–420.

39 Morris, E.R. & Ellis, R. (1976): Isolation of monoferric phytate from wheat bran and its biological value as an iron source to the rat. *J. Nutr.* **106**, 753–760.

40 Narasinga Rao, B.S. & Prabharathi, T. (1982): Tannin contents of foods commonly consumed in India and its influence on ionizable iron. *J. Sc. Fd Agric.* **33**, 89–96.

41 Saarinen, U.M. & Siimes, M.A. (1977): Iron absorption from infant formula and the optimal level of iron supplementation. *Acta Paed. Scand.* **66**, 719–722.

42 Saarinen, U.M., Siimes, M.A. & Dallman, P.R. (1977): Iron absorption in infants: high bioavailability of breast milk iron as indicated by extrinsic tag method for iron absorption and by the concentration of serum ferritin. *J. Pediat.* **91**, 36–39.

43 Sayers, M.H., Lynch, S.R., Charlton, R.W., Bothwell, T.H., Walker, R.B. & Mayet, F.G.H. (1973): The effect of ascorbic acid supplementation on the absorption of iron in maize, wheat and soya. *Br. J. Haemat.* **24**, 209–218.

44 Schricker, B.R. & Miller, D.D. (1983): Effects of cooking and chemical treatment of heme and nonheme iron in meat. *J. Fd Sci.* **48**, 1340–1344.

45 Taylor, P., Martínez-Torres, C., Romano, E. & Layrisse, M. (1985): The effect of cysteine containing peptides during meat digestion on iron absorption in humans. *Am. J. Clin. Nutr.* **43**, 68–71.

Iron in nutrition: use of stable isotopes

Susan J. FAIRWEATHER-TAIT
AFRC Food Research Institute, Colney Lane, Norwich NR4 7UA, UK.

Isotopic studies have long been recognized as the most versatile means of measuring absorption, metabolism and excretion of nutrients. The radioisotope ^{59}Fe was first used in animal studies[9] in investigations into the effect of anaemia on Fe absorption in dogs, and in humans[14], again in studies of anaemia. The application of radioisotopes in human studies (particularly pregnant women and infants), where the information obtained has no bearing on the medical management of the subject, is severely restricted because of the hazards associated with exposure to ionising radiation. More recently, however, there have been significant advances in methods employing stable isotopes of iron ([54]Fe, [57]Fe, [58]Fe) as biological tracers, involving neutron activation analysis (NAA) and mass spectrometry (MS).

In metabolic studies employing isotopes it is important that the body makes no distinction between naturally-occurring Fe and the Fe label. Isotope effects become a problem when the mass of an isotope is doubled or trebled (eg in the substitution of deuterium for hydrogen), but there is only a 3.4 per cent difference in weight between [58]Fe and [56]Fe. It proved impossible to demonstrate any biological effects of substituting [54]Fe for natural Fe in rats[15]. In dietary investigations it is essential that the isotope uniformly labels the endogenous Fe in the test meal. Several studies have shown that non-haem Fe in most foods is rapidly labelled by an extrinsic tag[10], thus supporting the common pool theory of Fe absorption[11].

In nutritional studies the same principles apply to stable isotopes as to radioisotopes, with the exception of quantity of label required. A greater quantity of stable isotope is required in absorption studies than radioisotope, the difference being several orders of magnitude; this mainly relates to the techniques by which the isotopes are measured. A further complication in the analysis of samples is the correction required to take into account the proportion of the isotope that is naturally-occurring and not derived from the enriched source. Clearly this is not generally necessary for radioisotopes, and the problem assumes increasing importance with isotopes of higher natural abundance. Furthermore, in absorption studies using the technique of faecal monitoring, the greater the apparent absorption, the smaller the relative standard deviation of the estimation of absorption. Unfortunately, Fe is usually poorly absorbed, especially non-haem Fe, which makes accurate sampling and precise determinations an absolute necessity.

Table. *Natural abundances of Fe isotopes and methods of measurement*

Isotope	*% Natural abundance*	*Method of measurement*
[54]Fe	5.82	Mass spectrometry
[56]Fe	91.66	Mass spectrometry
[57]Fe	2.19	Neutron activation analysis
[58]Fe	0.33	Mass spectrometry

Natural abundances of Fe isotopes and reported methods of measurements are shown in the Table. NAA has been successfully used to measure the [58]Fe content of biological samples for some time. When activated by thermal neutrons many radioactive nuclides are produced but with the high energy resolution of a Ge(Li) detector it is possible to separate the activity of the nuclide of interest from the other unwanted nuclides also formed. The procedure used by our group in collaboration with Imperial College Reactor Centre (Ascot, Berks.) is to irradiate samples and standards for two weeks in a 100 kW reactor at a flux of approximately

1.2×10^{16} neutrons/m^2/s. They are allowed to decay for 2 weeks to reduce the activity from short-lived radionuclides and analysed by gamma-ray spectrometry using a Ge(Li) semi-conductor detector (43 ml volume, resolution 1.81 KeV at 1332 KeV and 8.1 per cent counting efficiency) and a Nuclear Data (ND 6600) multi-channel analyser with dedicated computer and Fortran programs for spectral analysis. The capsules used to hold the sample take less than 1 g; sample size is therefore reduced by ashing dried material to remove organic matter, thereby increasing sample Fe concentration.

The detection limit for ^{58}Fe is 0.01 µg with a precision of about 1 per cent, depending on sample size, matrix and counting time (personal communication M. Minski, Imperial College Reactor Centre). It is also theoretically possible to measure ^{54}Fe by NAA, although the problems of separating and detecting the resultant ^{55}Fe free from all the other interferences are considerable. The other Fe isotopes cannot be measured by NAA as they do not form radionuclides.

Thermal ionisation mass spectrometry has long been accepted as the most precise method for isotope ratio measurements of inorganic elements, but when isotopic ratios of relatively volatile elements such as Fe are required, thermal ionization has been found to be particularly insensitive[6]. Considerable care is required in making proper corrections for isotopic fractionation effects. Nevertheless, isotope dilution thermal ionization[7] has been used to measure ^{58}Fe absorption in elderly men with acceptable precision and accuracy[17]. Unfortunately, thermal ionization mass spectrometers are not as readily available as conventional organic mass spectrometers which has led to the development of methods utilising electron ionization[13], gas chromatography[8] and fast atom bombardment mass spectrometry[2]. These methods are, in theory, applicable to all Fe isotopes, but are subject to a variety of inorganic interferences, eg from Cr with ^{54}Fe and Ni with ^{58}Fe measurement by FAB/MS. Such problems, however, can be overcome by chemical separations[16].

The application of stable isotopes to studies of Fe metabolism is still in its infancy. ^{58}Fe has been used successfully to determine the bioavailability of Fe in foods to human subjects, using the technique of faecal monitoring[3,12,18], and to study Fe utilization in pregnant women by measuring red blood cell incorporation[1]. In every experiment the advantage of using stable isotopes over radioisotopes, namely safety, must be weighed against the disadvantages (high cost, difficulty of measurement, poor analytical precision and high detection limits). A case can be argued for setting up hypotheses using animal models with radioisotopes, and then testing these in man using stable isotopes. For example, studies in our laboratory have shown clearly that in rats of similar Fe status the level of Fe in the diet given during the preceding 1–3 days dramatically influences Fe absorption from a subsequent test meal[4,5]. Preliminary studies in man, using ^{58}Fe (Fairweather-Tait, S.J. & Minski, M.J., unpublished results) lend support to our findings in the rat. When adult volunteers were given 50 mg Fe (as FeSO$_4$) or a placebo, followed 18 hours later by 10 mg Fe (as FeSO$_4$) labelled with 1.3 mg ^{58}Fe, there was a significant reduction ($P < 0.01$) in the proportion of Fe retained after the Fe-load (0.290 s.e.m. 0.051) compared with the placebo (0.354 s.e.m. 0.046), which suggests that previous Fe intake has a direct influence on subsequent Fe absorption from food or Fe preparations.

Another extremely useful application of stable isotopes is the assessment of Fe absorption in infants. A collaborative study is in progress with Dr Brian Wharton (Sorrento Maternity Hospital, Birmingham) in which Fe absorption in new-born infants from ^{58}Fe-labelled bovine lactoferrin, added to infant formulae, is being measured and compared with the well-absorbed Fe salt, ferrous sulphate.

The importance of stable isotopes in investigating Fe availability is beyond doubt. However, there is currently much discussion about the concept and measurement of availability. If it is defined as the proportion of the total in a foodstuff or diet that is digested, absorbed and metabolized by normal pathways, then the classical black box approach needs refining and improving. The suggestion that availability is assessed by measuring various indices of nutritional status requires further investigation, and should in fact be easily applied to Fe. Preliminary results from a study in non-anaemic men from the Gambia (in collaboration with the MRC Dunn Nutritional Laboratories) investigating Fe absorption from FeSO$_4$ or a typical Gambian meal, labelled with 690 µg ^{58}Fe, show a significant correlation between percentage absorption measured by faecal monitoring and [58]Fe-enrichment of the blood 10 days later. The fact that the relatively small dose of [58]Fe produced measurable enrichment by NAA (Imperial College Reactor Centre) in a small volume of blood is encouraging. Further studies are required to investigate the possibility of replacing the more time-consuming and potentially less accurate technique of faecal monitoring by measurements of [58]Fe-enrichment in red blood cells.

1 Dyer, N.C. & Brill, A.B. (1972): Use of the stable tracers [58]Fe and [50]Cr for the study of iron utilization in pregnant women. In *Nuclear activation techniques in the life sciences*, pp. 469–476. Vienna: International Atomic Energy Agency.
2 Eagles, J., Fairweather-Tait, S.J. & Self, R. (1985): Stable isotope ratio mass spectrometry for iron bioavailability studies. *Anal. Chem.* **57**, 469–471.
3 Fairweather-Tait, S.J., Minski, M.J. & Richardson, D.P. (1983): Iron absorption from a malted cocoa drink fortified with ferric orthophosphate using the stable isotope [58]Fe as an extrinsic label. *Br. J. Nutr.* **50**, 51–60.
4 Fairweather-Tait, S.J. & Wright, A.J.A. (1984): The influence of previous iron intake on the estimation of bioavailability of Fe from a test meal given to rats. *Br. J. Nutr.* **51**, 185–191.
5 Fairweather-Tait, S.J., Swindell, T.E. & Wright, A.J.A. (1985): Further studies in rats on the influence of previous Fe intake on the estimation of bioavailability of Fe. *Br. J. Nutr.* **54**, 79–86.
6 Fassett, J.D., Powell, L.J. & Moore, L.J. (1984): Determination of iron in serum and water by resonance ionization isotope dilution mass spectrometry. *Anal. Chem.* **56**, 2228.
7 Habfast, K. (1982): Application and measurement of metal isotopes. In *Stable isotopes*, ed H.-L. Schmidt, H. Förstel & K. Heinzinger, pp. 623–633. Amsterdam: Elsevier.
8 Hachey, D.L., Blais, J.-C. & Klein, P.D. (1980): High precision isotope ratio analysis of volatile metal chelates. *Anal. Chem.* **52**, 1131–1135.
9 Hahn, P.F., Bale, W.F., Laurence, E.O. & Whipple, G.H. (1939): Radioactive iron and its metabolism in anaemia. Its absorption, transportation and utilization. *J. exper. Med.* **69**, 739–753.
10 Hallberg, L. (1981): Bioavailability of dietary iron in man. *Ann. Rev. Nutr.* **1**, 123–147.
11 Hallberg, L. & Björn-Rasmussen, E. (1972): Determination of iron absorption from whole diet. A new two-pool model using two radioiron isotopes given as haem and non-haem iron. *Scand. J. Haematol.* **9**, 193–197.
12 Janghorbani, M. & Young, V.R. (1980): Use of stable isotopes to determine bioavailability of minerals in human diets using the method of fecal monitoring. *Am. J. Clin. Nutr.* **33**, 2021–2030.
13 Miller, D.D. & Van Campen, D. (1979): A method for the detection and assay of iron stable isotope tracers in blood serum. *Am. J. Clin. Nutr.* **32**, 2354–2361.
14 Ross, J.F. & Chapin, M.A. (1941): The selective absorption of radioactive iron by normal and non-deficient human subjects. *J. Clin. Invest.* **20**, 437.
15 Schricker, B.R., Gilbert, M.D., Miller, D.D. & Van Campen, D. (1982): Biological effects of substituting enriched [54]Fe for natural iron in rats. *J. Nutr.* **112**, 151–157.
16 Self, R., Fairweather-Tait, S.J. & Eagles, J. (1985): A double isotope labelling method for iron bioavailability studies using fast atom bombardment mass spectrometry. *Anal. Proc.* (In press).
17 Turnland, J.R., Michel, M.C., Keyes, W.R., King, J.C. & Margen, S. (1982): Use of enriched stable isotopes to determine zinc and iron absorption in elderly men. *Am. J. Clin. Nutr.* **35**, 1033–1040.
18 Young, V.R. & Janghorbani, M. (1981): Soy proteins in human diets in relation to bioavailability of iron and zinc: a brief overview. *Cereal Chem.* **58**, 12–18.

Assessment of iron status

J.D. COOK
University of Kansas Medical Center, 39th and Rainbow Boulevard, Kansas City, Kansas 66103, USA.

Epidemiologic evaluation of iron nutrition is the cornerstone of intervention programmes designed to combat iron-deficiency anaemia in developing countries. Estimates of iron status are required to determine the prevalence of nutritional anaemia, to confirm that iron lack is its prime cause, and to estimate the overall magnitude of the iron deficit. Iron status measurements are also needed to measure the improvement in iron nutrition resulting from intervention programmes initiated to alleviate iron-deficiency. Sensitive monitoring techniques are particularly important with iron fortification programmes where the improvement in iron status is modest in degree and occurs only after several months or years. Finally, the long-term monitoring of iron nutrition is important in detecting alterations that may occur independently of iron supplementation or fortification programmes. Recent surveys in industrialized countries indicate a pronounced reduction in the prevalence of iron-deficiency without obvious changes in the level or nature of dietary iron[6,8].

The usual approach for assessing iron nutrition is to determine the prevalence of anaemia using either the haematocrit or haemoglobin concentration. The limitations of surveys based solely on anaemia are now widely appreciated. There are many factors other than nutritional iron deficiency that impair haemoglobin production. Depending on the particular geographic region, chronic bacterial infection, haemoglobinopathies such as sickle cell anaemia and thalassaemia, malaria, and severe protein-energy malnutrition may all contribute to the prevalence of anaemia. Another major limitation of using only the haemoglobin or haematocrit level is the extensive overlap in values between normal and iron-deficient populations[7]. Even when the prevalence of iron-deficiency is high, the number of normal individuals with a haemoglobin value below the accepted cutoff level for anaemia may exceed the number with true iron deficiency anaemia[5]. Finally, haemoglobin measurements detect only severe iron-deficiency and provide no index of iron status in the non-anaemic segment of the population.

The assessment of iron nutrition has been greatly facilitated in recent years by the introduction of more specific and sensitive indices or iron status[1]. Three laboratory measurements that are particularly suited for use in the field are the transferrin saturation (serum iron expressed as a percentage of the transferrin concentration or total iron-binding capacity), erythrocyte protoporphyrin, and serum ferritin. The transferrin saturation and serum ferritin levels fall with iron deficiency whereas the erythrocyte protoporphyrin increases. The cutoff levels for these measurements are listed in the Table. The transferrin saturation and erythrocyte protoporphyrin detect iron-deficient erythropoiesis which is an impaired iron

Table. *Criteria of iron-deficiency in adult human subjects*

	Abnormal Value
Haemoglobin concentration (g/l)	
Men	< 130
Women	< 120
Serum iron* (µg/dl)	< 50
Transferrin saturation (per cent)	< 16
Erythrocyte protoporphyrin (µg/dl RBC)	> 70
Serum ferritin (µg/l)	< 12

*May be used in place of the transferrin saturation when total iron-binding capacity (TIBC) levels are not available.

supply to developing red cells[2]. These two measurements become abnormal prior to the development of overt anaemia and therefore detect a milder degree of iron-deficiency. This stage has been given a variety of other designations including iron-deficiency without anaemia, latent or masked iron-deficiency, impaired iron status, or iron-deficient erythropoiesis. Because this stage of iron lack is characterized by an inadequate supply of iron to the bone marrow and other body tissues, the term *iron-deficient transport* will be used. For its detection the transferrin saturation is more firmly established but has the disadvantages that the assay requires a larger blood sample than can be obtained by fingerstick and that the level in normal subjects is more labile than the erythrocyte protoporphyrin. In field studies the use of the latter measurement has been greatly facilitated by the haematofluorometer, an instrument capable of performing measurements on a single drop of blood. If lead poisoning, which also elevates the erythrocyte protoporphyrin, can be excluded in the sampled population and adequate methods for the long-term standardization of the instrument can be established, this assay offers distinct advantages over the transferrin saturation in field work.

Serum ferritin measurements during the past decade have provided an important new dimension to the assessment of iron status in population surveys. As an indirect measure of body iron stores, the serum ferritin provides information that could previously be obtained only by bone marrow examination[1]. Because iron-deficiency is the only disorder that depresses the serum ferritin, it is the most specific measure of iron deficiency. One drawback of serum ferritin measurements is that the detection of minute quantities of the circulating protein entail costly and complex immunoassays. However, the use of monoclonal antibodies has permitted the recent development of sensitive non-isotopic assays that will facilitate the use of serum ferritin measurements in developing countries. A major advantage of the serum ferritin is the small sample size required, permitting measurements on capillary blood. It has proved particularly valuable in assessing iron status in industrialized countries because it is the only parameter that detects changes in the iron-replete segment of the population. Furthermore, because the serum ferritin is invariably elevated when the anaemia is not caused by iron lack, it is useful for excluding disorders such as sickle cell anaemia, malaria, and chronic infection.

While there is little question about the importance of performing several iron measurements in tandem, there is little information about the most efficient method for analysing the data. Because of appreciable differences in sensitivity, the estimated prevalence of iron-deficiency varies considerably depending on whether it is defined as an abnormal serum ferritin, transferrin saturation, erythrocyte protoporphyrin, or haemoglobin. One approach to integrating this laboratory information is to employ multiple criteria. For example, the significance of an abnormal haemoglobin level has been enhanced by requiring that it be accompanied by an abnormality in at least two out of three iron parameters (transferrin saturation, erythrocyte protoporphyrin, or serum ferritin)[4,8]. Iron-replete individuals with an abnormal haemoglobin are largely excluded with this approach. The same approach can be used to refine the detection of iron-deficient transport by requiring abnormalities in at least two of the iron parameters. Reliable estimates of this milder form of iron lack are particularly important in regions where the prevalence of overt iron deficiency anaemia is low.

An alternative to relying solely on cutoff levels is to use these iron measurements to obtain a quantitative estimate of body iron in the population sample[3]. The serum ferritin level can be used to estimate iron stores in the iron-replete segment of the population, whereas in the severely iron-deficient segment the depression in haemoglobin can be used to estimate the iron deficit in circulating red cells. The transferrin saturation and/or erythrocyte protoporphyrin can be used to estimate body iron reserves between these two extremes. Application of this technique in an industrialized population has shown that body iron stores approach a Gaussian distribution when adult men or women are analysed separately[3]. This approach is feasible only with relatively large population surveys since it is still based on multiple cutoff levels. However, this analytical approach could be improved if it could be used to estimate body iron stores in small numbers of subjects.

It is important in a clinical setting to use a combination of laboratory measurements to estimate iron status in the individual patient. For example, in patients with iron-deficiency anaemia the haemoglobin level is used to monitor the repair of iron-deficiency following therapy. Similarly, the serum ferritin level is used during iron replacement to monitor the replenishment of storage iron. This same principle was applied epidemiologically to data collected in over 3000 adult subjects as part of the 2nd US National Health and Nutrition Examination Survey conducted between 1976 and 1980[8]. Values for haemoglobin, erythrocyte protoporphyrin, transferrin saturation, and serum ferritin were used to estimate iron stores in each sampled individual. When the frequency distributions were examined separately in adult men, pre-menopausal, and post-menopausal women, iron stores appeared normally distributed. Although average iron stores differed markedly in these three groups, the dispersion of the frequency distribution was very similar. Computer simulation studies indicate that this method will reduce the number of observations required to evaluate iron nutrition in population studies, permit on-going analysis of survey data, and facilitate evaluation of small, discrete segments of the population (Cook, J.D., Skikne, B.S., Lynch, S.R., unpublished observations).

1 Bothwell, T.H., Charlton, R.W., Cook, J.D. & Finch, C.A. (1979): *Iron metabolism in man*, pp. 1–576, Oxford: Blackwell Scientific.

2 Cook, J.D. (1982): Clinical evaluation of iron deficiency. *Semin. Hematol.* **19**, 6–18.

3 Cook, J.D. & Finch, C.A. (1979): Assessing iron status of a population. *Am. J. Clin. Nutr.* **32**, 2115–2119.

4 Cook, J.D., Finch, C.A. & Smith, N.J. (1976): Evaluation of the iron status of a population. *Blood* **48**, 449–455.

5 Cook, J.D., Alvarado, J., Gutniskey, A., Jamra, M., Labardino, J., Layrisse, M., Linares, J., Loria, A., Maspes, V., Restrepo, A., Reynafaije, C., Sanchez-Medal, L., Velaz, H. & Viteri, F. (1971): Nutritional deficiency and anemia in Latin America: a collaborative study. *Blood* **38**, 591–603.

6 Dallman, P.R., Yip, R. & Johnson, C. (1984): Prevalence and causes of anemia in the United States, 1976–1980. *Am. J. Clin. Nutr.* **39**, 437–445.

7 Garby, L., Irnell, L. & Werner, I. (1969): Iron deficiency in women of fertile age in a Swedish community. III. Estimation of prevalence based on response to iron supplementation. *Acta Med. Scand.* **185**, 113–117.

8 Pilch, S.M. & Senti, F.R. ed (1984): *Assessment of the iron nutritional status of the US population based on data collected in the Second National Health and Nutrition Examination Survey, 1976–1980*, pp. 1–66, Bethesda MD: Life Sciences Research Office, Federation of American Societies for Experimental Biology.

Studies on iron fortification

T.H. BOTHWELL

MRC Iron and Red Cell Metabolism Unit, Department of Medicine, University of the Witwatersrand Medical School, 7 York Road, Parktown 2193, Johannesburg, South Africa.

There are two ways in which nutritional iron-deficiency can be alleviated. *Supplementation* with medicinal iron is indicated in situations such as pregnancy, where rapid changes are required, while *fortification* of some dietary constituent with small quantities of iron is aimed at improving iron nutrition on a more long-term basis. From a theoretical standpoint fortification represents an attractive option. It is an approach which can be applied to large population groups at low cost, and it has the advantage that the identification and cooperation of actually or potentially deficient individuals is not a prerequisite as it is with supplementation[1,11].

Initial iron nutrition. In industrialized countries, iron nutrition is closely correlated with the total caloric intake, since the iron content in mixed Western diets is moderately constant, being about 6 mg/4.19 MJ (1000 kcal)[2]. In developing countries the situation is more complex, since more than one factor may be involved in the pathogenesis of the iron-deficiency. The single most important determinant is the low bioavailability in major staple foodstuffs, such as cereals and legumes[12]. For such iron to be adequately absorbed, enhancers of non-haem iron absorption, such as meat and ascorbic acid, must be present in the diet[4] but these are eaten only irregularly and in small quantities by many populations. Insofar as iron fortification is concerned these points have major relevance, since there is good evidence that fortification iron added to a diet of low bioavailability is equally poorly absorbed[12]. The other important cause of iron-deficiency in developing countries is hookworm infestation and it is important to establish its prevalence and the extent of blood losses caused by it before embarking on a fortification programme.

Choice of an iron compound. There are a number of iron compounds that have been used for fortification but there is no single one that is suitable for universal application. The reason is simple. Bioavailable sources of iron form complexes with food constituents and catalyse oxidative reactions. As a result, the colour and flavour of the vehicle may be changed and unpleasant odours may be produced. A number of *soluble iron compounds* are in current use. Ferrous sulphate, which is the cheapest, is widely used in bread and bakery products, since they are only stored for short periods[11]. Ferrous salts are also added to infant formulas. Elemental iron powders are widely used both in Europe and the USA for the fortification of bread and flour. Former problems relating to the absorbability of such compounds have been largely overcome by reduction in their particle size and surface area. For example, if the particle size of reduced iron is sufficiently small, it is absorbed as well as the iron in ferrous sulphate when baked into bread rolls[6]. *Chelated iron complexes* have also been tested in pilot studies. In this context, NaFeEDTA has been shown to be stable and to be less susceptible to the inhibitory ligands present in cereal based diets[13,14]. It is, however, relatively expensive. Another approach has been the use of relatively inert forms of iron, such as iron orthophosphate together with an enhancer of iron absorption, such as ascorbic acid[16]. Success in the fortification of common salt has been claimed using a modification of this approach in which a stabilizing agent was added to reduce the reactivity of the iron and an acidifying agent to enhance the availability of the iron at the time of ingestion[15,20].

Choice of vehicle. Major considerations include the pattern of consumption of the vehicle and the technical feasibility of fortifying it satisfactorily. Ideally it should be consumed by a high proportion of the population and there should be only small variations in individual consumption. From a technical standpoint it should be manufactured at relatively few production centres, it should have a limited storage time and it should lend itself to the unobtrusive addition of the fortificant at low cost[7]. The most widely fortified food items in Western countries are cereals such as flour. Most infant cereals and milk powders are also fortified with various forms of iron and there is good evidence that the iron in them is well absorbed, provided adequate amounts of ascorbic acid are also present[8].

In many developing countries the problems are more complex for several reasons. Food production is often decentralized, staple foodstuffs may not lend themselves easily to fortification and the intrinsic bioavailability of the iron in the diet may be low. Salt and sugar have both been explored as possible vehicles. However, bioavailable forms of iron tend to cause unacceptable colour changes in salt, especially when it is relatively unrefined and has a high moisture content. Such colour changes are even more pronounced when a promoter of iron absorption, such as ascorbic acid, is also present[16]. Success has, however, recently been reported using a combination of ferric orthophosphate and sodium acid sulphate[15]. Only slight discoloration was noted after prolonged storage and the iron proved bioavailable in a field trial[20]. Sugar has also been investigated as a vehicle. Available forms of iron darken the sugar and the iron also tends to segregate downwards. Furthermore, the fortification iron forms black complexes with tannins when the sugar is added to tea[9]. These problems can be overcome, in part at least, if the stable chelate NaFeEDTA is used as the fortificant[19]. It has been shown to be better absorbed than ferrous sulphate when added to a variety of meals[13,14] and sugar fortified with NaFeEDTA has been successfully used in an extensive field study[18].

A number of other vehicles may lend themselves to certain targetted programmes directed at certain groups within larger populations. These include condiments, such as fish sauce or paste, curry powders, monosodium glutamate and cool drinks. The fact that some of these vehicles are coloured and have strong tastes makes them particularly suitable for iron fortification. Perhaps the most novel of current approaches is one in which dried animal haemoglobin is being baked into chocolate biscuits in a school lunch programme involving 750 000 children in Chile[17].

Implementation of a fortification programme. It is important to know whether the prevalence of iron-deficiency is widespread or regional. If it is limited to certain segments of the population then a supplementation programme or some form of targetted fortification is indicated. If, however, a national programme is required them some dietary constituent must be identified that is centrally processed. When this is not feasible, several regional programmes may be required, with the vehicles tailored to the local diets. The presence in the diets of possible inhibitors and promoters of iron absorption must also be documented. It is also desirable to measure the absorption of iron from typical diets using an extrinsic radioiron label[11]. In this way the relative bioavailability of dietary iron can be assessed and hence the level of iron fortification that will be required. Having decided on the vehicle and the iron fortificant, it is essential to carry out storage tests, and to establish consumer acceptability, including the appearance and taste of typical meals[11]. If all the preliminary tests are satisfactory then some form of trial should if possible be done in order to confirm the efficacy of the iron fortification under field conditions.

The efficacy and safety of iron fortification. The results of several field trials indicate that current strategies of iron fortification can improve iron nutrition[7]. At a national level particularly persuasive evidence has been produced in Sweden, where a striking drop in the incidence of iron-deficiency in women was noted over a 10-year period during which time the level of fortification of flour with iron has been increased to 30 mg/lb[10]. However, it was also clear that the iron fortification was not the only factor responsible for the improvement. Over the same period there was an increase in the consumption of iron tablets and ascorbic acid tablets and in the use of the contraceptive pill.

A final consideration with regard to any fortification programme is the question of its safety. Two groups are particularly at risk of accumulating excessive amounts of iron, namely males who are homozygous for the HLA-linked mutant gene responsible for the iron storage disease, idiopathic haemochromatosis[5], and patients with chronic refractory anaemias, the most important of which is thalassaemia major[3]. Since the HLA-linked iron-loading gene occurs in the heterozygous state in about 10 per cent of some Caucasian populations, it is essential that careful monitoring of storage iron concentrations continues in countries such as Sweden where iron fortification levels are high. This can be done by serial measurements of the serum ferritin, since these provide a moderately accurate reflection of the size of the body iron stores.

1 Baker, S.J. & De Maeyer, E.M. (1979): Nutritional anemia: its understanding and control with special reference to the work of the World Health Organization. *Am. J. Clin. Nutr.* **32**, 368–417.

2 Beaton, G.H. (1974): The epidemiology of iron deficiency. In *Iron in biochemistry and medicine*, ed A. Jacobs & M. Worwood, pp. 477–528. New York: Academic Press.

3 Bothwell, T.H. & Charlton, R.W. (1982): A general approach to the problems of iron deficiency and iron overload in the population at large. *Sem. Hematol.* **19**, 54–67.

4 Bothwell, T.H., Charlton, R.W., Cook, J.D. & Finch, C.A. (1979): *Iron metabolism in man*, pp. 7–43. Oxford: Blackwell Scientific Publications.

5 Bothwell, T.H., Charlton, R.W. & Motulsky, A.G. (1983): Idiopathic hemochromatosis. In *The metabolic basis of inherited disease*, ed J.B. Stanbury, J.B. Wyngaarden, D.S. Frederickson, J.L. Goldstein & M.S. Brown, pp. 1269–1298. New York: McGraw-Hill.

6 Cook, J.D., Minnich, V., Moore, C.V., Rasmussen, A., Bradley, W.B. & Finch, C.A. (1973): Absorption of fortification iron in bread. *Am. J. Clin. Nutr.* **26**, 861–872.

7 Cook, J.D. & Reuser, M.E. (1983): Iron fortification: an update. *Am. J. Clin. Nutr.* **38**, 648–659.

8 Derman, D.P., Bothwell, T.H., MacPhail, A.P., Torrance, J.D., Bezwoda, W.R., Charlton, R.W. & Mayet, F.G.H. (1980): Importance of ascorbic acid in the absorption of iron from infant foods. *Scand, J. Haematol.* **25**, 193–201.

9 Disler, P.B., Lynch, S.R., Charlton, R.W., Torrance, J.D. & Bothwell, T.H. (1975): The effect of tea on iron absorption. *Gut* **16**, 193–200.

10 Hallberg, L. (1982): Iron nutrition and food iron fortification. *Sem. Hematol.* **19**, 31–41.

11 INACG (International Nutritional Anemia Consultative Group) (1977): *Guidelines for the eradication of iron deficiency anemia*, pp. 1-29. New York, NY: The nutritional Foundation.

12 INACG (International Nutritional Anemia Consultative Group) (1982): *Iron absorption from cereals and legumes*, pp. 1–14. New York, NY: The Nutrition Foundation.

13 Layrisse, M. & Martinez-Torres, C. (1977): Fe(111)-EDTA complex as iron fortification. *Am. J. Clin. Nutr.* **30**, 1166–1174.

14 MacPhail, A.P., Bothwell, T.H., Torrance, J.D., Derman, D.P., Bezwoda, W.R., Charlton, R.W. & Mayet, F. (1981): Factors affecting the absorption of iron from Fe(111)EDTA. *Br. J. Nutr.* **45**, 215–227.

15 Nadiger, H.A., Krishnamachari, K.A.V.R., Nadamuni, N., Rao, B.S.N. & Strikantia, S.G. (1980): The use of common salt (sodium chloride) fortified with iron to control anaemia: results in a preliminary study. *Br. J. Nutr.* **43**, 45.

16 Sayers, M.H., Lynch, S.R., Charlton, R.W., Bothwell, T.H., Walker, R.B. & Mayet, F. (1974): The fortification of common salt with ascorbic acid and iron. *Br. J. Haematol.* **28**, 483–495.

17 Stekel, A. (1981): Fortification from the laboratory to a national program. Two Chilean experiences. In *Proc. Annual Mtg Int. Nutr. Anemia Consultative Gp. (INACG)*. New York, NY: The Nutrition Foundation, Section VIII.

18 Viteri, F.E., Alvarez, E., Bulux, J., Pineda, O. & Batres, R. (1981): Iron fortification in developing countries. In *Nutrition in health and disease and international development*, ed A.E. Harper & G.K. Davis, pp. 345–354. New York: Alan R. Liss.

19 Viteri, F.E., Garcia-Ibanez, R. & Torun, B. (1978): NaFeEDTA as an iron fortification compound in Central America. Absorption studies. *Am. J. Clin. Nutr.* **31**, 961–971.

20 Working group on fortification of salt with iron. (1982): Use of common salt fortified with iron in the control and prevention of anemia: a collaborative study. *Am. J. Clin. Nutr.* **35**, 1442–1451.

Interactions involving inorganic nutrients

C.F. MILLS
Biochemistry Division, Rowett Research Institute, Bucksburn, Aberdeen AB2 9SB, UK.

The absorption, metabolism and physiological effects of many of the inorganic elements of Groups 2 to 6 of the Periodic Table are often modified by interactions involving other dietary constituents or their metabolites. It is now recognised that many such interactions influence requirements for the essential elements as well as modifying response to potentially toxic elements.

Some interactions, like those in which clinical expression of the effects of zinc deficiency can be governed by changes in protein or energy supply modifying the tissue redistribution of absorbed Zn, have complex metabolic origins that, in relation to their nutritional significance, have been very inadequately investigated. Much greater attention has been focused on interactions whose existence appears predictable from extrapolation of growing knowledge of the likely physicochemical behaviour of inorganic elements, when subjected to environments within the gut or tissues, which will promote either mutual precipitation or competition during incorporation into carriers or the functional sites of enzymes.

The literature describing such interactions is now substantial (for typical reviews see[7,9]). However, when viewed from the standpoint of those requiring guidance with dietary formulation much of it has important limitations. Firstly, many of the studies described are only of academic interest in that the experimentally imposed imbalances between antagonist and agonist exceed, often very substantially, those likely to be encountered in diets. While these data have produced biochemical evidence of the potential for competition between structurally similar inorganic ions[7], their nutritional relevance is frequently questionable. Of equal importance is the fact that much greater attention has been given to exploring the full panoply of possible interactions than to defining the circumstances under which the potency of a potential antagonist may change. It is now clear that potency can be influenced both by the form in which antagonist and agonist are present in the diet or external environment and by changes in such forms during digestion.

Table. *Dietary and metabolic interactions modifying susceptibility to inorganic element deficiency.* + *or* ++, *increased* dietary concentrations of component exacerbate biochemical or pathological manifestations of syndrome. −, low concentrations of component exacerbate. Observations awaiting confirmation are indicated in parentheses ( ).

Deficiency syndrome	Inorganic dietary component provoking or exacerbating syndrome
Co	$++CaCO_3$
Cu	$+Mo$, $+S$, $+Fe$, $+Cd$, $+Zn$, $+Ag$
I	$+Co$, $(+As)$, $(+F)$, goitrogens
Fe	$++PO_4^{3-}$, $+Cu$, $+Zn$, $+Cd$
	$-Cu$
Mn	$+Ca$, $+P_4^{3-}$
Mg	$++K$
Mo	$++W$
P	$++Fe+$
Se	$+S$ (in analogous chemical species), $+Cu$, $+Ag$
Zn	$++Ca$, $+Cu$, $+P$ (as phytate)

Rather than superficially reviewing the entire field of known dietary interactions influencing the metabolism of inorganic elements (briefly summarized in Table) I will concentrate here on two interactions for which there is abundant evidence of nutritional relevance, ie the apparently variable antagonistic effect of dietary phytate on the utilization of Zn by man and other non-ruminants and the, again variable, activity of molybdenum as an antagonist involved in the aetiology of copper-deficiency. Changes in the chemical form of the antagonist have an important bearing on its biopotency which must be taken into account when predicting its effects upon inorganic nutrient availability.

Determinants of the potency of phytate as a Zn antagonist. It is widely accepted in commercial agricultural practice that the Zn requirements of non-ruminant animals are increased substantially when diets based on cereals and soya products, rich in phytate are offered. Consistent indications of the importance of phytic acid as an inhibitor of Zn absorption have also been obtained in an extensive series of studies with rats. However, recent studies also indicate, in contrast to earlier proposals[14], that the potency of phytate as a Zn inhibitor is not constant and thus estimation of the phytate/Zn ratio of a food or diet is not a reliable criterion of the concentration of available Zn[12].

The inadequately defined effect of variables influencing phytate biopotency is clearly hindering attempts to assess its significance in the Zn nutrition of man. Such variables may well account for much of the controversy on the influence of cereal fibre-rich fractions of diets on Zn availability (for review see[5]), and have hindered the development of rational decisions on the need to monitor and, if necessary, to fortify with Zn, novel foods indigenously rich in phytate.

From evidence that phytate potency is directly relatable to dietary calcium[12] and suspicions that the less consistent antagonistic effect of phytate in the diet of man may be related to the normally lower Ca content of his diet than that of other species, it has been suggested that a more satisfactory prediction of the available Zn status of foods might be achieved by estimation of the molar concentration ratio $\dfrac{[\text{Ca}]\,[\text{Phy}]}{[\text{Zn}]}$ (mol/kg dietary D.M.)[11]. Evidence that rat growth is inhibited if this ratio exceeds a critical threshold of approximately 3 is convincing. The validity of this ratio for predicting Zn availability to man is being assessed. Indications from use of the more sensitive and rigorous criterion of the development of a negative Zn balance in man are that a ratio exceeding 0.3 may reduce the efficacy of Zn absorption (N.T. Davies & C.F. Mills, unpublished data).

However, before euphorically assuming that adoption of such a criterion may solve the problem, it is important to consider whether the synergistic influence of Ca itself is likely to bear a constant relationship to its dietary concentration, what factors may modify its effects, and how these may relate in significance to other relevant variables.

The effectiveness with which phytate inhibits Zn utilization is governed by events influencing the intraluminal stability of the phytate molecule against hydrolysis, by the extent to which hydrolytic attack proceeds beyond penta- or tetra-phosphorylated inositols and by both the timing and extent to which phytate and its partial degradation products have the opportunity to react with Ca and/or Zn.

The conditions most strongly potentiating the action of phytate as an antagonist of Zn absorption are assumed to be those which favour the reaction of ionic Ca^{2+} with free phytate to form an insoluble (Ca phytate) complex within which Zn is occluded[17]. Whether ingestion of preformed (Ca phytate) has a similar effect is controversial. Thus, while there is evidence that utilization of the *intrinsic* Zn|or Ca or Mg-precipitated, phytate-rich, isolates of soya protein is poor[4], other results suggest that ingested (Ca phytate) has remarkably little effect on the absorption of *extrinsic* Zn^{2+} [12]. That the basis for the inhibition of Zn absorption may not rest *per se* upon the formation of a (Zn phytate) complex but, rather, upon the physical occlusion of such a product within the matrix of an insoluble (Ca phytate) precipitate appears possible. Thus there is evidence that the Zn of (Zn_3 phytate) or (Zn_6 phytate) is readily utilized in situations in which dietary Ca exceeds requirements but no free phytate is present in the diet to permit formation of a (Ca phytate) precipitate[12].

If the above view of events is correct the apparently variable potency of phytate as a Zn inhibitor is likely to depend both upon factors modifying the form and intraluminal yield of precipitate and upon equilibria involving phytate and competing ligands which govern the yield of co-precipitable Zn.

Among the lower inositol polyphosphates produced by the stepwise hydrolysis of phytate by phytases of foods, the gut mucosa and gut microorganisms, precipitability by Ca^{2+} at near-neutral pH is inversely proportional to the remaining extent of phosphate substitution. Classical (Fe-sequestration) methods for 'phytate' analysis are insufficiently specific to distinguish between 'true' phytate (inositol hexaphosphate) and its less phosphorylated analogues[13]. Thus the recent introduction of highly specific ^{31}P-NMR techniques capable of distinguishing the individual products of phytate hydrolysis[6] is particularly welcome in the context of attempts to define the influence of ambient concentrations of Ca^{2+}, Mg^{2+} and other metals on the kinetics of phytate hydrolysis and on the yield of precipitable inositol polyphosphates in the small intestine. Results of an exploratory appraisal of the validity of this technique appear encouraging[18].

The value of attempts to define the effects of phytate on the availability of Zn from human diets may well have been improved by the inclusion in prediction equations of terms which allow for the potentiating effect of Ca. However it should not escape notice that this *ad hoc* approach takes account neither of the possibly similar potentiating effect of dietary Mg nor of the enhancing effect of dietary protein on Zn utilization from phytate-rich diets so clearly demonstrated by Sandström *et al.*[16].

For the present, such considerations merely indicate the importance of defining all likely relevant dietary variables in studies intended to clarify whether phytate limits Zn utilization by man. They also serve to caution against undue optimism that the effects of 'phytate' can be reliably predicted from data obtained with inadequately specific analytical methods and with remarkably superficial understanding of the factors that govern its capacity to limit the availability, not only of Zn, but of copper, manganese and iron[2].

Interactions involving copper, molybdenum and sulphur. In many areas of the world the development of copper-deficiency in ruminants can be related to the presence of elevated concentrations of molybdenum in their feed. Recent studies make it clear that expression of the adverse effects of Mo upon Cu utilization is contingent upon reactions within the gastrointestinal tract or occasionally in body tissues which yield reactive sulphide (S^{2-}) or hydrosulphide (HS^-) ions. Susceptibility to interactions involving Mo is thus greatest in ruminants in which S^{2-} generation is a normal feature of the intermediary metabolism of ingested sulphate and S-amino acids by rumen microorganisms. From a scientifically turbulent history of conflicting ideas on the mechanisms of this interaction, the view is now emerging that its basis lies in the modifying influence of dietary Mo upon the persistence within the g.i. tract of reactive species of S which, by virtue of their strong affinity for Cu, convert the latter into insoluble, unavailable forms.

The principal events in this process are summarized in the Figure compiled principally from published (eg[10]) and unpublished data from Rowett Institute studies. It includes data on the effects of Mo on the acid-labile S^{2-} 'profile' of g.i. tract contents (J.K. Chesters & M. Will, unpublished) and its relationship to the profile of physiologically available Cu determined by a rat bioassay technique[15].

The establishment of rumination is accompanied by a marked increase in rumen S^{2-} generation and by a concurrent decline in the physiological availability of Cu in rumen digesta. Even when dietary Mo is low, the molar excess of S^{2-} over Cu can exceed 100. Thus it must be assumed that the small component (usually 5 to 10 per cent) of dietary Cu remaining available under these conditions does so because of the existence on an as yet uncharacterized form of dietary Cu containing the element in a 'protected' core (as for example in the plant Cu protein, plastocyanin) inaccessible to reaction with S^{2-} at this stage. Because of the rapidity of their absorption and subsequent reoxidation in the reticulo-rumen, little S^{2-} or HS^- is normally detectable postruminally. Thus, within the duodenum and ileum, the proteolytic release of previously protected Cu proceeds uninhibited by reaction with sulphide to yield

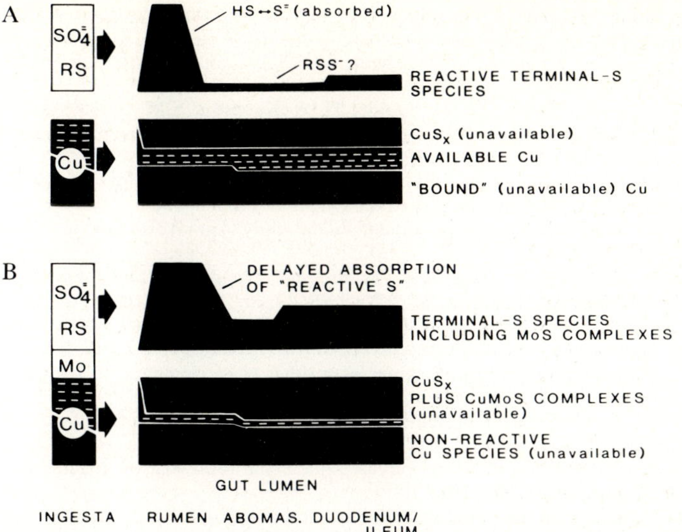

Fig. *Reactive sulphide and physiologically available copper profiles in the g.i. tract of ruminants offered low-molybdenum (A) or high-molybdenum diets (B).* Changes in available Cu concentration along the tract are indicated ▨. Note, in B, enhanced post-ruminal persistance of reactive S^{2-} species and additional post-ruminal decrease in available Cu.

physiologically available Cu which rises in concentration at these sites of maximal Cu absorption.

The principal changes noted when Mo is present in the diet at concentrations within the range 5 to 50 mg/kg D.M. are:- (1) a prolonged biological half life of rumen S^{2-}, (2) persistence of acid-labile (Cu-reactive) S species distal to the rumen, and (3) a marked decrease in the physiologically available Cu content of virtually all digesta fractions within which Mo is also sequestered.

There is strong presumptive evidence that Cu, Mo and S are all associated with the increased proportion of digesta Cu that becomes unavailable. However the intractability of the insoluble fractions formed has so far precluded chemical characterisation. Studies with the soluble phase of rumen contents indicate that thio- and oxythiomolybdate species are initially formed[1,3], but whether these react directly within the rumen to form insoluble Cu-derivatives, or form polymeric derivatives stable at rumen pH, but degrading under the more acid conditions of the abomasum and proximal duodenum, to yield Cu-reactive S^{2-} species is not yet known. The latter appears most likely since the most significant decreases in Cu availability occur within the duodenum and ileum.

Essentially, this view of events relegates Mo to a role in which, by extending the profile of Cu reactive sulphide species into regions of the gut at which Cu is most effectively released and absorbed, it is merely potentiating the inhibitory action of sulphur on Cu. If so, this property could be shared by elements such as Fe which, by forming sulphides stable at rumen pH, could restrict removal of free S^{2-} by absorption. Such events may well account for the additional inhibitory effect of high dietary Fe on Cu absorption by ruminants[8].

Better understanding of such processes is essential before the action of Mo and other metals on Cu availability can be reliably predicted. Currently, we are unable to explain why 3 to 4-fold differences in the inhibitory potency of Mo can exist between different diets. The answer may well lie in differences in the rates of rumenal S^{2-} generation and their effect on the yield of reactive Mo/S species clearly involved, at least as intermediates, in the processes inhibiting Cu utilization.

1 Bray, A.C., Suttle, N.F. & Field, A.C. (1982): The formation of tri- and tetra-thiomolybdates in continuous culture of rumen micro-organisms and their adsorption onto 'fibre'. *Proc. Nutr. Soc.* **41**, 67A.

2 Davies, N.T. & Nightingale, R. (1975): The effects of phytate on intestinal absorption and secretion of zinc, and whole-body retention of Zn, copper, iron and manganese in rats. *Br. J. Nutr.* **34**, 243–258.

3 El-Gallad, T.T.T., Mills, C.F., Bremner, I. & Summers, R. (1983): Thiomolybdates in rumen contents and rumen cultures. *J. Inorg. Biochem.* **18**, 323–331.

4 Forbes, R.M., Erdman, J.W., Parker, H.M., Kondo, H. & Ketelson, S.M. (1983): Bioavailability of zinc in congulated Soy protein (Tofu) to rats and effect of dietary calcium at a constant phytate:zinc ratio. *J. Nutr.* **113**, 205–210.

5 Frølich, W. (1984): Bioavailability of minerals from unrefined cereal products. PhD Thesis, University of Lund.

6 Frølich, W. & Drakenberg, T. (1984): Unpublished data cited by Frølich, 1984.

7 Hill, C.H. & Matrone, G. (1970): Chemical parameters in the study of in vivo and in vitro interactions of transition elements. *Fedn. Proc.* **29**, 1474–1481.

8 Humphries, W.R., Phillippo, M., Young, B.W. & Bremner, I. (1983): The influence of dietary iron and molybdenum on copper metabolism in calves. *Br. J. Nutr.* **49**, 77–86.

9 Kirchgessner, M., Schwarz, F.J. & Schnegg, A. (1982): Interactions of essential metals in human physiology. In *Clinical, biochemical and nutritional aspects of the trace elements*, ed A.S. Prasad, pp. 477–512, New York: Liss.

10 Mills, C.F. (1980): Metabolic interactions of copper with other trace elements. In *Biological roles of copper* ed D. Evered & G. Lawrenson, pp. 49–69. Amsterdam: Excerpta Medica.

11 Mills, C.F., Davies, N.T., Quarterman, J. & Aggett, P.J. (1985): Metal interactions in the aetiology of trace element deficiency and toxicity. *Nutr. Res. Suppl.* **1**, 471–473.

12 Morris, E.R. & Ellis, R. (1980): Effect of dietary phytate/zinc molar ratio on growth and bone zinc response of rats fed semi-purified diets. *J. Nutr.* **110**, 1037–1045.

13 Oberleas, D. (1971): The determination of phytate and inositol phosphates. *Meth. Biochem. Anal.* **20**, 87–101.

14 Oberleas, D. (1975): Factors influencing mineral availability. In *Proc. W. Hemisphere Nutr. Congr.* ed P.L. White & N. Selvey, pp. 156–161. Acton, Mass: Publishing Sciences Group.

15 Price, J. & Chesters, J.K. (1985): A new bioassay for assessment of copper availability and its application in a study of the effect of molybdenum on the distribution of available Cu in ruminant digesta. *Br. J. Nutr.* **53**, 323–336.

16 Sandström, B., Arvidson, B., Cederblad, A. & Bjorn-Rasmussen, E. (1980): Zinc absorption from composite meals. 1. The significance of wheat extraction rate, zinc, calcium and protein content in meals based on bread. *Am. J. Clin. Nutr.* **33**, 739–745.

17 Wise, A.H. (1983): Dietary factors determining the biological activities of phytate. *Nutr. Abstr. Rev.* **53**, 791–806.

18 Wise, A., Richards, C.P. & Trimble, M.L. (1983): Phytate hydrolysis in rat gastrointestinal tracts, as observed by ^{31}P Fourier transform nuclear magnetic resonance spectroscopy. *Appl. Environ. Microbiol.* **45**, 313–314.

Enriched stable isotopes of minerals and trace elements in nutritional research: a workshop report

M.J. JACKSON (Organizer)
Department of Medicine, University of Liverpool, PO Box 147, Liverpool L69 3BQ, UK.

This workshop was attended by approximately 50 delegates who considered the current state of research using these new techniques. Despite a large amount of interest in this area, there have been surprisingly few research groups utilizing these procedures. It was reported that a literature search revealed only 99 relevant publications, of which a surprisingly large number (18) have been reviews. The technique has been most widely used to study gastrointestinal absorption and blood dynamics of zinc, copper, iron, and selenium. Considerable discussion ensued on the appropriate circumstances in which radioactive or stable isotopes should be used, although it appears that in certain countries (eg USA) stable isotope studies have now virtually replaced those using radioactive isotopes because of the ethical problems associated with the use of radioactive materials in man.

Much of the discussion time was spent in examining the relative merits of the various different analytical techniques currently in use. There has been a move away from neutron activation analysis, which was almost exclusively used in early studies. Current interest is in the choice between different mass spectrometric techniques, each of which has advantages and disadvantages. Thermal ionization mass spectrometry offers excellent precision of analysis, but requires extensive clean-up prior to analysis. Some workers are using fast atom bombardment mass spectrometry which is more widely available than the other techniques, but currently suffers from a lack of precision. It was generally felt that inductively coupled plasma mass spectrometry is likely to become the method of choice for these analyses in future, but with present sampling systems it requires large volumes of sample to achieve suitable precision.

XI: Diet and disease

Nutrition and cardiovascular disease

Nutritional factors in carcinogenesis

NUTRITION AND CARDIOVASCULAR DISEASE

International trends in cardiovascular diseases in relation to dietary fat intake: inter-population studies

M.L. WAHLQVIST

Department of Human Nutrition, Deakin University, Geelong, Victoria 3217 Australia.

What is often not understood outside the scientific community is how important different lines of evidence are in arriving ultimately at a view about the aetiology and pathogenesis of a disease. This is nowhere more in evidence than in regard to coronary heart disease. Evidence comes from animal and human studies, epidemiological studies of various kinds and clinical studies, studies which are unifactorial or multifactorial in design and so on.

Furthermore, important as it is to resolve questions about the development of a particular disease, sight must not be lost of total mortality. That life expectancies are now increasing in developed countries is quite clear[7,29] (Table 1 and 2).

Nutritional pathways to coronary heart disease. The routes through which food intake might operate ultimately on the heart are several: (1) obesity (2) serum lipids (3) blood pressure[19] (4) platelet aggregation[8] (5) coagulation profiles (6) coronary vascular reactivity (7) cardiac membrane stability[3,17] and (8) cardiac substrate metabolism[26].

Thus, although much attention is correctly focused on the serum cholesterol as a particularly consequential pathway, other pathways should not be neglected. Moreover, some of the differences seen when a unifactorial approach is taken to inter-population studies, may be attributable to differences in the ways in which these different pathways are operative[4,25].

Table 1. *Life expectancy at birth*[7]

	m	f		m	f
Japan	74.2	79.2	Greece	71.0	75.0
Ireland	73.9	79.4	Australia	71.0	78.1
Netherlands	72.7	79.3	U.S.A.	70.8	78.2
Norway	72.5	79.2	New Zealand	70.4	76.6
Sweden	72.1	78.1	U.K.	70.4	76.7

Table 2. *Annual change (%) of the mortality from all causes and cardiovascular diseases, by sex, from 1968 to 1977*[29]. (Calculated from the average of the slopes of linear regressions for the six quinquennial age groups 40 to 69 years).

Country	All causes		Cardiovascular diseases		Cardiovascular diseases (excluding cerebrovascular disease)		Cerebrovascular disease		Ischaemic heart disease	
	m	f	m	f	m	f	m	f	m	f
Canada	−0.4	−0.9	−1.5	−1.8	−1.5	−1.7	−1.9	−2.2	−1.6	−0.9
United States of America	−2.2	−2.2	−3.0	−3.7	−2.8	−3.5	−4.5	−4.2	−3.0	−3.6
Japan	−2.9	−4.0	−3.5	−4.9	−1.5	−4.1	−4.8	−5.2	−2.6	−4.7
Austria	−1.2	−2.1	−0.8	−2.5	−0.6	−2.3	−1.3	−3.0	+0.6	+0.3
Belgium	−1.6	−1.4	−2.2	−2.4	−2.2	−2.6	−2.2	−2.3	−1.7	−1.1
Bulgaria	−1.7	−0.4	+3.7	−0.1	+4.0	−0.3	+3.3	+0.5	+5.6	+2.5
Czechoslovakia	+0.4	−0.7	+0.6	−0.4	−0.8	−1.8	+3.9	+3.0	+0.6	0.0
Denmark	0.0	−0.8	+1.0	−0.5	+1.1	−1.1	+0.6	+1.5	−1.7	+0.7
Finland	−2.1	−3.3	−2.3	−4.9	−2.1	−4.1	−3.3	−6.1	−1.8	−1.6
France	−0.7	−1.9	−1.1	−2.9	−0.5	−2.7	−2.8	−3.2	+1.1	+1.4
Germany, Federal Republic of	−0.8	−1.8	−1.1	−2.5	−0.9	−2.6	−2.2	−2.1	+0.4	+0.5
Hungary	+1.4	+0.8	−1.4	0.0	+1.0	−0.5	+3.6	+1.4	+2.6	+2.0
Ireland	−0.2	−1.5	+0.7	−2.8	+1.1	−3.2	−1.3	−2.2	+2.6	−0.4
Italy	−1.5	−2.6	−2.0	−4.3	−2.1	−5.0	−2.2	−2.2	−0.1	−2.0
Netherlands	−1.0	−1.9	−1.3	−1.7	−1.3	−1.7	−1.3	−1.8	−0.9	+0.8
Norway	−1.0	−1.6	−1.3	−2.6	−1.0	−1.9	−3.3	−5.1	−1.1	−0.3
Poland	+1.6	−1.3	+3.4	−0.4	+1.9	−1.5	+6.0	+4.2	+6.4	+5.2
Romania	0.0	−1.1	+1.0	−1.0	+1.4	−0.8	0.0	−1.3	+4.3	+3.8
Sweden	+0.5	−1.4	+0.5	−1.7	+0.6	−2.4	−0.2	−0.4	+2.0	+1.8
Switzerland	−1.9	−3.3	−0.4	−3.6	−0.2	−3.9	−1.8	−2.7	+0.2	−3.5
UK: England and Wales	−1.2	−0.9	−0.6	−1.5	−0.3	−1.1	−2.3	−2.6	+0.3	+1.1
Northern Ireland	+0.4	−0.7	+0.7	−1.3	+0.7	−1.0	+0.5	−2.3	+1.3	−0.2
Scotland	−0.6	−0.6	−0.5	−1.1	−0.4	−1.1	−1.0	−1.1	+0.1	+0.5
Yugoslavia	−0.7	−1.8	+1.8	−0.2	+2.0	−0.6	+1.2	+0.8	+0.6	+4.1
Australia & New Zealand	−1.4	−1.7	−2.3	−2.3	−2.3	−2.2	−2.4	−2.7	−2.1	−1.0

Food factors affecting the pathways to coronary heart disease. Putative food factors which may influence coronary heart disease include: (1) energy balance, (2) energy density, (3) intake of plant food (or dietary fibre), (4) dietary fat, (5) quality of fat, (6) cholesterol intake, (7) alcohol intake and (8) intake of minerals (eg selenium, magnesium, calcium, sodium, potassium).

It is often difficult to discern how factors which change with food intake might themselves contribute to coronary or any other kind of mortality[16,27]. This is exemplified by a recent report from Sweden, a prospective study of social influences on mortality where some of these social activities, at home and outside the home, clearly involve food[28]. Perhaps trends to eat outside the home in developed countries might have advantages.

There may be some merit in examining more nutritionally integrative measures of food intake than the commonly used nutrient approaches. At the very least, this would mean the use of food rather than nutrients. Specific food factors might interact synergistically, additively or antagonistically. An index of food variety could be particularly valuable, since with variety comes essential nutrient adequacy and the dilution of adverse factors. Variety is more achievable with an abundant food supply, food preservation beyond seasons by, for example, freezing, and the coexistence of several food cultures. Indeed, it could be reasonably hypothesized that, in countries showing the greatest fall in coronary mortality, USA, Japan and Australia, food variety has significantly increased.

It is particularly noteworthy that in at least two prospective studies of men, the greater the food energy intake and the greater the dietary fibre intake, the less the coronary mortality rates[12,18].

Changes in coronary heart disease mortality. Of particular value for hypothesis testing has been the different trends in coronary heart disease (CHD) mortality in different developed countries. In particular, rates have been falling for men in the USA, Australia, Canada, New Zealand, Belgium, Finland and Japan[20] (Table 2). In Sweden, the rates are increasing, although from rather lower initial rates than in other developed countries. In eastern Europe, rates are also increasing. There has been little change in coronary mortality rates in England and Wales[5,10,29] (Table 2).

For women, the trends in CHD mortality are different than for men. The decline in coronary mortality in several developed countries started earlier and led to a greater divergence in life expectancy between men and women[4,29] (Tables 1, 2). It may be that dietary factors operate differently for women. Could it be that women have watched their saturated fat and therefore their polyunsaturated/saturated fat ratio for longer than men? If so, this may have been not for concern about CHD, but for other reasons such as concern about obesity.

Explanation for changes in cardiovascular mortality. An important initial question is whether or not the improvement in coronary mortality rates reflects better treatment or management of established CHD or whether the disease process itself is less common. An important contribution to this field comes from Perth in Western Australia[11], set against data on declining mortality rates from ischaemic heart disease in Australia[15]. The Perth study indicates that the improvement in ischaemic heart disease mortality in Western Australia has been due mainly to a fall in the incidence of acute manifestations of ischaemic heart disease (sudden death and acute myocardial infarction), rather than improvements in case fatality. This kind of observation, along with analyses from the United States[9,23,25], make it worthwhile to take a closer look at lifestyle, presumably including dietary factors which might account for these changing coronary mortality rates.

Trends in food consumption. The most overall view of change in man's diet with time has been made by workers in the field of paleolithic nutrition[6] and a summary of these changes is given in Table 3. Man's original hunter-gatherer diet was probably higher in energy intake, related to higher levels of physical activity. It was lower in fat, leading to a higher polyunsaturated/saturated ratio, and lower in cholesterol. The other noteworthy assessment of paleolithic man is that he had the possibility of a reasonable life expectancy, in excess of 60 years.

The analyses of Dwyer and Hetzel[5,10], together with those of Oliver[22], indicate the importance of quality of fat in accounting for the trends in CHD mortality (Table 4). In the Dwyer and Hetzel study, a latent period for effect of a change in the proportion of vegetable to animal fat would appear to be 5 years.

This is even more relevant when one moves beyond the grosser relationships of total dietary fat and coronary mortality which have been reviewed by Stamler[24]. This is because there can be quite substantial differences in coronary rates for a percentage of total food energy from fat which is rather similar, say in the region 33 to 40 per cent for countries like the USA, Australia, the UK and Sweden. Between these countries there are, however, considerable differences in polyunsaturated fat intake (Table 5).

Of even greater interest in recent times are the differences in fish consumption between these countries (Table 5) which might partly account for any lack of relationship between percentage food energy from fat and even P:S ratio, and coronary morphology, morbidity or mortality[1,2,13,14,18,21].

It also needs to be noted that around the Mediterranean there can be contributions to food energy from fat comparable to those in other developed countries, although the quality of the fat is quite different, being more monounsaturated from olive oil (Table 6).

Table 3. *Comparison of the late paleolithic diet*, the current American diet, and US dietary recommendations. (From[6]: Modified Data).*

	Late paleolithic diet*	Current American diet	US Senate Select Committee recommendations
Percentage dietary energy as:			
Protein	34	12	12
Carbohydrate	45	46	58
Fat	21	42	30
Polyunsaturated: saturated fat ratio	1.41	0.44	1.00

(*assumed to contain 35 per cent meat and 65 per cent vegetables).

Table 4. *Changes with time in the consumption of vegetable fat, expressed as a percentage of animal fat[5].*

	UK	USA	Australia
1935	24	35	18
1950	40	35	21
1958	34	39	19
1962	34	32	16
1966	35	34	24
1970	35	38	25
1974	36	43	27

Table 5. *Polyunsaturated fat and fish and shell fish available in 20 countries 1954–1965. (Modified from[24]).*

Country	Polyunsaturated fat (g/person/d)	Fish & shell fish (as % total energy)
Finland	5	1.4
United States	16	0.7
New Zealand	7	0.7
Republic of Ireland	11	0.5
Australia	8	0.5
United Kingdom	14	0.9
Canada	10	0.8
Norway	37	2.2
Netherlands	31	0.7
Israel	21	0.8
Denmark	27	1.9
Belgium	22	0.9
German Federal Republic	26	0.8
Sweden	25	2.4
Austria	19	0.5
Venezuela[a]	8	1.7
Switzerland	24	0.5
Italy	13	0.8
France[a]	22	1.0
Japan	7	3.6

[a]Data for 1957–1965.

Table 6. *Dietary fat, serum cholesterol and 10-year CHD mortality rate for men originally age 40–59 years, in the Seven Countries Study[24].*

	Per cent of total energy as fat					Serum cholesterol (mg/dl)		10-year mortality (per 1000)	
	Total	Saturated (S)	Mono unsaturated	Poly- unsaturated (P)	2S-P	Median	90th centile	CHD	Total
Greece	36	7	26	3	11	201	258	9	57
Yugoslavia	31	5	21	5	5	171*	219*	12*	105*
Italy	26	9	14	3	15	198	253	21	126
Rome railroad workers	-	-	-	-	-	207	260	22	75
USA railroad workers	40	18	17	5	31	236	294	57	115
Finland	37	20	14	3	37	259	323	65	167
Netherlands	40	18	17	5	31	230	291	44	125

*Excludes Belgrade and Slavonia.

Cigarette-smoking and hypertension do not explain the trends in CHD mortality[5].

1 Arntzenius, A., Kromhout, D., Barth, J.D., Reiber, J.H.C., Bruschke, A.V.G., Buis, B., Van Gent, C.M., Kempen-Voogd, N., Strikwerda, S. & Van der Velde, E.A. (1985): Diet, lipoproteins, and the progression of coronary atherosclerosis. The Leiden Intervention Trial. *New Engl. J. Med.* **312**, 805–811.
2 Blankenhorn, D.H. (1985): Two new diet-heart studies. *New Engl. J. Med.* **312**, 851–853.
3 Charnock, J.S., McLennan, P.L., Abeywardena, M.Y. & Dryden, W.F. (1985): Diet and cardiac arrhythmia: effects of lipids on age-related changes in myocardial function in the rat. *Ann. Nutr. Metb. (In press)*
4 Department of Health & Social Security (1984): Report on health & social subjects 28. *Diet and cardiovascular disease.* Committee on Medical Aspects of Food Policy. Report of the Panel on Diet in Relation to Cardiovascular Disease. London: HMSO.
5 Dwyer, T. & Hetzel, B. (1980): A comparison of trends of coronary heart disease mortality in Australia, USA and England and Wales with reference to three major risk factors — hypertension, cigarette smoking and diet. *Int. J. Epidem.* **9**. 65–71.
6 Eaton, S.B. & Konner, M. (1985): Paleolithic nutrition. A consideration of its nature and current implications. *New Engl. J. Med.* **312**, 283–289.
7 Encyclopaedia Britannica (1985): *Book of the year*. Chicago: Encyclopaedia Britannica.
8 Glomset, J.A. (1985): Fish, fatty acids and human health. *New Engl. J. Med.* **312**, 1253–1254.
9 Goldman, L. & Cook, F. (1984): The decline in ischemic heart disease mortality rates. An analysis of the comparative effects of medical interventions and changes in lifestyle. *Ann. Int. Med.* **101**, 825–836.
10 Hetzel, B. & Dwyer, T. (1981): Soft fat — harder evidence. *Lancet* **1**, 1104.
11 Hobbs, M.S.T., Armstrong, B.K., Hockey, R.A., Thompson, P.L. & Martin, C.A. (1984): Trends in ischemic heart disease mortality and morbidity in Perth Statistical Division. *Aust. N.Z. J. Med.* **14**, 381–387.
12 Kromhout, D., Bosschieter, E.B. & De Lezenne Coulander, C. (1982): Dietary fibre and 10-year mortality from coronary heart disease, cancer and all causes. The Zutphen Study. *Lancet* **2**, 518–521.
13 Kromhout, D., Bosscheiter, E.B. & De Lezenne Coulander, C. (1985): The inverse relation between fish consumption and 20-year mortality from coronary heart disease. *New Engl. J. Med.* **312**, 1205–1209.
14 Kushi, L., Lew, R.A., Stare, F.J., Ellison, C.R., Lozy, M.E., Bourke, G., Daly, L., Graham, I., Hickey, N., Mulcahy, R. & Kevaney, J. (1985): Diet and 20-year mortality from coronary heart disease. The Ireland-Boston Diet-Heart Study. *New Engl. J. Med.* **312**, 811–818.
15 Leeder, S.R., Dobson, A.J., Gibberd, R.W. & Lloyd, D.M. (1984): Declining mortality rates from ischemic heart disease in Australia. *Aust. N.Z. J. Med.* **14**, 388–394.
16 Logan, R.L., Riemersma, R.A., Thomson, M., Oliver, M.F., Olsson, A.G., Walddius, G., Rosner, S., Kaijser, L., Callmer, F., Carlson, L.A., Lockerbie, L. & Lutz, W. (1978): Risk factors for ischaemic heart disease in normal men aged 40. *Lancet* **1**, 949–955.
17 McLennan, P., Abeywardena, M. & Charnock, J. (1985): Influence of dietary lipids on arrhythmia and infarction after coronary artery ligation in rats. *Can. J. Physiol. Pharm.* **64**, 1411–1417.
18 Morris, J.N., Marr, J.W. & Clayton, D.G. (1977): Diet and heart: a postscript. *Br. Med. J.* **2**, 1307–1314.
19 Moulds, R.F.W. (ed) (1983): NH & MRC Workshop on non-pharmacological methods of lowering blood pressure. *Med. J. Aust.* **2**, S1–23.
20 National Heart Foundation of New Zealand (1983): *Coronary heart disease*. A report on prevention and control in 1983. Auckland: The National Heart Foundation of New Zealand.
21 Nikkila, E.A., Viikinskoski, P., Valle, M. & Frick, M.H. (1984): Prevention of progression of coronary atherosclerosis by treatment of hyperlipidaemia: a seven year prospective angiographic study. *Br. Med. J.* **289**, 220–223.
22 Oliver, M.F. (1981): Diet and coronary heart disease. *Br. Med. Bull.* **37**, 49–58.
23 Pell, S. & Fayerweather, W.E. (1985): Trends in the incidence of myocardial infarction and in associated mortality and morbidity in a large employed population, 1957–1983. *New Engl. J. Med.* **312**, 1005–1010.
24 Stamler, J. (1979): Population Studies. In *Nutrition, lipids and coronary heart disease*, ed R. Levy, B. Rifkind, B. Dennis & N. Ernst, pp. 25–88. New York: Raven Press.
25 Stamler, J. (1985): Coronary heart disease: Doing the 'right things'. *New Engl. J. Med.* **312**, 1053–1054.
26 Thuesen, L., Nielsen, T.T., Thomassen, A., Bagger, J.P. & Henningsen, P. (1984): Beneficial effect of a low-fat low-calorie diet on myocardial energy metabolism in patients with angina pectoris. *Lancet* **2**, 59–62.
27 Wahlqvist, M.L. (1982): Social toxicants and nutritional status. In *Adverse effects of food*, ed E.F.P. Jelliffe, pp. 227–238. New York: Plenum Press.
28 Welin, L., Tibblin, G., Svardsudd, K., Tibblin, B., Ander-Peciva, S., Larsson, B. & Wilhelmsen, L. (1985): Prospective study of social influences on mortality. *Lancet* **1**, 915–918.
29 World Health Organization (1981): *World Health Statistics Quarterly* **34** (1).

Diets in communities with high and low incidence of coronary heart disease: intercommunity studies

F. FIDANZA

Istituto di Scienza dell'Alimentazione, Università degli Studi, Casella Postale 333, 06100 Perugia, Italy.

Findings on the relationship between dietary components and incidence of coronary heart disease (CHD) in man have not been consistent and unequivocal, particularly from within population studies, in which the unit of concern is the individual, rather than the group. The reasons for these problems are not widely understood. Basically the key problem has been inadequacy of methods of diet assessment, leading often to misleading data. That is, the method for dietary appraisal in many cases was not appropriate to the purpose, eg the 24-h recall was often used. This method is relatively simple and fast, but it has serious limitations at the individual level because of the large intra-individual variability in food intake. In several studies using this method, its reliability was not even assessed. Then there are problems of validity, including confounding. For example, in some studies the dietary survey was carried out during one of the follow-up visits of the epidemiological study, when other environmental factors (eg advertisements and information from mass media) had already induced modifications in the dietary habits of sizable numbers of people in the population under study in a non-random way, ie persons made aware they had hypercholesterolaemia were the ones making the greatest diet changes. As shown in the Chicago Western Electric study[12], this can produce serious defects in the data, obscuring true relationships. When such problems are taken into account and avoided, the relation within populations between the diet of individuals, especially dietary lipid (cholesterol, amount and type of neutral fat), emerges very clearly, as in the California Seventh-Day Adventist study, the Hawaiian Japanese-American study, the Irish brothers study, the Western Electric study, and the Zutphen study in The Netherlands.

The diets of a few communities with a high and low incidence of coronary heart disease will now be discussed. The past material has been reviewed previously[4,5] and only the most relevant data will be considered here.

In USA, a country with , in general, a high incidence of CHD, the results of the Western Electric study[12] are very interesting. The dietary assessment was not limited to a '…short dietary history of what the men usually ate or to a 24-hour recall'. Rather for 2 consecutive years, at baseline and at the first follow-up year, the habitual recent diet of the 1900 men was characterized in depth by the Burke method. With that method dietary cholesterol and saturated fatty acids were both significantly and independently related to serum cholesterol, dietary polyunsaturates nearly so. In contrast to other longitudinal studies, both univariate and multivariate analysis showed a positive relationship of dietary cholesterol and polyunsaturated fatty acids to 19-year risk of CHD. This was not the case for dietary saturated fatty acids in multivariate analysis. This relationship of dietary lipids to CHD risk in the multivariate analysis was independent of serum cholesterol, systolic blood pressure, cigarette-smoking and age. According to Stamler, other factors are also probably involved, needing further investigation. Studies comparing groups with different dietary habits within a single country have been useful in supporting the hypothesis of a relationship between dietary intake of macronutrients, CHD risk factors and CHD events. The Seventh-Day Adventists represent in this regard a very interesting experience, and have in fact been intensively studied. Their diet is mainly based on the use of whole grains, vegetables, nuts and soy products. Investigations both in USA and in Australia have shown that church members, both adults and children, have lower serum total cholesterol and LDL cholesterol than the general population of the country of residence. These low levels of serum cholesterol correlate with low intake of saturated fat and cholesterol[2,13]. To date only a few reports have been made on long-term follow-up studies. A 6-year follow-up study of 24 000 Seventh Day Adventists from California[10] showed that, overall, church members presented lower age-standardized CHD mortality rates than the general population of California. Among male church members aged 35 and over, a gradient was evident in CHD mortality in relation to the adoption of a vegetarian diet. According to the authors a key component of these lower mortality rates probably was the lower fat intake and the higher fibre intake of the Seventh-Day Adventists compared to the general population.

A good example of a country with a low incidence of CHD is Japan. In the Seven Countries Study, for the sample of middle-aged farmers of Tanushimaru (in the island of Kyushu), the age-standardized death rate from CHD in 15 years was only 144 per 10 000[8]. In the diet of these men, proteins, total fat and saturated fatty acids provided averages 12.3, 8.9 and 2.9 per cent of total energy respectively. For further details on the diet see[7]. To explain why the coronary death rate of Japanese men was so much lower than predicted by the logistic coefficients from each of the other regions (for age, blood pressure, serum cholesterol, and smoking habits) various hypotheses were formulated[8].

In this regard, the results of the Ni-Hon-San study are valuable, presenting comparisons between Japanese migrants to the United States and Japanese in Japan, with data on the possible influence of Americanization of eating habits on the traditionally low rate of CHD in Japanese people[6]. The study started in 1965 with middle-aged men of Japanese ancestry living in Hiroshima and Nagasaki, Japan, in Honolulu, Hawaii and in the San Francisco Bay area in the USA. Nutritional evaluation showed that Japanese men had a much lower mean intake of total fat, saturated fatty acids, animal protein, cholesterol, simple carbohydrates, total protein, and unsaturated fatty acids, than the Japanese-American men; on the contrary, intakes of total and complex carbohydrates, alcohol and salt were higher.

Marked differences were recorded in the incidence of myocardial infarction (MI) and CHD death for the three cohorts. The lowest incidence rate was observed in the Japanese; the Hawaiian was 2.1 times higher than the Japanese and the Californian 3.2 times.

Multivariate assessment of the relationship between baseline status for major risk factors and incidence of CHD for the Japanese and Hawaiian cohorts showed that serum cholesterol was significantly and independently related to risk in both populations.

In the Seven Countries Study the cohort with the lowest death rate for CHD in 15 years was the one in Crete (Greece). The rate per 10 000, standardized by age, of men aged 40–59 at entry, was only 38. For the other Greek cohort, in Corfu, the rate was higher, 202. The diets of these rural men were dominated by olive oil and bread (accounting for 50–60 per cent of total energy). Animal products contributed less than 10 per cent of total energy. Potatoes and vegetables were consumed in large amounts and legumes of various kinds formed an important part of the diet[3], but over the subsequent 20 years, dietary habits changed dramatically. In Corfu the total energy intake from fat increased 9.8 per cent, while in Crete over the same period there was a decrease of 7.7 per cent, with a great change in the fatty acid intake[1]. This may relate to the difference in incidence between the two cohorts. A new prospective study is now in progress to evaluate the health impact of these dietary changes.

In contrast to the Greek and Japanese cohorts, communities with a high incidence of CHD examined in the Seven Countries Study were USA, Finland and The Netherlands. The age-standardized 15-year death rate for men age 40–59 at entry, reached the maximum in East Finland, 1202 per 10 000, while in West Finland it was 741[8]. The main energy sources in the Finnish diet were cereals, milk and milk products, sugar, meat and potatoes. The consumption of other vegetables, fruits and berries, fish and eggs was relatively small[11]. In East Finland 39.2 per cent of total energy was derived from fats and in West Finland 35.4 per cent. In addition saturated fatty acid intake was higher in East than in West Finland. For the Zutphen cohort (The Netherlands), the 15-year CHD death rate was 637 per 10 000, very close to that in West Finland. The diet, assessed in depth[3], was characterized by frequent consumption of milk, cheese, fat meat, eggs, saturated visible fats, potatoes and sugar. Men of the Zutphen cohort consuming more than 30 g fish/d experienced a 50 per cent lower CHD death rate than men consuming no fish in the diet[9]. This finding may relate to altered haemostatic function, due to presence in the diet of eicosapentaenoic acid.

The comparisons of contrasting communities with high and low incidences of CHD show that the most relevant difference in the diet of these communities is their lipid content. From recent results, other nutrients also can play an important role, but their assessment in the diet is not yet comprehensive or satisfactory. There is also a need to take confounding factors into consideration, eg, blood pressure, smoking habit, obesity. But at least as important is to find and use more appropriate approaches to dietary appraisal, particularly at the metabolic level, especially since in general we do not find sizable correlations between nutrient intake and their status in the body.

1 Aravnais, C. (1983): The classic risk factors for coronary heart disease: experience in Europe. *Prevent. Med.* **12**, 16–19.

2 Cooper, R., Allen, A., Goldberg, R., Trevisan, M. *et al.* (1984): Seventh-Day Adventist adolescents — life-style patterns and cardiovascular risk factors. *West. J. Med.* **140**, 471–477.

3 Den Hartog, C., Buzina, R., Fidanza, F., Keys, A. & Roine, P. (1968): *Dietary studies and epidemiology of heart disease*, pp. 80, 84. Rotterdam: Wyt & Sons.

4 Fidanza, F. (1966): Dietary fat, obesity and coronary heart disease. *Nutr. Dieta* **8**, 200–209.

5 Fidanza, F. (1972): Epidemiological evidence for the fat theory. *Proc. Nutr. Soc.* **31**, 317–321.

6 Kato, H., Tillotson, J., Nichaman, M.Z., Rhoads, G.G. & Hamilton, H.B. (1973): Epidemiologic studies of coronary heart disease and stroke in Japanese men living in Japan, Hawaii and California. Serum lipids and diet. *Am. J. Epidemiol.* **97**, 372–385.

7 Keys, A. & Kimura, N. (1970): Diets of middle-aged-farmers in Japan. *Am. J. Clin. Nutr.* **23**, 212–223.

8 Keys, A., Menotti, A., Aravanis, C. *et al.* (1984): The Seven Countries Study: 2. 289 deaths in 15 years. *Prevent. Med.* **13**, 141–154.

9 Kromhout, D., Bosschieter, E.B. & de Lezenne Coulander (1985): The inverse relation between fish consumption and 20-year mortality from coronary heart disease. *New Engl. J. Med.* **312**, 1205–1209.

10 Phillips, R.L., Lemon, F.R., Beeson, W.L. & Kuzma, J.W. (1978): Coronary heart disease mortality among Seventh-Day Adventists with differing dietary habits: a preliminary report. *Am. J. Clin. Nutr.* **31**, S191–S198.

11. Roine, P., Pekkarinen, M. & Karvonen, M.J. (1964): Dietary studies in connection with epidemiology of heart disease: results in Finland. *Voeding* **25**, 383–393.

12. Shekelle, R.B., Stamler, J., Paul, O. *et al.* (1982): Dietary lipids and serum cholesterol level. Change in diet confounds the cross-sectional association. *Am. J. Epidemiol.* **115**, 506–514.

13. Webster, I.W. & Rawson, G.K. (1979): Health status of Seventh-Day Adventists. *Med. J. Aust.* **1**, 417–420.

Linoleic acid and coronary heart disease

D.A. WOOD, R.A. RIEMERSMA and M.F. OLIVER
Cardiovascular Research Unit, University of Edinburgh.

In 1956 Sinclair[3] asked the following question: 'The possibility exists that atherosclerotic heart disease results from a relative deficiency of the essential fatty acid arachidonic acid in relation to an excess of saturated fats; do such diets exist?'

While the Edinburgh group did not directly set out to answer this question, we incorporated methods which would enable us to accumulate data concerning this possibility in the Edinburgh-Stockholm study[1]. This study was conducted in men aged exactly 40 in the cities of Edinburgh and Stockholm in order to determine whether there were identifiable reasons as to why coronary heart disease (CHD) was three times more common in young Scotsmen compared with young Swedes; and precise information existed to indicate the threefold difference between the Edinburgh and Stockholm populations. The design of the study was a laboratory-based epidemiological survey and, in view of the extensive laboratory measurements made, the size of the two samples which were studied was deliberately restricted although at the same time randomly drawn and representative of the social class and life-style structure of the two cities under study. No inter-laboratory differences were possible, since all analyses were made in one laboratory: thus, all fatty acid analyses from Stockholm and Edinburgh were made in Edinburgh and, conversely all lipoprotein analyses were made in Stockholm. The principal findings were that Edinburgh men, in contrast to Stockholm men, had highly significantly less adipose linoleic acid, produced a greater concentration of insulin and more quickly in response to a glucose load, had higher very-low-density lipoprotein triglyceride and were shorter in height. There were, however, no significant differences in lipoprotein (LDL) cholesterol concentrations, blood pressure or uric acid between the populations.

The degree of difference in adipose linoleic acid between the Edinburgh and Stockholm population was highly significant ($P \pm 0.001$), whether considering the medians or the tails of distributions. Lower adipose arachidonic acid levels were also found in Edinburgh men, although the difference between the two populations was much less striking than for linoleic acid.

The possibility arose that the Stockholm men had been supplementing their diet with polyunsaturated oils and that the explanation of the striking differences was that the Swedish population was more health-conscious. Subsequent dietary analyses of the two populations did not, however, confirm this suspicion and therefore additional studies were made and at that time (1979) a collaborative study was conducted with Professor Nikkari in Finland and similar findings were observed in North Karelia, in contrast to Tampere (South-West Finland)[2]. The incidence of CHD in North Karelia is appreciably higher than that in South West Finland and there was significantly lower adipose linoleic acid concentrations in the North Karelian Finn.

The Edinburgh population study. A sample of 448 men was drawn at random from general practices representing the five social classes in the City of Edinburgh and surrounding districts and these practices had on their lists 6000 men aged 35–60 from which this random sample was drawn. All 448 men were examined and 28 were found to have coronary heart disease when they attended the clinic but none of these men had any previous history and none had attended their general practitioner on this account. There were a further 24 who had an identified and recognised previous history of CHD. In addition, there were 53 others who might have had CHD. This left a group of 343 in whom no features of CHD could be identified either by questionnaire or ECG.

Adipose tissue and platelet fatty acid compositions were determined in all 448 men. Adipose linoleic acid was significantly lower (7.8 per cent) in those with coronary heart disease compared with those who definitely had no CHD (8.9 per cent). The same trend was true for platelet linoleic acid (4.9 compared with 5.1 per cent). Additionally, dihomo-gamma-linolenic acid was significantly lower in the coronary patients (0.08 compared with 0.11 per cent). Adipose and platelet arachidonic acid showed the same trend, but this was not significant. These results have now been published[5].

The Edinburgh case-control study. In view of these findings of the Edinburgh population study, a case-control study was established and the fatty acid composition of adipose tissue and of platelets was contrasted in 125 men with angina pectoris, 92 men with acute myocardial infarction and 430 age-matched healthy controls. The men with angina were identified through the Rose angina questionnaire from a random population sample. The men with acute myocardial infarction were drawn randomly from those admitted acutely with their *first* myocardial infarct to one of the intensive care units in the City of Edinburgh and they were men who had not previously consulted their doctor or had any symptoms of CHD.

The results of this study, which will be published shortly, have shown that there is significantly lower adipose linoleic acid in the coronary patients. There was a progressive inverse relative risk of 3.2:1 in angina pectoris patients compared with controls and a similar progressive inverse relative risk of 3.3:1 for men with acute myocardial infarction compared with controls for the quintiles of distribution of adipose linoleic acid. While cigarette-smoking is an important confounding factor, the inverse relationship described also applies to the non-smoking CHD population. Comparable, but less strong, correlations were found with the analysis of platelet linoleic acid. As in the Edinburgh population study, an opposite trend applied for palmitoleic acid (16:1; n 7), coronary patients having high concentrations of this acid in their adipose tissue.

Multiple regression analysis has shown that low adipose linoleic acid concentrations in the case-control study phases out all other 'risk' variables, including cigarette-smoking although cigarette-smoking is the second most important of these variables. Indeed, low adipose linoleic acid is significantly more important as a risk factor than raised serum cholesterol or LDL cholesterol or low/high-density lipoprotein cholesterol.

Dietary studies. A 7-day prospective weighed record has been made in 164 healthy middle-aged Scotsmen drawn at random from 600 men drawn, in their turn, at random from general-practitioner lists. Analysis has been made of all nutrients and this has been based on the McCance & Widdowson tables but, in order to provide precise details of fatty acid composition, it was necessary to develop a new system of data analysis and computing. Some information concerning these nutrients has been published[4]. Data are available concerning dietary linoleic acid and the relationship between adipose and dietary linoleic acid, which shows a correlation coefficient of 0.58.

Cigarette-smokers were shown in this dietary analysis to consume significantly lower quantities of linoleic acid compared with non-smokers. The explanation of this is not entirely clear, except that non-smokers appear to consume more polyunsaturated oil possibly because they are more health conscious individuals.

It is to be expected, therefore, that the low consumption of dietary linoleic acid in cigarette smokers will be reflected by low adipose linoleic acid in those patients with CHD who are also smokers.

International study. A collaborative study of adipose linoleic acid concentrations in men in North Karelia, Kuopio, Edinburgh and Sapri (Calabria, Italy) has now been completed and shows results consistent with the above observations — namely, that the lowest levels of adipose linoleic acid are in North Karelia and in Edinburgh, whereas the highest levels are in the Italian population where the consumption of polyunsaturated oils is much higher. Interestingly, there were significantly low levels of vitamin C and vitamin E in the Edinburgh population compared with the others and 32 per cent of the apparently normal Edinburgh men had plasma ascorbic levels below the FAO/WHO recommended standard of 2 mg/l.

Conclusions. Sinclair's original proposition would, therefore, appear to be correct. Coronary-prone populations and patients with established CHD have lower adipose and, to a lesser extent, platelet linoleic acid compared with comparable controls. They also have higher palmitoleic concentrations, possibly indicating induced desaturation.

While cigarette-smoking certainly confounds the picture, it is not the sole explanation and the inverse relative risk that applies to the angina and myocardial infarct population is largely independent of cigarette smoking.

The full explanation of these findings is not yet clear.

1 Logan, R.L., Riemersma, R.A., Thomson, M., Oliver, M.F., Olsson, A.G., Rossner, A., Callmer, E., Walldius, G., Kaijser, L. & Carlson, L.A. (1978): Risk factors in ischaemic heart disease in normal men aged 40. *Lancet* **1**, 949–55.
2 Nikkari, T., Salo, M., Maatela, J. & Aromaa, A. (1983): Serum fatty acids in Finnish men. *Atherosclerosis* **49**, 139–48.
3 Sinclair, H.M. (1956): Deficiency of essential fatty acids and atherosclerosis etcetera. *Lancet* **1**, 381–3.
4 Thomson, M., Fulton, M., Wood, D.A., Brown, S., Elton, R.A., Birtwhistle, A. & Oliver, M.F. (1985): A comparison of the nutrient intake of some Scotsmen with dietary recommendations. *Hum. Nutr.: Appl. Nutr.* **39A**, 443–455.
5 Wood, D.A., Butler, S., Riemersma, R.A., Thomson, M., Oliver, M.F., Fulton, M., Birtwhistle, A. & Elton, R. (1984): Adipose tissue and platelet fatty acids and coronary heart disease in Scottish men. *Lancet* **2**, 117–21.

Dietary sodium intake in relation to hypertension

J.I.S. ROBERTSON
Medical Research Council, Blood Pressure Unit, Western Infirmary, Glasgow G11 6NT, UK.

Essential or primary hypertension is defined as high blood pressure without evident cause. This distinguishes essential hypertension from forms of high blood pressure where there is a distinct aetiological agent such as an aldosterone-secreting adenoma or renal artery stenosis. Despite however this rather negative definition of essential hypertension there has been no lack of industry in seeking aetiological factors in the pathogenesis of the condition. In particular there have been repeated suspicions of a connection between sodium chloride and essential hypertension.

First, it has long been considered probable that one reason for the high prevalence of essential hypertension in the Western world is an excessively high intake of dietary sodium chloride. Second, there is possibly in essential hypertension a renal abnormality which requires there to be an increased systemic arterial pressure in order to sustain sodium chloride excretion and hence to maintain sodium balance. Third, there is a mass of evidence now to show that in essential hypertension there is an abnormality of transmembrane electrolyte transport; again it is possible that this could underly the pathogenesis of the disease. These various notions are, of course, in no way mutually exclusive.

One further aspect needs emphasis and that is the close relationship between the renin-angiotensin system and both sodium balance and sodium intake. If, in a normal person, for any reason sodium is lost from the body, the kidney responds with an increased secretion of the enzyme renin. In turn this results in an increased concentration of the circulating pressor octapeptide angiotensin II which will help both to sustain arterial pressure and to stimulate aldosterone secretion. This latter mechanism will tend to restore sodium balance. When we consider modifications of dietary sodium chloride intake these changes necessarily involve the renin-angiotensin system.

The issues which I wish to address in this paper are: first, is sodium chloride intake in the diet an important initiating factor in essential hypertension?; second, can moderate and realistic dietary sodium chloride restriction, that is to say down to some 60–100 mmol (3.50–5.85 g)/d, prevent the development of essential hypertension or help to lower arterial pressure once it has been raised? These issues may well be illuminated by looking at the amount of sodium in the body in various hypertensive diseases.

This paper is based on a series of reports which have been published elsewhere and which give details of the various studies[1–4,6].

Methods. Some methodological considerations require to be touched upon before presenting the results. We have measured exhangeable sodium in the body by the standard technique of isotope dilution, that is by administering the radio-active isotope ^{24}Na, allowing a suitable time for equilibration, and then, from the dilution of the labelled isotope, calculating the amount of total exchangeable sodium in the body. The measurements of exchangeable sodium have been reinforced by measurements of total body sodium by a completely different method, namely by *in-vivo* neutron activation analysis employing a whole body counter.

It is necessary to express body sodium content in a form which permits comparisons between subjects of different sizes and shapes. We have found that leanness index or body surface area are each reasonably satisfactory in this regard. We have therefore expressed body sodium content as a percentage of the value expected for a normal subject of the same sex and either leanness index (height^3 ÷ weight) or body surface area. Thus, 100 per cent would be a strictly normal value.

Normal subjects. When a large series of normal subjects was examined no relationship could be discerned between either exchangeable sodium or total-body sodium expressed in the above fashion and the concurrent arterial pressure[1].

Aldosterone-secreting adenoma. The disease in which the clearest relationship between body sodium content and arterial pressure would be expected is Conn's syndrome (aldosterone-secreting adenoma). In this disease a tumour of the adrenal gland produces an excess of aldosterone; this results in sodium retention and potassium depletion with hypertension. Because of the sodium retention renin and angiotensin II are depressed. When a series of untreated patients with this condition was examined, a clear expansion of exchangeable sodium was seen[2]. Moreover, there was a close positive correlation between the extent of expansion of body sodium content and the level of arterial pressure. This relationship suggested, without of course proving, that the expansion of body sodium was aetiologically concerned with the genesis of the high blood pressure. The argument was carried a stage further by lowering the expanded body sodium content on giving a natriuretic and potassium-conserving drug, either spironolactone or amiloride. Each of these agents diminished the excess of body sodium and, in proportion to the reduction of sodium content, lowered arterial pressure. The same result was achieved by surgical excision of the aldosterone-secreting tumour. This again led to a reduction of the expanded body sodium content with a concomitant reduction of arterial pressure.

Thus Conn's syndrome, the classic form of mineralo-corticoid-induced hypertension, is seen to be a condition where one can plausibly invoke sodium retention in pathogenesis.

Renal artery stenosis. In sharp contrast to the findings in Conn's syndrome was the relationship between body sodium content and arterial pressure in hypertension with renal artery stenosis. In this condition we found that, untreated, there was a tendency to a diminution of body sodium content[4]. Moreover the relationship between blood pressure and body sodium was inverse. Those patients with renal artery stenosis and the highest levels of arterial pressure had the greatest tendency to sodium depletion; many were frankly sodium-deficient. These findings in renovascular hypertension clearly indicated that where we have a form of hypertension where sodium retention is not centrally involved in pathogenesis there is indeed a tendency to sodium depletion. The higher the arterial pressure the greater the tendency to sodium excretion and thus to sodium deficiency.

Essential hypertension. With these contrasting findings in Conn's syndrome and renovascular hypertension in mind, body sodium content in essential hypertension will be considered. When a large series of patients with untreated essential hypertension was examined we found that the mean level for exchangeable sodium was almost exactly 100 per cent, that is, indistinguishable from normal[1]. However, and in sharp contrast to normal subjects, there was in untreated essential hypertension a highly significant positive correlation between exchangeable sodium and the level of arterial pressure. The overall mean value arose because in mild (and presumably early) essential hypertension there was a tendency to sodium depletion, while in more severe hypertension exchangeable sodium was expanded.

It might have been that this relationship in essential hypertension was artefactual, arising as a result of the known abnormality of transmembrane electrolyte transport in that condition. The equilibration of the administered radio-active isotope necessary for the measurement of exchangeable sodium could have been affected in some way by these cell membrane abnormalities. However when, by the completely different technique of activation analysis we measured total body sodium, we found almost exactly the same as with exchangeable sodium; total body sodium had a mean value of 100 per cent. Overall there was a highly significant positive correlation between total body sodium and the level of arterial pressure, with mild hypertension having subnormal and more severe hypertension expanded body sodium content.

The subnormality of body sodium in mild essential hypertension deserves emphasis. When a group of 20 young untreated hypertensive subjects was matched for age, weight, sex and leanness index with a group of normal subjects, the hypertensives were found to have a clear, statistically significant deficiency of exchangeable sodium.

The full explanation of these very interesting findings in essential hypertension remains uncertain. One possibility which is certainly worthy of consideration is that essential hypertension is initiated by mechanisms which are independent of any tendency to sodium retention. Thus we see something akin to renovascular hypertension, where the elevated arterial pressure tends to promote the expulsion of sodium from the body. Perhaps only later in the course of the disease, and possibly because of hypertension-induced renal changes, there is a tendency to sodium retention and thus to a sodium-dependent factor in the high blood pressure. If these speculations have any validity, one might expect that dietary sodium restriction, while possibly effective in treating more severe essential hypertension, would be ineffective, or perhaps even adverse, in the early stages.

Effect of dietary salt restriction. Over the years moderate dietary salt restriction has been studied on a number of occasions in the treatment of essential hypertension. Several workers have found that overall this manoeuvre does produce a significant, albeit usually mild, blood pressure fall. By contrast other workers, who have apparently conducted their studies with no less diligence and efficiency, have found that such sodium restriction produces no significant overall blood pressure fall. It is of some interest that those authors who have found sodium restriction to be effective in lowering arterial pressure have in general studied older and more severe forms of hypertension than those who have had negative results.

As already mentioned, sodium restriction necessarily involves stimulation of the renin-angiotensin system: the extent of the rise in renin and hence of the pressor peptide angiotensin II can influence the final blood pressure achieved. Evidence of this was clearly shown by Richards *et al.*[5], changes in blood pressure induced by salt restriction being closely proportional (r = 0.75) to the concomitant changes in plasma renin activity. Thus, those persons in the trial whose blood pressure fell with sodium restriction had little or no change in plasma renin, whereas those whose blood pressure increased in response to sodium deprivation had the greatest corresponding rise in plasma renin.

Reinforcing these arguments are studies where dietary salt restriction has been tried in the prevention of essential hypertension. Several such trials have failed to show evidence of benefit.

On present evidence therefore it appears to me that the employment of dietary salt restriction in the treatment of hypertension should be circumspect. It is worth noting some of the conclusions of Richards *et al.*[5], who admitted they had embarked on their study expecting to show blood pressure reduction with salt restriction. Interpreting their negative results they made the following points: 'Proponents of widespread sodium restriction should be obliged to demonstrate (a) that the tiny overall reduction in blood pressure is of benefit to the patients; (b) that the increase in blood pressure in a sizeable minority of patients is not harmful; and (c) that the dietary manipulation is not in some unexpected way disadvantageous'.

Conclusions. My own views, in interpreting the present evidence, can be summarized as follows:- 1. Tolerable and realistic dietary salt restriction (i.e. down to some 60–100 mmol/day) probably is effective in lowering blood pressure in a substantial number of patients with moderately severe essential hypertension (i.e. with a fifth phase diastolic of around 110 mm Hg and upwards). This benefit is not seen in every case but is often useful and may reinforce the antihypertensive effect of drugs. I think that the value of such salt restriction in supervised patients is worthy of a strict long-term trial in which an assessment of morbidity and side-effects should be carried out, in much the same way as a study would be done using antihypertensive drugs. 2. The value of salt restriction in more mild hypertension is, as I have emphasised in this talk much more doubtful. Certainly the effects can vary greatly from one individual to another. This does not preclude a trial of such therapy provided the patient is kept under scrutiny and that appropriate action can be taken if there is a lack of response or an adverse effect. 3. The value of salt restriction as a preventive measure is quite uncertain. It is not supported by any controlled trial of which I am aware. Moreover it runs counter to strong theoretical arguments which I have advanced here. Thus although it has often been claimed that, even if salt restriction is without benefit, it is at least harmless, this claim is, I think, open to some doubt. In my view the application of salt restriction to whole unsupervised populations cannot be advocated with any confidence on present evidence.

1 Beretta-Piccoli, C., Davies, D.L., Boddy, K., Brown, J.J., Cumming, A.M.M., East, B.W., Fraser, R., Lever, A.F., Padfield, P.L., Semple, P.F., Weidmann, & P., Williams, E.D. (1982): Relation of arterial pressure with body sodium, body potassium and plasma potassium in essential hypertension. *Clinical Science* **63**, 257–270.
2 Beretta-Piccoli, C., Davies, D.L., Brown, J.J., Ferriss, J.B., Fraser, R., Lasaridis, A., Lever, A.F., Morton, J.J., Robertson, J.I.S., Semple, P.F., & Watt, R. (1983): Relation of blood pressure with body and plasma electrolytes in Conn's Syndrome. *Journal of Hypertension* **1**, 197–205.
3 Beretta-Piccoli, C., Boddy, K., Brown, J.J., Davies, D.L., East, B.W., Lever, A.F., McAreavey, D., Robertson, J.I.S. & Williams, E.D. (1984): Body sodium and potassium content in various hypertensive diseases: In ed Robertson, J.I.S., *Handbook of Hypertension, Vol. 1: Clinical Aspects of Essential Hypertension*. Elsevier, Amsterdam, pp. 267–277.
4 McAreavey, D., Brown, J.J., Cumming, A.M.M., Davies, D.L., Fraser, R., Lever, A.F., Mackay, A., Morton, J.J. & Robertson, J.I.S. (1983): Inverse relationship of exchangeable sodium and blood pressure in hypertensive patients with renal artery stenosis. *Journal of Hypertension* **1**, 297–302.
5 Richards, A.M., Nicholls, M.G., Espiner, E.A., Ikram, H., Maslowski, A.H., Hamilton, E.J. & Wells, J.E. (1984):

blood pressure response to moderate sodium restriction and potassium supplementation in essential hypertension. *Lancet* **1**, 757–761.

6 Robertson, J.I.S. (1984): The renin-aldosterone connection: past, present and future. *Journal of Hypertension* **2** (Suppl. 3): 1–14.

What have we achieved by changing dietary fat?

J.R.A. MITCHELL
Nottingham University Medical School, Nottingham, UK.

'The most costly of all follies is to believe passionately in the palpably-not true'. H.L. Mencken[4]

What matters to patients is death and disability, rather than mechanisms or theories. The studies which have linked diet and arterial disease have concentrated on coronary heart disease (CHD) and have virtually ignored stroke and limb artery disease despite the major contribution which these diseases make to the burden of suffering. Even in the field of CHD, we know less than many people think, so let us try to answer the questions our patients pose to us about the benefits which they can expect, in terms of prolongation of life and freedom from disability, if they follow the dietary advice which is now being so freely dispensed.

The theory. The chain of beliefs about diet and CHD runs as follows: — CHD is caused by atherosclerosis — Atherosclerotic plaques are cholesterol deposits in artery walls — A high serum cholesterol is a risk marker for CHD — Dietary lipids determine serum cholesterol…. Therefore: — Dietary lipids cause coronary heart disease — Dietary modifications will prevent coronary heart disease.

The facts. To those who keep saying that 'better eating prevents coronary disease' we can accept that anyone is entitled to his beliefs but that scientists should be expected to produce evidence. The only acceptable evidence is an adequately-conducted clinical trial in which the outcome of a group who were given dietary advice aimed at lowering their serum lipids can be compared with a group who were not. If coronary disease is very common and kills many of its victims, then a reduction in coronary disease should be reflected in a fall in total mortality. Valid trials which fulfil these criteria are few in number and can be divided into those which dealt only with lipids and those which aimed at changing multiple risk-factors.

Lipid-orientated studies. *The Los Angeles Veterans Administration (VA) Study*[1]. 846 men aged 55–89 living in a VA centre were randomly allocated to receive a low-cholesterol, low-saturated-fat, high-polyunsaturated diet, or to continue on the ordinary North American diet. The experimental group reduced their serum cholesterol by 13 per cent during the 8-year follow-up period; the total deaths were 177 in the control group and 174 in the cholesterol-lowered group although the total mortality concealed a suggestion of a reduction in CHD deaths and an increase of 12 per cent in non-cardiovascular system (CVS) deaths.

The Finnish Mental Hospitals Study[10]. Two mental hospitals were used; one continued its normal diet for 6 years while the other adopted a diet similar to the Los Angeles VA Trial. After 6 years, the hospitals switched their dietary styles, but a constant stream of patients had been moving through them for reasons which were nothing to do with the purposes of the trial. The calculations needed to relate the end-points to the exposure-period of the trial were therefore very complex. Cholesterol was reduced by 15 per cent in the experimental-diet periods but there was no significant effect on total mortality (34.8 per 1000 person-years in the cholesterol-reduced periods versus 39.5 in the control). As in the VA trial, within an unchanged total mortality there was reduction in CVS-attributed events which was balanced by an increase of 15 per cent in non-CVS deaths.

Multiple risk-factor trials. *The North Karelia Project*[8]. Because Finland had the highest CHD mortality in the world, a community-based multiple-risk factor reduction strategy was adopted in North Karelia while the adjacent province of Kuopio served as a non-intervention control. In North Karelia there was an aggregated reduction of the main risk factors by 17 per cent and the outcome is set out in Table 1. On their original trial design, the comparison between the designated test and control areas is non-significant; to get a difference which is significant, one has to go beyond the original design ('data-dredging') to show that men in Karelia fared better in respect of CHD than in the rest of the country, minus Karelia. Women were no different on any analysis. In respect of total mortality, no demonstrable benefit emerged for any group.

Table 1. *North Karelia Study*. Average annual regression-based percentage decline in age-standardised CHD mortality in 1974–1979 (95 per cent confidence limits)

Area	*Men*	*Women*
North Karelia	3.7 (1.5)	2.2 (3.4)
Control area — Kuopio	1.9 (2.3)	1.8 (1.4)
Finland except North Karelia	1.7 (2.2)	1.2 (2.4)

Table 2. *Results of MR FIT after 7 years.*

	Special intervention	*Usual care*
Total mortality/1000	41.2	40.4
CHD mortality/1000	17.9	19.3

The Oslo Study[2]. From 16 202 men aged 40–49, 1232 healthy men with elevated lipid levels were randomised into a 5-year study in which the intervention men were asked to stop smoking and to reduce their lipids by dietary means. During the trial, mean tobacco consumption per man fell 45 per cent more in the intervention than the control group while the fall in cholesterol was only 13 per cent greater in the intervention group. Had significant differences in outcome emerged, it would thus have been difficult to disentangle the benefit of stopping smoking from any effect of lipid reduction. However, the trial results were not conclusive (total mortality: control — 38 per 1000; intervention — 26 per 1000 which was not significant; fatal and non-fatal infarction plus sudden death was 47 per cent lower in the intervention group; $P < 0.03$).

The United States Multiple Risk-Factor Intervention Trial (MR FIT)[5] took 12 886 high-risk men and randomly allocated half to a special intervention group (SI) who had a programme of advice aimed to reduce blood pressure, smoking and plasma lipids, to conquer obesity and to increase physical activity. The comparative group, who knew of course that they were 'high risk' were simply sent back to their doctors for 'usual care' (UC), but as in Finland, this 'control, group changed their behaviour markedly, so both groups showed a fall in plasma lipids. Table 2 shows the end-result, in that the 'got-at' men did slightly worse in terms of overall mortality than the 'laissez-faire' men. As Oliver[6] observes of the trial: 'No amount of dredging of the data will turn it into a conclusive one. It is more honest to accept that multiple risk factor intervention, under the circumstances of this trial, did not work, than to say it might have worked.'

WHO European Collaborative Group Study[11]. 49 781 men aged 40–59 working in 66 factories were recruited. The factories were paired and one of each pair was randomly allocated to receive special intervention. Within an intervention factory the intention was to lower cholesterol by diet, to reduce smoking and weight, to increase physical activity and to control high blood pressure.

   Table 3 shows how the risk factors changed and the effect on the pre-determined end-points. Special intervention is clearly bad news for Britons in that they fared worse in all end-points than their fellows who were left alone. In the light of these findings it is astonishing that Rose *et al.*[9] 'reach the remarkable conclusion from the entirely negative UK section of the WHO study that effective multiple risk factor control probably works and that the problem now is how to get the message through to the public'[7].

Non-dietary trials. *The Lipid Research Clinics Program*[3]. Although a drug (oral cholestyramine) was used to lower serum lipids, the presentation of the results makes reference to the role of diet, so scrutiny of the trial is justifiable. They screened 480 000 men and identified the 3806 with cholesterol levels in the top 5 per cent of the distribution. These men were all given

Table 3. *Effects of intervention on risk factors and in outcome (per cent change compared with controls) in WHO factory study.*

Risk factors	UK	Belgium	Italy	Outcome	UK	Belgium	Italy
Cholesterol	−0.4	−0.9	−4.8	Fatal CHD	+8	−21	−30
Cigarettes/day	−15.6	−3.7	−5.5	Total CHD	+5	−24	−14
Weight	−0.4	+0.2	−1.9	Total mortality	+14	−17	−6
Systolic BP	−1.6	−2.3	−4.1				

cholesterol-lowering diets and only those whose serum lipids did not fall to predetermined levels went on into the drug-related phase of the study. Thus the trial results are based on diet-resistant patients who were then followed for a mean of 7.4 years. The total deaths in the cholestyramine-treated group ($n = 1906$) were 68 and 71 in the placebo group ($n = 1900$) so screening half-a-million men and subjecting nearly 2000 of them to 'treatment' for 7 years has 'saved' three lives. The trial organizers clearly perceived the unacceptability of a drug-based approach so wrote 'the LRC-CPPT results and those of similar trials thus suggest that the risk of an initial CHD episode in hypercholesterolaemic middle-aged men can be reduced by half with currently available appropriate cholesterol-lowering agents and diets' even though their trial offers no evidence on the value of diet.

The bottom line. What interests patients is staying alive and free from disability. They are not interested in risk-markers such as blood-lipids and blood pressure but only in their effect and in the benefit which modification of these risk factors will confer on them.

Once we have told our patients to stop smoking, then as scientists we have a duty to keep our mouths shut in terms of CHD prevention. If we do not do so, and our patients challenge us to produce evidence that by following the advice currently being given about diet they will live longer or stay free from clinical CHD, then we cannot do so.

1 Dayton, S., Pearce, M.L., Hashimoto, S., Dixon, W.J. & Tomiyasu, U. (1969): A controlled clinical trial of a diet high in unsaturated fat. *Circulation* **40** (Suppl. 2) 1–63.
2 Hjermann, I., Holme, I., Byre, K.V. & Leren, P. (1981): Effect of diet and smoking intervention on the incidence of coronary heart disease. *Lancet* **2**, 1303–1310.
3 Lipid Research Clinics Program (1984): The lipid research clinics coronary primary prevention trial results I. Reduction in incidence of coronary heart disease. *J. Am. Med. Ass.* **251**, 351–74.
4 Mencken, H.L. (1980): *Quotations for our time*, ed L. Peter, p. 41. London: Magnum.
5 Multiple Risk Factor Intervention Trial Research Group. (1982): Multiple risk factor intervention trial. Risk factor changes and mortality results. *J. Am. Med. Ass.* **248**, 1465–1477.
6 Oliver, M.F. (1983): Should we not forget about mass control of coronary risk factors? *Lancet* **2**, 37–38.
7 Oliver, M.F. (1983): Targeting coronary risk factor control. *Lancet* **2**, 449–450.
8 Puska, P., Salonen, J.T., Tuomilehto, J., Issinen, A. & Koskela, K. (1983): Mass control of coronary risk factors. *Lancet* **2**, 406–407.
9 Rose, G., Tunstall-Pedoe, H.D. & Heller, R.F. (1983): UK Heart Disease Prevention Project: incidenece and mortality results. *Lancet* **1**, 1062–1065.
10 Turpeinen, O., Karvonen, M.K., Pekkarinen, M., Miettinen, M., Eluoso, R. & Paavilainen, E. (1979): Dietary prevention of coronary disease; the Finnish Mental Hospital Study. *Int. J. Epidemiol.* **8**, 99–118.
11 WHO European Collaborative Group. (1983): Multifactorial trial in the prevention of coronary disease 3. Incidence and mortality results. *Eur. Heart. J.* **4**, 141–147.

Effects of saponins in legumes on plasma lipids: a workshop report

D. G. OAKENFULL (Organizer)
CSIRO Division of Food Research, Food Research Laboratory, PO Box 52, North Ryde, NSW 2113, Australia.

The discussion centred on two basic question: (1) Do the saponins present in many legumes significantly lower plasma cholesterol concentrations and has this effect nutritional significance — particularly for those at risk from heart disease? (2) Which are the areas where more research is most urgently needed?

A brief review was given of the experimental evidence that purified saponins fed to animals produce lower concentrations of cholesterol and triglycerides in the blood plasma. The mechanism of the effect depends on the detailed chemical structure of the saponin. Some saponins form non-absorbable complexes with cholesterol; others block reabsorption of bile acids by forming large mixed micelles.

The possible toxicity of saponins was discussed. We agreed that, although large doses of purified saponins could be harmful, saponins are clearly not detrimental when consumed as normal components of foods such as soya beans and chickpeas. Also in this connection, the food use of mahua flowers (*Bassia latifolia*) was discussed. These saponin-containing flowers are rich in carbohydrate. They are used as an 'emergency' food in India but often produce adverse reactions. We agreed that the traditional practice of not giving them to small children or pregnant women was very sound.

Some areas suggested for further research were: (1) the dose-response relationships, (2) the effects of saponins on the various secretions of the gastro-intestinal tract, (3) the possible synergistic interactions of saponins with other dietary components, and (4) the use of isotopically labelled saponins to explore their metabolic fate and check the extent to which they remain within the gastro-intestinal tract. A point that we felt should be emphasised, though, is that saponins are an enormous and diverse class of compounds. It is important not to generalise. In conclusion, we agree that beans are excellent food. Their consumption in Western countries should be encouraged!

Diet and blood pressure: a workshop report

P. BURSZTYN (Organizer)
University of Southampton, U.K.

Participants: Elizabeth Barrett-Connor, University of California, La Jolla, USA; G. Beevers, University of Birmingham, UK; M. Burr, MRC Epidemiology Unit, Cardiff, UK; P. Dodson, University of Birmingham, UK; A. Gairard, Universite Louis Pasteur, Strasbourg, France; J. Iacono, USDA Human Nutrition Center, San Francisco, USA; N. Karanja, Oregon Health Sciences, University, Portland, USA; A. Klatsky, Permanente Medical Group, Oakland, California, USA; B. Margetts, MRC Epidemiology Unit, Perth, Australia; J. Swales, University of Leicester, UK and J. Villar, Instituto de Nutricion de Centro America y Panama.

The influence of diet on blood pressure was recognised early in this century with two observations: (a) blood pressure was found to be related to salt intake, and (b) vegetarians' blood pressures increased when they were given an omnivore diet. These observations have since been repeated and expanded.

Today, we recognise that other dietary constituents may influence blood pressure. The workshop discussed: vegetarian diets, fibre, fats and fatty acids, alcohol, sodium, calcium, and the use of dietary treatment for hypertension.

Vegetarian diets. The effects of vegetarian diets on blood pressure are well-documented. People habitually consuming vegetarian diets have lower blood pressures than their omnivore neighbours[1], and omnivores taking a vegetarian diet experimentally exhibit a decrease in blood pressure. Some of the constituents of a vegetarian diet which might be responsible for this effect are a high fibre intake, less energy from fats, more of which are polyunsaturated, and the type of protein consumed.

Swales adds that vegetarians are typically leaner and lighter than omnivores, and this might be partly responsible for their lower blood pressures. There is also a possibility that cultural or religious factors often associated with vegetarian diets may play a role in maintaining their low blood pressures, although the results of Armstrong *et al.*[1] suggest that this effect is not very important.

Fibre. *Burr's* recent survey of patrons of health-food shops indicated that blood pressures were related to total fibre intake and cereal fibre intake, but not to vegetarianism[2]. In a companion survey of the general population, blood pressures were found to be related to vegetarianism and to fibre intake. Both surveys also uncovered an independent association between fibre intake and heart rate.

Dietary manipulation experiments have shown that increasing fibre intake lowers the blood pressure and *vice versa*[3]. However, dietary manipulations carried out independently by *Burr's* group in Cardiff and *Margetts'* group in Perth have failed to confirm this effect.

Margetts emphasised that a vegetarian diet is not just high in fibre. Other factors could be responsible, singly or in combination, for lowering blood pressure.

Protein. Dietary protein differs markedly between vegetarians and omnivores. *Bursztyn* presented data which showed that changes in protein source (casein, fish meal, or soya meal) had no effect on the blood pressures of rabbits, either in low fat or high fat (mildly hypertensive) diets[4]. In addition, substituting textured vegetable protein (soya) for a quarter of the protein intake of omnivore human volunteers for 6 weeks had no effect on their blood pressures. Although these results are not conclusive, because of the large number of proteins which might be tested, it is felt that protein type is unlikely to have an effect on blood pressure.

Fats and fatty acids. *Iacono* has shown that reducing dietary fat intake and replacing some saturated fat with polyunsaturated fat together reduce blood pressures in normo-tensive volunteers[5]. He suggests that this is partly due to changes in prostaglandin metabolism resulting from the changed P/S ratio in the diet.

Margetts criticised this point because he found that replacing saturated fat with polyunsaturated fat for periods of 6 weeks had no effect either on thromboxane release from stimulated platelets, or on the blood pressures of normotensive volunteers[6].

Several workers have suggested that dietary linoleic and γ-linolenic acid lower blood pressure in rats with various types of experimental hypertension. *Bursztyn* presented data showing that four fat-enriched diets differing in linoleic and linolenic acid content were almost equally hypertensive in rabbits. Although the diet containing both linoleic and γ-linolenic acid was marginally less pressor than the others, it could not be called antihypertensive.

Alcohol. Most of the epidemiological evidence agrees that alcohol intake correlates positively with blood pressure. *Klatsky* estimated that a minimum of 5 per cent of American hypertension is alcohol-related[7]. A relatively modest intake of 3–4 drinks per day is sufficient to increase the blood pressure, although lower intakes of alcohol may have no effect, or even reduce blood pressure. It was also noted that alcohol intake estimated from population surveys is half that estimated from sales data.

The mechanism by which moderate alcohol ingestion may increase blood pressure has been difficult to discover, although a relationship was found between plasma cortisol concentrations and systolic pressure in heavy drinkers[8]. Most workers have failed to find any associations between pressor hormones and either chronic or acute alcohol ingestion in moderate drinkers. *Beevers* presented evidence that both renin and noradrenalin were elevated in hypertensive subjects consuming alcoholic beer compared to those consuming alcohol-free beer.

Sodium. *Swales* asked whether we ought to recommend population education on sodium intake. Realistic reductions in sodium intake will generally lower only high blood pressures. The reduction which can be achieved is likely to be modest. However, even if mean population blood pressures drop by only 5 per cent over 20–30 years this should have a beneficial effect on mortality. This will operate by preventing or attenuating the development of high blood pressure among salt-sensitive individuals in the population. A reduction in the sodium intake of hypertensive patients will probably not replace drug treatment, but it may control modest elevations of blood pressure, and reduce the amount of medication required for control of more severe hypertension.

The point was raised that low sodium intakes have been shown to increase blood pressure in experimental animals. However, it was agreed that the relatively modest reduction in sodium intake proposed by *Swales* would not have this effect.

Calcium. Hypertensives tend to have lower calcium intakes than normotensives. *Barrett-Connor*[9] and others[10] have shown that blood pressure is negatively related to calcium intake in random samples of the population. The bulk of American calcium intake is obtained from dairy products, much of which is taken as whole milk. Although milk consumption is inversely related to age and to alcohol intake, the negative association between dietary calcium and blood pressure remains when the data are corrected for age and alcohol intake, and for other factors.

Gairard, working on spontaneously hypertensive rats, showed that hypertension is enhanced by a calcium-free diet and reduced (though not prevented) by a high calcium diet[11]. He suggests that the hypertension may be associated with high concentrations of intracellular calcium in arterial smooth muscle. Low calcium diets stimulate parathyroid calcium concentrations and blood pressure. Moreover, parathyroid ablation lowers both intracellular calcium and blood pressure.

Karanja argued that the relationship between blood pressure and calcium intake may be due to an associated factor, such as a class of food. To test this, hypertensive rat pups were born to dams which were fed either high or low calcium diets. The pups were then given to either high or low calcium dams, giving four groups of pups. Pups from high calcium dams had lower blood pressures than those from low calcium dams. Pups suckled by high calcium dams had lower blood pressure than those suckled by low calcium dams.

Karanja also described a clinical trial in which hypertensive patients were given calcium supplements. Blood pressures fell in those receiving additional calcium, but only after 6 weeks.

Several years ago, a clinical trial showed that the blood pressures of normotensive volunteers could be reduced by the ingestion of calcium supplements[12]. *Villar* presented new results in which the blood pressures of pregnant women given calcium supplements were decreased. The effect was seen only in women given 2 g/d or 1.5 g/d. Those given 1 g/d had similar blood pressures to women not given calcium.

Dietary treatment for hypertension. Dietary manipulations may reduce blood pressures in hypertensive as well as normotensive individuals. However, the effects of a particular dietary manoeuvre are generally small and inadequate as an antihypertensive treatment. *Dodson* compared the effects of a dietary regime combining raised fibre and reduced fat and sodium intake, with the results of thiazide therapy in 50 diabetic hypertensives. Both the dietary regime and thiazide therapy produced comparable reductions in blood pressure. Moreover, thiazide treatment worsened glycaemic control while the modified diet improved it, and also promoted weight loss[13].

The main benefit of diet modifications as a treatment for hypertension lies in the absence of adverse side-effects and low cost. Even if the diet-induced reduction in blood pressure is small, it is likely that smaller doses of drugs will be required to control hypertension.

Recommendations. A low salt diet will often reduce high blood pressures, but genetic sensitivity plays a role in this response. On the other hand, diets low in fat-energy appear to decrease blood pressures in all individuals. High-fibre diets are associated with low blood pressures, although the evidence that adopting such a diet will reduce pressure is disputed. Reduction in alcohol consumption will reduce blood pressure, but only in heavy drinkers. There is also evidence that modest alcohol intake will lower blood pressure in teetotalers. Increased calcium intake reduces blood pressure, but in 'Western diets' calcium is often associated with fat and one must be wary of recommending any increase in our already high fat intake.

In conclusion, diet may play a role in determining the antihypertensive treatment. Hypertension is uncommon among vegetarians. However, apart from vegetarians, there is little evidence that prolonged adherence to a 'hypotensive' diet will prevent the development of hypertension.

Reference has been made to relevant work by participants in this workshop. The list is not intended to be comprehensive, but only to introduce the reader to the subject.

1 Armstrong, B.K., van Merwyk, A.J. & Coates, H. (1977): Blood pressure in Seventh-Day Adventist vegetarians. *Am. J. Epidemiol.* **105**, 444–449.
2 Burr, M.L., Sweetnam, P.M. & Barsai, M.E. (1985): Dietary fibre, blood pressure and plasma cholesterol. *Nutr. Res.* **5**, 465–472.
3 Wright, A., Bursztyn, P.G. & Gibney, M.J. (1979): Dietary fibre and blood pressure. *Br. Med. J.* **2**, 1541–1543.
4 Bursztyn, P.G. & Vas Dias, F.W. (In press): Dietary protein and blood pressure. *Clin Expt. Hypert.*
5 Iacono, J.M., Puska, P., Dougherty, R.M., Pietinen, P., Vartiainen, E., Leino, U., Mutanen, M. & Moisio, S. (1983): Effect of dietary fat on blood pressure in a rural Finnish population. *Am. J. Clin. Nutr.* **38**, 860–869.
6 Margetts, B.M., Beilin, L.J., Armstrong, B.K., Rouse, I.L., Vandongen, R., Croft, K.D. & McMurchie, E.J. (1985): Blood pressure and dietary polyunsaturated and saturated fats: a controlled trial. *Clin. Sci.* **69**, 165–175.
7 Friedman, G.D., Klatsky, A.L. & Steiglaub, M.S. (1982): Alcohol, tobacco and hypertension. *Hypertension* **4**, 43–50.
8 Bannan, L.T., Potter, J.F., Beevers, D.G., Saunders, J.B., Walters, J.R.F. & Ingram, M.C. (1984): Effect of alcohol withdrawal on blood pressure, plasma renin activity, aldosterone, cortisol and dopamine B-hydroxylase. *Clin. Sci.* **66**, 659–663.
9 Ackley, S., Barrett-Connor, E. & Suarez, L. (1983): Dairy products, calcium and blood pressure. *Am. J. Clin. Nutr.* **38**, 457–461.
10 McCarron, D.A., Morris, C.D. & Cole, C. (1982): Dietary calcium in human hypertension. *Science* **217**, 267–269.
11 Schleiffer, R., Pernot, F., Berthelot, A. & Gairard, A. (1984): Low calcium diet enhances development of hypertension in the spontaneously hypertensive rat. *Clin. Expt. Hypert.* **6**, 783–793.
12 Belizan, J.M., Villar, J., Pineda, O., Gonzalez, A.E., Sains, E., Garrera, G. & Siberiam, R. (1983): Reduction of blood pressure with calcium supplementation in young adults. *J. Am. Med. Ass.* **249**, 1161–1165.
13 Pacey, P.J., Dodson, P.M., Kubicki, A.J., Fletcher, R.F. & Taylor, K.G. (1984): Comparison of the hypotensive and metabolic effects of Bendrofluazide therapy and a high fibre, low fat, low sodium diet in diabetic subjects with mild hypertension. *J. Hypert.* **2**, 215–220.

★   ★   ★

NUTRITIONAL FACTORS IN CARCINOGENESIS

Nutrition and cancer — the research problems

K.K. CARROLL
Department of Biochemistry, University of Western Ontario, London, Ontario, Canada N6A 5C1.

Evidence relating nutrition to cancer. The first clear evidence that nutrition can significantly influence carcinogenesis came from experiments on animals carried out more than 40 years ago[22]. These showed that factors such as energy intake and level of fat in the diet had very marked effects on tumour incidence in animals.

The recent resurgence of interest in nutrition and cancer stems largely from epidemiological data that have shown large intercountry variations in cancer incidence and mortality[19,23]. Studies on migrating populations have indicated that these variations are due mainly to environmental factors rather than heredity, since the pattern of cancer in emigrants tends to change from that of their country of origin to that of their newly-adopted country[12].

Nutrition is thought to be one of the more important factors influencing carcinogenesis because of the results obtained from experiments on animals and because of correlations between nutrition and cancer observed in epidemiological studies[10]. One should be cautious in extrapolating results of experiments on animals to humans, but such results can help to decide whether correlations observed in epidemiological data are meaningful or merely fortuitous. Experiments with animals can also provide guide-lines for further epidemiological studies and clinical trials related to cancer, and can give clues to mechanisms by which specific components of the diet may influence carcinogenesis. It would be difficult to determine the details of mechanisms of action solely from studies on humans.

Nature of the process of carcinogenesis. Experiments on skin cancer in the 1940s by Berenblum and others led to the concept of cancer as a two-stage process[4]. The first stage, initiation, is believed to involve the transformation of a normal cell to a pre-neoplastic cell, due to a change in its genome, as a result of interaction with a carcinogenic agent. This change is thought to occur rapidly and to be essentially irreversible. Initiation is followed by a second stage, referred to as promotion, during which the pre-neoplastic cell and others derived from it are greately influenced by environmental factors which may either enhance or impede their proliferation to form a tumour. This concept is now generally accepted and is probably characteristic of many kinds of cancer[13].

It seems probable that tumours arise in each case from a single cell and diversify during development. This diversification can lead to changes that alter the characteristics of the tumour in what has been referred to as progression[11]. This diversification in tumours may be a result of cell–cell interactions that influence gene expression, or of further changes in the genome of cells forming part of the clone derived from the original transformed cell. Such changes could be caused by exposure to mutagenic agents. It is also possible that the original transformation imparts an instability to the genome that makes it more susceptible to additional changes.

Nutritional modification of carcinogenesis. As outlined briefly above, it now appears that carcinogenesis is a multistage process, and it is pertinent to consider how the different stages of this process may be influenced by nutrition. In the past, much attention has been given to environmental carcinogens and mutagens in the environment, including the food supply. This is appropriate since the development of a cancer requires some type of initiating event.

A number of naturally-occurring carcinogens and mutagens have been identified in foodstuffs[2,10]. Others can be formed during cooking or other processing of foods for consumption[21].

It is important to know as much as possible about the carcinogens and mutagens to which people are exposed, but intervention at the promotional stage of carcinogenesis may be a more hopeful approach than attempting to prevent formation of initiated cells. So many mutagenic agents are known to exist that it is difficult to see how they can be avoided, or to identify those that are mainly responsible for initiating the kinds of cancer that lead to high mortality.

The promotional stage of carcinogenesis occupies a much longer time span during which the process is considered to be potentially reversible, particularly in the early stages after initiation. The evidence that is accumulating indicates that nutritional factors, particularly fat, fibre, retinoids and salt, may play an especially important role during this phase of carcinogenesis.

Aims of research on nutrition and cancer. A major incentive for research on nutrition and cancer is the hope that it will provide means of reducing the high morbidity and mortality due to cancer. Effects of dietary components on carcinogenesis in experimental animals can suggest leads to possible means of influencing cancer in humans. It is desirable to consider the results of such studies in relation to epidemiological data on human populations, because of uncertainties in extrapolating from animal models to humans. If the results of experimental and epidemiological data both lead to the same conclusion, the evidence is obviously much stronger than if they point to different conclusions with respect to the effects of any particular dietary ingredient.

Another goal of research on nutrition and cancer is to determine the mechanism involved. Studies on experimental animals appear to offer the most promising approach to this objective. A brief consideration of studies dealing with effects of dietary fat on mammary carcinogenesis will serve to illustrate progress in this direction.

Dietary fat and mammary carcinogenesis. High-fat diets clearly promote mammary tumorigenesis in experimental animals, provided that the fat contains a sufficient level of polyunsaturated fatty acids[8,14] and various mechanisms have been suggested[7,15]. Hormonal mechanisms have been studied extensively[24] but now appear less likely. The requirement for polyunsaturated fatty acids suggests that promotion of mammary carcinogenesis may be mediated by prostaglandins or other biologically-active eicosanoids derived from such fatty acids. This idea has received support from experiments showing that the effect of dietary fat can be counteracted by inhibitors of prostaglandin biosynthesis[1,9].

Recent experiments have shown that polyunsaturated fish oils have a suppressive effect rather than promoting mammary tumorigenesis[5,16,17]. The polyunsaturated fatty acids of fish oil belong mainly to the n-3 linolenate family whereas linoleate (n-6) is the main polyunsaturated fatty acid in vegetable oils. The n-3 and n-6 fatty acids are precursors of two different series of eicosanoids with differing biological properties and compete for enzymes that catalyze the formation of these compounds[20]. The fact that fish oils and vegetable oils have differing effects on mammary carcinogenesis is another indication that eicosanoids may be involved.

Theories are also being proposed with regard to the mechanism of action at the cellular level. There appear to be important interactions between the glandular tissue and the adipose tissue of the mammary gland[6]. A mechanism by which the transfer of polyunsaturated fatty acids from adipose tissue to epithelial tissue may lead to proliferation of the latter has recently been suggested[18]. Another possibility, involving alterations in intercellular communication, has been suggested[3]. Further experimental work should help to elucidate the mechanism of action of dietary fat in animal models. Such knowledge will be useful in attempts to reduce breast cancer incidence and mortality in human populations by dietary means.

Acknowledgement. Studies on nutrition and cancer in our laboratory are supported by the National Cancer Institute of Canada.

1 Abraham, S. & Hillyard, L.A. (1983): Lipids, lipogenesis, and the effects of dietary fat on growth in mammary tumor model systems. In *Dietary fats and health*, ed E.G. Perkins & W.J. Visek, pp. 817–853. Champaign, IL: American Oil Chemists' Society.

2 Ames, B.N. (1983): Dietary carcinogens and anticarcinogens. *Science* **221**, 1256–1264.

3 Aylsworth, C.F., Jone, C., Trosko, J.E., Meites, J. & Welsch, C.W. (1984): Promotion of 7,12-dimethylbenz(a)anthracene-induced mammary tumorigenesis by high dietary fat in the rat: possible role of intercellular communication *J. Nat. Cancer Inst.* **72**, 637–645.

4 Berenblum, I. (1979): Theoretical and practical aspects of the two-stage mechanism of carcinogenesis. In *Carcinogens: identification and mechanisms of action*, ed A.C. Griffin & C.R. Shaw, pp. 25–36. New York: Raven Press.

5 Carroll, K.K. & Braden, L.M. (1985): Dietary fat and mammary carcinogenesis. *Nutr. Cancer* **6**, 254–259.

6 Carroll, K.K., Gammal, E.B. & Plunkett, E.R. (1968): Dietary fat and mammary cancer *Can Med. Ass. J.* **98**, 590–594.

7 Carroll, K.K., Hopkins, G.J., Kennedy, T.G. & Davidson, M.B. (1981): Essential fatty acids in relation to mammary carcinogenesis. *Prog. Lipid Res.* **20**, 685–690.

8 Carroll, K.K. & Khor, H.T. (1971): Effects of level and type of dietary fat on incidence of mammary tumors induced in female Sprague-Dawley rats by 7,12-dimethylbenz(α)anthracene. *Lipids* **6**, 415–420.

9 Carter, C.A., Milholland, R.J., Shea, W. & Ip, M.M. (1983): Effect of the prostaglandin synthetase inhibitor indomethacin on 7,12-dimethylbenz(a)anthracene-induced mammary tumorigenesis in rats fed different levels of fat. *Cancer Res.* **43**, 3559–3562.

10 Committee on Diet, Nutrition, and Cancer (1982): *Diet, nutrition, and cancer*. Washington DC: National Academy Press.

11 Foulds, L. (1969): *Neoplastic development*, Vol. 1. New York: Academic Press.

12 Gori, G.B. (1978): Diet and nutrition in cancer causation. *Nutr. Cancer* **1**, 5–8.

13 Hecker, E., Fusenig, N.E., Kunz, W., Marks, F. & Thielmann, H.W. (1982): *Carcinogenesis: a comprehensive survey, Vol. 7. Cocarcinogenesis and biological effects of tumor promoters*. New York: Raven Press.

14 Hopkins, G.J. & Carroll, K.K. (1979): Relationship between amount and type of dietary fat in promotion of mammary carcinogenesis induced by 7,12-dimethylbenz(a)anthracene *J. Nat. Cancer Inst.* **62**, 1009–1012.

15 Hopkins, G.J. & West, C.E. (1976): Possible roles of dietary fats in carcinogenesis. *Life Sci.* **19**, 1103–1116.

16 Jurkowski, J.J. & Cave, W.T. Jr. (1984): Dietary effects of a n-3 polyunsaturated lipid (menhaden oil) on the growth and membrane composition of rat mammary tumors. *Proc. Am. Assoc. Cancer Res.* **25**, 210.

17 Karmali, R.A., Marsh, J. & Fuchs, C. (1984): Effect of omega-3 fatty acids on growth of a rat mammary tumor. *JNCI* **73**, 457–461.

18 Kidwell, W.R. & Shaffer, J. (1984): Growth stimulatory activity of unsaturated fatty acids for normal and neoplastic breast epithelium. *J. Am. Oil Chemists' Soc.* **61**, 1900–1904.

19 Kurihara, M., Aoki, K. & Tominaga, S. (1984): *Cancer mortality statistics in the world*. Nagoya: Univ. of Nagoya Press.

20 Oliw, E., Granstrom, E. & Anggard, E. (1983): The prostaglandins and essential fatty acids. In *New comprehensive biochemistry. Vol. 5. Prostaglandins and related substances*, ed C. Pace-Asciak & E. Granstrom, pp. 1–44. Amsterdam: Elsevier.

21 Sugimura, T., Kawachi, T., Nagao, M. & Yahagi, T. (1981): Mutagens in food as causes of cancer. In *Nutrition and cancer: etiology and treatment*, ed G.R. Newell & N.M. Ellison, pp. 59–71. New York: Raven Press.

22 Tannenbaum, A. (1947): The role of nutrition in the origin and growth of tumors. In *Approaches to tumor chemotherapy*, ed F.R. Moulton, pp. 96–127. Washington DC: American Association for the Advancement of Science.

23 Waterhouse, J., Muir, C., Shanmugaratnam, K., Powell, J., Peacham, D., Whelen, S. and Davis, W. (1982): *Cancer incidence in five continents, Vol. IV. IARC Sci. Publ. No. 42*. Lyon: International Agency for Research on Cancer.

24 Welsch, C.W. & Aylsworth, C.F. (1983): Enhancement of murine mammary tumorigenesis by feeding high levels of dietary fat: a hormonal mechanism? *J. Nat. Cancer Inst.* **70**, 215–221.

Carcinogenicity of mutagens formed during cooking

S. SATO

Biochemistry Division, National Cancer Center Research Institute, 1–1, Tsukiji 5-chome, Chuo-ku, Tokyo 104, Japan.

We found that when fish or meat were broiled or fried, they exert marked mutagenicity detected by *Salmonella typhimurium* TA98 with metabolic activation[1,2]. Mutagen formation was also observed when various amino acids or proteins were pyrolysed[4]. From these cooked foods and amino acid and protein pyrolysates, a series of mutagenic heterocyclic amines have been isolated[13,14]. This article presents data on the carcinogenicity of these mutagenic heterocyclic amines in mice and rats.

Mutagenicity of heterocyclic amines. These heterocyclic amines show marked mutagenicity as shown in Table 1. They exert mutagenicity especially on *S. typhimurium* TA98 with metabolic activation[13,14].

Table 1. *Mutagenic activities of heterocyclic amines towards two strains of* S. typhimurium *with S9 mix.*

Mutagen (abbreviations: below)	Mutagenic activity (revertants/µg)	
	Strain TA98	Strain TA100
IQ	433 000	7000
MeIQ	661 000	30 000
MeIQx	145 000	14 000
Trp-P-1	39 000	1700
Trp-P-2	104 200	1800
Glu-P-1	49 000	3200
Glu-P-2	1900	1200
AαC	300	20
MeAαC	200	120

IQ, 2-amino-3-methylimidazo[4,5-*f*]quinoline; MeIQ, 2-amino-3,4-dimethylimidazo[4,5-*f*]quinoline; MeIQx, 2-amino-3,8-dimethylimidazo[4,5-*f*]quinoxaline; Trp-P-1, 3-amino-1,4-dimethyl-5*H*-pyrido[4,3-*b*]indole; Trp-P-2, 3-amino-1-methyl-5*H*-pyrido[4,3-*b*]indole; Glu-P-1, 2-amino-6-methyldipyrido[1,2-*a*:3′,2′-*d*]imidazole; Glu-P-2, 2-aminodipyrido[1,2-*a*:3′,2′-*d*]imidazole; AαC, 2-amino-9*H*-pyrido[2,3-*b*]indole or 2-amino-α-carboline; MeAαC, 2-amino-3-methyl-9*H*-pyrido[2,3-*b*]indole or 2-amino-3-methyl-α-carboline.

Carcinogenicity of heterocyclic amines in mice and rats. Carcinogenicity of IQ, MeIQ and MeIQx (see Table 1 for abbreviations) in mice is summarized in Table 2[5,6,10]. Induced tumours in the liver were, histologically, hepatocellular carcinomas and hepatocellular adenomas. Squamous cell carcinomas and papillomas in the forestomach were also induced by IQ and MeIQ. Lung tumours induced by IQ were adenocarcinomas and adenomas. About half of squamous cell carcinomas in the forestomach induced by MeIQ metastasized to the liver.

Table 2. *Carcinogenicity of IQ, MeIQ and MeIQx (abbreviations as in Table 1) in CDF$_1$ mice.*

Compound	Sex	No. of animals examined	Liver	Forestomach	Intestine	Lung
IQ	M	39	16	16	3	27
(0.03%)	F	36	27	11	0	15
MeIQ	M	38	7	35	15	12
(0.04%)	F	39	27	34	6	7
MeIQx[a]	M	37	14	1	0	12
(0.06%)	F	38	30	0	1	14
None	M	33	3	1	0	7
	F	38	3	0	0	7

The "No. of mice with tumours" spans the Liver, Forestomach, Intestine and Lung columns.

[a]Result of macroscopical observation.

In F344 rats fed 0.3g IQ/kg diet, hepatocellular carcinomas, adenocarcinomas in the small and large intestines, as well as their corresponding benign tumours and squamous cell carcinomas in the Zymbal gland, clitoral gland, skin and oral cavity, were induced as shown in Table 3[10,17]. When IQ was administered into SD rats by gavage, it was found to induce mammary carcinomas[18].

Table 3. *Numbers of F344 rats fed 0.3 g IQ/kg diet that developed tumours.*

Compound	Sex	Effective No. animals	Liver	Intestine Small	Intestine Large	Zymbal gland	Clitoral gland	Skin	Oral cavity
IQ	Male	40	27	12	25	36	–	17	2
	Female	40	18	1	9	27	20	3	1
None	Male	50	1	0	0	0	–	0	0
	Female	50	0	0	0	0	0	0	0

The results in CDF$_1$ mice with Trp-P-1, Trp-P-2, Glu-P-1, Glu-P-2, AαC are shown in Table 4[3,7,10]. The common target of their carcinogenicity is the liver where hepatocellular carcinomas and hepatocellular adenomas were induced by all these compounds. Blood vessel tumours were haemangioendothelial sarcomas and haemangioendotheliomas in the brown adipose tissue mainly at the interscapular region as well as in the pleural and abdominal cavities and axilla.

So far, our experiments in F344 rats have established the carcinogenicity of Trp-P-1, Glu-P-1 and Glu-P-2 as shown in Table 5[10,15,16]. Trp-P-1 induced hepatocellular carcinomas and hepatocellular adenomas. The spectrum and histological appearances of tumours by Glu-P-1 and Glu-P-2 were very similar to those by IQ. Tumourigenicity of Trp-P-2 in the liver of ACI rats has been reported[2].

Comments. All the heterocyclic amines so far tested proved carcinogenic in mice or rats or in both. In mice, liver tumours were induced by all the heterocyclic amines with a higher incidence in females than in males. The mechanisms of this sex difference are not yet clear, but the induction of enzymes involved in the metabolic activation of Trp-P-1 in the mouse liver by its feeding was found to be higher in females[1]. It is also noteworthy that IQ, Glu-P-1 and Glu-P-2 induced intestinal tumours in high frequency in rats. We have found a marked excretion of the metabolites of Glu-P-1 into the bile when it was administered into rats by gavage. Among the metabolites, N-acetyl-Glu-P-1, which is also mutagenic, was identified as well as the unchanged Glu-P-1[9]. A high rate of excretion of Glu-P-1 and its metabolites into the bile may somehow be involved in the development of intestinal tumours by this compound in rats.

The average TD$_{50}$ value for heterocyclic amines, ie the dose sufficient to give tumours in 50 per cent of animals when fed over their whole lives[8], was around 8 mg/kg per day[11]. The estimated human intake of heterocyclic amines through cooked food is much less than that and cannot by itself explain the occurrence of human cancers. For the evaluation of risk of these carcinogens for human cancer development, the effect of co-administration with other various

Table 4. *Carcinogenicity of Trp-P-1, Trp-P-2, Glu-P-1, Glu-P-2, AαC and MeAαC (see Table 1 for abbreviations) when fed to CDF$_1$ mice*

			No. mice with tumours	
Compound (g/kg)	Sex	No. animals	Liver	Blood vessel
Trp-P-1	M	24	5	0
(0.2)	F	26	16	0
Trp-P-2	M	25	3	0
(0.2)	F	24	22	0
Glu-P-1	M	34	4	30
(0.5)	F	38	37	31
Glu-P-2	M	37	10	27
(0.5)	F	36	36	20
AαC	M	38	15	20
(0.8)	F	34	33	6
MeAαC	M	37	21	35
(0.8)	F	33	28	28
None	M	39	0	0
	F	40	0	0

Table 5. *Carcinogenicity of Trp-P-1, Glu-P-1 and Glu-P-2 (see Table 1 for abbreviations) when fed to F344 rats*

				No. rats with tumours			
					Intestine			
Compound (g/kg)	Sex	Effective No.	Liver	Small	Large	Zymbal gland	Clitoral gland
Trp-P-1							
(0.15)	Male	40	30	1	2	0	–
(0.2)	Female	40	37	1	0	0	0
Glu-P-1	Male	42	35	26	19	18	–
(0.5)	Female	42	24	10	7	18	5
Glu-P-2	Male	42	11	14	6	1	–
(0.5)	Female	42	2	8	8	7	11
None	Male	50	2	0	0	0	–
	Female	50	0	0	0	0	0

environmental carcinogens or after treatment with various tumour promoters, simulating the human conditions should be carefully evaluated. The presence of exogenous and endogenous factors which inhibit the mutagenicity of heterocyclic amines should also be considered.

Acknowledgements — Our work was supported by grants from the Ministry of Health and Welfare and the Ministry of Education, Science and Culture, Japan.

1. Degawa, M., Kojima, M., Hishinuma, T. & Hashimoto, Y. (1985): Sex-dependent induction of hepatic enzymes for mutagenic activation of a tryptophan pyrolysate components, 2-amino-1,4-dimethyl-5*H*-pyrido[4,3-*b*]indole, by feeding in mice. *Cancer Res.* **45**, 96–102.
2. Hosaka, S., Matsushima, T., Hirono, I. & Sugimura, T. (1981): Carcinogenic activity of 3-amino-1-methyl-5*H*-pyrido[4,3-*b*]indole(Trp-P-2),. a pyrolysis product of tryptophan. *Cancer Lett.* **13**, 23–28.
3. Matsukura, N., Kawachi, T., Morino, K., Ohgakai, H., Sugimura, T. & Takayama, S. (1981): Carcinogenicity in mice of mutagenic compounds from a tryptophan pyrolyzate. *Science* **213**, 346–347.
4. Nagao, M., Yahagi, T., Kawachi, T., Seino, Y., Honda, M., Matsukura, N., Sugimura, T., Wakabayashi, K., Tsuji, K. & Kosuge, T. (1977): Mutagens in foods, and especially pyrolysis products of protein. In *Progress in genetic toxicology*, ed D. Scott, B.A. Bridges & F.H. Sobels, pp. 259–264. Amsterdam: Elsevier/North-Holland Biomedical Press.
5 Ohgaki, H., Hasegawa, H., Kato, T., Suenaga, M., Ubakata, M., Sato, S., Takayama, S. & Sugimura, T. (1985): Induction of tumors in the forestomach and liver of mice by feeding 2-amino-3,4-dimethylimidazo[4,5-*f*]quinoline (MeIQ). *Proc. Jpn Acad.* **61B**, 137–139.

6 Ohgaki, H., Kusama, K., Matsukura, N., Morino, K., Hasegawa, H., Sato, S., Sugimura, T. & Takayama, S. (1984): Carcinogenicity in mice of a mutagenic compound, 2-amino-3-methylimidazo[4,5-*f*]-quinoline, from broiled sardine, cooked beef and beef extract. *Carcinogenesis* **5**, 921–924.

7 Ohgaki, H., Matsukura, N., Morino, K., Kawachi, T., Sugimura, T. & Takayama, S. (1984): Carcinogenicity in mice of mutagenic compounds from glutamic acid and soybean globulin pyrolysates. *Carcinogenesis* **5**, 815–819.

8 Peto, R., Pike, M.C., Bernstein, L., Gold, L.S. & Ames, B.N. (1984): The TD_{50}: A proposed general convention for the numerical description of the carcinogenic potency of chemicals in chronic-exposure animal experiments. *Environmental Health Perspectives* **58**, 1–8.

9 Sato, S., Negishi, C., Umemoto, A. & Sugimura, T. (1985): Metabolic aspects of pyrolysis mutagens in foods. *Environmental Health Perspectives*. (In press).

10 Sugimura, T. (1985): Carcinogenicity of mutagenic heterocyclic amines formed during the cooking process. *Mutation Res.* **150**, 33–41.

11 Sugimura, T. (1985): Past, present and future on mutagens in cooked foods. *Environmental Health Perspectives*. (In press).

12 Sugimura, T., Nagao, M., Kawachi, T., Honda, M., Yahagi, T., Seino, Y., Sato, S., Matsukura, N., Matsushima, T., Shirai, A., Sawamura, M. & Matsumoto, H. (1977): Mutagen-carcinogens in food, with special reference to highly mutagenic pyrolytic products in broiled foods. In *Origins of human cancer*, Book C, ed H.H. Hiatt.

13 Sugimura, T. & Sato, S. (1983): Mutagens-carcinogens in foods. *Cancer Res. (Suppl.)* **43**, 2415s–2421s.

14 Sugimura, T. & Sato, S. (1983): Bacterial mutagenicity of natural materials, pyrolysis products and additives in foodstuffs and their association with genotoxic effects in mammals. In *Developments in the science and practice of toxicology*, ed A.W. Hayes, R.C. Schnell & T.S. Miya, pp. 115–133. Amsterdam: Elsevier.

15 Takayama, S., Ishikawa, T., Nakatsuru, Y., Sato, S. & Sugimura, T. (1985): Carcinogenicity in rats of a mutagenic compound from tryptophan pyrolysate. *Jpn J. Cancer Res. (Gann)* **76**, 815–817.

16 Takayama, S., Masuda, M., Mogami, M., Ohgaki, H., Sato, S. & Sugimura, T. (1984): Induction of cancers in the intestine, liver and various other organs of rats by feeding mutagens from glutamic acid pyrolysate. *Gann* **75**, 207–213.

17 Takayama, S., Nakatsuru, Y., Masuda, M., Ohgaki, H., Sato, S. & Sugimura, T. (1984): Demonstration of carcinogenicity in F344 rats of 2-amino-3-methylimidazo[4,5-*f*]quinoline from broiled sardine, fried beef and extract. *Gann* **75**, 467–470.

18 Tanaka, T., Barnes, W.S., Weisburger, J.H. & Williams, G.M. (1985): The fried food mutagen 2-amino-3-methyli-midazo[4,5-*f*]quinoline (IQ) is a powerful carcinogen for rat mammary gland. *Jpn J. Cancer Res. (Gann)* **76**, 570–576.

The modulation of carcinogenesis by retinoids

D.L. McCORMICK and R.C. MOON
Laboratory of Pathophysiology, IIT Research Institute Chicago, Illinois 60616, USA.

The potential for use of natural and synthetic vitamin A compounds (retinoids) to modify cancer induction in humans may best be addressed as three separate issues, determined by the vitamin A status and risk of tumour development in a particular population. These issues can be summarized as follows: (1) Can reversal of vitamin A deficiency reduce cancer incidence in underdeveloped areas of the world, where high rates of cancer are associated with marginal vitamin A status? (2) Can increased intake of vitamin A compounds reduce cancer incidence in populations which have no clinical evidence of vitamin A deficiency? (3) Can administration of retinoids at pharmacologic levels inhibit cancer induction in high-risk individuals whose vitamin A status is normal?

Data relevant to the first question, whether cancer rates can be lowered through reversal of vitamin A deficiency, comes from both experimental and epidemiological investigations. In general, such studies have found an increased susceptibility to carcinogenesis in individuals whose vitamin A intake is deficient or marginally deficient. In the 1920s, several investigators demonstrated independently that animals maintained on a diet deficient in vitamin A developed neoplastic and pre-neoplastic lesions in epithelial tissues; these lesions were not observed in parallel control groups maintained on a diet adequate in vitamin A[5,19,23]. Other workers have since reported reversal of such pre-neoplasias through the reversal of vitamin A deficiency[3]. Similarly, an increased tumour response has been found in experiments in which carcinogens were administered to animals maintained on diets deficient in vitamin A[4,21]; this general inverse relationship between vitamin A intake and cancer risk has been confirmed in epidemiologic studies conducted in populations whose vitamin A intake is low or marginal[20]. These data suggest that administration of vitamin A may reduce cancer risk in populations whose vitamin A status is deficient or marginal. It should be noted, however, that other disorders associated with vitamin A deficiency, such as night blindness and growth retardation, are likely to be more immediate and serious consequences of vitamin A deficiency in such populations than is a statistical increase in cancer risk.

The relationship between vitamin A intake and cancer risk in populations without frank vitamin A deficiency has been the subject of numerous epidemiological investigations over the past decade (for review, see[12]). In general, these studies have found that individuals with a relatively high intake of foods containing vitamin A or precursors are at a decreased risk of cancer in comparison to individuals consuming less of these foods. However, several limitations to the protective effects of vitamin A should be noted: First, the protection conferred is organ-specific: while consumption of high levels of vitamin A compounds appears to reduce risk of cancer induction in the lung, oral cavity, larynx, oesophagus, stomach, urinary bladder, prostate, ovary, and cervix, no such protection is seen against cancer of the colon. The source of such protection has not been identified with certainty; although several studies have noted protection conferred by consumption of preformed vitamin A, most evidence indicates that vitamin A precursors such as β-carotene are the most likely protective dietary component(s). Finally, due to homoeostatic regulation, serum retinol alone is unlikely to be an adequate indicator of vitamin A status in terms of predicting cancer risk. These limitations notwithstanding, a large body of epidemiological evidence suggests that increased consumption of vitamin A compounds can provide protection against cancer induction in specific target organs.

The final issue is whether synthetic retinoids will be effective in preventing cancer in individuals at high risk for the disease. In this instance, the requirement for retinoid administration, and the doses used, are essentially unrelated to nutritional requirements for vitamin A; synthetic retinoids are being used pharmacologically, at doses far in excess of requirements for normal physiologic function. In fact, certain synthetic retinoids may have no 'classical' vitamin A activity, as defined by maintenance of normal visual and growth processes.

Although clinical trials to determine the activity of synthetic retinoids in cancer prevention in humans are only in preliminary stages, the inhibition of carcinogenesis by synthetic vitamin A analogues has been studied extensively in experimental animals[16,17]. These experiments have demonstrated that a number of retinoids are effective in preventing tumours induced by agents as diverse as chemical carcinogens, radiation, and viruses. As was seen in the epidemiologic data regarding vitamin A intake and cancer, chemoprevention by retinoids is an organ-specific process: while apparently ineffective in preventing tumorigenesis in the colon, certain retinoids are highly active in cancer prevention in the skin, urinary bladder, oral cavity, pancreas, and mammary gland. Furthermore, individual retinoids show organ specificity in their activity; for example, while 13-*cis*-retinoic acid is highly effective in the prevention of experimental bladder cancer, it has little inhibitory activity against mammary carcinogenesis[17].

Retinoid chemoprevention has been studied extensively in carcinogen-induced adenocarcinoma of the rat mammary gland and the inhibition of retinyl acetate of mammary carcinogenesis induced by 7,12-dimethylbenz(a)anthracene (DMBA) has been reported[15]. While the levels of retinyl acetate used to achieve this inhibition were non-toxic, they were at least 40 times greater than the animals' normal physiological requirements. Several other retinoids have since been demonstrated to have chemopreventive activity in this target tissue[17]; notable among these compounds is the synthetic analogue, N-(4-hydroxyphenyl)-retinamide (4-HPR), an agent which has significant anticarcinogenic activity, but which is less toxic than natural vitamin A compounds[18].

Several experiments have been conducted in order to identify temporal requirements for retinoid modulation of mammary carcinogenesis. Retinoids can inhibit both the 'early' and 'late' stages of mammary cancer induction, phases which correspond to the period of carcinogen metabolism and target cell interaction, and tumour development and growth, respectively.

Chemoprevention of post-carcinogen tumour development appears to be a reversible phenomenon[8,22], since cessation of retinoid exposure is followed by loss of protection. Conversely, however, retinoid administration can be delayed significantly beyond carcinogen exposure and retain most or all of its anticarcinogenic activity[11]. These data suggest that retinoids may act to stabilize or reverse existing pre-neoplastic lesions, thereby preventing their progression into carcinoma.

Current work centres on mechanisms of retinoid anticarcinogenesis, delineation of retinoid metabolic pathways, and 'combination chemoprevention' studies which seek to increase the activity of cancer preventive regimens. Retinoids may act to prevent cancer through a variety of mechanisms, including influences on tissue differentiation, cell kinetics, host immune function, and a variety of biochemical pathways. Although retinoic-acid-binding protein (RABP) and retinol-binding protein (RBP) are present in many normal and neoplastic tissues[14], retinoids can influence growth, differentiation, and transformation in some cell lines which lack these binding proteins[6]. This suggests that, while RABP and RBP may be involved in the normal physiological and nutritional roles of vitamin A, levels of retinoid-binding proteins in a tissue or lesion may not be predictive of retinoid pharmacological activity in that tissue.

Pharmacological studies have focused on patterns of retinoid metabolism in various target tissues, in the effort to identify metabolites which may be involved in retinoid anticarcinogenesis. A novel polar metabolite has been isolated from mammary glands of rats treated with 4-HPR, and from mouse mammary glands exposed to 4-HPR in organ culture. Structural identification of this metabolite is being attempted.

Combination chemoprevention studies have been conducted in an effort to increase the efficacy of chemoprevention above that which has been achieved by retinoids alone. In addition, such studies can provide insight into mechanisms of anticarcinogenesis of the agents involved. Administration of retinyl acetate or 4-HPR in combination with bilateral ovariectomy resulted in a synergistic inhibition of mammary cancer induction[9,17]; an additive, but not synergistic, interaction was observed when 4-HPR was combined with the antiestrogen, tamoxifen[13]. Similarly, a retinoid administered with the phenolic antioxidant, BHT, resulted in an enhanced inhibition of carcinogenesis[10]. However, no such interaction was observed when 4-HPR was given in combination with MVE-2, an inducer of interferon biosynthesis[7]; this lack of activity may be due to retinoid transcriptional control of interferon synthesis, or inhibition of its activity[1,2]. These results indicate that retinoid chemopreventive activity can be increased through combined administration with other chemopreventive regimens. However, the data from the 4-HPR/MVE-2 study indicate that to obtain optimal anticarcinogenic efficacy, considerations of possibly confounding biological effects, as well as the putative anticarcinogenic mechanism(s) of both agents must be included in the design of such protocols.

1 Blalock, J.E. & Gifford, G.E. (1975): Inhibition of interferon action by vitamin A. *J. Gen. Virol.* **29**, 315–324.

2 Blalock, J.E. & Gifford, G.E. (1977): Retinoic acid (vitamin A acid) induced transcriptional control of interferon production. *Proc. Nat. Acad. Sci. USA* **74**, 5382–5386.

3 Chopra, D.P. & Wilkoff, L.J. (1976): Inhibition and reversal by β-retinoic acid of hyperplasia induced in cultured mouse prostate tissue by 3-methylcholanthrene or N-methyl-N-nitrosoguanidine. *J. Nat. Cancer Inst.* **56**, 583–589.

4 Cohen, S.M., Wittenberg, J.F. & Bryan, G.T. (1976): Effect of avitaminosis A and hypervitaminosis A on urinary bladder carcinogenicity of N-[4-(5-nitro-2-furyl)-2-thiazolyl] formamide. *Cancer Res.* **36**, 2334–2339.

5 Fujimaki, Y. (1926): Formation of gastric carcinoma in albino rats fed on deficient diets. *J. Cancer Res.* **10**, 469–477.

6 Lotan, R., Ong, D.E. & Chytil, F. (1980): Comparison of the level of cellular retinoid-binding proteins and susceptibility to retinoid-induced growth inhibition of various neoplastic cell lines. *J. Natl. Cancer Inst.* **64**, 1259–1262.

7 McCormick, D.L., Becci, P.J. & Moon, R.C. (1982): Inhibition of mammary and urinary bladder carcinogenesis by a retinoid and a maleic anhydride-divinyl ether copolymer (MVE-2). *Carcinogenesis* **3**, 1473–1477.

8 McCormick, D.L., Burns, F.J. & Albert, R.E. (1980): Inhibition of rat mammary carcinogenesis by short dietary exposure to retinyl acetate. *Cancer Res.* **40**, 1140–1143.

9 McCormick, D.L., Mehta, R.G., Thompson, C.A., Dinger, N., Caldwell, J.A. & Moon, R.C. (1982): Enhanced inhibition of mammary carcinogenesis by combined treatment with N-(4-hydroxyphenyl)retinamide and ovariectomy. *Cancer Res.* **42**, 508–512.

10 McCormick, D.L., May, C.M. & Moon, R.C. (1985): Temporal patterns of retinoid and antioxidant modulation of rat mammary carcinogenesis. *Proc. Am. Ass. Cancer Res.* **26**, 119.

11 McCormick, D.L. & Moon, R.C. (1982): Influence of delayed administration of retinyl acetate on mammary carcinogenesis. *Cancer Res.* **42**, 2639–2643.

12 McCormick, D.L. & Moon, R.C. (1985): Vitamin A deficiency and cancer. In *Vitamin A deficiency and its control*, ed J .C. Bauernfeind. New York: Academic Press. (In press).

13 McCormick, D.L. & Moon, R.C. (1985): Retinoid-tamoxifen interaction in mammary cancer chemoprevention. *Carcinogenesis*. (In press).

14 Mehta, R.G., Cerny, W.L. & Moon, R.C. (1980): Distribution of retinoic acid-binding proteins in normal and neoplastic mammary tissues. *Cancer Res.* **40**, 47–49.

15 Moon, R.C., Grubbs, C.J. & Sporn, M.B. (1976): Inhibition of 7,12-dimethylbenz(a)anthracene-induced mammary carcinogenesis by retinyl acetate. *Cancer Res.* **36**, 2626–2630.

16 Moon, R.C. & Itri, L.M. (1984): Retinoids and cancer. In *The retinoids, Vol. 2*, ed M.B. Sporn *et al.*, pp. 327–371. New York: Academic Press.

17 Moon, R.C., McCormick, D.L. & Mehta, R.G. (1983): Inhibition of carcinogenesis by retinoids. *Cancer Res.* **43**, 2469s–2474s.

18 Moon, R.C., Thompson, H.J., Becci, P.J., Grubbs, C.J., Gander, R.J., Newton, D.L., Smith, J.M., Phillips, S.L., Henderson, W.R., Mullen, L.T., Brown, C.C. & Sporn, M.B. (1979): N-(4-hydroxyphenyl)retinamide, a new retinoid for prevention of breast cancer in the rat. *Cancer Res.* **39**, 1339–1346.

19 Mori, S. (1922): The changes in the paraocular glands which follow the administration of diets low in fat-soluble A; with notes of the effects of the same diets on the salivary glands and the mucosa of the larynx and trachea. *Johns Hopkins Hosp. Bull.* **33**, 357–359.

20 Peto, R., Doll, R., Buckley, J.D. & Sporn, M.B. (1981): Can dietary beta-carotene materially reduce human cancer rates? *Nature* **290**, 201–208.

21 Rowe, N.H. & Gorlin, R.J. (1959): The effect of vitamin A deficiency upon experimental oral carcinogenesis. *J. Dent. Res.* **38**, 72–83.

22 Thompson, H.J., Becci, P.J., Brown, C.C. & Moon, R.C. (1979): Effect of the duration of retinyl acetate feeding on inhibition of l-methyl-l-nitrosourea-induced mammary carcinogenesis in the rat. *Cancer Res.* **39**, 3977–3980.

23 Wolbach, S.B. & Howe, P.R. (1925): Tissue changes following deprivation of fat-soluble A vitamin. *J. Exp. Med.* **42**, 753–778.

Dietary fibre as a protective factor in human large bowel cancer

Sheila A. BINGHAM
Medical Research Council and University of Cambridge Dunn Clinical Nutrition Centre, 100 Tennis Court Road, Cambridge CB2 1QL, UK.

Overview of fibre intakes. Elsewhere[2] we have made some limited observations on the amount of fibre eaten in Britain, Europe, America and parts of rural Africa and there are some more recent data for New Zealand and Australia, based on the British Food Tables, which show that fibre intakes of these other 'westernized' countries are similar to those found in USA and Britain, about 20 g per day.

These studies have shown that it is quite true to say that fibre intakes are higher in some parts of rural Africa than in westernized populations[6]. This, however, is not the only difference between the diet of rural Africans, and that eaten in the USA. The rural African eats minimal fat and meat which have also been associated epidemiologically with large bowel cancer[1]

Some recent and interesting data from Japan[17] show that rates for colon cancer and diverticular disease are still, despite recent post-war changes, among the lowest in the world: in migrants, rates for this cancer change to those of the host country within one or two generations[12]. Fibre, however, cannot be the reason for these low rates. Intakes in Japan are 20 g per day, no greater than in countries such as Britain, USA and New Zealand with the highest colon cancer rates in the world.

The reason for this is that the fibre content of rice is low, whatever method of analysis is used, and as a consequence, despite the recent trends towards westernization of the Japanese diet, there have been no major changes in the Japanese fibre intake over the past 50 years[17]. However, intakes of fat and animal protein are low, and, despite recent changes, the Japanese still only eat 70 g meat/d, compared with about 160 g in Britain, and half the fat. It is, therefore, necessary to look at the role of dietary fibre in countries that can otherwise be supposed to be at high risk of colon cancer from a 'westernized' type of diet or lifestyle.

Time trends. A cornerstone of the hypothesis relating fibre intake to the aetiology of colon cancer was the suggested decline in intakes following the introduction of roller milling of wheat in Britain, Europe and the USA around 1880. However, the most striking feature in Britain during the 20th century was a probable doubling of total dietary fibre intake due to an increase in the extraction rate of flour and increases in consumption of bread to conserve food supplies during World War II. Time trends in colon cancer mortality rates may be associated in Britain and the USA with changes in crude fibre intakes, particularly in Britain where there was a marked post-war fall in mortality[15]. This analysis has recently been extended[18] by more accurate analyses for non-starch polysaccharide (NSP) consumption, based on the data of Englyst *et al.*[9] to include four other countries. The estimated war-time increases in NSP from flour were 15 g in Ireland, 12 g in England and Wales, 10 g in Switzerland, 4 g in New Zealand, with virtually no change in Australia and the USA. In these two latter countries the ratio of observed to expected mortality 11 to 15 years after the increase, extrapolating from pre-war trends, was about 0.8, but 0.6 in Ireland, the population which had experienced the greatest increase in NSP consumption. Over the six populations studied, the correlation coefficient between these two variables was -0.88. The most obvious problem with this type of analysis, however, is that changes in dietary habits rarely occur in isolation; in Britain for example, fat consumption fell from 39 per cent of total energy in the 1930s to 33 per cent of total energy in 1947[11].

Correlation studies. *Household surveys.* In Britain, regional household intakes of foodstuffs have been documented every year by the British National Food Survey, under the auspices of the Ministry of Agriculture, Fisheries and Food[16]. Since intake of meat and fat are comparatively high in Britain, regional NSP intake was investigated and compared with regional death rates for colo-rectal cancer.

To determine regional NSP intake, composite diets were made up of all fibre-containing foods for the years 1969–73, and analysed by the method of Englyst & Cummings[10]. When intakes were compared with age and sex-standardized truncated colon and rectal cancer rates for 1969–73 a significant ($P < 0.05$) and negative association ($r = -0.74$) between NSP intake and colon cancer emerged[5]. We were, however, unable to confirm the strong inverse relationship between the pentose fraction of dietary fibre and colon cancer[4] although the association with vegetable consumption ($r = -0.940$) remains.

Geographical comparisons of diet and cancer incidence between representative groups of individuals. Established cancer registries in Scandinavia show a three to four-fold range in colon cancer incidence within an area with a fairly homogenous population. Age standardized truncated colon cancer incidence rates per 100 000 men are lowest in rural Finland (6.7) and highest in Copenhagen (22.8). Rates in rural Denmark and Helsinki are intermediate (12.9 and 17.0). In collaboration with the International Agency for Research on Cancer, a study was undertaken to characterize the diets eaten by representative population samples in each area, with particular reference to the consumption of NSP using the method of Englyst & Cummings. Thirty men aged 50–59 were randomly selected from population registers in each of the four areas: Parikkala in the Kymi region of South-East Finland; Them, in Jutland; Helsinki, and Copenhagen. Response rates among those approached were Parikkala 83.3 per cent, Helsinki 74.4 per cent, Copenhagen 75 per cent and Them 62.5 per cent[13].

Each of the 120 men were asked to keep a weighed food record for 4 d, in order to assess nutrient intake from local food tables. Because analyses for dietary fibre are generally not available in food tables, the amounts of NSP eaten in each of the four areas had to be established from direct chemical analysis of duplicate diets in Cambridge. It is, however, notoriously difficult to collect complete duplicates of food eaten from free living individuals, and a number of methodological checks were built into the protocol. These suggested that the food samples were complete duplicates and the normal dietary habits had not been interfered with[3].

Average intakes of fat and animal protein were high, fat ranging from 102 to 146 g per day, and meat consumption from 148 to 214 g per day. There were no significant associations with fat, cholesterol or meat consumption and large bowel cancer incidence. The simple correlation coefficient between non-starch polysaccharide consumption and large bowel cancer incidence was −0.776, although more sophisticated statistical techniques demonstrated a significant relationship[13].

Case-control studies. Out of 12 westernized population samples studied since 1966, no case-control studies have supported a role for dietary fibre. However, colo-rectal cancer patients are likely to alter their food intake at the onset of symptoms such as altered bowel habit and abdominal pain[8]. Authors have attempted to control for this by asking all subjects to give information only concerning food intake by up to 3 years previously but this in fact is probably not possible[7,14,19]. In addition, numerical comparisons are difficult because of the problems with systematic bias in methods of assessing food consumption and the analysis of dietary fibre. No case-control study to date has assessed non-starch polysaccharide consumption.

Conclusions. The epidemiological examination of the fibre hypothesis has been hampered by the absence of data on the fibre content of most of the world's foods. In Scandinavia and Britain where the consumption of the major chemical fraction of dietary fibre, the non-starch polysaccharides, has been measured using accurate methods, significant negative associations have been shown with the incidence of colon cancer. These studies suggest that non-starch polysaccharides may be protective in populations at otherwise high risk of colon cancer from an excess of meat and fat. However, methodological problems in the assessment of non-starch polysaccharide consumption in individuals preclude the use of case control studies in verifying these associations within a single homogeneous population.

1 Armstrong, B. & Doll, R. (1975): Environmental factors and cancer incidence in different countries, with special reference to dietary practices. *Int. J. Cancer* **15**, 617–631.

2 Bingham, S. & Cummings, J.H. (1980): Intakes and sources of dietary fiber in man. In *Medical aspects of dietary fibre*, ed G.A. Spiller & R.M. Amen, pp. 261–284. New York: Plenum.

3 Bingham, S., Wiggins, H.S., Englyst, H., Seppanen, R., Helms, P., Strand, R., Burton, R., Jorgensen, I.M., Poulsen, L., Paerregaard, A., Bjerrum, L. & James, W.P.T. (1982): Methods and validity of the dietary assessments in four Scandinavian populations. *Nutr. Cancer* **4**, 23–33.

4 Bingham, S., Williams, D.R.R., Cole, T.J. & James, W.P.T. (1979): Dietary fibre consumption and regional large bowel cancer mortality in Britain. *Br. J. Cancer* **40**, 456–463.

5 Bingham, S., Williams, D.R.R. & Cummings, J.H. (1985): Dietary fibre consumption in Britain; new estimates and their relation to colon cancer mortality. *Br. J. Cancer* **52**, 399–402.

6 Burkitt, D.P. (1969): Related disease-related cause. *Lancet* **2**, 1229–1231.

7 Byers, T.E., Randall, I., Marshall, J.R., Rzepka, T.F., Cummings, K.M. & Graham, S. (1983): Dietary history from the distant past. *Nutr. Cancer* **5**, 69–77.

8 Cummings, J.H. (1981): Dietary fibre and large bowel cancer. *Proc. Nutr. Soc.* **40**, 7–14.

9 Englyst, H.N., Anderson, V. & Cummings, J.H. (1983): Starch and non-starch polysaccharides in some cereal foods. *J. Sci. Fd Agric.* **34**, 1434–1440.

10 Englyst, H.N. & Cummings, J.H. (1984): Simplified method for the measurement of total NSP by GLC of constituent sugars as alditol acetates. *Analyst* **109**, 937–942.

11 Greaves, J.P. & Hollingsworth, D.F. (1966): Trends in food consumption in the United Kingdom. *Wld Rev. Nutr. Diet.* **6**, 34–89.

12 Haenszel, W. & Kurihara, M. (1968): Studies of Japanese migrants. Mortality from cancer and other diseases among Japanese in the United States. *J. Nat. Cancer Inst.* **40**, 43–68.

13 Jensen, O.M., MacLennan, R. & Wahrendorf, J. (1982): Diet, bowel function, fecal characteristics and large bowel cancer in Denmark and Finland. *Nutr. Cancer* **4**, 5–19.

14 Jensen, O.M., Wahrendorf, J., Rosenquist, A. & Geser, A. (1984): The reliability of questionnaire-derived historic dietary information and temporal stability of food habits in individuals. *Am. J. Epid.* **120**, 281–290.

15 McMichael, A.J., Potter, J.D. & Hetzel, B.S. (1979): Time trends in colorectal cancer mortality in relation to food and alcohol consumption. *Int. J. Epid.* **8**, 296–303.

16 Ministry of Agriculture, Fisheries and Food (1953–1983): *Household food consumption and expenditure 1950–1981*. Annual Reports of the National Food Survey Committee. London: HMSO.

17 Minowa, M., Bingham, S. & Cummings, J.H. (1983): Dietary fibre intake in Japan. *Hum. Nutr: Appl. Nutr.* **37A**, 113–119.

18 Powles, J. & Williams, D.R.R. (1984): Trends in bowel cancer in selected countries in relation to war-time changes in flour-millingssment of dietary intake. *Am. J. Epid.* **120**, 876–877.

19 Rohan, T.E. & Potter, J.O. (1984): Retrospective assessment of dietary intake. *Am. J. Epid.* **120** 876–877.

Interactions between dietary fat and fibre in relation to colon cancer: experimental studies in the rat

E.J. SINKELDAM, C.F. KUPER and M.C. BOSLAND
TNO-CIVO Toxicology and Nutrition Institute, Department of Biological Toxicology, Utrechtseweg 48, PO Box 360, 3700 AJ Zeist, The Netherlands; MCB (present address): Institute of Environmental Medicine, New York University Medical Center, 550 First Avenue, New York, NY 10016, USA.

Epidemiological studies indicate that diet is a major aetiological factor in cancer of the large bowel ([9]for review). Diets high in fat and low in fibre are generally associated with a high incidence of large bowel cancer in humans, whereas diets low in fat and high in fibre, which are common in most countries of Africa, Asia and Latin America, are in most cases coupled with a low incidence of colon cancer.

On the basis of epidemiological studies, however, it is hardly, if at all, possible to discriminate between fat and fibre as separate factors in colon carcinogenesis. In one case-control study an interrelationship between dietary fibre and fat was found[2], highest risk of developing colorectal cancer being associated with a diet both high in fat and low in fibre. An evaluation of the results of several experimental studies in animals concluded that dietary fibre inhibits colon carcinogenesis only when the fat content of the diet is not excessive[7]. The purpose of the present study was to examine how dietary fibre and fat interactively affect the genesis of both 1,2-dimethylhydrazine (DMH)- and N-methyl-N'-nitro-N-nitrosoguanidine (MNNG)-induced colon cancer in rats.

Experimental. Newly-weaned, random-bred Wistar male rats (Cpb:WU), obtained from the Central Institute for the Breeding of Laboratory Animals TNO, Zeist, The Netherlands, were divided randomly into nine groups of 30 animals each and fed on of the diets presented in Table 1 for 9 months. The animals were kept in groups of five in stainless steel wire mesh cages in a well-ventilated room (10 airchanges/h) having a stationary temperature of $23 \pm 1\,^\circ C$, a relative humidity of 40–70 per cent and a light/dark cycle of 12 h. After 4 weeks of feeding the various diets all animals were treated with either MNNG (first study) or DMH (second study). MNNG was freshly dissolved in a 1 per cent carboxymethylcellulose solution of saline and given intrarectally in five weekly dosages of 6 mg/kg b.wt. DMH was injected subcutaneously in ten weekly dosages of 50 mg/kg b.wt. Before injection DMH was freshly dissolved in saline and the pH was adjusted to 6.5. The animals were maintained on their respective diets before, during and after the carcinogen administration. Body weight of each individual rat and food intake per cage of five rats were determined weekly during the whole experimental period of 9 months. After 9 months, the surviving animals were killed by decapitation under slight ether anaesthesia and subjected to detailed gross examination. The colon was examined carefully for the presence

Table 1. *Approximate composition of the diets.* The basal low-fat- low-fibre diet, composed of white flour, casein and lard, was modified to give the medium and high-fibre diets by the addition of wheat bran and to give the medium and high-fat diets by increasing the lard. L-F/M-F/H-F: low-/medium-/high-fibre.

	Low fat			Medium fat			High fat		
	L-F	M-F	H-F	L-F	M-F	H-F	L-F	M-F	H-F
Per cent energy as protein	24.6	24.7	24.9	24.5	24.6	24.8	24.5	24.5	24.7
Per cent energy as fat	15.6	15.7	15.8	27.6	27.8	27.9	39.6	39.8	40.4
Fibre g per 420 kJ (100 kcal)	0.8	2.2	3.7	0.7	2.4	3.8	0.5	2.2	3.9
Energy content (kJ/100 g)	1499	1420	1341	1637	1521	1435	1805	1665	1544

of tumours and lesions suspected of being a tumour. The number of tumours, their gross appearance and the distance from the anal orifice were recorded. Each tumour and tumourlike lesion was fixed in formalin and examined histopathologically.

Results. Mean body weights, energy intake data, and the colon tumour response are presented in Table 2. For body weight and energy intake only the results with MNNG are given, since similar results were obtained with DMH. The fastest growth rate was observed for the animals on the hig-fat-low fibre diet. Body weights on the low-fibre diets increased with increasing level of fat in the diet. On the medium and high-fibre diets the effect of fat was, on the other hand, less clear. Increasing the fat content from low to medium generally resulted in higher body weights, whereas a further increase from medium to high fat was associated with a decline in body weight.

Table 2. *Body weight, energy intake and colon tumour response in rats (30 in each group) fed diets with various fat/fibre combinations and treated with either MNNG or DMH.*

		MNNG			DMH	
Dietary group	*B.wt (g) at wk 37*	*Total energy intake wk 0–37 (MJ/rat)*	*Animals with colon tumours (%)*	*No. of colon tumours per tumour-bearing rat*	*Animals with colon tumours (%)*	*No. of colon tumours per tumour-bearing rat*
Low fat — low fibre	485.4	64.7	40	1.4	57	1.8
Low fat — medium fibre	496.2	61.9	60	1.8	40	1.5
Low fat — high fibre	490.7	60.9	43	1.6	30	1.6
Medium fat — low fibre	521.7	62.1	60	1.4	62	1.7
Medium fat — medium fibre	520.3	61.8	80***	1.8	69	1.5
Medium fat — high fibre	486.4	60.2	40	1.8	47	1.4
High fat — low fibre	535.9*	64.3	73**	3.0	64	2.9
High fat — medium fibre	517.5	61.9	57	3.0	66	2.2
High fat — high fibre[a]	479.9	63.2	55	1.6	24**	1.9

[a]In the MNNG experiment the effective No. of animals was 29 in this group.
*Significantly different from the group fed the low fat-low fibre diet by Dunnett's Multiple Comparison's test ($P < 0.01$); **Significantly different from the group fed the low fat-low fibre diet by Fisher Exact Probability test ($P < 0.05$); ***Significantly different from the group fed the low fat-low fibre diet by Fisher Exact probability test ($P < 0.01$).

The total energy intake showed some variation amongst the groups, but the difference between the highest and the lowest figure amounted to 8 per cent at most. On the low and medium fat diets there was a decrease in energy intake with an increasing level of fibre, whereas on the high fat diets the decrease in energy intake was not dose-related, but with a minimum on the medium-fibre diet.

The colon tumour response for both the MNNG and the DMH experiment showed that the percentage of animals with colon tumours (incidence) and the number of tumours per tumour-bearing rat (multiplicity) was high in the groups fed the high-fat-low-fibre diet (Western type diet), independent of the type of carcinogen used. An enhancing effect of fat on both the incidence and the multiplicity was clearly present for the low-fibre diets, when MNNG was applied as carcinogen. In the low-fibre groups treated with DMH, no effect of fat was observed on the tumour incidence, but the multiplicity was almost twice as high in the group fed the high fat-low fibre diet as compared to the other two groups fed a low-fibre diet. A protective effect of fibre on the incidence of DMH-induced tumours was found only when the level of fat was high in the diet.

In general, the results showed a non-linear dose-response relationship for fibre and fat. Non-linearity for the level of fat occurred in particular at the medium fibre level. For the medium-fibre diets, the highest tumour incidence was seen in the medium-fat group. The lowest tumour incidence among the high-fibre diets was observed in the high-fat-high-fibre group, when DMH was applied as carcinogen. It is remarkable that in both studies a similar non-linear pattern of tumour incidences occurred.

Discussion and conclusion. The three-by-three factorial design of the present studies enables evaluation of the individual effects of fat and fibre as well as the interactions of these nutrients on MNNG and DMH colon carcinogenesis From the results obtained it is clear that both fibre and fat affect chemically induced colon carcinogenesis in rats. Moreover, a fibre and fat interaction was apparent.

The inhibiting effect of fibre (from wheat bran) on colon carcinogenesis found in the present studies has been shown also by other investigators ([4] for review). In the present studies, this effect was especially seen in combination with the high-fat diets, whereas the low-fat diets did not result in a noticeable inhibiting effect of fibre on MNNG-induced colon cancer. In this respect, the findings are not in agreement with Nigro's[7], who stated that dietary fibre inhibits colon carcinogenesis only when fat content of the diet is not excessively high.

In most animal studies on the effects of fat on colon carcinogenesis, an enhancing effect of fat was found ([8] for review), but in some studies[5,6] no effect of fat was seen. In the present study a clear increase in tumour incidence with an increasing level of fat was found only when the fibre content of the diet was low and only when MNNG was applied as carcinogen. These results indicate that the effect of fat on colon carcinogenesis depends on the fibre content of the diet as well as on the type of carcinogen used.

It is not easy to account for the fat-fibre interaction found nor for the non-linear dose-response relationship, resulting for instance in the highest tumour incidence for the medium-fat-medium-fibre group, both with MNNG and DMH. The fact that the fibre diets were given during the entire experimental period may have influenced the results. In DMH-treated rats it was actually noticed that wheat bran given during the carcinogen administration enhanced colon carcinogenesis, whereas it inhibited colon carcinogenesis, when given after carcinogen administration[3]. Since fat exhibits its effect on colon carcinogenesis mainly after the carcinogen administration, in the promotion phase[1], it is reasonable to assume that the interactive effect of fat and fibre is the result of a complex interaction of opposite and augmenting effects of fat and fibre in both the initiation and promotion phase of colon carcinogenesis.

It can be concluded that the present studies demonstrated that dietary fat and fibre effect colon carcinogenesis, both independently as well as in an interactive manner, indicating that dietary influences on colon carcinogenesis are the result of a complex multifactorial process. It may be too easy to formulate dietary recommendations in the sense that more fibre and less fat will be beneficial in the case of colon cancer prevention. Non-linearity of the effects, interactions and differential effects of types of fibre may be decisive factors.

Acknowledgements. We wish to thank the animal-house staff, especially Wim Riebeek and Gerrit de Kruijf, Nel Somer and co-workers for their technical assistance and Mrs L.M.H. Nieuwenhuijsen for editorial help. This study was financially supported by the Netherlands Cancer Foundation, the Koningin Wilhelmina Fonds.

1 Bull, A.W., Soullier, B.K., Wilson, P.S., Hayden, M.T. & Nigro, N.D. (1979): Promotion of azoxymethane-induced intestinal cancer by high-fat diet in rats. *Cancer Res.* **39**, 4956–4959.

2 Dales, L.G., Friedman, G.D., Ury, H.K., Grossman, S. & Williams, S.R. (1979): A case-control study of relationships of diet and other traits to colorectal cancer in American blacks. *Am. J. Epidemiol.* **109**, 132–144.

3 Jacobs, L.R. (1983): Enhancement of rat colon carcinogenesis by wheat bran consumption during the stage of 1,2-dimethylhydrazine administration. *Cancer Res.* **43**, 4057–4061.

4 Kritchevsky, D. (1983): Fiber, steroids, and cancer. *Cancer Res. (Suppl.)* **43**, 2491S–2495S.

5 Nauss, K.M., Locniskar, M. & Newberne, P.M. (1983): Effect of alterations in the quality and quantity of dietary fat on 1,2-dimethylhydrazine-induced colon tumorigenesis in rats. *Cancer Res.* **43**, 4083–4090.

6 Nauss, K.M., Locniskar, M., Sondergaard, D. & Newberne, P.M. (1984): Lack of effect of dietary fat on N-nitrosomethylurea (MNU)-induced colon tumorigenesis in rats. *Carcinogenesis* **5**, 255–260.

7 Nigro, N.D. (1981): Animal studies implicating fat and fecal steroids in intestinal cancer. *Cancer Res.* **41**, 3769–3770.

8 Reddy, B.S. (1981): Dietary fat and its relationship to large bowel cancer. *Cancer Res.* **41**, 3700–3705.

9 Zaridze, D. (1983): Environmental etiology of large-bowel cancer. *J. Natl. Cancer Inst.* **70**, 389–399.

Salt and gastric cancer

J. GEBOERS and J.V. JOOSSENS
Division of Epidemiology, School of Public Health, University of Leuven, Kapucijnenvoer 33, B-3000 Leuven, Belgium.

About 80 per cent of all cancer deaths may be attributed to exogenous factors, among which tobacco and diet are the most important[5]. Gastric cancer (GC), although generally conceived as of environmental causation, is a multi-stage process, each step of which may have different causes and modifying factors[4]. Here we will briefly review the epidemiology of GC, thereby focusing on the role of salt in the aetiology of GC and its precursor lesions.

General aspects of GC epidemiology. There is a marked variation on GC morbidity and mortality throughout the world. Levels are particularly high in Japan, South Korea, Chile, Colombia, Iceland, Finland and Eastern Europe; they are low in the USA, Australia and New Zealand. This between-countries variation is accompanied by variation within countries, the general rule being that northern and/or colder regions have the highest risk. Such regional differences were observed in Japan, Chile, Colombia, Belgium and the USA[1,13]. GC has been declining continuously for several decades, first in the USA, later in England, Western Europe, and, only recently also in Eastern Europe[13].

GC occurs twice as frequently in males than in females, and is inversely related to socioeconomic status. No consistent urban-rural gradient could be observed[1].

Migrants from high-risk areas to low-risk areas have GC levels comparable to those of their homeland, while their offspring adapt to levels similar to those of native born. This has been observed in Japanese migrants in Hawaii and California, in East European migrants to Australia and the USA, as well as in migrants within Chile and Colombia, and suggests exposure early in life to an exogenous (dietary) agent. Migrant studies have therefore enabled epidemiologists to establish the predominant role of environmental factors in GC aetiology[10].

Yet, since gastric cancer is a multi-stage process, each step having its own characteristics, it is unlikely that epidemiology may reveal all the secrets of its pathogenesis. A multidisciplinary approach is required for this purpose. For the last two decades, the synergism between epidemiology and pathology had a major impact on the understanding of the mechanism of gastric carcinogenesis, beginning with the description of two types of GC: the diffuse or genetic type and the intestinal or environmental type[17]. It is the latter type of GC that is likely to be caused by environmental factors. Evidence for this has arisen from the observations that the difference in GC incidence between Japanese living in Hawaii and in Japan was entirely due to a difference in the environmental type of GC[3], and that the decline in GC incidence in Norway[19] and in the USA[20] could be primarily ascribed to a decline in the intestinal type of GC with no change at all in the diffuse type.

Another key event was the postulation of a histopathological model for gastric carcinogenesis, particularly for the environmental type of GC[4]. The first stage is gastric atrophy resulting from the irritation of the gastric mucosa. This results in gastric achlorhydria and consequently bacterial overgrowth in the stomach. Bacteria reduce dietary nitrate to nitrite, which may then combine with secondary amines to nitrosamines and with amides to nitrosamides[6]. Those N-nitroso compounds are then responsible for the intestinalization of the gastric mucosa and subsequent stages, ie dysplasia and carcinoma. Although this hypothesis has already generated a lot of research, the first stage of generating gastric atrophy is still poorly understood.

The salt hypothesis. Salt intake has been suspected as a possible factor in GC aetiology since the late 1950s when salt intake was compared with GC death rates in Japanese prefectures[22]. Further epidemiologic work in Japan gave substance to this hypothesis[11]. Salted and smoked fish and meat products, and pickled vegetables have emerged as aetiological risk factors of GC from case-control studies carried out in Japan and Hawaii[9]. In all countries where salt intake has been documented to be high, ie more than 15 g/day, as for instance in Japan, South Korea, the People's Republic of China, Colombia, Finland, and Eastern Europe, GC mortality levels are high as well. In the few countries where salt intake has been monitored over time, there is also a good within-country correlation between salt consumption and GC. Salt intake is also much higher in lower social classes[14,15].

Further epidemiological evidence may result from the close relationship observed between GC and stroke mortality, with salt as the common aetiological factor[13]. This relationship was present between and within countries, and for changes in rates of both diseases. Chronic atrophic gastritis (CAG), a precursor of GC, has a very high prevalence (50–90 per cent) in populations living on a high salt intake as has been observed in Colombia[2] and Finland. Salted foods have been associated with intestinal metaplasia in case-control studies in Japan[21] and Colombia.

When high amounts of salt are used from an early age, CAG may be induced resulting from the irritant properties of hypertonic salt solutions. This process may be enhanced by a high-starch diet[16]. The deleterious nature of salt has been demonstrated in animal experiments[7], but it has never been tested in humans. Experimentally it has been shown that hypertonic salt solutions delay the emptying of the stomach due to osmotic receptors in the duodenum[12], and as a result of which potential carcinogens may be in longer contact with the gastric mucosa.

The acute effect of salt intake on the gastric mucosa is dose-dependent and induces a marked ornithine decarboxylase activity and an increased DNA-synthesis[8], just as nitrosocarcinogens do. Hypertonic salt solutions are also acting as a co-carcinogen during induction with nitrosamides and significantly promotes GC in rats[23]. Vitamin C, on the other hand, blocks the synthesis of nitrosocarcinogens[18].

Results from animal experiments are fully compatible with the major impact which the introduction of the refrigerator may have had on GC incidence. Indeed, refrigeration makes the use of salt and nitrates for food presentation less necessary, and has increased the availability of fresh fruits and vegetables throughout the year[13–15,18].

Conclusion. Although a substantial amount of epidemiological and experimental data are available which may help to explain the pathogenesis of GC, further research is still required, especially on the aetiology of precursors of GC.

1 Boyd, J., Langman, M. & Doll, R. (1964): The epidemiology of gastrointestinal cancer with special reference to causation. *Gut* **5**, 196–200.

2 Correa, P., Cuello, C. & Duque, E. (1970): Carcinoma and intestinal metaplasia of the stomach in Colombian migrants. *J. Natl. Cancer Inst.* **44**, 297–306.

3 Correa, P., Sasano, N., Stemmerman, G.N. & Haenszel, W. (1973): Pathology of gastric carcinoma in Japanese populations: comparisons between Miyagi Prefecture, Japan, and Hawaii. *J. Natl, Cancer Inst.* **51**, 1449–1459.

4 Correa, P., Haenszel, W., Cuello, C., Tannenbaum, S. & Archer, M. (1975): A model for gastric cancer epidemiology. *Lancet* **2**, 58–60.

5 Doll, R. & Peto, R. (1981): The causes of cancer: quantitative estimates of avoidable risks of cancer in the United States today. *J. Natl. Cancer Inst.* **66**, 1191–1308.

6 Fraser, P., Chilvers, C., Beral, V. & Hill, M.J. (1980): Nitrate and human cancer: a review of the evidence. *Int. J. Epidemiol.* **9**, 3–11.

7 Frenning, B. (1973): The effects of large osmolality variations on the gastric mucosa surface ultrastructure. *Scand. J. Gastroent.* **8**, 185–192.

8 Furihatu, C., Sato, Y., Hosaka, M., Matsushima, T., Furukawa, F. & Takahashi, M. (1984): NaCl induced ornithine decarboxylase and DNA synthesis in rat stomach mucosa. *Biochem. Biophys. Res. Comm.* **121**, 1027–1032.

9 Haenszel, W., Kurihara, M., Segi, M. & Lee, R.K.C. (1972): Stomach cancer among Japanese in Hawaii. *J. Natl. Cancer Inst.* **49**, 969–988.

10 Haenszel, W. & Correa, P. (1975): Developments in the epidemiology of stomach cancer over the past decade. *Cancer Res.* **35**, 3452–3459.

11 Hirayama, T. (1971): Epidemiology of stomach cancer. *Gann Monogr.* **11**, 3–19.

12 Hunt, J.N. & Pathak, J.D. (1960): The osmotic effect of some simple molecules and ions on gastric emptying. *J. Physiol.* **154**, 254–269.

13 Joossens, J.V. & Geboers, J. (1981): Nutrition and gastric cancer. *Nutr. Cancer* **2**, 250–261.

14 Joossens, J.V. & Geboers, J. (1983): Epidemiology of gastric cancer: a clue to etiology. In *Precancerous lesions of the gastrointestinal tract*, ed P. Sherlock, B.C. Morson, L. Barbara & U. Veronesi, pp. 97–113. New York: Raven Press.

15 Joossens, J.V. & Geboers, J. (1984): Diet and environment in the etiology of gastric cancer. In *Frontiers of gastrointestinal cancer*, ed B. Levin & R.H. Riddell, pp. 167–183. New York: Elsevier.

16 Kodama, M., Kodama, T., Suzuki, H. & Kondo, K. (1984): Effect of rice and salty rice diets on the structure of the mouse stomach. *Nutr. Cancer* **6**, 135–147.

17 Laurén, P. (1965): The two histological main types of gastric carcinoma: diffuse and so-called intestinal type carcinoma. An attempt at a histo-clinical classification. *Acta Pathol. Microbiol. Scand.* **64**, 31–49.

18 Mirvish, S.S. (1983): The etiology of gastric cancer. Intragastric nitrosamide formation and other theories. *J. Natl. Cancer Inst.* **71**, 629–647.

19 Munoz, N. & Asvall, J. (1971): Time trends of intestinal and diffuse types of gastric cancer in Norway. *Int. J. Cancer* **8**, 144–157.

20 Munoz, N. & Connolly, R. (1971): Time trends of intestinal and diffuse types of gastric cancer in the United States. *Int. J. Cancer* **8**, 158–164.

21 Nomura, A., Yamakawa, H., Ishidate, T., Kamiyama, S., Masuda, H., Stemmerman, G.N., Heilbum, L.K. & Hankin, J.H. (1982): Intestinal metaplasia in Japan: association with diet. *J. Natl. Cancer Inst* **68**, 401–405.

22 Sato, T., Fukuyama, T., Suzuki, T., Takayagami, J., Murukami, T., Shiotshuki, N., Tanaka, R. & Tsuji, R. (1959): Studies on the causation of gastric cancer. 2. The relation between gastric cancer mortality rate and salted food intake in several places in Japan. *Bull. Inst. Pub. Hlth* **8**, 187–198.

23 Takahashi, M., Kokubo, T., Furukawa, F., Kurokawa, Y. & Hayashi, Y. (1984): Effects of sodium chloride, saccharin, phenobarbital and aspirin on gastric carcinogenesis in rats after initiation with N-methyl-N′-nitro-N-nitrosoguanidine. *Gann* **75**, 494–501.

Methodological aspects of nutrition in cancer epidemiology: a workshop report

J. WAHRENDORF (Organizer)
International Agency for Research on Cancer, 150, cours Albert-Thomas, F-69372 Lyon Cedex 08, France.

The possibility that diet plays a role in the aetiology of human cancers has led to several epidemiological investigations of this question. The resulting cooperation of nutritionists and epidemiologists should be supported by a thorough understanding by each side of the principles and concepts of the scientific approach of the other side. It had been frequently observed that this is not always the case, and this workshop was organized in order to improve interdisciplinary communication.

The essential point in the cooperation between nutritionists and epidemiologists is the choice of the appropriate method to assess people's dietary habits. There is a general tendency for nutritionists to propose methods which place a higher burden on the participants in epidemiological studies than epidemiologists would like to see. To highlight these contrasting attitudes, workshop participants were asked in advance to address very specific questions in a stimulating, even provocative way.

'Why are epidemiologists interested in nutrition?' *M. Ewertz* (Danish Cancer Registry, Copenhagen). First, the speaker answered this question 'to prevent diseases caused by dietary factors'. While an involvement of dietary factors in the aetiology of digestive tract cancers may be self-evident, she illustrated the possible role of nutrition in breast cancer aetiology.

'Why do nutritionists prefer longer methods?' *J.W. Marr* (University of London, UK). In order to classify individuals correctly into thirds of a study population in respect of their average daily consumption of certain nutrients prolonged recording of food habits would be required due to the large intra-individual variations. Whereas for some nutrients a duration of recording of 4–7 d would be required, for other nutrients a much longer period is necessary. The discussion of this presentation made it very clear that the emphasis in cancer epidemiology is on correctly classifying individuals into subgroups of the study population rather than measuring an individual's personal dietary habits as correctly as possible.

'Why do nutritionists prefer shorter methods?' *P. Pietinen* (National Public Health Institute, Helsinki, Finland). The speaker discussed a large intervention trial with vitamins in male smokers comprising some 20 000 men. The size of this study, including financial aspects, led to the development of an instrument to assess an individual's dietary habits which could be self-administered, but at the same time would provide a picture of long prevailing habits. A self-administered diet history was developed and underwent validation. The desirability to have a glossary of terms of dietary methodology became very apparent in the discussion.

'Why do epidemiologists prefer longer methods?' *E. Riboli* (IARC, Lyon, France). When studying diet as a whole too few items should not be addressed, it should always be possible to investigate the complex interrelationships between different aspects of the diet and a study should not be initiated with preconceived ideas. A certain shift of scale between nutritionists and epidemiologists for categorizing methods was brought to light by noting the use of terms such as 'rudimentary' by nutritionists for short methods devised by epidemiologists and 'prohibitive' by epidemiologists for long methods devised by nutritionists.

'Why do epidemiologists prefer shorter methods?' *J.R. Marshall* (State University of New York, Buffalo, NY, USA: read by J. Wahrendorf). Epidemiologists, in general, prefer longer methods, but there are exigencies which force them to bow to practicalities and that the clues derived so far on nutritional aspects of cancer aetiology may make it worthwhile to concentrate future studies on sharpened hypotheses addressing only a few nutrients, which could be investigated through a limited number of food items. It was questioned whether single nutrients may be appropriate to focus on since preventive measures could only address more general behavioural dimensions. Some investigators have attempted to identify such factors in people's dietary pattern and whereas this appeared to be very promising in an US investigation, studies in southern Europe were less conclusive.

The general discussion made it clear that in a given epidemiological investigation the claims towards the method(s) for assessing dietary habits should very closely be spelt out in advance; this refers not only to the items to be investigated but also to the precision anticipated. In addition, the nutritional method of choice will depend on various aspects of practicability including the experience with certain instruments in a population similar to the one under investigation. Adequate surrogates should be considered for dietary items which are difficult to assess. Assessment of reliability and validity of the instruments seems to be a particular aspect of nutritional epidemiology. The quantitative information generated by this was deemed to be very important in interpreting the results of epidemiological studies.

Nutritional modulators of carcinogenesis: a workshop report

B.S. REDDY (Organizer)
Division of Nutrition and Endocrinology, Naylor Dana Institute for Disease Prevention, Valhalla, NY 10595 USA.

Participants. *K. Carroll* (Canada), *D.P. Rose* (USA), *B. Reddy* (USA), *E. Mahboubi* (Saudi Arabia), *J. Chen* (China), *T.K. Basu* (Canada), *E. Castro* (USA), *P.P. Nair* (USA) and *D.R. Rao* (USA).

During the last 15 years, a substantial amount of progress has been made in the understanding of nutritional factors as they relate to the development of cancer of the large bowel and breast that predominate in the developed Western countries and of cancer of the stomach which is high in Japan. However, little progress has been made in the understanding of the nutritional modulation of cancer of the oral cavity, oesophagus, liver, and cervix, to cite a few, that predominate in the developing countries. The purpose of this workshop was to present the objective and up-to-date brief review of the role of diet and specific nutrients in the development of various types of cancer and to gain some collective insight on future research direction. With this in mind, we discussed the role of nutritional factors in cancer of the breast, colon and oesophagus, nutritional factors as they relate to cancer mortality in China, the relationship of vitamin A and cancer, nutritional and biochemical endpoints in colon carcinogenesis, diet and processes of genome, and nutritional inhibitors of carcinogenesis. The discussions during the workshop made it possible to formulate the recommendations for the future study.

Carroll summarized his latest results on the effect of type of fat in mammary carcinogenesis. Polyunsaturated fats, such as corn oil and sunflower seed oil, promote 7,12-dimethyl-benz(a)anthracene (DMBA)-induced mammary carcinogenesis in rats. A blend of fats containing about 18 per cent polyunsaturated fatty acid (as linoleate) which approximated the fatty acid composition of the American diet increased the DMBA-induced mammary tumours in Sprague-Dawley rats fed on a semi-purified diet about as effectively as sunflower seed oil (containing 75 per cent linoleate) when the fats were fed at a dietary concentration of 200 g/kg. In another study, DMBA-induced tumorigenesis was promoted by feeding a diet containing 200 g American fat blend/kg. After 9–10 weeks on the diet, the level of dietary fat was decreased by varying amounts to determine the effect on tumour yield. Reducing the level of fat to 50 g/kg significantly decreased the number of tumours that subsequently developed, but reduction of fat to 100 or 150 g/kg had little effect. These results suggest that it may be desirable to decrease the degree of polyunsaturation as well as the level of fat in the diet to maximize the reduction in risk of developing breast cancer. This forms the basis for clinical trials in breast cancer patients.

Rose reported that Japanese post-mastectomy breast-cancer patients have a better prognosis than their American counterparts, and that this is true regardless of disease stage at the time of surgery, because Japan is a country with a low dietary-fat intake. This difference appears to apply specifically to post-menopausal patients. A number of investigators have reported that obesity and consumption of a high-fat diet are associated with a poor prognosis after mastectomy. With this background, and supporting data from animal model studies, clinical trials are underway to evaluate the efficacy of a low-fat diet (15 per cent of total energy) as an adjunct to surgery in breast-cancer patients, and of another low-fat diet (20 per cent of total energy) for reducing the incidence of breast-cancer in women previously identified as being at high risk for this disease.

The role of diet in colon cancer was discussed by *Reddy*. The bulk of nutritional epidemiological evidence suggests that diets high in total fat and low in certain fibres are associated with an increased risk of colon cancer in man. In several populations consuming diets high in fat, increased consumption of certain dietary fibres acts as a protective factor. Studies of animal models indicate that diets high in polyunsaturated fats of vegetable origin (corn oil and safflower oil) and saturated fats of animal origin (lard and beef tallow) increased chemically-induced colon tumour incidence in rats, whereas diets high in monounsaturated and saturated fats of vegetable origin (olive oil and coconut oil) and in fish oil had no tumour-promoting effect. The varied effects of different types of fat on colon cancer suggest that the fatty acid composition is one of the important factors in determining the modifying effect of various fats in colon tumour promotion. It was recommended that clinical trials to evaluate the efficacy of low fat/high fibre diets be performed in patients with colon cancer and in patients with adenomatous polyps with the aim of reducing the incidence of new polyps or carcinomas. It was also suggested that additional prospective studies should be carried out to address issues of specificity not resolved in epidemiologic studies. The advantage of encouraging the public at large to alter their dietary pattern is that these measures have no obvious adverse effects, but would go beyond colon cancer in that a reduction of fat intake might also influence the risk for other diet-related cancers and, in particular, could reduce the rate of coronary heart disease.

Junshi Chen presented some preliminary results on the relationship between the dietary and nutritional status and cancer mortality in China. Sixty-five rural counties with a population over 100 000 were selected from a total of about 2000 counties in China. A three-stage random cluster sampling procedure was used to select the survey commune and production teams. The household and individual subjects were also randomly selected. Information on intakes of foods and nutrients was collected on 30 households per county. Assays on blood, urine and food were performed for various biochemical parameters. Multiple regression analysis showed that plasma cholesterol, ascorbic acid and selenium, lignin intake and urinary N-nitroso compounds are synergistically significantly correlated with oesophagus and stomach cancer mortality. Single correlation analysis (Pearson method) suggested the following: a positive correlation of plasma cholesterol with cancer of liver, colon, and lung; negative correlation of plasma carotene with stomach cancer; negative correlation of plasma selenium with cancer of oesophagus and stomach; and positive correlation of protein intake with cancer of oesophagus, stomach, colon and lung.

T.K. Basu reported the results of studies from his laboratory on the relationship between vitamin A and epithelial cancer in man. The overall retrospective and prospective biochemical data indicate that vitamin A deficiency may be one of the predisposing factors to epithelial cancer. Considering this evidence, the public at large should be advised to take a well-balanced diet containing vitamin A to meet the recommended dietary allowances.

Mahboubi summarized the results suggesting a relationship between dietary factors and risk of oesophageal cancer in man.

Nair reported that the levels of faecal coprostanol and coprostanone and faecal secondary bile acids, (deoxycholic and lithocholic acid) were higher in non-vegetarians who are at high risk for colon cancer as compared to vegetarians who are at low risk for colon cancer. He suggested that these parameters can be used as biochemical endpoints in screening populations for colon cancer.

The role of diet on the processes of the genome was illustrated by *Elizabeth Castro*, who discussed early work which suggested that the accessibility of chromatin in rat liver to micrococcal nuclease can be diet-dependent. She reported that liver nuclear chromatin from zinc- and magnesium-deficient rats is less accessible to micrococcal nuclease than chromatin from rats fed the respective supplemental diets. Deficiency of either micronutrient alters the H1 class of histones quantitatively and qualitatively. The interaction of nutritional factors and genome structure is an immensely important basic concept worthy of further research effort. The knowledge generated should offer a unified view of how nutrition alters the functions of the genome.

The role of fermented milk products in the inhibition of carcinogenesis was discussed by *Rao*. Although there is no direct epidemiological evidence, recent studies on the faecal enzymes incriminated in the conversion of procarcinogens to carcinogens indicate that cultured or culture-containing dairy products have a protective role. Recently, extracts from fermented milk have been shown to possess potent antimutagenic activity in the Ames *Salmonella* assay system. Thus, future research should be aimed at confirming the anticarcinogenic activity of fermented milk and isolation and identification of anticarcinogenic compound(s) of fermented milk.

Nutrition and dental health: a workshop report

T.H. GRENBY (Organizer)
Guy's Hospital Medical & Dental School, London, UK.

Principal participants. *H.A.B. Linke* (New York University Dental Center, USA), *G. Siebert* and *S.C. Ziesenitz* (Universitäts-Zahnklinik, Würzburg, W. Germany), *A.F. Hackett* (University of Newcastle-upon-Tyne, UK).

Aims and discussion. This workshop was arranged because in recent congresses the effects of over- and under-nutrition on many different body tissues and functions have been examined, but the importance of diet in relation to dental health has been overlooked. The main purposes were: (1) to focus attention on the state of dental health in the Western world and developing countries; (2) to emphasise both the very high prevalence and destructive action of dental caries in Western nations and its rising incidence in some developing countries and to discuss its aetiology, with particular reference to different kinds of foods and eating patterns, and (3) to outline possible preventive measures, including changes in eating habits and the use of alternative sweeteners in place of sugars, and to make practicable recommendations for improvements in these matters.

To set the scene, some general comments were made initially on the current level of dental caries and the recent decrease in certain areas in developed countries. This was followed by a brief explanation of the reasons for the widespread attack of the disease, including epidemiological links with sugar consumption and other dietary habits, such as the frequency of intake of sugary foods and drinks, and the form and texture of different foods. Views on the mechanism of the tooth-destructive action of sucrose were discussed, with reference to current theories on the role of acidogenic oral bacteria, which produce both acid and polysaccharide from sucrose in the dental plaque and in the fissures of molar and pre-molar teeth, where food residues and the bacteria become impacted.

These matters generated a lively discussion from representatives of the food industry, academic life, clinical dental practitioners and members of the public health professions. Many different points of view were expressed: an attempt has been made to summarize constructive measures put forward, in the recommendations at the end of this report.

Hackett described the changing dental disease patterns in developing countries, and reviewed some evidence on how an increase in the consumption of refined carbohydrates and sucrose, coupled with the loss of protective factors, could be linked to rising caries prevalence and severity, particularly in urban areas. The presentation of some data on *per caput* sugar intake and the declining dental state of populations in different parts of the world led to an animated exchange of ideas on this and other aspects of the caries process.

The role of sugars in the onset of dental disease was considered in more detail by *Siebert*, bringing in biochemical aspects of the metabolism of fermentable carbohydrates by oral micro-organisms, and experimental data on acidogenesis and polysaccharide synthesis. This theme was continued by *Linke*, whose specialised knowledge of oral microbiology enabled him to evaluate the importance of *Streptococcus mutans* and its particular metabolic pathways in the dental caries process, in comparison with other micro-organisms.

Amid continuing broad audience participation, *Hackett* presented data he had gathered in a survey of diet in relation to eating and drinking habits in adolescents in North-East England. He again emphasized the influence of frequent sugar intake, correlating measurements of the sugar consumed with the increment in dental caries over 2 years. The difficulties of conducting surveys such as this, and interpreting the data so as to exclude the effects of other features of the diet, were brought out.

Attention then switched to altering the composition of the diet to diminish the risk of dental caries. One approach which is now the subject of much active research, is the replacement of sugars by other sweeteners. *Ziesenitz's* data on the use of bulk sweeteners (carbohydrate derivatives that provide energy and bulk as well as sweetness) were then presented. Topics covering the assessment of cariogenicity, digestion, utlization and microbial fermentation were raised and discussed, with particular reference to the polyols and the newer disaccharide derivatives.

Finally *Linke* gave details of dental research on the properties of the intense sweeteners, which are non-caloric non-carbohydrates with no bulking properties, and therefore particularly suitable for blending with the bulk sweeteners and for use in drinks. He concentrated on the inhibitory action of saccharin on the metabolism of oral bacteria, especially *mutans*, and on its modest influence in curbing experimental caries in laboratory animals. It was pointed out that aspartame, but not the other intense sweeteners currently approved for use in various Western countries, also shows some inhibitory effects on oral micro-organisms.

Recommendations. These summarize the presentations of the key participants and the valued contributions from a cross-section of the audience expressing a wide variety of views. (1) The predominant aetiologic factor in the initiation and development of dental caries is frequency of sugar (sucrose) intake, with confectionery, sweetened cereal foods, soft drinks and other sweetened snack foods high on the list of dentally unsafe products. (2) Other dietary factors that need to be taken into account include the texture and adhesiveness of foods. 'Natural' sugar can do as much damage as added sugar. Another source that can increase the frequency of intake, is the sugar included as an ingredient of many savoury foods not normally bought for their sweetness. (3) It should be the role of better health education, which should receive a higher priority than at present, to inform the public of these matters, and to counsel a reduction in sucrose intake and frequency, with the derivation of an increased proportion of energy requirements from starchy foods rather than from fermentable carbohydrates. (4) Another approach is the re-formulation by the manufacturers of cariogenic foods and drinks with less harmful sweetening agents than sucrose. A widening range of products is now available for this, including among the bulk sweeteners starch hydrolysates, polyols and related materials, and among the intense sweeteners, saccharin, aspartame, acesulfam-K, Talin and cyclamate (in some countries). The intense sweeteners also have a role in the formulation of reduced-energy foods and drinks to assist weight control, and together with certain polyols, in diabetic products. (5) Although a caries-inhibitory action of fluoride and various phosphates (especially glycerophosphate) added to certain foods has been shown experimentally, the use of these and the alternative sweeteners to sucrose always has to await full evaluation and approval by the regulatory authorities in the countries where they are proposed for use. (6) Many further aspects of the connection between diet and dental disease remain to be investigated. The advice customarily given on tooth-brushing and what to eat is sometimes misguided, and does not have the desired effect of subduing dental caries. The need for further research with adequate funding and improved communication on these matters is apparent. (7) Although dental caries is a clinically treatable disease, and although various control measures such as improved oral hygiene, immunization, tooth fissure sealing and the wider use of fluoride have been put forward, it remains highly destructive to dental health — the most widespread disease in developed countries. Its origins are dietary. Major improvements could be made, particularly in childrens' dental health, by attention to the measures summarized here.

What is the calcium requirement for optimal bone health? a workshop report

E.W. SPECKMANN
National Dairy Council, Rosemont, Illinois, USA.

Primary contributors. *John J.B. Anderson* (University of North Carolina at Chapel Hill, N. Carolina, USA), *Robert P. Heaney* (Creighton University, Omaha, Nebraska, USA), *A.M.C. Laval-Jeantet* (University of Paris VI, Paris, France), *B.E.C. Nordin* (Royal Adelaide Hospital, Adelaide, Australia), *M. Peacock* (The General Infirmary, Leeds, UK), *C.J. Robinson* (University of Newcastle, Newcastle upon Tyne, UK), *G. Schaafsma* (Netherlands Institute for Dairy Research, Ede, The Netherlands).

The workshop discussion focused on four basic questions. A brief summary is presented for each of the questions.

For optimal bone health, what is the calcium requirement in childhood, adolescence, young adulthood, pregnancy, lactation, perimenopausal and post-menopausal years, and later life? The calcium requirement for non-pregnant, non-nursing, healthy adults is the amount of dietary calcium necessary to achieve calcium equilibrium. For an individual to be in calcium equilibrium, absorption (the difference between dietary and faecal calcium) must equal obligatory dermal and urinary losses. Assuming average calcium absorption efficiency, a dietary calcium intake of 550 mg/d is the mean dietary requirement necessary to achieve calcium equilibrium in young adults, but the recommended dietary allowance has to be much higher.

The recommended dietary allowance (RDA) for a nutrient is intended to provide for individual variation among most normal healthy persons as they live in a given population under usual environmental stresses. Thus it may exceed the actual requirement of many individuals, but it remains a realistic goal to achieve the requirement of almost all healthy individuals in that population.

The calcium requirements and suggested calcium allowances in Table 1 were presented by *B.E.C. Nordin.*

Table 1

	Mean minimal dietary requirement to achieve calcium balance (mg/d)	Suggested dietary allowance (mg/d)	Median value for 50 countries that publish allowances (mg/d)
Infant — breast milk	225	300	500
cow's milk	350	500	500
Children	500	800	500
Puberty	1000	1200	800
Adult	550	800	575
Postmenopausal female			
— no oestrogen replacement	700	1000	
Pregnancy	800	1100	1200
Lactation	1100	1300	1200

Table 2

Age (year)	Recommended calcium intake (mg/d)
0–0.5	90– 100
0.5–6.0	400– 650
6–10	600– 850
10–16 (F)	700–1000
10–13 (M)	750–1000
13–16 (M)	1100–1500
16–20	900–1200
Adult	700– 900
50+	800–1000
Pregnancy	800–1000
Lactation	1000–1200

The 1984 National Institutes of Health Concensus Development Conference on Osteoporosis recommended that oestrogen-replete, perimenopausal women receive 1000 mg calcium/d and oestrogen-deprived post-menopausal women, 1500 mg calcium/d.

New provisional data from the Dutch Nutrition Board were presented by *G. Schaafsma* (Table 2).

In general, Blacks achieve higher 'peak' bone mass than Whites (peak bone mass is the point at which the skeleton has its greatest mass and density). In fact, US Blacks have a greater bone mass than Whites at virtually every age onwards from birth. The efficiency of calcium absorption declines with age but is high during pregnancy and lactation. Sustained high producers of milk during lactation may require 1200–1800 mg calcium/d in the diet to remain in calcium balance. Calcium intake generally is lower in females than males and is lower in lower social classes than in higher social classes.

Mean and median calcium intakes in males and females, 1976–1980 as revealed by the National Health and Nutrition Examination Survey in the United States (HANES II) compared to the current RDA (9th edn, 1980) for calcium were presented by *E.W. Speckmann* and are illustrated in Figs (*a*) and (*b*) respectively.

In males, at least 50 per cent do not ingest the RDA for calcium on any given day at ages 12–17 and over 34 years of age. In females, more than 50 per cent do not ingest the RDA for calcium on any given day after 10 years of age. Furthermore, there has been a significant decline in calcium intake for teenage girls from the first (1971–1974) to the second (1976–1980) HANES. During the years of 'peak' bone mass development, 18–30 years of age, more than 66 per cent of all US women fail to consume recommended amounts of calcium on any given day; and after age 35 years of age this percentage increases to over 75 per cent. A strong educational programme is needed for individuals 11–35 years of age, particularly females, so that they eat at least the RDA for calcium daily for maximum bone development and achievement of a high 'peak' bone mass. Dairy foods represent the most important source of calcium in the diet.

What is the effect of habitual calcium intake on bone mass and bone integrity? Does this effect differ with age? Does the effect differ with skeletal size? Does habitual calcium intake influence the rate of age-related or menopausal bone loss? Individuals consuming more than 800 mg calcium/d have increased density of the radius compared to individuals

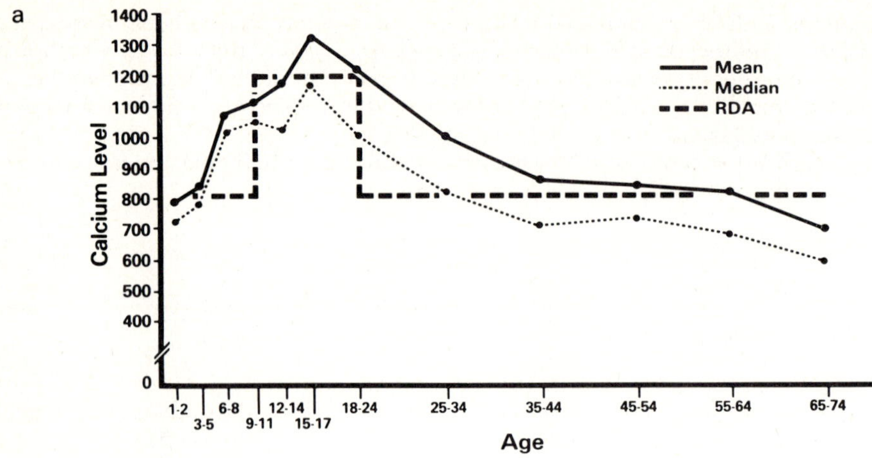

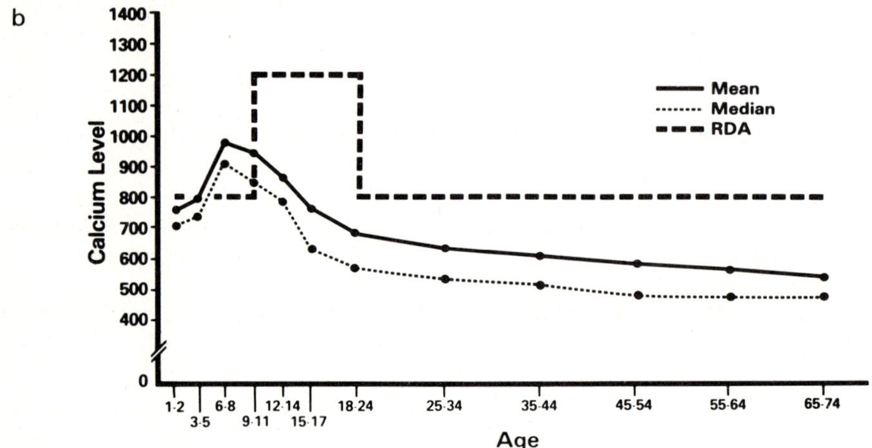

Fig. (a). *Daily calcium intake (mg) for males in USA 1976–1980, as shown by HANES II, and RDA for calcium (DHSS Publication No. [PHS]83–1681, March 1983). (b): Similar data for females.*

consuming less than 600 mg/d. A recommended dietary intake of 500–600 mg calcium/ 1000 kcal would achieve 1000–1200 mg calcium per day on a dietary intake of 2000 kcal. Individuals consuming less than 2000 kcal per day must be particularly mindful of the calcium content of their diets.

Bone mass in the normal healthy perimenopausal woman may be dependent more on biological than on chronological age. The mean rate of forearm bone loss in the perimenopausal woman is about 1.9 per cent of bone mass each year. Some data were presented suggesting that the rate of loss of bone in the distal radius is not influenced by habitual dietary calcium intake between 500–1800 mg/d and widely varying calcium to phosphorus ratios but other data refuted this and showed a relationship between bone density and calcium intake in post-menopausal women. Much discussion focused on whether the distal forearm responds to factors altering bone mass as do other skeletal sites of the body. It appears that the distal forearm is *not* useful in the assessment of calcium intake on bone mass.

What is the relationship between calcium balance and bone mass? (The relationship between bone mass and fracturability, and measures of bone density or mass). **Does a greater peak bone mass result in protection from fracture later in life?** A Yugoslav study found that persons living in a community distinguished by a traditionally high calcium intake (800–1100 mg/d) had a greater 'peak' bone mass at age 40, as reflected in improved metacarpal density; and a 75 per cent reduction in the prevalence of hip fracture compared to those in an area of lower calcium intake (350–500 mg/d). The two communities were similar in all respects except for calcium intake. There was no difference in age-related bone loss between the two communities, but because 'peak' bone mass was greater for the inhabitants of the high-calcium district, their bone mass continued to be greater in the ensuing years resulting in fewer hip fractures.

R.P. Heaney presented data revealing that calcium absorption efficiency falls with age. Despite a fall in calcium intake, data on the frequency distribution for true fractional absorption (adjusted to a mean intake of 800 mg/d) of 273 oestrogen-deprived, non-osteoporotic, post-menopausal women, mean age 53.8 years, revealed that more than half of the women were not absorbing enough calcium to offset the calcium loss from endogenous secretions plus obligatory non-intestinal losses and were in negative calcium balance. Thus the problem of bone loss in the middle years is not only a question of inadequate intake, but also of the failure of the adaptive mechanism to make better use of the calcium in the diet.

What other nutritional factors have significant influence on the calcium requirement of humans? Of all the nutritional factors influencing calcium absorption, a failure in the vitamin D-hormonal system and possibly in the absorption apparatus itself, may have the most significant adverse affect on the adaptive mechanism for calcium absorption. It is known, for example, that plasma 25(OH)D, renal function and fractional calcium absorption fall with age and it appears that vitamin D deficiency may be a widespread problem in the elderly. The vitamin D status of an individual can be defined by measuring the change in plasma $1,25(OH)_2D_3$ when its precursor $25(OH)D_3$ is administered. From such data the following definitions of vitamin D status, ie plasma concentration of 25(OH)D, were recommended — nmol/l(ng/ml): deficiency 0–10 (0–4); insufficiency 10–60 (4–24); sufficiency 60–120 (24–48), and toxicity > 120 (> 48).

To achieve a sufficient level of plasma 25(OH)D from intake and/or body production dietary intake of vitamin D might have to be in the range of 25–50 µg/day (1000–2000 IU/day), a level higher than most elderly persons receive.

Future research directions. The workshop participants recommended that the following areas merited future research emphasis: longitudinal data of nutrient intake and bone status of females throughout life at different levels of physical activity; precise measurement of the calcium requirement for optimal bone mass under defined metabolic conditions where vitamin D, protein, phosphate and other nutritional factors can be independently varied; precise measurement of the bone loss occurring with age and that which occurs as a result of oestrogen loss at the menopause; precise measurement of the influence of dietary calcium on 'peak' bone mass, rate of bone loss and fracture risk at different skeletal sites, including the alveolar bone of the jaw, and studies to define optimal vitamin D status and calcium balance performance in the vitamin D replete individual.

XII: Free radicals

New concept of the importance of free radicals in nutrition

NEW CONCEPT OF THE IMPORTANCE OF FREE RADICALS IN NUTRITION

Free radicals in medicine and the biological role of selenium

A.T. DIPLOCK
Division of Biochemistry, The United Medical and Dental Schools of Guy's and St Thomas's Hospitals, Guy's Hospital, London SE1 9RT, UK.

Oxygen radicals in biological systems. The generation of oxygen radicals in biological systems is a normal process in the reduction of dioxygen to water. The possible detrimental effects of these events are kept in check by a sophisticated and complex multifactorial protective mechanism which has been reviewed extensively recently[3,6]. The monovalent reduction of dioxygen involves the sequential addition of four single electrons, which at each intermediate stage results in the production of a potentially damaging molecular species:

$$O_2 \xrightarrow{\varepsilon} O_2^{\cdot-} \quad \text{(superoxide anion radical)}$$
$$O_2^{\cdot-} \xrightarrow{\varepsilon} O_2^{--} \quad \text{(peroxy anion)}$$
$$O_2^{--} \xrightarrow{H^+} [O_2H^-] \quad \text{(hydrated peroxy anion)}$$
$$[O_2H^-] \xrightarrow{H^+} H_2O_2 \quad \text{(hydrogen peroxide)}$$
$$\left. \begin{array}{l} H_2O_2 \xrightarrow{\varepsilon} OH^{\cdot} + OH^- \\ OH^{\cdot} \xrightarrow{\varepsilon} OH^- \end{array} \right\} 2\,OH^- \xrightarrow{2H^+} 2\,H_2O$$

Overall: $O_2 + 4H^+ + 4\varepsilon \rightarrow 2H_2O$

The accumulation of the superoxide anion radical is prevented by enzymes called superoxide dismutases, that contain Mn or Cu and Zn at their active site. In mammalian cells, the Mn-containing enzyme is localized in the mitochondria, and the Cu/Zn- containing enzyme is located in the cytoplasm so that both the inner mitochondrial membrane and the cytoplasmic (endoplasmic reticulum, outer mitochondrial and nuclear) membranes are protected from attack by the superoxide anion radical. The selenoenzyme glutathione peroxidase catalyses the reduction of hydrogen peroxide to water by the addition of reducing equivalents derived from glutathione, and this enzyme is also capable of catalysing the reduction of a wide range of lipid hydroperoxides to the corresponding hydroxyacids. Catalase, which is largely sequestered in peroxisomes, catalyses the disproportionation of H_2O_2 to H_2O and O_2 but it cannot catalyse the reduction of lipid hydroperoxides because the active site of the enzyme is inaccessible to an hydrophobic substrate.

It will be clear, therefore, from the foregoing that in situations where there is likely to be dietary restriction of manganese, copper, zinc and/or selenium, accumulation of $O_2^{\cdot-}$ and H_2O_2 may result in generation of the highly reactive $OH^{\cdot}$ radical in significant quantities, particularly since this process may be catalysed by iron.

$$O_2^{\cdot-} + Fe^{3+} \longrightarrow Fe^{2+} + O_2$$
$$H_2O_2 + Fe^{2+} \longrightarrow OH^{\cdot} + OH^- + Fe^{3+}$$

$OH^{\cdot}$ generation will occur principally in regions of high oxygen reduction in cells, namely the mitochondria and smooth endoplasmic reticulum. The main likely target for $OH^{\cdot}$ attack will be the unsaturated fatty acids of intracellular membrane phospholipids, in particular those located in the inner mitochondrial and smooth endoplasmic membranes that are closest to the point of origin of the $OH^{\cdot}$. The consequent disruption of the architecture of the membranes, with loss of metabolic control and compartmentation, is probably the biochemical lesion that leads to the pathology of selenium-and vitamin-E-responsive diseases in animals.

A further control on the pathogenesis of free-radical-initiated damage is provided by vitamin E. The unique lipid antioxidant activity of the vitamin, which is superior to that of most synthetic antioxidants, probably derives from its molecular properties, since its amphipathic nature enables it to be orientated in biological membranes. In this location, it is able to prevent the generation of free-radical-initiated chain reactions among the polyunsaturated fatty acyl chains (PUFA) of membrane phospholipids.

$$R-CH_2-CH{=}CH-CH_2-CH{=}CH-(CH_2)_n-COOH \qquad \text{(PUFA molecule in phospholipid)}$$

$$\Big\downarrow OH^{\cdot}$$

$$R-CH_2-CH{=}CH-{\cdot}CH-CH{=}CH-(CH_2)_n-COOH + H_2O \qquad \text{(PUFA from which H has been abstracted to form a free radical)}$$

$$\Big\downarrow O_2$$

$$R-CH_2-CH{=}CH-CH{=}CH-{\cdot}CH-(CH_2)_n-COOH \qquad \text{(molecular re-arrangement)}$$

$$\Big\downarrow$$

$$R-CH_2-CH{=}CH-CH{=}CH-CH-(CH_2)_n-COOH \qquad \text{(peroxide free radical)}$$
$$\underset{O-O}{\big|}$$

vitamin E

Either
$$R-CH_2-CH{=}CH-CH{=}CH-CH-(CH_2)_n-COOH$$
$$\underset{O-OH}{\big|}$$
(fatty acid hydroperoxide)
+ vitamin E radical

Or, when vitamin E is absent, attack on another PUFA

PUFA free radical

In the absence of vitamin E, however, a further unsaturated fatty acid residue in an adjacent phospholipid provides the hydrogen atom necessary to quench the lipid peroxyl radical, and a chain reaction is thereby initiated with widespread detrimental consequences in the membrane structure. The peroxidised unsaturated fatty acids are removed from the membrane by the action of phospholipase A_2 and the liberated fatty acid hydroperoxide is reduced to the corresponding hydroxy acid under the catalytic activity of glutathione peroxidase. In the absence of dietary selenium, when glutathione peroxidase levels will be low, accumulation of fatty acid hydroperoxides will lead to the formation of fatty acid peroxyl radicals or oxy radicals, under the catalytic activity of complexed iron.

$$\text{Lipid} - OOH + (Fe^{2+}\ \text{complex}) \longrightarrow \text{Lipid} - O^{\cdot} + (Fe^{3+}\ \text{complex}) + OH^-$$
$$\text{Lipid} - OOH + (Fe^{3+}\ \text{complex}) \longrightarrow \text{Lipid} - OO^{\cdot} + (Fe^{2+}\ \text{complex}) + H^+$$

Detrimental effects of free radicals in man. The potential detrimental effects of oxygen radicals in the pathogenesis of disease states in man will be self-evident from the previous section. There are many examples in which either oxygen radicals, or some other free radical species, are of significance in medicine and these have been reviewed[6]. Some examples of particular interest are as follows.

The eye. Retrolental fibroplasia is a condition that arises principally in low-birth-weight infants that have been resuscitated by the use of elevated oxygen concentrations in their incubators. Such babies usually have low circulating concentration of α-tocopherol, because the placenta transfers α-tocopherol poorly during the second trimester, and it is believed that the underlying cause of the retinal damage, which may lead to irreversible blindness, is the generation of oxygen-free radicals that cause peroxidation of membrane structures within the retina[4,7]. Certainly, treatment with vitamin E has proved to be an effective preventive measure. Similar considerations apply to the aetiology of intraventricular brain haemorrhages in low-birth-weight babies, and treatment with α-tocopherol also appears to be successful in the condition[2].

In toxicology. The toxicity of many xenobiotic chemicals involves, or may involve, free-radical events at some stage of the process. Thus, the bipyridyl herbicides paraquat and diquat, which have been extremely valuable in agriculture, are remarkably toxic to mammals, and there are many reported instances of paraquat poisoning in farm and domestic animals and in man (eg[5]). The action of the herbicides in plants is the generation of $O_2^{\cdot-}$, which involves the action of light on the chloroplasts, and, following the formation of H_2O_2 by chloroplast superoxide dismutase, the CO_2 fixation process is inhibited because all the available GSH and ascorbate are utilized in the ascorbate-glutathione cycle which removes H_2O_2 and the Calvin cycle cannot proceed. In mammalian organisms, the lung is the principal organ affected and here it is presumed that the accumulation of the herbicide results in accelerated formation of $O_2^{\cdot-}$.

Several drugs such as paracetamol, phenacetin and phenyl hydrazine and its acetyl derivative, also involve free-radical events in their toxicological mechanisms, although the precise nature of this may be subject to some debate. Ethanol toxicity, in particular the biochemical events leading to the characteristic liver degeneration in this condition in man, is thought to involve free-radical mechanisms and the well substantiated role of free-radical intermediates in the toxicology of halogenated hydrocarbons is of particular interest:

$$CCl_4 \longrightarrow CCl_3^{\cdot} + Cl^-$$

and the $CCl_3^{\cdot}$ is thought to initiate lipid peroxidation of membrane lipids by abstraction of hydrogen from the methylene carbon between two double bonds.

Ageing. The free-radical theory of ageing suggests that progressive and accumulative defects in protection against free-radical events allows tissue damage to occur. The principal evidence that favours this theory is the accumulation of 'age pigments' in older animals, and the observation that certain antioxidants prolong the life-span of some small mammals and of invertebrate organisms.

Cancer. The induction of the cancer process involves *inter alia* the production of damage to DNA. There is much evidence that oxygen radicals can cause breakage or other changes in bacterial and mammalian DNA, and, in the latter case, cultured mammalian cells in the presence of phagocytosing neutrophils have been shown to have fragmented DNA and, indeed, the neutrophils themselves often have DNA damage following the phagocytic oxygen burst. Thus, the possible role of oxygen radicals must be considered seriously as a factor in the initiation of the cancer process.

Many cancers in man are caused by chemical carcinogens. In addition to the range of polycyclic hydrocarbons in cigarette smoke, consideration must also be given to the nitrogen oxides present which can act as free-radical initiators of peroxidation. There is, however, a large range of chemicals that are carcinogenic because they undergo metabolic transformation in the liver microsomal mixed function oxidase system, and without doubt free-radical events are involved in many of these processes.

Selenium-deficiency diseases in man. Deficiency of selenium in forages and feedstuffs of domestic farm animals has been recognized worldwide for many years and in territories such as the South Island of New Zealand and in certain parts of Australia and the United States of America it has presented a serious economic problem. Supplementation of pastures with selenium seems an obvious remedy, but the toxicity of selenium at levels not much greater than those needed to satisfy the nutritional need, indicates that great caution is required before indiscriminate selenium supplementation is carried out. In general, the selenium requirement in the diet of most animals is about 0.1 mg/kg, whereas toxicity may be seen at around 2.0 mg/kg.

It might be expected that, in those regions where selenium deficiency disease occurs in farm animals, some parallel deficiency disease might be expected to occur in human populations in the same location. Until quite recently there have been no reports of an association of selenium deficiency with disease states in man; two reasons may provide a possible explanation for this. First, there is evidence that man can tolerate a lower level of selenium intake than can most other animals. Thus, a low blood selenium level in man (around 15–20 ng Se/ml) which apparently is without serious detrimental effect in human subjects, would, if observed in many farm animals, inevitably lead to disastrous consequences in terms of a selenium deficiency disease. Secondly, the food of man is more diverse than that of farm animals and, whereas farm animals frequently eat only food derived from a particular region, or even from one single small farm, human dietary intake will include food brought to the area from many different sources, some of which may provide moderate or even high levels of selenium.

The first description of a selenium-deficiency state associated with disease in human populations arose in the People's Republic of China, where large tracts of land in a broad belt stretching from the north-east to the south-west have been shown to contain extremely low levels of selenium, which in farm livestock gives rise to selenium deficiency disease states. In man, two diseases that are prevalent in these areas, although not always together in the same region, are Keshan disease and Kaschin-Beck disease. These diseases are normally seen in remote areas where the peasant populations affected by disease eat food derived exclusively from their own small-holdings, or from the adjacent communes where soil selenium levels are extremely low. Keshan disease was first described in 1935 and is a cardiomyopathy that affects children and young women, and is normally found in regions where the staple grain content of selenium is less than 0.025 mg/kg[1]. The first reports of the preventive effect of selenium in this condition were published in the Chinese literature, the clue to the involvement of selenium being the close association between the incidence of the disease in human populations and a high incidence of selenium-deficiency disease in farm livestock[8–10]. Intervention with weekly doses of about 1 mg of sodium selenite has been successful in reducing the incidence of the disease to a very low level; there is, however, some doubt whether Keshan disease can be classified as a pure selenium-deficiency disease and the present view is that the disease has a multiple aetiology, one factor in which is a very low dietary intake of selenium.

Kaschin-Beck disease is an endemic osteoarthropathy with disturbance of endochondral ossification and deformity of the affected joints. The most prominent pathological changes, characterized by multiple chondronecrosis, occur in the hyaline cartilage in epiphyses, in articular cartilage and in the epiphyseal growth plates at the end of the long bones[12]. The Kaschin-Beck disease areas in the north of China overlap with the Keshan disease areas, whereas in the south-west they tend to occur separately. The susceptible inhabitants are children in the age-group 5 to 13, usually in peasant families in rural communities[13]. While some reports indicate a close relationship between the incidence of the disease[11] and selenium status, others report only a poor correlation or no correlation at all. Intervention trials with sodium selenite are reported to be successful, however[11,12]. At the present time, it seems that, as in the case of Keshan disease, Kaschin-Beck disease cannot be regarded as a human selenium-deficiency disease, but rather that it is a disease in the aetiology of which a low intake of dietary selenium is an important factor.

1 Chen, X., Yang, G., Chen, J., Chen, X., Wen, Z. & Ge, K. (1980): *Biol. Trace Elem. Res.* **21**, 91.

2 Chiswick, M.L., Johnson, M., Woodhall, C., Gowland, M., Davies, J., Toner, N. & Sims, D. (1983): In *Biology of vitamin E*, ed R. Porter & J. Whelan. Ciba Found. Symp. No. 101, p. 186. London: Pitman.

3 Diplock, A.T. (1984): *Med. Biol.* **62**, 78.

4 Finer, N.N., Peters, K.L., Schindler, R.F. & Grant, G.D. (1983): In *Biology of vitamin E*, ed R. Porter & J. Whelan. Ciba Found. Symp. No. 101, p. 147. London: Pitman.

5 Frank, L. (1981): *Biochem. Pharmacol.* **30**, 2319.

6 Halliwell, B. & Gutteridge, J.M.C. (1985): In *Free radicals in biology and medicine*. Oxford: Clarendon Press.

7 Hitner, H.N. & Kretzer, F.L. (1983): In *Biology of vitamin E*, ed R. Porter & J. Whelan. Ciba Found. Symp. No. 101, p. 165. London: Pitman.
8 Keshan Disease Laboratory of Xi'an Medical College (1965): *Collected papers of Xi'an Medical College* **13**, 94.
9 Keshan Disease Laboratory of Xi'an Medical College (1969): *Collected papers on Keshan disease, Xi'an Medical College* **1**, 10.
10 Keshan Disease Laboratory of Xi'an Medical College (1979): *Zhonghua Yixue Zazi* **59**, 457.
11 Li, J-Y. (1982): *Acta Scientifica Circumstantiae* **2**, 91.
12 Mo, D-X. (1985): *Acta Acad. Med. Xi'an* **6**, 32.
13 Xu, G-L. & Jiang, Y-F. (1985): *Proc. Symp. Geochem. Health, London* (In press).

The toxicity of oxidized fats: lipid hydroperoxides, their decomposition products and their co-oxidation products

W.A. PRYOR
Department of Chemistry and Biochemistry, Louisiana State University, Baton Rouge, LA 70803–1804, USA.

The heating of fats and fat-containing foods is so common, and the polyunsaturated fatty acids (PUFA) in fats are so easily oxidized, that the ingestion of the oxidized products from fats cannot be avoided. In recent years, considerable interest has been shown in the association between fatty diets and a number of pathological conditions, including heart and artery diseases and cancer[35] but there has been relatively little scientific study of the toxicity and physiological effects of the products of autoxidized fats and PUFA, although several recent publications have discussed particular aspects of the problem[1,10,11,13,15,39].

A conceptual framework. PUFA readily undergo oxidation in air, leading to the production of conjugated diene hydroperoxides[26,29]. Carefully purified PUFA undergo spontaneously-initiated autoxidation only after being exposed to air for several days[34]; however, in the presence of transition metals (such as iron) and nitrogenous materials (such as proteins and nucleic acids), PUFA undergo autoxidation with little or no induction period. Since fats of biological origin are almost always contaminated with iron (complexed in haem compounds and other biological chelators), commercial fats and oils used in food production and fatty foods can be expected to undergo autoxidation at a very rapid rate at cooking temperatures. Even at room temperature, oxidation of fats occurs with relative ease.

The effects of co-oxidation on a biological material also must be appreciated. When easily autoxidized materials such as PUFA undergo autoxidation in the presence of more slowly-oxidized materials such as proteins, the proteins are also oxidized[7,26,30] to give an extremely complex mixture of co-oxidation products.

Lipid hydroperoxide toxicity. The LD_{50} values in mice for a number of hydroperoxides and peroxides are shown in the Table[17]. As can be seen, all of these materials are modestly toxic, and autoxidized linoleic acid is the most toxic. The toxicity of these peroxidic materials appears to parallel the ease with which they are reduced; hydroperoxides are reduced quite easily, benzoyl peroxide is reduced reasonably easily, and tert-butyl peroxide is reduced only with considerable difficulty. One-electron reduction of these materials (for example, by ferrous ions or by cytochrome P450) would lead to oxy-radicals.

Table. *The toxicity of some peroxides in various strains of mice injected intra-peritoneally expressed as LD_{50} (µmol).*

Autoxidized linoleic acid 7	Benzoyl peroxide 20	Tetralin hydroperoxide 40
Disuccinoyl peroxide 10	Autoxidized squalene 20–50	tert-Butyl hydroperoxide 60–70
3-Cyclohexene hydroperoxide 15–20	Autoxidized ethyl linoleate 45–60	tert-Butyl peroxide 1080

The LD_{50} for methyl linoleate hydroperoxide-1-C-14 is approximately 1–2 mg when the hydroperoxide is injected into rabbits' ears[9]. The lungs (3 per cent), liver (7 per cent), and blood (3 per cent) retained most of the radioactivity after 2 h. Radioactivity was excreted as carbon dioxide (78 per cent) and in the urine (4 per cent) in 22 h. Lipids in the lung, liver, and kidney were found to contain both tri- and di-enoic PUFA and their hydroxyl derivatives, suggesting the presence of a reductase. In a similar study, the same group found no evidence for hydroxy acids in rats, although a trienoic acid was recovered that could have resulted from dehydration of the dienoic alcohol[3].

A number of other workers have also found that lipid alcohols appear in organs after the ingestion of lipid hydroperoxides and they too have suggested the presence of a reductase. Clearly, such a reductase would be of considerable importance as a detoxification pathway, but any reductase present in the digestive tract has not been characterized. Enzymes that can convert linoleic hydroperoxide (LOOH) to LOH are known. There is, for example, the reductase associated with the prostaglandin endoperoxide synthetase that converts PGG_2 to PGH_2[21].

The cytochrome P450 system can act as a reductase toward lipid hydroperoxides and it has been shown[22] that a reconstituted P450 system can effect the reduction of LOOH to LOH. Furthermore, there is P450 activity in the intestine. but little or none in the stomach[38].

Thirty mg per 100 g B.Wt. of methyl-LOOH is lethal when injected i.v. in the rat[6] and the ozonide of methyl linoleate has a very similar toxicity. Ten times this dose of hydroperoxide taken orally does not cause death, again consistent with the presence of a reductase (or other detoxification pathway) in the gut. The lung is the principal organ showing morphological change probably because it is highly aerated and, therefore, unusually susceptible to autoxidation. Lipid hydroperoxides of course would be expected to initiate autoxidation of lung lipids, and lipid ozonides can also have this effect[31,32,34].

The effects of diets containing oxidized fats on rats deficient or replete in vitamin E were such that vitamin-E-deficient animals showed more extensive haemolysis of red blood cells[25]. Furthermore, larger yields of thiobarbituric acid-reactive materials (TBARM) were obtained from the liver mitochondria of animals fed on diets that contained PUFA than in animals fed hydrogenated coconut oil. Also, the TBARM values for rats fed diets high in PUFA were very much elevated for the group that was vitamin-E-deficient; in contrast, difference in TBARM values between the vitamin E sufficient and vitamin-E-deficient groups fed hydrogenated coconut oil was less. These data suggest, to the extent that TBARM values correctly measure lipid autoxidation *in vivo*[27], that PUFA hydroperoxides can initiate radical-induced damage, particularly in animals that are vitamin-E-deficient.

When methyl linoleate hydroperoxide (10 mg per 100 g) was injected (i.v.) into rats the lung was again the principal organ affected, and a deficiency of vitamin E increased the damage[2]. The alcohol has been reported to be the initial reduction product produced in the rat from 2-ethylbenzene hydroperoxide-C-14[5]. The metabolism of hydroperoxides has been reviewed[38], concentrating particularly on the enzymatic reactions *in vitro* of hydroperoxides produced by the oxidation of PUFA and of steroids.

Secondary products of lipid autoxidation. The decomposition of lipid hydroperoxides produces a variety of products, including malondialdehyde, α-β-unsaturated aldehydes, 4-hydroxy-unsaturated aldehydes, cyclic peroxides, saturated and unsaturated acids of reduced chain length, and saturated and unsaturated hydrocarbons[4,12]. The toxicity of all of these products should be studied, but relatively little data are available. Malondialdehyde (MDA) is a moderate mutagen in bacterial assays and is genotoxic toward mammalian cells. Its metabolism has been investigated[40]. Other aldehydes, unsaturated aldehydes and 4-hydroxy unsaturated aldehydes are also produced on autoxidation of PUFA and are more toxic than MDA. In particular, 4-hydroxynonenal is highly cytotoxic[36].

In a study of oxidized rapeseed oils[18], which are used to manufacture fried fish paste in Japan, rats were fed a diet that contained 150 g oil/kg, and TBARM was increased significantly in the liver of the rats fed oxidized oils as compared with fresh oil. The TBARM values correlated extremely well with the yields of oxidation products that could be extracted from the oils.

In a recently published study a diet containing 100 g unsaturated lipids/kg was heated ten times, for 9 min each, at 180 °C in the presence of potato sticks[14]. This diet and an unoxidized control diet were fed to rats. The heated oils lost 90 per cent of their vitamin E and polar oxidation products were formed. Despite the loss in vitamin E, the heated diet remained nutritionally adequate in vitamin E. However, the rats fed the heated diet showed some elevation of arachidonate in plasma and heart compared with the controls, suggesting the presence of an inflammatory response. Thromboxane B_2 production from platelets was doubled and prostacyclin (PGI_2) from arterial walls was elevated by 20 per cent; thus a higher ratio of TXB_2 to PGI_2 was produced by the autoxidized fats, suggesting that these diets might lead to higher risk of thrombin production. Vitamin E supplementation (300 mg/kg) was found to protect against the changes in the prostaglandin-thromboxane levels.

[^{14}C]-linoleic acid (LA) was heated for 7 d at 37 °C and the mixture separated into LOOH and secondary products (SP)[19]. LA, LOOH, and SP were then fed, in one 100 mg dose intragastrically, to Wistar rats. All animals were found to be clinically normal. When SP was fed, 25 per cent of the radioactivity was excreted in urine and 25 per cent as carbon dioxide. About 3 per cent of the activity accumulated in the liver 12–24 h after feeding, a larger amount than was found for LA or LOOH. The feeding of SP also produced some elevation in serum transaminase activities (GOT and GPT) and slight hypertrophy of the liver.

These reports suggest that peroxides containing secondary oxidation products, while more toxic than pure lipid hydroperoxides, are not so very toxic. However, the suggested relationship between the TXB_2/PGI_2 ratio and the ability of vitamin E to moderate these changes is worthy of further study, since this implies a mechanism by which a high-fat diet might lead to conditions producing atherosclerosis. Furthermore, the long-term effects of these products, as opposed to their acute toxicity, has hardly been studied at all.

Co-oxidation. The powerful effect of co-oxidation in increasing the complexity of product mixtures formed during the oxidation of fatty foods has already been noted. Autoxidation chain reactions involve peroxyl radicals, ROO˙, as the chain-carrying radical[29]. Peroxyl radicals are relatively unreactive and are reasonably selective; thus, they tend to attack the most easily oxidized material that is present in a mixture. However, autoxidation systems always have pathways in which peroxyl radicals are converted to alkoxyl radicals; for example, ROO˙ radicals react with olefines, sulphides, and a number of other types of materials to transfer an oxygen atom, themselves being converted to RO˙ radicals. Alkoxyl radicals are very much more reactive and less selective than are peroxyl radicals[29]. Thus, autoxidation chain reactions lead to the formation of reactive, unselective RO˙ radicals, which attack not only the most autoxidizable material present but also less oxidizable species. The types and toxicities of the products resulting when complex biological materials undergo autoxidation have received relatively little study.

Brown pigments are formed when PUFA undergo autoxidation in the presence of amino acids[20,24]. These pigments are similar to the Maillard compounds produced when sugars and amino acids are heated together[8,41]. Maillard reaction products are extremely important in forming the colours and flavours that are associated with cooked foods[8,41] and they give stable free radical signals detected by electron spin resonance[16]. The toxicological effects of these stable free radicals have not been studied.

During lipid autoxidation polynuclear aromatic hydrocarbons (PAH) could be converted to arene oxides, a carcinogenic derivative of some PAH[28]. Autoxidizing PUFA can convert benzo(a)pyrene (BaP) to mutagenic products that cause sister chromatid exchange in CHV79 cells[23]. The yield of TBARM from PUFA is reduced in the presence of BaP, a result that could be predicted if ROO˙ radicals were the precursor of endoperoxides that lead to TBA reactive materials[33].

1 Ames, B.N. (1984): Dietary carcinogens and anticarcinogens. *Science* **224**, 659–660.

2 Anderson, W.R., Tan, W.C., Takatori, T. & Privett, O.S. (1976): Toxic effects of hydroperoxide injections on rat lung. *Archs Pathol. Lab. Med.* **100**, 154–162.

3 Bergan, J.G. & Draper, H.H. (1970): Absorption and metabolism of 1^{14}C-methyl linoleate hydroperoxide in the rat. *Lipids* **5**, 976–982.

4 Bird, R.P., Draper, H.H. & Basrur, P.K. (1982): Effect of malonaldehyde and acetaldehyde on cultured mammalian cells. Production of micronuclei and chromosomal aberrations. *Mutation Res.* **101**, 237–246.

5 Climie, I.J.G., Hutson, D.H. & Stoydin, G. (1983): The metabolism of ethylbenzene hydroperoxide in the rat. *Xenobiotica* **13**, 611–618.

6 Cortesi, R. & Privett, O.S. (1972): Toxicity of fatty ozonides and peroxides. *Lipids* **7**, 715–721.

7 Desai, I.D. & Tappel, A.L. (1963): Damage to proteins by peroxidized lipids. *J. Lipid Research* **4**, 204–207.

8 Eriksson, C. (1981): Maillard Reactions in Food, In *Progr. Fd Nutr. Sci.* Vol. 5, Numbers 1–6. New York: Pergamon Press.

9 Findlay, G.M., Draper, H.H. & Bergan, J.G. (1970): Metabolism of 1^{14}C-methyl linoleate hydroperoxide in the rabbit. *Lipids* **5**, 970–975.

10 Finley, J.W. & Schwass, D.E. eds (1983): *Xenobiotics in foods and feeds*, ACS Symp. Ser. 234.

11 Finley, J.W. & Schwass, D.E. ed.s (1985): *Xenobiotic metabolism: nutritional effects*, ACS Symp. Ser. 277.

12 Frankel, E.N., Neff, W.E. & Selke, E. (1984): Analysis of autoxidized fats by gas chromatography-mass spectrometry. IX. Homolytic vs heterolytic cleavage of primary and secondary oxidation products. *Lipids* **19**, 790–800.

13 Friedman, M. ed (1984): *Nutritional and toxicological aspects of food safety*. New York: Plenum Press.

14 Giani, E., Masi, I. & Galli, C. (1985): Heated fat, vitamin E and vascular eicosanoids. *Lipids* **20**, 439–448.

15 Grobstein, C. *et al.* (1982): *Diet, nutrition, and cancer*, Washingtom, DC: National Academy Press.

16 Hayashi, T., Ohta, Y. & Namiki, M. (1977): Electron spin resonance spectral study on the structure of the novel free radical products formed by the reactions of sugars with amino acids or amines. *J. Agric. Fd Chem.* **25**, 1282–1287.

17 Horgan, V.J., Philpot, J.St.L., Porter, B.W. & Roodyn, D.B. (1957): Toxicity of autoxidized squalene and linoleic acid, and of simpler peroxides, in relation to toxicity of radiation. *Biochem. J.* **67**, 551–558.

18 Izaki, Y., Yoshikawa, S. & Uchiyama. M. (1984): Effect of ingestion of thermally oxidized frying oil on peroxidative criteria in rats. *Lipids* **19**, 324–331.

19 Kanazawa, K., Kanazawa, E. & Natake, M. (1985): Uptake of secondary autoxidation products of linoleic acid by the rat. *Lipids* **20**, 412–419.

20 Kawamura, S. (1983): Seventy years of the Maillard reaction. In *The Maillard reaction in foods and nutrition* ed G.R. Waller & M.S. Feather, pp. 3–18, ACS Symp. Ser. 215.

21 Lands, W.E.M., Kulmacz, R.J. & Marshall, P.J. (1984): Lipid peroxide actions in the regulation of prostaglandin biosynthesis. In *Free radicals in biology*, Vol. 6, ed W.A. Pryor, pp. 39–61. New York: Academic Press.

22 Lindstrom, T.D. & Aust, S.D. (1984): Studies on cytochrome P450-dependent lipid hydroperoxide reduction. *Archs Biochem. Biophys.* **233**, 80–87.

23 McNeill, J.M. & Wills, E.D. (1985): The formation of mutagenic derivatives of benzo[a]pyrene by peroxidising fatty acids. *Chem.-Biol. Interactions* **53**, 197–207.

24 Pokorny, C. (1981): Browning from lipid-protein interactions. *Prog. Food Nutr. Sci.* **5**, 421–428.

25 Privett, O.S. & Cortesi, R. (1972): Observations on the role of vitamin E in the toxicity of oxidized fats. *Lipids* **7**, 780–787.

26 Pryor, W.A. (1976): Free radical reactions in biological systems. In *Free Radicals in Biology*, Vol. I (W.A. Pryor, ed), pp. 1–43. New York: Academic Press.

27 Pryor, W.A. (1980): Methods of detecting free radicals and free radical-mediated pathology in environmental toxicology. In *Molecular Basis of Environmental Toxicity* (R.S. Bhatnagar, ed), pp. 3–36. Ann Arbor Science Publishers, Inc., Ann Arbor, Michigan.

28 Pryor, W.A. (1982): Free radical biology: Xenobiotics, cancer, and aging. In *Vitamin E: Biochemical Hematological and Clinical Aspects* (eds B. Lubin and L.J. Machlin), pp. 1–22, New York Academy of Sciences, New York (1982).

29 Pryor, W.A. (1984): Free radicals in autoxidation and in aging. In *Free Radicals in Molecular Biology, Aging, and Disease* (eds D. Armstrong, R.S. Sohol, R.G. Cutler & T.F. Slater), Raven Press, New York.

30 Pryor, W.A. (1984): Free radical involvement in chronic diseases and aging. In *Xenobiotic Metabolism: Nutritional Effects* (eds J.W. Finley & D.E. Schwass), pp. 77–96, American Chemical Society, Washington, DC.

31 Pryor, W.A., Lightsey, J.W. & Prier, D.G. (1982): The production of free radicals *in vivo* from the action of xenobiotics: The initiation of autoxidation of polyunsaturated fatty acids by nitrogen dioxide and ozone. In *Lipid Peroxides in Biology and Medicine* (eds K. Yagi), pp. 1–21, Academic Press, New York.

32 Pryor, W.A., Prier, D.G. & Church, D.F. (1981): Radical production from the interaction of ozone and PUFA as demonstrated by electron spin resonance spin trapping techniques. *Environ. Res.* **24**, 42–52.

33 Pryor, W.A., Stanley, J.P. & Blair, E. (1976): Autoxidation of polyunsaturated fatty acids: II. A suggested mechanism for the formation of TBA-reactive materials from prostaglandin-like endoperoxides. *Lipids* **11**, 370–379.

34 Pryor, W.A., Stanley, J.P., Blair, E. & Cullen, G.B. (1976): Autoxidation of polyunsaturated fatty acids. Part I. Effect of ozone on the autoxidation of neat methyl linoleate and methyl linoleate. *Arch. Environ. Health* **31**, 201–210.

35 Roe, D.A. ed. (1983): *Diet, Nutrition, and Cancer: From Basic Research to Policy Implications*, Alan R. Liss, Inc., New York.

36 Schauenstein, E., Esterbauer, H. & Zollner, H. (1977): *Aldehydes in Biological Systems*, Academic Press, London.

37 Seitz, H.K., Garro, A.J. & Lieber, C.S. (1978): Effect of chronic ethanol injestion on intestinal metabolism and

mutagenicity of benzo(a)pyrene. *Biochem. Biophys. Res. Comm.* **85**, 1061–1066.

38 Sies, H., Wendel, A. & Bors. W. (1982): Metabolism of organic hydroperoxides. In *The Metabolic Basis of Detoxification* (W.B. Jakoby, J.R. Bend & J. Caldwell, eds), pp. 307–321, Academic Press, New York.

39 Simic, M.G. & Karel, M. eds. (1980): *Autoxidation in Food and Biological Systems*, Plenum Press, New York.

40 Siu, G.M. & Draper, H.H. (1982): Metabolism of malonaldehyde *in vivo* and *in vitro*. *Lipids* **17**, 349–355.

41 Waller, G.R. & Feather, M.S. eds. (1983): *The Maillard Reaction in Foods and Nutrition*, ACS Symp. Ser. 215.

Role of toxic oxygen metabolites in tissue ischaemia: an overview of recent progress in laboratory models of human disease

G.B. BULKLEY and J.B. MORRIS

Department of Surgery, The Johns Hopkins Medical Institutions, Baltimore, Maryland, USA.

Tissue damage due to the loss of blood flow constitutes a major cause of death and suffering, particularly in industrially advanced societies. As such, ischaemic injury is the fundamental cause of stroke, heart attack, renal failure, and a number of other common diseases to which modern man is vulnerable. Recent advances in our understanding of the fundamental mechanisms of post-ischaemic injury, however, suggest that this whole group of apparently disparate diseases, affecting several different organs, may be caused by a similar mechanism.

By far the most important discovery has been the realization that a major proportion of the injury that results from an episode of ischaemia is sustained not during the ischaemic period itself, but at the time of re-perfusion. This means that what has heretofore been considered an irreversible injury at the time of the first opportunity for therapeutic intervention, may not even yet have taken place. Moreover, the mechanism that mediates this injury is a remarkably simple one, which easily lends itself to therapeutic intervention.

Free radical generation at re-perfusion: studies in the intestine. Since the discovery of the free-radical scavenging function of superoxide dismutase (SOD)[26] there has been rapid progress in our understanding of free-radical-mediated tissue injury[24]. Although much of this work has focused on superoxide production by neutrophils using an NADPH oxidase system[23], it had previously been discovered that superoxide could also be generated in other cells as a byproduct of the oxidation of hypoxanthine and xanthine by xanthine oxidase[25]. McCord's group, responsible for these studies, had found that under non-ischaemic conditions the activity of xanthine oxidase in many tissues was quite low, but that it increased rapidly after the onset of ischaemia. This was due to the proteolytic conversion of another enzyme, xanthine dehydrogenase, which was normally present in many tissues[40]. The activation of xanthine oxidase by ischaemia thus provided a potential mechanism for free-radical generation in parenchymal tissues following ischaemia/re-perfusion.

Knowing that the intestinal mucosa contained particularly high levels of xanthine dehydrogenase[4], with rapid conversion to xanthine oxidase following the onset of ischaemia[27,39] this principle was applied[10] to a standard model of ischaemic mucosal injury in the cat small intestine[2]. Using the osmotic reflection coefficient, a rather precise measure of capillary permeability, as an index of post-ischaemic injury, they found that the administration of SOD prior to re-perfusion prevented most of the injury caused by a 1 h period of hypotensive perfusion (ischaemia). Of particular importance was the fact that SOD was effective when it was administered near the end of the ischaemic period, shortly prior to re-perfusion. This was the first demonstration that much of the injury due to a period of ischaemia was sustained afterwards, during the period of re-perfusion.

Granger *et al.*[10] proposed that with the onset of ischaemia there is a rapid proteolytic conversion of xanthine dehydrogenase to xanthine oxidase, and an accumulation of the substrate hypoxanthine from the breakdown of adenine nucleotides (ATP). The actual oxidation of hypoxanthine cannot take place, however, in the absence of oxygen. When this missing substrate is suddenly available in great excess, as it is at the moment of re-perfusion, the oxidation proceeds rapidly, with the parallel reduction of molecular oxygen. This reduction results in the generation of superoxide radicals as a byproduct. Although somewhat cytotoxic themselves, these superoxides can then go on to form hydrogen peroxide, and secondarily the extremely cytotoxic hydroxyl radical through the Haber-Weiss reaction[12]. These toxic oxygen metabolites cause cellular damage primarily through the peroxidation of lipids in the membranes of cells and mitochondria[23]. It is presumably this injury to the endothelial cell that is first manifest as an increase in capillary permeability.

Since the original proposal, a great deal of subsequent work has supported this mechanism. In the cat intestine, SOD was also found to protect the mucosa from frank epithelial necrosis after 3 h of partial ischaemia[34]. Moreover, allopurinol, a specific inhibitor of xanthine oxidase, provided equivalent protection. Since then, the same group has demonstrated that a similar mucosal injury (measured by the leakage of labelled albumin from the intravascular space into the bowel lumen) can be produced by either ischaemia/re-perfusion or by the perfusion of the lumen with hypoxanthine and xanthine oxidase in the absence of ischaemia[11]. The latter injury could be prevented with SOD. Furthermore, pre-treatment with either allopurinol or the hydroxyl radical scavenger dimethylsulfoxide (DMSO) blocked the aforementioned capillary permeability injury following 1 h of ischaemia[35]. Similarly, this injury could be mimicked by the intra-arterial infusion of hypoxanthine and xanthine oxidase, and this effect could be blocked by SOD or DMSO[38]. Finally, both the capillary and the mucosal injury following 3 h of partial arterial occlusion could be blocked by pretreatment with soybean trypsin inhibitor, a serine protease inhibitor that blocks the proteolytic activation of xanthine oxidase from xanthine dehydrogenase[37]. Although based on indirect evidence employing specific (SOD, catalase), somewhat specific (allopurinol, soybean trypsin inhibitor) and relatively nonspecific (mannitol, DMSO) inhibitors of particular biochemical processes, these data comprise an overwhelming body of circumstantial evidence for the above scheme as the primary mechanisms of post-ischaemic re-perfusion injury[32].

There have been noteworthy negative results, however. Despite extensive efforts, we have been unable to demonstrate protection by SOD or allopurinol in the cat or rat small intestine following varying periods of *total* vascular occlusion[32,36]. Indeed, more serious degrees of intestinal injury seem uninfluenced by manipulation of the free-radical mechanism. This is disappointing, because it suggests that this approach is unlikely to benefit most patients suffering from *ischaemic bowel disease*, who primarily die of a much more advanced transmural infarction, which is far more severe than the superficial mucosal lesion described above. Apparently, most of this advanced injury is due to ischaemia itself, and cannot be substantially ameliorated by modification of the events at re-perfusion. Only in young animals is there a suggestion that an injury leading to full thickness necrosis can be prevented with free radical scavengers[8,30]. This has provided some basis for hope that the application of the above principles may at least prove fruitful in the treatment of *neonatal necrotizing enterocolitis*[3,32].

Studies in models of human disease. *Gastrointestinal tract.* Studies based upon the above mechanism have proliferated rapidly since its first proposal in 1981. In the gastrointestinal tract, in addition to the studies in the small intestine, two separate groups have provided evidence that the superficial gastric mucosal ulceration seen in response to severe physiological stress (*stress gastric ulceration*) can be prevented by treatment with SOD[18]. Studies in the isolated, perfused canine pancreas show that in models of *acute pancreatitis*, caused not only by ischaemia, but also by gallstones or by hyperlipidaemia, the injury is markedly ameliorated by either SOD or allopurinol[41,42]. This has led us to suggest that the final common pathway in acute pancreatitis might be the proteolytic activation of xanthine oxidase from xanthine dehydrogenase by a pancreatic protease, probably chymotrypsin[42,43]. Finally, recent studies in the rat liver have shown that much of the injury that has previously been attributed to *liver ischaemia* may well be mediated by free radicals at re-perfusion[1]. This is also supported by a study which shows substantial protection of the rat liver from ischaemic injury by pretreatment with allopurinol[29]

Skin. A number of studies conducted here at Johns Hopkins suggest an important role for this mechanism in post-ischaemic injury to the skin. Both SOD and allopurinol substantially protect both island skin flaps and free flap transfers from necrosis following the ischaemia necessitated by their creation[16,17,21,22,28]. In these studies, biochemical assays of xanthine oxidase activity also support the proposed mechanism.

Heart. Certainly the most fashionable area for the study of ischaemic injury has been the heart. Indeed, some of the earliest evidence for the above proposed mechanism was provided by McCord in the rat heart (McCord *et al.*, personal communication). There is presently a substantial body of evidence to suggest that there may be extensive clinical application of these principles for the treatment of global cardiac ischaemia, as seen in *cardioplegic arrest* for cardiopulmonary bypass[5,6,19,44–46], and in regional myocardial ischaemia, as seen in *myocardial infarction*[7,9]. Furthermore, the quantitative impact of free-radical injury modification was quite large. One of the most interesting aspects of these studies is the finding that allopurinol substantially reduced infarct size in the canine myocardium following embolization of the coronary artery, whether or not the embolus was subsequently removed to provide for gross re-perfusion[7]. These findings suggest that the events of ischaemia and of re-perfusion may not be completely separated temporally in all cases. Indeed, in these experiments the two appeared to be taking place simultaneously. If this is true, it would mean that therapy directed at free-radical-mediated re-perfusion injury may well be beneficial as *primary* treatment of acute myocardial infarction. Moreover, this therapy might be expected to be effective after the onset of infarction.

Organ transplantation. Aside from the well-known immunologic barriers, a major limitation in the use of transplantation techniques is the availability of suitable organs. Many centres in the USA and Europe are forced to depend upon very wide catchment areas for kidney donors. This necessitates long delays between harvest and grafting. In many places, delays of 24–36 h are common, and many otherwise good kidneys have to be discarded after longer periods of ischaemia. Unfortunately, current techniques of organ preservation are far from optimal and we have approached this problem as one of free-radical-mediated re-perfusion injury. Although treatment by free-radical removal significantly ameliorates injury due to periods of warm ischaemia[13–15,31,33], Baker & Corry, personal communication, the beneficial effect is even more dramatic following periods of cold ischaemia, that minic conditions of organ preservation[20]. Based upon our current understanding, it is not unreasonable to expect use of these techniques to substantially increase the numbers of usable organs, and to thereby significantly improve the overall results of organ transplantation in man.

1 Adkinson, D., Hollworth, M.E., Benoit, J.N., Parks, D.A., McCord, J.M. & Granger, D.N. (1986): Role of free radicals in ischemia-reperfusion injury to the liver. *Acta Physiol. Scand.* **126**, (Suppl. 548), 101–108.

2 Ahren, C. & Haglund, U. (1973): Mucosal lesions in the small intestine of the cat during low flow. *Acta Physiol. Scand.* **88**, 541–50.

3 Bailey, R.W. & Bulkley, G.B. (In press): Role of the circulation in neonatal necrotizing enterocolitis. In *Pathophysiology of the splanchnic circulation*, ed P.R. Kvietys, J.A. Barrowman, and D.N. Granger. Boca Raton, FL: CRC Press.

4 Battelli, M.G., Della Corte, E. & Stirpe, F. (1972): Xanthine oxidase type D (dehydrogenase) in the intestine and other organs of the rat. *Biochem. J.* **126**, 747–749.

5 Burton, K.P., McCord, J.M. & Ghai, G. (1984): Myocardial alterations due to free-radical generation. *Am. J. Physiol.* **246**, H776–H783.

6 Casale, A.S., Bulkley, G.B., Bulkley, B.H., Flaherty, J.T., Gott, V.L. & Gardner, T.J. (1983): Oxygen free–radical scavengers protect the arrested, globally ischaemic heart upon reperfusion. *Surg. Forum* **34**, 313–316.

7 Chambers, D.E., Parks, D.A., Patterson, G., Yoshida, S., Burton, K., Parmley, L.F., McCord, J.M. & Downey, J.M. (1983): Role of oxygen derived free radicals in myocardial ischemia. *Fed. Proc.* **47**, 1093.

8 Dalsing, M.C., Sieber, P., Grosfeld, J.L., Hasewinkel, J., Hull, M. & Weber, T.R. (1983): Ischemic bowel: the protective effect of free-radical anion scavengers. *J. Ped. Surg.* **18**, 360–364.

9 Gardner, T.J., Stewart, J.R., Casale, A.S., Downey, J.M. & Chambers, D.E. (1983): Reduction of myocardial ischemic injury with oxygen-derived free radical scavengers. *Surgery* **94**, 423–427.

10 Granger, D.N., Rutili, G. & McCord, J.M. (1981): Superoxide radicals in feline intestinal ischemia. *Gastroenterology* **81**, 22–29.

11 Grogaard, B., Parks, D.A., Granger, D.N., McCord, J.M. & Forsberg, J.O. (1982): Effects of ischemia and oxygen radicals on mucosal albumin clearance in intestine. *Am. J. Physiol.* **242**, G448–G454.

12 Haber, F. & Weiss, J. (1934): The catalytic decomposition of hydrogen peroxide by iron salts. *Proc. R. Soc.* **147**, 332–351.

13 Hansson, R. (1983): Postischemic renal damage. PhD thesis, pp. 59–107, University of Goteborg.

14 Hansson, R., Gustafsson, B., Jonnson, O., Lundstam, S., Petterson, S., Schersten, T. & Waldenstrom, J. (1982): Effect of xanthine oxidase inhibition on renal circulation after ischemia. *Transplant. Proc.* **14**, 51–58.

15 Hansson, R., Jonnson, O., Lundstam, S., Petterson, S., Schersten, T. & Waldenstrom, J. (1983): Effects of free radical scavengers on renal circulation after ischemia in the rabbit. *Clin. Scien.* **65**, 605–610.

16 Im, M.J., Manson, P.N., Bulkley, G.B. & Hoopes, J.E. (1985): Effects of superoxide dismutase and allopurinol on the survival of acute island skin flaps. *Ann. Surg.* **201**, 357–359.

17 Im, M.J., Shen, W., Pak, C.J., Manson, P.N., Bulkley, G.B. & Hoopes, J.E. (1984): Effect of allopurinol on the survival of island skin flaps: prevention of ischemic and reperfusion injury. *J. Plast. Reconstr. Surg.* **73**, 276–278.

18 Itoh, M. & Guth, P.H. (1985): Role of oxygen-derived free radicals in hemorrhagic shock-induced gastric lesions in the rat. *Gastroenterology* **88**, 1162–1167.

19 Jolly, S.R., Kane, W.J., Bailie, M.B., Abrams, G.D. & Lucchesi, B.R. (1984): Canine myocardial reperfusion injury: its reduction by the combined administration of superoxide dismutase and catalase. *Circ. Res.* **54**, 277–285.

20 Koyama, I., Bulkley, G.B., Williams, G.M. & Im, M.J. (1985): The role of oxygen free radicals in mediating the reperfusion injury of cold preserved ischemic kidneys. *Transplantation* **40**, 590–595.

21 Manson, P.N., Anthenelli, R.M., Im. M.J., Bulkley, G.B. & Hoopes, J.E. (1983): The role of oxygen-free radicals in ischemic tissue injury in island skin flaps. *Ann. Surg.* **198**, 87–90.

22 Manson, P.N., Narayan, K.K., Im, M.J., Bulkley, G.B. & Hoopes, J.E. (1986): Improved survival in free skin flap transfers in rats. *Surgery* **99**, 211–215.

23 McCord, J.M. (1983): The superoxide free radical: its biochemistry and pathophysiology. *Surgery* **94**, 412–414.

24 McCord, J.M. (1985): Oxygen-derived free radicals in postischemic tissue injury. *New Engl. J. Med.* **312**, 159–163.

25 McCord, J.M. & Fridovich, I. (1968): The reduction of cytochrome c by milk xanthine oxidase. *J. Biol. Chem.* **243**, 5753-60.

26 McCord, J.M. & Fridovich, I. (1969): An enzymatic function for erythrocuprein (hemocuprein). *J. Biol. Chem.* **244**, 6049–55.

27 McCord, J.M. & Roy, R.S. (1982): The pathophysiology of superoxide: roles in inflammation and ischemia. *Can. J. Physiol. Pharmcol.* **60**, 1346–52.

28 Narayan, K.K., Im, M.J., Manson, P.N., Bulkley, G.B. & Hoopes, J.E. (In press): Mechanism and prevention of ischemia/reperfusion injury in island skin flaps. *Surg. Forum.*

29 Nordstrom, G., Seeman, T. & Hasselgren, P.O. (1985): Beneficial effect of allopurinol in liver ischemia. *Surgery* **97**, 679–684.

30 Oshima, A., Bulkley, G.B. & Hamilton, S.R. (1984): Role of oxygen-derived free radicals in the development and progression of reperfusion necrosis in the rat small intestine, a model of neonatal necrotizing enterocolitis. *Gastroenterology* **86**, 1202.

31 Paller, M.S., Hoidal, J.R. & Ferris, T.F. (1984): Oxygen free radicals in ischemic acute renal failure in the rat. *J. Clin. Invest.* **74**, 1156–1164.

32 Parks, D.A., Bulkley, G.B. & Granger, D.N. (1983): Role of oxygen-derived free radicals in digestive tract diseases. *Surgery* **94**, 415–422.

33 Parks, D.A., Bulkley, G.B. & Granger, D.N. (1983): Role of oxygen free radicals in shock, ischemia, and organ presentation. *Surgery* **94**, 428–432.

34 Parks, D.A., Bulkley, G.B., Granger, D.N., Hamilton, S.R. & McCord, J.M. (1982a): Ischemic injury in the cat small intestine: role of superoxide radicals. *Gastroenterology* **82**, 9–15.

35 Parks, D.A. & Granger, D.N. (1983): Ischemia-induced vascular changes: role of xanthine oxidase and hydroxyl radicals. *Am. J. Physiol.* **245**, G285–G289.

36 Parks, D.A., Granger, D.N. & Bulkley, G.B. (1982): Superoxide radicals and mucosal lesions in the ischemic small intestine. *Fed. Proc.* **41**, 1742.

37 Parks, D.A., Granger, D.N., Bulkley, G.B. & Shah, A.K. (1985): Soybean trypsin inhibitor attenuates ischemic injury to the feline small intestine. *Gastroenterology* **89**, 6–12.

38 Parks, D.A., Shah, A.K. & Granger, D.N. (1984): Oxygen radicals: effects of intestinal vascular permeability. *Am. J. Physiol.* **247**, G167–G170.

39 Roy, R.S. & McCord, J.M. (1982): Ischemia-induced conversion of xanthine dehydrogenase to xanthine oxidase. *Fed. Proc.* **41**, 767.

40 Roy, R.S. & McCord, J.M. (1983): Superoxide and ischemia: conversion of xanthine dehydrogenase to xanthine oxidase. In *Oxy radicals and their scavenger systems: cellular and medical aspects, II*, ed Greenwald, R.A. & Cohen, G., pp. 145–153. New York: Elsevier Science.

41 Sanfey, H., Bulkley, G.B. & Cameron, J.L. (1984): The role of oxygen-derived free radicals in the pathogenesis of acute pancreatitis. *Ann. Surg.* **200**, 405–413.

42 Sanfey, H., Bulkley, G.B. & Cameron, J.L. (1985): The pathogenesis of acute pancreatitis: the source and role of oxygen-derived free radicals in three different experimental models. *Ann. Surg.* **201**, 633–639.

43 Sanfey, H., Sarr, M.G., Bulkley, G.B. & Cameron, J.L. (In press): Oxygen-derived free radicals and acute pancreatitis: a review. *Acta. Physiol. Scand.*

44 Shlafer, M., Kane, P.F. & Kirsh, M.M. (1982): Superoxide dismutase plus catalase enhances the efficacy of hypothermic cardioplegia to protect the globally ischemic, reperfused heart. *J. Thorac. Cardiovasc. Surg.* **83**, 830–839.

45 Shlafer, M., Kane, P.F., Wiggins, V.Y. & Kirsh, M.M. (1982): Possible role for cytotoxic oxygen metabolites in the pathogenesis of cardiac ischemic injury. *Circulation* **66**, I85–I92.

46 Stewart, J.R., Blackwell, W.H., Crute, S.L., Loughlin, V., Greenfield, L.J. & Hess, M.L. (1983): Inhibition of surgically induced ischemia/reperfusion injury by oxygen free radical scavengers. *J. Thor. Cardiovasc. Surg.* **86**, 262–272.

Free radicals in the pathogenesis of kwashiorkor

M.H.N. GOLDEN and D. RAMDATH
Wellcome Trace Element Research Group, Tropical Metabolism Research Unit, University of the West Indies, Kingston, 7, Jamaica.

The skeletal spectre of the marasmic child clearly results from a lack of intake of the bulk nutrients. Marasmus can be reproduced easily and consistently in any convenient species of experimental animal.

In stark contrast, the other major form of malnutrition — kwashiorkor — has only once been convincingly reproduced in experimental animals. Coward & Whitehead[3] produced oedema, fatty liver, skin lesions, hair discolouration and friability, hypoproteinaemia and mental changes in baboons by feeding the animals exactly the same diets that children with kwashiorkor received in Uganda. Why should the kwashiorkor syndrome be so difficult to reproduce experimentally? Why have the programmes designed to prevent kwashiorkor been so uniformly unsuccessful? The obvious first answer to be considered is that all the hypotheses that have been proposed, tested experimentally and used as the conceptual framework for the programmes, are incorrect. Certainly the extant hypotheses do not adequately explain more than a few of the features of kwashiorkor. These features must all be reconciled in any unifying hypothesis. Recently we have proposed that kwashiorkor results from an imbalance between the production of free radicals and their safe disposal[9]. It is the purpose of this paper to examine the evidence for such a hypothesis.

The hypothesis, illustrated in Fig. 1, states that in kwashiorkor various noxa are imposed upon the subject. These noxa produce free-radical-mediated lipid peroxides and toxic carbonyls. Under normal metabolic and nutritional circumstances, provided that the flux of radicals is not too intense, the radicals are scavenged and dissipated through the appropriate

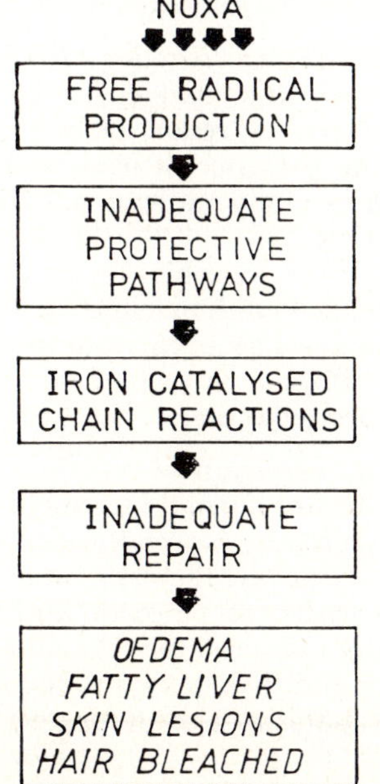

Fig. 1. Proposed steps in the pathogenesis of kwashiorkor.

protective pathway. The flux of radicals is increased with abundant storage iron, or at least in the absence of iron deficiency. This is because iron, being a redox catalyst, both multiplies the number of radicals produced and creates more reactive and damaging species, unless it is strictly compartmentalized and bound to a restrictive chelator.

The reason why the radicals and their products result in kwashiorkor is that there is a relative, and probably also an absolute general deficiency of the protective mechanisms. Most of the protective pathways require micronutrients. A severe dietary deficiency of any one of these nutrients will lead to loss of free radical protection in some cellular compartment. Even a mild deficiency of several of the micronutrients is likely to lead to a general lack of protection. The balance between radical production and dissipation, repair of damage and safe disposal of the toxic products of free radical action, cannot be redressed. The resulting damage then gives rise to the oedema, fatty liver, pigmentary changes, diarrhoea, immunoincompetence and mental changes that are typical of kwashiorkor. The steps of the hypothesis are discussed below.

Free-radical-producing noxa in kwashiorkor. *Infection* is almost ubiquitous in kwashiorkor[20] being frequently precipitated for example by measles[21]. The body's defence against invading organisms is to produce free radicals in quantities sufficient to kill the organisms. The body relies upon its own protective mechanisms to limit the extent of self-damage and to repair the unavoidable damage after the organism is killed. Thus, stimulated white cells produce large quantities of superoxide and hydrogen peroxide[7] which they release into the surrounding medium. Peroxy lipids are formed which stimulate further white cells[15]. Infections and inflammatory toxins are thus potent stimulators of free radical formation.

Toxins. Kwashiorkor occurs in areas with inadequate food handling and storage facilities, and in times of food shortage when spoilt foods are likely to be consumed. In these areas most weaning foods are heavily contaminated with toxogenic bacteria[23]. In addition, a whole range of toxogenic fungi grow on stored foods in Third World communities. Attention has been focused upon one of these, aflatoxin, which should probably be regarded as an index of general mycotoxin exposure rather than as a specific intoxication. Furthermore, the overgrowth of the child's small intestine with bacteria constitutes an uncontrolled biochemical powerhouse capable of producing numerous products[4], many of them toxic. Small bowel overgrowth[13] and endotoxaemia (unpublished) are usual in kwashiorkor. Fatty liver, a hallmark of hepatic free radical damage, is produced by small bowel overgrowth both clinically and experimentally.

Catalysis of free radical production. The major catalyst of free-radical reactions *in vivo* is iron[11]. This is because of its relative abundance and the ease with which it changes its valency state under *in-vivo* conditions of Eh and pH. Iron acts as a catalyst by redox cycling with reducing equivalents such as ascorbic acid and NADPH. In the presence of iron a single radical can readily initiate a chain reaction with the formation of many radicals and their peroxy and carbonyl products[19].

The hepatic iron concentrations in Jamaican children dying from kwashiorkor is much higher than in controls and similarly high hepatic iron has been found in children from Lebanon[17], India[22] and South Africa[8]. Furthermore, when marrow has been examined in these countries it has been found to contain abundant iron[1]. Plasma ferritin in severely malnourished children is increased[10], particularly in those children who die.

Protective mechanisms against free radicals in kwashiorkor. Free-radical reactions are one of the basic biochemical mechanisms of the body: free radicals are normal intermediates in metabolism. Thus all mono-oxygenases, and several dehydrogenases, especially xanthine oxidase, cytochromes P450 and B6, prostaglandin and leucotriene synthetases, and the mitochondrial respiratory chain, normally generate superoxide, hydrogen peroxide and free radicals. Radical production is purposely increased as part of any inflammatory reaction by the activity of specific NADPH-dependent lipo-oxygenases. They and their toxic products do not normally cause damage because a whole range of defence mechanisms exist to protect the different parts of the cell.

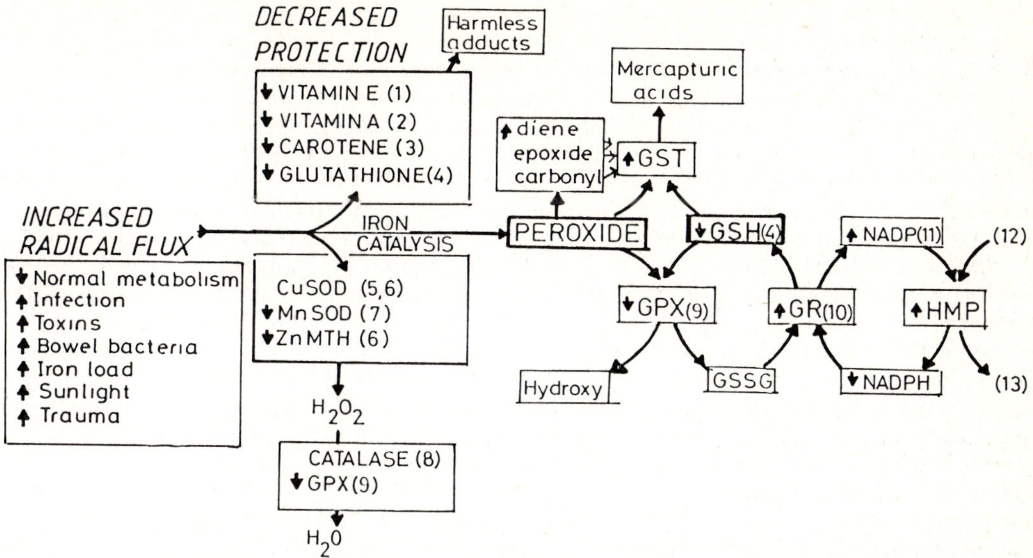

Fig. 2. *Diagram showing the mechanisms of radical production and subsequent metabolism.* The arrows BESIDE the substrates, products and enzymes show whether they have been demonstrated to be increased or decreased in children with kwashiorkor. The numbers refer to the essential nutrients involved: (1) vitamin E: (2) vitamin A: (3) carotene: (4) sulphur amino acids, CYS: (5) copper: (6) zinc: (7) manganese: (8) iron: (9) selenium: (10) riboflavin: (11) nicotinic acid: (12) magnesium and phosphorus: (13) thiamin. Abbreviations: CuSOD — Copper-zinc superoxide dismutase: MnSOD — Manganese superoxide dismutase: GST — Glutathione-S-transferase: GPX — Glutathione peroxidase: GSH — Glutathione (reduced): GSSG — Glutathione (oxidized): GR — Glutathione reductase: NADP — Nicotine adenine dinucleotide phosphate (oxidized): NADPH — Nicotine adenine dinucleotide phosphate (reduced): HMP, Hexose-monophosphate-shunt (G6PD and 6-phosphogluconic acid dehydrogenase).

Figure 2 summarizes the major protective pathways, the nutrients involved and the changes that occur in kwashiorkor.

Dismuting pathways. In malnutrition, plasma vitamin E, vitamin A and carotene are each severely reduced, both absolutely and relative to lipid concentrations. Vitamins E and A are specifically related to the prognosis and are useful in the classification of malnourished children[18]. In Jamaica we find that vitamins E and A are reduced in both oedematous and non-oedematous malnutrition. These nutrients are bleached and consumed when they dismute a free radical.

Zinc, in the form of zinc metallothionein, is a very effective free radical sink *in vitro*, and probably also *in vivo*. Although the concentration of intracellular zinc metallothionein has not yet been measured in malnutrition, circulating zinc levels are uniformly low in kwashiorkor (unpublished results).

Removal of radical-induced toxic products. The radicals that escape safe dissipation generate peroxides, particularly in cell membranes. The organic peroxides are substrates for the selenium containing enzyme, glutathione peroxidase (GPX), which reduces the peroxide to hydroxyl with oxidation of glutathione. This enzyme is reduced in malnutrition, particularly in children with more severe disease. Selenium, itself, has also been shown to be reduced in the blood of children with kwashiorkor from Guatemala[2], Thailand[14] and Zaire[6]. Presumably GPX is reduced in all these populations. The result will be an inefficient removal of organic peroxide. The peroxides will then break down to form toxic aldehydic products such as 4-hydroxynonenal[5], which may be the most damaging species produced[24].

Glutathione. This is the central component of the whole protective repertoire. Not only is glutathione an effective aqueous free radical scavenger in its own right, but it also functions to maintain protein sulphydryl groups in the reduced state and is the cofactor for both of the major detoxification pathways, GST and GPX. Clearly, the GSH status of the malnourished child will be crucial to his ability to withstand a free-radical stress, and may indeed determine whether or not kwashiorkor, as opposed to marasmus, will supervene.

We have found that the concentration of glutathione is specifically reduced in the red cells of children with kwashiorkor, with or without concomitant marasmus, whereas glutathione levels are normal in pure marasmus. The sensitivity and specificity of red cell GSH to differentiate oedematous from non-oedematous malnutrition (93 subjects) were both over 91 per cent. Furthermore, the few 'false negatives' had equivocal or minimal oedema, which disappeared in a day or so; they did not lose any weight on refeeding, they also did not have the skin, hair or liver changes associated with kwashiorkor. They were classified as kwashiorkor, however, because we use the Wellcome classification in which the presence or absence of oedema has primacy in differentiating the conditions. All the children with unequivocal kwashiorkor syndrome had very low levels of glutathione and the very sick children had profoundly reduced glutathione concentrations. One can certainly successfully differentiate between kwashiorkor and marasmus on the basis of the red cell glutathione concentration alone and we believe that the red cell glutathione is reduced *in vivo* predominantly because of increased consumption rather than decreased production. The glutathione is almost certainly consumed in detoxifying peroxides and carbonyls that enter the circulation from the tissues. This itself implies that in kwashiorkor there is a greatly increased flux of peroxides requiring disposal.

Damage produced by unsuppressed radical peroxidation. That oedema can result from free-radical-mediated mechanisms is demonstrated by the oedema that occurs in vitamin-E-deficient premature infants stressed by a diet high in poly-unsaturated fats[12]: indeed, this oedema is very similar in behaviour and distribution to the oedema of kwashiorkor. However, if free-radical-mediated damage is the cause of oedema, the precise mechanisms is not clear.

Fatty liver is the hallmark of all forms of peroxidation reaction in the liver, the distribution of fat depending upon the mode of production of the radical. The hepatic mitochondrial membrane will be particularly vulnerable if there is a reduction in manganese superoxide dismutase and GPX because these two enzymes provide the major protection from the intense oxygen metabolism in the mitochondria.

Nausea, diarrhoea, vomiting and immunoincompetence, all characteristic albeit nonspecific signs commonly found in kwashiorkor, are the cardinal symptoms of radiation injury — an unequivocal example of generalized free radical formation.

We conclude that, although there are individually other plausible aetiologies for the clinical features of kwashiorkor, each can be caused by an excess free radical stress in the face of inadequate protection, and that none of the other candidate hypotheses adequately account for the association between the different clinical features.

Death from malnutrition. Examination of the results we have described shows that those children who die have the lowest levels of vitamin E, glutathione peroxidase, zinc, and glutathione; they have the highest levels of plasma ferritin and hepatic iron[25]. It was only in these desperately ill children who died that the proportion of GSSG to total glutathione was raised (up to 20 per cent). At the same time, these children had extraordinarily high activities of their hexose-monophosphate-shunt enzymes (up to five times normal). In other words, the features which distinguish the children with kwashiorkor are all exaggerated in those who die from kwashiorkor.

Figure 3 shows the admission red cell GPX activity plotted against the admission plasma ferritin concentrations from a series of malnourished children. All the children who, on admission, had a GPX of below 17 IU/gHb and a ferritin of above 250 µg/l subsequently died. All except one child who did not fulfil these criteria survived. Thus we were able to predict accurately which children would subsequently die and which would survive on the basis of measuring two of the integral components of the free radical scheme. This is particularly

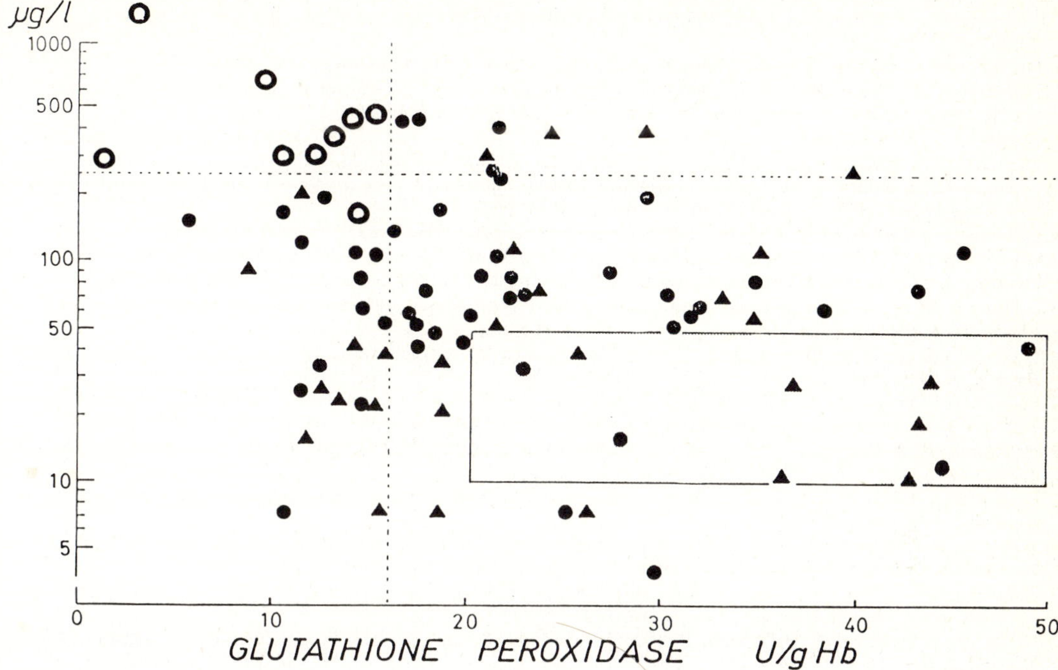

Fig. 3. Admission red blood cell glutathione peroxidase vs plasma ferritin in malnourished children. The area within the box is the normal range. ▲, marasmus: ●, kwashiorkor; ○, children who subsequently died. The dashed lines are arbitrarily drawn at GPX = 17 U/gHb and ferritin = 250 µg/l.

impressive as most of the children did not succumb for a considerable time after the measurements were made. This opens the way for rational treatment to be instituted before the children become moribund.

Clearly many of the therapeutic manoeuvres that have been tried are inappropriate or even dangerous if the free radical hypothesis is correct. For instance, on the basis of the assumption that the children have an energy deficit as part of their syndrome, we have in the past advocated adding oil to the children's diet: it would be hazardous to give a child without free radical protection a diet high in polyunsaturated fatty acids. It is probably relevant that giving iron to children with kwashiorkor resulted in a very high mortality rate[16] while giving protein hydrolysates intravenously also results in an extraordinarily high mortality rate[8].

On the other hand, if the present hypothesis is correct, there are a number of new therapeutic lines that could be very effective in treating and preventing kwashiorkor. They are all open to experimental testing and if they are found to be effective will provide very strong evidence in favour of the hypothesis.

We conclude that trials of iron chelation, anti-oxidant therapy with both water and fat-soluble agents, possibly allopurinol, as well as selenium, manganese, zinc, copper and vitamin replacement therapy, with the avoidance of polyunsaturated fats, suppression of small bowel flora and active treatment of infections, are warranted in children with kwashiorkor.

Acknowledgements. This work would not have been possible without the continued support of the Wellcome Trust. Professor J.C. Waterlow, Dr A.A. Jackson and Dr B.E. Golden provided the atmosphere in which these ideas were germinated. We thank Mrs L. Charley and Miss J. Foreman for their technical assistance and the nursing staff for their loving care of our unfortunate patients.

1 Adams, E.B. & Scragg, J.N. (1965): Iron in the anaemia of kwashiorkor. *Br. J. Haematol* **11**, 676–681.

2 Burk, R.F., Pearson, W.N., Wood, R.P.II. & Viteri, F. (1967): Blood selenium levels and in-vitro red cell uptake of 75 Se in kwashiorkor. *Am. J. Clin. Nutr.* **20**, 723–733.

3 Coward, D.G. & Whitehead, R.G. (1972): Experimental protein-energy malnutrition in baby baboons. *Br. J. Nutr.* **28**, 223–237.

4 Drasar, B.S. & Hill, M.J. (1974): *Human intestinal flora.* New York: Academic Press.

5 Esterbauer, H. (1982): Aldehydic products of lipid peroxidation. In: *Free radicals, lipid peroxidation and cancer*, ed D.C.H. McBrian & T.F. Slater, pp. 101–128. New York: Academic Press.

6 Fondu, P., Hariga-Muller, C., Mozes, N., Neve, J., Van Steirteghem, A. & Mandekbaum, I.M. (1978): Protein-energy malnutrition and anaemia in Kivu. *Am. J. Clin. Nutr.* **31**, 46–56.

7 Gabig, T.G. & Babior, B.M. (1982): Oxygen-dependent microbial killing by neutrophils. In *Superoxide dismutase*, Vol. 2, ed Oberly, L.W., pp. 1–15. Boca Raton: C.R.C. Press.

8 Gillman, J. & Gillman, T. (1951): *Perspectives in human nutrition.* New York: Grune & Stratton.

9 Golden, M.H.N. (1985): The consequences of protein deficiency in man and its relationship to the features of kwashiorkor. In *Nutritional adaptation in man*, ed K. Blaxter & J.C. Waterlow pp. 169–187 London: John Libbey.

10 Golden, M.H.N., Golden, B.E. & Bennett, F.I. (1985) High ferritin values in malnourished children. In *Trace element metabolism in man and animals-5*, ed C.F. Mills. (In press)

11 Halliwell, B. & Gutteridge, J.M.C. (1984): Oxygen toxicity, oxygen radicals, transition metals and disease. *Biochem. J.* **219**, 1–14.

12 Hassan, H., Hashim, S.A., Van Itallie, T.B. & Sebrell, W. H. (1966): Syndrome in premature infants associated with low plasma vitamin E levels and high polyunsaturated fatty acid diet. *Am. J. Clin. Nutr.* **19**, 147–157.

13 Heyworth, B. & Brown, J. (1975): Jejunal microflora in malnourished Gambian children. *Archs Dis. Child.* **50**, 27–33.

14 Levine, R.J. & Olson, R.E. (1970): Blood selenium in Thai children with protein-calorie malnutrition. *Proc. Soc. Expt. Biol. Med.* **134**, 1030–1034.

15 McCord, J.M. & Petrone, W.F. (1982). A superoxide activated lipid-albumin chemotactic factor for neutrophils. In *Lipid peroxides in biology and medicine*, ed K. Kagi, pp. 123–131. New York: Academic Press.

16 McFarlane, H., Reddy, S., Adcock, K.J., Adeshina, H., Cooke, A.R. & Akene, J. (1970): Immunity transferrin and survival in kwashiorkor. *Br. Med. J.* 268–720.

17 McLaren, D.S., Faris, R. & Zekian, B. (1968): The liver during recovery from protein-calorie malnutrition. *J. Trop. Med. Hyg.* **71**, 271–281.

18 McLaren, D.S., Shirajian, E., Loshkajian, H. & Shadarevian, S. (1969): Short term prognosis in protein-malnutrition. *Am. J. Clin. Nutr.* **22**, 863–870.

19 Mead, J.F., Wu, G.-S. & McElhaney, R.N. (1982): Mechanism of protection against membrane peroxidation. In *Lipid peroxides in biology and medicine*, ed K. Kagi, pp. 161–178. New York: Academic Press.

20 Morehead, C.O., Moorehead, M., Allen, D.M. & Olson, R.E. (1974): Bacterial infections in malnourished children. *J. Trop. Paed.* **20**, 141–147.

21 Morley, D. (1964): The severe measles of West Africa. *Proc. Roy. Soc. Med.* **57**, 846–849.

22 Mukherjee, K.L. & Sakar, N.K. (1958): Liver enzymes in human undernutrition. *Br. J. Nutr.* **12**, 1–7.

23 Rowland, M.G.M., Barrel, R.A.E. & Whitehead, R.G. (1978): Bacterial contamination of traditional Gambian weaning foods. *Lancet* **1**, 136–138.

24 Slater, T.F. (1984): Free-radical mechanisms in tissue injury. *Biochem. J.* **222**, 1–15.

25 Waterlow, J.C. (1948): *Fatty liver disease in infants in the British West Indies.* MRC Spec. Rep. Ser. No. 263. London: HMSO.

XIII: Maternal and infant nutrition

Nutrition in pregnancy and lactation

Adequacy of breast-feeding and maternal nutritional status

Workshop

Nutritional management of the preterm infant

Nutritional and developmental factors affecting performance of newborn babies and piglets

NUTRITION IN PREGNANCY AND LACTATION

Incremental dietary needs to support pregnancy

R.G. WHITEHEAD, M. LAWRENCE and A.M. PRENTICE
MRC Dunn Nutrition Laboratory, Cambridge, UK and Keneba, The Gambia.

Each pregnancy is associated with short-term but dramatic changes in a woman's nutritional physiology. Over a period of 9 months she gains an average of 12–13 kg in weight, most of this during the last 5 months. Such a rapid phase of tissue growth and energy storage never occurs at any other stage in adult life: the rate of weight gain is swifter than in the most rampant developing obesity.

The dietary situation in affluent countries. It is not surprising therefore that all expert committees have judged it necessary to recommend substantial increases in energy and nutrient intakes at this time. For example, in the United Kingdom[1] we recommend during the last two trimesters of pregnancy a 12 per cent increase in dietary energy consumption. For many of the individual nutrients the recommended rise is much greater being 67 per cent in the case of folate, 100 per cent for vitamin C and 140 per cent for calcium. Britain, in fact, tends to be a rather conservative country where recommendations for vitamins and minerals are concerned and the corresponding increased allowances for the USA are even more marked.

Generous recommendations to provide optimum protection for both the mother and her unborn baby are readily defensible. The embarrassment comes when one compares such recommendations with actual measured intakes. In affluent Western countries it is now common for nutritionists to report either no increases, or only slight increases, in food consumption during pregnancy[12]. Investigators have not been able to come up with any really convincing reason for this discrepancy but a woman's concern about not putting on too much fat during pregnancy, so that she can get rid of it quickly afterwards, has been suggested as one explanation. Alternatively it is suspected that many doctors too are over-worried about weight matters during pregnancy and caution the mother accordingly.

For many of the vitamins and minerals one could argue that a lack of an increased food consumption during pregnancy is unlikely to be of pathophysiological significance, as in countries like the UK the customary diet is relatively rich in protein and the micronutrients. For example our National Food Survey[9] suggests the average person ordinarily consumes 89 per cent above his physiological needs for vitamin C and 57 per cent in the case of calcium. Be this as it may, one is still left with the enigma of how women accommodate the extra energy needs as there is no evidence of a widespread and substantial over-eating with respect to this dietary component: indeed the consumption figures for 1984 estimate the average UK citizen selects a level of energy intake 8 per cent *below* the physiologically-based recommendation.

The third world. In the third world the lack of correlation between our recommendations and what women actually eat during pregnancy is even more marked[12]. Again there is little evidence of a general increase in overall food consumption and, furthermore, baseline energy intakes are generally set well below those in more affluent countries. A comparative compilation of energy consumption among pregnant women from different parts of the third world suggests a typical intake of around 1700 kcal (7.11 MJ)/d in contrast with the recommended intake of 2400 kcal (10.04 MJ)/d[3], a deficit of 700 kcal (2.93 MJ)/d. This difference is so great that many investigators have cast doubt on the validity of the food intake measurments. It is to be hoped that the newer technologies now available to us, such as those involving doubly-labelled water, will clarify the situation but for the time being we are left with a substantial literature all firmly indicating that pregnancy in the third world is being met without anything approaching the recommended level of increase in energy intake.

Since the overall quality of the food customarily eaten by deprived people in the third world is also generally much poorer than that of the West, and there is rarely any demonstrable switch towards more nutritious foods during pregnancy, one is left bemused as to how it is that the physiology of a woman can possibly cope with so many nutrient as well as energy deficiencies. Our own work in the The Gambia puts the pathophysiological limit for dietary energy accommodation at around 1500–1600 kcal (6.27–6.69 MJ)/d: above this value fetal development is relatively satisfactory, below it the incidence of babies born weighing less than 2.5 kg rises rapidly to unacceptable proportions[10].

It is quite clear that such low dietary intakes during pregnancy must be avoided at all costs. Our laboratory in The Gambia has developed a locally produced, highly nutritious biscuit, to correct particularly the food shortage which occurs every year there during the hungry season[10]. From a national and international health planning point of view, however, we need to know, more precisely, the minimum amount by which we really must boost the energy and nutrient intakes of active women during pregnancy. One has to be economically realistic: if we set our recommendations too high it may well be impossible for the poorer countries of the world to meet them, whatever the political will. An uncritical overenthusiasm on the part of nutritionists, we fear, has often resulted in our achieving just the opposite of what we have set out to do, not only in the third world! Before we can unequivocally advise the national and international agencies we must have a more complete understanding of the ways the body metabolizes energy and nutrients in pregnancy. We also need to know the range of energy and nutrient intakes, which at both an individual and a community level, can safely be accommodated. Within the time constraints it is necessary to concentrate on the key dietary component, energy.

Nutritional metabolism during pregnancy. What precisely is known about the changes in nutritional metabolism needed to support the dramatic physiological events which accompany pregnancy? Hytten & Leitch[5], in their classic work, have suggested that the total energy cost of the average pregnancy is of the order of 80 000 kcal (334.6 MJ). The energy value of the protein deposited in the fetus and in the various maternal reproductive organs represents only a small proportion of this, around 5–7000 kcal (20.9–29.3 MJ). The bulk of the energy needs are almost equally divided between two principal functions, the laying down of about 4 kg of maternal body fat and supporting theoretical increases in maintenance metabolism. The latter are believed to be necessary because of an enhancement of a number of physiological processes relating both to the mother and her growing fetus. Additionally, in setting the net total energy cost of pregnancy at only 80 Mcal (334.6 MJ), scientists have tacitly assumed that either the considerably heavier woman needs no extra to perform her normal daily work and leisure pursuits, or that these are accommodated by a reduced activity.

To reconcile the fact that most investigators fail to observe anything like such major rises in energy intake during pregnancy, it is obvious we have to examine by direct measurement what is currently happening to the three major components listed above, fat deposition, maintenance metabolism and activity patterns, in women living under differing environmental circumstances. This is exactly what an international collaborative team set out to do a few years ago. We have been studying women from various industrialized countries, Scotland (Professor Durnin) the Netherlands (Professor Hautvast) as well as England. In the third world we have been working with women from The Gambia (The Dunn, Cambridge), from Thailand (Professor Valyasevi) and from the Philippines (Dr Barba). The overall project is coordinated by the Nestlé Foundation, an independent Swiss charity established 20 years ago to study nutritional problems, mainly of the developing countries.

The project is not yet complete and it would be inappropriate to attempt any comparative analysis. To provide some insight into the sorts of results we are obtaining, however, and the scientific challenges they represent, we will discuss some of the Gambian results.

Maternal fat storage. The most obvious component to look at in the hope of discovering a major way of cutting down on energy costs is perhaps body fat. The accepted gynaecological norm derived from the literature is for 4 kg of fat to be laid down and recent findings from studies carried out in Cambridge[13] are identical with these data. This indicates, interestingly, that current day Western women are not saving energy by this process even if they are consciously or unconsciously tempted to weight-watch by moderating their food intake.

In The Gambia, however, our findings are quite different. The average woman in our cohort, not receiving the dietary biscuit supplement, actually lost 0.32 kg of fat during the course of her pregnancy. The fact that this was due to a dietary energy deficit and not some other factor, is established by results from the supplemented women who laid down 1.68 kg of fat. An even more dramatic demonstration is provided by an examination of seasonal variations. Elsewhere in these proceedings[7], it has been shown that unsupplemented women who conceive during February and who thus have much of their critical second and third trimesters during the hungry season, July–September, actually *lose* 4 kg of fat during their pregnancy, a net difference of 8 kg of fat from Cambridge women or a massive 75 Mcal (313.7 MJ).

It would be premature to come to any definitive conclusion at this time but it might prove that a mother does not reduce fat deposition during pregnancy except in extreme dietary circumstances. We have to look elsewhere for a complete understanding of energy balance, particularly if we are to explain the position prevailing in the Western world.

Activity during pregnancy. The next most obvious facet to look at is activity. To what extent do the energy costs of routine activities rise as the women get heavier and, if this does occur, are they compensated for by alterations in the pattern of activity? Such information is so elementary it is astonishing that so few objective data are available to us. Clearly there will be major differences from country to country and we would plead that this information gap be filled as a matter of urgency.

As far as our Gambian data are concerned no activity except walking, which is load-bearing, exhibited any increased energy cost in the second and third trimesters over that found in non-pregnant, nonlactating women. Even the walking values only increased by an amount which was barely statistically significant[8]. At the present time it is impossible to say how universal this general finding will prove; it is always possible that women in countries like The Gambia, living on marginal energy intakes, might be responding subconsciously by carrying out their same daily duties with a greater economy of effort in the latter two trimesters. What it certainly means for women in The Gambia is that any reductions in the *time* spent on active occupations will result in net savings in energy expenditure. In some early work from The Gambia it was estimated that after standardization for season the average time occupied on work, as opposed to leisure, activities fell from around 550 min/d at the onset of pregnancy to 400 min/d by the ninth month[11]. These changes in activity pattern are currently being investigated in much greater detail, but if they are confirmed they clearly afford considerable opportunity for energy saving.

In the Western world, where most women are not involved in anything like so much manual work, the potential for energy saving from a modification of activity patterns clearly cannot be so great as in countries like The Gambia. Never-the-less, both Durnin in Glasgow[2] and the Dunn team in Cambridge have described progressive trends during pregnancy in which more time is spent lying down and carrying out seated activities and less on walking or standing activities. Small though these changes may be, when integrated over pregnancy as a whole, they make a worthwhile contribution towards the estimated total 80 000 kcal (334.6 MJ) required.

Maintenance metabolism. The final energy consuming component is maintenance metabolism. Because the different physiological processes involved had differing development patterns, it was predicted[5] that overall maintenance requirements would increase in an essentially linear manner during pregnancy (Fig. 1). The direct way to determine exactly what happens in practice is to monitor progressive changes in resting metabolic rate (RMR) during the course of pregnancy. This was the approach adopted by the Nestlé Foundation Collaborative Group. We do not have data from all the centres but in The Gambia the pattern of change was quite different from that predicted on theoretical grounds[6]. There was no rise in RMR during the first half of pregnancy indeed the tendency was for a reduction. The ultimate rise during the last trimester was also much smaller than that predicted. The net result was that instead of an estimated extra 40 Mcal (167.3 MJ) being spent on supporting a raised maintenance metabolism,

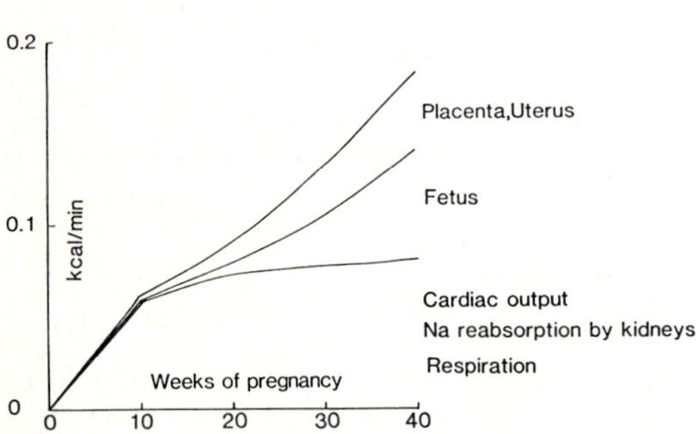

Fig. 1 *Estimated increases in maintenance energy needed to support various physiological processes during the course of pregnancy (drawn from Hytten & Leitch[5]). The lower line represents the estimated amount of energy required for increased cardiac, respiratory and renal function. The middle line is the sum of the latter three functions plus the needs imposed by the fetus. The upper line is as the middle line but with placental and uterine metabolic needs also added. 1 kcal = 4.18 kJ.*

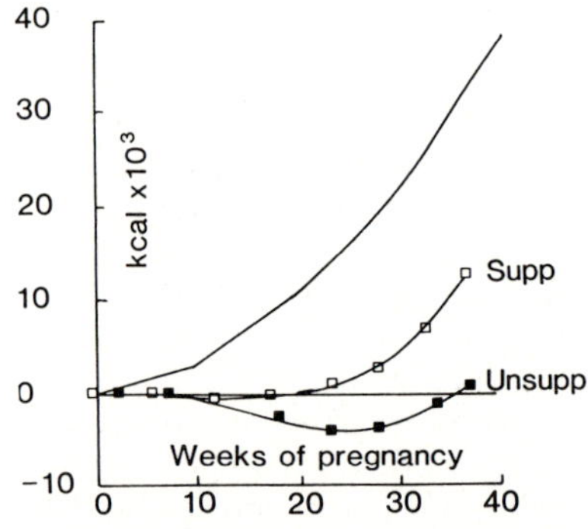

Fig. 2. *Accumulative extra cost of maintenance metabolism (RMR) in supplemented and unsupplemented Gambian mothers during pregnancy contrasted with theoretical estimates[5]. The lower two lines are calculated from RMR data collected in The Gambia (see script) the uppermost line relates to the accumulative amount of energy theoretically required for the sum of all the activities in Fig. 1.*

only 628 kcal (2.63 MJ) were expended in the average unsupplemented women. In supplemented women, on the other hand, the net energy cost of increased maintenance was 10 Mcal (41.83 MJ) (Figure 2).

Preliminary published results by Durnin[2] from Glasgow are remarkably similar to those in supplemented women from The Gambia, but a recent publication from Sweden[4], commenting on our Gambian results, pointed out that patterns of change in RMR among the women they had studied during pregnancy were much closer to those predicted by Hytten & Leitch[5]. One clue as to an explanation for this variability could come from the observation that in The Gambia the pattern of change was dependent on maternal energy intake and could be influenced by maternal dietary supplementation. Whatever the explanation ultimately proves to be, it is clear that in The Gambia at least the net amount of energy spent on increased rates of resting metabolism is far less than 40 Mcal (167.3 MJ).

Net energy costs of pregnancy in The Gambia. If we put the three components together, fat deposition, acitivity and resting metabolic rate we clearly come up with something quite startling. Again we will concentrate upon The Gambia as these data are the most complete of those available to us. The average unsupplemented women in our cohort spent only an extra 600 kcal (2.51 MJ) on RMR and minus 2900 kcal (12.13 MJ) on fat storage a net cost of minus 2300 kcal (9.62 MJ). Additionally, one should allow for modifications to the pattern of activity. It thus becomes easy to appreciate how our mothers have been balancing their energy expenditure on little or no increase in intake.

Conclusions. Finally, some important words of warning. To achieve energy balance is one thing, to do so *safely* is another. Mothers in The Gambia live on very marginal intakes and during the hungry season the high incidence of low-birth-weight babies clearly indicates that energy accommodation has been carried out well beyond acceptable limits. One must ask why the Gambian pattern of RMR changes should be sensitive to dietary intake? Might not this too indicate that what is occurring in unsupplemented women is far from ideal? Furthermore, what significance do our low fat deposition figures have?

Clearly there are a lot of important questions still to answer. It would be quite unwise to alter dietary recommendations for the developing world until we are much wiser. We must also not forget needs for the individual nutrients, protein, vitamins and minerals. The processes which may enable the mother to accommodate variations in energy intake would have little bearing on the physiological mechanisms necessary to overcome marginal nutrient deficiencies. With all the current interest and concern about maternal nutrition in pregnancy it is important we do not allow oversimplified concepts to lead to precipitous action.

1 Department of Health and Social Security (1979): Recommended daily amounts of food energy and nutrients for groups of people in the United Kingdom. *Rep. Hlth Soc. Subj. No. 15.* London: HMSO

2 Durnin, J.V.G.A. (1982): Energy requirements of lactating women. *Nestlé Foundation Ann. Rep.*, pp. 13–22.

3 FAO/WHO. (1973): Energy and protein requirements, p. 522 *WHO Tech. Rep. Ser./FAO Nutr Meetings Rep Ser; No. 52.*

4 Forsum, E., Sadurskis, A. & Wager, J. (1985): Energy maintenance cost during pregnancy in healthy Swedish women. *Lancet* **1**, 107–108.

5 Hytten, F.F. & Leitch, I. (1971): *The physiology of human pregnancy.* Oxford: Blackwell Scientific Publications.

6 Lawrence, M., Lawrence, F., Lamb, W.H. & Whitehead, R.G. (1984): Maintenance energy cost of pregnancy in rural Gambian women and influence of dietary status. *Lancet* **1**, 363–365.

7 Lawrence, M., Coward, W.A., Lawrence, F., Cole, T.J. & Whitehead, R.G. (1986): Pregnancy fat gain in rural Gambian women. Abstracts of XIIIth International Congress of Nutrition, p. 154.

8 Lawrence, M., Singh, J., Lawrence, F. & Whitehead, R.G. (1985): The energy cost of common daily activities in African women: Increased expenditure in pregnancy? *Am. J. Clin. Nutr.* **42**, 753–763.

9 NFS (1984): *Household food consumption and Expenditure: 1984.* London: HMSO.

10 Prentice, A.M., Whitehead, R.G., Watkinson, M., Lamb, W.H. & Cole, T.J. (1983): Prenatal dietary supplementation of African women and birthweight. *Lancet* **1**, 489–492.

11 Roberts, S.B., Paul, A.A., Cole, T.J. & Whitehead, R.G. (1982): Seasonal changes in activity, birthweight and lactational performance in rural Gambian women. *Trans Roy. Soc. Trop. Med. Hyg.* **76**, 668–678.

12 Whitehead, R.G. (1983): Maternal diet, breast feeding capacity and lactational infertility. Report of a UNU/WHO/IPPF/UNICEF Workshop held in Cambridge, UK on 9, 10, 11 March 1981, ed R.G. Whitehead. *UNU Fd Nutr. Bull.* Suppl. 6, pp 1–107.

13 Whitehead, R.G., Paul, A.A., Black, A.E. & Wiles, S.J. (1981): Recommended dietary amounts of energy for pregnancy and lactation in the United Kingdom. *UNU Fd Nutr. Bull.* Suppl. 5, 259–264.

The role of the placenta in fetal nutrition

S. HAUGUEL and J. GIRARD
Centre de Recherches sur la Nutrition, CNRS, 9, rue Jules Hetzel, 92190 Meudon-Bellevue, France.

In mammals, the function of the placenta is to ensure optimal nutrition of the fetus. This involves transmission of nutrients, oxygen and water to the fetus, excretion of waste products of fetal metabolism (CO_2, urea) into the maternal circulation and the adaptation of maternal metabolism to different stages of pregnancy by secreting specific hormones[30]. The flux of nutrients from the maternal circulation to the fetal circulation is affected by various factors: (1) substrate and hormone concentrations in maternal circulation, (2) the uteroplacental blood flow, (3) placental transfer mechanisms, (4) placental metabolism. In this short review, we will discuss briefly the contribution of these different factors to fetal nutrition, focusing mainly on data collected in the chronically catheterized sheep preparation and in the human.

(1) Substrate and hormone concentrations in maternal circulation. During gestation, an appropriate environment must be achieved to provide sufficient supply of nutrients to the growing fetus and maternal metabolic adjustments are necessary to face this situation. In mammals, glucose is the principal fuel of fetal metabolism[2,10,12], and its placental uptake and transfer are major determinants of fetal growth. In sheep and in man, placental glucose uptake and transfer are dependent upon maternal blood glucose concentration[14,16]. By contrast, umbilical amino acid uptake is not directly related to maternal plasma amino acid concentration[28,39]. The uptake and transfer of fatty acids by the placenta varies among species. In sheep it is very limited[2], but a correlation between umbilical FFA uptake and maternal plasma FFA concentration has been observed in man[9].

The placenta also modulates the nature of fuels available to the fetus by synthesizing hormones which modify maternal substrates concentration. *Human chorionic somatomammotropin* (HCS or human placental lactogen) has both lipolytic and insulinotropic effects ([21]in review). *Progesterone and oestrogens* stimulate insulin secretion by the pancreas and are involved in the hypertriglyceridaemia which appears in late pregnancy[21]. The hormones secreted by the placenta could be involved in the action of insulin on maternal tissues. A sequential change in maternal metabolism has been suggested in regard to advancing gestation[22]. An early anabolic phase favouring the action of insulin on adipose tissue and skeletal muscles is followed by a late catabolic phase opposing the effect of insulin on glucose metabolism in maternal tissues[11]. Thus, by increasing maternal plasma FFA and triglycerides and by decreasing the sensitivity of maternal tissues to insulin, the placental hormones could be involved in sparing glucose utilization in maternal tissues and in directing glucose preferentially towards the fetoplacental unit[11,22].

(2) Uteroplacental blood flow. Blood flow to the uteroplacenta increases markedly during pregnancy. In the pregnant ewe near term it is 50-fold higher than in non-pregnant animals[27]. In women, the uteroplacental blood flow ranges from 500 to 700 ml/min near term[36] but its value is not precisely known in early pregnancy. The formation and rapid development of new placental vessels is the *primum movens* of the increase of blood flow, but the large increase of maternal cardiac output and of uterine vascular resistance are also implicated in this process[27]. Since the transfer of oxygen and amino acids is dependent upon uteroplacental blood flow[38,39] the increase in uteroplacental blood flow in later pregnancy obviously enhances the transfer of these nutrients to the fetus. By contrast, placental glucose uptake is mainly dependent upon maternal glucose concentration (see above), and the umbilical glucose uptake is affected only when blood flow is severely reduced[33], such as during severe vascular restriction[7].

(3) Placental transfer mechanisms. Mechanisms by which maternal nutrients enter and cross the placenta are now well characterized[18]. Three types of transfer mechanisms have been described: (1) passive diffusion, highly dependent upon uteroplacental blood flow; (2)

facilitated diffusion which is carrier mediated, and (3) active transport acting against a concentration gradient which is an energy-dependent process.

In the human placenta, glucose is transported by facilitated diffusion and the glucose carrier of placental membranes has been characterized[4,20,33]. The placental glucose transport system is similar to that described in adipocytes and skeletal muscles.

In mammals, the concentration of amino acids in fetal blood is higher than in maternal blood due to an active transport of L-amino acids across the placenta. Similar characteristics of amino acid transport have been reported for sheep[24] and for man[8,39]. Neutral amino acids are transferred in excess to the fetus, whereas the supply of basic amino acids approximates their rate of accretion in fetal tissues[23]. The maternal acidic amino acids (glutamic and aspartic acids) are not taken up by the placenta. Glutamic acid is even excreted through the placenta from the fetal side. Variations of uteroplacental blood flow can modify specifically the transport of different amino acids. The transfer of basic amino acids is markedly reduced by a vascular restriction[39]. By contrast, the placental transfer of amino acids is marginally affected by changes in umbilical blood flow or in amino acid concentration in maternal blood.

FFA enter and cross the human placenta by a gradient-dependent diffusion process[9]. *In-vitro* studies indicate that there is little evidence for a selective transfer of different FFA and the net transfer of FFA from mother to fetus seems to be related to FFA concentration in maternal circulation[19]. Maternal triglycerides do not cross the placenta. A lipoprotein lipase activity has been found in placental homogenates[25] which could be responsible for the hydrolysis of maternal triglycerides and for the transfer of liberated FFA across the placenta. However, the physiological role of this enzyme remains to be clarified.

With regard to transfer mechanisms, it may also be that as pregnancy progresses, the human placenta undergoes marked structural changes. The thickness of the placental membrane is reduced from 25 to 2 μ whereas the villous branching more than doubles the villous surface area from 5 m^2 at 28 wk to 11 m^2 at term[1], both processes tending to improve transfer efficiency. In addition, the increase of uteroplacental blood flow may also be a factor contributing to the increase in the transfer of nutrients in late pregnancy.

(4) Placental metabolism. The placenta should no longer be considered as an inert membrane between the mother and the fetus. On the contrary, it is a very active metabolic tissue which develops rapidly. The trophoblast is the most metabolically active tissue but it represents only 13 per cent of total placental mass. To satisfy its own metabolic requirements, the placenta retains a part of the substrates circulating in the uterine artery. Only 30 to 40 per cent of glucose taken up by the placenta is transferred to the sheep or human fetus[13,26]. The remaining glucose is metabolized within the placental tissue. Near term the glucose requirement of the fetoplacental unit represents as much as 33 per cent of total maternal glucose production in sheep[15] and about 30 to 40 per cent in man[14]. In both species the placenta has a high glycolytic capacity. Lactate production represented 37 to 38 per cent of total glucose utilization[13,26]. However, there is a striking difference between humans and the sheep concerning placental lactate output. In sheep, placental lactate is delivered both in maternal and fetal circulations whereas in the human very little lactate is excreted in to the fetal circulation.

Data concerning placental lipid metabolism are scarce, but it is obvious that a small part of FFA taken up by the placenta is metabolized within the trophoblast. Enzymes necessary for *de-novo* fatty acid synthesis and esterification, triglyceride hydrolysis and FFA oxidation have been characterized. Fatty acid synthesis seems of minor importance when compared with the transfer of FFA from the mother to the fetus[40]. In addition, fatty acid oxidation in term placenta is quantitatively more important than fatty acid synthesis[40]. Fatty acids can also be esterified *in situ* to form triglycerides and phospholipids[35]. As late human pregnancy is associated with an endogenous maternal hypertriglyceridaemia this could potentially induce an increased placental FFA uptake and transfer to the fetus. Furthermore placental triglyceride accumulation could be an intermediary step in the FFA transport to the fetus.

The human placenta plays an important role in regulating fetal amino acid concentration. Amino acid transfer to the fetus occurs after an intraplacental accumulation of amino acids to a level exceeding maternal and fetal plasma concentrations[32]. In sheep, it has been estimated that 14 per cent of the amino acid nitrogen entering the uteroplacenta is returned to maternal and fetal circulation as ammonia[3,26]. In the human placenta, ammonia is mostly secreted in maternal circulation[13].

Protein synthesis within the placenta near term is mostly devoted to hormone synthesis. It represents 12 to 16 per cent of amino acid transferred[5]. The placentas of various species are richly endowed with insulin receptors[31], located on the maternal surface of microvillous membranes[37]. However, maternal insulin does not increase glucose transport and metabolism either in the sheep[17] or in the human placenta[6]. In addition insulin does not enhance placental amino acid transport[34]. Thus, the physiological significance of placental insulin receptors remains to be elucidated, although they could be involved in insulin degradation. In the perfused human placenta the rate of insulin disappearance is 10 mU/min for a 500 g placenta at plasma insulin level of 100 µU/ml[6]. It was estimated to be 40 mu/min in sheep[29].

Conclusions. The placenta is able to influence fetal nutrition and growth directly by conditioning nutrient transport and availability to the fetus. It can also act indirectly by means of hormones to induce large metabolic readjustments in the mother in order to direct important metabolic fuels, such as glucose, and amino acids to the fetus. Thus, it is evident that the placenta is strongly implicated in fetal development and further investigations would help to elucidate some of the unsolved question raised in this review.

1 Aherne, W. & Dunhill, M.S. (1966): Quantitative aspects of placental structure. *J. Path. Bact.* **91**, 123–131.

2 Battaglia, F.C. & Meschia, G. (1978): Principal substrates of fetal metabolism. *Physiol. Rev.* **58**, 499–527.

3 Battaglia, F.C. & Meschia, G. (1981): Foetal and placental metabolisms, their interrelationships and impact upon maternal metabolism. *Proc. Nutr. Soc.* **40**, 99–113.

4 Bissonnette, J.M., Black, J.A., Thornburg, K.L., Acott, K.M. & Koch, P.L. (1982): Reconstitution of D-glucose transporter from human placental microvillous plasma membranes. *Am. J. Physiol.* **242**, C166–C171.

5 Carroll, M.J. & Young, M. (1983): The relationship between placental protein synthesis and transfer of amino acids. *Biochem. J.* **210**, 99–105.

6 Challier, J.C., Hauguel, S. & Desmaizieres, V. (1985): Effect of insulin on glucose transport and metabolism in the human placenta. (In prep).

7 Clapp, J.F., Szeto, H.H., Larrow, R., Hewitt, J. & Mann, L.I. (1981): Fetal metabolic response to experimental placental vascular damage. *Am. J. Obstet. Gynecol.* **140**, 446–450.

8 Dancis, J., Money, W.L., Springer, D. & Levitz, M. (1968): Transport of aminoacids by placenta. *Am. J. Obstet. Gynecol.* **101**, 820–829.

9 Dancis, J., Jansen, S., Kayden, H.J., Schneider, H. & Levitz, M. (1973): Transfer across perfused human placenta. II Free fatty acids. *Pediat. Res.* **7**, 192–197.

10 Girard, J., Pintado, E. & Ferré, P. (1979): Fuel metabolism in the mammalian fetus. *Ann. Biol. Anim. Bioch. Biophys.* **19**, 181–187.

11 Girard, J.R., Leturque, A., Burnol, A-F., Ferré, P., Satabin, P. & Gilbert, M. (1984): Glucose homeostatis during pregnancy in the rat. In *Lessons from animal diabetes*, ed E. Shafrir & A.E. Renold, pp. 667–675. London & Paris: John Libbey.

12 Girard, J. (1985): Carbohydrate and amino acid metabolism in the fetus. In *Pediatrics*, ed J. Metcoff & J.C. Arneil, vol 3, pp. 3–24. London: Butterworth.

13 Hauguel, S., Challier, J.C., Cedard, L. & Olive, G. (1983): Metabolism of the human placenta perfused in vitro: glucose transfer and utilization, O_2 consumption, lactate and ammonia production. *Pediat. Res.* **17**, 729–732.

14 Hauguel, S., Desmaizieres, V. & Challier, J.C. (1985): Placental glucose uptake, transfer and utilization as functions of maternal glucose concentration. (In prep.)

15 Hay, W.W., Sparks, J.W., Wilkening, R.B., Battaglia, F.C. & Meschia, G. (1983): Partition of maternal glucose production between conceptus and maternal tissues in sheep. *Am. J. Physiol.* **245**, E347–350.

16 Hay, W.W., Sparks, J.W., Wilkening, R.B., Battaglia, F.C. & Meschia, G. (1984): Fetal glucose uptake and utilization as functions of maternal glucose concentration. *Am. J. Physiol.* **246**, E237–E242.

17 Hay, W.W., Sparks, J.W., Gilbert, M., Battaglia, F.C. & Meschia, G. (1984): The effect of insulin on glucose uptake by the maternal hindlimb and uterus and by the fetus in conscious pregnant sheep. *J. Endocr.* **100**, 119–124.

18 Hill, E.P. & Longo, L.D. (1980): Dynamics of maternal-fetal nutrient transfer. *Fed. Proc.* **39**, 329–344.

19 Hull, D. & Elphick, M.C. (1979): Transfer of fatty acids. In *Placental transfer* ed G.V.R. Chamberlain, A.W. Wilkinson, pp. 159–166. London: Pitman.

20 Johnson, L.W. & Smith, C.H. (1980): Monosaccharide transport across microvillous membrane of human placenta. *Am. J. Physiol.* **238**, C160–C168.

21 Kalkhoff, R.K., Kissebah, A.H. & Kim, H.J. (1978): Carbohydrate and lipid metabolism during normal pregnancy: relationship to gestational hormone action. *Semin. Perinatol.* **2**, 291–307.

22 Knopp, R.H., Montes, A., Childs, M., Li, J.R. & Mabuchi, H. (1981): Metabolic adjustments in normal and diabetic pregnancy. *Clin Obstet. Gyncecol.* **24**, 21–48.

23 Lemons, J.A., Adcock, E.W., Jones, M.D., Naughton, M.A., Meschia, G. & Battaglia, F.C. (1976): Umbilical uptake of amino acids in the unstressed fetal lamb. *J. Clin. Invest.* **88**, 1428–1434.

24 Lemons, J.A. (1979): Fetal-placental nitrogen metabolism. *Sem. Perinatol.* **3**, 177–190.

25 Mallow, S. & Alousi, A.A. (1965): Lipoprotein lipase activity of rat and human placenta. *Proc. Soc. Exp. Biol. Med.* **119**, 301–306.

26 Meschia, G., Battaglia, F.C., Hay, W. & Sparks, W. (1980): Utilization of substrates by the ovine placenta in vivo. *Fed. Proc.* **39**, 245–249.

27 Meschia, G. (1984): Circulation to female reproductive organs. In *Handbook of physiology. The cardiovascular system III*, ed pp. 241–269. Bethesda (Md): The American Physiological Society.

28 Morriss, F.H., Adcock, E.W., Paxson, C.L. & Greeley, W.J. (1979): Uterine uptake of aminoacids throughout gestation in the unstressed ewe. *Am. J. Obstet. Gynecol.* **135**, 601–609.

29 Morriss, F.H. (1981): Placental factors conditioning fetal nutrition and growth. *Am. J. Clin. Nutr.* **34**, 760–768.

30 Munro, H.N., Pilistine, S.J. & Fant, M.E. (1983): The placenta in nutrition. *Ann. Rev. Nutr.* **3**, 97–124.

31 Posner, B.I. (1974): Insulin receptors in human and animal placental tissue. *Diabetes* **23**, 209–214.

32 Ruzycki, S.M., Kelley, L.M. & Smith, C.H. (1978): Placental aminoacid uptake. IV. Transport by microvillous membrane vesicles. *Am. J. Physiol.* **234**, C27–C36.

33 Simmons, M.A., Battaglia, F.C. & Meschia, G. (1979): Placental transfer of glucose. *J. Dev. Physiol.* **1**, 227–243.

34 Steel, R.B., Mosley, J.D. & Smith, C.H. (1979): Insulin and placenta: degradation and stabilization, binding to microvillous membrane receptors and aminoacid uptake. *Am. J. Obstet. Gynecol.* **135**, 522–529.

35 Szabo, A.J., Lellis, R. & Grimaldi, R.D. (1973): Triglyceride synthesis in human placenta. I. Incorporation of labeled palmitate into placental triglycerides. *Am. J. Obstet. Gynecol.* **115**, 257–262.

36 Van Lierde, M., Oberweis, D. & Thomas, K. (1984): Ultrasonic measurement of aortic and umbilical blood flow in the human fetus. *Obstet. Gynecol.* **63**, 801–805.

37 Whitsett, J.A. & Lessard, J.L. (1978): Characteristics of the microvillus brush border of human placenta: insulin receptor localization in brush border membranes. *Endocrinol.* **103**, 1488–1468.

38 Wilkening, R.B., Anderson, S., Martensson, L. & Meschia, G. (1982): Placental transfer as a functions of uterine blood flow. *Am. J. Physiol.* **242**, H429–436.

39 Young, M. (1981): Placental aminoacids transfer and metabolism. *Placenta* Suppl. 1, 125–138.

40 Zimmerman, T., Hummel, L., Möller, U. & Kinzl, U. (1979): Oxidation and synthesis of fatty acids in human and rat placental and fetal tissues. *Biol. Neonate* **36**, 109–119.

Partition of nutrients in the pregnant and lactating dairy cow

J.D. OLDHAM
Edinburgh School of Agriculture, West Mains Road, Edinburgh EH9 3JG, UK.

The metabolic fate of nutrients in cows depends on their amounts and relative proportions and on the physiological state of the cow. In order to make clear the types of metabolic control which govern this interaction between current nutritional status and physiological state, the terms 'homoeostasis' and 'homoeorhesis' have been applied[3]. The former (homoeostatis) is familiar and refers to controls which maintain physiological equilibrium or constant (metabolic) conditions in the internal environment. The other term, homoeorhesis, is less familiar and refers to controls which govern the co-ordinated changes in metabolism which are necessary to support a physiological state, or which guide modifications in metabolism as physiological state changes. Both types of control have consequences for nutrient partitioning in pregnancy and lactation.

Partition as influenced by physiological state. *Pregnancy.* The process of pregnancy has been considered biphasic, the first two trimesters being anabolic, the third catabolic[30]. Fat and protein accumulate in the anabolic phase in well-nourished animals[17,31,46]. These reserves of fat and protein are important for the fetus during its rapid growth phase particularly when maternal nutrition is poor.

The extent to which fat stores are mobilized depends on the balance between plane of nutrition and fetal burden. Thus, the highest rates of loss of body fat from pregnant sheep were found among those bearing quadruplets and on a low plane of nutrition[39]. The highest rate of utilization was 176 g/d equivalent to a net fractional rate of 0.016/d. The importance of fatty acid metabolism in late gestation is seen in a comparative study which showed that as much as 85 per cent of CO_2 produced by muscle in fasted pregnant sheep comes from NEFA and ketone bodies[38]. The equivalent figure for fed non-pregnant sheep is 23 per cent. Glucose oxidation in contrast contributes 50–60 per cent of muscle CO_2 production in fed non-pregnant sheep muscle, but only 10 per cent in fasted pregnant sheep muscles. Thus the advantage of maternal fat mobilization is to give to maternal tissues an alternative metabolic fuel not available to the fetus.

Maternal protein stores can also be depleted in late gestation. Net rates of maternal protein loss are small in animals offered diets which are not deficient in dietary protein — fractional rates of 0.002/d and 0.004/d can be calculated for ewes[39] and rats[32] near term. These net rates of whole-body protein depletion hide the transfer of protein from non-mammary to mammary tissue. Allowing for the deposition of protein in mammary tissue it is more likely that for the ewes referred to[39] maternal non-mammary loss was closer to 0.004/d still, however, a relatively low rate. These rates can be increased substantially when dietary protein content is low. Losses in ewes on a low-protein diet equivalent to 0.033/d over the whole of gestation have been observed[43]. Oxidation of ^{14}C-tyrosine is reduced in the catabolic phase of pregnancy, especially when the diet has a low protein content[27]. In pregnant sheep, oxidation of, or glucose formation from, U-^{14}C-threonine depended more on plane of nutrition than stage of pregnancy[12]. These observations might imply that the primary purpose of protein mobilization in late gestation is to supply amino acids for fetal metabolism.

In the fetus, amino acid uptake exceeds net rates of amino acid accretion by a considerable amount[23,28]. There is, therefore, considerable scope for the fetus to use amino acids as a fuel. Amino acid catabolism might account for 20 per cent of oxygen consumption in well-fed sheep near term, but might be as much as 60 per cent in fasted sheep[17]. From studies of placental clearance of urea, it has been[40] suggested the figure might be as high as 80 per cent in fasting. It has been found[15] that both previous and current states of maternal nutrition influence urea production, and by inference, amino acid oxidation in the fetus, estimates ranging from 30–55 per cent of oxygen consumption attributable to amino acid catabolism in fetal sheep.

The extent to which amino acids are used as glycogenic substrates by the fetus is still not clear[35]. It seems that net fetal gluconeogenesis from amino acids is usually a minor contributor to the fetal glucose economy, although the net contribution might increase when maternal undernutrition is severe.

Partition of nutrients in pregnancy, especially late pregnancy, is clearly controlled so as to enable 'normal' development of the conceptus, even to the extent that maternal tissues undergo net depletion. The picture which emerges gives an indication (perhaps *in extremis* as regards dairy cows) that the emphases on nutrient use can adjust, so that there can be increased use of maternal fat as a metabolic fuel, with a possibility of net protein mobilization from non-mammary maternal tissues — which is partly to allow increased protein accretion of mammary tissue, and partly to increase supply of amino acids to the fetus, where they may be used substantially to fuel metabolic processes as well as to support increased rates of net protein accretion. In late pregnancy, amino acids may become less quantitatively important as oxidative substrates in maternal tissues.

Lactation. For many cows in early lactation milk production increases much more rapidly than food intake. To maintain lactation, tissues are mobilized and cows lose weight and 'condition'. Both fat and protein can be lost from body tissue[34], but in general it seems that body tissue which is mobilized in early lactation contains a high proportion of fat and a low proportion of protein[1]. In this early phase of lactation a number of changes in nutrient use occur which appear to be coordinated (homoeorhetic control) so as to minimise the catabolic metabolism of glucose and amino acids, both of which are often in relatively short supply in relation to the high demand for milk production.

An important adaptation is hypertrophy of the gut[16] which is perhaps more to do with increasing food intake consequent on changes in lactational output than a direct effect of lactation itself, although the possibility has been hinted at that prolactin may be implicated in the hypertrophy and increased absorptive capacity which occurs in the GI tract of rats at the onset of lactation[3]. The effect of the hypertrophy is to create an increased absorptive area in the GI tract which should facilitate nutrient extraction in support of productive processes.

As shown indirectly by energy balance studies[29], and measurement of fatty acid 'turnover'[20] and directly by slaughter[8,22] substantial amounts of fat can be mobilised in early lactation. The extent of fat mobilisation seems largely to be determined by the amount of fat tissue which has been accumulated by the time of parturition[13]. Not only does fatty acid mobilization/flux change with time post-partum, but also the metabolic fate of fatty acids changes. Early in lactation a greater proportion of triglyceride flux is oxidised with a reduced proportion being incorporated into body fat[18]. In adipose tissue, rates of lipogenesis are decreased and lipolysis increased[45] with associated, and reciprocal changes in fatty acid metabolism in the mammary gland[4]. The control of these processes is governed, to a considerable extent, by the influence of insulin relative to that of those hormones which chronically inhibit aspects of tissue deposition, most notably growth hormone, glucagon and glucocorticoids[19].

Glucose oxidation is reduced in early lactation[5] independently of changes in food intake, and there is indirect evidence (from changes in urea synthesis) that amino acid oxidation is also reduced[6]. Whether or not there is always net mobilization of tissue protein in support of lactation is debatable[24] but it does seem that amino acid incorporation into muscle protein is reduced in the early phase of lactation[7]. It may be that there is increased amino acid incorporation into gut protein as part of the recognised hypertrophy of the gut[16] so that, even though total body protein synthesis may not change much in lactation[36], there may be substantial redistribution of amino acid use between organs for protein synthesis.

Net use of amino acids for glucose-synthesis is low when milk protein secretion is high[6] although when capacity for net protein accretion is low in ruminants there may be a substantial contribution to net glucose synthesis from amino acid catabolism[24].

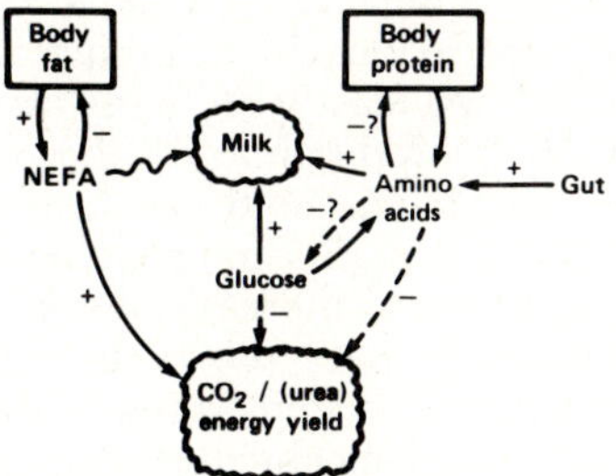

Figure. *Changes in use of maternal tissues and certain, potentially 'limiting', nutrients in early lactation.*

For early lactation (as compared with late lactation) we might therefore summarise the organization of nutrient partition as in the Figure, which shows reduced emphasis on glucose and amino acids as metabolic fuels (but enhanced use for milk synthesis), and increased use of fatty acids as energy substrate, facilitated by enhanced adipose lipolysis and reduced adipose lipogenesis resulting in net body-fat mobilisation. Amino acid use for glucose synthesis may be reduced (proportionately) and there may also be alterations in the extent or site of amino acid incorporation into tissue proteins.

Mechanisms of partition. Much attention, currently, is being given to roles of different hormones in the control of nutrient partition, in lactation especially[3,10,19,26]. The role which growth hormone (bovine somatotropin) plays in the control of nutrient use for milk production has attracted particular attention in recent years. Circulating concentrations of GH are positively correlated with milk yield and, over the lactation cycle, blood GH concentrations fall progressively as lactation progresses and milk yield diminishes[19]. Blood insulin concentration follows the reverse pattern. Daily injection of GH (either pituitary extracted or recombinantly derived) have been found to stimulate milk yield substantially[14,19] and to alter partition of nutrients between use for tissue accretion and milk secretion. In the short term, GH injections stimulate milk secretion at the expense of tissue (induced net lipolysis) but partial efficiencies of the various metabolic conversions are as normal[44], hence the effects of GH on milk secretion result in enhanced gross efficiency of food use (defined as milk net energy divided by metabolizable energy of food consumed) which is achieved by nutrients being diverted to use via pathways with a relatively high energetic efficiency (milk) and not by changing the energetic efficiency of any particular pathway. In the long term[14] food intake rises in response to the increase in milk yield following GH injection. This is a particularly important observation as it demonstrates that nutrient (metabolite) disposal into milk is a major force controlling food consumption and that food intake is as much a *result*, as a *cause*, of milk secretion.

The relationships between changes in nutrient use, hormone action and blood flow with changing physiological (or nutritional state), are by no means clear; but indications are that the fraction of cardiac output which perfuses the udder of dairy cows plays an important role in the partitioning of nutrients between milk and body tissues[10,11].

Partition as influenced by nutrition. In lactation the most dramatic effects of changing diet are seen in the partition of fat metabolism between secretion via the mammary gland or accumulation in adipose tissue. The effect of diet on relative amounts of acetic, propionic and butyric acids (A, P and B) absorbed from the rumen is particularly important in this regard. Where change in diet affects milk lactose secretion there may also be changes in nutrient use in order to supply glucose for lactose formation. Effects on milk protein secretion can usually be attributed to changes in amino acid supply from the gut in a relatively simple fashion, but there are numerous instances of change in protein/amino acid supply from the GI tract having effects on nutrient use/partition additional to the simple effects on milk protein yield[34].

Rumen VFA and milk fat. The amount and pattern of propionate supplied from the gut seems to have marked effects on the partition of fat metabolism between secretion in milk and deposition in body fats. Cows offered rations which contain relatively little fibre but substantial proportions of starch are likely to yield milk which contains a low concentration of fat ('low-milk-fat syndrome'). Such rations are characterised by a low molar ratio of (acetic + butyric acids) to propionic acid (ratio (A + B)/P) in rumen VFA. Milk fat concentration falls with decreasing (A + B)/P when (A + B)/P is caused to vary by changing concentrate:forage ratio in the diet, or plane of feeding or meal pattern[41]. At least with high-starch, low-roughage diets it seems that change in the ratio (A + B)/P is predominantly the result of enhanced propionate production which increases glucose entry in the body[2] and, probably, induces a change in insulin status. Blood insulin concentration is sensitive to propionate supply from the rumen and enhanced insulin status would be expected to increase uptake of nutrients into adipose tissue while suppressing lipolysis[19]. Mammary tissue is, relatively, insulin-insensitive[19] so a reasonable, though yet to be fully confirmed, hypothesis concerning control of fat partition would be that propionate supply plays a major role by altering glucose and insulin status so as to alter the competitive advantage between mammary and adipose tissue for use of triglyceride precursors. Sutton *et al*[42] have produced results which raise the intriguing possibility that it is not just the amount of propionate produced which is important for the control of fat partition but also its pattern of production over the day. It may be that a certain threshold in either/both rumen propionate/blood insulin needs to be exceeded to trigger the mechanism which perpetuates the reduction in milk fat synthesis.

Interactions between protein and energy-yielding nutrients. On some occasions changing dietary protein will increase milk energy secretion by more than can be accounted for by any change in energy intake[34]. When this happens the change in protein status must have altered nutrient partition, with the main emphasis being a change in fat utilization. The mechanism whereby a change in amino acid supply to the body influences fat metabolism is not fully understood.

We have sometimes, but not always, found that changing protein status of cows alters blood GH concentration[34]. Work done by others has, similarly, failed to show consistent effects of protein supplementation on blood GH[11]. The hypothesis that effects of protein feeding on nutrient partition are mediated via a change in GH status is therefore (though appealing) not an adequate explanation.

Some part of the response may be the result of the particular effects of methionine, which, by acting as a methyl-group donor, might facilitate lipid flux through the liver[33]. Methionine supplements have been found to increase milk fat secretion in cows[9]. It has been suggested[25] that the dispensable amino acids aspartic and glutamic acids might be important facilitators of acetate disposal in dairy cattle, with consequent effects on lipid metabolism. Casein supplements given *per abomasum* did increase whole-body flux of acetate and palmitate in cows during early lactation[21], but a superficial test of the MacRae & Lobley hypothesis[37] failed to substantiate it.

Net conversion of amino acid carbon to glucose is generally low in high-yielding cows[6], but increasing protein supply to the intestines consistently increases whole body glucose flux[21] so it is possible that some of the effects of protein on nutrient partition are related to changes in glucose economy of the animal but the precise nature of this link has not been documented.

 1 Alderman, G., Broster, W.H., Strickland, M.J. & Johnson, C.L. (1982): The estimation of the energy value of liveweight change in the lactating dairy cow. *Livestock Prod. Sci.* **9**, 665–673.
 2 Annison, E.F., Bickerstaffe, R. & Linzell, J.L. (1974): Glucose and fatty acid metabolism in cows producing milk of low fat content. *J. Agric. Sci.* Camb. **82**, 87–95.
 3 Bauman, D.E. & Currie, W.B. (1981): Partitioning of nutrients during pregnancy and lactation: A review of mechanisms involving homeostasis and homeorhesis. *J. Dairy Sci.* **63**, 1514–1529.
 4 Bauman, D.E. & Elliot, J.M. (1983): Control of nutrient partitioning in lactating ruminants. In *Biochemistry of lactation* ed, T.B. Mepham, pp. 437–468. London: Academic Press.
 5 Bennink, M.R., Mellenberger, R.W., Frobish, R.A. & Bauman, D.E. (1972): Glucose oxidation and entry rate as affected by the initiation of lactation. *J. Dairy Sci.* **55**, 712–713.
 6 Bruckental, I., Oldham, J.D. & Sutton, J.D. (1980): Glucose and urea kinetics in cows in early lactation. *Br. J. Nutr.* **44**, 33–45.
 7 Bryant, D.T.W. & Smith, R.W. (1982): The effect of lactation on protein synthesis in ovine skeletal muscle. *J. Agric. Sci.*, Camb. **99**, 319–323.
 8 Butler-Hogg, B.W., Wood, J.D. & Bines, J.A. (1985): Fat partitioning in British Fresian cows: the influence of physiological state on dissected body composition. *J. Agric. Sci.* Camb. **104**, 519–528.
 9 Chamberlain, D.G. & Thomas, P.C. (1982): Effect of intravenous supplements of L-methionine on milk yield and composition in cows given silage-cereal diets. *J. Dairy Res.* **49**, 25–28.
10 Collier, R.J., McNamara, J.P., Wallace, C.R. & Dehoff, M.H. (1984): A review of endocrine regulation of metabolism during lactation. *J. Anim. Sci.* **59**, 498–510.
11 Davis, S.R. & Collier, R.J. (1985): Mammary blood flow and the regulation of substrate supply for milk synthesis. *J. Dairy Sci.* **68**, 1041–1058.
12 Egan, A.R. & MacRae, J.C. (1983): Threonine metabolism in sheep. 2. Threonine catabolism and gluconeogenesis in pregnant ewes. *Br. J. Nutr.* **49**, 385–393.
13 Emmans, G.C. & Neilson, D.R. (1985): A sufficient description of a cow and its feed requirements to attain its potential. *Livestock Prod. Sci.* (In press)
14 Eppard, P.J. & Bauman, D.E. (1984): The effect of long-term administration of growth hormone on performance of lactating dairy cows. In *Proc. 1984 Cornell Nutr. Conf. Feed Manufacturers.* pp. 5–12. Ithaca: Cornell University.
15 Faichney, G.J. (1981): Amino acid utilisation by the fetal lamb. *Proc. Nutr. Soc. Aust.* **6**, 48–53.
16 Fell, B.F. (1977): The gut in reproduction. *Report of the Rowett Research Institute.* 97–108. Aberdeen: Rowett Research Institute.
17 Girard, J., Pintado, E. & Ferre, P. (1979): Fuel metabolism in the mammalian fetus. *Ann. Biol. Anim. Bioch. Biophys.* **19**, 181–197.
18 Glascock, R.F., Smith, R.W. & Walsh, A. (1983): Partition of circulating triglycerides between formation of milk fat and other metabolic pathways in sheep. *J. Agric. Sci.*, Camb. **101**, 33–38.
19 Hart, I.C. (1983): Endocrine control of nutrient partition in lactating ruminants. *Proc. Nutr. Soc.* **42**, 181–194.
20 König, B.A., Parker, D.S. & Oldham, J.D. (1979): Acetate and palmitate kinetics in lactating dairy cows. *Ann. Rech. Vet.* **10**, 368–370.
21 König, B.A., Oldham, J.D. & Parker, D.S. (1984): The effect of abomasal infusion of casein on acetate, palmitate and glucose kinetics in cows during early lactation. *Br. J. Nutr.* **52**, 319–328.
22 Lamont, D.I., Neilson, D.R., Emmans, G.C., Fraser, J. & Prescott, J.H.D. (1984): The relationship between live animal measurements and the physical and chemical composition of dairy cows. *Anim. Prod.* **38**, 529–530.
23 Lemons, J.A., Adcock, E.W., Jones, D., Naughton, M.A., Meschier, G. & Battaglia, F.C. (1976): Umbilical uptake of amino acids in the unstressed fetal lamb. *J. Clin. Invest.* **58**, 1428–1434.
24 Lindsay, D.B. (1978): Gluconeogenesis in ruminants. *Biochem. Soc. Trans* **8**, 1152–1156.
25 MacRae, J.C. & Lobley, G.E. (1985): Interactions between energy and protein. *Can. J. Anim. Sci.* (In press)
26 McDowell, G.H. (1983): Hormonal control of glucose homeostasis in ruminants. *Proc. Nutr. Soc.* **42**, 149–166.
27 Mayel-Afshar, S., Grimble, R.F. & Taylor, T.G. (1981): Tyrosine oxidation during pregnancy in normal and protein deficient rats. *Proc. Nutr. Soc.* **40**, 36A.
28 Meier, P., Teng, C., Battaglia, F.C. & Meschia, G. (1981): The rate of amino acid nitrogen and total nitrogen accumulation in the fetal lamb. *Proc. Soc. Exp. Biol. Med.* **167**, 463–468.
29 Moe, P.W., Tyrell, H.F. & Flatt, W.P. (1971): Energetics of body tissue mobilisation. *J. Dairy Sci.* **54**, 548–553.
30 Naismith, D.J. (1980): Maternal nutrition and the outcome of pregnancy — a critical appraisal. *Proc. Nutr. Soc.* **39**, 1–11.
31 Naismith, D.J., Richardson, D.P. & Pritchard, A.E. (1982): The utilisation of protein and energy during lactation in the rat, with particular regard to the use of fat accumulated in pregnancy. *Br. J. Nutr.* **48**, 435–441.
32 Niiyama, Y., Endo, S., Kainori, K. & Inone, G. (1973): Body composition and nitrogen balance in malnourished pregnant sows. *Nutr. Rep. Int.* **8**, 61–70.

33 Oldham, J.D. (1981): Amino acid requirements for lactation in high-yielding dairy cows. In Recent advances in animal nutrition — 1980, Ed W. Haresign, pp. 33–65. London: Butterworths.

34 Oldham, J.D. (1984): Protein-energy interrelationships in dairy cows. *J. Dairy Sci.* **67**, 1090–1114.

35 Oldham, J.D. & Lindsay, D.B. (1983): Interrationships between protein-yielding and energy-yielding nutrients. In *IVth Int. Symp. Protein metabolism and nutrition*, pp. 183–209. Les Colloques de l'INRA (Paris).

36 Oldham, J.D., Lobley, G.E., König, B.A., Parker, D.S. & Smith, R.W. (1980): Amino acid metabolism in lactating dairy cows early in lactation. In *Proc. 3rd E.A.A.P. Symp. protein metab. and nutr.*, ed H.J. Oslage & K. Roler, pp. 458–463. E.A.P.P. Publ. No. 27.

37 Oldham, J.D., Bines, J.A. & MacRae, J.C. (1984): Milk production in cows infused abomasally with casein, glucose or aspartic and glutamic acids early in lactation. *Proc. Nutr. Soc.* **43**, 65A.

38 Pethic, D.W., Lindsay, D.B., Barker, P.J. & Northrup, A.J. (1983): The metabolism of circulating non-esterified fatty acids by the whole animal, hind-limb muscle and uterus of pregnant ewes. *Br. J. Nutr.* **49**, 129–143.

39 Robinson, J.J., McDonald, I., McHattie, I. & Pennie, K. (1978): Studies on reproduction in the prolific ewe. 4. Sequential changes in the maternal body during pregnancy. *J. Agric. Sci.* Camb. **91**, 291–304.

40 Simmons, M.A., Meschia, G., Makowski, E.L. & Battaglia, F.C. (1974): Fetal metabolic response to maternal starvation. *Pediat. Res.* **8**, 830–836.

41 Sutton, J.D. (1984): Feeding and fat production. *Occ. Publ. Br. Soc. Anim. Prod.* **9**, 43–52.

42 Sutton, J.D., Hart, I.C. & Broster, W.H. (1982): The effect of feeding frequency on energy metabolism in milking cows given low-roughage diets. In *Energy metabolism in farm animals*, ed A. Ekern & F. Sundstol, pp. 26–29. Aas: Agricultural University of Norway.

43 Sykes, A.R. & Field, A.C. (1972): Effects of dietary deficiencies of energy, protein and calcium on the pregnant ewe. 1. Body composition and mineral content of the ewes. *J. Agric. Sci.* Camb. **78**, 109–117.

44 Tyrrell, H.F., Brown, A.C.G., Reynolds, P.J., Haaland, G.L., Peel, C.J., Bauman, D.E. and Steinhour, W.D. (1982): In *Energy metabolism of farm animals*, ed A. Ekern & F. Sundstol, pp. 46–49. EEAP Publication No. 29.

45 Vernon, R.G. (1981): Lipid metabolism in the adipose tissue of ruminant animals. pp. 279–362 *in* Lipid metabolism in Ruminant Animals, ed W.W. Christie Oxford: Pergammon Press.

46 Widdowson, E.M. (1976): Changes in the body and its organs during lactation: nutritional implications. *In Breast-feeding and the Mother*, pp. 103–118. Ciba Fdn Symp 45 (New Series). Amsterdam: Elsevier.

Comparative aspects of milk composition and quantity

O.T. OFTEDAL
National Zoological Park, Smithsonian Institution, Washington DC 20008, USA.

All mammals produce milk as a source of nutrients for their young, but the amount and composition of milk varies greatly, as does the frequency of suckling and the duration of lactation. These differences in the pattern of nutrient output during lactation imply that the nutrient requirements of the lactating animal differ from one species to another. One must question whether species commonly used in lactation studies are appropriate models for human lactation.

In this paper inter-specific differences in the composition and yield of milk will be examined in relationship to such biological characterics as phylogenetic origin, body size, number of young, developmental state at birth and nursing pattern.

Milk composition. *The major constituents.* Although the major constituents (water, lipid, protein, sugar and ash) have been reported for the milks of more than 200 species, many of these data cannot be considered reliable[18,29]. In only about one-fourth of these species have as many as ten samples been assayed, and the confounding effects of sampling bias and lactation stage undoubtedly influence the results reported for many species. Sampling bias is especially problematic with respect to milk fat content, since fat levels increase several fold over the course of a milking session in most species that have been examined.[17,20,27,40]. Large compositional changes occur in early and late lactation in many species, although the degree and direction of change vary among species. For example, in primates, carnivores and ungulates, the initial secretion (colostrum) typically has an elevated content of protein (especially immunoglobulins), whereas the colostrum of rodents, rabbits, and seals does not appear to be particularly high in protein[29]. A late lactation rise in dry matter, fat and protein content, and a concurrent decline in sugar level, are commonly observed in a wide variety of species.

Table 1. *Composition of mid-lactation milk in selected mammals.*(From[29])

Species	Energy[a] content (kJ/g)	Dry matter (%)	Total lipid (%)	Total[b] protein (%)	Total sugar (%)
Black rhino	1.5	8.8	0.2	1.2	6.6
Horse	2.1	10.5	1.3	1.9	6.9
Human	2.9	12.4	4.1	0.8	6.8
Goat	2.9	12.0	3.8	2.9	4.7
Cow	3.0	12.4	3.7	3.2	4.6
Sheep	4.6	18.2	7.3	4.1	5.0
Rat	6.0	22.1	8.8	8.1	3.8
Dog	6.1	22.7	9.5	7.5	3.8
Reindeer	6.9	26.3	10.9	9.0	3.4
Mouse	7.7	29.3	13.1	9.0	3.0
Rabbit	8.5	31.2	15.2	10.3	1.8
Brown bear	9.5	33.6	18.5	8.5	2.3
Calif. sealion	13.8	41.0	30.7	8.6	0.3
Elephant seal	20.4	64.4	48.8	7.6	0.3

[a]Calculated gross energy; [b]true protein except rabbit, bear and elephant seal for which only crude protein data are available.

Compositional data for mid-lactation milks of a selected set of species are presented in Table 1. Although some sampling or analytical error may remain in these data, it is apparent that very large differences exist between species in all constituents. Degree of dilution by water accounts for much of the variability, with dry matter levels ranging from less than 10 per cent to more than 60 per cent (Table 1). By comparison with other mammals, most species that are bred and milked for commercial purposes (cow, goat, buffalo, sheep, horse) produce dilute milks (10–18 per cent dry matter). Perhaps this reflects human preference for milk of similar dry matter composition to human milk (12 per cent), or it may simply be that species with dilute milks tend to compensate by producing large amounts.

Milk energy. The range in dry matter levels of milk is paralleled by an even wider range in energy content. Milks vary in gross energy content more than 10 fold, from 1.5 kJ/g (0.35 kcal/g) in the black rhinoceros to about 20 kJ/g (5 kcal/g) in some seals (Table 1). An increase in energy content is largely accomplished by an increase in milk lipids and a decrease in milk sugars. The proportion of milk energy derived from lipid rises from 5 per cent in the black rhino to 91 per cent in the elephant seal while the energy contributed by sugar drops from 75 per cent in the rhino to 0.3 per cent in seal. Milks of most species fall in an intermediate range of 40–70 per cent lipid energy and 5–40 per cent sugar energy[29]. For example, human, cow, dog and mouse milks contain 54, 48, 59 and 65 per cent lipid energy and 39, 26, 11 and 6 per cent sugar energy respectively. Protein content typically increases with energy content (Table 1) such that the percentage of milk energy supplied by protein remains at 20–35 per cent in most species[29]. Both the dilute milks of primates and the very concentrated milks of seals and sealions are lower in protein energy (7–19 per cent), however. Human milk contains the least protein reported for any species, whether compared on a fresh weight (0.8 per cent) or an energetic basis (7 per cent).

The osmotic role of lactose. The inverse relationship between dry matter content and sugar level (Table 1) can be attributed in part to the osmotic role of the principal milk sugar, lactose, in secretory physiology. As a low-molecular-weight solute, lactose draws water osmotically into Golgi vesicles which subsequently discharge their contents into the lumina of mammary alveoli by exocytosis[36]. Milks high in lactose such as primate, equine and rhino milks are thus inevitably dilute milks. Some marsupial milks contain oligosaccharides rather than lactose, however, such that the osmotic consequences of a small molecule are avoided[14]. Thus in mid-lactation tammar wallaby milk contains more than 12 per cent sugar and yet is moderately high (24 per cent) in dry matter. The osmotic mechanisms by which milks of negligible sugar content (eg, seal and sealion milks) are secreted remain a mystery[35].

Adaptive significance of dilution. Concentrated milks reduce the water burden of lactation on the female. Species that neither eat nor drink during lactation, such as many true seals[7] and hibernating bears[26], might not be able to derive sufficient water from body water stores or metabolic sources to sustain production of a dilute milk. The milks of these species are especially concentrated (Table 1). Low sugar levels may also serve a protein-sparing function by limiting gluconeogenesis. Contrary to expectation, camels and many other desert species do not produce milks particularly low in water, perhaps because the young requires water for thermoregulatory purposes. These animals must adopt other behavioural and physiological strategies to economize in their water budgets[23].

Milk concentration is also correlated with suckling frequency: neonates consuming dilute milks appear to suckle frequently[4]. Conversely, species with intervals of one or more days between suckling bouts, such as rabbits, hares, tree shrews, sea lions and fur seals[7,39] produce particularly concentrated milks (30–60 per cent) dry matter[29]. In this case high dry matter content may reflect a need to minimize the volume occupied by milk during prolonged accumulation, whether due to restricted mammary capacity or inability of the young to ingest an unlimited amount at the infrequent feedings. Even so the amounts transferred from mother to young at a suckling session can be phenomenal. A newborn tree shrew, for example, may ingest up to 40 per cent of body weight at each suckling period[24].

Several authors[5,6] have maintained that milk concentration is inversely correlated to body weight, yet it is clear that many medium-sized and large animals (including the very largest living animals, baleen whales) defy this trend by secreting highly concentrated milks. It is possible that the young of very small animals require relatively energy-rich milks because of their high energy requirements per unit body weight.

It is commonly assumed that differences in milk composition between species reflect differences in the nutrient requirements of the young. Long ago[1] a correlation of milk protein content with time to double birthweight among various domestic and laboratory species was shown. Since protein content is related to dry matter and energy content, however, this correlation is confounded by milk concentration. When protein content is expressed as a percentage of milk energy, there is no clear relationship to rate of growth[3,28,37]. Related species with similar milk protein levels can have quite different growth rates[28]. As a group, primates exhibit both low-protein milks and low rates of growth, however[34].

The proportions of the major milk proteins (alpha-, beta-, and kappa-caseins, beta-lactoglobulins, alpha-lactalbumins) vary among species with consequent differences in total amino acid profile[19]. The low sulphur amino acid content of casein implies that these amino acids will be limiting in milks with a preponderence of casein, such as cow's milk[13,38]. Conversely, the amino acid pattern of milks containing a high proportion of whey proteins (eg, horse milk, human milk) is apt to be more balanced[28].

Milk minerals. The nutritional significance of inter- and intra-species variation in milk minerals is poorly understood. The ratio of potassium to sodium in most milks is similar to that of intracellular fluids, about 3:1; deviations from this ratio are thought to reflect paracellular ion movement in mammary alveoli[35,36] and may be unrelated to nutrient requirements of the young.

Milk calcium and phosphorus contents vary more than 10 fold among species, with calcium ranging from less than 50 mg/100g to more than 500 mg/100g and phosphorus from about 20 to 280 mg/100g[28]. Much of this variation can be explained by varying casein concentration, since casein micelles provide a major vehicle for calcium and phosphorus transfer from mother to young[28]. Nutritional interpretation of calcium and phosphorus data is complicated by the effects of lactation stage. In horses, for example, calcium and phosphorus levels decline steadily over the first four months of lactation, such that levels at 4 months are but 52 and 57 per cent of the levels in the first week (H.F. Schryver, unpublished). By contrast the calcium and phosphorus contents of black bear milk increase 4-fold and 2.5-fold, respectively, over the first two months of lactation (O.T. Oftedal, unpublished).

The milks of many species are low in iron content, forcing the suckling neonate to draw on iron stores accumulated *in utero*[5]. Species bearing very small or undeveloped young (eg, monotremes, marsupials) may be unable to transfer sufficient iron prenatally to cover requirements during lactation. These species tend to produce milks of much higher iron content, at least in early lactation[14,15].

Although there has been an increased interest in the vitamin content of human milk, relatively little is known about interspecies variation in milk vitamin levels of non-domestic animals.

Milk yield. *Problems in methodology.* The nutritional consequences of lactation depend as much on the quantity as on the composition of milk. Methods of measuring yield that are suitable in one species may produce erroneous results in another.

In studies of human and domestic ruminant lactation, weight differential or test-weighing procedures involving repeat weighings of young both before and after suckling are common. Interference with the normal behaviour and timing of suckling can cause reduced milk transfer and underestimation of yield, especially in untrained or easily stressed animals[10,11,29].

Measurement of yield by milk collection will be an accurate estimate for non-dairy animals only if a high and replicable degree of mammary evacuation is achieved at each milking, and the amount removed is comparable to what the young would take. This may be difficult in stressed animals or in species without spacious storage cisterns. Removal of residual milk may cause overestimation of milk yield in the initial period after birth[11].

Estimates of water turnover in the young permit calculation of milk yield as long as incorporation of hydrogen isotopes into non-exchangeable sites is negligible and water from metabolic or non-milk sources can be accounted for[8,25,29]. Isotope recycling and increasing pool size must also be corrected for[2,12].

The various procedures provide for useful comparison and validation since the sources of error and direction of expected bias differ. While good correspondence has been obtained in some species, in others the yield estimates are quite divergent[8,11,21,30,32].

Interspecific trends. Values of peak milk yields (Table 2) were obtained by weight-differential or isotope dilution methods with animals that were apparently well-nourished. Peak milk output generally rises as body size increases, but represents a declining percentage of maternal weight. Daily milk production can equal as much as 20 per cent of body weight in the rat and as little as 1.5 per cent in reindeer. Milk production also varies in relation to number of offspring: species with litters of several young produce more milk, relative to body weight, than species with a single offspring.

Milk production represents a major metabolic effort and as such would be expected to vary in proportion to maternal metabolic size (weight $^{0.75}$). If milk energy output (EO, MJ) at peak

Table 2. *Milk and milk energy output at peak lactation in selected mammals.* Energy values represent gross energy (From[29]).

Species	Body weight (kg)	Milk output (MO) (g/d)	MO as % weight (%)	Energy output (EO) (MJ/d)	EO per maternal mass (MJ/kg$^{.75}$/d)	EO per litter mass (MJ/kg$^{.83}$/d)
Species with litters:						
Rat	0.20	41	20.5	0.24	1.01	0.89
Mink	0.96	119	12.4	0.59	0.60	0.89
Guinea-pig	0.98	77	7.9	0.35	0.35	0.64
Skunk	2.22	151	6.8	1.24	0.69	1.05
Rabbit	4.40	270	6.1	2.32	0.77	1.01
Dog	12.7	1050	8.3	6.44	0.96	1.11
Pig	120	7160	6.0	37.3	1.03	0.95
Ungulates with one young:						
Gazelle	20.6	560	2.7	3.6	0.37	0.88
Sheep	52.6	1610	3.1	7.5	0.38	1.05
Red deer	85.3	1570	1.8	9.0	0.32	0.95
Reindeer	107	1590	1.5	11.0	0.33	1.19
Beef cow	340	7240	2.2	22.1	0.29	0.82
Horse	515	17600	3.4	37.2	0.34	0.89
Primates						
Baboon	16.7	400	2.4	1.34	0.16	0.85
Human	57	1050	1.8	3.03	0.15	0.72

lactation is compared with body weight (W, kg) by the relationship $EO = aW^b$, the exponent b has been estimated as 0.65–0.79 and the coefficient a as 0.52–0.61 (124–146 for energy in kcal[16,22,31]. Most species with litters secrete milk energy at a level ($0.6–1.0\,MJ/kg^{0.75}/day$) several fold higher than that of ungulates with single young ($0.3–0.4\,MJ/kg^{0.75}/day$). The guinea-pig provides an interesting exception in that the lactating female with three young produces milk energy at a level ($0.35\,MJ/kg^{0.75}/day$) equivalent to that of an ungulate with one offspring. During the first few weeks neonatal guinea-pigs must draw upon fat reserves deposited prior to birth to supplement the limited amount of energy supplied as milk[28,41]. Milk energy yields of baboons and humans are lower still, and presumably reflect the low rates of postnatal growth that are characteristic of primates[9].

In an analysis of milk energy intakes of neonates of 14 species[28] energy intake was proportional to neonatal weight to the power 0.83 rather than 0.75, and energy intakes (MJ per day) were within 15 per cent of $0.94\,W^{0.83}$ in most species. It is not surprising, therefore, that maternal milk energy output is more closely tied to litter metabolic mass (ie litter size multiplied by neonatal weight$^{0.83}$) than to maternal metabolic mass. Energy output per litter metabolic mass falls within the narrow range of $0.8–1.2\,MJ/kg^{0.83}/day$ in most species; once again both the human and the guinea-pig are below the usual range.

Most comparative analyses of lactation performance have been restricted to examination of peak yields since data on total milk yields are much more difficult to obtain from animals with offspring. Peak yield does provide an indication of total yield over the course of lactation in ungulates[33]. Total milk energy output over lactation appears to be about 80–114 times peak energy output in ungulates weighing 20–500 kg and suckling single offspring. In smaller species total energy output is a smaller multiple of peak output since lactation is of shorter duration[33].

Animals with highly divergent lactation patterns may not have similar total to peak yield ratios, however. The shortest lactation among mammals apparently belongs to the hooded seal, which lactates for 3–5 d. The rate of energy transfer from mother to pup must be phenomenal in this seal since the pups gain 7 kg/d (Bowen, Oftedal & Boness, in preparation). By contrast in primates a prolonged lactation period may result in total milk output similar to other species even though peak production is low. Thus peak milk yield is a valuable indicator of total milk production only among species with comparable lactation patterns.

Conclusion. *Use of animal models.* Animal models of lactation must be approached with an appreciation of interspecific variation in lactation patterns. Nutritional, physiological and biochemical aspects of lactation are apt to differ among species in ways that can influence experimental results.

Application of results from animal studies to the human context can be especially misleading. Human lactation is characterized by secretion of relatively small amounts of a dilute, low protein milk over a long lactation period. None of the common laboratory or domestic rodents, carnivores or ungulates exhibit a similar lactation pattern. Human lactation is probably fairly typical of the pattern found in primates, and especially the great apes. Unfortunately relatively little lactation research has been conducted on primates, and next to nothing on great apes. It would be especially valuable to develop a small primate model that would be suitable to lactation research.

1 Abderhalden, E. (1898): Die Beziehungen der Wachsthumsgeschwindigkeit des Sauglings zur Zusammensetzung der Milch beim Kaninchen, bei der Katz und beim Hunde. *Hoppe-Seyler's Z. Physiol. Chem.* **26**, 487–497.
2 Baverstock, P. & Green, B. (1975): Water recycling in lactation. *Science* **187**, 657–658.
3 Bernhart, F.W. (1961): Correlation between growth-rate of the suckling of various species and the percentage of total calories from protein in the milk. *Nature Lond.* **191**, 358–360.
4 Ben Shaul, D.M. (1962): The composition of the milk of wild animals. *Int. Zoo Yearbk.* **4**, 333–342.
5 Blaxter, K.L. (1961): Lactation and the growth of the young. In: *Milk: the mammary gland and its secretion*, ed S.K. Kon & A.T. Cowie, pp. 305–361. New York: Academic Press.
6 Blaxter, K.L. (1964): Protein metabolism and requirements in pregnancy and lactation. In *Mammalian protein metabolism*, ed H.W. Munro & J.B. Allison, pp. 173–223. New York: Academic Press.
7 Bonner, W.N. (1984): Lactation strategies in pinnipeds: problems for a marine mammalian group. *Symp. Zool. Soc. Lond.* **51**, 253–272.
8 Butte, N.F., Garza, C., Smith, E.O. & Nichols, B.L. (1983): Evaluation of the deuterium dilution technique against the test-weighing procedure for the determination of breast milk intake. *Am. J. Clin. Nutr.* **37**, 996–1003.

9 Case, T.J. (1978): On the evolution and adaptive significance of postnatal growth rates in the terrestrial vertebrates. *Q. Rev. Biol.* **53**, 243–282.

10 Coombe, J.B., Wardrop, I.D. & Tribe, D.E. (1960): A study of milk production of the grazing ewe, with emphasis on the experimental technique employed. *J. Agric. Sci., Camb.* **54**, 353–359.

11 Doney, J.M., Peart, J.N., Smith, W.F. & Louda, F. (1979): A consideration of the techniques for estimation of milk yield by suckled sheep and a comparison of estimates obtained by two methods in relation to the effect of breed, level of production and stage of lactation. *J. Agric. Sci.*, Camb. **92**, 123–132.

12 Dove, H. & Freer, M. (1979): The accuracy of tritiated water turnover rate, as an estimate of milk in lambs. *Aust. J. Agric. Res.* **30**, 725–739.

13 Foldager, J., Huber, J.T. & Bergen, W.G. (1977): Methionine and sulfur amino acid requirement in the preruminant calf. *J. Dairy Sci.* **60**, 1095–1104.

14 Green, B. (1984): Composition of milk and energetics of growth in marsupials. *Symp. Zool. Soc. Lond.* **51**, 369–387.

15 Griffiths, M., Green, B., Leckie, R.M.C., Messer, M. & Newgrain, K.W. (1984): Constituents of platypus and echidna milk, with particular reference to the fatty acid complement of the triglycerides. *Aust. J. Biol. Sci.* **37**, 323–329.

16 Hanwell, A. & Peaker, M. (1977): Physiological effects of lactation on the mother. *Symp. Zool. Soc. Lond.* **41**, 297–312.

17 Jaouen, J.C. & Mens, P. (1981): Change in the composition of goat milk during milking. *Dairy Sci. Abstr.* **43**, 376.

18 Jenness, R. (1974): The composition of milk. In *Lactation: a comprehensive treatise*, ed B.L. Larson & V.R. Smith, vol. 3, pp. 3–107. New York: Academic Press.

19 Jenness, R. (1979): Comparative aspects of milk proteins. *J. Dairy Res.* **46**, 197–210.

20 Labussiere, J., Combaud, J., Petrequin, P., Tessonniere, R. & Gouget, R. (1969): Importance, composition et significance des differentes fractions de lait obtenus successivement au cours de la traite mecanique des bresbis. *Annls Zootech.* **18**, 185–196.

21 LeDu, Y.L.P., MacDonald, A.J. & Peart, J.N. (1979): Comparison of two techniques for estimating the milk production of suckler cows. *Livestock Prod. Sci.* **6**, 277–281.

22 Linzell, J.L. (1972): Milk yield, energy loss in milk, and mammary gland weight in different species. *Dairy Sci. Abstr.* **34**, 351–360.

23 Maltz, E. & Shkolnik, A. (1984): Lactational strategies in desert ruminants: the Bedouin goat, ibex and desert gazelle. *Symp. Zool. Soc. Lond.* **51**, 193–213.

24 Martin, R.D. (1968): Reproduction and ontogeny in tree shrews (*Tupaia belangeri*) with reference to their general behavior and taxonomic relationships. *Z. Tierpsychol.* **25**, 409–495, 505–532.

25 Nagy, K.A. & Costa, D.P. (1980): Water flux in animals: Analysis of potential errors in the tritiated water method. *Am. J. Physiol.* **238**, R454–465.

26 Nelson, R.A., Beck, T.D.I. & Steiger, D.L. (1984): Ratio of serum creatinine in wild black bears. *Science* **226**, 841–842.

27 Neville, M.C., Keller, R.P., Seacat, J., Casey, C.E., Allen, J.C. & Archer, P. (1984): Studies on human lactation. I. Within-feed and between-breast variation in selected components of human milk. *Am. J. Clin. Nutr.* **40**, 635–646.

28 Oftedal, O.T. (1981): Milk, protein and energy intakes of suckling mammalian young: a comparative study. Ph.D. thesis, Cornell University Press.

29 Oftedal, O.T. (1984): Milk composition, milk yield and energy output at peak lactation: a comparative review. *Symp. Zool. Soc. Lond.* **51**, 33–85.

30 Oftedal, O.T. (1984): Body size and reproductive strategy as correlates of milk energy yield in lactating mammals. *Acta Zool. Fenn.* **171**, 183–186.

31 Oftedal, O.T. (1984): Lactation in the dog: milk composition and intake in puppies. *J. Nutr.* **114**, 803–812.

32 Oftedal, O.T., Hintz, H.F. & Schryver, H.F. (1983): Lactation in the horse: milk composition and intake by foals. *J. Nutr.* **113**, 2096–2106.

33 Oftedal, O.T. (In Press): Pregnancy and lactation. In *The bioenergetics of wild herbivores*, ed R.J. Hudson & R.G. White. Boca Raton, Florida: CRC Press.

34 Payne, P.R. & Wheeler, E.F. (1968): Comparative nutrition in pregnancy and lactation. *Proc. Nutr. Soc.* **27**, 129–138.

35 Peaker, M. (1977): The aqueous phase of milk: ion and water transport. *Symp. Zool. Soc. Lond.* **41**, 113–134.

36 Peaker, M. (1978): Ion and water transport in the mammary gland. In *Lactation: a comparative treatise*, ed B.L. Larson & V.R. Smith, vol. 4, pp. 437–462. New York: Academic Press.

37 Powers, G.F. (1933): The alleged correlation between the rate of growth of the suckling and the composition of the milk of the species. *J. Pediat.* **3**, 201–216.

38 Walker, D.M. (1979): Nutrition of preruminants. In *Digestive physiology and nutrition of ruminants*, ed D.C. Church, pp. 258–280. Corvallis, Ore.: O & B Books.

39 Walser, E.S. (1977): Maternal behaviour in mammals. *Symp. Zool. Soc. Lond.* **41**, 297–312.

40 Whittlestone, W.G. (1953): Variations in the fat content of milk throughout the milking process. *J. Dairy Res.* **20**, 146.

41 Widdowson, E.M. & McCance, R.A. (1955): Physiological undernutrition in the newborn guinea-pig. *Br. J. Nutr.* **91**, 316–321.

ADEQUACY OF BREAST-FEEDING AND MATERNAL NUTRITIONAL STATUS

Growth faltering of exclusively breast-fed infants in Manipur (India)

N.C. LUWANG
3/IV Babupara, Imphal 795001, India.

In developing countries, infants are invariably breast-fed for prolonged periods[7] and weaning is delayed. Prolonged, exclusive breast-feeding and delayed weaning are among the most important factors contributing to the high prevalence of malnutrition. At some point in the first year of life, breast-milk alone will not meet the infant's energy requirements for the maintenance of proper growth and health and supplementary food is then needed. The important question to decide is how long breast-milk alone is adequate as the sole source of food for the infant. There are conflicting reports on this important issue[1,2,5-8] and in the present study an attempt was made to answer the question by studying growth of exclusively breast-fed infants by measuring their weight gain at fortnightly intervals for up to 7 months.

Material and methods. The study covered a period from November, 1981 to November, 1983 and was carried out at the Well Baby Clinic, Regional Medical College Hospital and the Urban Health Centre Field Practice Area, Regional Medical College. The study population came from the Imphal Municipality. The aim of the study was to observe healthy infants from healthy mothers who were representative of the community. However, selection of a true random sample was not feasible. Mothers included in the study belonged to the typical Manipuri community of the middle socioeconomic group. Mothers of the age group 18–30 years and with 0–3 child births who were not sick or anaemic were selected for the study. Babies of both sexes with birth-weight of 2500g or more which were well-established on breast-feeding were selected for the study. Registration and weighing of the infants were done within 3 days of delivery, together with a collection of detailed information about the mother, and her family, socioeconomic and environmental background. The infants were followed up at fortnightly intervals for weighing and for collecting information about feeding practices and about any sickness experienced by infants or mothers. Weight measurements were done accurateley on a beam balance which can measure up to 10 g accuracy (manufactured by the CMS Weighting Equipments Ltd., London). A field worker appointed for the purpose contacted the mothers by home visits whenever necessary and made sure that measurement and examination of the infants were done regularly. A deficit of an absolute weight gain by more than 2 S.D. from the expected figure[4] for two successive fortnightly periods was the criterion for growth faltering.

During the period of study 80 infants (44 male and 36 female) were followed-up from birth till the faltering of growth. Attempts were made to check that the faltering was due to insufficient food and not to some infection or sickness.

Results. The distribution of ages at which growth faltering occurred is shown in the Table. The

Table. *Numbers and proportions of exclusively breast-fed infants showing growth faltering at different ages*

Age	Number faltering		% Faltering
(months)	No.	Cumulative	(Cumulative)
1–2	7	7	8.75
2–3	4	11	13.75
3–4	17	28	35.00
4–5	19	47	58.75
5–6	20	67	83.75
6–7	8	75	93.75
7–8	5	80	100.00

incidence of growth faltering increased progressively from 8.75 per cent at the end of the first month to 100 per cent at the end of the 7th month. By the 5th month nearly 60 per cent of the infants had an unsatisfactory rate of weight gain.

Discussion. The faltering of growth observed in the present study and reported by other authors could be due to an inadequate supply of breast-milk or to infection, although the latter cause of growth faltering was unlikely. Taking growth rate as the indicator, the present study showed that a high proportion of infants failed to get adequate energy from breast-milk alone from about 4–5 months of age or even earlier. Lactation failure of mothers at 3 months of age[6], and incidence of failure to thrive at the breast in the UK[3] has also been reported. An investigation of the adequacy of breast milk as a sole source of food concluded that breast-milk alone fails to cover the energy needs of many infants after about 3 months[8]. Whitehead *et al* also came to the same conclusion from their study at the Gambia[9]. A prospective study of the growth pattern of infants, concluded that breast-milk alone is nutritionally adequate as the only source of food for the majority of healthy infants up to 8 months[2]. In a retrospective analysis of the weight and height curves of 96 infants who had been exclusively breast fed for at least 6 months within the past 2 years, it was observed that breast-milk alone provided adequate nutrition for growth through 9 months[1], but Gopalan[5] reported that breast-milk alone will not be able to sustain growth at an adequate level beyond about 20 weeks of age.

The main conclusion from this study is that breast-fed infants require supplementary food from 4 to 5 months of age if proper growth is to be maintained.

1 Ahn, C.H. & MacLean, Jr. W.C. (1980): Growth of the exclusively breast fed infants. *Am. J. Clin. Nutr.* **33**, 183–192.
2 Chandra, R.K. (1981): Breast feeding, growth and morbidity. *Nutr. Res.* **1**, 25–31.
3 Davies, D.P. & Evans, T.I. (1976): Failure to thrive at the breast. *Lancet* **2**, 1194–1195.
4 Fomon, S.J. (1974): *Infant nutrition*, 2nd ed, Philadelphia: W.B. Saunders.
5 Gopalan, C. (1958): Studies on lactation in poor Indian communities. *J. Trop. Pediat.* **4**, 87–97.
6 Kimmance, K.J. (1972): Failure to thrive and lactation failure in Jordanian villages in 1970. *Env. Child Hlth.* **18**, 313–320.
7 Waterlow, J.C., Ashworth, A. & Griffiths, M. (1980): Faltering in infant growth in less developed countries. *Lancet* **2**, 1176–1177.
8 Waterlow, J.C. & Thomson, A.M. (1979): Observations on the adequacy of breast feeding. *Lancet* **2**, 238–241.
9 Whitehead, R.G., Rowland, M.G.M., Hutton, M., Prentice, A.M., Muller, E. & Paul, A. (1978): Factors influencing lactation performance in rural Gambian mothers. *Lancet*, **2**, 178–181.

Interventions to improve lactational performance. A practical proposition?

A.M. PRENTICE, R.G. WHITEHEAD, Ann PRENTICE and T.J. COLE
Dunn Nutrition Unit, Milton Road, Cambridge, CB4 1XJ, UK and Keneba, The Gambia.

In considering the adequacy of breast-feeding and its possible relationship to maternal nutritional status it is important to distinguish between factors which *control* and those which *limit* milk output. The amount of milk received by the baby of a well-nourished mother is influenced by a combination of stimulatory and inhibitory *controls*. In an undernourished mother, although the amount of breast-milk received by the baby will be controlled in a similar way, it may also be *limited* by a direct or indirect limitation of substrate supply to the breast. This may be caused by a combination of acute or chronic shortfalls in food intake, the absence of maternal energy and nutrient reserves to subsidize lactation, or the stresses of a heavy agricultural work load and maternal infections. The purpose of this paper is to examine whether nutritional interventions can improve lactational performance either by modifying the controls or by removing the presumed limits to milk secretion.

Lactational performance in affluent and developing countries — the consensus a decade ago. In 1975 the Dunn Nutrition Unit began a detailed study of lactational performance among women in the rural village of Keneba, The Gambia. A review of the literature on breast-milk intakes available at that time is summarized in Fig. (a) which demonstrates a striking difference between milk intakes reported for exclusively breast-fed infants from affluent and developing countries at 3 months of age. Although it was appreciated that many of the very high values from the affluent societies were obtained from professional wet-nurses such values encouraged the belief that mean outputs in excess of 1 litre per day should be easily achievable in well-fed women. The exceptionally low energy intakes reported for lactating women in many areas of the developing world seemed to provide an obvious explanation for the apparent difference in lactational performance, and this suggestion was strengthened by seasonal decreases in milk output which coincided with the hungry period of the year in The Gambia, Kenya and Zaire.

However, in spite of all this circumstantial evidence, the only way to obtain conclusive proof that the level of energy restriction observed in The Gambia, which is representative of many areas of the developing world, was sufficient to impair lactation was to increase the mothers' energy intake and observe a positive effect on milk output. We undertook a study to test this in Keneba.

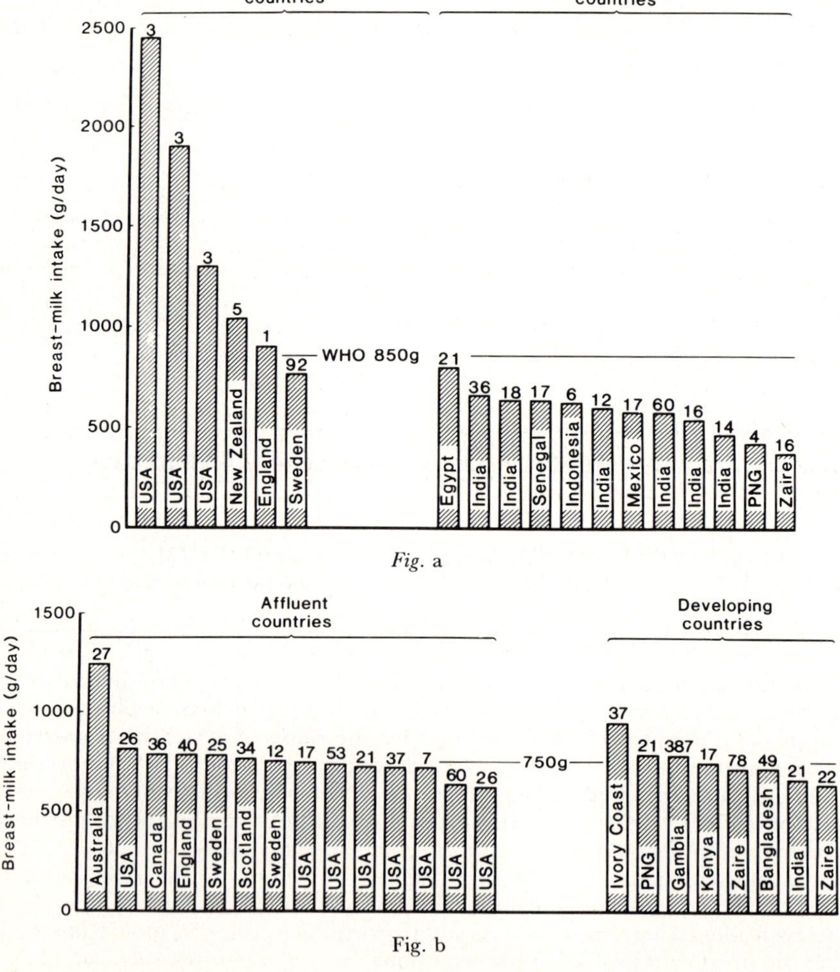

Figure. Data on breast-milk volume at 3 months post-partum: (a) pre-1975, (b) post-1975
Numbers above each column represent number of subjects

Dietary supplementation of lactating women. An energy-dense and nutritionally balanced supplement of groundnut-based biscuits and a vitamin-fortified tea drink succeeded in raising the energy intake of 130 women in Keneba by a net amount of 720 kcal (3.01 MJ)/d once the small replacement effect on the home diet was accounted for[3]. The gross energy intake after supplementation was still lower than WHO/FAO recommendations, but exactly matched observed intakes in well-nourished women from Cambridge, UK. However, in spite of achieving such a large increase in energy intake and largely correcting deficits of protein, riboflavin, vitamin A and calcium, dietary supplementation had no effect on breast-milk output. This conclusion is based on over 1700 12-h and over 100 24-h measurements of breast-milk output. A detailed analysis of the data failed to reveal any selective effect in the hungry season, in mothers with lower than average milk outputs or in mothers with lower than average nutritional status or food intakes. Milk protein content was slightly improved together with certain vitamins, but the energy content remained unchanged.

A number of other community-based studies from Zaire, India, Mexico, Colombia and Guatemala have also attempted to boost lactational performance by maternal dietary supplementation, but none of them have provided convincing evidence of a positive effect on milk output and even in the few studies where there has been a suggestion of an effect the magnitude could not be considered cost-effective. Ashworth and Feachem[1] have reached a similar conclusion in a recent review of this topic. In addition there may be adverse consequences of supplementation such as the reduction in the period of post-partum amenorrhoea observed in our study[2].

Why does dietary supplementation appear to be so unsuccessful? The most likely explanation appears to be that our original conclusion that milk output was limited by substrate supply was incorrect.

Lactational performance in affluent and developing countries — a reappraisal. In the decade since we started our studies there have been more data published on breast-milk outputs than in the preceding century. These data, summarised in Fig. (b) reveal no difference between affluent and developing countries. The reasons for the difference between the old and new data are the care taken to be non-selective in subject recruitment in affluent countries and the much greater care not to disturb traditional patterns of demand feeding and not to impose psychological stresses on the mothers in developing countries. Many of the earlier studies from the developing world had been performed in metabolic wards.

A provisional conclusion based on the new data is that in most nutritional circumstances studied so far in the developing world there is a strong drive towards milk synthesis, and that milk output is not *limited* by food intake but is *controlled* by the characteristics of the mother-infant pair. However, it should be stressed that this conclusion should not be extended to conditions of famine and possibly not to areas where protein deficiency may cause pathophysiological adjustments of nutrient partitioning which may compromise milk synthesis.

Might other interventions be effective? Since attempts to improve lactational performance by improving substrate supply to the breast seem to be ineffective in most circumstances research should now concentrate on attempts to modify any of the *controls* which may be down-regulating milk output. The main possible areas for consideration are: (1) improving the infant's appetite, which may be achieved by producing a bigger baby by prenatal supplementation; (2) improving feeding practices both in the early post-partum period and during established lactation. This may be particularly important in the agricultural season in developing countries when contact between a mother and her infant is reduced and standards of child-care deteriorate; (3) avoiding unnecessarily early introduction of complementary feeds which inhibit milk production.

1 Ashworth, A. & Feachem, R.G. (1985): Interventions for the control of diarrhoeal diseases among young children: improving lactation. *Bull. Wld Hlth Org.* **63**, 165–184.
2 Lunn, P.G., Austin, S., Prentice, A.M. & Whitehead, R.G. (1984): The effect of improved nutrition on plasma prolactin concentrations and post-partum infertility in lactating Gambian women. *Am. J. Clin. Nutr.* **39**, 227–235.
3 Prentice, A.M., Roberts, S.B., Prentice, A., Paul, A.A., Watkinson, M., Watkinson, A.A. & Whitehead, R.G. (1983): Dietary supplementation of lactating Gambian women. I. Effect on breast-milk volume and quality. *Hum. Nutr.: Clin. Nutr.* **37C**, 53–64.

Effect of traditional feeding practices on breast-milk production

K. TONTISIRIN
Ramathibodi Hospital and Institute of Nutrition, Mahidol University, Bangkok, Thailand.

It is currently held that milk production from well-nourished mothers is 700–900 ml/24 h and that breast-feeding alone can be nutritionally adequate for the first 3–6 months of an infant's life[7,8,18]. There is sufficient evidence from widely scattered areas, including such diverse sources as the United States[5], The People's Republic of China[14] and India[2] that breast-feeding with little or no supplementation resulted in excellent growth for about the first 5 to 6 months of life.

However, breast-milk alone does not assure adequate nutrition for the first full year, and usually not beyond the first 6 months, even under favourable circumstance. Many infants show evidence of a faltering rate of weight gain or other consequences of undernutrition because appropriate complementary feeding is not given when needed[13]. This may occur as early as 3 to 4 months in infants in some populations[16–19], or as late as 5 to 6 months in others[2,9,10,12]. The variations are due primarily to differences in the health, nutrition and life-style of the mother, all of which may affect milk production and to the overall burden on the infant from diarrhoeal, respiratory and other infectious disease.

The relationship between breast-feeding and the introduction of supplementary foods can be illustrated as in Fig. 1.

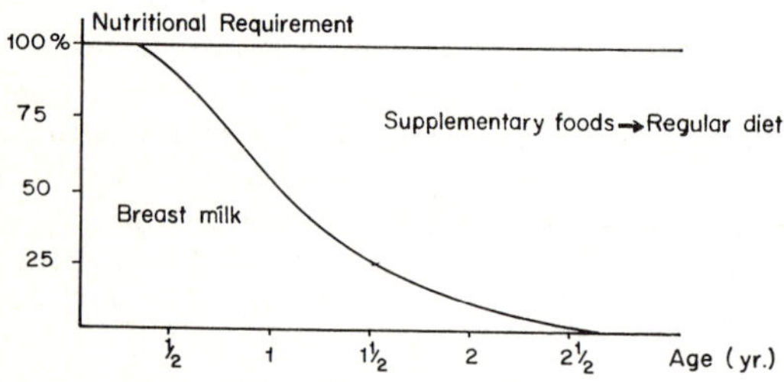

Fig. 1. Relationship between breast milk and supplementary food during infancy and early childhood.

Supplementary feeding practices. In many traditional societies breast-feeding is a common practice for 18 months or longer, but there is a widespread practice of early supplementary feeding. The reasons vary with societies but mainly due to their cultures and socioeconomic status. Traditional feeding practices that are widely observed in most of the rural areas of developing countries are the early weaning practices. For example, a short breast-feeding was frequently observed in Chilean mothers, and infants were given thin rice-water or barley-water. In Indian communities, supplementary feeding of infants is started by 5 or 6 months but the supplements are mostly modified poor adult diets[6].

In Thailand, an early introduction of semi-solid food is very common among rural families. Chewed glutinous rice and or banana are usually given to the baby at the age of 3–7 d. By the first 3 months of life, 70–90 per cent of the infants already obtained these supplements in considerable amount[15]. The infants fed semi-solid foods at an early age tend to have distended stomachs which will result in decreased suckling reflexes and which in turn reduce the stimulation for milk production. As the child approaches the weaning age (6–18 months) food supplements are gradually increased and become the main meals, breast milk serving as a supplement. Most of rural children get mainly rice with banana or a small piece of fish or meat. Fat intake was only 6–10 per cent of total energy intake as compared to the recommended level of 30 per cent.

Evidence of infant-feeding in the United States in the 1960s showed that at least 90 per cent of infants were receiving supplementary food below 3 months and often during the first week of life[3]. Most infants were fed commercially prepared formulas and supplementary foods other than milk, eg cereal, vegetables and fruits were frequently introduced during the 1st month of life. However, a strong return to breast-feeding is now evident in North America, Scandinavia and in other European countries[13].

Supplementary feeding, suckling stimuli, prolactin and breast-milk production. It is generally accepted that the maintenance of successful lactation depends upon a continuing adequate stimulus provided by the feeding infant[20]. The ejection of breast-milk is mediated by the psychosomatic let-down reflex, resulting from nipple stimulation ('prolactin reflex') and to the degree of intra-alveolar tension, related to emptying. The prolactin response to suckling declines with time post-partum, but if suckling frequency is maintained, a high level of milk output may well remain for 18 months or more[1]. Thus, complete weaning is associated with a reduction in feeding frequency and the reduction in the duration of lactation results in a decrease in the total quantity of milk produced.

Breast-feeding is associated with high plasma concentration of prolactin, at least at the onset of lactation, the level correlating to some extent with the number of suckling episodes[1]. Studies have shown that a gradual introduction of supplementary food does not have an effect on the level of prolactin unless the baby's suckling ceases; otherwise, prolactin levels remain above normal for 18 months[1,4,11].

The relationships between the various factors influencing the production of breast-milk are shown in Fig. 2.

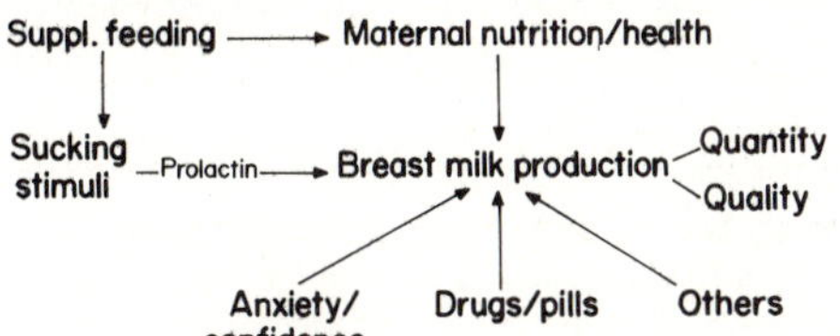

Fig. 2. *The relationships between the various factors influencing breast-milk production.*

A study was performed attempting to examine the volume of breast-milk produced by mothers in rural communities in north-east Thailand. The data showed that breast-feeding and early supplementary feeding represent their habitual pattern. Infants' ages ranged from 0–18 months and some were fed with the supplements only 9 d after birth. The supplements were low in energy and density of nutrients. The volume of milk produced by the mothers was somewhat below that of data from WHO Collaborative Study on Breast-feeding 1981. This might be due to the poor maternal nutrition and maternal health in rural populations since prolactin measurement was not performed in this study. However, the fact that those mothers were all fully breast-feeding implied that the suckling episodes may well have remained normal.

Conclusion. Supplementary food has much relevance to breast-feeding in traditional communities. First, the foods taken need to be considered as being complemented nutritionally by the small, but significant, continuing amount of breast milk secreted. Secondly, the time at which foods are introduced is relevant to milk production as they may have the effect of decreasing the suckling stimulus and prolactin secretion, and hence diminishing milk output.

Overdilute, frequently contaminated, traditional weaning foods of low nutritional value are introduced too soon. The approach should be to improve lactation by attention to the mother's diet and health in pregnancy and during breast-feeding, to persuade parents to delay the introduction of weaning foods to 4–6 months and to make them more concentrated, more nutritious, and less likely to be contaminated.

1 Delvoye, P., Demaegd, M., Delogne-Desnoeck, J. & Robyn, C. (1977): The influence of the frequency of nursing and of previous lactation experience on serum prolactin in lactating mothers. *J. Biosoc. Sci.* **9**, 447–451.
2 Gopalan, C. (1958): Studies on lactation in poor Indian communities. *J. Trop. Pediat.* **4**, 87–97.
3 Gyorgy, P. (1961): Orientation in infant feeding Nutrition in maternal and infant feeding. *Fed. Proc* **20**, 169–175.
4 Howie, P.W., McNelly, A.S., Houston, M.J., Cook, A. & Boyle, H. (1981): Effect of supplementary food on suckling patterns and ovarian activity during lactation. *Br. Med. J.* **283**, 757–759.
5 Jackson, R.L., Westerfield, R., Flynn, M.A., Kimball, E.R. & Lewis, R.B. (1964): Growth of well born American infants fed human and cow's milk. *Pediatrics* **33**, 642–652.
6 Jelliffe, D.B. (1962): Culture, social change and infant feeding. *Am. J. Clin. Nutr.* **10**, 19–45.

7 Jelliffe, D.B. & Jelliffe, E.F.P. (1978): The volume and composition of human milk in poorly nourished communities. A review. *Am. J. Clin. Nutr.* **31**, 492–515.
8 Jelliffe, D.B. & Jelliffe, E.F.P. (1978): *Human milk in the modern world.* London: Oxford University Press.
9 Lauber, E. & Reinhardt, M. (1979): Studies on the quality of breast milk during 23 months of lactation in a rural community of the Ivory Coast. *Am. J. Clin. Nutr.* **32**, 1159–1173.
10 Lee, K.Y., Band, S. & Yun, D.J. (1963): Dietary survey of weanling infants in south Korea. *J. Amer. Diet. Ass.* **43**, 457–461.
11 Lunn, P.G., Prentice, A.M., Austin, S. & Whitehead, R.G. (1980): Influence of maternal diet on plasma-prolactin levels during lactation. *Lancet* **1**, 623–625.
12 Rajalakshmi, R. (1971): Reproductive performance of poor Indian women on a low plane of nutrition. *Trop. Geogn. Med.* **23**, 117–125.
13 Scrimshaw, N.S. & Underwood, B.A. (1980): Timely and appropriate complementary feeding of the breast-fed infant an overview. *Fd Nutr. Bull.* **2**, 19–22.
14 Shanghai Child Health Coordination Group (1975): Measurement of the growth and development of children up to 20 months in Shanghai. *J. Trop. Pediat. Environ. Child Hlth* **21**, 284–289.
15 Tontisirin, K. & Valyasevi, A. (1981): Protein energy malnutrition related to diarrhea in Thai children. *J. Nutr. Sci. Vitaminol.* **27**, 513–520.
16 Venkatachalam, P.S., Sushula, T.P. & Rare, P. (1967): Effect of nutritional supplementation during early infancy on growth of infants. *J. Trop. Pediat.* **13**, 70–76.
17 Waterlow, J.C. (1979): Adequacy of breast-feeding. *Lancet* **2**, 897–898.
18 Waterlow, J.C. & Thomson, A.M. (1979): Observations on the adequacy of breast-feeding *Lancet* **2**, 238–242.
19 Whitehead, R.G. (1976): The infant food industry. *Lancet* **2**, 1192–1194.
20 Whitehead, R.G., Rowland, M.G.M. & Hutton, M. (1978): Factors influencing lactation performance in rural Gambian mothers. *Lancet* **2**, 178–181.

The nutritional status of the infants of working and non-working mothers in Central Java

SOEKIRMAN
Bureau of Health and Nutrition, National Development Planning Agency, Jakarta, Indonesia.

The major objective of this study was to investigate how maternal employment away from home affects infant nutritional status and how this effect relates to infant feeding practices in low-income urban and semiurban households in Semarang municipality, Central Java. In addition, the mothers' decision to fully or partially breast-feed or bottle-feed was explored: What factors influenced mothers in their decision? The study was also interested in the nature of the relationship between infant feeding practices, infection, and infant nutritional status.

The general hypothesis generated from this study is that: In low-income households, with a given level of other socioeconomic conditions mothers' work status away from home indirectly and inversely affects infants' nutritional status. The effect is assumed to work through infant-feeding practices and infection.

The objectives of the study were achieved by interviewing a sample of mothers from low-income households who were working in factories away from home and non-working mothers as comparison. Both groups of mothers had infants 0–6 months of age and met other criteria set for the study[4].

Definitions. (1) Breast-feeding: infants are given only breast milk, with or without solid food and/or other fluids. (2) Mixed-feeding: infants are given both breast-milk and infant formula in a bottle or in some other way, with or without solid food and/or other fluids. (3) Bottle-feeding: infants are only given a formula made of milk or milk products, with or without solid food and/or other fluids. (4) Solid food: any food given to infants in nonfluid form. (5) Fluids: any fluid other than breast-milk or milk formula. (6) Diarrhoea: loose, watery, and greenish stools which occurred more than 3 times/d for at least 2 d and which were unusual for the particular child. Sometimes it is accompanied by blood and/or mucus. (7) Working women: mothers with infants of 0–6 months of age who worked in factories (away from home), at least 2 years. (8) Socioeconomic status: represented by two indicators — income and education. The information collected on income was grouped to put the households into three main levels: lower, middle, and upper. (9) Infant nutritional status: measured as the percentage of weight for age relative to the median value of the WHO/NCHS standard[5].

Methods. The study is a quasi-experiment which is a cross-sectional study with a comparison group[1]. The sampling units are mothers, infants and households. The sampling frame for the working mothers were low-income women working in factories. The comparison group were randomly selected from non-working mother-infant pairs with a similar socio-economic background.

Results and discussion. The Table presents some of the variables employed in the analysis and its summary statistics for working and non working mothers. The statistical analysis is a multiple regression using OLS and Logit technique employing infants' nutritional status as dependent variable and working mothers' age, sex of infant, family income, mothers' and fathers' education, and breastfeeding pattern as independent variables. Breast-feeding pattern and diarrhoea were employed as dependent variables in Logit technique[3]. The main findings were as follows. (a) When mothers work in factories the nutritional status of the infants is negatively affected. The variation in the nutritional status of infants can be partly explained by differences in breast-feeding practices and the prevalence of diarrhoea. Non-working mothers breast-feed more than working mothers. For non-working mothers, breast-feeding has a positive and significant effect, and the prevalence of diarrhoea has no significant effect on infants' nutritional status. Conversely, among working mothers, the negative effect of diarrhoea is significant, whereas there is no significant effect of breast-feeding. (b) There is a negative effect of the time a mother spends at work on infant nutritional status. For employed mothers, the effect of breast-feeding on the infant's nutritional status is significant and positive only if the mothers work less than 40 hours, if they work longer hours than this they do not have adequate time left for infant care. Even if these mothers attempted to breast-feed, the frequency of breast-feeding and the volume of breast-milk would not be adequate to have a positive effect on their infant's weight. (c) For working mothers, the distance to work and wage level have significant negative effects on their infants' nutritional status, but these effects are too small to be physiologically meaningful. In addition, these effects are not related either to breastfeeding or to diarrhoea. The wage effect on breastfeeding and nutritional status is dependent on the length of the mother's hours of work. (d) There is an interaction between time and wage effects and infant nutritional status. The negative effect of the mother's employment is only significant if the mothers work more than 40 hours per week and earn less than the basic minimum wage (Rp. 16,000/month). (e) If the mothers work more than 40 hours per week but are adequately paid, the negative effect is no longer significant. However, this phenomenon cannot be attributed to the effect of breast-feeding or diarrhoea. (f) When mothers have to work more than 40 hours per week and are not adequately paid, the role of the father's education is positive and significant. This suggests that, in this situation, the father shares responsibility for infant care.

Table. *Mean values and their standard deviations (s.d.) for the variables studied in the investigation on the nutritional status of infants of working and non-working mothers.*

	Non-working			Working		
Variables	*n*	*Mean*	*s.d.*	*n*	*Mean*	*s.d.*
1 Infant's nutritional status (% weight for age)	121	87.8	11.6	117	84.5	11.8
2 Infant's weight (kg)	121	5.3	1.2	117	5.4	1.2
3 Infant's height (cm)	121	59.7	4.5	117	59.8	5.0
Frequency of breastfeeding						
4 — day	122	7.4	2.9	117	4.1	2.8
5 — night	122	2.9	1.3	117	2.2	1.5
6 Family income (Rp/month)	120	49 135	23 211	112	52 744	19 471
7 Father's education (years)	120	7.9	3.3	113	7.4	3.0
8 Mother's education (years)	122	4.8	2.8	116	4.7	2.8
9 Infant's age (months)	122	3.2	1.6	117	3.4	1.6

If, on the other hand, the mothers work more than 40 hours and are adequately paid, the family's income has a positive and significant effect on the infant's nutritional status. It can be speculated that, when mothers earn more than the basic minimum wage, this allows more of the family's income to be spent on supplementary food and health care for their infants. Unfortunately, only about 25 per cent of the working mothers in this sample were in this situation. Most of them had to work long hours and still earned wages below the basic minimum. (g) The probability that a mother will exclusively breast-feed is negatively related to her work status, her education, and her infant's age. Thus, on average, the probability is lowest if the mother works, is more educated and has an older infant (3–6 months). (h) The probability of an infant having diarrhoea is positively related to the infant's age and the mother's work status. On average, the probability is highest when the infant is older and the mother works. The mechanism by which a mother's employment influences diarrhoea is through feeding practices: ie the greater use of foods and utensils that can be easily contaminated by diarrhoea-causing organisms.

Conclusion and recommendations. The main conclusion of the study is that mothers' employment in factories is incompatible with desirable breastfeeding practices. However, this incompatibility does not necessarily have a negative effect on the nutritional status of infants. The mother's working hours and wages and the father's education are also likely to influence the nutritional status of the infants of employed mothers[2].

Among the recommendations suggested here are: Appropriate policies should be formulated to give special attention to low-income working women at their work place and at home. A joint programme to promote working women's welfare among government and nongovernment agencies should be encouraged.

1 Cook, T.D. & Campbell, D.T. (1979): *Quasi-experimentation design and analysis issues for field settings*. Chicago: Rand McNally.
2 Engel, P.L. (1980): The intersecting needs of working women and their young children. Ford Foundation (Mimeo).
3 Pindyck, D.S. & Rubinfeld, D.L. (1976): *Econometric models and economic forecast*. New York: McGraw Hill.
4 Soekirman, (1983): The effect of maternal employment on nutritional status of infants from low-income households in Central Java. Ph.D. Thesis, Cornell University.
5 WHO (1979): *Measurement of nutritional impact*. Geneva: WHO.

Maternal nutritional status and breast-milk production in rural and urban areas

H.L. VIS
Université Libre de Bruxelles, Hôpital Universitaire St. Pierre, Clinique Pédiatrique, Rue Haute 320, B-1000 Bruxelles, Belgium.

To evaluate the possible influence of maternal nutritional status on breast-milk production in rural and urban areas of developing countries, we studied the situation in the interlacustrian highlands of Central Africa (Kivu-Zaire) and in the main city of the same area (Bukavu). As a rule the population of black Africa is better fed in urban than in traditional rural areas, especially when the rural population is living in a nearly self-sufficient economic system.

In developing countries the nutritional status of the lactating mother is influenced by four main factors: (1) food intake and food reserves (fat storage before and during pregnancy); (2) infections and parasitosis; (3) energy out-put (physical work at home and in the field) and (4) breast-feeding. It may be erroneous to think that changing one of the four factors would affect any other one. For example, an increase in food intake would not necessarily improve production. A supplementary energy intake by the mother may be diverted to her energy output in her work, or it may be directed toward her fertility cycle and reduce the duration of post-partum amenorrhoea. Two independent factors, the mother's nutritional status and the suckling pattern, influence primarily the quantity and quality of the milk production by the

Table *Comparisons between rural and urban mothers in their nutritional status and in the amount of breast-milk produced at different stages of lactation.*

General data referring to the mothers at birth	Rural (n = 337)	Urban (n = 176)
Weight (kg)	52.1 ± 0.7	55.8 ± 9.0
Height (cm)	151.2 ± 0.7	154.0 ± 6.9
W/H^2 (kg/m^2)	22.7 ± 3.9	23.5 ± 3.5
Parity	5.0 ± 1.0	3.2 ± 2.5
Number of feeds per 24h	13.0 ± 1.0	12.9 ± 3.2

Quantity of milk versus age of infant	*n*	*Quantity of milk (g/24h)[a]*	*Wt of mother (kg)[a]*	*Prolactin level ($\mu U/ml$)[a]*	*n*	*Quantity of milk (g/24h)[a]*	*Wt of mother (kg)[a]*	*Prolactin level ($\mu U/ml$)[a]*
1 month ± 1 week	8	517	50.6	1141	32	775	54.2	1080
3 months ± 2 weeks	22	605	54.4	853	46	681	56.8	806
6 months ± 2 weeks	29	525	52.0	789	28	675	59.7	686
9 months ± 4 weeks	39	580	52.0	833	21	655	54.1	689
12 months ± 4 weeks	43	582	51.8	743	23	576	54.1	701
18 months ± 4 weeks	38	532	52.8	584	4	386	52.6	613
24 months ± 8 weeks	22	473	51.8	513	–	–	–	–

[a]values are means

mother. Both these two factors are influenced by the socio-economic environment. The suckling pattern depends upon the mother's behaviour[8].

The suckling pattern influences milk secretion not only through hormonal stimulation (prolactin-oxytocin) but perhaps also through a direct action on the mammary gland as well. In order to study the specific action of one of these two factors, however, the other must remain constant. Thus, at one extreme is the mother who breast-feeds on demand (more than six to eight times a day) and who by so doing, maximizes the effect of the suckling pattern. In such a case, the quantity and quality of milk depend solely upon her nutritional status. At the other extreme is the mother who breast-feeds only a few times a day, but is in a good nutritional state; in this case, the effect of her nutritional status is maximized and the quality and quantity of milk depend upon the possible variations in the suckling pattern.

The suckling pattern is itself influenced by the introduction of supplementary food into the infant's diet, a step which depends not only on the socio-economic environment, but also on the mother's nutritional status. The suckling pattern can also influence the length of post-partum amenorrhoea, which in turn determines in some traditional populations the duration of breast-feeding by controlling the time intervals between births, since a new pregnancy signals the end of breast-feeding. The socio-economic environment, while acting on both the mother's nutritional status and the suckling pattern, diversely affects these two factors[6].

Breast-feeding in the traditional milieu[4,8]. In the rural area of Kivu the population lives in an economy which is still very close to self subsistence, the entire diet being produced from their own fields. For the breast-fed child, there is no dietary substitute for the mother's milk. Consequently, all mothers breast-feed, and a child can be weaned after 1 year of age, and then only in a progressive manner, so that at 2 years of age, 60 per cent of the children are still breast-fed.

Malnutrition in Kivu mothers is attested by several facts. (1) Weight gain overall during pregnancy is seldom more than 5 kg; there is not even the accumulation of subcutaneous fat which normally serves as a source of energy for milk production. (2) The mean weight of the newborn is notably below that in Western Europe: 2.9 kg for males and 2.8 kg for females. (3) Serum albumin levels in the mothers are significantly lower than in the men of the same community. (4) Characteristic signs of kwashiorkor in nursing mothers are by no means rare.

At an early age, 15 d to 3 weeks, the mothers introduce a supplement consisting of boiled bananas, sorghum or even cassava, although formerly supplemenation was apparently not given before 2 or 3 months of age. When asked why, the mothers usually reply that it is because the breast-fed child cries with hunger.

Measurements have shown that milk production is low and that it fluctuates with the seasons.

This is understandable since the mother feeds on her own family's harvest. In an 'abundant' period, when the beans are harvested, nursing mothers produce a daily average of 600–650 g of milk. This quantity remains constant during the first 12–14 months, after which it declines. In the period of a protein gap, the quantity is 100–150 g less, 400–450 /day, and it remains constant until the 12th–14th month[4].

The introduction of a supplement is necessary, due to the small quantity of milk produced. It should be noted that the introduction of this additional food to the infant's diet does not result in a decrease in the mothers' milk production.

In the rural areas of Central Africa, the mothers never leave their babies; they sleep beside them at night and during the day and when they travel or when they are working, they carry their babies on their hips or on their back. This enables them to nurse at any time. On the average in rural Kivu, the infant is breast-fed 13 times per 24 hours (with at least three or more night feeds) during the first 12 months. The high number of feedings per 24 hours has, as a corollary, an increased baseline for serum prolactin in the mother[1]. Indeed, each feeding causes a discharge of prolactin in the beginning of the post-partum period, but this effect falls rapidly in intensity and is practically abolished by the 3rd month. In the later post-partum period, after 3 months, there is no longer a sharp increase in prolactin secondary to a feeding, but the baseline level remains elevated if breast-feeding is still continued on demand. The post-partum amenorrhoea continues as long as baseline prolactin level remains elevated. This suggests that the baseline level of prolactin plays a role in the maintenance of post-partum amenorrhoea.

In rural Kivu the nutritional status in women is poor. As an average, the mothers have the same weight after delivery as before pregnancy. Weight changes during the whole lactation period are negligible. As a consequence, if there is no weight loss during lactation, the extra nutrition necessary for milk production and for energy expenditure will come only from the daily food intake. In some marginal circumstances, the mother has to make a choice between energy expenditure and lactation[3], a choice which can be made by changing the suckling frequency. However it is also possible, but still not proven by the data in the literature, that energy expenditure may directly influence the duration of lactional amenorrhoea by hormonal changes in the hypothalamus[9]. In most poor third-world regions (at least in rural African areas) during the period of seasonal food scarcity, extra physical work is demanded from the women. In such conditions the food intake is spent either on physical labour or on lactation. Among African nursing mothers in rural Kivu, no difference was found in body weight/ height^2 ratio or serum albumin level between those who recovered their menses and those who remained amenorrhoeic, and lactating women have the weight/height^2 criteria for ovulation.

In certain parts of the Kivu (Kabare and Ngweshe region), in opposition to the pattern prevailing in the other regions studied, the mothers, on whom rests the greatest part of the agricultural workload, breast-feed their infants only in the mornings and evenings. During the day they leave their children under the care of a grandmother or sister who can only feed them boiled manioc, bananas or sorghum. As a result, the infant contracts infections very quickly and dies from a classic case of marasmus complicated mostly by gastro-enteritis. In that area, the nutritional situation is precarious and food shortages occur periodically. Sooner or later, the lactating mother upon whose shoulders rest the burdens of crop cultivation, meal preparation for the entire family, and the care of her latest born, must make a choice. She ends by leaving her child at home because her poor nutritional status makes it impossible for her to adequately fulfil all the functions imposed upon her. The conclusion is a gradual abandon-ment of breast-feeding, a drop in the serum prolactin level and menstruations resume. The weight/height^2 index of the mother remains constant because less energy is needed for the diminishing lactation, so that the mothers are able to become pregnant again. In this case, the control of post partum amenorrhoea is not so much the nutritional status but the suckling pattern.

Breast-feeding, suckling behaviour and nutritional status in the city[5,7]. When tradi-tional populations, living in a subsistence economy, migrate to the cities, several aspects of their life-style change. The subsistence economy is transformed for the most part to a money-based one. The large cyclic variations in available food, which are dependent on the seasons, are lessened so that, in the urban environment, the adult population frequently is better nourished. Childbirth no longer occurs at home, but in maternity hospitals. The organization found in these is based on the Western model, even with separation of mother and child, the introduction of the crib, and a certain rigidity in feeding times. All this more or less inhibits the reflex secretion of prolactin and oxytocin. When the mother and her newborn baby leave the hospital she no longer finds the protective social environment of the traditional rural community. On the contrary, she will have to resume her domestic chores, go shopping, take the other children to school, and go to work herself. All this leads, as soon as they leave hospital, to a separation between the mother and her infant child, for several hours, even days. The situation, thus, is set for a failure to breast-feed. A study we did in the city of Bukavu illustrates this.

Results. The nutritional status of the mothers is better in the city than in the rural area (Table). All mothers nursed their infants at birth and urban mothers produced more milk than rural ones: on the other hand, post-partum amenorrhoea was of shorter duration than in the rural environment and complete weaning occurred earlier[2]. Of interest was the fact that in Bukavu there were no commercial infant foods available. The tendency to abandon breast-feeding existed without the introduction of commercial substitutes for mother's milk.

1 Delvoye, P., Delogne-Desnoeck, J., Uwayitu-Nyampeta & Robyn, C. (1977): Time-course of physiological hyperprolactinemia during two years lactation. *Clin. Endocrinol.* **7**, 257–259.
2 Delvoye, P. & Robyn, C. (1980): Breast-feeding and post partum amenorrhoea in Central Africa. 2. Prolactin and post partum amenorrhoea. *J. Trop. Pediatr.* **26**, 184–189.
3 Hennart, Ph. (1983): Allaitement maternel en situation nutritionnelle critique: adaptations et limites (Thesis). Université Libre de Bruxelles — Brussels.
4 Hennart, Ph. & Vis, H.L. (1980): Breast-feeding and post partum amenorrhoea in Central Africa. 1. Milk production in rural areas. *J. Trop. Pediatr.* **26**, 177–183.
5 Hennart, Ph., Ruchababisha, M. & Vis, H.L. (1983): Breast-feeding and post partum amenorrhoea in Central Africa. 3. Milk production in an urban area. *J. Trop. Pediatr.* **29**, 185–189.
6 Vis, H.L. (1985): Commentaries made on the paper of R.E. Frisch 'Maternal nutrition and lactation amenorrhoea: perceiving the metabolic costs' In *Maternal nutrition and lactational infertility*, ed J. Dobbing, pp. 80–84. Nestlé Nutrition workshop series vol. 9. New York: Raven Press.
7 Vis, H.L. & Hennart, Ph. (1978): Decline in breast-feeding (About some of its causes). *Acta Paediatr. Belg.* **31**, 195–206.
8 Vis, H.L., Hennart, Ph. & Ruchababisha, M. (1981): Some issues in breast-feeding in deprived rural areas. Assignment Children (UNICEF) **55/56**, 183–200.
9 Warren, M.P. (1983): Effects of undernutrition on reproductive function in the human. *Endocr. Rev.* **4**, 363–377.

The relationship of breast-feeding practices to amenorrhoea and contraception: the case of Indonesia and Kenya

M.C. LATHAM, Beverly WINIKOFF, G. SOLIMANO and Virginia H. LAUKARAN
Program in International Nutrition, Division of Nutritional Sciences, Savage Hall, Cornell University, Ithaca, New York 14853 (MCL); The Population Council, One Dag Hammarskjold Plaza, New York, New York 10017 (BW, VHL); Center for Population and Family Health, School of Public Health, Columbia University, New York, New York 10032, USA (GS).

This paper examines the relationship of infant feeding practices to amenorrhoea in Indonesia and Kenya. The data used are from a major study of the determinants of infant-feeding practices in four countries — Indonesia, Thailand, Colombia and Kenya. The preliminary findings have been published[5] and other papers will follow.

The exact physiological mechanisms by which breast-feeding influences fertility remain unknown[7]. It has, however, been well demonstrated that nipple stimulation, mainly resulting from breast-feeding, results in higher blood levels of the anterior pituitary hormone prolactin, which in turn are associated with amenorrhea and anovulation. There are many other factors which may influence human fertility[3]. Here we concentrate on how amenorrhoea might be influenced by infant-feeding practices because this has important policy implications.

Two recent WHO papers[9,10] describe a typology which it is suggested may be useful for classifying countries in respect to current breast-feeding practices. An important problem with the WHO typology is that it is based entirely on breast-feeding prevalence and duration. This ignores the situation where breast-feeding is prevalent and prolonged, but where these mothers commonly also feed breast-milk substitutes to their infants at a dangerously early age while continuing to breast-feed. We believe this is a common practice in many countries. In Kenya we find that even in Nairobi there is a pattern of widespread and long duration breast-feeding. We have coined the term 'triple nipple infant feeding' to describe this situation[4] where on the same day young infants are fed both from a feeding bottle and the mothers' breasts.

Reports on breast-feeding duration without information on its frequency and on the extent to which other foods are provided to the infant may mask major individual or community differences in fertility. Mothers who breast-feed, but who also feed substantial quantities of formula or cow's milk from a bottle during the early months of the infant's life, may have a shorter duration of amenorrhoea, and a narrower interval between births. Prolactin levels in mothers who are partially breast-feeding are lower than in mothers totally or near totally breast-feeding their young infants, and there is probably a level of blood prolactin or other hormones which triggers the resumption of ovulation and menstruation. Our main emphasis here is on the pattern of infant-feeding.

The data presented in this paper refer mainly to findings from 1092 mother-child pairs in the city of Semarang in Indonesia and 981 in Nairobi, Kenya. The sampling and other methods used, and details of the ethnographic and marketing studies, have been provided elsewhere[5].

Breast-feeding pattern and amenorrhoea in Semarang and Nairobi. The feeding pattern is compared in Fig. 1 in the period from 0–4 months and 5–9 months for women in Semarang and Nairobi. These data are based on those mothers currently breast-feeding. In Nairobi, compared with Semarang, there is a much greater use of breast-milk substitutes, mainly infant formula and cow's milk, from a feeding bottle (45 vs 23 per cent at 0–4 months and 58 vs 18 per cent at 5–9 months of age). In both cities solid foods were commonly introduced early; the amounts fed are believed to be relatively small up to 6 months of age, and then become an increasingly important contribution to the young child's diet. Our data show that 38 per cent of Nairobi infants between 1 and 2 months of age are already receiving breast-milk substitutes, and these are infants from the lower socioeconomic classes. In both Semarang and Nairobi the median length or duration of breast-feeding is considerably longer in those not using, compared with those using, commercial milk. So the feeding of commercial milk preparations is associated with a markedly shorter length of breast-feeding in both cities[11].

Our data have shown that in both Semarang and Nairobi the mean duration of breast-feeding is relatively long, but is longer in Semarang. Figure 2 shows the median duration of amenorrhoea in Semarang and Nairobi for those women in our study breast-feeding for different lengths of time. As in almost all other studies, a strong relationship between duration of breast-feeding and length of post-partum amenorrhoea was found. Very striking differences are seen between the two cities.

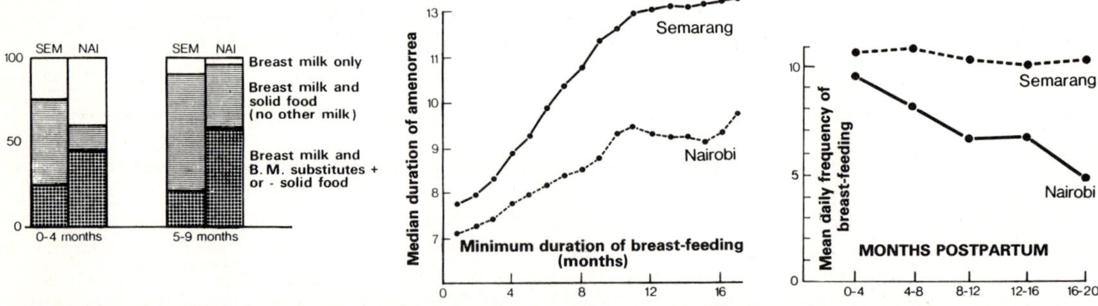

Fig. 1 (above, left). Patterns of infant-feeding in Semarang (Sem) and Nairobi (Nai) among mothers currently breast-feeding. The percentage values are of total energy intake.

Fig. 2 (above, centre). Median duration of amenorrhoea in relation to length of breast-feeding in Semarang and Nairobi.

Fig. 3 (above, right). Mean daily frequency of breast-feeding in relation to age of infant in Semarang and Nairobi.

The findings on frequency of breast-feeding in the last 24 h for currently breast-feeding women in Semarang and Nairobi are shown in Fig. 3. It can be seen that mothers in Semarang breast-fed their infants more frequently than did Nairobi mothers. In Nairobi there was a marked decline in breast-feeding frequency as the child grew older, but this phenomenon was not observed in Semarang. The difference in frequency of breast-feeding in the two countries is probably due to the higher prevalance of bottle-feeding in Nairobi compared with Semarang.

A number of studies have found correlations between, on the one hand, duration of breast-feeding and amenorrhoea, and on the other, factors such as mother's age, parity, educational level and economic status. In our data we find all four of these are related to breast-feeding duration and length of amenorrhoea in the expected direction. The data were further examined[6] using both a multivariate and a hazards analysis. After accounting for the effects of breast-feeding, the effects of socioeconomic variables remain as significant covariates. For example, women with more schooling still seem to have a shorter duration of amenorrhoea. Depite this we believe that breast-feeding and the pattern of other feeding are the most important determinants of length of amenorrhoea in these women.

In the women interviewed in our study 24 per cent in Semarang and 23 per cent in Nairobi reported using contraceptives at the 6 month postpartum. However, at the 12th month the figures were 48 and 12 per cent respectively. The World Bank[1] reports that 26 per cent of women 15–49 years of age in Indonesia and only 7 per cent in Kenya are using contraceptives. The annual population increase is projected at 1.5 per cent in Indonesia and 4.1 per cent in Kenya.

Discussion and conclusions. We believe that in both countries breast-feeding is playing an important role in influencing birth-spacing. In Indonesia the duration of breast-feeding is longer, frequency of suckling is higher, and there is a lower use of breast-milk substitutes than in Kenya. This, together with greater use of contraceptives reduces fertility.

Using the WHO typology of breast-feeding, Kenya, like Indonesia, would be placed in the 'traditional phase with high prevalence and duration of breast-feeding'. But our data show that even though breast-feeding prevalence and duration are high, there is a pattern of triple nipple infant-feeding. In the first few months of life a majority of Nairobi babies are fed breast-milk substitutes often from a bottle, there is a declining frequency of breast-feeding, and as a result amenorrhoea is reduced in length and birth intervals may be markedly shortened.

A diagrammatic model (Fig. 4) shows what might be the common pattern of infant-feeding in Indonesia and Kenya. It is postulated that when more than about 750 ml of breast-milk is being consumed in the first 18 months then prolactin levels remain high enough to maintain amenorrhoea. This level of milk would provide about 2.3 MJ (550 kcal), 100 per cent of energy needs for infants at 2 months; 62 per cent for infants at 6 months; 53 per cent for infants at 12 months; and 49 per cent for infants at 18 months of age.

The contrast between Semarang and Nairobi is strikingly revealed in this study. National differences in breast-feeding duration (22 vs 16 months), birth intervals (36 vs 29 months), and contraceptive use (33 per cent vs 7 per cent in 2nd year postpartum) were also shown in the World Fertility Survey[8].

We conclude that the pattern of infant feeding is having an important influence on fertility in Nairobi, and probably elsewhere in Kenya. If this pattern of infant feeding persists or becomes more extensive, then Kenya's fertility can be expected to increase above its currently alarmingly high levels. We believe that in both countries great efforts are needed to protect, support and promote breast-feeding[2]. Such actions if successful will have important effects on child spacing

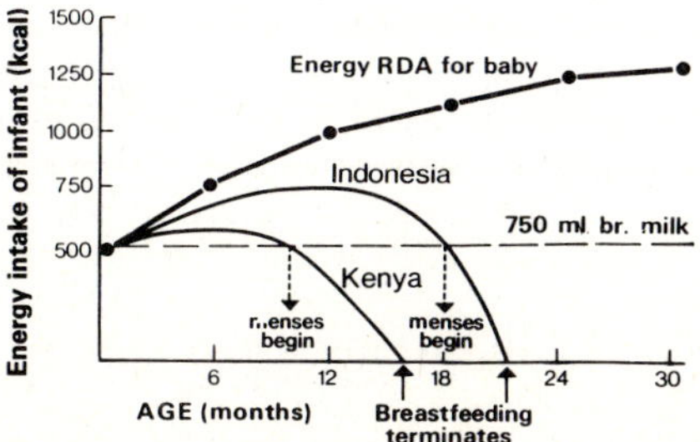

Fig. 4. Schematic relationship between the volume of breast milk sucked by infants and the end of amenorrhoea in Kenya and Indonesia, which it is suggested, occurs when the volume falls below 750 ml/d.

and at relatively low cost. They need to be regarded as the partner of each country's programmes to control family size using modern contraceptive methods.

Acknowledgements. We appreciate financial assistance provided by AID (Contract AID/DSAN-C-0211) and funds from the Rockefeller Foundation, IDRC and UNICEF. We are particularly grateful for the collaboration of many individuals in Indonesia and Kenya. In Indonesia Prof. Moeljono Trastotenojo and Dr F. Muis of Diponegoro University, and in Kenya Mr K. O. Agunda, Mr J. Kekovole and Dr C. Wood from CBS and AMREF, were key leaders in the research. Much of the data analysis used in the paper was done by Dr L. Lee. Figures 2 and 3 are based on her work[6]. The field work in Kenya was ably directed by Mr T. Elliott. We are also grateful for the help of Dr P. Van Esterik, Dr R. Smith, Dr J. Bongaarts, Dr J. Post, Dr L. Stephenson, Ms J. Spicehandler, Ms M. Shekar and Ms D. Doty.

1 Anon (1984): *World development report 1984*, pp. 51–185. Published for World Bank, IBRD by Oxford University Press: Oxford.

2 Elliott, T.C., Agunda, K.O., Kigondu, J.G., Kinoti, S.N. and Latham, M.C. (1985): Breastfeeding versus infant formula: the Kenyan case. *Fd Policy* **10**, 7–10.

3 Latham, M.C. (1982):The relationship of breastfeeding to human fertility. In *The Decline of the breast*, ed M.C. Latham, pp. 1–21. Cornell International Nutrition Monograph No. 10, Cornell University, Ithaca, NY.

4 Latham, M.C., Elliott, T.C., Winikoff, B., Kekovole, J. & Van Esterik, P. (1986): Infant feeding in urban Kenya: a pattern of early triple nipple feeding. *J. Trop. Pediatr.* (In press).

5 Latham, M.C., Laukaran, V.H., Post, J.E., Smith, R.A., Solimano, G., Van Esterik, P. & Winikoff, B. Research Consortium for the Infant Feeding Study (1984): The determinants of infant feeding practices: preliminary results of a four-country study, pp. 1–97. *International Programs Working Papers*. New York: The Population Council.

6 Lee, L.W. (1985): Postpartum amenorrhea: behavioral and social-demographic correlates. Ph.D. Dissertation, University of California, Berkeley.

7 McNeilly, A.S., Glasier, A. & Howie, P.W. (1985): Endocrine control of lactational infertility. In *Maternal nutrition and lactational infertility*. ed. J. Dobbing, pp. 1–24. New York: Raven Press.

8 Smith, D. (1985): Breastfeeding, contraception, and birth intervals in developing countries. *Studies in Family Planning* **16**, 154–163.

9 WHO (1982): The prevalence of breast-feeding: a critical review of available information. *WHO Stat. Quart.* **2**, 92–116.

10 WHO (1983): The dynamics of breast-feeding. *WHO Chron.* **37**, 6–10.

11 Winikoff, B. & Lee, L.W. (1985): Breast feeding patterns and postpartum amenorrhea. Presented at Annual Meeting of the American College of Obstetrics and Gynecologists, Washington DC, May.

Fertility and nutrition: a workshop report

O. DARWISH (Organizer)
Nutrition Department, High Institute of Public Health, University of Alexandria, Alexandria, Egypt.

Participants: *O. Galal* (Nutrition Institute, Ministry of Health, Cairo, Egypt); *K. Amatayakul* (Research, Institute for Health Sciences, Chiang Mai, University Thailand); *Rose Frisch* (Centre for Population Studies Harvard University, USA); *Beverly Winikoff* (The Population Council, New York, USA); *P. Lunn* (Dunn Nutritional Laboratory, Cambridge, UK).

The main thrust of our discussion was the problems raised when increasing nutritional status in a developing country appears to contribute to an increase in population. Of course, the contribution of nutritional factors to the increase in population is only one facet of the problem. In under-developed countries relatively stable populations have existed for many years and it is usually with the onset of development as a whole that population increase is associated. The stable population of an under-developed country remains so because there is a balance between the birth-rate and death-rate (largely due to infant and childhood mortality). Quite rightly one of the first priorities of development is to reduce the suffering associated with high mortality by improving public health. Thus the introduction of clean water supplies, adequate sewage disposal, the elimination of insect vectors associated with parasitic diseases and the use of immunization programmes to eradicate diseases such as smallpox have all contributed to a considerable reduction in mortality in these countries.

Where these measures have not been associated with an adequate birth-control programme, the imbalance created between birth-rate and death-rate has led to large increases in population.

The above consequences all follow when the birth-rate remains stable but in developing countries, in addition to improvements in public health, there are also improvements in agriculture associated with land drainage or irrigation, mechanisation, use of fertilizers and new seed varieties and pest control. Taken together these improvements can lead to increasing nutritional status even in the face of the population increase. However, there is clearly a maximum level to which food supplies can be increased (the effect tends to be hyperbolic) whereas population growth without constraint is exponential (ie has no upper limit).

We are concerned here with the evidence that increasing nutritional status in a population exacerbates the problem set out above by actually increasing female fertility, and hence the birth-rate, above the level maintained prior to development. This evidence was presented in the workshop.

The results of studies presented in the workshop. *Rose Frisch* presented her evidence for a close association between the amount of bodily adipose tissue and female fertility, based on her studies of anorexics and female athletes and on population studies of the age of menarche and its association with national nutritional status. Her conclusions indicate that increasing the nutritional status of a population lowers the age of the menarche and raises the age of menopause so extending the fertile life of the female and reducing the number of mature infertile females.

Beverly Winikoff's studies showed that the length of lactational amenorrhoea in developing countries is greatly influenced by breast-feeding patterns, especially the introduction of supplementary feeding of infants. This leads to the conclusion that, again, the increase in food supply and the changing social customs associated with development cause increased female fertility, by changing breast-feeding patterns and reducing the duration of lactational infertility and hence increasing the number of fertile females in the population at any given time.

Lunn and *Darwish* both described work in which the period of lactational infertility in women of different nutritional status had been studied by measurement of various parameters of hormonal status. These studies indicated that increasing nutritional status reduces the length of the period of lactational amenorrhoea and so increases the potential fertility of the population. *Darwish* showed that although some women had some infertile cycles, preceding their return to full fertility, this was by no means universal and that some lactating women showed a sudden return to fertility without prior indication.

Conclusions. The major conclusions of the Workshop was that increasing nutritional status in a country can contribute to an increase in population by increasing the proportion of fertile females in a population. This effect is due to three factors. Increasing nutritional status leads firstly to an increase in the length of a woman's fertile lifespan and secondly to a reduction in the length of lactational infertility and so to a reduction of the interval between children. The third factor is the availability of feed supplements for infants which changes the established patterns of breast feeding and leads to a reduction of the period of lactational infertility.

Recommendations. The main recommendation of the workshop was that its conclusions should be drawn to the attention of the governments of those developing countries which had been successful in increasing the nutritional status of their population with the strong recommendation that adequate birth-control programmes should be maintained or where necessary introduced.

However, our discussions also led us to the conclusion that contraception for lactating women is a neglected area of research. The problems in this area arise from several factors. First, it is inadvisable to prescibe synthetic steroids to a lactating mother. Secondly, there is an unwillingness on the part of mothers to take 'pills'. Thirdly, there are now reservations about the use of IUDs. Fourthly, lactating women often only seek contraceptive advice when their periods return, and as we have seen above this may be too late if they have a sudden return to full fertility. We therefore recommend that urgent attention be given to developing new approaches to contraception for lactating women. The following proposals are suggested.

The use of progesterone as an oral contraceptive for lactating women should be investigated. There would, of course, still be maternal resistance to taking this but the risks of using a natural steroid seem low when it is considered that progesterone is present in the milk of women whose menstrual cycles have returned.

More long-term projects are suggested by the observation that the return to fertility is preceded by a fall in prolactin secretion. If this fall could be prevented, infertility could be maintained throughout lactation. Recent studies suggest that the gonadotrophin-releasing-hormone gene associated peptide is a prolactin-release inhibiting factor. We therefore suggest a programme to develop antagonists to this peptide (cf GnRH antagonists) which could be tested as agents for suppressing the return to fertility during lactation. Also, as the fall in prolactin precedes the return to fertility, research to develop a simple home-use test to detect this change should be undertaken with a view to predicting the return to fertility in time to initiate the use of conventional contraceptives.

★   ★   ★

NUTRITIONAL MANAGEMENT OF THE PRETERM INFANT

Strategies in the nutritional management of the preterm infant

H.K.A. VISSER
Department of Paediatrics, Erasmus University and University Hospital/Sophia Children's Hospital, Gordelweg 160, 3038 GE Rotterdam, The Netherlands.

The aim of the nutritional management of the preterm infant is to achieve the best possible growth and to avoid specific deficiencies. For a long time paediatricians thought that the preterm infant had a low milk tolerance and that only the mother's milk was suitable. Gordon & Levine[3] questioned the low protein content of human milk and from then until the early 70s the generally accepted protein requirement for preterm infants was 2.5–4.0 g/kg per day. During the last 10 years the use of human milk for feeding preterm infants has increased considerably. This is mainly due to the findings of cellular and humoral immune factors in human milk and the suggestion that they may be protective against infections.

The intra-uterine increments of various nutrients during normal growth of a 'reference fetus' have been calculated[6]. When one extrapolates these data to estimate the nutritional requirements of the preterm infant, one has to take into account the physiological and metabolic changes which occur after birth. On the basis of such calculations human milk is inadequate in meeting nutritional requirements for energy, protein, calcium, phosphorous, sodium, iron and possibly vitamins and trace elements. A number of artificial formulas based on cow's milk and adapted to the calculated nutritional requirements of the preterm infant have become available recently.

The controversy concerning the best type of feeding — human milk or adapted formula — for the preterm infant remains. Those who emphasize the importance of continuation of normal intra-uterine growth rate recommend the use of adapted formulas. Those who emphasize the 'natural' character of human milk, its immune factors and other, beneficial factors, known or unknown, recommend the use of human milk. Further studies are needed to answer many questions and some of these studies are now underway.

Strategies in nutritional management. A variety of dietary regimens is available for feeding the low-birth-weight infant.

1. Human milk. Atkinson and coworkers[1] were the first to report a difference in nitrogen concentration in milk from mothers of term and preterm infants during the early weeks of lactation. Lemons *et al*[4] studied the composition of human milk from mothers delivering preterm and at term during the first weeks of lactation. Complete 24-h milk expressions were obtained. Preterm milk contained significantly higher concentrations than term-milk of total nitrogen, protein nitrogen, sodium, chloride, magnesium and iron. No differences were found for non-protein nitrogen, volume, solids, total energy, lactose, fat, fatty acids, potasssium, calcium and phosphorus. The nutrients supplied to a 33-week preterm infant fed 200 ml/kg per day of 'average' preterm milk were in excess of calculated intrauterine requirement for protein and minerals except calcium, phosphorus and iron.

In practice only a limited number of preterm mothers are able to continue their lactation for some weeks. If one decides to feed all preterm infants on human milk, one is forced to organize a milk bank. Disadvantages or hazards of such a system are microbial contamination, the possible presence of drugs and environmental contaminants and the nutritional value of pooled milk. Rapid high temperature treatment or pasteurization, freeze-thawing and storage at $-70\,°C$ is recommended to minimize bacterial and viral contamination. The effects of these procedures on immune factors, nutrients and enzymes have been studied extensively, but further studies are needed.

2. Fortified human milk. The variability of the composition of human milk is well known. Some nutrient concentrations, eg protein, sodium, potassium and zinc, decrease during the first weeks of lactation. Milk composition varies between women, and between the beginning and end of a breast-feed. It is evident that with individual milk samples, but also with pooled samples, it may be difficult to obtain feeds of standardized composition.

Ideally one would like to analyse nutrient concentrations in 24-h milk samples from individual mothers or in pooled milk samples before feeding the preterm infants, but obviously the practical problems are formidable. When the milk composition is not suitable for the nutrient needs of the infants receiving the milk, one may add fat, protein, carbohydrates, minerals and trace elements. Some studies are being done, but results are not available. Another possibility is to add a nutritional supplement to the mother's own milk for the preterm infant without chemical analysis. Considering the variability of the composition of human preterm milk, it is theoretically possible that by adding such 'fortifier' supplements to milk samples without previous chemical analyis, an excess of some nutrients may be provided.

Lucas *et al*[5] have undertaken a large multicentre study on the short- and long-term clinical and developmental outcome of low-birth-weight infants randomized to different diets. An important dietary effect on the number of days taken to regain birth-weight and subsequent gains in weight, length and head circumference was observed. Only infants fed a preterm formula as their sole diet had maintained their birth centile by discharge from hospital. Growth performance of infants fed expressed breast-milk supplemented with preterm formula was better than with either banked breast-milk or expressed breast-milk supplemented with banked breast-milk. By the time they reached 2000 g, infants of birthweights 1200 to 1849 g fed on banked breast-milk and infants below 1200 g fed on banked breast-milk or maternal milk supplemented with banked milk had weights less than 2 s.d. below the mean for age and fulfilled the criteria for failure to thrive.

3. Adapted preterm formulas. Preterm formulas have a great variability in composition, but there are some common characteristics. Compared with human milk, the preterm formulas contain higher concentrations of energy, protein, (fat), sodium, calcium, phosphorus, trace elements (as zinc, copper, iodine) and vitamins (particularly vitamin D). Composition of fat mixtures in the preterm formulas is highly variable; some formulas contain up to 40 per cent medium-chain triglycerides. Carbohydrates vary from lactose only to mixtures of lactose, dextrin-maltose and glucose.

Many questions concerning the nutritional composition of preterm formulas have to be answered. What is the role of taurine? What mixture of animal and vegetable fats should be chosen to replace butterfat, and should medium chain triglycerides be added or not? Do preterm infants require nutrition with chain elongated desaturation products of essential fatty acids? What concentrations of sodium, calcium, phosphorus, iron and other minerals as well as trace elements and vitamins should be recommended? Our knowledge on absorption and retention of various nutrients in preterm infants of different gestational ages is limited. The practical and methodological problems of balance studies are enormous, and such studies should be ethically justified. Stable isotope methodology can now be used to study the absorption of calcium and other nutrients in preterm infants.

Long-term effects of low growth rates in the preterm infant. Numerous studies have evaluated the short-term effects of preterm formulas on growth and metabolism. There is now convincing evidence that the incidence of necrotizing enterocolitis is not different in infants fed human milk or preterm formulas. Long-term studies on the effects of different feeding regimens of the preterm infant on morbidity, growth (including body composition) and neurological development are not available. Obviously such studies are difficult to design, because of the many and complex factors involved. There is very good evidence that growth restriction during early life, the intra uterine period and the first years of extra uterine life, will permanently reduce growth potential and affect ultimate height[2]. The question whether undernutrition during early life has any important influence on brain growth and development, behaviour and higher mental functions has become very controversial. Brain growth is closely linked with body growth and a greater part of brain growth after birth takes place in the first 2 years of life. It seems evident that promotion of the best somatic growth in the intra-uterine period and the first years of life will be the best we can do to ensure good brain growth. Long term follow-up studies have to be designed[5] to provide answers to the many questions raised and particularly on whether or not undernutrition or low growth rates in the preterm infant will have ultimate effects.

1 Atkinson, S.A., Bryan, M.H. & Anderson, G.H. (1978): Human milk: difference in nitrogen concentration in milk from mothers of term and premature infants. *J. Pediatr.* **93**, 67–69.
2 Dobbing, J. (1981): Vulnerable periods in somatic growth. In *Infant and child feeding*, ed J.T. Bond, L.J. Filer Jr., G.A. Leveille, A.M. Thomson & W.B. Weil, pp. 399–411. New York, London, Toronto, Sydney, San Francisco: Academic Press.
3 Gordon, H.H. & Levin, S.Z. (1944): The metabolic basis for the individualized feedings of infants, premature and full-term. *J. Pediatr.* **25**, 464–475.
4 Lemons, J.A., Moye, L., Hall, D. & Simmons, M. (1982): Differences in the composition of preterm and term human milk during early lactation. *Pediatr. Res.* **16**, 113–117.
5 Lucas, A., Gore, S.M., Cole, T.J., Bamford, M.F., Dossetor, J.F.B., Barr, I., Dicarlo, L., Cork, S. & Lucas, P.J. (1984): Multicentre trial on feeding low birthweight infants: effects of diet on early growth. *Arch Dis. Child.* **59**, 722–730.
6 Ziegler, E.E., O'Donnell, A.M., Nelson, S.E. & Fomon, S.J. (1976): Body composition of the reference fetus. *Growth* **40**, 329–341.

Metabolic and endocrine responses in enteral and parenteral feeding of the preterm infant

R.D.G. MILNER
Department of Paediatrics, University of Sheffield, Children's Hospital, Sheffield S10 2TH, UK.

Enteral nutrition. Those preterm infants who are strong enough to suck effectively at a nipple or teat are unlikely to arouse enough professional curiosity to warrent ethical study. Infants in whom measurements have been made have been fed by a tube passed into the stomach or duodenum. Nasogastric (NG) feeding may be intermittent or continuous, whereas transpyloric (TP) feeding is always continuous. The lack of oral sucking might be expected to reduce the secretion of lingual lipase, but infants fed via a tube appear to digest fat as well as those fed by mouth; perhaps the presence of a tube in the pharynx is an adequate stimulation to salivary secretion and swallowing.

There are theoretical reasons why milk delivered directly into the duodenum or jejunum should not be digested and absorbed as efficiently as that delivered into the mouth or stomach of a preterm infant. Exocrine pancreatic function is deficient by adult standards and lingual lipase which has a pH optimum of 3.0–5.0 is inactive at pH 7.0[5]. TP feeding might thus be expected to result in poorer lipid absorption than NG feeding and increased steatorrhoea has been reported in babies fed TP[13]. We studied the effects of these different routes of milk administration by measuring plasma glucose, alanine, pyruvate, hydroxybutyrate, glycerol, insulin, pancreatic glucagon and total glucagon (the sum of pancreatic and gut glucagon) in a group of 20 infants on the last day of TP feeding and, under exactly the same circumstances, the following day when the tube had been pulled back to delivered milk NG[11]. Further measurements were made on the 5th day of NG feeding. Five blood samples were collected at hourly intervals during TP feeding. Glucose and alanine concentrations were relatively stable, but pyruvate and hydroxybutyrate fluctuated markedly. The important findings from this study were that: (a) there was no significant difference in the concentration of any metabolite or hormone between NG and TP feeding; (b) the infants gained weight at a similar and satisfactory rate on both TP and NG regimens despite having plasma insulin and pancreatic glucagon levels that, in the adult, would be characteristic of a catabolic state.

The plasma concentrations of a number of gut hormones at 0, 30, 60 and 120 min after a gastric bolus of milk was given to preterm infants aged 2, 6, 13 or 24 d have been described[9]. Only one blood sample was taken from each baby, so the results are not suitable for the dynamic interpretation given them by the authors. Nonetheless, it appears that plasma levels of motilin, neurotensin, gastric inhibitory polypeptide (GIP), enteroglucagon and secretin may change in response to a feed and with postnatal age. The plasma concentrations of motilin, neurotensin and GIP appear to increase with age, whereas that of gastrin falls. No clear change is seen in enteroglucagon or secretin. It has been pointed out[8] that the preprandial concentrations of motilin, neurotensin, GIP, enteroglucagon and pancreatic polypeptide (PP) rise with age from low levels in cord blood to values often far in excess of those found in the fasting adult. Plasma gastrin by contrast is high at birth and falls with increasing age. A direct comparison of fed and non-fed preterm infants was made by measuring metabolites and hormones in 6-d-old preterm infants fed by NG bolus and in those who had received only i.v. dextrose from birth on account of hyaline membrane disease[10]. The two groups of babies had similar preprandial levels of glucose, pyruvate, acetoacetate and vasoactive intestinal peptide (VIP). The infants on i.v. dextrose had significantly lower levels of alanine, glycerol, hydroxybutyrate, GIP, neurotensin, motilin, gastrin, glucagon and enteroglucagon, but significantly higher levels of secretin than those who had been fed. The authors' deduction that the differences were due to feeding is plausible, but it is also possible that some of the effect was due to one group being sick and the other being well.

It has been shown[1], using the same blood samples, that the preprandial plasma growth hormone appears to fall with increasing age, but that a prandial rise in growth hormone appears to develop with increasing age. In the same way an increasing insulinaemic response to milk feeding has been reported with increasing age[2], despite the preservation of a stable glycaemic response.

Parenteral nutrition. The umbilical nutrition of the fetus has led some to argue simplistically that it would be desirable to feed all very immature infants in the first instance by a parenteral route. In this way the complications of enteral feeding such as aspiration pneumonia and necrotising enterocolitis may be avoided. But parenteral nutrition has its own complications such as systemic infection and metabolic imbalance and in addition is both costly and labour intensive. Parenteral feeding should be reserved for those preterm infants with medical or surgical gut problems that prevent enteral feeding for more than 3 d.

The early parenteral regimens for use in the newborn delivered glucose and amino acid then lipid fractions sequentially (SR)[6], but in 1977 it was reported[7] that it was feasible to infuse glucose, amino acids and Intralipid concurrently (CR). This prompted a controlled comparison of SR and CR regimens of parenteral nutrition[14]. Each delivered the same amount of nutrient per kg in 24 h: 2.8 g amino acids, 4.8 g fat and 12.0 g glucose. In the SR regimen, Vamin-glucose and Intralipid were given together over a 3 to 10 h period followed by a glucose infusion for the rest of the day. In the CR regimen all three nutrient sources were infused continuously over the 24 h. Infants fed by SR had wide fluctuations of blood alanine, glycerol, hydroxybutyrate, acetoacetate and insulin throughout the 24 h. Ketone body and glycerol levels in particular were high at the end of the glucose-Vamin-Intralipid period and low just before it started. Peak ketone levels fell with advancing postnatal age. The fluctuation of blood metabolite levels was less in infants fed by the CR regimen and resembled the variation in infants fed enterally. The rate of weight gain was similar and satisfactory in both SR and CR groups, and there was no difference in the incidence of complications such as jaundice and infection. While it can be argued that fluctuating metabolite levels are desirable to promote optimal growth the values found in SR were excessive, particularly for ketone bodies. The CR regimen was less work to control and for these reasons the SR regimen was abandoned.

Discussion. It is clear that different feeding regimens can promote widely different metabolic and endocrine responses in the preterm infant and it could be argued biochemical changes are relatively unimportant if the baby thrives. Up to a point this is true and it is noteworthy that clinically acceptable rates of weight gain were achieved on all the regimens reviewed here. But weight gain should not be taken uncritically as a yardstick of growth. It has been shown[12] that preterm infants fed by gavage or bottle laid down protein at a similar rate to a fetus of similar gestational age, but deposited fat at twice the intrauterine accretion rate; in other words the preterm baby becomes chubby. In this respect the infant resembles the term baby more closely than the fetus he might have remained. Is this important? I am of the view that different patterns of weight gain in the early weeks of preterm extrauterine life are remodelled in the later months of infancy and that the clinician should not try obsessionally to mimic what was happening *in utero* when he feeds a preterm infant.

Of more importance is the route of administration. The work of Aynsley-Green, Lucas, Bloom and their colleagues reviewed here has shown clearly that enteral feeding provokes gut endocrine turbulence. Lucas[8] argued for the continuance of at least minimal enteral feeding whenever possible because of the belief that the hormonal surges stimulated by luminal nutrient are trophic to gut growth, maturation and motility. Animal experiments endorse this view. Widdowson[15] showed a dramatic development of the gut and related viscera in the piglet in response to enteral feeding. More recently intestinal mucosal enzyme development in the rat was shown to depend on the route and nature of the nutrient[4] and it has been reported that epidermal growth factor which is contained in breast-milk stimulates the intestinal growth of neonatal rats fed enterally[3].

Conclusions. Enteral feeding of preterm infants is associated with large changes in plasma concentration of a wide variety of gut hormones. Nasogastric and transpyloric feeding regimens each produce similar metabolite and hormonal profiles. A continuous parenteral regimen results in less metabolic fluctuation than a sequential regimen and is to be preferred. Clinically acceptable rates of weight gain can be achieved on both parenteral and enteral feeding regimens, but enteral feeding is preferable because is stimulates gut growth and maturation. Enteral feeding is also less costly and labour intesive than parenteral feeding.

1 Adrian, T.E., Lucas, A., Bloom, S.R. & Aynsley-Green, A. (1983): Growth hormone response to feeding in term and preterm neonates. *Acta Paediatr. Scand.* **72**, 251–254.
2 Aynsley-Green, A. (1985): Metabolic and endocrine interrelations in the human fetus and neonate. *Am. J. Clin. Nutr.* **41** (Suppl 2), 399–417.
3 Berseth, C.L. (1985): EGF-mediated breast milk-enhanced intestinal growth in neonatal rats. *Ped. Res.* **19**, 213A
4 Castillo, R.O., Pittler, A., Costa, F. (1985): Role of enteral nutrients in intestinal maturation. *Ped. Res.* **19**, 215A.
5 Hamosh, M., Scanlon, J.W., Ganot, D., Likel, M., Scanlon, K.B., Hamosh, P. (1981): Fat digestion in the newborn —characterization of lipase in gastric aspirates of premature and term infants. *J. Clin. Invest.* **67**, 838–847.
6 Harries, J.T. (1971): Intravenous feeding in infants. *Archs Dis. Childh.* **46**, 855–863.
7 Lindblad, B.S., Settergren, G., Feychting, H., Persson, B. (1977): Total parenteral nutrition in infants. *Acta Paediatr. Scand.* **66**, 409–419.
8 Lucas, A. (1983): Endocrine aspects of enteral nutrition. In *New aspects of clinical nutrition*, ed G. Kleinberger and E. Deutsch, pp. 581–594. Basel: Karger.
9 Lucas, A., Bloom, S.R., Aynsley-Green, A. (1980): Development of gut hormone responses to feeding in neonates. *Archs Dis. Childh.* **55**, 678–682.
10 Lucas, A., Bloom, S.R. & Aynsley-Green, A. (1983): Metabolic and endocrine consequences of depriving preterm infants of enteral nutrition. *Acta Paediatr. Scand* **72**, 245–249.
11 Milner, R.D.G., Minoli, I., Moro, G., Rubecz, I., Whitfield, M.F., Assan, R. (1981): Growth and metabolic and hormonal profiles during transpyloric and nasogastric feeding in preterm infants. *Acta Paediatr. Scand.* **70**, 9–13.
12 Reichman, B., Chessex, P., Putet, P., Verellen, G., Smith, J.M., Heim, T., Swyer, P.R. (1981): Diet, fat accretion and growth in premature infants. *New Engl. J. Med.* **305**, 1495–1500.
13 Roy, R.N., Pollnitl, R.P., Hamilton, J.R., Chance G. (1977): Impaired assimilation of nasojejunal feeds in healthy LBW infants. *J. Pediat.* **90**, 431–434.

14 Whitfield, M.F., Spitz, L., Milner, R.D.G. (1983): Clinical and metabolic consequences of two regimens of total parenteral nutrition in the newborn. *Arch Dis. Childh.* **58**, 168–175.
15 Widdowson, E.M., Colombo, V.E., Artavanis, C.A. (1976): Changes in the organs of pigs in response to feeding for the first 24 hours after birth. II The digestive tract. *Biol. Neonat.* **28**, 272–281.

Protein requirements and metabolism in the preterm infant

P.B. PENCHARZ
The Research Institute, The Hospital for Sick Children, The Departments of Paediatrics and Nutritional Sciences, The University of Toronto, Toronto, Ontario, Canada.

The objective, when considering the protein requirements for neonates, is how to provide the optimal mixture of amino acids for growth and development, taking into account their metabolic and neurological immaturities. The most widely used benchmark for protein requirements is intra-uterine accretion rate[9]. Whilst it is possible to provide neonates with sufficient protein or amino acids to achieve intra-uterine accretion rates without major perturbations in plasma amino acid profiles or acid base status[8,10], it is by no means certain that these levels of intake are optimal.

Various methods have been used to study protein needs of preterm infants. These include: growth in length, weight and head circumference[8]; estimates of body composition; nitrogen balance and measurement of plasma amino acid profiles in response to feeding different protein levels and sources[8,10]. The most widely used method to date has been nitrogen balance since it is the most direct way of determining whether or not intra-uterine accretion rates are achieved. Various authors have shown that there are marked perturbations in plasma amino acid profiles, blood urea nitrogen and acid base status once the protein intake exceeds 4–6 g/kg per d[2,8]. Our own data and those of others have suggested that nitrogen equilibrium is achieved in premature infants receiving approximately 1.1 g protein/kg per d[3]. However, neonates are growing rapidly and in order to gain nitrogen at intra-uterine levels, requirements have been estimated at approx. 3 g/kg/d in neonates weighing $<$1500 g[1,10]. In larger infants, the amounts required diminish progressively so that we have been able to achieve intrauterine accretion rates with approximately 2.25 g protein/kg per d in infants weighing 2 kg[5].

Because of the various limitations and problems with the classical methods used in studying protein requirements, we decided to study the dynamic aspects of whole body protein metabolism in neonates and to determine the effects of various physiological and nutritional factors.

Experimental. A modification of the constant infusion approach described by Picou & Taylor-Roberts[7] was used. Briefly, this involves administration of a ^{15}N labelled amino acid, usually glycine, either as a constant infusion or in repeated equal doses and the measurement of a urinary nitrogenous end-product, usually urea. We have carried out a series of studies examining questions such as the effects of birth-weight, intra-uterine nutritional status, postnatal age, route of feeding (ie intravenous feeding vs enteral feeding) as well as energy intake and protein quality.

1. Effects of birth-weight and intrauterine nutritional status[4]. We have studied the effect of birth-weight ($>$ and $<$ 1500 g) and intra-uterine nutritional status on the whole-body protein metabolism of 40 neonates divided into 14 equal groups by birth-weight and nutritional status. We were unable to show any effects of birth-weight on the parameters of whole-body protein turnover; however, as shown in Table 1, babies who were small-for-gestational age (SGA) had approximately 30 per cent higher rates of amino nitrogen flux, protein synthesis and breakdown. We were able to study 24 of these children a second time, approximately 2 weeks after the initial study. At the time of the second study, although turnover rates in the SGA infants were still numerically higher than those of the appropriate-for-gestational age (AGA) infants, the differences were no longer statistically significant.

Table 1. *Effect of intrauterine nutritional status on total body N-flux, protein synthesis and breakdown.* (Mean values for 20 infants ± s.e.m.)

Study group†	N-flux (mgN/kg/h) (Q)	Synthesis (g/kg/d) (S)	Breakdown (g/kg/d) (B)
AGA	103.3 ± 5.9	14.4 ± 0.9	10.9 ± 0.9
SGA	129.9 ± 7.3**	18.3 ± 1.0**	14.7 ± 1.0**

**Significantly greater than corresponding AGA mean ($P < 0.01$)

†AGA: appropriate-for-gestational age; SGA: small-for-gestational age

Table 2. *Effects of energy intake and protein quality on protein synthesis (S) and breakdown (B) in relation to whole body nitrogen flux (Q).* (Mean values for 6 infants ± s.e.m.).

Aminoacid source	Energy level	S/Q × 100	B/Q × 100
Amigen	high	90.4 ± 1.3[a]	77.9 ± 1.9[c]
	low	85.6 ± 2.2[b]	76.3 ± 2.2[c]
Vamin	high	92.3 ± 0.9[a]	72.0 ± 2.3[d]
	low	88.5 ± 1.3[b]	70.3 ± 1.8[d]

a > b $P < 0.01$; c > d $P < 0.025$ — by two-way analysis of variance.

2. Effects of energy and protein quality on the protein metabolism of parenterally fed neonates[1]. Twenty-four premature infants, weight <1500 g, were studied during the 1st week of life. All infants were fed approx. 3 g of amino acids/kg per d and those on the glucose only received approx. 60 kcal (250 kJ)/kg per d. Those receiving the additional lipid received approx. 85 kcal (355 kJ)/kg per d. Nitrogen balance and net nitrogen utilisation were significantly better by the addition of the fat. Two different amino acid sources were used: one, a casein hydrolysate (Amigen, Baxter-Travenol Labs); the other, a crystalline L-amino acid mixture (Vamin, KabiVitrum, Sweden). Nitrogen balance and net nitrogen utilization were shown to be significantly better with Vamin than with Amigen, as predicted from their respective amino acid patterns. We carried out protein turnover studies in order to elucidate the mechanism by which the better nitrogen utilisation was achieved. Inspection of the rates of whole-body amino nitrogen flux, synthesis and breakdown did not show any statistically significant effects of either energy intake or protein quality, although there was a trend for higher rates of turnover in the infants receiving the higher energy intake. When, however, the economy of nitrogen utilization was examined (Table 2), it was clear that energy improved nitrogen utilization by enhancing whole-body protein synthesis. The higher quality amino acid mixture appeared to improve nitrogen utilization by reducing endogenous protein breakdown.

3. Effect of route of feeding on whole body protein turnover[6]. In considering the absolute rates of protein turnover determined in the first two studies, it was evident that the rate of protein synthesis — for example, in enterally-fed infants — averaged about 14 g/kg per d, whereas in the intravenously-fed neonates, average values were approximately 8 g/kg per d. These values were, however, derived from totally separate studies. We therefore decided to compare the intravenous and oral routes of feeding in the same subjects, using 12 neonates who were on parenteral nutrition following surgery. They were studied first when they were stable and completely recovered from the effects of the surgery but still on parenteral nutrition and again later when on a full oral intake. On both occasions, the protein intake was adequate and averaged 2.7 g/kg per d. Energy intake during the intravenous study was 85 ± 4 kcal (355 ± 17 kJ)/kg per d, which meets the estimated requirement for parenterally fed neonates. These same neonates were taking 111 ± 7 kcal (465 ± 29 kJ) when orally fed and this was also within the requirement range for orally fed premature infants. The rates of protein turnover are shown in Table 3 and it is clear that the same differences in protein turnover are seen in this study, carried out with the same subjects, as in the two earlier studies. We suggest that these

Table 3. *Effect of intravenous (i.v.) and oral feeding on estimates of whole body protein turnover* (Mean values for 12 infants ± s.e.m.)

Parameter	i.v.	Oral
Nitrogen flux (mgN/kg per h)	65 ± 4	91 ± 5*
Protein synthesis (g/kg per d)	8.7 ± 0.6	12.6 ± 0.7*
Protein breakdown (g/kg per d)	7.5 ± 0.6	11.2 ± 0.8*

*Significantly greater than corresponding i.v. mean ($P < 0.05$) by paired t-test.

differences reflect the additional protein metabolism involved in the rapidly growing and developing gastrointestinal tract of the orally-fed infant.

1 Duffy, B., Gunn, T., Collinge, J. & Pencharz, P.B. (1981): The effect of varying protein quality and energy intake on the nitrogen metabolism of parenterally fed very low birthweight (<1600 g) infants. *Pediatr. Res.* **15**, 1040–1044.
2 Goldman, H.T., Freudenthal, R., Holland, B. & Karelitz, S. (1969): Clinical effects of two different levels of protein intake on low-birth-weight infants. *J. Pediatr.* **74**, 881–889.
3 Pencharz, P.B., Steffee, W.P., Cochran, W., Rand, W., Scrimshaw, N.S. & Young, V.R. (1977): Protein metabolism in human neonates: nitrogen balance studies, estimated obligatory N losses and whole body N turnover. *Clin. Sci.* **52**, 485–498.
4 Pencharz, P.B., Masson, M., Desgranges, F. & Papageorgiou, A. (1981): Total body protein turnover in human premature neonates: effects of birth weight, intra-uterine nutritional status and diet. *Clin. Sci.* **61**, 207–215.
5 Pencharz, P.B., Farri, L. & Papageorgiou, A. (1983): The effects of human milk and low protein formulae on the rates of total body protein turnover and urinary 3MH excretion of preterm infants. *Clin. Sci.* **64**, 611–616.
6 Pencharz, P.B. & Duffy, B. (1986): Effect of feeding route on the protein metabolism of neonates. *Am. J. Clin. Nutr.* **43**, 108–111.
7 Picou, D. & Taylor-Roberts, T. (1969): The measurement of total protein synthesis and catabolism and nitrogen turnover in infants in different nutritional states and receiving different amounts of dietary protein. *Clin. Sci.* **36**, 283–296.
8 Raiha, N.C.R., Heinonen, K., Rassin, D.K. & Gaull, G.E. (1976): Milk protein quality and quality in low-birthweight infants. 1. Metabolic response and effects of growth. *Pediatrics* **57**, 659–674.
9 Widdowson, E.M. (1981): Changes in body composition during growth. In *Scientific foundations of paediatrics*, 2nd edn, ed J. Davis & J. Dobbing, pp. 330–342. London: Heinneman Medical.
10 Zlotkin, S.H., Bryan, M.H. & Anderson, G.H. (1981): Intravenous nitrogen and energy intakes required to duplicate in utero nitrogen accretion in prematurely born human infants. *J. Pediatr.* **99**, 115–120.

Some physiological aspects of energy metabolism in low-birth-weight infants

J. MESTYÁN
Department of Paediatrics, University Medical School of Pécs, József Attila u.7., 7623 Pécs, Hungary.

Activity and energy expenditure. *Activity quota of maintenance energy expenditure.* It was reported[9] that the contribution of physical activity to daily energy expenditure of premature infants maintained at thermoneutrality did not exceed 10 per cent. Later, quite similar results were obtained in dysmature infants[15], supporting the previous suggestion that the activity fraction of total heat production at neutral temperatures is very small indeed. This is also true for very-low-birth-weight infants as shown by recent energy balance studies[4,12,16] summarized in Table 1. When a sizeable activity quota was reported it was certainly due to the very short periods during which oxygen consumption was measured.

The characteristics of activity and energy metabolism relationship. An analysis was attempted[15] of data on the relationship between energy expenditure and different activity levels in 30 low-birth weight-infants appropriate (AGA) and small (SGA) for gestational age. The mean scores of successive 10 minute intervals were used to quantify the changes in activity during an observation period of 6 to 12 h. The following conclusions could be drawn. (1) Mean activity score increased with postnatal age. (2) A correlation between activity and heat production was observed. (3) The energy cost corresponding to identical activity ratings increased with postnatal age. (4) Maximum increments above the resting rates of oxygen consumption in different age periods were significantly related to the activity scores despite the wide individual differences.

Postprandial thermogenesis vs thermic cost of growth. *Postprandial thermogenesis in low and very-low-birth-weight infants.* A study some years ago[10] in formula-fed premature infants

Table 1. *Activity quota of the daily energy expenditure at thermoneutrality in low and very-low-birth-weight infants reported by different investigators.*

Investigators (Ref. No.)	Birth weight range or mean (g)	Gestational age range or mean (wk)	Postnatal age at investigation range or mean (days)	Observation period range or mean (hours)	Activity quota		
					(kcal/kg/day)	(kJ/kg/day)	Percentage of total heat production
9	1100–2120	–	2–31	4–11	3	12.5	6
			2–15		3	12.5	
14	1070–2400	34–40		6–13			6.9
			16–39		8	33	
2	990–2030	29–35	10–29	5–10 min.	23	96	26
12	1155	29.3	21	6	4.3	16.7	6.8
4	1532	31	19.3	6	4.6	19.2	9.7
			1–7		4.4	18	10
16	920–1750	29–35		4–24			
			7–58		11.4	48	17

maintained at thermoneutrality found that oxygen consumption 30 min after the ingestion of formula was already higher than the BMR, and at 90–120 min the increase amounted to about 30 per cent above the preingestion level (Fig. 1).

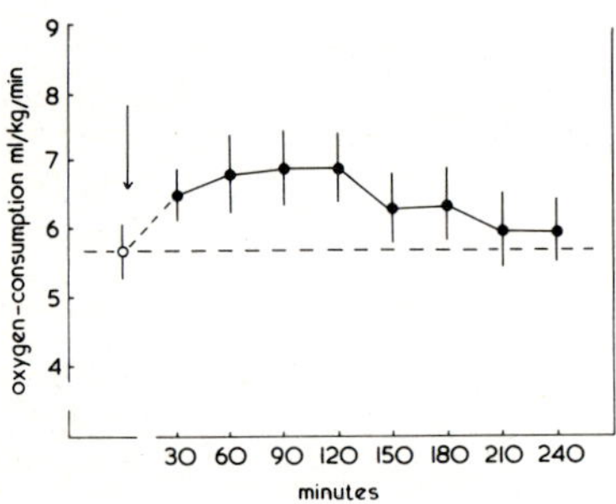

Fig. 1. *Oxygen consumption of premature infants before (○) and at half-hour intervals (●) after the ingestion of an artificial formula at thermoneutrality[10].*

Two later studies reported on the magnitude of dietary-induced thermogenesis in formula-fed low and very-low-birth-weight infants. They measured a postprandial increase of 6.4 kcal (26 kJ)/kg per d[2] and 3.6 kcal (15 kJ)/kg per d[12] respectively. The latter group noted that in two infants fed every 3 h the postprandial metabolic increase amounted to 8.15 and 8.75 kcal (34 and 36.5 kJ)/kg per d, indicating that with longer feeding intervals the increase in postprandial metabolism would be even greater. Thus, avoiding underestimation, the authors used a calculated value of 11.3 kcal (47.2 kJ)/kg per d.

Postprandial thermogenesis and the energy cost of tissue synthesis. Observations in rapidly growing older infants and children recovering from malnutrition suggested that postprandial energy expenditure reflects the cost of synthetic processes[1,2,8]. Recent investigations in low and very-low-birth-weight infants also refer to the dietary induced thermogenesis as a cause of the postnatal increase in energy expenditure associated with the increasing energy intake and body weight[2,4,6].

The partition of maintenance energy expenditure in growth retarded newborn infants before and during recovery revealed, in an earlier study[14], that growth was associated with an increase in resting heat production comprising basal metabolism, slight activity and postprandial thermogenesis.

Table 2. *The thermic cost of 1 g weight gain in low and very-low-birth-weight infants observed by different groups of investigators.*

Investigators	Thermic cost of 1 g weight gain	
	(kcal/g)	(kJ/g)
14, 15	1.10	4.60
17	0.8	3.34
2	1.72	7.20
4	0.67	2.80
6	0.54	2.25
16	0.26	1.10

Six recent contributions stand out for their effect on the present day concept concerning the mechanism of postprandial thermogenesis in low and very-low-birth-weight infants (Table 2). Brooke[2] reported a positive relationship between postprandial metabolism and the rate of weight gain. The high value of 1.72 kcal (7.2 kJ)/g for the energy cost of weight gain was probably an overestimate, since very short periods of measurements of energy expenditures were used for extrapolation. Chessex[4] obtained a value of 0.67 kcal (2.8 kJ)/g similar to that observed earlier[17]. Gudinchet *et al*[6] also found a significant correlation between weight gain and energy expended with an estimate of 0.54 kcal (2.26 kJ)/g concluding that the increase in energy expenditure for the 1st postnatal week to the 3rd is mainly due to the energy cost of synthetic processes. Sauer *et al.*[16] observed some high values for the energy cost of growth during the second week of life, but thereafter the results were constant, 0.26 kcal (1.1 kJ)/g weight gain. It can be inferred from these data that the energy cost of synthesis of new tissues represents 10–13 per cent of the energy expenditure, which compares well with that (11.4 per cent) found earlier[3] for the same rate of growth in children recovering from malnutrition.

Early compositional growth in very-low-birth-weight infants. *Recent energy and nutrient balance studies.* As to the percentage composition of weight gain in breast-fed and formula-fed very-low-birth-weight infants the comparison of the observations of three groups of investigators revealed interesting, but in some respects conflicting information[11,13,18]. In Fig. 2 the percentage composition of weight gain observed in the two dietary groups of very-low-birth weight-infants is depicted together with the composition of weight gain in the human fetus at gestational periods comparable to the postconceptional age of the infants investigated[19]. The similarities and differences of the observations made in the three comparative studies are the following. (1) The percentage of protein accretion was not very much different in the two dietary groups and was of similar magnitude as that for the fetus from 28 to 32 and 33–35 weeks gestation. (2) The contribution of fat to energy storage exceeded the lipid content of the transplacentally-nourished fetus; (3) While in Reichman's *et al.*[13] study fat stored/g weight gain

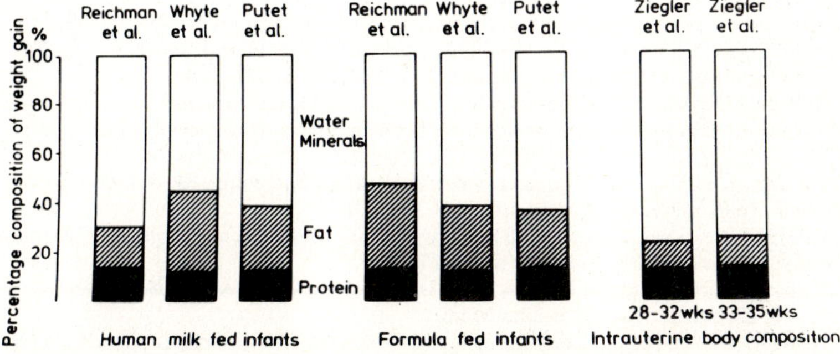

Fig. 2. *Percentage composition of weight gain of human-milk and formula-fed very-low-birth-weight infants reported by different groups of investigators and compared with intrauterine body composition at similar postconceptional ages*[11,13,18].

was significantly higher in formula-fed than in breast-fed infants, in the studies of Whyte *et al.*[18] and Putet *et al.*[11] both dietary groups exhibited an increased percentage weight gain as fat. Since Whyte *et al.*[18] and Reichman *et al.*[13] observed identical weight gains the contribution of fat to energy storage in infants maintained on breast-milk was twice as high in the former (33.8 per cent) as in the latter study (16.6 per cent). Feeding banked human milk Putet *et al.*[11] obtained a fat weight gain ratio of 26 per cent.

Energy intake and compositional growth. Energy intake, postnatal age and growth rate are important variables affecting partitioning of the deposited energy between fat and protein. It would be interesting to know to what extent accretion of these two fractions change with increasing energy intake at a fixed postnatal age, and inversely, at fixed level of nutrition with increasing age. Under both conditions it has been observed in animals[5,7] that a decreasing fraction of growth energy goes into protein synthesis resulting in an increasing rate of fat gain. Such a reciprocal relationship between lean and fat gain in very-low-birth-weight infants has been observed[18].

To assess the growth-promoting effects of energy intake in very-low-birth-weight infants it would be important to know the range of energy intake associated with growth. Particularly useful would be the knowledge of the lowest energy intake producing an acceptable growth rate. Research in this line would also be helpful in estimating the 'true' energy requirement about which there is still inconsistency.

1 Ashworth, A. (1969): Metabolic rates during recovery from protein calorie malnutrition. The need for a new concept of specific dynamic action. *Nature* **223**, 407–409.

2 Brooke, O.G., Alvear, J. & Arnold, M. (1979): Energy retention, energy expenditure and growth in healthy immature infants. *Pediatr. Res.* **13**, 215–220.

3 Brooke, O.G. & Ashworth, A. (1972): The influence of malnutrition on postprandial metabolic rate and respiratory quotient. *Br. J. Nutr.* **27**, 407–415.

4 Chessex, P., Reichman, B.L., Verellen, G.J.E., Putet, G., Smith, J.M., Heim, T. & Swyer, P.R. (1981): Influence of postnatal age, energy intake and weight gain on energy metabolism in the very low birth weight infant. *J. Pediatr.* **99**, 761–766.

5 Close, W.H. & Mount, L.E. (1978): The effects of plane of nutrition and environmental temperature on the energy metabolism of the growing pig. 2. growth rate including protein and fat deposition. *Br. J. Nutr.* **40**, 423–431.

6 Gudinchet, F., Schutz, Y., Micheli, J., Stettler, E. & Jéquier, E. (1982): Metabolic cost of growth in very low birth weight infants. *Pediatr. Res.* **16**, 1025–1030.

7 Koch, A. (1982): Partition of energy for growth in the steer. *Growth* **46**, 60–75.

8 Krieger, I. & Whitten, C.F. (1969): Energy metabolism in infants with growth failure due to maternal deprivation, undernutrition or causes unknown. II. Relationship between nitrogen balance, weight gain and postprandial excess heat production. *J. Pediatr.* **75**, 374–379.

9 Mestyán, J., Járai, I. & Fekete, M. (1968): The total energy expenditure and its components in premature infants maintained under different nursing and environmental conditions. *Pediatr. Res.* **2**, 161–171.

10 Mestyán, J., Járai, I., Fekete, M. & Soltész, Gy. (1969): Specific dynamic action in premature infants kept at and below the neutral temperature. *Pediatr. Res.* **3**, 41–50.

11 Putet, G., Senterre, J., Rigo, J. & Salle, B. (1984): Nutrient balance, energy utilization and composition of weight gain in very low birth weight infants fed pooled human milk or a preterm formula. *J. Pediatr.* **105**, 79–85.

12 Reichman, B.L., Chessex, Ph., Putet, G., Verellen, G.J.E., Smith, J.M., Heim, T. & Swyer, P.R. (1982): Partition of energy metabolism and energy cost of growth in the very low birth weight infant. *Pediatr.* **69**, 446–451.

13 Reichman, B., Chessex, Ph., Verellen, G., Putet, G., Smith, J.M., Heim, T. & Swyer, P.R. (1983): Dietary composition and macronutrient storage in preterm infants. *Pediatr.* **72**, 322–328.

14 Rubecz, I. & Mestyán, J. (1975): The partition of maintenance energy expenditure and the pattern of substrate utilization in intrauterine malnourished newborn infants before and during recovery. *Acta Paediatr. Acad. Sci. Hung.* **16**, 335–350.

15 Rubecz, I. & Mestyán, J. (1975): Activity, energy metabolism and postnatal age relationship in low birth weight infants. *Acta Paediatr. Acad. Sci. Hung.* **16**, 351–362.

16 Sauer, P.J.J., Dane, H.J. & Visser, H.K.A. (1984): Longitudinal studies on metabolic rate, heat loss and energy cost of growth in low birth weight infants. *Pediatr. Res.* **18**, 254–259.

17 Sinclair, J.C. (1978): Energy balance of the newborn. In *Growth and development of the full term and premature infant.* ed J.H.P. Jonxis, pp. 19–22. Amsterdam, Excerpta Medica.

18 Whyte, R.K., Haslam, R., Vlainic, C., Shannon, S., Samulski, K., Campbell, D., Bayley, H.S. & Sinclair, J.C. (1983): Energy balance and nitrogen balance in growing low birth weight infants fed human milk or formula. *Pediatr. Res.* **17**, 891–898.

19 Ziegler, E.E., O'Donnel, A.M., Nelson, J.E. & Fomon, S.J. (1976): Body composition of the reference fetus. *Growth* **40**, 329–341.

Requirements of the preterm infant for some vitamins and trace elements and for carnitine and taurine

O.G. BROOKE
Department of Child Health, St. George's Hospital, Cranmer Terrace, London SW17 0RE, UK.

The purpose of this paper is to review the principal micronutrients which have been claimed to be of special significance for the preterm infant, either because disease due to deficiency has been identified, or because growth has been found to improve when supplements of the nutrient are given. It is worth reflecting at this point that the sum of improved growth claimed for various dietary manipulations in the preterm infant should, when expressed in a particular infant, result in a weight gain of magnificently unlikely proportions, and one should regard growth comparisons made in small numbers of infants with healthy scepticism.

Vitamin A. Vitamin A (retinol) is transported across the placenta down a concentration gradient. It is stored in the liver and is released from the liver and carried in the plasma bound to a transport protein, retinol binding protein (RBP). There is evidence that liver stores of retinol are low in preterm infants[18], and from work in other mammalian species[25] it seems that RBP synthesis does not occur to any great extent until quite late in pregnancy. Plasma concentrations of retinol and RBP are low in preterm compared with term infants[17], and considerably lower than in maternal plasma[2]. Absorption of the vitamin from the premature gut may be poor because of fat malabsorption. For all these reasons there is cause to be concerned about vitamin A nutrition in preterm infants, although overt signs of deficiency seem to be rare. Nevertheless, a recent publication[19] points to the very low plasma concentrations of retinol found in infants with bronchopulmonary dysplasia and speculates on the possible effect of retinol deficiency on lung growth and development. More work is necessary, but all preterm infants should receive vitamin A supplements as a matter of course.

Vitamin D. Like vitamin A, vitamin D is transported to the fetus down a concentration gradient. It is also stored in the liver and transported in the plasma on a special binding protein, vitamin D binding globulin (VDBG). The main circulating form of vitamin D is the principal liver metabolite, 25-OH Vit D. There is no evidence that the availability of vitamin D in preterm infants is limited by deficient synthesis of VDBG, and the main problems of vitamin D nutrition are related to its relatively poor absorption, and possibly to limitation in the capacity for hepatic hydroxylation[16]. There is little evidence that the renal hydroxylation of 25-(OH)D to 1,25-$(OH)_2$D, the main active metabolite, is implicated in disturbances of vitamin D nutrition in preterm infants. Optimal calcium retention in infants less than 34 weeks gestation requires vitamin D intakes of 1000–2000 IU/day, and on such intakes plasma concentrations of 25-(OH)D are within the normal range for adults[11]. Nevertheless, metabolic bone disease of prematurity occurs quite often in infants <1000g at birth, especially when fed on breast milk[11]. Substrate deficiency is the likely cause in these cases, and supplements of phosphorus and calcium are necessary[5].

Vitamin E. The role of vitamin E in neonatal nutrition is controversial. Vitamin-E-deficiency in preterm infants has been described[15] and causes haemolytic anaemia. This is rare and appears to be related to the use of unsuitable formulas with a low ratio of vitamin E to polyunsaturated fatty acids. Under these circumstances toxic free radicals accumulate, causing cell membrane damage. There is little evidence that preterm infants, even very small ones, develop clinical evidence of vitamin-E-deficiency when fed on breast milk or one of the current low birthweight formulas, although their plasma tocopherol concentrations are low[9] and it is known that ante-natal transfer across the placenta is minimal[2]. Large doses of vitamin E (100 mg per day) may, however, protect the immature neonate from retinal damage due to oxygen toxicity[14], and may also reduce the incidence of intraventricular haemorrhage[6,22], perhaps by improving the stability of the capillary vessels in the germinal matrix of the brain. It is beginning to look as though it may be advisable to give such supplements to all very immature infants, though it will be important to establish that there is no risk of toxicity.

Folic acid. Folate requirements are increased during rapid growth, and megaloblastic anaemia due to folate deficiency sometimes occurs in premature infants[23]. Subclinical evidence of deficiency is common, however[24], and the vitamin has such an important role in purine and pyrimidine synthesis that routine supplementation is reasonable. An intake of 50 µg/day or more will prevent the development of abnormal blood cell morphology and will maintain plasma folate concentrations within the normal adult range[20]. Fresh human milk will only supply about 5–10 µg per day for a 1 kg infant and less if it has been heated. Most formulae designed for premature infants provide 20–25 µg per kg per d at currently recommended feed intakes.

Zinc. Zinc is an essential nutrient and deficiency causes growth failure, skin lesions and defects of cell mediated immunity inter alia. Disease due to zinc-deficiency is rare but well recognised in premature infants[1] and occurs mainly in breast-fed infants. Most preterm infants are in negative zinc balance during their first month. It is likely that zinc-deficiency, even if not clinically apparent, will also produce sub-optimal growth, although definite evidence for this is lacking. There is at present no real justification for suggesting zinc supplements for premature infants as a routine but we should keep an open mind on this.

Copper. Copper deficiency causes bone defects, anaemia, neutropenia and hypopigmentation. It has been described in a few preterm infants, some of whom had a fish odour[5]. It has not been seen in breast-fed infants. Some formulas designed for full-term infants have very low copper concentrations and are therefore unsuitable for use with premature infants. Formulas designed for preterm infants usually have added copper, which should probably be in the range of 60–90 µg/100 ml for minimum risk of deficiency.

Carnitine. Carnitine is a quarternary amine which has an important function in the metabolism of lipids to facilitate the transport of long-chain fatty acids across the mitochondrial membrane[12]. It is synthesized in the body but there is evidence that synthesis may be deficient in neonates[13]. It has been reported that underweight infants show increased weight gain if fed a formula supplemented with carnitine[4]. There is, however, no evidence that preterm infants suffer clinical illness as a result of carnitine-deficiency, although a disorder attributed to this cause has been described in a full-term infant[21]: there seems no good reason to supplement feeds with carnitine, which is present naturally in both breast and cow's milk.

Taurine. The amino acid taurine is present in breast milk but only very small amounts are found in cow's milk. This accounts for the fact that bile acids in formula-fed infants are mainly glycine-conjugated, while those of breast-fed infants are predominantly taurine-conjugated. Infants fed on breast-milk excrete taurine in the urine, while those fed on formula do not[7]. There appears to be no difference in bile salt function, as judged by fat absorption and weight gain, between infants fed taurine-supplemented formulas and those fed taurine-deficient formulas[26].

Cats fed on a diet containing no taurine develop retinal damage[10] and retinal lesions possibly due to taurine deficiency have been described in children during parenteral feeding[8]. Infants, both preterm and full-term, have been fed on taurine-deficient formulas for generations without problems of visual development coming to light so it seems very unlikely that taurine supplementation is necessary.

1 Aggett, P.J., Atherton, D.J., More, J., Davey, J., Delves, H.T. & Harries, J.T. (1980): Symptomatic zinc deficiency in a breast-fed preterm infant. *Archs Dis. Child* **55**, 547–550.
2 Baker, H., Frank, O. & Thompson, D. (1975): Vitamin profiles of 174 mothers and newborns at parturition. *Am. J. Clin. Nutr.* **28**, 59–65.
3 Blumenthal, I., Lealman, G.T. & Franklyn, P.P. (1980): Fracture of the femur, fish odour, and copper deficiency in a preterm infant. *Archs Dis. Child* **55**, 229–231.
4 Borniche, P. & Canlorbe, P. (1960): Action clinique et humorale de la carnitine dans les syndromes de denutrition post-infectieux de l'enfance. *Clin. Chim. Acta* **5**, 171–176.
5 Brooke, O.G. & Lucas, A. (1985): Metabolic bone disease in preterm infants. *Archs Dis Child.* **60**, 682–685.
6 Chiswick, M.L., Johnson, M., Woodhall, C. *et al.* (1983): Protective effect of vitamin E against intraventricular haemorrhage in premature babies. *Br. Med. J.* **287**, 81–84.

7 Gaull, G.E., Rassin, D.K., Raiha, N.C.R. & Heinoren, K. (1977): Milk protein quantity and quality in low birthweight infants. *J. Pediat.* **90**, 348–355.

8 Geggol, H.S., Ament, M.E., Heckenlively, J.R. *et al.* (1982): Evidence that taurine is an essential aminoacid in children receiving total parenteral nutrition. *Clin. Res.* **30**, 486A.

9 Haga, P. & Lunde, G. (1978): Selenium and vitamin E in cord blood from preterm and full term infants. *Acta Paediat. Scand.* **67**, 735–739.

10 Hayes, K.C., Carey, R.E. & Schmidt, S.Y. (1975): Retinal degeneration associated with taurine deficiency in the cat. *Science* **188**, 949–951.

11 McIntosh, N., Livesey, A., Brooke, O.G. (1982): Plasma 25-hydroxyvitamin D and rickets in infants of extremely low birthweight. *Archs Dis Child* **57**, 848–850.

12 Mitchell, M.E. (1978): Carnitine metabolism in human subjects. 1. Normal metabolism. *Am. J. Clin. Nutr.* **31**, 293–306.

13 Penn, D., Schmidt-Sommerfeld, E. & Pascu, F. (1981): Decreased tissue carnitine concentration in newborn infants receiving total parenteral nutrition. *J. Pediat.* **98**, 976–978.

14 Phelps, D.L. (1982): Vitamin E and retrolental fibroplasia in 1982. *Pediatrics* **70**, 420–425.

15 Ritchie, J.H., Fish, M.B., McMasters, V. & Grossman, M. (1968): Edema and hemolytic anaemia in premature infants: a vitamin E deficiency syndrome. *New Engl. J. Med.* **279**, 1185–1190.

16 Senterre, J. & Salle, B. (1982): Calcium and phosphorus economy of the preterm infant and its interaction with vitamin D and its metabolites. *Acta Paediat. Scand* Suppl. **296**, 85–92.

17 Shenai, J.P., Chytil, F., Jhavesi, A. & Stahlman, M.T. (1981): Plasma vitamin A and retinol-binding protein in premature and term neonates. *J. Pediat.* **99**, 302–305.

18 Shenai, J.P., Chytil, F. & Stahlman, M.T. (1982): Liver vitamin A reserves of very low birth-weight infants. *Pediat. Res.* **16**, 177.

19 Shenai, J.P., Chytil, F. & Stahlman, M.T. (1985): Vitamin A status of neonates with bronchopulmonary dysplasia. *Pediat. Res.* **19**, 185–188.

20 Shojania, A.M. & Gross, S. (1964): Folic acid deficiency and prematurity *J. Pediat.* **64**, 323–326.

21 Slonim, A.E., Borum, P.R., Tanaka, K. *et al.* (1981): Dietary dependent carnitine deficiency as a cause of non-ketotic hypoglycaemia in an infant. *J. Pediat.* **99**, 551–556.

22 Speer, M.E., Blifield, C., Rudolph, A.J. *et al.* (1984): Intraventricular haemorrhage and vitamin E in the very low-birth-weight infant: Evidence for efficacy of early intramuscular Vitamin E administration. *Pediatrics* **74**, 1107–1112.

23 Strelling, M.K., Blackledge, D.G., Goodall, H.B. & Walker, C.H.M. (1966): Megaloblastic anaemia and whole-blood folate levels in premature infants. *Lancet* **1**, 898–900.

24 Strelling, M.K., Blackledge, D.G. & Goodall, H.B. (1979): Diagnosis and management of folate deficiency in low birthweight infants. *Archs Dis. Child* **54**, 271–277.

25 Takahashi, Y.I., Smith, J.E. & Goodman, D.S. (1977): Vitamin A and retinol-binding protein metabolism during fetal development. *Am. J. Physiol.* **233**, E263–272.

26 Watkins, J.B., Jarvenpaa, A.L., Szczepanik Van-Leenwen, P. *et al.* (1983): Feeding the low birth weight infant. *Gastroenterology* **85**, 793–800.

★   ★   ★

NUTRITIONAL AND DEVELOPMENTAL FACTORS AFFECTING PERFORMANCE OF NEWBORN BABIES AND PIGLETS

Comparative aspects of the developmental physiology and endocrinology of the human and pig fetus

A.A. MACDONALD
Department of Anatomy, Royal (Dick) School of Veterinary Studies, University of Edinburgh, Edinburgh EH9 1QH, Scotland.

Neonatal infant mortality has declined in a number of countries throughout the world during the last 30 years. The uneven spread of success in reducing mortality has provoked analyses of the various factors placing infants at risk. It is accepted that children may be born a number of weeks earlier than the normal length of gestation but it is only recently that it has been appreciated that the physiology and endocrinology of babies at birth differ according to the amount of time spent *in utero*[22–24].

The pig is a domestic species which has a long history in biomedical and fetal research[11]. It offers opportunities and potential for the study of problems related to fetal and neonatal development[4,12,19]. The fetus is relatively large (1 kg) at birth after a gestation length of 114 ± 1 d, and naturally occurring intrauterine growth retardation may be found within the average litter size of 10–11 piglets. Techniques for chronic catheterization of the fetus have been developed (for review[16,18]) and the litter size means that studies can be cost effective by allowing one or more experimental treatments and controls to be examined within the environment of the same uterus[13]. It is also clear that despite a number of obvious differences in anatomy there are many similarities in organ systems and physiology between the human and pig fetus[8,9].

The pattern of growth in body weight is similar in human and pig fetuses. Glycogen is an important energy reserve in both species and it is mobilized to aid survival during labour and immediately after birth. Various pancreatic, adrenal, thyroid and pituitary hormones contribute towards the development and mobilization of energy reserves, and the maintenance of fetal nutrition during the fetal and perinatal period[4,19]. This brief review highlights a few examples of studies on the first two of these glands in the human and pig fetus. More detailed information is presented in a number of the reviews mentioned above.

Pancreatic hormones. The human B-cell is recognizable from the 10th week of gestation[10] and insulin is detected in the fetal circulation from the 12th week[1]. In the pig fetus, small numbers of insulin containing cells have been located by immunohistochemistry as early as the 4th week of gestation. Initially found only in the dorsal pancreatic primordia, by 90 d gestation they are numerous and randomly distributed throughout the growing exocrine parenchyma[2]. At about this time the glucose sensitivity of insulin release becomes apparent. By 100 d, plasma insulin concentrations are demonstrably increasing and exogenous infusions of insulin reduce circulating glucose concentrations and increase tissue glycogen deposition[4,5,7,20].

Little is known about the other pancreatic hormones of the human and pig fetus[4]. Glucagon is present in the pancreas of the human fetus by the 6th week and is found in the circulation by the 11th week of gestation[3]. Recent studies of the pig fetus revealed glucagon immunoreactive cells in the dorsal pancreatic primordia and adjacent proximal small intestine at 4 weeks of gestation. By term they are found predominantly in the pancreatic islets, and also in the distal small intestine and colon[2]. Plasma concentrations of glucagon increase during gestation and are responsive to catecholamine stimulation inducing liver glycogen mobilization[5]. Pancreatic polypeptide- and somatostatin-containing cells are present respectively in the ventral and dorsal primordia of the pig pancreas at 4 weeks of gestation[2]. By the end of gestation the former are present in large numbers in the duodenal portion of the pancreas but relatively few are found elsewhere in the gland. The numbers of somatostatin cells increase during gestation and by about 70 d are concentrated in small nests of cells[2]. Further studies are required to define the roles played by these hormones in fetal growth and carbohydrate metabolism. Recently developed techniques of fetal pancreatectomy[4] and fetal pancreas transplantation[17] promise new experimental possibilities for the study of pancreatic endocrinology in the pig fetus.

Adrenal hormones. The adrenal of the human fetus has been more completely studied than that of the pig. However recent work has indicated that the pig adrenal is very mature structurally and is capable of responding to stimulation earlier in gestation than in a number of other species[6,21]. Adrenal and circulating corticosteroid concentrations increase during the last week of gestation[13,15], and recent studies have shown that cortisol, like insulin, has a marked positive effect on the glycogen content of liver and skeletal muscle[6]. Catecholamines induce the secretion of glucagon which has the opposite effect on liver glycogen[4]. At 60 d of gestation only noradrenaline-containing cells are present in the adrenal medulla[21] but by the end of gestation both adrenaline and noradrenaline are in circulation and plasma levels are responsive to stimulation[14]. Further studies are needed before the extent of adrenal involvement in fetal energy metabolism is fully appreciated.

Conclusions. In this short review attention was drawn to a number of recent studies which indicate that the pig fetus has a number of interesting characteristics useful to the study of fetal physiology and endocrinology. Recent reviews of literature relevant to the developing pig fetus have been highlighted to guide the interested reader to further sources of information. The examples of recent studies on the pancreas and adrenal of the pig fetus indicate that experiments relevant to a further understanding of the physiology and endocrinology of the prenatal human infant may be carried out on the pig fetus. It is also worth bearing in mind that in addition to this, the results of studies involving the pig fetus are likely to be information of direct relevance to our understanding of the physiology of a domestic species which is a major world source of animal protein in the human diet.

1 Adam, P.A.J., Teramo, K., Raiha, N., Gitlin, D. & Schwartz, R. (1969): Human fetal insulin metabolism early in gestation. Response of acute elevation of fetal blood glucose concentration and placental transfer of human insulin I 131. *Diabetes* **18**, 409–416.

2 Alumets, J., Hakanson, R. & Sundler, F. (1983): Ontogeny of endocrine cells in porcine gut and pancreas. *Gastroenterology* **85**, 1359–1372.

3 Assan, R. & Boillot, J. (1973): Pancreatic glucagon and glucagon-like material in tissues and plasma from human infants 6–26 weeks old. *Pathol. Biol.* **21**, 149–155.

4 Fowden A.L. (1985): Pancreatic endocrine function and carbohydrate metabolism in the fetus. In *Research in perinatal medicine, IV. Perinatal endocrinology*, ed E. Albrecht & G. Pepe, Ithaca, NY: Perinatology Press. (In press).

5 Fowden, A.L., Bloom, S.R., Comline, R.S. & Silver, M. (1985): The endocrine pancreas of the fetal pig. In *Swine in biomedical research*, ed M.E. Tumbleson. (In press).

6 Fowden, A.L., Comline, R.S. & Silver, M. (1985): The effects of cortisol on the concentration of glycogen in different tissues in the chronically catheterised fetal pig. *Quart. J. Exp. Physiol.* **70**, 23–35.

7 Garssen, G.J., Specenr, G.S.G., Colenbrander, B., Macdonald, A.A. & Hill, D.J. (1983): Lack of effect of chronic hyperinsulinaemia on growth and body composition in the fetal pig. *Biol. Neonate* **44**, 234–242.

8 Hausman, G.J. & Martin, R.J. (1985): Regulation of adipose tissue development in the fetus: the fetal pig model. In *Swine in biomedical research*, ed M.E. Tumbleson (In press).

9 Hill, D.E. (1985): Swine in perinatal research: an overview. In *Swine in biomedical research*, ed M.E. Tumbleson (In press).

10 Like, A.A. & Orci, L. (1972): Embryogenesis of the human pancreatic islets. *Diabetes* **21**, 511–534.

11 Macdonald, A.A. (1981): Studies on the anatomy and physiology of the pig fetus and placenta: an historical review. In *Adv. Physiol. Sci. 21. History of physiology*, ed E. Schultheisz, pp. 53–60, Oxford: Pergamon Press.

12 Macdonald, A.A. (1985): Cardiovascular physiology of the pig fetus. In *Swine in biomedical research*, ed M.E. Tumbleson (In press).

13 Macdonald, A.A., Colenbrander, B. & van Vorstenbosch, C.J.A.H.V. (1982): Physiology and endocrinology of the fetus in late gestation. In *Control of pig reproduction* ed D.J.A. Cole & G.R. Foxcroft, pp. 377–404. Oxford: Butterworth.

14 Macdonald, A.A., Colenbrander, B., Versteeg, D.H.G., Heilhecker, A. & Wensing, C.J.G. (1984): Catecholamines in fetal pig plasma and the response to acute hypoxia and chronic fetal decapitation. *Roux's Archs. Dev. Biol.* **193**, 19–23.

15 Randall, G.C.B. (1983): Changes in the concentrations of corticosteroids in the blood of fetal pigs and their dams during late gestation and labor. *Biol. Reprod.* **29**, 1077–1084.

16 Randall, G.C.B. (1985): Chronic implantation of catheters and other surgical techniques in fetal pigs. In *Swine in biomedical research*, ed M.E. Tumbleson (In press).

17 Sasaki, N., Yoneda, K., Bigger, C., Brown, J. & Mullen, Y. (1984): Fetal pancreas transplantation in miniature swine. *Transplantation* **38**, 335–340.

18 Silver, M. (1980): Intravenous catheterization and other chronic preparations in the mare and the sow. In *Animal models in fetal medicine*, ed P.W. Nathanielsz, pp. 107–132. Amsterdam: Elsevier/North-Holland Biomedical Press.

19 Spencer, G.S.G. (1985): Hormonal influence on growth of the fetal pig in utero. In *Swine in biomedical research*, ed M.E. Tumbleson (In press).

20 Spencer, G.S.G., Garssen, G.J., Colenbrander, B., Macdonald, A.A. & Bevers, M.M. (1983): Glucose, growth hormone, somatomedin, cortisol and ACTH changes in the plasma of unanaesthetised pig foetuses following intravenous insulin administration in utero. *Acta Endocr.* **104**, 240–245.

21 Stadnicka, A. & van Wynsberghe, D. (1982): Cytochemistry and ultrastructure of the prenatal porcine adrenal medulla. Z. Mikrosk. Anat. Forsch. **96**, 103–112.

22 Stanley, C.A., Anday, E.K., Baker, L. & Delivoria-Papadopolous, M. (1979): Metabolic fuel and hormone responses to fasting in newborn infants. *Pediatrics* **64**, 613–619.

23 Van Assche, F.A., De Prins, F., Aerts, L. & Verjans, M. (1977): The endocrine pancreas of the small-for-dates infants. *Br. J. Obstet. Gynaecol.* **84**, 751–753.

24 Williams, P.R., Fiser, R.H., Sperling, M.A. & Oh. W. (1975): Effects of oral alanine feeding on blood glucose, plasma glucagon and insulin concentrations in small-for-gestational age infants. *New Engl. J. Med.* **292**, 612–614.

Development of the stomach and gastric secretions in the baby and the piglet

P.D. CRANWELL
School of Agriculture, La Trobe University, Bundoora, Victoria 3083, Australia.

Although the neonatal pig can be a satisfactory model of some aspects of protein metabolism in infants[29], there is little comparative information in the literature on many aspects of protein digestion. This paper summarizes recent information on the development of gastric acid secretion and gastrin physiology in pigs and humans, including some unpublished data from the author's laboratory. Reviews of earlier work on the development of gastric function in the human and pig are to be found in[2,3,8–11,22].

Gastrin. In the fetal pig (gestation period 115 ± 3 d) gastrin cells are present in the stomach and duodenum at 28–42 d gestation and reach adult frequency at 105–112 d[32]. In the human fetus (gestation period 280 ± 21 d) gastrin cells have been found in the duodenum at 70 d and in the antrum at 98 d gestation[15]. By 120–154 d gestation the concentration of gastrin in the duodenum exceeds adult levels[8]. Gastrin has been detected in the blood of the human fetus at 126–147 d gestation[3] and reaches adult concentrations during the final 56 d of gestation[30]. Although comparative information is not available for the fetal pig, studies in the fetal lamb (gestation period 150 ± 2 d) show[4] that gastrin can be detected in fetal blood at 90 d gestation and concentrations are similar to and often exceed maternal concentrations during the final 21 d of gestation. Results of infusion studies in the sheep show that maternal gastrin does not cross the placenta to the fetus[4].

At birth gastrin concentrations in the blood of both piglets and babies are significantly greater than those found in adults and are often greater than those in the maternal circulation at delivery[1,6,8,12]. In the period immediately after birth, transient decreases in blood gastrin concentrations have been found to occur in human babies before the first feed[25] and in piglets 150 min after the first feed[6]. However, in both older pigs and babies, fasting blood gastrin concentrations remain greater than adult fasting levels for up to 6 weeks of age in the pig[13] (Xu & Cranwell, unpublished) and 22 months in the human infant[8]. The significance of the high levels of gastrin and other regulatory peptides during gestation and early life and their effects on development of the gastrointestinal tract 'have just begun to be explored'[22,23].

It has been reported that the first feed of milk given 3–6 h after birth to term infants caused a significant increase in plasma gastrin concentrations[2,34]. However, a similar study[31] found no significant rise above fasting concentrations of serum gastrin 30 min after the first feed at 3–5 h of age or after a feed given at 48–60 h. In pigs, serum gastrin concentrations 30–45 min after the first sucking were slightly but not significantly greater than at birth[12].

In pre-term infants it has been found that gastrin responses to feeding occur by 13 d of age but in both term and pre-term infants there was no evidence of a response at 6 d[2,24]. Other reports indicate that significant gastrin secretory responses to feeding occur in infants by 3 weeks of age[8]. In contrast other authors[27] did not observe significant responses in infants less than 3 months of age. In pigs 3–6 weeks old both sucking and eating a meal of solid food evoke significant gastrin responses[10,11]. The response to solid food was comparable with that seen in adult pigs, and was significantly greater and longer than in those receiving milk. Another study however, did not detect a response to a liquid meal given by orogastric tube in pigs 4–28 d old[28].

Gastric acid secretion. Both new-born pigs and infants are capable of secreting acid soon after birth and before their first feed[8,9]. Gastric secretory responses to feeding have also been demonstrated at an early age, 21–48 h in humans[17] and 48 h in pigs[14]. Responses to the synthetic secretagogues betazole HCl (Histalog) and pentagastrin have not been convincingly demonstrated in human infants in the 1st week of life[8].

In older infants, 1–12 months, several authors have reported gastric secretory responses to histamine and pentagastrin[19–21]. The maximal acid outputs in these infants (range 0.221–0.280 mmol/kg per h) are similar to the acid secretory response to feeding (0.236 ± 0.049 mmol/kg per h) found by Cavell[7]. Also, they are considerably greater than the responses to pentagastrin reported in the preterm infant during the 1st month of life (0.021–0.044 mmol/kg per h)[18], and the responses to a meal in 21 to 48-h-old full-term infants (0.064 mmol/kg per h)[1]. In infants and children 0–15 years and approx 2–60 kg B.Wt., significant linear correlations between maximal or peak acid output and body weight (kg) have been reported[20,21,26].

Significant gastric secretory responses to histalog and histamine in new-born unsuckled and suckled piglets have been demonstrated[16,33]. Also significant linear correlations between maximal acid output and body weight have been reported in weaned and sucking pigs using histalog as the secretagogue[13]. In this study maximal acid outputs in new-born pigs < 24 h old (0.41 ± 0.05 mmol/kg per h) were significantly lower than those in 25 to 42-d-old sucking pigs (0.68 ± 0.07 mmol/kg per h) which in turn were significantly lower than those in 25 to 42-d-old pigs which had been weaned on to solid food at 21 d (1.13 ± 0.09 mmol/kg per h).

Information on the response to pentagastrin in the new-born pig is limited to a report that, in *in vitro* experiments, it does not significantly stimulate the gastric mucosa to secrete acid[16]. Recently a study on basal and pentagastrin induced gastric acid secretion was done using 30 pigs, 0 to 26-d-old and 1.1–8.9 kg B.Wt. by Xu & Cranwell (unpublished). The procedure followed, gastric perfusion under barbiturate anaesthesia, was similar to that described by Cranwell[10] except that pentagastrin (0.5–8.0 µ/kg per h) was used as the secretagogue. Acid was found in the perfusate from all pigs during the basal period. In pigs 2 to 43-h-old basal secretion of acid (0.021 ± 0.002 mmol/kg per h) was significantly lower ($P < 0.02$) than in pigs 3 to 26-d-old (0.097 ± 0.027 mmol/kg per h).

For all pigs maximal acid secretory responses to pentagastrin occurred at the dose rates of 4 and 8 µg/kg per h and were the same, 0.53 ± 0.05 mmol/kg per h. There were significant correlations between maximal acid output and (i) age (r^2 0.79; $P < 0.001$), (ii) body weight (r^2 0.94, $P < 0.001$) and (iii) stomach weight (r^2 0.94, $P < 0.001$). There were also significant correlations between maximal acid output per unit stomach weight and age in pigs up to 50 h, and in pigs 50 to 624-h-old (Figure). The slope of the regression line for the younger pigs was significantly different from that for the older pigs ($P < 0.001$). The lower relative acid secretory response to pentagastrin in the first 48 h of life could be due to the immaturity of parietal cells in new-born pigs[33] and to the immaturity of mechanisms involving receptors[22,23].

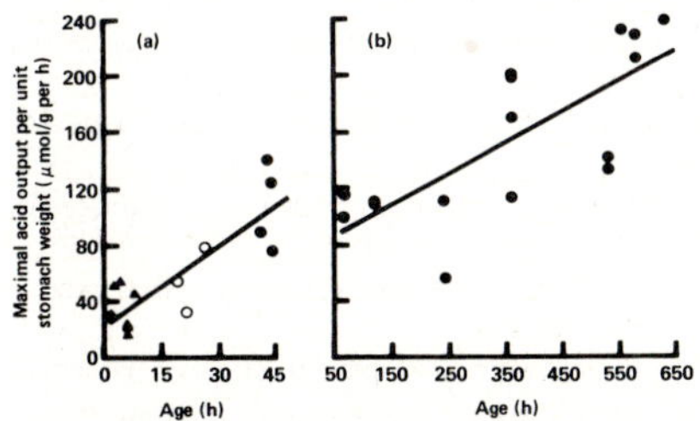

Figure. *Linear regressions of maximal acid output per unit stomach weight (µmol/g per h) against age (h).* (a). The regression equation was: $Y = 1.9 X + 22.1$, r^2 0.69, $P < 0.01$. (▲) unsuckled pigs ($n = 7$); (○) pigs suckled for 3 h and fasted for 16–23 h ($n = 3$); (●) pigs with unlimited access to the sow and fasted for 24 h ($n = 4$). (b). The regression equation was: $Y = 0.22 X + 74.8$, r^2 0.58, $P < 0.05$. (●) as in (a). ($n = 16$).

Conclusions. From the work reviewed here it is evident that in humans and pigs: (1) the fetus secretes its own gastrin at quite an early stage during gestation; (2) the neonate is hypergastrinaemic and remains so for a considerable period after birth; (3) gastric acid secretion occurs within a few hours of birth; (4) acid secretory responses to feeding occur in the first 2 d of life; and (5) acid secretory capacity increases with body weight.

It is also apparent that in the pig: (1) acid secretory responses to gastrin and histamine develop at an earlier age; (2) acid secretory capacity develops more rapidly; and (3) acid secretory capacity relative to body size is always greater than in the human infant.

Some of the differences in gastric development between the two species could be due to the larger size of the porcine stomach relative to body weight and the much faster growth rate of the pig compared with the human infant[5].

1 Attia, R.R., Ebeid, A.M., Fischer, J.E. & Goudsouzian, N.G. (1982): Maternal fetal and placental gastrin concentrations. *Anaesthes.* **37**, 18–21.

2 Aynsley-Green, A. (1982): The control of the adaptation to postnatal nutrition. *Monogr. Paediatr.* **16**, 59–87.

3 Aynsley-Green, A. (1985): Metabolic and endocrine interrelationships in the human fetus and neonate. *Am. J. Clin. Nutr.* **41**, Suppl. No. 2, 399–417.

4 Bell, A.W., Cranwell, P.D. & Hansky, J. (1984): Plasma gastrin in the fetal and neonatal lamb, and the pregnant and lactating ewe. *Can. J. Anim. Sci.* **64**, (Suppl.), 97–99.

5 Braude, R. (1981): Symposium on the function of the gastrointestinal tract in health and disease: introduction. *Progr. Clin. Biol. Res.* **77**, 841–846.

6 Bunn, C.M. & Titchen, D.A. (1984): Plasma gastrin in the pig from birth to weaning. *Res. Vet. Sci.* **37**, 362–363.

7 Cavell, B. (1983): Postprandial gastric acid secretion in infants. *Acta Paediatr. Scand.* **72**, 857–860.

8 Christie, D.L. (1981): Development of gastric function during the first month of life. In *Textbook of gastroenterology and nutrition in infancy*, ed E. Lebenthal, pp. 109–120. New York: Raven Press.

9 Cranwell, P.D. (1984): Gastric digestion in the young pig. *Proc. Austr. Soc. Anim. Prod.* **15**, 145–157.

10 Cranwell, P.D. (1985): The development of acid and pepsin (EC3.4.23.1) secretory capacity in the pig; effects of age and weaning. 1. Studies in anaesthetized pigs. *Br. J. Nutr.* **54**, 305–320.

11 Cranwell, P.D. (1985): The development of the stomach in the pig: the effect of age and weaning. II. Acid and proteolytic enzyme secretory capacity. In *Digestive physiology in the Pig*, ed A. Just, H. Jørgensen & J.A. Fernandez, pp. 116–119. Report No. 580. Copenhagen: Nat. Inst. Anim. Sci.

12 Cranwell, P.D. & Hansky, J. (1980): Serum gastrin in newborn, sucking and weaned pigs. *Res. Vet. Sci.* **29**, 85–88.

13 Cranwell, P.D. & Hansky, J. (1980): Effect of parturition, age and feeding on serum gastrin levels in the pig. *Proc. IPVS 6th Congr.* (Copenhagen) p. 76.

14 Cranwell, P.D., Noakes, D.E. & Hill, K.J. (1976): Gastric secretion and fermentation in the suckling pig. *Br. J. Nutr.* **36**, 71–86.

15 Dubois, P.H., Paulin, C. & Chayvialle (1976): Identification of gastrin-secreting cells and cholecystokinin-secreting cells in the gastrointestinal tract of the human fetus and adult man. *Cell Tiss. Res.* **175**, 351–356.

16 Forte, J.G., Forte, T.M. & Machen, T.E. (1975): Histamine-stimulated hydrogen ion secretion by *in vitro* piglet gastric mucosa. *J. Physiol.* **244**, 15–31.

17 Harada, T., Hyman, P.E., Everett, S. & Ament, M.E. (1984): Meal-stimulated gastric acid secretion in infants. *J. Pediatr.* **104**, 534–538.

18 Hyman, P.E., Clarke, D.D., Everett, S.L., Sonne, B., Stewart, D., Harada, T., Walsh, J.H. & Taylor, I.L. (1985): Gastric acid secretory function in preterm infants. *J. Pediatr.* **106**, 467–471.

19 Hyman, P.E., Feldman, E.J., Ament, M.E., Byrne, W.J. & Euler, A.R. (1983): Effect of enteral feeding on the maintenance of gastric acid secretory function. *Gastrenterol.* **84**, 341–345.

20 Kopel, F.B. & Barbero, G.J. (1967): Gastric acid secretion in infancy and childhood. *Gastroenterol.* **52**, 1101.

21 Lari, J., Lister, J. & Duthie, H.L. (1968): Response to gastrin pentapeptide in children. *J. Pediatr. Surg.* **3**, 682–690.

22 Lebenthal, E. (1982): Gastrointestinal ontogeny and its impact on infant feeding. *Monograph. Paediatr.* **16**, 17–38.

23 Lichtenberger, L. (1984): A search for the origin of neonatal hypergastrinaemia. *J. Pediatr. Gastroenterol. Nutr.* **3**, 161–166.

24 Lucas, A., Blackburn, A.M., Aynsley-Green, A., Sarson, D.L., Adrian, T.E. & Bloom S.R. (1980): Breast *vs* bottle: endocrine responses are different with formula feeding. *Lancet* **1**, 1267–1269.

25 Lucas, A., Bloom, S.R. & Aynsley-Green, A. (1982): Postnatal surges in plasma gut hormones in term and preterm infants. *Biol. Neonate* **41**, 63–67.

26 Micheli, H. (1969): La stimulation gastrique maximale a l'histamine chez l'enfant normal. *Helvet. Paediatr. Acta* **24**, 278–292.

27 Moazam, F., Kirby, W.J., Rodgers, B.M. & McGuigan, J.E. (1984): Physiology of serum gastrin production in neonates and infants. *Annl. Surg.* **199**, 389–392.

28 Moazam, F., Miller, R.L., Rodgers, B.M., Talbert, J.L. & McGuigan, J.E. (1980): Fasting and postprandial serum gastrin in neonatal swine, and changes following antrectomy. *J. Surg. Res.* **28**, 39–43.

29 Newport, M.J. & Henschel, M.J. (1984): Evaluation of the neonatal pig as a model for infant nutrition: effects of different proportions of casein and whey protein in milk on nitrogen metabolism and composition of digesta in the stomach. *Pediatr. Res.* **18**, 658–662.

30 Ogawa, S. (1979): An investigation of the dynamics of immunoreactive gastrin in pregnant women and their fetuses. *Nichidae Igaku Zasshi* **38**, 1739–1749.

31 Rodgers, B.M., Dix, P.M., Talbert, J.L. & McGuigan, J.E. (1978): Fasting and postprandial serum gastrin in normal human neonates. *J. Pediatr. Surg.* **13**, 13–16.

32 Sundler, F. & Håkanson, R. (1984): Gastro-entero-pancreatic endocrine cells in higher mammals, with special reference to their ontogeny in the pig. In *Evolution and tumour pathology of the neuroendocrine system*, ed S. Falkner, R. Håkanson & F. Sundler, pp. 111–135. Amsterdam: Elsevier.

33 Tudor, E.McI. (1983): Studies on the gastric mucosa of young pigs. PhD Thesis, Monash University.

34 Von Berger, L., Henrichs, I., Raptis, S., Heinze, E., Jonatha, W., Teller, W.M. & Pfeiffer, E.F. (1976): Gastrin concentration in plasma of the neonate at birth and after first feeding. *Pediatr.* **58**, 264–267.

Perinatal nutrition in baby and piglet

P. H. DUÉE, C. SIMOES-NUNES and J. P. PÉGORIER
Centre de Recherches sur la Nutrition CNRS, 9, rue J. Hetzel 92190 Meudon-Bellevue; C.S-N. Laboratoire de Physiologie de la Nutrition INRA - CNRZ 78350 Jouy-en-Josas, France.

For ethical considerations, experimental research on babies appears somewhat difficult and the pig has always been considered as an adequate animal model[3,7].

Prenatal nutrition. *Fetal growth.* Several features are important before considering fetal nutrition and the effect of maternal conditions upon the growth of the fetus: (1) the fetal mass produced by the mother, (2) the time over which this fetal mass is built, (3) the composition of the fetal mass at term and, particularly, the water content (higher in pig: 81 per cent compared with 70 per cent) and the fat content (higher in babies: 16 per cent compared with 1 per cent). This last point may be used to estimate the fetal energy requirement of the fetus[36]. The energy accretion near term has been estimated to be 170 kJ (40 kcal)/kg per d, which is higher than in pigs, (125 kJ [31 kcal]/kg per d). In humans, the deposition of fat accounts for over 90 per cent of the energy accumulated by the fetus (FFA placental transfer and lipogenesis); in pigs, the value amounts to only 15 per cent.

Another component of energy requirement is represented by the energy expenditure for fetal oxidative metabolism which can be estimated indirectly from the oxygen consumption. It has been pointed out that fetal oxygen consumption expressed per kg B.Wt. was relatively constant among different species (7–8 ml/min per kg)[1]. In both species, the relative contribution of glucose in the fetal oxidative metabolism is high, which allows this component of energy requirement to be estimated approximately to 210–230 kJ (50–55 kcal)/kg B.Wt. per d.

Thus the total energy requirement near term amounts to 380–400 kJ/kgB.Wt. per d in the human fetus, 15 per cent lower in the pig fetus.

Maternal nutrition and fetal growth. Maternal nutrition is often considered as an important regulator of human fetal growth but this is based on epidemiological studies, some food intervention programmes or morphological studies[24]. In the pig, the reduction of energy intake slowly affects the weight of the fetus (review[21]): the weight of the new-born pig is decreased by 2 per cent when energy intake is reduced by 15 per cent.

This moderate effect can be justified by the above calculations. Human fetus at term requires 1500 kJ (650 kcal)/d ie 15 per cent of the energy intake of the pregnant woman. The requirement for a pig litter amounts to 3500 kJ (800–850 kcal)/d, ie nearly 15 per cent of the energy intake of the pregnant sow.

The effect of maternal nutrition could operate in two ways — (1) a lower nutrient availability, (2) a decreased placental blood flow — which, in turn, reduces the nutrient transfer to the fetus. In the pig, a reduced food intake does not seem to affect the uterine blood flow, but the weight heterogeneity in the litter at term could represent a model for the study of human intra-uterine growth retardation.

Fetal growth retardation does not only result from a reduced maternal food intake. In primiparous gilts, which exhibit an intensive growth rate, lysine imbalance induces fetal hypotrophy[10], comparable to obstetric problems found in adolescent pregnancy[25].

Hormonal control of fetal growth. The role of hormones in the regulation of fetal growth remains little understood, although insulin and various peptide factors, are often considered as candidates[26]. The few experiments carried out on pigs have shown a lack of effect of fetal decapitation or chronic hyperinsulinaemia on fetal growth and body composition and the hormonal control of the fetal growth in this species needs further experiment.

These observations suggest that pregnancy does represent a challenge to maternal glucose homoeostasis. Indeed, glucose utilization by the conceptus represents 35 to 40 per cent of the maternal glucose utilization near term in both species;[15,22] Duée (unpublished data). Such stress on maternal carbohydrate metabolism can lead to a pathological status typical of diabetes. Nevertheless it seems difficult in the pig to produce any effect of streptozotocin-diabetes on the fetus[12].

Postnatal metabolism and nutrition. At birth, the sudden interruption of the maternal supply completely alters the metabolic environment of the new-born. From a nutritional point of view, intake of the first meal, ie colostrum, does not represent the same meaning in both species since placental transfer of immunoglobulins is deficient in the pig. By contrast, intake of milk or formulas correspond, in both species, to the ingestion of a low-energy diet (290 kJ [70 kcal]/100 ml in man; 500 kJ [120 kcal]/100 ml in the pig) with a large part of total energy represented by fat 50 to 60 per cent[18]. Three aspects of this metabolic adaptation will now be described.

Development of digestive enzymes and of the gut flora. An efficient digestion and absorption of milk constituents is a prerequisite for the supplying of available nutrients to the organism and for normal growth. The picture of the digestive adaptation during the neonatal period[19,35] suggests that the pig represents a good model for human. Another aspect of neonatal adaptation is represented by the implantation of the gut flora. It seems that the dominant bacterial genera (facultatively or strictly anaerobic) which become established in the gut are similar in both species[8].

Regulation of fuel homoeostasis during the first days of life. While glucose appears to be the major energy fuel during fetal development, the new-born pig or human rapidly develops the capacity to oxidize fatty acids as a fuel alternative to glucose[17]. Nevertheless, several tissues are dependent on glucose for their energy metabolism and the glucose turnover rate (10 to 15 g/kg B.Wt. per d) in the human neonate or the piglet[2,13,31], appears to be two to three-fold higher than in the adult.

Glucose supplied from the milk only covers one-third of this glucose requirement so that endogenous glucose production is initiated after birth. Since liver glycogen stores are rapidly exhausted, hepatic gluconeogenesis seems crucial for the regulation of glucose homoeostasis of sucklings.

In the pig, studies performed *in vitro* with isolated hepatocytes have shown that the rates of gluconeogenesis profoundly increase within the 1st day of life[29]. In humans, there are several direct[16], or indirect[34,38] lines of evidence of an active gluconeogenesis in this period. The development of gluconeogenesis in the newly-born animal results from several factors: (1) the development of key enzymes of gluconeogenesis in the liver; (2) an appropriate hormonal environment (low plasma insulin and high plasma glucagon), which characterizes the neonatal transition, and (3) the supply of gluconeogenic precursors and FFA to the liver.

The sucking newborn receives FFA from milk but only breast-fed new-born infants have a marked hyperketonemia[23], and ketone bodies represent an important alternative fuel for brain metabolism. By contrast, fatty acid oxidation in the pig liver is reduced[30] and its role in the regulation of gluconeogenesis appears limited[9]. This discrepancy between the two species is not explained by a lower supply of carnitine or by a carnitine acyltransferase deficiency. Thus the pig does not represent an appropriate model for studying these related situations in humans[4].

This species difference becomes more evident when the first milk intake has been delayed. The new-born pig develops profound hypoglycaemia during 48 h fasting beginning at birth[28] whereas the normal human baby at term, endowed with large fat stores, can survive prolonged starvation without hypoglycaemia[11]. By contrast, the small-for-gestational age (SGA) new-born has a low body-fat content at birth and develops hypoglycaemia after a short fast[6]. A defect in gluconeogenesis has been proposed to explain hypoglycaemia in SGA babies and it has been shown that infusion of triglycerides into hypoglycaemic SGA neonates raises their blood glucose levels[33]. However the relevance of such a situation in the new-born pig remains to be demonstrated.

Postnatal growth. The species difference in post natal growth appears obvious and related to the difference in the nutrient intake from the milk. A higher growth rate in the piglet corresponds to an equal increase in protein and fat deposition. In the human neonate, the daily growth rate

— corresponding first to fat deposition and secondly to protein deposition — decreases progressively within the first months of life[14], illustrating the competition between maintenance metabolism and the process of energy deposition (growth). In babies, the maintenance process plays an even more important role than in the growing pig[37]. Nevertheless, the partition of energy expenditure between growth and maintenance functions may be modified in very-low-birth-weight infants[20] exhibiting a higher protein synthesis rate than normal babies, which then corresponds to the protein turnover value seen in growing pigs[32].

In taking into account these metabolic peculiarities of pig growth, the neonatal pig may be a useful model for an assessment of the nutritional value of various food formulas[27] since piglets survive early weaning[5].

1 Battaglia, F.C. & Meschia, G. (1978): Principal substrates of fetal metabolism. *Physiol. Rev.* **58**, 499–527.

2 Bier, D.M., Leake, R.D., Haymond, M.W., Arnold, K.J., Gruenke, L.D., Sperling, M.A. & Kipnis, D.M. (1977): Measurement of 'true' glucose production rates in infancy and childhood with 6,6-dideuteroglucose. *Diabetes* **26**, 1016–1023.

3 Book, S.A. & Bustad, L.K. (1974): The fetal and neonatal pig in biomedical research. *J. Anim. Sci.* **38**, 997–1002.

4 Bougnères, P.F., Saudubray, J.M., Marsac, C., Bernard, O., Odieve, M. & Girard, J.R. (1981): Fasting hypoglycemia due to hepatic carnitine palmitoyl transferase deficiency. *J. Pediatr.* **98**, 742–746.

5 Braude, R., Mitchell, K.G., Newport, M.J. & Porter, J.W.G. (1970): Artificial rearing of pigs. *Br. J. Nutr.* **24**, 501–516.

6 Cornblath, M. & Schwartz, R. (1976): Hypoglycemia in the neonate. In *Disorders of carbohydrate metabolism in infancy* 2nd edn, ed A.J. Schaffer & M. Markowitz, pp. 72–111. Philadelphia: Saunders.

7 Dodds, W.J. (1982): The pig model for biomedical research. *Fed. Proc.* **41**, 247–256.

8 Ducluzeau, R. (1983): Implantation and development of the gut flora in the newborn animal. *Ann. Rech. Vét.* **14**, 354–359.

9 Duée, P.H., Pégorier, J.P., Péret, J. & Girard, J. (1985): Separate effects of fatty acid oxidation and glucagon on gluconeogenesis in isolated hepatocytes from newborn pigs. *Biol. Neonate* **47**, 77–83.

10 Duée, P.H. & Rérat, A. (1975): Etude du besoin en lysine de la truie gestante nullipare. *Ann. Zootech.* **24**, 447–464.

11 Elphick, M.C. & Wilkinson, A.W. (1981): The effects of starvation and surgical injury on the plasma levels of glucose, free fatty acids and neutral lipids in newborn babies suffering from various congenital anomalies. *Pediatr. Res.* **15**, 313–318.

12 Ezekwe, M.O., Ezekwe, E.I., Sen, D.K. & Ogolla, F. (1984): Effects of maternal streptozotocin — diabetes on fetal growth, energy reserves and body composition of newborn pigs. *J. Anim. Sci.* **59**, 974–980.

13 Flecknell, P.A., Wootton, R. & John, M. (1980): Total body glucose metabolism in the conscious, unrestrained piglet and its relation to body-and organ weight. *Br. J. Nutr.* **44**, 193–203.

14 Fomon, S.J., Haschke, F., Ziegler, E.E. & Nelson, S.E. (1981): Body composition of reference children from birth to age 10 years. *Am. J. Clin. Nutr.* **35**, 1169–1175.

15 Ford, S.P., Reynolds, L.P. & Ferrell, C.L. (1984): Blood flow, steroid secretion and nutrient uptake of the gravid uterus during the periparturient period in sows. *J. Anim. Sci.* **59**, 1085–1091.

16 Frazer, T.E., Karl, I.E., Hillman, L.S. & Bier, D.M. (1981): Direct measurement of gluconeogenesis from [2,3 - $^{13}C_2$] alanine in the human neonate. *Am. J. Physiol.* **240**, E615–E621.

17 Girard, J., Duée, P.H., Ferré, P., Pégorier, J.P., Escriva, F. & Decaux, J.F. (1985): Fatty acid oxidation and ketogenesis during development. *Reprod. Nutr. Dévelop.* **25**, 303–319.

18 Girard, J. & Ferré, P. (1982): Metabolic and hormonal changes around birth. In *Biochemical development of the fetus and neonate*, ed C.T. Jones, pp. 517–551. Amsterdam: Elsevier.

19 Hamosh, M. (1982): The development of the metabolic and transport function of the gastrointestinal system. In *Biochemical development of the fetus and neonate*, ed C.T. Jones, pp. 591–619. Amsterdam: Elsevier.

20 Heim, T., Verellen, G., Chessex, P., Putet, G., Reichman, B.L., Swyer, P.R. & Smith, J.M. (1983): Partition of energy metabolism in the very-low-birth-weight infant. In *Intensive care in the newborn*, ed L. Stern, H. Bard & B. Friis-Hansen, pp. 169–181. New York: Masson.

21 Henry, Y. & Etienne, M. (1978): Alimentation énergétique du porc. *Journ. Rech. Porcine en France.* **10**, 119–165.

22 Kalhan, S.C., D'Angelo, L.J., Savin, S.M. & Adam, P.A.J. (1979): Glucose production in pregnant women at term gestation. Sources of glucose for human fetus. *J. Clin. Invest.* **63**, 388–394.

23 Melichar, V., Drahota, Z. & Hahn, P. (1965): Changes in the blood levels of acetoacetate and ketone bodies in newborn infants. *Biol. Neonate* **8**, 348–352.

24 Metcoff, J., Costiloe, J.P., Crosby, W., Bentle, L., Seschachalam, D., Sandstead, H., Bodwell, C.E., Weaver, F. & McClain, P. (1981): Maternal nutrition and fetal outcome. *Am. J. Clin. Nutr.* **34**, 708–721.

25 Miller, K.A. & Field, C.S. (1984): Adolescent pregnancy: a combined obstetric and pediatric management approach. *Mayo Clin. Proc.* **59**, 311–317.

26 Milner, R.D.G. & Hill, D.J. (1984): Fetal growth control: the role of insulin and related peptides. *Clin. Endocrinol.* **21**, 415–433.

27 Newport, M.J. & Henschel, M.J. (1984): Evaluation of the neonatal pig as a model for infant nutrition. *Pediatr. Res.* **18**, 658–662.

28 Pégorier, J.P., Duée, P.H., Assan, R., Péret, J. & Girard, J. (1981): Changes in circulating fuels, pancreatic hormones and liver glycogen concentration in fasting or suckling newborn pigs. *J. Dev. Physiol.* **3**, 203–217.

29 Pégorier, J.P., Duée, P.H., Girard, J.R. & Péret, J. (1982): Development of gluconeogenesis in isolated hepatocytes from fasting or suckling newborn pigs. *J. Nutr.* **112**, 1038–1046.

30 Pégorier, J.P., Duée, P.H., Girard, J. & Péret, J. (1983): Metabolic fate of non-esterified fatty acids in isolated hepatocytes from newborn and young pigs. *Biochem. J.* **212**, 93–97.

31 Pégorier, J.P., Duée, P.H., Simoes-Nunes, C., Péret, J. & Girard, J. (1984): Glucose turnover rate and recycling in unrestrained and unanesthetized 48-h-old fasting or post-absorptive newborn pigs. *Br. J. Nutr.*, **52**, 277–287.

32 Reeds, P.J. & Harris, C.I. (1981): Protein turnover in Animals: Man in his context. In *Nitrogen metabolism in man*, ed J.C. Waterflow & J.M.L. Stephen, pp. 391–408. London: Applied Science Publishers.

33 Sabel, K.G., Olegard, M., Mellander, M. & Hildingsson, K. (1982): Interrelation between fatty acid oxidation and control of gluconeogenic substrates in small-for-gestational-age (SGA) infants with hypoglycemia and with normoglycemia. *Acta Paediatr. Scand.* **71**, 53–61.

34 Saudubray, J.M., Marsac, C., Charpentier, C., Cathelineau, L., Besson Leaud, M. & Leroux, J.P. (1976): Neonatal congenital lactic acidosis with pyruvate carboxylase deficiency in two siblings. *Acta Paediatr. Scand.* **65**, 717–724.

35 Simoes-Nunes, C. (1982): Quelques aspects de l'évolution avec l'âge et de l'adaptation à la composition du régime alimentaire des enzymes digestives. In *Physiologie digestive chez le porc (n° 12)*, pp. 133–151. Paris: INRA.

36 Sparks, J.W., Girard, J.R. & Battaglia, F.C. (1980): An estimate of the caloric requirements of the human fetus. *Biol. Neonate* **38**, 113–119.

37 Van Es, A.J.H. (1977): The energetics of fat deposition during growth. *Nutr. Metab.* **21**, 88–104.

38 Vidnes, J. & Sovik, O. (1976): Gluconeogenesis in infancy and childhood. III. Deficiency of the extramitochondrial form of hepatic phosphoenolpyruvate carboxykinase in a case of persistent neonatal hypoglycaemia. *Acta Paediatr. Scand.* **65**, 307–312.

Baseline biochemical and haematological parameters of neonatal miniature piglets: model for perinatal toxicology

M.A. KHAN*, Arlen O.SAGER*, Zia R. KHATTAK†, R.C. BRAUNBERG*, T.J. SOBOTKA*, and G.S. TRAVLOS‡ (with technical assistance of Vira L. Olivito*)
Beltsville Research Facility, Metabolism Branch (HFF-169), Division of Toxicology, US Food and Drug Administration, Beltsville, MD 20811; †Department of Pediatrics, Union Memorial Hospital, Baltimore, MD 21218; ‡Vetpath, 1 Malcolm Avenue, Teterboro, NY 07608, USA.

The development of various strains of miniature pigs has increased interest in the use of pig models in research because of their physiological and anatomic similarities to humans[8], particularly in infancy[12]. Pigs are particularly useful in nutrition research because of their rapid growth[19] and ability to feed soon after birth. Piglets have been used to evaluate the efficacy of nutrients and to assure nutritional quality of infant feeds[14,15]. Reliable data are needed on the normal physiological and biochemical parameters of pigs at various stages of growth and development, yet only limited data have been published[3,18]. Therefore we decided to collect baseline data for biochemical, physiological, and growth parameters for the strain of miniature pigs kept by the US Food and Drug Administration (FDA).

Materials and methods. Miniature pigs of the FDA's strain (Hormel:Hanford) were used. Sows were farrowed at the Beltsville Research Facility. Piglets older than 6 h received 1 ml of iron dextran within 24 h of birth and again at 21 d. Non-fasted blood samples (15–20 ml) were obtained in Vacutainers through the superior vena cava from the colostrum-free new-born piglets within 1 h of |birth, between 6–8 h, 3 d ± 4 h, 7 d ± 4 h, or 28 d ± 1 d. Blood specimens were obtained between 9 and 11 am except at birth and 6 h of age.

A separate sample (1–2 ml) for haematological parameters was taken in a Vacutainer with NaEDTA as anticoagulant. Two smears were prepared from the anticoagulated blood at the time of bleeding. Blood specimens and smears were picked up the same day by Vetpath Laboratories, where all biochemical and haematological measurements were carried out.

Biochemical measurements of serum were performed on the Prisma automated biochemical profiler (Clinicon, Bromma, Sweden) based on established methods for glucose, cholesterol, blood urea nitrogen (BUN), creatinine, sodium and potassium by flame photometry using internal lithium standards, chloride, phosphorus, calcium, total protein, albumin, globulin, total and direct bilirubin, alkaline phosphatase, lactic dehydrogenase (LDH), gamma-glutamyl transpeptidase (GGTP), glutamic oxaloacetic transaminase (SGOT), and glutamic pyruvic transaminase (SGPT). Complete blood counts were performed on a Coulter-S counter (Coulter Electronics, Hialeah, FL). Differential counts were made by standard manual methods of examination of a blood smear. Statistical analyses were performed by the Student's *t*-test to determine sex differences. Differences among means were considered significant at $P < 0.05$.

Results and discussion. The Table gives data for baseline biochemical and haematological parameters of the FDA strain of miniature pigs during the early phases of growth and development. The progressive rise with age in serum glucose, cholesterol, total protein, and albumin levels may be due to nutrient passage from the gut into the circulation. Humans do not exhibit such a rise at comparable ages[4,7,9]. These data are consistent with findings by others[2,5,11]. A dramatic rise in serum globulin for the first 3 d may reflect unabated absorption of large molecules from the gut for 36 h[19]. BUN values in the piglet are lower than those in the human, possibly due to the pig's more efficient utilization of protein. Mean serum creatinine concentration decreased about 50 per cent in the piglet after birth. The FDA strain has about 50

Table. *Serum biochemical parameters and haematological parameters in miniature pigs.*

Parameter	Birth	6–8 h	3 d	7 d	28 d
Glucose (mmol/l)	4.56 ± 0.44	6.91 ± 0.96	7.14 ± 0.47	9.24 ± 0.3	8.11 ± 0.31
Cholesterol (mmol/l)	1.75 ± 0.10	1.66 ± 0.13	2.93 ± 0.18	3.51 ± 0.03	4.36 ± 0.25
Total protein (g/dl)	2.54 ± 0.07	5.82 ± 0.3	5.88 ± 0.33	6.15 ± 0.13	5.56 ± 0.15
Albumin (g/dl)	0.95 ± 0.07	0.96 ± 0.03	1.53 ± 0.04	2.43 ± 0.08	3.60 ± 0.09
Globulin (g/dl)	1.59 ± 0.08	4.87 ± 0.31	4.35 ± 0.32	3.73 ± 0.12	1.96 ± 0.09
A/G ratio	0.62 ± 0.07	0.21 ± 0.02	0.37 ± 0.03	0.66 ± 0.03	1.88 ± 0.10
BUN (mmol/l)	4.65 ± 0.29	7.80 ± 0.48	6.77 ± 0.48	5.64 ± 0.66	1.72 ± 0.13
Creatinine (μmol/l)	187 ± 11	104 ± 4	83 ± 4	90 ± 4	90 ± 6
Total bilirubin (μmol/l)	4.58 ± 0.47	11.89 ± 1.14	13.4 ± 2.16	14.8 ± 1.24	9.14 ± 0.96
Direct bilirubin (μmol/l)	1.61 ± 0.20	3.46 ± 0.50	2.66 ± 0.44	3.0 ± 0.69	3.15 ± 0.27
Serum enzymes					
Alkaline phosphatase (IU/l)	489 ± 57	651 ± 62	304 ± 26	302 ± 24	125 ± 12
GGTP (U/l)	34 ± 4	91 ± 15	34 ± 2	27 ± 3	24 ± 3
SGOT (IU/l)	88 ± 7	166 ± 14	55 ± 5	52 ± 3	58 ± 9
SGPT (IU/l)	17 ± 1	33 ± 4	42 ± 2	28 ± 3	32 ± 2
LDH (IU/l)	611 ± 27	771 ± 55	751 ± 34	805 ± 53	828 ± 76
Serum electrolytes					
Sodium (mmol/l)	144 ± 0.5	139 ± 1	140 ± 0.6	140 ± 0.8	142 ± 1
Potassium (mmol/l)	5.5 ± 0.24	4.9 ± 0.65	5.4 ± 0.24	5.0 ± 0.18	4.8 ± 0.2
Chloride (mmol/l)	98 ± 0.7	98 ± 1	98 ± 0.7	95 ± 1.6	99 ± 0.5
Calcium (mmol/l)	2.67 ± 0.03	2.54 ± 0.13	3.00 ± 0.04	3.09 ± 0.07	2.72 ± 0.34
Phosphorus (mmol/l)	1.84 ± 0.12	2.20 ± 0.12	3.46 ± 0.20	3.64 ± 0.13	3.03 ± 0.16
Haematological parameters					
Leukocyte count ($\times 10^3$ cells/mm^3)	11 ± 1.1	11 ± 1.2	9 ± 0.7	22 ± 4	13.8 ± 0.9
Erythrocyte count ($\times 10^6$ cells/mm^3)	6.9 ± 0.19	5.4 ± 0.28	4.6 ± 0.26	4.3 ± 0.32	6.7 ± 0.2
Haemoglobin (g/dl)	14.3 ± 0.44	11.8 ± 0.68	9.2 ± 0.41	8.3 ± 0.55	12.5 ± 0.3
Packed cell colume (%)	46 ± 1	38 ± 2	31 ± 2	28 ± 2	40 ± 1
Mean corpuscular volume (fl)	67 ± 1	68 ± 2	67 ± 2	66 ± 1	61 ± 1
Mean corpuscular haemoglobin (pg)	21 ± 0.3	21 ± 0.3	20 ± 0.6	19 ± 0.5	19 ± 0.3
Mean corpuscular haemoglobin conc. (%)	31 ± 0.5	31 ± 0.5	30 ± 0.5	29 ± 0.7	31 ± 0.3
Polymorphonuclear leukocytes (%)	56 ± 4	69 ± 4	49 ± 6	27 ± 3	50 ± 4
Lymphocytes (%)	43 ± 5	27 ± 4	50 ± 7	70 ± 4	47 ± 4
Monocytes (%)	2.4 ± 0.3	2.4 ± 0.2	4.3 ± 0.5	2.7 ± 0.4	2.8 ± 0.3

per cent lower levels of serum creatinine at 28 d of age than Sinclair miniature pigs[6]. The rise in the total and direct bilirubin may reflect immaturity of the piglet's haematopoietic and hepato-biliary systems[1]. No comparative data for these parameters are available for any other strain of miniature pig at these ages.

The high activity of serum enzymes at birth and the significant increase 6–8 h after birth are consistent with observations of other investigators in crossbred domestic pigs[17,20]. The significant decline in the activities of alkaline phosphatase, GGTP, and SGOT beyond the 3rd day of life may represent an adaptation by the piglet to the postnatal environment. A progressive increase in LDH activity agrees with data from miniature[5] and crossbred domestic pigs[18]. Comparative data for GGTP are not available.

Low variability of serum electrolytes may indicate a relatively well developed homoeostatic regulation of electrolyte balance. The rise in serum calcium and phosphorus observed in this study may reflect the electrolyte content of sow's milk[13].

Dynamic changes in the haemogram take place during early growth and development. The decrease in RBC, PCV, and haemoglobin during the first 3 d after birth were similar to reported data[10,11,16,17]. Haemoglobin concentration and PCV were lower in the piglet than in the human. Supplemental iron must be provided to stimulate erythropoiesis in postnatal life of the fast-growing piglet[11].

The data on baseline biochemical and haematological parameters of the neonatal piglet presented in this report will be of value for scientists in making logical selections of experimental models for research in development biology and will enhance the validity of the pig model in biomedical research.

Acknowledgements. The authors thank Roger Mathews, Widmark Johnson, Rusty Long, and Helen Reynolds, without whose help this project could not have been completed.

1 Behrman, R.E. & Vaughan, V.C. (1983): *Nelson's Textbook of pediatrics.* 12th edn. p. 380. Philadelphia: W.B. Saunders.

2 Brooks, C.C. & Davis, J.W. (1969): Changes in haematology of the perinatal pig. *J. Anim. Sci.* **28**, 517–522.

3 Burks, M.F., Evans, P.S. & Tumbleson, M.E. (1974): Haematologic values of malnourished Sinclair (S-1) miniature swine. *Lab. Anim. Sci.* **24**, 84–89.

4 Cloherty, J.P. (1982): *Manual of neonatal care.* pp. 435–437. Boston: Little, Brown.

5 Earl, F.L., Melveger, B.E., Reinwall, J.E. & Wilson, R.L. (1971): Clinical laboratory values of neonatal and weanling miniature pigs. *Lab. Anim. Sci.* **21**, 754–759.

6 Hutcheson, D.P., Tumbleson, M.E. & Middleton, C.C. (1979): Serum electrolyte concentrations in Sinclair (S-1) miniature swine from 1 through 36 months of age. *Growth* **43**, 62–70.

7 Kenp, C.H., Silver, K.H. & O'Brien, D. (1982): *Current pediatrics: diagnosis and treatment.* pp.1062–1070. Los Altos: Lang Publications.

8 Khan, M.A. (1984): Minipig: advantages and disadvantages as a model in toxicity testing. *J. Am. Coll. Toxicol.* **3**, 337–342.

9 Klans, M.H. & Fanaroff, A.A. (1979): *Care of high risk neonate.* pp. 395–399. Philadelphia: W.B. Saunders Co.

10 McCance, R.A. & Widdowson, E.M. (1959): The effect of colostrum on the composition and volume of plasma of newborn piglets. *J. Physiol.* **145**, 547–550.

11 Miller, E.R., Ullrey, D.E., Ackerman, I., Schmidt, D.A., Hoefer, J.A. & Luecke, R.W. (1961): Swine haematology from birth to maturity. I. Serum proteins. *J. Anim. Sci.* **20**, 31–35.

12 Newport, M.J. & Henschel, M.J. (1984): Evaluation of the neonatal pig as a model for infant nutrition: Effects of different proportions of casein and whey protein in milk on nitrogen metabolism and composition of digesta in the stomach. *Pediatr. Res.* **18**, 658–662.

13 Perrin, D.R. (1955): Chemical composition of the colostrum and milk of the sow. *J. Dairy Res.* **22**, 103–107.

14 Schneider, D.L. & Sarett, H.P. (1966): Use of hysterectomy-obtained SPF pig for nutritional studies of the neonate. *J. Nutr.* **89**, 43–48.

15 Schneider, D.L. & Sarett, H.P. (1966): Nutritional studies on hysterectomy-obtained SPF baby pigs fed infant formula products. *J. Nutr.* **89**, 158–164.

16 Tegeris, A.S., Earl, F.L. & Curtis, J.M. (1966): Normal haematological and biochemical parameters of young miniature swine. In *Swine in biomedical research,* ed L.K. Bustad & R.O. McClellan, pp. 575–596. Seattle: Frayn Publishing.

17 Tumbleson, M.E., Hutcheson, D.P. & Fogg, T.J. (1970): Serum biochemic values of fetal and neonatal crossbred swine. In *Advances in automated analysis,* Vol. 2, pp. 149–156. Miami: Thurman.

18 Tumbleson, M.E. & Kalish, P.R. (1972): Serum biochemical and haematological parameters in crossbred swine from birth through eight weeks of age. *Can. J. Comp. Med.* **36**, 202–209.

19 Widdowson, E.M., Colombo, V.E. & Artavanis, C.A. (1976): Changes in the organs of pigs in response to feeding for the first 24 h after birth. II. The digestive tract. *Biol. Neonate* **28**, 272–281.

20 Young, G.A., Jr. & Underdahl, N.R. (1948): Phosphatase activity in suckling pig. *J. Biol. Chem.* **172**, 759–761.

Factors influencing the intestinal absorption of protein in the neonatal piglet and infant

*B. KARLSSON, †I. JAKOBSSON, *B. WESTRÖM, ‡J. SVENDSEN, †T. LINDBERG
Department of Zoophysiology, University of Lund, Helgonavägen 3B, S-22362 Lund; † Departments of Pediatrics and Experimental Research, University of Lund, Malmö General Hospital, S-21401 Malmö; ‡Department of Farm Buildings, Swedish University of Agricultural Sciences, Box 624, S22006 Lund, Sweden.

The complete digestion of food macromolecules is considered to be the normal role of the gastrointestinal tract, but there is increasing experimental and clinical evidence that undigested or partially digested proteins may be absorbed into the systemic circulation of mammals. During fetal and neonatal development a period characterized by enhanced absorption is followed by a period with markedly reduced transport — intestinal (or gut) closure.

The aim of this presentation is to consider a selected number of intracellular and extracellular factors contributing to the physiological regulation of absorption of macromolecules, especially proteins, from the gut lumen to the blood by the epithelium of the small intestine in the neonatal piglet and infant, with emphasis on the piglet.

The cellular basis for absorption of proteins. Enterocytes apparently transport intraluminal proteins to the circulation in two main steps: (a) endocytosis, internalization and intracellular processing of the proteins, and (b) release of these intracellular products to the circulation.

In the fetal pig, the structural apparatus necessary for endocytosis has been observed in the enterocytes, with a well-developed system of apical vesicles, tubules and vacuoles present. In the neonatal pig, endocytosis of proteins and other macromolecules can be detected, at least in the most distal part of the small intestine, from birth up to the age of 3 weeks. However, the endocytosed macromolecules are transported further into the blood in large amounts only in the preclosure piglet. The prominent apical tubular and vacuolar system present in the ileum disappears by the age of 3 weeks[3] and these fetal-type enterocytes are replaced by adult-type enterocytes not capable of endocytosing macromolecules in appreciable amounts[8].

During the growth of the human fetus the enterocytes undergo maturational processes similar to those observed in the postnatal pig, and by term the human small intestine is replete with adult-type enterocytes[5]. It appears as if the process of uptake of macromolecules and their internalization in the enterocyte of the human fetus is well developed, whereas the extent of further transmission of the macromolecules from the enterocytes into the circulation is at the moment unclear.

The endocytosis of proteins may be affected by many factors, and these, in turn will affect the rate of transport of macromolecules to the circulation. Factors in colostrum may enhance the uptake and further absorption of macromolecules by acting directly on the charge of the intestinal membrane. Another factor influencing macromolecular transport at the cellular level is the ability of the microvilli of the enterocyte to change the speed of their movement, thus possibly affecting endocytosis. During the intracellular digestion of endocytosed proteins the lysosomal membrane might be affected, leading to changes in the amount of protein released into the circulation.

Characteristics of intestinal transport. The overall absorption of proteins in the preclosure piglet can reach levels of 50 per cent of the orally-administered protein as compared with levels of about 0.1 per cent for the neonatal term infant and the postclosure piglet.

Using markers in the molecular range of 3 to 70 kD, it was recently shown[9] that the maximum levels of the massive macromolecular transport to the blood in the preclosure pig, were obtained 4 to 12 h after feeding. After this time, there was a steady decrease in absorption, with intestinal closure well developed by 18 h in more than 50 per cent of the piglets, and in all piglets by 36 h. Intestinal closure by the pig appears to exclude molecules larger than about a few kD. The markedly reduced absorption noted at closure was independent of the presence of intestinal proteolytic activity, since the transport of the non-proteolytic susceptible marker FITC-D also ceased at closure.

It has been suggested that the ability of the human gastrointestinal tract to exclude antigenically intact food proteins increases with gestational age, and that gut closure occurs normally before birth. This is illustrated by studies in preterm neonates, particularly those of less than 33 weeks of gestation, who had higher concentrations of β-lactoglobulin in their sera after receiving a formula based on cow's milk than did neonates that had been born at term[7]. Prior feeding with breast-milk did not diminish the amounts of β-lactoglobulin absorbed.

Recent studies have shown that the human neonate is capable of transmitting antigenically intact human α-lactalbumin (isolated from human milk), from the gut into the blood for period of at least 3 months after birth. Moreover, certain food proteins eg, bovine β-lactoglobulin can be transported into the circulation and then to the milk of lactating mothers, resulting in hypersensitivity symptoms appearing in the full-term breast-fed infants[4].

Effect of extracellular factors on absorption. In a series of experiments, we have used the new-born preclosure pig for studying the effects on intestinal macromolecular absorption by sow colostrum, bovine colostrum, sow colostrum trypsin inhibitor, soyabean trypsin inhibitor, a commercial sow milk replacer, protease/protease inhibitor complexes or trypsin[10].

The efficiency of transport appears to be governed by colostrum factors, such as the protease inhibitors and the total protein content. High colostrum protein content probably enhances macromolecular transport by stimulating endocytosis in the enterocytes[1]. The enhancing effect of the protease inhibitors in sow and bovine colostrum is probably due to their reducing gastrointestinal proteolysis leading to an increased amount of proteins in the gut and thus increased endocytosis[2]. However, it should be noted that colostrum alone had a greater enhancing effect on transport than did the addition of both protein and protease to the test-marker system. Therefore, colostrum contains additional factors important for the enhancement of macromolecular intestinal absorption.

There is some question as to whether intraluminal proteases can be transported into the circulation of the neonate. This is of great significance for the neonatal infant, since a specific trypsin inhibitor is not present in human colostrum, although serum-type protease inhibitors have been detected[6]. In the postnatal pig, proteases have been shown to be present in the blood serum as shown in some preliminary experiments. The role of the proteases in the intestinal absorption of proteins and other macromolecules is of considerable interest and is at present under investigation.

Conclusions. On the structural level, the enterocytes of the small intestine in the fetal and neonatal pig and infant have much in common. Species differences are primarily to be sought in the changing proportions between fetal-type and adult-type enterocytes during the ontogeny. For the new-born pig, the most important extracellular factors influencing the intestinal transport of proteins are to be found in homologous colostrum, with the high total protein content and high activity of trypsin inhibitors, especially the specific sow colostrum trypsin inhibitor.

The greatest difference between the neonatal pig and man is that intestinal closure, with its markedly reduced macromolecular absorption, is evident at 18 to 36 h after birth in the sucking pig, whereas closure in man appears to be a more drawn-out process.

The preclosure pig corresponds to fetal stages of development in man that are not available for experimental studies, and may be used for the studies of factors influencing massive intestinal protein absorption. The postclosure piglet appears to be a promising model for studying factors influencing intestinal absorption of proteins in the neonatal infant.

1 Burton, K.A. & Smith, M.W. (1977): Endocytosis and immunoglobulin transport across the small intestine of the newborn pig. *J. Physiol. Lond.* **270**, 473–488.

2 Carlsson, L.C.T., Weström, B.R. & Karlsson, B.W. (1980): Intestinal absorption of proteins by the neonatal piglet fed on sow's colostrum with either natural or experimentally eliminated trypsin-inhibiting activity. *Biol. Neonate.* **38**, 309–320.

3 Clarke, R.M. & Hardy, R.N. (1971): Histological changes in the small intestine of the young pig and their relation to macromolecular uptake. *J. Anat.* **108**, 63–77.

4 Jakobsson, I., Lindberg, T., Benediktsson, B. & Hansson, B.G. (1985): Dietary bovine β-lactoglobulin is transported to human milk. *Acta Paediatr. Scand.* **74**, 342–345.
5 Lecce, J.G. (1984): Absorption of macromolecules by mammalian intestinal epithelium. In *Intestinal toxicology*, ed C.M. Schiller, pp. 33–44. New York: Raven Press.
6 Lindberg, T., Ohlsson, K. & Weström, B. (1982): Protease inhibitors and their relation to protease activity in human milk. *Pediatr. Res.* **16**, 479–483.
7 Roberton, D.M., Paganelli, R., Dinwiddie, R. & Levinsky, R.J. (1982): Milk antigen absorption in the preterm and term neonate. *Archs. Dis. Childh.* **57**, 369–372.
8 Smith, M.W. & Peacock, M.A. (1980): Anomalous replacement of foetal enterocytes in the neonatal pig. *Proc. Roy. Soc. Lond. B* **206**, 411–420.
9 Weström, B.R., Svendsen, J., Ohlsson, B.G., Tagesson, C. & Karlsson, B.W. (1984): Intestinal transmission of macromolecules (BSA and FITC-labelled dextrans) in the neonatal pig. Influence of age of piglet and molecular weight of markers. *Biol Neonate* **46**, 20–26.
10 Weström, B.R., Ohlsson, B.G., Svendsen, J., Tagesson, C. & Karlsson, B.W. (1985): Intestinal transmission of macromolecules (BSA and FITC-dextran) in the neonatal pig: enhancing effect of colostrum, proteins and proteinase inhibitors. *Biol. Neonate* **47**, 359–366.

Dietary hypersensitivity and protective mechanisms in the new-born

F.J. BOURNE
Department of Veterinary Medicine, Langford House, Langford, Bristol BS18 7DU, UK.

A well-developed mucosal immune system exists in mature mammals that is able to protect against infectious disease and to distinguish dietary antigens. The latter is critical in order to avoid the development of tissue damaging allergic reactions and is effected by the mechanisms of immune exclusion, immune elimination and immune tolerance.

I shall address myself in this paper to the question — how well developed the mucosal immune system is in the young animal and how is it influenced by colostrum and milk and also by diet particularly at weaning?

The limited amount of research carried out on immune development in the young pig poses more questions than it has provided answers — nonetheless some interesting findings are emerging. It is evident from early work[12] that the young pig is able to respond to an antigenic challenge *in utero* and that piglets are immmuno-competent at birth. However they are immunologically naive, as a result of the protective effect of the placenta, and rely for early immune protection on colostrum and milk antibody[3]. Following antigenic challenge in the post-natal period, plasma cell development quickly occurs, appearing in the gut at 4 to 5 days of age, a little earlier in tonsils, and a mature profile in the gut lamina propria in terms of cell density is obtained at 3 to 4 weeks of age. Our own work has also shown that a protective immune response can be stimulated in the week-old pig by oral immunization with live *E. coli*.

The above studies indicate that the young pig is capable of B-cell differentiation and of mounting an antibody response. However there is considerable evidence of active suppression of these responses in the young pig[5,10]. The causes include (1) high cortisol levels persisting for the first few days of life, (2) specific suppression by colostrum derived passive antibody (this effect may persist for many weeks), and (3) colostrum deprivation. It is the latter observation that indicates that colostrum can have an immune-enhancing as well as suppressive effect on immune development. In summary, research findings indicate the presence of active populations of both B and T lymphocytes in the new-born pig and that a humoral response can be stimulated although immune suppression may occur in some circumstances.

Much less is known about the development of cell-mediated immunity in the young pig. It has been shown that all elements of the cellular immune system are represented at birth[1] but changes in cell numbers[7] and functional activity[2] do occur in the first few weeks of life. The importance of cell-mediated immune defence mechanisms to viruses has been shown in older pigs by a number of workers but others[4] were unable to demonstrate cytotoxic cells to transmissible gastroenteritis virus in pigs during the first 3 weeks of life. Similarly we have recently shown that while intra epithelial lymphocytes (IELs) in the mature pig are able to respond to mitogens no response could be stimulated in young pigs (3 weeks of age). The functional significance of this is not clear but it is known that IELs have important immune effector activities and it is suggested they may be involved in antigen presentation and immune regulation. We have also shown that early weaning delays the maturation of responsiveness of IELs (7 weeks in unweaned pigs; 10 weeks in pigs weaned at 3 weeks). This observation that weaning suppresses T lymphocyte activity has also been made by other workers. Thus suppression of the humoral immune response to parenteral vaccination in early weaned pigs has been shown[6] and CMI responses have been shown to be reduced in pigs weaned at less than 5 weeks of age[2]. The cause of this suppression is not known and the relative importance of milk withdrawal or dietary change is unclear. Interestingly, our own observations in mice have shown that the inclusion of nutritionally insignificant levels of a novel protein in the diet can result in an altered capacity to present antigen that persists for several days[13].

The relationship between dietary antigens and the mucosal immune response involving the development of oral tolerance to dietary antigens has been widely researched[11]. Studies in the mouse[14] have shown that a short period of hypersensitivity precedes the development of tolerance during which an alteration in dietary presentation can lead to a hypersensitivity response resulting in increased crypt cell division and the appearance of immature enterocytes on the villus. Immune studies have shown this response to be T-cell mediated.

These observations led us to hypothesize that post weaning diarrhoea in the pig associated with a morphologically altered gut with maldigestion and malabsorption may be caused by a dietary hypersensitivity. Early pig experiments stimulating an immune response in the gut of pre-weaned animals and subsequent studies on dietary manipulation and the use of hypoantigenic diets suggest that this hypothesis is correct although the immune mechanisms in the pig have not yet been established[8,9].

The post-weaning changes are seen to result from a crypt cell hyperplasia with immature enterocytes coating the villus. Besides reduced digestive and absorptive capacity, secondary *E. coli.* growth may occur, subsequent to the changes in villous structure, and the increased sensitivity of immature enterocytes to enterotoxin leads to severe diarrhoea.

The influence of the age of the piglet on these events or the influence of colostral and/or milk antibody is not known but experimental evidence from rabbits and guinea pigs have shown that offspring may be tolerized by components of their mothers' milk. These are both areas that require further study.

1 Binns, R.M. (1973): Cellular immunology in the pig. *Proc. R. Soc. Med.* **66**, 1155–1160.
2 Blecha, F., Pollmann, D.S. & Nichols, D.A. (1983): Weaning pigs at an early age decreases cellular immunity. *J. Anim. Sci.* **56**, 396–400.
3 Bourne, F.J. (1977): The mammary gland and neonatal immunity. *Vet. Sci. Comm.* **1**, 141–151.
4 Cepica, A. & Derbyshire, J.B. (1983): Antibody dependent cell cytotoxicity and spontaneous cell mediated cytotoxicity against cells infected with porcine transmissible gastroenteritis virus. *Can. J. Comp. Med.* **47**, 298–303.
5 Cortier, G. & Charley, B. (1978): Influence of colostral antibodies on pig immunisation against hog cholera virus. *Ann. Rech. Vet.* **9**, 245–253.
6 Haye, S.N. & Kornegay, E.T. (1979): Immunoglobulin G, A and M and antibody response in sow reared and artificially reared pigs. *J. Anim. Sci.* **48**, 1116–1122.
7 McCauley, I. & Hartmann, P.E. (1984): Changes in piglet leucocytes, B lymphocytes and plasma cortisol from birth to three weeks after weaning. *Res. Vet. Sci.* **37**, 234–241.
8 Miller, B.G., Newby, T.J., Stokes, C.R. & Bourne, F.J. (1984): Influence of diet on postweaning malabsorption and diarrhoea in the pig. *Res. Vet. Sci.* **36**, 187–193.
9 Miller, B.G., Newby, T.J., Stokes, C.R., Hampson, D.J., Brown, P.J. & Bourne, F.J. (1984): The importance of dietary antigen in the cause of postweaning diarrhoea in pigs. *Am. J. Vet. Res*, **45**, 1730–1733.
10 Muscoplatt, C.C., Setcavage, T.M. & Kim, Y.B. (1977): Regulation of the immune response in neonatal piglets by maternal antibody. *Int. Archs. Allergy Appl. Immunol.* **54**, 165–170.
11 Newby, T.J. & Stokes, C.R. (1984): *Local immune responses of the gut.* Boca Raton USA: CRC Press.
12 Sterzl, J. & Silverstein, A.M. (1967): Developmental aspects of immunity. *Adv. Immunol.* **6**, 337–459.
13 Stokes, C.R., Newby, T.J. & Bourne, F.J. (1983): The influence of oral immunisation on local and systemic immune responses to heterologous antigens. *Clin. Exp. Immunol.* **52**, 399–406.
14 Stokes, C.R., Newby, T.J., Miller, B. & Bourne, F.J. (1984): The immunological significance of transient cell mediated immune reactions to dietary antigens. In *Cell mediated immunity* ed P.J. Quinn, pp. 249–259. Luxembourg: CEC.

RECENT ADVANCES IN FEEDING DURING ORGAN FAILURE

Nutrition in liver failure

I.R. CROSSLEY and R. WILLIAMS

The Liver Unit, King's College Hospital and School of Medicine & Dentistry, Denmark Hill, London SE5 8RX, UK.

In recent years increasing attention has been drawn to the malnutrition associated with the syndromes of liver cell failure with an emphasis on both the clinical importance of nutritional deficiency and the practical difficulties of giving nutritional support to patients.

Incidence and sequelae of malnutrition. The recent nutritional surveys from the Liver Unit at King's College Hospital serve to highlight the frequency of PEM in the patient with chronic liver disease. Between 40 and 60 per cent of 66 cirrhotic patients were found to be malnourished and immuno-incompetent[17], whilst in a further study of 64 patients with acute alcoholic hepatitis, with or without cirrhosis, 23 and 34 per cent, respectively, had a mid-arm muscle circumference and triceps skin-fold thickness below the 5th centile[1].

Impaired host defence mechanisms have long been recognised in the patient with cirrhosis in whom spontaneous bacterial infection is common and a major cause of mortality. In an early study from the Liver Unit[17] 50 per cent of anergic patients died in hospital compared with 18 per cent of those who were reactive to one or more recall antigens, and of those who died while anergic, 91 per cent had a documented bacterial infection of blood, ascites, urine or sputum in the preceding week. Whilst impaired host defence to infection is an undoubted result of underlying liver disease, the close association between anergy and evidence of malnutrition suggest a potentially reversible component to this abnormality.

Nutritional support. The anorexia and nausea often associated with chronic liver disease are frequently compounded by the lack of palatability of food imposed by dietary restriction of sodium needed for control of ascites and protein restriction as part of the management of hepatic encephalopathy. In recent years increasing attention has also been drawn to an additional catabolic state probably induced by hyperglucagonaemia which, with impaired utilization of both carbohydrate and fat, leads to mobilization of amino acids from muscle as an energy source.

In cases with inadequate dietary intake a liquid diet supplement is of particular value. For inpatients with access to a diet kitchen we use a specially formulated 'low-sodium milk shake' of which 1 litre daily provides 96 g protein and 1300 kcal (5.4 MJ) with only 6 mmol sodium. There will remain, however, a proportion of patients with severe anorexia who are unable to take in adequate nutrients even with the use of supplements, and in such cases feeding via a fine-bore naso-enteric tube is next tried.

Enteral nutrition. Most of the proprietary tube feeds readily available are too high in sodium for general use in liver disease. In conjunction with the dietetic department, we have devised a nutritionally complete liquid diet which is suitable for tube-feeding. The available low-sodium constituents are relatively high in viscosity and osmolality and, in order to pass through a fine-bore tube and to lower osmotic load on the gut, a relatively high fluid volume is needed to administer this formula, which provides 35 g protein, 1000 kcal (4.2 MJ) and only 9 mmol sodium per litre. The liquid diet is administered by continuous infusion 2 to 3 l/d over 24 h starting with a half-strength regimen for the first 2 d to prevent osmotic diarrhoea. Of the proprietary tube feeds, Clinifeed ISO (Roussell) or low-sodium Fortison (Cow & Gate) have the highest protein to sodium ratio. One litre of the latter provides 36 g protein, 1000 kcal (4.2 MJ) and 11 mmol sodium.

In the patient with encephalopathy precipitated by dietary protein, or with signs of chronic portal systemic encephalopathy, it is difficult to supplement dietary intake of protein and efforts should be directed towards increasing energy intake with preparations such as Hycal or Fortical, which provide 1700 kcal (7.1 MJ)/l, to improve utilization of whatever protein can be tolerated. There may be a place for branched-chain amino acid (BCAA)-enriched nitrogen sources such as Hepaticaid (Boots) which may be both better tolerated than conventional protein and have specific anti-catabolic effects. This compound may be used as a dietary supplement, but it is not a nutritionally complete diet and does not contain electrolytes, minerals, trace elements or vitamins.

Parenteral nutrition and use of branched-chain amino acids. Decompensated cirrhosis is characterized by an abnormal amino acid profile which has been implicated in the pathogenesis of encephalopathy and has led to the suggestion that BCAA may be the preferred source of nitrogen in such patients. Raised plasma concentrations of glycogen stimulate muscle catabolism with release of amino acids for gluconeogenesis[10]. When hepatic function is poor, however, the uptake and metabolism of the aromatic amino acids in impaired and plasma levels rise[18]. In contrast, with BCAA, valine, leucine and isoleucine are preferentially metabolized in muscle and fat and their concentrations fall, in part due to enhanced uptake as a result of hyperinsulinism[10,16]. These two groups of amino acids compete for entry through the blood-brain barrier and transport of the toxic aromatic amino acids tyrosine and phenylalanine may be facilitated by the low concentrations of BCAA giving rise to an imbalance of cerebral neurotransmitters and the development of encephalopathy[14,19].

Infusion of BCAA lowers the plasma concentrations and decreases the brain uptake of the toxic aromatic amino acids[5,22]. Their use, either intravenously or in oral form, has been advocated on the grounds that correction of this abnormal plasma amino acid profile in patients with liver failure would be beneficial for encephalopathy. In addition BCAA are thought to play a regulatory role in the efflux of amino acids from muscle[16] and as endogenous protein catabolism is enhanced in cirrhosis and contributes significantly to the plasma amino acid imbalance, suppression of muscle catabolism would be beneficial not only to nutritional status but also to encephalopathy.

Nevertheless, controversy continues to surround which type of amino acid formulation, conventional or branched-chain-enriched, is better for parenteral nutrition in liver failure. Many conventional solutions are available and a branched-chain-enriched preparation containing decreased amounts of phenylalanine, tyrosine and tryptophan is available as FO80 (McGaw). A similar product is marketed by Travenol.

Although several studies have suggested that conventional amino acid solutions are poorly tolerated and precipitate encephalopathy in the cirrhotic[6,7] and while this may indeed be so in some patients with end-stage disease, it is not so in other groups of patients. In those with acute alcoholic hepatitis and cirrhosis, for example, our experience that intravenous infusion of 70–85 g conventional amino acids daily does *not* exacerbate encephalopathy has been confirmed by others[15].

BCAA-enriched preparations can achieve positive nitrogen balance, although 80–100 g daily are frequently required, and recent reports have suggested that formulations such as FO80 may not be a complete protein source when used alone since hypotyrosinaemia and hypocystinaemia occur in cirrhotic patients following the use of such parenteral nutrition solutions devoid of these amino acids and are associated with failure to achieve metabolic balance[13,21]. Although the theoretical advantage of ameliorating encephalopathy is attractive, from the controlled studies currently available[2,12,20,24] no clear picture has emerged as to the value of formulations such as FO80 with respect to encephalopathy.

Our current practice is therefore based on the use of conventional amino acids initially. The Synthamin range (Travenol) is chosen on the grounds of flexibility of concentration and availability, both with and without electrolytes, as sodium restriction is commonly required. The patient is started on a regimen providing 7 g nitrogen daily via a 3 litre bag administration system, and is subsequently increased to 14 g nitrogen/24 h, depending upon nitrogen balance, providing there is no neurological deterioration. Should this occur the amino acid content is temporarily reduced by half and reintroduced with half of the nitrogen supplied as a BCAA source. Glucose is given to provide a minimum energy: nitrogen ratio of 150 kcal (628 kJ)/g. Calcium, magnesium and trace element requirements are provided by the substitution of a daily dose of electrolyte solution A (Travenol) for a bottle of 20 per cent glucose or by the addition of a concentrate (eg, Addamol, Kabivitrum). High potency B and C vitamins (Parenterovite HP — ampoules 1 and 2, Bencard) and folic acid 5 mg and vitamin K 10 mg are added to the TPN solution. Although we use a maximum volume of 2500 ml TPN solution daily, volume restriction is not infrequently required because of hyponatraemia. Concentrations of amino acid solutions and glucose are easily adjusted with this regimen to provide the required solutes in the desired volume.

Current studies in chronic encephalopathy and alcoholic hepatitis. Recent studies have focused principally upon the therapeutic effect of either vegetable protein or BCAA supplementation upon encephalopathy rather than nutritional status. Three studies[3,8,23] now suggest that vegetable-protein diets are better tolerated than animal protein. In addition it has been shown[3] that nitrogen balance is greater with vegetable than with meat protein. A vegetarian diet is unlikely to hold favour with many, however, because of gastrointestinal side-effects. Although BCAA supplementation appears to have little beneficial effect upon encephalopathy in some studies[5,11] its use has not been detrimental and may provide a way of increasing nitrogen intake without exacerbating encephalopathy. A recent study of 37 protein-intolerant patients fed conventional protein or Hepaticaid[9] showed that with a comparable nitrogen intake only one of 17 in the BCAA group developed encephalopathy compared to seven of 20 in the conventional protein group. Nitrogen balance studies obtained in 11 patients were not significantly different.

A significant reduction in mortality in patients with acute alcoholic hepatitis treated with parenteral nutrition has been demonstrated[15]. The control group were offered a conventional diet whilst the treatment group received an additional 70–85 g of intravenous amino acid daily. These results are at variance with our own controlled study[1] in 64 patients with acute alcoholic hepatitis and cirrhosis. A further controlled randomized study of parenteral nutrition in alcoholic hepatitis[4] for one month did not demonstrate any clinical advantage at the end of the study, although initial improvement was more rapid in the treated group.

1 Calvey, H., Davis, M. & Williams, R. (1985): Controlled trial of nutritional supplementation, with and without branched chain amino acid enrichment in treatment of acute alcoholic hepatitis. *J. Hepatol.* **1**, 141–145.

2 Cerra, F.B., Cheung, N.K., Fischer, J.E., Kaplowitz, N., Schiff, E.R., Dienstag, J.L., Mabry, C.D., Leevy, C.M. & Kiernan, T. (1982): A multi-center trial of branched chain enriched amino acid infusion FO80 in hepatic encephalopathy (Abstr). *Hepatology* **2**, 699.

3 De Bruijn, K.M., Blendis, L.M., Zilm, D.H., Carlen, P.L. & Anderson, G.M. (1983): Effect of dietary protein manipulations in sub-clinical portal systemic encephalopathy. *Gut* **24**, 53–60.

4 Diehl, A.M., Bortnoff, J.K., Herlang, F. Potter, J.J., Van Duyn, M.A., Chandler, E. & Mezey, E. (1985): Effect of parenteral amino acid supplementation in alcoholic hepatitis. *Hepatology* **5**, 57–63.

5 Eriksson, L.S., Persson, A., Wahren, J. (1982): Branched-chain amino acids in the treatment of chronic hepatic encephalopathy. *Gut* **23**, 801–806.

6 Freund, H., Dienstag, J., Lehrieh, J., Yoshimura, N., Bradford, R.R., Rosen, H., Atarnian, S., Slemmer, E., Holroyde, J., Fischer, J. (1982): Infusion of branched chain enriched amino acid solution in patients with hepatic encephalopathy. *Ann. Surg.* **196**, 208–220.

7 Galambos, J.T., Hersh, T., Fulenwider, J.T., Ansley, J.D. & Rudman, D. (1979): Hyperalimentation in alcoholic hepatitis. *Am. J. Gastroenterol.* **72**, 535–41.

8 Greenberger, N.J., Carley, J. & Schenker, S. (1977): Effects of vegetable and protein diets in chronic hepatic encephalopathy. *Am. J. Dig. Dis.* **22**, 845–55.

9 Horst, D., Grace, N.D., Conn, H.O., Schiff, E., Schenker, S., Viteri, A., Law, D. & Atterbury, C.E. (1984): Comparison of dietary protein with an oral branched-chain-enriched amino acid supplement in chronic portal-systemic encephalopathy. *Hepatology* **4**, 279–287.

10 Marchesini, G., Forlani, G., Zoli, M.N., Angiolini, A., Scolari, M.P., Bianchi, F.B., Pisi, E. (1979): Insulin and glucogen levels in liver cirrhosis. Relationship with plasma amino acid imbalance of chronic hepatic encephalopathy. *Dig. Dis. Sci.* **24**, 594–601.

11 McGhee, A., Henderson, M., Millikan, W.J., Blerer, J.C., Vogel, R., Kassouny, M., Rudman, D. (1983): Comparison of the effects of hepatic aid and a casein modular diet on encephalopathy, plasma amino acids and nitrogen balance in cirrhotic patients. *Ann. Surg.* **197**, 288–93.

12 Michel, H., Pomier-Layrargues, G., Duhamel, O., Lacombe, B., Cuilleret, G. & Bellet, H. (1980): Intravenous infusion of ordinary and modified amino acid solutions in the management of hepatic encephalopathy. *Gastroenterology* **79**, 1038 (Abstr.).

13 Millikan, W.J., Henderson, J.M., Warren, W.D., Riepe, S.P., Kitner, M.H., Wright-Bacon, L., Epstein, C. & Parks, R.B. (1983): *Ann. Surg.* **197**, 294–304.

14 Munro, W.J., Fernstrom, J.D. & Wurtman, R.S. (1975): Plasma neutral amino acids and hypertrophy in cirrhosis. *Lancet* **2**, 419–21.

15 Nasrallah, S.M. & Galambos, A.S.L. (1980): Amino acid therapy of alcoholic hepatitis. *Lancet* **2**, 1276–77.

16 Odessey, R. & Goldberg, A.L. (1972): Oxidation of leucine by rat skeletal muscle. *Am. J. Physiol.* **223**, 1376–83.

17 O'Keefe, S.J., El Zayadi, A.R., Carraher, A.R., Davis, M., Williams, R. (1980): Malnutrition and immuno incompetence in patients with liver disease. *Lancet* **2**, 615–17.

18 O'Keefe, S.J., Abraham, R. El Zayadi, A.R., Marshall, W., Davis, M. & Williams, R. (1981): Increased plasma tyrosine concentrations in patients with cirrhosis and fulminant hepatic failure associated with increased plasma tyrosine flux and reduced hepatic oxidation capacity. *Gastroenterology* **81**, 1017–24.

19 Oldendorf, W.H. & Szabo, J. (1976): Amino acid assignment to one of the three blood-brain barrier amino acid carriers. *Am. J. Physiol.* **230**, 96–106.

20 Rossi-Fanelli, F., Riggio, O., Cengiano, C., Cascino, A., De Conciliis, D., Merli, M., Stortom, M., Giunchi, G. & Capacaccia, L. (1982): Branched chain amino acids vs Lactulose in the treatment of hepatic coma. A controlled study. *Dig. Dis. Sci.* **27**, 929–35.

21 Rudman, D., Kitner, M. & Ansley, J.D. (1981): Hypotyrosinaemia, hypocystinaemia and failure to retain nitrogen during total parenteral nutrition of cirrhotic patients. *Gastroenterology* **81**, 1025–35.

22 Sato, Y., Eriksson, S., Hagenfeldt, L. & Lahren, J. (1981): Influence of branched chain amino acid infusion on arterial concentrations and brain exchange of amino acids in patients with hepatic cirrhosis. *Clin. Physiol.* **1**, 151–65.

23 Uribe, M., Marquez, M.A., Mata, J., Guevara, L., Garcia-Ramos, G. & Ramos, C. (1980): Treatment of chronic portal systemic encephalopathy with vegetable protein diets. *Gastroenterology* **79**, 1128–32.

24 Wahren, J., Denis, J., Desurmont, P., Eriksson, L.S., Escoffier, J., Gauthier, A.P., Hagenfeldt, L., Miehel, H., Opolon, P., Paris, J.C. & Veyrae, M. (1983): Is intravenous administration of branched chain amino acids effective in the treatment of hepatic encephalopathy? A multi-center study. *Hepatology* **3**, 475–80.

Recent advances in feeding during renal failure

P-O. ATTMAN
Department of Nephrology, University of Göteborg, Sahlgrenska Sjukhuset, S-413 45 Göteborg, Sweden.

Treatment of uraemia. The role of diet in the treatment of patients with chronic renal failure is now well established[8]. Protein restriction reduces the accumulation of nitrogenous metabolites and uraemic symptoms and may thereby postpone dialysis.

The potential of the dietary treatment is demonstrated by our results from 1978–1982 when 105 patients with uraemic symptoms and a glomerular filtration rate (GFR) below 10 ml/min per 1.73 m² began treatment. The median time of diet was 7.6 months with one-third of the patients being treated for 12 months or more. When GFR had decreased to around 4 ml/min, the uraemic intoxication could no longer be controlled by diet and dialysis became mandatory.

The extent of protein restriction required to affect the symptoms and to reduce the urea levels depends on the residual renal function and only when the GFR is below 10 ml/min is it necessary to reduce the dietary protein intake to 20–25 g/d. With such a low protein intake the diet has to be supplemented with the essential amino acids and histidine to achieve nitrogen balance.

Amino acid supplementation. The essential amino acids have hitherto generally been provided in proportions according to the classical work of Rose but there is now mounting evidence that the requirements for uraemic patients are different. Studies of intra and extracellular amino acid patterns have revealed marked abnormalities[1]. Patients treated with protein-restricted diet supplemented with the conventional amino acid preparations even in large amounts still have low intracellular concentrations of valine, tyrosine and serine. This can partly be corrected by increasing the amounts of valine and tyrosine, showing that the amino acid abnormalities in uraemia can be influenced by nutritional means. Thus, histidine, tyrosine and possibly serine may be considered to be essential amino acids in uraemia. The beneficial effect of the correction of these amino acid abnormalities is demonstrated by a concomitant improvement in nitrogen balance.

Keto- or hydroxy- analogues of certain essential amino acids have been introduced to maintain nitrogen balance at a lower total nitrogen intake than with conventional supplementation. There are, however, divergent opinions as to the superiority of the keto acids and at present amino acids remain the first choice for supplementing a 20 g protein diet.

Nutritional status. The clinical benefit of the diet depends on whether the long-term treatment carries a risk of malnutrition or worsening of the metabolic abnormalities inherent in chronic renal failure. The dietary treatment might then be an inferior substitute for dialysis that would otherwise have to be instituted.

There are considerable difficulties in identifying early malnutrition in renal failure patients since many of the parameters commonly used to determine nutritional status are influenced by the renal failure itself and, thus, of little or no value for assessment of nutritional status in uraemic patients. The net result of anabolic and catabolic influences on the individual is reflected in body composition. Determination of total body potassium is a reliable assessment of body cell mass in both normal individuals and in patients with chronic renal failure. Our studies on body composition indicate that it is possible to maintain body cell mass even after 12 months or more of treatment[2].

Lipid and carbohydrate metabolism. One aspect of the provision of considerable amounts of carbohydrate and fat in the diet in renal failure is a possible derangement of lipid and carbohydrate metabolism that resembles type IV hyperlipoproteinaemia. These disturbances appear to be a consequence of a reduced plasma lipolytic activity, with accumulation of triglyceride-rich lipoproteins of low or intermediate density and a reduced clearance of exogenous triglycerides. Our extensive investigations of lipid and carbohydrate metabolism during dietary treatment do not, however, indicate such a detrimental influence[3,5].

Diabetic patients with uraemia can also be treated with as good results as for non-diabetics[4].

Dietary treatment in children. In children the first manifestation of uraemic toxicity is a retardation of growth, which may persist during dialysis. We have recently found that, if treatment with a low-protein diet is instituted early, when the retardation of growth has already begun, children can continue to grow and, in some instances, even catch up to normal growth for age. These results indicate that diet influences basal pathophysiological mechanisms of uraemia[11].

Dietary factors and progression of renal disease. In recent years new evidence has emerged that treatment with low-protein diets may be beneficial not only in symptomatic renal failure but also in influencing the rate of progression of earlier stages of renal disease[10].

In experimental renal failure in rats it has been found that a reduction of protein intake results in a considerable prolongation of life. It has been postulated that a normal protein intake, which initially increases GFR in experimental renal failure, contributes to an increase in glomerular pressure and flow. This hyperfiltration in the remnant glomeruli could then wear them out to produce a progressive glomerulosclerosis. Such haemodynamic changes may be prevented by a reduction in protein intake, thus protecting the individual with the compromized renal function[7]. It is, however, important to point out that, although this hypothesis may be applicable to experimental renal failure, there is so far less evidence of its relevance in man with renal failure from chronic disease.

A clinical counterpart to the experimental situation may be found in kidney donors. We have investigated 44 donors 10–18 years after nephrectomy and found no deterioration of renal function in the remaining kidney. There was even a positive correlation between the actual protein intake and the compensatory increase in GFR after nephrectomy. Thus, a normal protein intake does not seem harmful to glomerular performance in healthy human kidneys on a long-term basis even after 50 per cent reduction of renal mass[9].

Patients with diabetes mellitus often develop progressive nephropathy, but the rate of progression varies considerably in different individuals. We have studied the protein intake in three groups of juvenile diabetic patients with similar duration of disease: patients with no evidence of nephropathy, patients with a reduced but stable renal function over several years, and patients with progressive deterioration of renal function. There was no difference in protein intake between the groups and no correlation between the rate of progression and the protein intake of individual patients (Nyberg *et al.*, submitted for publication).

These findings do not support reports of the beneficial effects of early protein reduction in experimental and human renal disease[6]. The matter is thus far from settled and prospective studies are needed to separate the effect of protein reduction, if any, from that of other factors known to influence the progression of renal disease, such as control of blood pressure, phosphate metabolism, and also the well-known effect of paying more attention to the patient.

Conclusion. The supplemented low-protein diet is a safe treatment for the patient with advanced renal failure. More research is however needed to define the optimal composition of both diet and supplement to ensure adequate nutrition. Further studies may also indicate a role for protein restriction in the earlier stages of the disease, which would be a major breakthrough in our efforts to prevent renal failure.

1 Alvestrand, A., Furst, P. & Bergström, J. (1982): Plasma and muscle free amino acids in uremia: influence of nutrition with amino acids. *Clin. Nephrol.* **18**, 297–305.

2 Attman, P-O., Ewald, J. & Isaksson, B. (1980): Body composition during long-term treatment of uremia with amino acid supplemented low protein diet. *Am. J. Clin. Nutr.* **33**, 801–810.

3 Attman, P-O. & Gustafson, A. (1980): Lipid and carbohydrate metabolism in uremia. Influence of treatment with protein-reduced diet and essential amino acids. *Nutr. Metab.* **24**, 261–280.

4 Attman, P-O., Bucht, H., Larsson, O. & Uddebom, G. (1983): Protein-reduced diet in diabetic renal failure. *Clin. Nephrol.* **19**, 217–220.

5 Attman, P-O., Gustafson, A., Alaupovic, P. & Wang, C-S. (1984): Effect of protein-reduced diet on plasma lipids, apolipoproteins and lipolytic activities in patients with chronic renal failure. *Am. J. Nephrol.* **4**, 92–98.

6 Bergström, J. (1984): Discovery and rediscovery of low protein diet. *Clin. Nephrol.* **21**, 29–35.

7 Brenner, B.M., Meyer, T.W. & Hostetter, T.H. (1982): Dietary protein intake and the progressive nature of kidney disease: the tole of hemodynamically mediated injury in the pathogenesis of progressive glomerular sclerosis in aging, renal ablation, and intrinsic renal disease. *New Engl. J. Med.* **307**, 652–659.

8 Giovanetti, S. (1985): Dietary treatment of chronic renal failure: Why is it not used more frequently? *Nephron* **40**, 1–12.

9 Mathillas, Ö., Attman, P-O., Aurell, M., Blohmé, I., Brynger, H., Granerus, G. & Westberg, G. (1984): Long-term outcome of renal function and proteinuria in kidney transplant donors. *Proc. EDTA-ERA* **21**, 574–578.

10 Rosman, J.B., Meijer, S., Sluiter, M.J., Ter Wee, P.M., Piero-Becht, T.P. & Doncker, A.J.M. (1984): Prospective randomised trial of early dietary protein restriction in chronic renal failure. *Lancet* **2**, 1292–1296.

11 Sigström, L., Attman, P-O., Jodal, U. & Odenman, I. (1984): Growth during treatment with low-protein diet in children with renal failure. *Clin. Nephrol.* **21**, 152–158.

Nutritional support in pancreatic failure

R.K. TANDON
Department of Gastroenterology, All India Institute of Medical Sciences, New Delhi — 110 029, India.

Nutritional support in pancreatic failure can best be discussed under two headings: acute pancreatitis and chronic pancreatic failure.

Acute pancreatitis. Intensive nutritional support is required in this setting to: (a) compensate for the catabolic state; (b) tide the patient over a prolonged period of starvation following nasogastric suction and/or the inability to consume normal meals because of abdominal pain and ileus; and (c) provide rest to the pancreas. A special requirement is that exocrine pancreatic stimulation should be minimal.

Total parenteral nutrition (TPN). One of the major advances in therapeutics has been the development of TPN. This form of nutritional support has been widely shown to cause minimal pancreatic stimulation[15,19,25] and is not affected by the state of the bowel (ileus, improper digestion or assimilation). TPN has therefore been extensively used in the early stages of acute pancreatitis[1,10,21] and has been shown to provide significant benefit to many patients — one study showing[2] that addition of TPN to the treatment regimen led to a reduction in mortality from 22.4 to 15.6 per cent in patients with acute pancreatitis undergoing surgery.

Elemental diet (ED). Because of the high cost and frequent complications of TPN, a parallel development in clinical nutrition has been the perfection of chemically-formulated, partially-predigested, residue-free liquid diets for oral administration[7,18]. Experimental and clinical observations have consistently shown that enteral diets provide greater energy and nitrogen supplies and hence a better and faster re-establishment of body weight and muscle mass than TPN[19,20,27]. Their effect on pancreatic stimulation is, however, controversial as is their role in acute pancreatitis. Some authors have found elemental diets to be stimulatory for the exocrine pancreas[5,18,28] while others disagreed[18,23,27]. The consensus of opinion at the present is that bypassing the stomach and duodenum and delivering the ED into the jejunum is associated with minimal pancreatic stimulation[18,20,23,25]. Hence, ED fed through a jejunostomy tube is being widely used for providing nutrition in acute pancreatitis. Its relatively lower cost and better tolerance as compared with TPN are factors in its favour. Its successful use by the oral route is also on record[21].

Polymeric diets. Elemental diets still remain costly and much scepticism has appeared lately as to their reputation of increased efficacy over simpler polymeric diets[7,18]. In one study[26], pancreatic secretions of lipase and chymotrypsin in response to ED and a crushed food homogenate were studied in normal subjects. The results indicated that both diets stimulated pancreatic enzyme secretion in proportion to their nitrogen content and that ED had no advantage over polymeric diets. Recently, enteral nutrition by alimentation jejunostomy using mixed diets has been shown to be successful in severe acute pancreatitis[20]. Enteral nutrition begun on the 6th or 7th post-operative day provided 2500–3000 kcal (10.5–12.5 MJ)/d for 30–45 d and was well tolerated.

The following therapeutic scheme would thus appear rational for acute pancreatitis[21]: (1) TPN for the first 6–10 d; (2) From 6th to 30th d ED is added, preferably through a jejunostomy tube, and (3) thereafter, gradual alimentation is carried out, first using medium-chain fatty acids and then a balanced oral diet.

Chronic pancreatitis. Nutritional support to the patient with chronic pancreatitis is a long-term measure since this disease is usually irreversible and incurable. The most logical mode of therapy is pancreatic enzyme replacement but nutritional support on a long-term basis is necessary in many patients with severe malabsorption and cachexia.

Enzyme replacement. When malabsorption is manifest, about 90 per cent of the exocrine pancreas is believed to have been destroyed, so that 5–10 per cent of the normal pancreatic enzyme output should reach the duodenum to abolish the malabsorption[6]. Lipase is the most vulnerable and important of the pancreatic enzymes. It has been estimated that about 30 000 i.u. of this enzyme will be required daily for correcting the compromised lipid digestion. Even if we estimate the lowest possible enzyme requirement, the daily requirement of lipase would be about 10 000 i.u.[6]. To deliver this amount of lipase in an active form into the duodenum, the gastric pH must be maintained above 4 for 60 min and the duodenal pH above 4 for 90 min. Antacids and cimetidine have been used extensively for achieving and maintaining this level of pH and the results so far suggest that cimetidine may be the best drug for this purpose because of the ease of administration and lack of side effects[2,5,14]. Aluminium hydroxide and sodium bicarbonate may be equally effective but with prolonged use carry certain objectionable side effects[3]. Magnesium and calcium based antacids do not provide much benefit and, they may even aggravate steatorrhoea[14]. Calcium salts form precipitates with glycine-conjugated bile acids and cause a depletion of the bile acid pool which may in turn compromise further lipid digestion. Antacids have to be administered at the beginning as well as the end of each meal.

Another approach to bypass the acid induced destruction of the pancreatic enzymes has been to provide the enzymes in an enteric coated tablet form[11,13]. Such tablets, however, pose the problem of delayed exit from the stomach and hence of creating a discordance between the delivery of the enzymes into the duodenum and the peak of intraluminal digestion[4,12]. Also, if the enteric coated tablets stay in the stomach for a prolonged period and the pH in the stomach rises above 5.5 the enteric coat is released and the enzymes destroyed. To obviate all these problems, particularly the prolonged gastric retention, the enteric coated pancreatic preparations have been provided in microsphere form[11,13]. At least in cystic fibrosis patients, the microsphere preparations have been shown to be more effective than the ordinary enteric coated preparations in terms of reducing steatorrhoea[11].

Another novel method employed for supplementing the pancreatic enzymes has been the use of bromelains, a mixture of proteolytic plant enzymes prepared from the fresh fruits and stalk of the pineapple. Bromelains added to pancreatin and ox bile have been shown to increase significantly the digestive capacity of the pancreatic preparations[8,9,17].

Dietary therapy. TPN is obviously impractical in the chronic condition. Reliance has therefore to be placed on enteral feeding. Medium-chain triglycerides (MCT), ie caproic and capric acids, could be a very useful nutritional supplement because they are acted on more readily by the pancreatic enzymes than long-chain triglycerides, and they can enter directly into the portal vein or mucosal cells without undergoing hydrolysis because of their small molecular size. However, MCT are unpalatable and may produce dumping and, occasionally, hepatic encephalopathy[15].

Polymeric diets have been shown to be equally effective, if not superior to elemental diets in providing nutrition to chronic pancreatitis patients. In fact, nitrogen utilization might be better with polymeric than with elemental diets[22].

Lastly, in a specific condition such as exocrine pancreatic insufficiency secondary to protein-energy malnutrition, correction of the latter has been shown to correct the deranged exocrine functions of the pancreas[24].

1 Bazan, P., Agnello, G. & Lanza, V. (1982): The role of artificial nutrition in the treatment of acute pancreatitis. In *Controversies in acute pancreatitis*, ed L.F. Hollander, pp. 288–292. Berlin, Heidelberg and New York: Springer-Verlag.
2 DiMagno, E.P. (1979): Medical treatment of pancreatic insufficiency. *Mayo Clin. Proc.* **54**, 435–442.
3 DiMagno, E.P. (1982): Controversies in the treatment of exocrine pancreatic insufficiency. *Dig. Dis. Sci.* **27**, 481–484.
4 DiMagno, E.P., Malagelada, J.R., Go, V.L.W. and Moertel, C.G. (1977): Fate of orally ingested enzymes in pancreatic insufficiency: a comparison of two dosage schedules. *New Engl. Jour. Med.* **296**, 1318–1322.
5 Duric, P.R., Bell, L., Linton, W., Corey, M. and Forstner, G.G. (1980): Effect of cimetidine and sodium bicarbonate on pancreatic replacement therapy in cystic fibrosis. *Gut* **2**, 778–786.
6 Dutta, S.K., Rubin, J. & Harvey, J. (1983): Comparative evaluation of the therapeutic efficacy of a pH-sensitive enteric-coated pancreatic enzyme therapy in the treatment of exocrine pancreatic insufficiency. *Gastroenterology* **84**, 476–482.

7 Freeman, J.B. & Egan, M.C. (1976): The elemental diet. *Surg. Gynaecol. Obstet.* **143**, 925–982.
8 Geevarghese, P.J. & Kutty, M.A. (1980): Pancreatic extracts in pancreatic steatorrhoea. *Indian Practitioner* **33**, 73–79.
9 Goebell, H. & Bode, C. (1969): Untersuchungen zur Substitutionsbehandlung mit Pankreasenzym — Preparaten. *Med. Welt (Stuttg.)* **20**, 877–84.
10 Goodgame, J.T. & Fischer, J.E. (1977): Parenteral nutrition in the treatment of acute pancreatitis. *Ann. Surg.* (Suppl. 5) **186**, 651–658.
11 Gow, R., Francis, P., Bradbear, R. & Shepherd, R. (1981): Comparative study of varying regimes to improve steatorrhoea and creatorrhoea in cystic fibrosis: effectiveness of an enteric-coated preparation with and without antacids and cimetidine. *Lancet* **2**, 1071–1074.
12 Graham, D.Y. (1977): Enzyme replacement therapy of exocrine pancreatic insufficiency in man: Relation between in vitro enzyme activities and in vivo potency in commercial pancreatic extracts. *New. Engl. J. Med.* **296**, 1314–1317.
13 Graham, D.Y. (1979): An enteric-coated pancreatic enzyme preparation that works. *Dig. Dis. Sci.* **24**, 906–909.
14 Graham, D.Y. (1982): Pancreatic enzyme replacement: the effect of antacids or cimetidine. *Dig. Dis. Sci.* **27**, 485–490.
15 Greenberger, N.J. & Skillman, T.G. (1969): Medium-chain triglycerides: physiologic considerations and clinical implications. *New. Engl. J. Med.* **280**, 1045–1058.
16 Kelly, G.A. & Nahrwold, D.L. (1976): Pancreatic secretion in response to an elemental diet and intravenous hyperalimentation. *Surg. Gynaecol. Obstet.* **143**, 87–91.
17 Knill-Jones, R.P., Pearce, H., Batten, J. & Williams, R. (1970): Comparative trial of Nutrizyme in chronic pancreatic insufficiency. *Br. Med. J.* **4**, 21–24.
18 Koretz, R.L. & Meyer, J.H. (1980): Elemental diets — facts and fantasies. *Gastroenterology* (Suppl 7) **78**, 398–410.
19 Lickley, H.L.A., Track, N.S., Vranic, M. & Bury, K.D. (1978): Metabolic responses to enteral and parenteral nutrition. *Am. J. Surg.* **135**, 172–176.
20 Maillet, P. (1982): Enteral nutrition by alimentation jejunostomy in 11 cases of severe acute pancreatitis. In *Controversies in acute pancreatitis*, ed L.F. Hollander, pp. 283–287 Berlin, Heidelburg and New York: Springer-Verlag.
21 Motton, G., Pistorelli, C., Fracastoro, G. *et al.* (1982): Role of complete parenteral treatment nutrition in acute pancreatitis. In *Controversies in acute pancreatitis*, ed L.F. Hollander, pp. 293–296. Berlin, Heidelberg and New York: Springer-Verlag.
22 Nasrallah, S.M. & Martin, D.M. (1984): Comparative effects of Criticare HN and Vivonex HN in the treatment of malnutrition due to pancreatic insufficiency. *Am. J. Clin. Nutr.* **39**, 251–254.
23 Ragins, H., Levenson, S.M., Signer, R., Stamford, W. & Seifter, E. (1973): Intrajejunal administration of an elemental diet at neutral pH avoids pancreatic stimulation: Studies in dog and man. *Am. J. Surg.* **126**, 606–614.
24 Tandon, B.N., Banks, P.A., George, P.K., Sama, S.K., Ramachandran, K. & Gandhi, P.C. (1970): Recovery of exocrine pancreatic function in adult protein-calorie malnutrition. *Gastroenterology* **58**, 358–362.
25 Towne, J.B., Hamilton, R.F. & Stephenson, D.V. (1973): Mechanism of hyperalimentation in the suppression of upper gastrointestinal secretions. *Am. J. Surg.* **126**, 714–716.
26 Vindon, N., Hecketsweiter, P., Butel, J. and Bermer, J.J. (1978): Effect of continuous jejunal perfusion of elemental and complex nutritional solutions on pancreatic enzyme secretion in human subjects. *Gut* **19**, 194–198.
27 Voitk, A., Brown, R.A., Echave, V., McArdle, A.H. *et al.* (1973): Use of elemental diet in the treatment of complicated pancreatitis. *Am. J. Surg.* **125**, 223–227.
28 Wolfe, B.M., Keltner, R.M. & Willman, V.L. (1972): Intestinal fistula output in regular, elemental and intravenous alimentation. *Am. J. Surg.* **124**, 803–806.

Small intestine failure

V.I. MATHAN
The Wellcome Research Unit, Christian Medical College Hospital, Vellore 632 004, India.

The optimum digestion and absorption of ingested food is essential for the maintenance of healthy life. The failure of this fundamental function, which follows massive small intestinal resection for diseases such as superior mesenteric arterial or venous occlusion can rapidly lead to death due to severe acute malnutrition[7]. However, while this form of small intestinal failure is probably the most dramatic in its effect, a variety of conditions associated with maldigestion and malabsorption of nutrients can produce different degrees of small intestinal failure which leads to malnutrition and impaired quality of life. The assessment of the functional status of the intestinal tract and its impact on the nutritional status of the individual and of the community is an area which has been relatively neglected. Currently available methods can make physiologically meaningful evaluations.

Short bowel. The best example of intestinal failure is the short-gut syndrome, where removal of part or all of the intestine has been necessitated by trauma or diseases such as regional enteritis, mesenteric vascular occlusion and bowel infarction. It has now been clearly established that the outcome after intestinal resection will depend on the extent of the resection, the area of the small bowel involved, disease in the remaining small bowel, the preservation of the ileocaecal valve and the ability of the remaining small intestine to undergo morphologic and functional adaptation. Resection of one-third to half the small bowel is consistent with the adequate oral maintenance of nutrition. If less than 25 per cent of the small bowel only remains the patient needs special management. The ileum acts as a large functional reserve area for the jejunum, but absorption of vitamin B_{12} and bile salts can be affected by even small resections of the ileum. Malabsorbed bile salts alter colonic water and electrolyte absorption, lead to choleraic diarrhoea, depletion of bile-acid pool, fat malabsorption due to lack of micelle formation, hyperoxaluric urolithiasis (by increasing oxalate solubility) and mucosal permeability, and the bile may become lithogenic.

Small intestinal resection for conditions such as Crohn's disease or scleroderma usually results in severe malabsorption as the disease may affect the remaining bowel. Other concomitant diseases of the liver, pancreas or even right-sided heart failure may further impair the function of the remaining small intestine. Preservation of the ileocaecal valve seems to decrease the incidence of diarrhoea following small intestinal resection, possibly by an intact valve protecting against bacterial overgrowth in the remaining small intestine. The integrity of the colon is also important as resections involving colon cause more severe diarrhoea as the reserve capacity to absorb water is reduced[8].

Adaptation of the intestine to resection has been studied extensively in a variety of animal models[9]. In the rat, resection of the proximal and mid-small bowel results in a true increase in the size of the villi in the remaining ileum. This process, with hyperplasia of the epithelial cells and expansion of the proliferative zone in the crypt region, appears to occur within 2 days of the resection. Concomitant with these morphological adaptations, improvement in nutrient absorption over several months has been described. Luminal nutrients have been shown to be important for adaptation in a variety of animal experiments but their role has been questioned in the human. It is not clear whether it is the food itself or trophic factors such as bile acids, pancreatic enzymes, or gut hormones released by food which are important[2]. Gastrin and enteroglucagon are considered to be enterotrophins, mediators of the adaptive response. Cholecystokinin may also play such a role[13]. Gastric acid hypersecretion following small bowel resection occurs in almost 50 per cent of patients and is mediated by increase in circulating gastrin levels[1]. This has to be managed medically as any surgical intervention increases the problems of short bowel.

Management. In the immediate postoperative period watery diarrhoea with stool volumes as high as 10 litres makes it essential to ensure that dehydration, electrolyte losses and acid-base disturbances are adequately corrected. The pathogenesis of this diarrhoea is multifactorial, loss of mucosal area, osmotic effects of unabsorbed nutrients, damaging effect of unabsorbed fatty acids and bile acids in the colon and possibly gastric hypersecretion. Intravenous alimentation with all essential nutrients in a readily tolerated fluid volume (usually 2000 to 3500 ml/d) should be adminstered into a high flow vessel. Glucose and fats will provide most of the energy requirements while amino acid mixtures in the ratio of 1 g nitrogen to every 600 to 1000 kJ (143–239 kcal) of glucose and fat need to be given.

When oral feeding is initiated the diarrhoea may be aggravated and restriction of oral feeds reduces diarrhoea significantly at this stage. The rate of gastric emptying and presentation of fluid to the intestine is related to the intragastric volume. This dictates that frequent meals of small size is the ideal to aim for. Theoretically it would be ideal if the patient eats at a very slow rate constantly, but from the clinical point of view this is impractical! Chemically defined liquid diets are useful, particularly early in the course of oral feedings, but the high osmolality of many of these preparations may cause osmotic diarrhoea and most of them have a bad taste. A diluted form of these elemental diets can be used for supplementary feeding if given by a transnasal, duodenal or jejunal feeding tube. Elemental diets prepared from oligopeptides and glucose polymers may not have the problem of bad taste and increased osmolality. Since di- and tri-peptides can be absorbed without prior hydrolysis in the gastrointestinal tract such diets are valuable for nitrogen supplementation. In patients with a major problem of fluid and electrolyte losses, a modification of the oral rehydration solution which contains sodium chloride and glucose can maintain fluid and electrolyte balance, but is not a nutritional supplement. Specific parenteral replacements to be considered in the short term include calcium, vitamin D, magnesium, fat soluble vitamins and vitamin B_{12}. In some patients reduction of fat intake or replacing dietary fat by medium-chain triglycerides may reduce the diarrhoea[4]. Antimotility drugs may be of importance in increasing the contact time of nutrients with the mucosa, thus increasing net absorption per unit surface area. Oral agents such as loperamide are preferable[5]. If choleraic diarrhoea is diagnosed cholestyramine may reduce stool volume, but may increase steatorrhoea. Bacterial overgrowth should be treated by appropriate antibiotics.

Prolonged parenteral nutrition and permanent parenteral nutrition at home have been used successfully for the management of these patients[10,12]. Experience gained in such studies have indicated the necessity for many trace nutrients such as zinc, copper and essential fatty acids which have to be added to the infusate which should contain all nutrients, minerals, vitamins and trace elements. Unfortunately, the technology involved in this and the necessity for the patient and his relatives to understand and comply with the protocol makes it relatively unavailable to vast segments of the worlds population especially in tropical developing countries.

Reversal of a segment of the lower small bowel in an attempt to prolong transit and enhance absorption has not been very successful and has inherent risks[15].

Other causes of small intestine failure. Massive intestinal resection and the resultant failure of function are emergency clinical situations. The process of adaptation to loss of intestinal surface area is challenging to understand and modify. This has led to the relative neglect of problems associated with less dramatic malabsorption syndromes, especially diseases associated with primary enterocyte lesions like tropical sprue. There was an era when diet therapy was considered to be the answer to many of these problems and with diseases like coeliac sprue and cow's-milk-protein enteropathy this still holds true. However, the dietary considerations in most other malabsorption syndromes are similar. The pattern of nutrient absorption should be studied and it may be particularly useful to determine the capacity of the intestine to absorb energy by energy balance studies[11]. Adequate intake of nutrients should maintain the nutritional status of the individual and enhancing the total nutrient intake may be necessary. Many of these diseases are associated with severe anorexia which is a constraint in increasing nutrient intake and such patients would benefit by a period of parenteral alimentation. In many parts of the world where malabsorption syndromes are widely prevalent economic factors operate against parenteral nutrition.

Public health implications of small intestinal failure. Nutritionists and gastroenterologists are primarily concerned with clinically dramatic small intestinal failure and the battle for preserving the life of an individual whose capacity to absorb food is almost totally lost. However, minor degrees of small intestinal failure which are widespread may have a significant impact on the nutritional status of population groups. It has now been shown that in several areas of the tropical developing world the structure and function of the small intestine is abnormal compared to residents in the temperate zones[3]. This condition has been designated as 'tropical enteropathy' and in a study in southern India 10 per cent of apparently healthy asymptomatic village adults were malabsorbing fat and nearly 50 per cent had xylose malabsorption. In a smaller proportion vitamin B_{12} malabsorption was also present. Quantification of energy absorption in this population showed that the faecal energy excretion was more than twice that in a comparable population in UK and that only 91 per cent of the ingested energy was absorbed[6]. It has been suggested that this tropical enteropathy is an adaptation to a variety of environmental factors[14] and it is exciting to speculate that if the enteropathy can be eliminated up to 9 per cent more of nutrients may be available for the population without an actual increase in the availability of food grains. This idea at present is purely speculative, but detailed research on the pathogenesis of tropical enteropathy and its nutritional significance is clearly required.

1 Aber, G.M., Ashton, F., Carmalt, M.H.B. & Whitehead, T.P. (1967): Gastric hypersecretion following massive small bowel resection in man. *Am. J. Dig. Dis.* **12**, 785–794.
2 Altman, G.G. (1971): Influence of bile and pancreatic secretions on the size of the intestinal villi in the rat. *Am. J. Anat.* **132**, 167–178.
3 Baker, S.J., Mathan, V.I. (1972): Tropical enteropathy and tropical sprue. *Am. J. Clin. Nutr.* **25**, 1047–1055.
4 Bochenek, W., Rodgers, J.B. & Balint, J.A. (1970): Effects of changes in dietary lipids on intestinal fluid loss in the short bowel syndrome. *Ann. Int. Med.* **72**, 205–213.
5 Cameron, J.L., Gayler, B.W. & Hendrix, T.R. (1976): The use of intramuscular propantheline in the short bowel syndrome. *John. Hop. Med. J.* **138**, 91–95.
6 Chacko, A., Begum, A. & Mathan, V.I. (1984): Absorption of nutrient energy in southern Indian control subjects and patients with tropical sprue. *Am. J. Clin. Nutr.* **40**, 771–775.
7 Compston, J.E. & Creamer, B. (1977): The consequences of small intestinal resection. *Quart. J. Med.* **46**, 485–497.
8 Cummings, J.H., James, W.P.T. & Wiggins, H.S. (1973): Role of the colon in ileal-resection diarrhoea. *Lancet* **1**, 344–347.
9 Dowling, R.H. (1982): Small bowel adaptation and its regulation. *Scand. J. Gastroenterol.* **17**, (Supp. 74), 53–74.
10 Dudrick, S.J. & Ruberg, R.L. (1971): Principles and practice of parenteral nutrition. *Gastroenterology.* **61**, 901–910.
11 Heymsfield, S.B., Smith, J., Kasriel, S. *et al.* (1981): Energy malabsorption: measurement and nutritional consequences. *Am. J. Clin. Nutr.* **34**, 1954–1960.
12 Jeejeebhoy, K.N., Zohrab, W.J., Langer, B. *et al.* (1973): Total parenteral nutrition at home for 23 months, without complication, and with good rehabilitation. A study of technical and metabolic features. *Gastroenterology* **65**, 811–820.
13 Johnson, L.R. (1982): Effect of exogenous gut hormones on gastrointestinal mucosal growth. *Scand. J. Gastroenterol.* **17**(Supp. 17), 89–92.
14 Mathan, V.I., Ponniah, J. & Mathan, M. (1982): Tropical enteropathy: an adaptation of the small intestine to accelerated cell loss in 'contaminated' environments. In *Mechanisms of intestinal adaptation*, ed J.W.L. Robinson, R.H. Dowling, E.O. Reicker, pp. 690–691. Lancaster, PA: MTP Press.
15 Rygick, A.N. & Nasarov, L.U. (1969): Antiperistaltic displacement of an ileal loop without twisting its mesentery. *Dis. Colon. Rectum.* **12**, 409–411.

An overall view of nutrition in organ failure

H.A. LEE
Department of Renal Medicine, University of Southampton, St. Mary's Hospital, Milton Road, Portsmouth PO3 6AD, UK.

Clearly, the nutritional approach used will depend upon whether there is relative or absolute end organ failure, eg, acute pancreatitis as opposed to chronic pancreatitis or acute renal failure versus chronic renal failure. Whereas formerly too little attention was paid to the nutritional support of patients, a mystique has now arisen that very special nutritional approaches are required for specific organ failure, eg, kidney, liver, gut, singly or in combination. Usually, many critically-ill patients will have multiple organ failure and fortunately current nutritional support therapies cater for such patient needs. Choices can be made between enteral, assuming the gut is functional, and parenteral nutrition. The latter, if combined with continuous arteriovenous haemfiltration (CAVH) can obviate the problem of fluid volume constraint. The old adage of 'starvation in the midst of plenty' should no longer apply to hospital patients. Many such patients will have associated sepsis but they too can use energy and nitrogen substrates like non-septic patients.

Gastro-intestinal failure. This is a common accompaniment in many critically-ill patients following trauma or intra-abdominal operations where adynamic ileus develops and there may be multiple entero-cutaneous fistulae. With modern, safe, central venous catheterisation techniques, total parenteral nutrition (TPN) can maintain such patients for weeks, months or even years. The total daily nutrients of fat, carbohydrate, amino acids, trace elements, vitamins, electrolytes and fluids can be given in a 3-litre bag over a 12 to 16 h period. The energy is provided equally between carbohydrate and fat, rarely exceeding 2200 kcal (9.2 MJ)/d and on average most patients require between 12–14 g of amino acid nitrogen daily. There cannot be any justification for giving more that 21 g nitrogen daily. Clearly, after massive gut resection for whatever reason, patients have to be maintained in the long term and world-wide there are many patients who have been treated with home TPN and have survived for more than 5 years. Problems relating to trace element metabolism need to be resolved, eg, selenium, manganese and chromium requirements and the potential problems of TPN-related bone disease.

In terms of diarrhoeal disease in Third World countries where there has been an appallingly high mortality rate, there can be no doubt that the greatest break-through has been with simple oral rehydration therapy — basically, glucose and salt mixtures which are easily given, cheap to provide and rapidly effective and can save millions of lives.

Renal disease. The mortality rate in acute renal failure still remains unacceptably high and nutritional problems abound. There is growing agreement that patients with acute renal failure can receive exactly the same nutritional substrates as their non-renal-failure counterparts, be they enteral or parenteral. Fluid volume constraints need not preclude adequate treatment with the use of CAVH. There is little support now for giving low-protein diets in acute renal failure in the hope of reducing dialysis frequency. The aim must be to dialyse patients as frequently as is necessary to ensure they receive full nutritional requirements. There is no need for special enteral or parenteral preparations in acute renal failure. It has been clearly shown that these patients, adequately dialysed, metabolize glucose and fat substrates enterally or parenterally in the same way as their counterparts. It has been shown in some series that by applying TPN principles immediately to all patients with acute renal failure, the mortality rate can be reduced by some 20 per cent.

There has been a resurgence of interest in the application of low-protein diets in chronic renal failure. Hitherto, it has been customary to reserve low-protein diets (0.25 g/kg B.Wt.) until the GFR has decreased to 10 ml/minute or less. Many recent studies have shown that the application of low-protein diets (30–40 g/d) when the GFR has decreased to about 40 per cent normal, ie serum creatinine between 200 and 300 µmol/l, can dramatically reduce the rate of deterioration in renal function. Allied to the treatment of associated hyperlipidaemia, hyperuricaemia and hyperphosphataemia, and with control of hypertension such diets can lead to a delay of months or years in a patient requiring end-stage renal failure management with dialysis. Nevertheless, the management of end-stage renal failure patients with ultra-restricted protein intake (protein 6 g dietary equivalents — P6) can still be successful in patients who may not be suitable for any form of end-stage renal failure replacement management or for patients changing from one form of treatment to another because of intercurrent problems, eg, infection. It must be emphasized that severe protein restriction is not a substitute for starting diabetic end-stage nephropathy patients early on dialysis. Many patients have been kept in good health on P6 diets for between 6 months and 3 years. Finally, more attention to the hyperlipidaemias associated with chronic renal disease will reduce the number of patients dying from premature coronary artery disease when they may be otherwise successfully dialysed or transplanted.

Liver disease. Caution must be exercised about grouping all patients together. Much has been written in the past 10 years about the value of i.v. branched-chain amino acid (leucine, isoleucine and valine) formulations in the management of encephalopathic patients. One must differentiate between the chronic cirrhotic patient with or without encephalopathy and hypoalbuminaemia and those who have fulminating hepatitis with encephalopathy. For the cirrhotic patient who is encephalopathic there may be a place for a modified protein intake (enterally or parenterally), with the emphasis on branched-chain amino acids because of the known altered plasma amino acid profile with respect to increased aromatic and decreased branched-chain amino acids. This altered ratio is thought to lead to alterations of intra-cerebral concentrations of false neuro-transmitters. Some evidence suggests that enteral diets with the emphasis on milk are more effective than those which are either fish or meat-based.

Nevertheless, very few controlled trials have been done in such patients and recently the first satisfactory trial from Italian workers suggests that branched-chain amino acid preparations given orally or i.v. convey no benefits. As in acute renal failure, so in acute liver disease, one must be wary of protein restriction. For a chronic, cirrhotic, non-encephalopathic hypoalbuminaemic patient with fluid retention, the emphasis must be on fluid removal, high protein intake, anti-aldosterone agents and electrolyte correction, eg low sodium intake whilst ensuring adequate potassium repletion. For patients with acute fulminant hepatitis (viral or alcohol-induced) there is no indication for using specific amino acid formulations but high protein and energy intakes are required, with carbohydrate as the main source of energy, although some fat may be given. Here the protein turnover may exceed 100 g daily and the emphasis on giving high biological value protein cannot be overstressed.

Pancreatic disease. In acute pancreatitis malnutrition rapidly ensues and this is often further accentuated by the use of the standard 'drip and suck regimen'. The idea of enteral rest for the pancreas has been inappropriately transferred to 'intravenous rest' in the mistaken belief that i.v.-administered energy and amino acids stimulate the pancreas. Whilst this is certainly not true for glucose or amino acids, there is a minor doubt concerning i.v. fat provision and pancreatic lipase stimulation. Nevertheless, a few trials, most of them poorly controlled, have shown that TPN can significantly reduce the mortality rate in acute pancreatitis. There is no need for specifically designed amino acid solutions or for the use of different energy substrates.

The malnutrition associated with chronic pancreatitis remains a challenge and a number of approaches have been used such as enteric-coated microspheres, the use of elemental diets and the provision of pre-digested nutrients with enzyme replacement. Here, the results have been variable and thus far not very encouraging.

Respiratory failure. Many critically-ill patients have respiratory failure, sometimes with a 'white lung syndrome'. The latter may be due to fluid overload, intra-alveolar DIC, lung infection or intra-pulmonary haemorrhage, but has never been truly described as secondary to TPN. Thus, for any patient with acute respiratory failure, irrespective of the associated end-organ problem, standard i.v. amino acid solutions can be used together with fat and carbohydrate substrates in the usual proportions.

Cardiac failure. Patients who have undergone major cardiac surgery, eg, valve replacement, coronary artery by-pass surgery or cardiac transplantation often require aggressive supportive management in the post-operative period when liver, kidney and lung function may all be compromised. Once again, there is no evidence to suggest that such patients require specifically tailored enteral or parenteral nutritional support preparations. They can be managed in exactly the same way as other patients. Where there may be the extra problems of fluid and sodium overload these patients can be nicely managed by CAVH which allows for complete control of fluid and electrolyte replacement as well as provision of nutritional support.

End-organ failure and sepsis. After some 15 years of debate, there is an increasing body of opinion that suggests that specific enteral or, in particular, parenteral preparations are not required for the management of septic patients. Hitherto, it has been considered that the septic patient could not utilize intravenously administered fat. Much evidence supports the view that such patients not only metabolize i.v. fat usefully but may actually do so preferentially over glucose when compared to non-infected counterparts. This, therefore, makes the management of these patients easier without a need to give large doses of i.v. soluble insulin to cover large doses of glucose given because fat was thought non-utilisable. Previously, there has been a tendency to give such patients far too much energy, 3000–4000 kcal (12.5–16.7 MJ)/d whereas, in fact, they rarely require more than 2500 kcal (10.5 MJ)/d. This error has been further compounded by the provision of far too much i.v. nitrogen often 30–40 g daily, whereas, in fact, the liver cannot cope with a load of more than 21 g daily.

Conclusion. It is clear from the forgoing there is very considerable rationalization in the management of patients with organ failure. This has led to simplification in design of their nutritional support. In general terms one is providing less nitrogen, on average 12–14 g daily, less energy, 2200 kcal (MJ) daily and rarely any insulin. Clearly, few clinicians need have any worries about the nutritional support of their patients irrespective of whether they are infected, what organ is mainly involved or what combination of organs. Obviously, more patients will die from end-organ failure and associated complications if they are not fed than if they are.

★   ★   ★

PARENTERAL NUTRITION

A comparison of the enteral and parenteral provision of micronutrients

A. SHENKIN
Department of Biochemistry, Royal Infirmary, Glasgow, Scotland.

A fundamental principle of i.v. nutrition is to supply nutrients in the same amount and chemical form as would be absorbed from an adequate oral diet. Particularly with regard to micronutrients, the basic knowledge is often not available to meet such a specific objective. Here I will, however, attempt to compare the provision of micronutrients by enteral and parenteral routes and show how the amount present in the 'food' may differ from that finally available to the tissues.

Micronutrients is a convenient 'umbrella' title, but the area covered is vast, essential inorganic elements (with the exception of sodium, potassium, calcium, magnesium and phosphorus) and essential organic micronutrients, ie vitamins. The substances which should therefore be provided i.v. are: inorganic — Zn, Fe, Cu, Mn, I, Co, Se, Cr, Mo; organic — all water-soluble (nine) and fat-soluble (four) vitamins.

In addition, fluoride is known to be beneficial and certain inorganic elements are possibly essential although not yet proven (Si, Ni, V, Sn, As, Li). Only a few selected examples can therefore be given.

Enteral nutrition. In enteral nutrition, a major variable is the bioavailability of each micronutrient present. Despite chemical analysis demonstrating the presence of an element, it may be absorbed only in reduced amounts[16]. Complexing to other food components is of particular importance. Dietary fibre reduces absorption of copper, zinc and magnesium[7], whereas the phytate content is the major reason for the reduced zinc absorption from soy products[14]. By contrast, combination with more complex substances may also improve absorption relative to the inorganic salts eg the organic complex of chromium[5]. Similarly, the naturally occurring chemical form may influence absorption, iron in haem being more effectively absorbed than inorganic iron, and ferrous iron better absorbed than ferric.

The proportion absorbed may also depend upon interactions with other elements with similar absorption pathways. For example, zinc absorption can be inhibited by inorganic iron or tin[19] whereas zinc supplements may reduce copper status[9]. Interaction may also occur with vitamins, eg folic acid supplements reduce zinc absorption, possibly by formation of insoluble chelates, but do not alter iron or copper absorption[15], whereas ascorbic acid improves iron absorption but reduces that of copper[18].

The above factors are probably equally relevant to oral or synthetic enteral feeds. Specific to oral diets are the variable losses during cooking, especially due to oxidation of ascorbic acid and extraction of other water-soluble nutrients.

During enteral nutrition, the absorption mechanism itself may be controlled by specific carriers. In iron-deficiency mucosal transport of iron increases so that a higher proportion is absorbed, and greater quantities of transferrin are present in blood to permit maximal transport to the bone marrow. In the process, a change of valency may occur from Fe^{+++} to Fe^{++}. Similar mechanisms may exist for other elements.

Intravenous nutrition (IVN). Thus in enteral nutrition, although absorption may be variable, the micronutrient is finally presented to the blood stream in the 'correct' physiological form and in an amount regulated to the requirement of the individual. By contrast, IVN bypasses these mechanisms. Whatever is present in the infusate enters the bloodstream. The chemical nature of the element is still important for its utilization. Complexes may occur between elements and individual amino acids or with amino sugars which are present as a result of a Maillard reaction[12]. For example, we found that if 100 μmol zinc was supplied i.v. to post-operative surgical patients in crystalloid dextrose/saline only 10 per cent was excreted in urine, whereas during complete IVN approximately 47 per cent of the zinc input was found in urine.

Alternatively, certain forms of an element may be better utilized. The requirement of cobalt can only be met from cobalamin, and not from the inorganic element. Sodium selenite has also been widely used as a source of selenium but it is liable to reduction by ascorbate to elemental selenium, whereas selenomethionine is more effectively retained by the body but possibly in an unavailable protein pool. Sodium selenate has recently been suggested as a more suitable form of selenium supplement[13].

There is a theoretical risk of precipitation of certain micronutrients. Folate is relatively insoluble at pH < 5. Excess zinc has been observed to cause precipitation in one amino acid preparation[8] whereas precipitation with iron has been observed in phosphate-rich amino acid solutions[2]. At the concentrations of inorganic micronutrients normally used, we have not observed significant losses due to precipitation.

The amount of vitamins provided may be significantly reduced as a result of chemical changes within the infusate. Depending upon the brightness and duration, ultraviolet light may cause almost total degradation of retinol[1] and riboflavin[6]. The presence of fat emulsion may reduce this effect. Adsorption of fat-soluble vitamins on to the infusion bag and sets may occur: this can be as much as 75 per cent of retinol acetate in PVC bags and 35 per cent in vitamins D and E over 24 h[11].

Interaction between trace elements and vitamins is likely in complete nutritive mixtures of all nutrients in one bag. Copper oxidizes ascorbic acid and this may lead to rapid loss of vitamins[2]. However, this may be of limited practical importance since we have observed that provision of IVN from such a mixture leads to virtually identical blood concentrations of vitamins and essential elements, in comparison with provision of trace elements and vitamins in separate infusions.

Biological differences between oral and i.v. provision. Provision of nutrition intravenously bypasses the control mechanisms for inorganic micronutrients present in the gut. There is therefore a theoretical risk of overprovision. Enterally absorbed elements also pass directly to the liver in the portal vein, whereas parenterally infused nutrients are delivered directly into the systemic circulation. This may be relevant to the potentially harmful effects of elements such as iron in infection[20]. In acute sepsis, iron is taken up rapidly by the liver bound to ferritin, whereas zinc is complexed to hepatic thionein. It can be speculated that parenteral provision of excess of these elements may exacerbate severe infections. The dosage of intravenous trace elements must therefore be carefully regulated so that binding proteins in serum are not saturated.

Provision of micronutrients. Clinical deficiency states during IVN have now been reported for most inorganic micronutrients and vitamins. It is probable also that many patients have a subclinical deficiency or depletion state of uncertain clinical relevance. In a recent study, we observed that in patients referred for nutritional support, those who subsequently died had poorer nutritional status, not only in terms of protein-energy status, but also in biochemical indices of status of vitamins (A, thiamin and riboflavin) and trace elements (zinc and copper). It seems logical therefore to provide all micronutrients from the commencement of IVN.

The major problem is deciding how much of each micronutrient to provide. Without even discussing the possible effects of disease states on requirements, the above discussion highlights the difficulties in extrapolating from oral/enteral recommendations to requirements in IVN regimens. This has been further complicated by the recent trend to use complete nutritive mixtures of all nutrients in one large plastic bag in which interactions are likely. Based upon the available literature, recommendations have been reached for enteral and parenteral nutrition and these are compared and contrasted in the Table. Particularly with regard to inorganic micronutrients these recommendations must be used with caution: certain preparations of

Table. *Recommended dietary allowances (RDA) of micro-nutrients for enteral nutrition compared with recommendations for parenteral nutrition and with amounts actually provided by solutions in clinical use*

| | | Inorganic micronutrients | | | | | Organic micronutrients | |
| | | Enteral | Parenteral | | | | Enteral | Parenteral |
		RDA^a	AMA^b	GRI 1*			RDA^a	AMA^c (GRI 2)*
Iron	μmol	180	n.s.	20	Retinol	i.u.	2500–3300	3300
	mg	10	n.s.	1.1	Ergocalciferol	i.u.	200–400	200
Zinc	μmol	230	38–92	100	α Tocopherol	i.u.	10	10
	mg	15	2.5–6.0	6.4	Vitamin K	μg	70–140	(150)
Copper	μmol	32–48	8–24	20	Ascorbic acid	mg	30–60	100
	mg	1.0–3.0	0.5–1.5	1.3	Thiamin	mg	1.0–1.4	3.0
Iodine	μmol	1.2	–	1.0	Riboflavin	mg	1.6	3.6
	mg	150	–	127	Pyridoxine	mg	2.2	4.0
Manganese	μmol	46–91	3–15	5	Niacin	mg	18	40
	mg	2.5–5.0	0.15–0.8	0.27	B_{12}	μg	3.0	5.0
Fluoride	μmol	79–210	–	50	Pantothenic acid	mg	4–7	15
	mg	1.5–4.0	–	0.95	Biotin	μg	100–200	60
Chromium	μmol	1–4	0.2–0.3	0.2	Folic acid	μg	300–400	400
	mg	0.05–0.2	0.01–0.15	0.01				
Selenium	μmol	0.6–2.5	–	0.4				
	mg	0.05–0.2	–	0.03				
Molybdenum	μmol	1.6–5.2	–	0.2				
	mg	0.15–0.5	–	0.02				

*Prepared by Kabi Vitrum, Stockholm, Sweden. n.s. — Recommended but amount not specified. [a]Food & Nutrition Board (1980); [b,c]American Medical Association, Nutrition Advisory Board (1979)[3,4] respectively.

amino acids may already contain sufficient chromium as contaminant, for example, so that additional provision is not necessary[17]. Most other elements are also present as contaminants to varying extents. Monitoring of blood and possibly urine levels should therefore be performed, especially in long-term IVN. Most micronutrients are now given as part of a multi-nutrient mixture, although to meet special requirements, individual supplements may be required. In our experience, the mixtures shown in the Table (GRI 1 and 2) have been able to correct or maintain normal blood levels of vitamins and inorganic micronutrients in most patients requiring IVN. Considerable further progress will be necessary to characterize the level of provision to achieve optimal tissue metabolism in different disease states.

1 Allwood, M.M. (1982): The influence of light on vitamin A degradation during administration. *Clin. Nutr.* **1**, 63–70.
2 Allwood, M.C. (1984): Compatibility and stability of TPN mixtures in big bags. *J. Clin. Hosp. Pharm.* **9**, 181–198.
3 American Medical Association (1979a): Guidelines for essential trace element preparations for parenteral use. A statement by the Nutrition Advisory Group. *J. Parent, Ent. Nutr.* **3**, 263–267.
4 American Medical Association (1979b): Multivitamin preparations for parenteral use. A statement by the Nutrition Advisory Group. *J. Parent. Ent. Nutr.* **3**, 258–262.
5 Anderson, M., Riley, D., Rotrick, J. (1980): Chromium III trisacetylacetonate — an absorbable bioactive source of chromium. *Fed. Proc.* **39**, 787.
6 Chen, M.F., Boyce, H.W. & Triplett, C. (1983): Stability of the B vitamins in mixed parenteral nutrition solution. *J. Parent, Ent. Nutr.* **7**, 462–4.
7 Drews, L.M., Kies, H.M. & Fox H.M. (1979): Effect of dietary fibre on copper, zinc and magnesium utilisation by adolescent boys. *Amer. J. Clin. Nutr.* **32**, 1893–7.
8 Earnshaw, M. (1980): Mixtures and compatibilities in total parenteral nutrition solutions. *Acta. Chir. Scand.* **507**, 364–70.
9 Fischer, P.W.F., Giroux, A. & Abbe, M.R.L. (1984): Effect of zinc supplementation on copper status in adult man. *Amer. J. Clin. Nutr.* **40**, 743–6.
10 Food and Nutrition Board. (1980): Recommended dietary allowances. *National Acad. Sci.* Washington.
11 Gillis, J., Jones, G. & Pencharz, P.B. (1983): Delivery of vitamins A, D, and E in total parenteral nutrition solutions. *J. Parent. Ent. Nutr.* **7**, 11–14.
12 Hallman, P.S., Perrin, D.D. & Watt, A.E. (1971): The computer distribution of copper and zinc ions among seventeen amino acids present in human plasma. *Biochem. J.* **121**, 549–55.
13 Levander, O.A. (1984): The importance of selenium in total parenteral nutrition. *Bull. N.Y. Acad. Med.* **60**, 144–55.
14 Lonnerdal, B., Cederblad, A., Davidsson, L. & Sandstrom, B. (1984): The effect of individual components of soy

formula and cows milk on zinc bioavailability. *Am. J. Clin. Nutr.* **40**, 1064–70.

15 Milne, D.B., Canfield, W.K., Mahalko, J.R. & Sandstead, H.H. (1984): Effect of oral folic acid supplements on zinc, copper and iron absorption and excretion. *Am. J. Clin. Nutr.* **39**, 535–9.

16 Rosenberg, I.H. & Solomons, N.W. (1982): Biological availability of minerals and trace elements: a nutritional overview. *Am. J. Clin. Nutr.* **35**, 781–2.

17 Shenkin, A., Fell, G.S., Halls, D.J., Dunbar, P.M., Holbrook, I.B. & Irving, M. (1985): Essential trace element provision to patients receiving home IVN in the United Kingdom. *Br. Med. J.* (In press).

18 Solomons, N.W., Viteri, F.E. (1982): Biological interactions of ascorbic acid with mineral nutrients. In *Ascorbic acid chemistry, mechanism and uses*, ed P. Seib & B. Tolbert. *Amer. Chem. Soc. Press*, 557–69.

19 Valberg, L.S., Flanagan, P.R. & Chamberlain, M.J. (1984): Effects of iron, tin and copper on zinc absorption in humans. *Am. J. Clin. Nutr.* **40**, 536–41.

20 Weinberg, E.D. (1984): Iron with-holding: a defence against infection and neoplasia. *Physiol. Rev.* **64**, 65–102.

Changes in body composition and muscle function and effect of nutritional support

K.N. JEEJEEBHOY
Department of Medicine, University of Toronto, Canada.

Studies in animals have shown that starvation results in reduced weight gain and growth. In contrast the intake of nutrients sufficient to meet requirements promotes growth and weight gain. In consequence the optimal nutritional status was defined in anthropometric terms[3]. Unfortunately in adult humans a number of non-nutritional factors may alter the anthropometric[15], biochemical[7] and immunological status of the individual[6]. In addition, nutritional support does not influence body composition to the same extent as it does in growing children and animals. This is because, in adults, the size of muscles and the skeleton is dependent on exercise. In this communication the difficulties of equating changes of body composition with malnutrition in patients and the evidence that nutritional support primarily alters function will be presented.

Spectrum of effects of nutritional deficiency. Disequilibrium between intake and needs results in a succession of changes which start with altered metabolism[14], followed by altered function[9,17] and finally wasting[2]. Hence loss of body components is the final stage of malnutrition. Thus it is not surprising that body composition does not accurately reflect the risks of morbidity and mortality in malnourished subjects[1,12,23]. By contrast loss of muscle power does predict for morbidity and mortality[9].

Effect of nutritional support on body composition. While short-term nitrogen retention can be shown by nitrogen balance during nutritional support, by contrast body nitrogen measurements have shown little change in total body nitrogen (TBN) in patients during nutritional support[8,21]. However there is a gain in body fat, potassium and water. Plasma proteins often fall during nutritional support because of dilution[21,22]. In addition changes in body potassium correlate poorly with plasma transferrin[16].

Clinical assessment. In the present climate of relying on data obtained from techniques using laboratory data it is unfashionable to rely on clinical judgment. However, controlled studies have clearly shown that clinical judgment was superior to single objective parameters in predicting the development of nutritionally associated complications based on a careful evaluation of conditional probabilities and the sensitivity and specificities of the various clinical and objective parameters[2,4]. Clinical judgment was superior to measurement of DCH in predicting post-operative infection[13].

Functional tests of malnutrition. Because of these problems we examined muscle function as a specific measure of the effect of withdrawing nutrients and refeeding. The problem previously of assessing muscle function has been the inability to use methods which did not involve exercising on treadmills or bicycles. In order to study critically-ill patients we had to develop a method which did not require the cooperation of the patient and was not non-specifically affected by sepsis, drugs, trauma, surgical intervention and anaesthesia. In order to do this we selected a method used to study muscle fatigue[5,11]. It consisted of measuring the contraction of the *adductor pollicis* muscle in response to an electrical stimulus of the ulnar nerve at the wrist. When the nerve is stimulated at the above site with unidirectional square wave pulses lasting only 50–70 microseconds at a range of frequencies from 10 to 50 Hz there is a progressive increase in force with a maximal attained at 50 Hz. This is called the Force-frequency curve. In addition, if the nerve is stimulated at 20 Hz for 2 sec and then the stimulus is switched off, the muscle relaxes and the rate of relaxation can be measured. Finally if the stimulus at 20 Hz is continued any loss of power represents fatigue of an objective nature (not due to voluntary relaxation)[10]. By studying two pure models of human starvation and refeeding, namely the obese subject starving and the anorexia patient being refed, we showed that starvation causes the ratio of the force at 10 Hz/50–100 Hz to double and the relaxation rate to slow from a mean of about 10 per cent of maximal force lost/10 ms to 5–6 per cent. In addition we showed the development of fatigue. Refeeding corrected these changes. We demonstrated these changes in rats fed on a low energy diet[17–20]. Thus we showed that the force frequency curve of the *adductor pollicis* muscle is a sensitive and specific measure of the nutrient intake or withdrawal in both humans and animals. It is not nonspecifically rendered abnormal by surgery, anasthaesia, steroids, sepsis, and only mildly and temporarily altered by severe trauma (crush injuries). We also showed that neither muscle power nor the force frequency spectrum is dependent on body nitrogen, potassium or muscle bulk as assessed by arm muscle circumference. In addition we showed that muscle power in the *adductor pollicis* can be doubled simply by nutritional support without any change in the arm muscle circumference. In addition using muscle biopsies we showed that there was fibre atrophy and Z-band degeneration during the reduction of dietary intake to 400 kcal (1674 kJ) in otherwise healthy subjects without gross change in body composition. Hence it is obvious that a more relevant and specific way of assessing nutritional status in the future may be through a study of muscle function.

1 Anderson, C.F., Moness, K., Meister, J. & Burritt, M.F. (1984): The sensitivity and specificity of nutrition related variables in relationship to the duration of hospital stay and the rate of complications. *Mayo Clin. Proc.* **59**, 477–483.

2 Baker, J.P., Detsky, A.S., Wesson, D.E., Wolman, S.L., Stewart, S., Whitewell, J., Langer, B., Jeejeebhoy, K.N. (1982): Nutritional assessment: a comparison of clinical judgement and objective measurements. *New. Engl. J. Med.* **306**, 969–972.

3 Blackburn, G.L., Bistrian, B.R., Maini, B.S., Schlamm, H.T. & Smith, M.F. (1977): Nutritional and metabolic assessment of the hospitalized patient. *J. Parent Ent. Nutr.* **1**, 11–22.

4 Detsky, A.S., Baker, J.P., Mendelson, R.A., Wolman, S.L., Wesson, D.A. & Jeejeebhoy, K.M. (1984): Evaluating the accuracy of nutritional assessment techniques applied to hospitalized patients: methodology and comparisons. *J. Parent. Ent. Nutr.* **8**, 153–159.

5 Edwards, R.H.T.(1978): Physiological analysis of skeletal muscle weakness and fatigue. *Clin. Sci. Mol. Med.* **54**, 463–470.

6 Howard, R.J. & Simmons, R.L. (1974): Viral infections and the surgical patient. *Surg. Gynecol. Obstet.* **139**, 771–782.

7 Jeejeebhoy, K.N. (1962): Cause of hypoalbuminaemia in patients with gastrointestinal and cardiac disease. *Lancet* **1**, 343–348.

8 Jeejeebhoy, K.N., Baker, J.P., Wolman, S.L., Harrison, J.E. & McNeill, K.G. (1982): Critical evaluation of the role of clinical assessment and body composition studies in patients with malnutrition and after total parental nutrition. *Am. J. Clin. Nutr.* **35**, 1117–1127.

9 Klidjian, A.M., Foster, K.J., Kammerling, R.M. (1980): Relation of anthropometric and dynamometric variables to serious postoperative complications. *Br. Med. J.* **281**, 899–901.

10 Lopes, J., Russell, D. McR., Whitwell, J. & Jeejeebhoy, K.N. (1982): Skeletal muscle function in malnutrition. *Am. J. Clin. Nutr.* **36**, 602–610.

11 Merton, P.A. (1954): Voluntary strength and fatigue. *J. Physiol.* **123**, 555–564.

12 Mullen, J.L., Gertner, M.H., Buzby, G.P., Goodhart, G.L., Rosato, E.F. (1979): Implications of malnutrition in the surgical patient. *Arch. Surg.* **114**, 121–125.

13 Ottow, R.T., Bruining, H.A. & Jeekel, J. (1984): Clinical judgement versus delayed hypersensitivity skin testing for the prediction of post-operative sepsis and mortality. *Surg. Gynecol. Obstet.* **159**, 475–477.

14 Owen, O.E., Reichart, G.A., Patel, M.S. (1979): Energy metabolism in feasting and fasting. *Adv. Expt. Med. Biol.* **111**, 119–188.

15 Rich, A.J. (1982): The assessment of body composition in clinical conditions. *Proc. Nutr. Soc.* **41**, 389–403.

16 Roza, A.M., Tuitt, D. & Shizgal, H.M. (1984): Transferrin — a poor measure of nutritional status. *J. Parent. Ent. Nutr.* **8**, 523–528.

17 Russell, D.McR., Leiter, L.A., Whitwell, J., Marliss, E.B. & Jeejeebhoy, K.N. (1983): Skeletal muscle function during hypocaloric diets and fasting: a comparison with standard nutritional assessment parameters. *Am. J. Clin. Nutr.* **37**, 133–138.

18 Russell, D.McR., Pendergast, P.J., Darby, P.L., Garfinkel, P.E., Whitwell, J. & Jeejeebhoy, K.N. (1983): A comparison between muscle function and body composition in anorexia nervosa: the effect of re-feeding. *Am. J. Clin. Nutr.* **38**, 229–237.

19 Russell, D.McR., Atwood, H.L., Whittaker, J., Itakura, T., Walker, P.M., Mickle, D.A.G. & Jeejeebhoy, K.N. (1984): The effect of fasting and hypocaloric diets on the functional and metabolic characteristics of rat gastrocnemius muscle. *Clin. Sci.* **67**, 185–194.

20 Russell, D.McR., Walker, P.M., Leiter, L.A., Sima, A.A.F., Tanner, W.K., Mickle, D.A.G. and Jeejeebhoy. K.N. (1984): Metabolic and structural changes in skeletal muscle during hypocaloric dieting. *Am. J. Clin. Nutr.* **39**, 503–513.

21 Shike, M., Russell, D.R., Detsky, A.S., Harrison, J.E., McNeil, K.G., Shephard, F.A., Feld, R., Evans, W.K. & Jeejeebhoy, K.N. (1984): Changes in body composition in patients with small-cell lung cancer. *Ann. Int. Med.* **101**, 303–309.

22 Starker, P.M., Gump, F.E., Askanazi, J., Elwyn, D.H. & Kinney, J.M. (1982): Serum albumin levels as an index of nutritional support. *Surgery* **91**, 194–199.

23 Symreng, T., Anderberg, B., Kagedal, B., Norr, A., Schildt, B. & Sjödahl, R. (1983): Nutritional assessment and clinical course in 112 elective surgical patients. *Acta. Chir. Scand.* **149**, 657–662.

XV: Nutrition and ageing

Life span, metabolic age and genetics

St.C.S. TAYLOR

AFRC Animal Breeding Research Organisation, West Mains Road, Edinburgh EH9 3JQ, UK.

Each mammalian species has its own genetically-controlled characteristic life span and rate of ageing. The basis of this control is a key question in gerontological research. We also know that life span is strongly genetically correlated with adult body size. How this genetic relationship is controlled also remains both a mystery and a challenge. Yet the relationship is clear, and much more use should be made of it.

The inter-species relationship of time traits to body size. *Life span and body size.* The regression of the natural logarithm of the life span on the natural logarithm of adult body weight has been given for mammalian species as 0.291 ± 0.054^5, 0.198 ± 0.021^9, 0.310 ± 0.025^8, which is significantly higher than[9], and 0.267 ± 0.023^{14}. None of the estimates differ from the weighted mean of 0.255 ± 0.013. Estimates over more restricted ranges have been 0.27 ± 0.027 for artiodactyls, 0.17 ± 0.026 for carnivores and 0.24 ± 0.038 for primates[15]. Most coefficients are in line with the 0.27 originally found for metabolic processes in mammals and birds[2].

Time and age traits in general. Pseudo-significant differences among published estimates of regression on adult body size are fairly typical for many age and time traits other than life span. Samples taken from the highly diverse population of mammalian species may be neither normal nor random. Critical examination of collections of estimates[5,7,10,11,14] suggest that virtually all the regression coefficients are consistent with a single common value of 0.25 to 0.27.

Metabolic age. This conclusion, or assumption, of uniformity has led me to advocate universal use of a single common value of 0.27 (or 0.25) for all age and time traits[12,13]. Using one universal value allows a much wider and more comprehensive application of the concept of metabolic age which is age, measured from an origin near conception, divided by adult body weight to the power of 0.27. Such an age scale allows different species to be compared on a fairly precise quantitative basis.

Developmental events in the life of a mammal. The general temporal life-plan of a mammal is outlined in terms of metabolic age in the Table. This life-plan is the same as that given in Taylor (1985)[14] but with one or two additional events included.

Prenatal. Implantation occurs on average at about 4 metabolic days of age. The first somites appear at about 7 metabolic d and the last somites at about 14 metabolic d at the end of metamorphosis. Fetal eyelids close at about 17 metabolic d, and open at twice that age. Birth occurs at about 50 metabolic d. These developmental horizons show a great deal of genetic variation.

Table. *Expected life-plan of a mammal in relation to metabolic age ($\pm$ 20 per cent) (age in days from conception divided by adult body weight, g, to the power of 0.27).*

Metabolic age	Developmental event	Metabolic age	Developmental event
0	egg enters uterus (3.5 d after ovulation)	110	becomes sexually mature
		115	is 0.5 mature in body weight
4	implants	150	breeds for the first time and starts lactating
7	first somites appear		
10	mammal becomes 0.00001 mature in body weight	200	ends first lactation
		270	tibial epiphyses fuse
14	end of metamorphosis	440	0.98 mature in body weight
17	fetal eyelids close	500	is fully mature in body weight
40	is 0.04 mature in body weight and heavier than all mammals of the same age	700	end of prime of life
		1000	first onset of cancer ($P>10^{-3}$)
50	is born 0.05 mature in body weight	2000	dies
90	is weaned		
100	is 0.4 mature in body weight		

Postnatal. In postnatal life, weaning occurs on average at a metablic age of about 100 d (that is, about 50 metabolic d after birth so that gestation length and lactation length are in general roughly equal). Sexual maturity occurs roughly at about 110 metabolic d (when animals are about 0.45 to 0.50 mature in body weight). First parturition is normally expected at about 200 metabolic d but is prone to outside influences such as seasonal cycles in feral species or human intervention in domestic species. Epiphyseal fusion of the proximal extremity of the tibia occurs at about 270 metabolic d. Animals are on average about 0.98 mature in body weight at about 440 metabolic d so that normal growth is over by about 500 metabolic d. The prime of life is from 500 to 700 metabolic d, after which senescence begins. Eventually death is expected at about 2000 metabolic d of age.

Metabolic processes can be described in a similar way. For example, the heart beat lasts 0.3 metabolic s and the entire blood volume circulates every 0.3 metabolic min.

Mean mammalian curves for biosenescent traits. In relation to intake, metabolism and growth, mammalian species are known to have common physiological and biochemical characteristics, but show large quantitative differences because of differences in body size. On a metabolic age scale, all the genetic variation between species associated with differences in adult body size is automatically removed. In this way, mean mammalian curves were produced for growth, food intake, heat production and body composition[14]. Mammalian species also have common biosenescent processes: they undergo senescence in the same way qualitatively but at different rates[3]. Mean curves similar to those for growth traits could therefore be produced for traits associated with senescence. These mean curves would quantitatively combine information from different species on the time course of senescent processes, and would allow deviant species to be recognized and their deviations to be quantified.

Among the many traits that might usefully be examined, compared and summarized in terms of metabolic age are (1) population mortality curves for different species, (2) incidence of disease (especially tumours and atherosclerosis) and frequency of chromosomal aberations, (3) rates of mineralisation in tissue, (4) rate of accumulation of age pigments, (5) amount of collagen cross-linking, (6) dopamine depletion in normal brain — similar in humans and mice[4], (7) number of oocytes and ovarian follicles[1], (8) rate of decline in male and female sexual activity and reproductive capacity[1], (9) the capacity of cells for dividing repeatedly *in vivo* (number of 'doublings'[6]) and (10) physiological function including maximum cardiac output, vital capacity and renal clearance rates (eg[3]). Mean mammalian life curves for five of these biosenescent traits are tentatively illustrated in the Figure.

Conclusion. The concept of metabolic age, which furnishes the measure for a common temporal life plan for mammals, would also appear to furnish a most useful basis on which to compare species for biosenescent traits.

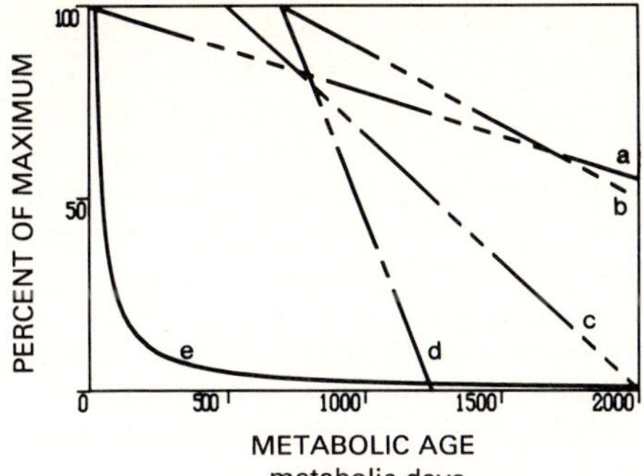

Figure. *Mean mammalian curves describing the common pattern of ageing in mammals.* Five different aspects of biological senescence are illustrated. Each trait is expressed as a percentage of its maximum value: (a) proliferative capacity of cell cultures (decline is 1 unit every 60 metabolic d starting from early fetal stage), (b) maximum output of heart, lungs and kidneys (decline is 1 unit every 30 metabolic d starting at 700), (c) male reproductive activity (1 unit every 15 metabolic d starting from 500), (d) female reproductive capacity (decline is 1 unit every 5 metabolic d starting at 700), (e) number of oocytes remaining (expected proportion at metabolic age θ ($\geqslant 25$) is $25/\theta$).

1 Adams, C.E. (1985): Reproductive senescence. In *Reproduction in mammals. Book 4. Reproductive fitness*, ed C.R. Austin & R.V. Short, pp. 210–233. London: Cambridge University Press.
2 Clark, A.J. (1927): *The Comparative physiology of the heart*. London: Macmillan.
3 Cutler, R.G. (1984): Evolutionary biology of aging and longevity in mammalian species. In *Aging and cell function*, ed J.E. Johnson, pp. 1–147. New York: Plenum Press.
4 Finch, C.E. (1978): The brain and aging. In *The biology of aging*, ed J.A. Behnke & C.E. Finch, pp. 301–309. New York: Plenum Press.
5 Gunther, B. & Guerra, E. (1955): Biological similarities. *Acta Physiol. Latinoam.* **5**, 169–186.
6 Hayflick, L. (1973): Programmed number of possible cell divisions of fibroblasts. *Am. J. Med. Sci.* **265**, 433.
7 Lindstedt, S.L. & Calder, W.A. (1981): Body size, physiological time and longevity in homeothermic animals. *Quart, Rev. Biol.* **56**, 1–16.
8 Mallouk, R.S. (1975): Longevity in vertebrates is proportional to relative brain weight. *Fed. Proc.* **34**, 2102–2103.
9 Sacher, G.A. (1959): Relation of lifespan to brain weight and body weight in mammals. In *Ciba Foundation Colloquium on Aging*, 1, ed G.E.W. Wolstenholme, pp. 115–141. London: Churchill.
10 Schmidt-Nielsen, K. (1984): *Scaling. Why is animal size so important?* London: Cambridge University Press.
11 Stahl, W.R. (1962): Similarity and dimensional methods in biology. *Science* **137**, 205–212.
12 Taylor, St.C.S. (1965): Time taken to mature in relation to mature weight in domesticated mammals. *Anim. Prod.* **7**, 203–220.
13 Taylor, St.C.S. (1980): Genetic size-scaling rules in animal growth. *Anim. Prod.* **30**, 161–165.
14 Taylor, St.C.S. (1985): The use of genetic size-scaling in evaluation of animal growth. *J. Anim. Sci.* (Suppl. 2), **61**, 118–143.
15 Western, D. (1979): Size, life history and ecology in mammals. *Afr. J. Ecol.* **17**, 185–204.

Nutrition and the ageing rat

E.J. MASORO
Department of Physiology, University of Texas Health Science Center, 7703 Floyd Curl Drive, San Antonio, TX 78284, USA.

The report by McCay & Crowell (1934)[17], which showed that restricting food intake increases the longevity of rats, provided the first strong evidence pointing to nutrition as an important factor in their ageing. Since then, a broad spectrum of ageing characteristics have been found to be influenced by food restriction, thus further establishing nutrition as an important modulator of ageing in rats[14]. Current research is aimed at defining the mechanism by which food restriction influences the ageing processes and at learning whether specific nutrients are involved and, if so, which.

Ageing characteristics of rats modulated by food restriction. A striking aspect of the effects of food restriction is that the life span (ie, the maximum length of life) of a cohort of rats is extended as effectively as life expectancy (ie, the mean length of life)[31]. Moreover, life span is extended as much by food restriction started in young adult life (at 6 months of age) as when it is initiated soon after weaning[30]. These findings serve to focus the action of food restriction on adult ageing rather than on maturation processes. Further, on the basis of the analysis of survival curves by the method of Gompertz, it has also been concluded that food restriction influences the longevity of rats by slowing the rate of ageing[2]. Many and varied age changes occur in the physiological systems of mammals and most are deteriorative in nature[14] and this physiological deterioration in rats is retarded or partially prevented by food restriction.

A third line of evidence supporting the concept that food restriction acts by slowing ageing processes is its effect on age-related disease processes. Food restriction started soon after weaning or in young adult rats markedly retards the development of chronic nephropathy and cardiomyopathy and delays the occurrence of neoplastic disease[30].

For food restriction to modulate so many ageing characteristics of rats, it must act on one or more basic cellular ageing process. Indeed, uncovering the mechanism of action of food restriction should further our understanding of the fundamental nature of ageing and furnish clues to interventions capable of delaying or preventing the deleterious aspects of ageing.

Mechanism by which food restriction modulates ageing in rats. The first view proposed for the mechanism of action of food restriction on ageing was that it did so by slowing growth and development[18]. This hypothesis held sway for many years and is still often cited. However, recent studies show that food restriction initiated in adult life[11,29,30] also increases life expectancy. These data provide strong evidence against the growth and development hypothesis.

It has been hypothesized[2] that food restriction increased longevity by preventing the accumulation of excess body fat. However, food restriction during the first years of life, followed by *ad-libitum* feeding, resulted in obesity and also an increased longevity[29]. It was found that there was no correlation between adiposity and longevity in *ad-libitum* fed rats and there was a positive correlation between adiposity and longevity in food-restricted rats[3].

It was proposed that food restriction slows the ageing process by inhibiting the secretion of a pituitary ageing factor[7], and the same author developed the following model for his hypothesis: food restriction modulates hypothalamic neurotransmitter metabolism so as to decrease the secretion of a hypothalamic-releasing hormone which results in a decreased secretion of a pituitary hormone[8]. In support of this hypothesis, it was shown[9] that both food-restricted rats and hypophysectomized rats receiving only cortisone replacement therapy have an increased life expectancy and life span, a delayed onset of renal and neoplastic disease and a retarded ageing of collagen. However, these few findings in common do not provide strong support of this hypothesis. Moreover, there is little information on the effects of food restriction on pituitary hormone secretion or on whether a reduction in the secretion of a particular pituitary hormone influences the ageing processes.

It was proposed (by Sacher) that food restriction modulates ageing by reducing the metabolic rate[27]. That metabolic rate influences ageing was first suggested by Rubner[26] and formalized by Pearl in his 'Rate of living theory of ageing'[20]. Sacher supported his hypothesis by an analysis of the data from a study in which five different diets causing a range of longevity characteristics were studied[24]. Sacher calculated caloric expenditure to be within 5 per cent of 0.43 MJ (102 kcal) per gram B.Wt. per life time for each of the dietary groups. He concluded that by decreasing the metabolic rate, food restriction increases the time required for the rat to reach the life time limit of energy expenditure, thereby increasing the length of life. Harman[12] expanded this theory by postulating that this decrease in metabolic rate decreases the rate of free radical generation and by this mechanism slows the ageing processes. Although this metabolic hypothesis is attractive, recent evidence does not support it: I have reported[15] that food restricted rats consumed more energy per day per g B.Wt. than *ad-libitum* fed rats and that the life time energy consumption per g B.Wt. was much greater for food-restricted than for *ad-libitum* fed rats[15]. McCarter *et al.*[16] measured oxygen consumption of rats throughout the 24 h under usual living conditions and found that 6-month-old *ad-libitum* fed rats had a metabolic rate of 0.57 MJ (136 kcal) and rats food restricted from 6 weeks of age on had a metabolic rate of 0.60 MJ (143 kcal) per kg lean body mass per day. These studies show that food restriction can markedly increase longevity without reducing the metabolic rate.

Recently, it has been suggested that food restriction influences ageing processes by retarding the progressive age-related decrease in the rate of protein turnover[22]. They pointed out that a decline in protein turnover reduces the ability of the organism to respond to changes such as environmental challenges and that such a blunting of responses is a hallmark of ageing. Experimental support for this hypothesis came when it was reported that food restriction retards the age-related decline in protein synthesis in many tissues of the rat[28]. Much more experimental data are needed before this provocative hypothesis can be accepted or rejected.

Specific nutrients and the ageing of rats. The findings on the effects of specific nutrients on the ageing of rats have been much less consistent and striking than those just described for food restriction. Decreasing the intake of protein increases the longevity of rats[1,23] and it has been suggested that extension of life span by food restriction may in part be due to the restriction of protein. However, other studies[19,25] have yielded data contradicting this view. When this problem was addressed by authors who controlled for food intake by restricting it so that energy intake was the same irrespective of the protein content of the diet it was found that reducing the dietary protein decreased longevity[4]. Recently it was found that moderate protein restriction in *ad-libitum* fed rats in the absence of energy restriction resulted in a significant increase in longevity, but that the extent of this increase was much less than that obtained with a similar level of protein restriction accompanied by energy restriction[30].

High-fat diets decreased life expectancy but not life span[10]. In a more recent study, increasing the fat content of the diet or altering its nature had only marginal effects on the survival characteristics of rats[13]. There is some evidence that specific carbohydrates can influence longevity. Longevity was decreased in male Wistar rats in which sucrose was increased from 15 to 30 per cent of the diet by weight, replacing starch[5]. Similar results were obtained with male BHE rats, but there was no statistically significant effect of dietary sucrose on longevity in male Wistar rats[6]. Clearly, much more data are needed on the effects of dietary carbohydrate and fat on longevity and ageing processes.

The design of some food restriction studies (eg,[31]) indicates that the restriction of vitamins and minerals are not involved in the longevity effects but more work is needed on this point. Supplementation of the diet with vitamin E has been shown to increase the life span of rats fed diets containing high levels of unsaturated fat, but the interpretation of this study and others on the effects of vitamin E and other antioxidants is clouded by the fact that when fed such diets rats reduce their food intake[21].

1 Barrows, C.H., Jr. & Kokkonen, G. (1975): Protein synthesis, development, growth and life span. *Growth* **39**, 525–533. .

2 Berg, B.H. & Simms, H.S. (1960): Nutrition and longevity in the rat. II. Longevity and the onset of disease with different levels of intake. *J. Nutr.* **71**, 255–263.

3 Bertrand, H.A., Lynd, F.T., Masoro, E.J. & Yu, B.P. (1980): Changes in adipose mass and cellularity through adult life of rats fed ad libitum or a life-prolonging restricted diet. *J. Gerontol.* **35**, 827–835.

4 Davis, T.A., Bales, C.W. & Beauchenne, R.E. (1983): Differential effects of dietary caloric and protein restriction in the aging rat. *Exp. Gerontol.* **18**, 427–435.

5 Dolderup, L.M. & Visser, W. (1969): Influence of extra sucrose in the daily food on the life-span of Wistar Albino rats. *Nature* **222**, 1050–1052.

6 Durand, A.M.A., Fischer, M. & Adams, M. (1968): The influence of type of dietary carbohydrate. *Archs. Path.* **85**, 318–324.

7 Everitt, A.V. (1973): The hypothalamic-pituitary control of aging and age-related pathology. *Exp. Gerontol.* **8**, 265–277.

8 Everitt, A.V. (1982): Nutrition and the hypothalamic pituitary influence of aging. In *Nutritional approaches to aging research*. ed B.G. Monet, pp. 245–256. Boca Raton, FL: CRC Press.

9 Everitt, A.V., Seedsman, N.J. & Jones, F. (1980): The effects of hypophysectomy and continuous food restriction begun at age 70 or 400 days on collagen aging, proteinuria, incidence of pathology and longevity in the male rat. *Mech. Age. Dev.* **12**, 161–172.

10 French, C.E., Ingram, R.H., Uram, J.A., Barron, G.P. & Swift, R.W. (1953): The influence of dietary fat and carbohydrate on growth and longevity of rats. *J. Nutr.* **51**, 329–339.

11 Goodrick, C.L., Ingram, D.K., Reynolds, M.A., Freeman, J.R. & Cider, H.L. (1983): Differential effects of intermittent feeding and voluntary exercise on body weight and life span in adult rats. *J. Gerontol.* **38**, 36–45.

12 Harman, D. (1981): The aging process. *Proc. Natl. Acad. Sci.* **78**, 7124–7128.

13 Harman, D., Hendricks, S., Eddy, D.E. & Siebold, J. (1976): Free radical theory of aging: Effect of dietary fat on central nervous system function. *J. Am. Geriat. Soc.* **24**, 301–307.

14 Masoro, E.J. (1984): Nutrition as a modulator of the aging process. *Physiologist* **27**, 98–101.

15 Masoro, E.J., Yu, B.P. & Bertrand, H.A. (1982): Action of food restriction in delaying the aging process. *Proc. Natl. Acad. Sci. (USA)* **79**, 4239–4241.

16 McCarter, R.J.M., Masoro, E.J. & Yu, B.P. (1985): Does food restriction retard aging by reducing the metabolic rate? *Am. J. Physiol.* **248**, E488–490.

17 McCay, C.M. & Crowell, M.F. (1934): Prolonging the life span. *Sci. Monthly* **39**, 405–414.

18 McCay, C., Crowell, M. & Maynard, L. (1935): The effect of retarded growth upon the length of life span and upon ultimate body size. *J. Nutr.* **10**, 63–79.

19 Nakagawa, I. & Masano, Y. (1971): Effect of protein nutrtion of growth and life span in the rat. *J. Nutr.* **101**, 613–620.

20 Pearl, R. (1928): *The rate of living*. New York: Alfred Knopf.

21 Porta, E.A., Joun, N.S. & Nitta, R.T. (1980): Effects of the type of dietary fat at two levels of vitamin E in Wistar male rats during development and aging. I. Lifespan, serum biochemical parameters and pathological changes. *Mech. Age. Dev.* **13**, 1–39.

22 Richardson, A. & Cheung, H.T. (1982): The relationship between age-related changes in gene expression, protein turnover and the responsiveness of the organism to stimuli. *Life Sci.* **31**, 605–613.

23 Ross, M.H. (1961): Length of life and nutrition in the rat. *J. Nutr.* **75**, 197–210.

24 Ross, M.H. (1969): Aging, nutrition and hepatic enzyme activity in the rat. *J. Nutr.* **97**, Suppl. Pt II, 563–602.

25 Ross, M. & Bras, G. (1973): Influence of protein under- and over-nutrition on spontaneous tumor prevalence in the rat. *J. Nutr.* **103**, 944–963.

26 Rubner, M. (1908): *Das Problem der Lebensdauer und Seine Beziehungen zum Wachstum und Ernabrung*. Munich: Oldenbourg.

27 Sacher, G.A. (1977): Life table modification and life prolongation. In *Handbook of the biology of aging*, ed C.E. Finch & L. Hayflick, pp. 582–638. New York: Van Nostrand Reinhold.

28 Sparks, M.B., Rickett, W.G., Rehwaldt, C.A., Cheung, H.T. & Richardson, A. (1983): Effect of dietary restriction on gene expression. *Fed. Proc.* **42**, 1307.

29 Stuchlikova, E., Juricova-Horakova, J. & Deyl, Z. (1975): New aspects of the dietary effects of life prolongation in rodents. What is the role of obesity in aging. *Exp. Gerontol.* **10**, 141–144.

30 Yu, B.P., Maeda, H., Murata, I. & Masoro, E.J. (1984): Nutritional modulation of longevity and age-related disease. *Fed. Proc.* **43**, 858.

31 Yu, B.P., Masoro, E.J., Murata, I., Bertrand, H.A. & Lynd, F.T. (1982): Life span study of SPF Fischer 344 rats fed ad libitum or restricted diets: longevity, growth, lean body mass and disease. *J. Gerontol.* **37**, 130–141.

Ageing, nutrition and the endocrine system

B.J. MERRY and Anne M. HOLEHAN
Wolfson Institute, University of Hull, Hull, HU6 7RX, UK.

It has been recognized from the early work of Osborne *et al.* (1917)[8] that controlled underfeeding will extend maximum life span in several rodent species. A number of physiological and biochemical indices suggest that such underfed rodents are retained in a physiologically younger condition than their fully-fed age-matched controls[4].

The biochemical mechanism by which chronic underfeeding extends life span is unknown but it has been proposed that the neuroendocrine system which integrates gene expression during development and maturation may also function to control the timing of senescence changes[3].

Experimental model. Growth was retarded in experimental animals by limiting the intake of the normal diet so that the body weight was maintained at 50 per cent that of the *ad-libitum*-fed control animals[5,6]. This procedure will extend maximum life span in the male by 42 per cent and in the female by 36 per cent.

Endocrine response of male rats to chronic underfeeding. Dietary restricted male rats showed a delay of 10 to 20 d in the timing of puberty as evident from both fertility studies and the timing of the peak of plasma testosterone,[6,7]. While *ad-libitum*-fed animals maintained high plasma FSH

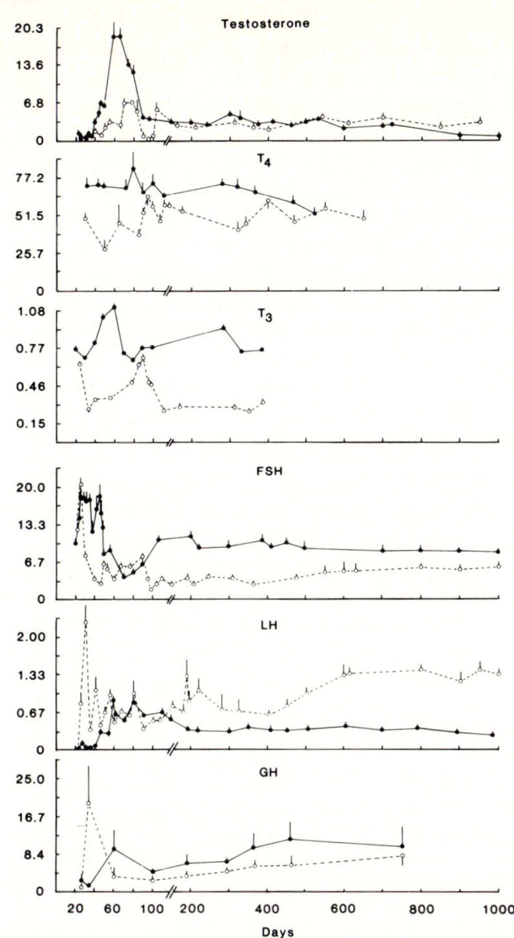

Figure. *Age profiles for plasma testosterone, T_4, T_3, FSH, LH and GH for male* ad-libitum-(●) *fed and dietary restricted (○) rats.* Each point represents the mean ± s.e.m. for 10 rats. Data for testosterone, FSH and LH redrawn from Merry & Holehan (1981). Data for T_4 and T_3 redrawn from Merry & Holehan (1985).

values until the onset of puberty at 35–40 d, chronic underfeeding resulted in a premature decline in the plasma levels of this hormone and is thought to be the major cause of delayed puberty[5]. In contrast, elevated but unstable plasma concentrations of luteinising hormone (LH) were recorded in the prepubertal dietary restricted rat.

Since prolonged underfeeding may be associated with depressed adrenocortical function, the ability of fully-fed and dietary restricted rats to respond to an environmental stress was assessed throughout the 1st 2 years of life,[7]. During the 1st year of life the ability to respond to stress was impaired but partially recovered after refeeding for 7 d. In 148 d rats bearing indwelling cannulae, elevation of plasma corticosterone was observed in response to infused ACTH, indicative of a pituitary origin for the modified stress response.

Within 2–3 d of restricted feeding circulating T_4 levels fall to about 65 per cent and T_3 levels are severely depressed to approximately 40 per cent of control values. Although the depressed plasma T_4 levels are probably indicative of reduced thyroid stimulating hormone (TSH) release, the greatest effect is on the peripheral conversion of T_4 to T_3 which contributes 85–90 per cent of the overall thyroidal status of the target tissues.

GH in rats is released episodically with a periodicity of approximately 3.3 h and plasma levels were examined in free-moving conscious rats bearing in-dwelling atrial cannulae. A restriction in peak duration was observed in the underfed animals, but decreased GH levels are not the primary cause of the retarded growth for injection of ovine GH over a 3-week period did not accelerate growth[7].

Endocrine response in the female: effect on reproduction. Female rats fed a restricted diet from weaning showed a retention of normal vaginal cyclicity for more than 18 months[5]. Rats retained on a restricted diet were fertile, bearing multiple live litters to as late as 920 d, in comparison to 500 d in the fully-fed animals. The decline in litter size which accompanies ageing in fully-fed rats was not evident in the dietary restricted animals although maximum litter size in this group was significantly smaller. A comparison of the hormone profiles from weaning to puberty revealed significantly depressed FSH levels while a 2 to 3-fold elevation of circulating oestradiol-17β and depressed levels of progesterone were recorded[1]. The ovary of underfed prepubertal rats is responsive to gonadotropin stimulation as shown by elevated plasma progesterone levels after priming with a regime known to induce superovulation in control animals[7].

At an age, (180–200 d), when fully-fed animals were beginning to show the first age-related perturbations in the cycle, the hormonal profile of the oestrous cycle demonstrated significantly higher levels of plasma FSH in underfed rats associated with an early release of the preovulatory peak of LH. The peak of oestradiol-17β occurred 6 h later in the cycle and the total amount of hormone released was 46 per cent that recorded in the fully-fed rats. The retention of a hormonal profile in female dietary restricted rats characteristic of a chronologically younger animal is supported by studies on the steroidogenic pathways of individual follicles.

Conclusion. Fundamental to the neuroendocrine theories of ageing is the postulate that the neuroendocrine axis which is central to other ontogenetic processes, is also involved in the timing of senescence. Clearly hypothalamic-pituitary ageing in the female rat is proceeding at a slower rate as is evident from the extension of reproduction in these animals but the most persistent change in hormone status is observed in the T_3 plasma levels. While the endocrine system may amplify the physiological changes associated with underfeeding, the primary response of the animal may be decreased total protein synthesis with enhanced protein turnover, the endocrine response observed being secondary to this general cellular adaptation[2].

1 Holehan, A.M. (1984): The effect of ageing and dietary restriction upon reproduction in the female CFY Sprague Dawley rat. PhD Thesis, University of Hull.
2 Lewis, S.E.M., Goldspink, D.F., Phillips, J.G., Merry, B.J. & Holehan, A.M. (1985): The effects of ageing and chronic dietary restriction on whole body growth and protein turnover in the rat. *Exp. Geront.* (In press)
3 Meites, J., Hylka, V.W. & Sonntag, W.E. (1984): Cellular-molecular versus neuroendocrine concepts of aging: a need for integration. In *Molecular basis of aging*, ed A.K. Roy & B. Chatterjee, pp. 187–207. London: Academic Press.
4 Merry, B.J. (1985): Dietary manipulation of ageing in rodents. In *Ageing and longevity*, ed J.K. Collins, Society for the Study of Human Biology Symposium volume. Cambridge: University Press. (In press).
5 Merry, B.J. & Holehan, A.M. (1979): Onset of puberty and duration of fertility in rats fed a restricted diet. *J. Reprod. Fert.* **57**, 253–259.
6 Merry, B.J. & Holehan, A.M. (1981): Serum profiles of LH, FSH, testosterone and 5α-DHT from 21 to 1000 days of age in *ad libitum* fed and dietary restricted rats. *Exp. Geront.* **16**, 431–444.
7 Merry, B.J. & Holehan, A.M. (1985): The endocrine response to dietary restriction in the rat. In *The molecular basis of aging*, ed A.V. Woodhead & A. Blackett, Brookhaven Symposium in Biology, no. 33. (In press).
8 Osborne, T.B., Mendel, L.B. & Ferry, E.L. (1917): The effect of retardation of growth upon the breeding period and duration of life in rats. *Science* **45**, 294–295.

Calcium homoeostasis in ageing

H.H. DRAPER
Department of Nutrition, College of Biological Science, University of Guelph, Guelph, Ontario, Canada NIG 2W1.

The capacity of animals to adapt to a range of calcium intakes by altering the efficiency of calcium absorption was demonstrated by Norwegian investigators[9,13]. The mechanism of this adaptation has been elucidated, mainly through the work of DeLuca and co-workers[2] in the United States and of Fraser & Kodicek[3] in Britain, in terms of a parathyroid hormone

(PTH)-calcitriol axis regulating the synthesis of calcium-binding protein(s) in the intestinal mucosa.

This mechanism presumably accounts for the ability of adults in some countries to maintain calcium homoeostasis on a calcium intake that is little more than half that of adults in other countries. The WHO/FAO recommendation (400–500 mg/d) reflects the calcium content of cereal-based diets. However, national agencies have recommended intakes as high as 1000 mg/d, and recently it has been suggested that the recommended daily allowance (RDA) for postmenopausal women in the USA be raised from the current 800 mg/d to 'at least 1200 to 1500 mg/d'[7]. An international comparison of calcium recommendations reveals an influence of Parkinson's Law, ie the intake recommended rises to meet the supply available.

The demonstration that the requirement of adults for calcium homoeostasis is variable led to the conclusion that calcium deficiency is unlikely to be a significant factor in bone diseases of children and adults. This view was reinforced by the report that ageing bone loss in adults was similar in countries with markedly different calcium intakes (El Salvador, Guatemala and the United States)[4]. However, it has become apparent that the capacity of adults to adapt to a low calcium intake is not universal and that full adaptation is not achieved by most older adults. Malm's early study revealed a cohort of adults who failed to reestablish calcium homoeostasis over weeks or months following a reduction in calcium intake. A negative calcium balance, reflected in osteopenia, is a general (though probably not inevitable) accompaniment of ageing. Superimposed on ageing osteopenia there is, in women, a marked acceleration of bone loss following the menopause which is clearly associated with the cessation of oestrogen production, and which predisposes to postmenopausal osteoporosis, the most prevalent bone disease of older women.

Calcium intake and bone disease. Epidemiological evidence for the relationship between calcium intake, ageing bone loss and osteoporotic bone fractures among Yugoslavian adults has been obtained[10]. Osteopenia was more extensive in middle-aged adults living in a region with a low calcium intake (400–500 mg/d) than in adults inhabiting a high calcium area (approximately 900 mg/d), and the occurrence of osteoporotic bone fractures, particularly among women, was markedly greater. It is noteworthy that a difference in metacarpal bone mass existed at 30 years of age, the earliest age at which subjects were examined. This observation reinforces the view that the most important determinant of osteoporotic bone disease in the aged is the mass of bone accumulated at skeletal maturity. This factor accounts for the lower susceptibility of blacks than of whites and for familial differences in vulnerability to osteoporosis.

Further epidemiological evidence for a relationship between chronic calcium intake and ageing osteopenia has been obtained on a cohort of women in Nebraska[6]. Longitudinal assessments of diet and bone density indicated that calcium balance in postmenopausal women required an average intake of 1200 mg/d. These investigators concluded that an intake of 1500 mg would prevent osteoporosis in essentially all postmenopausal women.

Ingestion of 1500 mg calcium day from natural sources would require major diet modification on the part of a segment of the population with entrenched food habits and a declining requirement for energy. Since the average calcium intake of middle-aged women in the United States is about 200 mg below the current RDA of 800 mg, it appears likely that the main effect of raising the RDA would be to increase the percentage of women who fail to comply with it. The alternative is to prescribe a calcium supplement of about 1000 mg/d. Despite the prevalence of osteoporosis among postmenopausal women, however, only a minority of women ever incurs a bone fracture. To recommend that the entire female population take a calcium supplement three times a day for one or two decades is an extreme solution to the problem. It would seem more practicable to limit this recommendation to menopausal women diagnosed for vulnerability to osteoporosis on the basis of an assessment of inherited bone mass, physical activity and food habits.

Vitamin D and calcium homoeostasis. Calcium supplements presumably exert their effect of calcium homoeostasis by producing a rise in serum calcium ion concentration and a consequent reduction in the synthesis of PTH, the main stimulator of bone resorption, thereby removing the imbalance between osteoclastic bone resorption and osteoblastic bone formation which otherwise exists during the postmenopausal period. Serum calcium is also depressed by a deficiency of vitamin D which is necessary for normal calcium absorption. Evidence that a significant number of adults are in questionable vitamin D status (defined as having a serum calcidiol level of < 10 ng/ml) has been found in several countries. Low calcidiol levels appear to be due mainly to lack of solar radiation resulting from indoor living or envelopment with clothing. Serum calcidiol levels are generally higher in the United States and Canada than in Britain, where there is less exposure to sunlight and less fortification of foods with vitamin D. It has been recommended that the RDA for vitamin D be raised from 400 IU to 800 IU/d[14], postulating that vitamin D deficiency may be responsible for the decrease in calcium absorption during ageing.

Phosphorus intake and calcium metabolism. Serum calcium is also depressed in the presence of excess phosphate, producing an increase in PTH-mediated bone resorption. An adverse effect of excess dietary phosphorus on calcium homoeostasis in adult animals has been recognized for many years, and recently there has been an interest in whether the calcium requirement of adults in some Western countries in increased by a high intake of phosphorus from natural sources and phosphate additives. Evidence for increased parathyroid activity, including increased hydroxyproline and cyclic AMP excretion and reductions in serum and urinary calcium, has been obtained in adults fed experimental diets high in phosphorus[1,17]. However, balance studies have indicated that, at least in young adults, calcium homoeostasis is maintained over the normal range of phsophorus intakes. For example, it was found that calcium balance was maintained by young adults consuming 500 mg calcium/d and over 2000 mg phosphorus[8]. These findings indicate that any increase in bone resorption in these subjects caused by their high phosphorus intake was fully compensated by an increase in bone formation, ie that their high phosphorus diet produced an increase in bone turnover rate but no bone loss.

While these observations are reassuring, it has not been demonstrated whether postmenopausal women respond to a high phosphorus intake in the same way as do younger adults. Ageing in women has been reported to be associated with a decreased capacity for bone formation, a decline attributable to lack of oestrogen. If so, the ability of postmenopausal women to maintain calcium homoeostasis in the face of an increase in bone resorption caused by ingestion of excess phosphate cannot be assumed from studies on young adults. It is also not clear why a decrease in serum calcium caused by a low calcium or vitamin D intake should cause bone loss if a similar decrease caused by excess dietary phosphorus does not.

Protein intake and calcium balance. The high protein content of the diets consumed by many adults in Western countries also has come under investigation as a possible cause of osteoporotic bone disease. Excess dietary protein leads to an increase in endogenous acid production, the excretion of which (mainly as ammonium ions and acid phosphates) is associated with a decrease in the renal reabsorption of calcium. Acid production by adults consuming a high protein diet is derived mainly from the oxidation of excess sulphur amino acids. The complete oxidation of 1 mol of sulphur amino acids generates 2 mol of hydrogen ions.

It has been shown that a high intake of purified proteins increases urinary calcium and the amount of dietary calcium required to maintain homoeostasis[8]. However, failure to observe either hypercalciuria or a negative calcium balance in adults fed a high protein diet (2 g/kg per d) as meat has also been reported[15].

The protein-phosphorus-calcium interaction. The discrepancy between these two findings apparently lies in the increase in phosphorus intake that is associated with a high meat diet. Urinary calcium is reduced on a high phosphorus diet as a result of increased calcium reabsorption from the renal tubules induced by parathyroid stimulation. The calciuretic effect of excess protein in a high meat diet is counteracted by the hypocalciuric effect of excess phosphorus. The influence of dietary protein on calcium metabolism recently has been reviewed[16].

Whether the counterbalancing effects of excess protein and phosphorus intakes are always conducive to calcium homoeostasis in adults is unknown. It is of interest, however, that Alaskan and Canadian Eskimos consuming a semi-carnivorous diet have an unusually rapid rate of ageing bone loss[11,12]. The diet of the Alaskan Eskimos involved in this study was derived mainly from land and sea mammals. In addition to being extraordinarily high in protein and phosphorus, it was unusually low in calcium, since bone-chewing is no longer extensively practised by this population. Hence it is impossible to determine whether their accelerated osteopenia is attributable to their high protein and phosphorus intake, their low calcium intake, or to a combination of these factors. In this context, Eskimos examined in the course of the Canadian nutrition survey were found to have a lower calcium intake (about 400 mg/d in adult females), higher serum phosphorus and lower serum calcium than the national sample[5].

1 Bell, R.R., Draper, H.H., Tzeng, D.T.M., Shin, H.K. & Schmidt, G.R. (1977): Physiological responses to foods containing phosphate additives. *J. Nutr.* **107**, 42–50.
2 DeLuca, H.F. (1978): Vitamin D metabolism and function. *Archs Int. Med.* **138**, 836–847.
3 Fraser, D.R. & Kodicek, E. (1970): Unique biosynthesis by kidney of a biologically active vitamin D metabolite. *Nature* **228**, 764–766.
4 Garn, S.M., Rohmann, C.G. & Wagner, B. (1967): Bone loss as a general phenomenon in man. *Fed. Proc.* **26**, 1729–1736.
5 Health and Welfare Canada (1975): *Nutrition Canada. The Eskimo Survey Report.* Ottawa: Information Canada.
6 Heaney, R.P., Recker, R.R. & Saville, P.D. (1978): Menopausal changes in calcium balance performance. *J. Lab. Clin. Med.* **92**, 953–963.
7 Heaney, R.P., Gallagher, J.C., Johnston, C.C., Neer, R., Parfitt, A.M. & Whedon, G.D. (1982): Calcium nutrition and bone health in the elderly. *Am. J. Clin. Nutr.* **36**, 986–1003.
8 Linkswiler, H.M., Zemel, M.B., Hegsted, M. & Schuette, S.A. (1981): Protein induced hypercalciuria. *Fed. Proc.* **40**, 2429–2433.
9 Malm, O.J. (1958): *Calcium requirement and adaptation in adult men.* Oslo: Oslo University Press.
10 Matkovic, V., Kostial, K., Simonovic, I., Buzina, R., Brodarec, A. & Nordin, B.E.C. (1979): Bone status and fracture rates in two regions of Yugoslavia. *Am. J. Clin. Nutr.* **32**, 540–549.
11 Mazess, R.B. & Mathur, W. (1974): Bone mineral content of northern Alaskan Eskimos. *Am. J. Clin. Nutr.* **27**, 916–925.
12 Mazess, R.B. & Mathur, W. (1975): Bone mineral content of Canadian Eskimos. *Hum. Biol.* **47**, 45–63.
13 Nicolaysen, R. (1953): Physiology of calcium metabolism. *Physiol. Rev.* **33**, 424–444.
14 Parfitt, A.M., Gallagher, J.C., Heaney, R.P., Johnston, C.C., Neer, R. & Whedon, G.D. (1982): Vitamin D and bone health in the elderly. *Am. J. Clin. Nutr.* **36**, 1014–1031.
15 Spencer, H., Kramer, L., Debartolo, M., Norris, C. & Osis, D. (1983): Further studies on the effect of high protein diet as meat on calcium metabolism. *Am. J. Clin. Nutr.* **37**, 924–929.
16 Yuen, D.E., Draper, H.H. & Trilok, G. (1985): The effect of dietary protein on calcium metabolism in man. *Nutr. Abst. Rev.: Rev. Clin. Nutr.* **54**, 447–459
17 Zemel, M.B. & Linkswiler, H.M. (1981): Calcium metabolism in young adult males as affected by level and form of phosphorus intake and level of calcium intake. *J. Nutr.* **111**, 315–324.

Guide-lines for the elderly: a workshop report

Louise DAVIES (Organizer)
Gerontology Nutrition Unit, Royal Free Hospital School of Medicine, 21 Pond Street, London NW3 2PN, UK.

An invited speaker on each topic was asked to consider national and international guide-lines for the general population and to submit a suggested guide-line specifically for the elderly. These preliminary guide-lines were presented to the Workshop participants and summarized below.

Fats. (*M.A. Crawford* Nuffield Laboratories of Comparative Medicine, London, UK.) The deterioration of the nervous and vascular systems are common features associated with ageing. Consequently, the general principles recently outlined by the Committee on Medical Aspects of Food Policy (1984) and the National Advisory Committee on Nutrition Education (1983) should apply.

Essential fatty acid requirements are likely to be heightened as the desaturase system operates at reduced rates with ageing. The requirement for preformed 20 and 22-carbon-chain-length derivatives of linoleic and linolenic acids may be accentuated. As brain cell deterioration accelerates in the elderly, nutritional strategy should aim towards the conservation of the 20 and 22 carbon chain lengths derivatives of the parent essential fatty acids. It should be noted that the brain only uses the long-chain derivatives. This would mean improved intake of the trace elements zinc and selenium together with foods rich in vitamins E and C. It would also be desirable to set high standards of vitamin B_6 which is involved in the conversion of the parent essential fatty acids to their long-chain derivatives.

In practical terms, this would imply a focus on food such as fish, together with sea food such as mussels and oysters, very lean meat and game, dark green vegetables, an abundance of fresh salads employing French dressing, whole seed foods, nuts and fresh fruit, in particular, strongly coloured and seed-containing fruits.

The speaker made it clear that his approach is speculative and derives from his research on patients with multiple sclerosis. He agreed that there is no evidence that diets such as he proposes are associated with measurable differences in intellectual performance. Nevertheless, he reiterated his view that guide-lines on fats for the elderly need to pay more attention to the *quality* of fats in the diet.

Refined carbohydrates (*I. MacDonald* Guy's Hospital, London, UK.). Refined carbohydrates in the diet of the elderly have the advantage of being cheap, convenient, satisfying hunger and being psychologically rewarding. The disadvantage of dental caries does not apply, but refined carbohydrates have low nutrient density, may be conducive to overweight, encourage constipation and giver rise to reactive hypoglycaemia.

Although it is relatively easy to change the amount of sugar consumed by the elderly, eg in beverages, this should not be attempted unless there is some good reason, such as overweight, or reactive hypoglycaemia which might cause those already unsteady to stumble or fall.

Dietary fibre and complex carbohydrates (*Patricia A. Judd* King's College, Kensington, London, UK.). For 'younger', active older people the recommendations should be similar to those for the adult population, ie a gradual changeover to food high in complex carbohydrates and dietary fibre.

In older age groups, especially if housebound or immobile, energy intakes may be low and increasing dietary fibre intake difficult without resorting to supplements such as bran. This may have undesirable effects on mineral and trace element absorption and may also further limit food intake.

Increased dietary fibre intake should be achieved by increasing intakes of wholegrain cereals, potatoes, vegetables and fruits at the expense of 'refined' cereals and sucrose-containing foods; this should have the effect of decreasing nutrient density of the diet and counteract effects on mineral and trace element absorption.

The speaker felt that guide-lines suggested for younger adults (eg 25–30 g dietary fibre per day) would be impractical for elderly people with low energy intakes to achieve without supplementation. When increasing dietary fibre it is important to maintain intakes of fluid, calcium and other minerals. Supplements were deemed expensive. A wide variety of food sources of dietary fibre is needed to achieve benefits in addition to the relief of constipation.

Salt (*P. Dodson* Dudley Road Hospital, Birmingham, UK.). Unless there are specific clinical indications, the elderly population should not be recommended to reduce salt intake.

There is no direct evidence that a high sodium intake produced high blood pressure in the elderly; however the speaker would support the recommendation of a lower salt intake in the management of patients with hypertension or mild cardiac failure. In his view there may be grounds for a general reduction in salt intake for those in their 50s but not for those aged seventy plus, particularly as such a reduction may lessen the palatability of food. However it was pointed out that a high sodium intake promotes urinary calcium loss; a reduction of salt intake might therefore be important in delaying the development of metabolic bone disease. Interaction of sodium with other nutrients also needs to be taken into account when producing dietary guide-lines.

Protein (*V. Young* Massachussetts Institute of Technology, USA.). The minimum physiological requirements for protein and the individual indispensable amino acids in the healthy elderly (70s +) are based on limited and contradictory findings.

For the healthy elderly we have proposed that a safe protein intake should be equivalent to about 12–14 per cent of an adequate energy intake.

Because the elderly frequently experience conditions likely to increase protein (and amino acid) needs, relative to those for healthy young adults, there is an urgent need to establish more precisely the protein nutritional requirements for elderly populations.

The need for protein is increased under conditions of stress, disease and rehabilitation. Dr Young suggested that for the institutionalized, frail or bedridden elderly, the protein:energy ratio of the diet would need to be higher than the 12–14 per cent proposed for the free-living generally healthy population. The nutritionally indispensable amino acids can be supplied equally well from plant or animal sources (although other nutrients such as highly bioavailable iron from meat are of importance when devising dietary guide-lines). There is a need for further research on the advisability of restricting dietary protein where there is a reduction in kidney function, particularly in diabetics.

Alcohol (*Marsha Morgan* Royal Free Hospital, London, UK.). Alcohol should be avoided in elderly patients with known cerebral disease and in those taking regular medication particularly psychoactive drugs. No amount of alcohol taken daily can be considered safe. However, amounts of alcohol = 30–40 g in males (2–2½ pints of beer) and = 10–20 g in females (½–1 pint of beer) may be safely taken on 3 to 4 occasions per week. Alcohol should be avoided as a 'nightcap'.

Dr Morgan pointed out that excessive drinking is often a cry for help from those who are lonely or ill in their retirement. Her main recommendation was to avoid *daily* alcohol consumption. When challenged, she referred to findings that even at a relatively low level, daily drinking is likely to lead to physical disease. However, if an elderly person has habitually taken a daily drink, and there is no other reason for him to stop, he should be left to continue the habit. Alcohol as a nightcap can cause the sedated elderly to awake confused; it is an addictive drug, not a safe alternative to other drugs.

The problems of producing RDAs for the elderly (*H. Munro* Tufts University, Boston, USA.). There are few data for most nutrients on the requirements of the over 60s, and especially for those of 75 or 80+. Present RDAs do not sufficiently take into account disabilities and immobility, nutrient consumption in relation to reduced energy intake, socio-economic risk factors, drug nutrient interaction, digestion and absorption. RDAs need to be related to the retention of function in the elderly.

Obesity (*J. Garrow* Clinical Research Centre, Harrow, Middlesex, UK.). Old age is associated with decreased exercise tolerance, and obesity makes matters even worse. However other hazards of obesity, such as heart disease, affect old people less than young ones. Since metabolic rate decreases with age it is difficult for obese old people to lose weight. In many cases the effort of dieting is not repaid by commensurate benefit from weight loss.

The speaker agreed that if osteoarthritis has developed, weight reduction is often more effective in restoring mobility than the use of drugs; even a relatively small weight loss can lead to a noticeable improvement. However, he stressed that, in general, severe dietary restrictions which may be of benefit to younger adults would not necessarily achieve an improved standard of life for elderly people.

Exercise (*E. Joan Bassey* The University of Nottingham Medical School, UK.). The 'normal' patterns of exercise to which we aspire should be set by the healthy, active elderly, not those unfortunates with marked pathology nor those who have drifted into inactivity without good cause. Inevitable age-related deterioration *per se* is modest, especially in relation to stamina for rhythmic activities such as walking; therefore the advice must be, 'keep going; if you could do it yesterday, you can do it tomorrow'.

Although there may be physical hazards in encouraging increasing activity in the elderly, the dangers of remaining unnecessarily inactive may be greater. It is important to maintain stamina in old age and it is essential not to discourage personal effort, even when the pace is slow. Exercise is important in the maintenance of appetite and the management of disease such as osteoporosis. Gardening can do harm if it involves maintaining a crouched or bent posture for long periods. Dr Bassey agreed that walking can be boring and that exercise regimes for the elderly call for an imaginative approach. For instance, the embarrassment of swimming can be overcome by encouraging elderly people, good swimmers together with beginners, to join together as a group in a sheltered environment.

Nutrition education (*M. Diane Holdsworth and Louise Davies* Gerontology Nutrition Unit, London, UK.). Nutrition education for the elderly needs to take into account their widely differing mental and physical capabilities. It should be targeted either direct to the elderly themselves or indirectly to those looking after them or providing their meals. An essential aim should be to encourage elderly men and women to keep up an interest in food; thus social problems affecting dietary intake are relevant to this type of nutrition education.

Non-nutritional intervention, eg provision of a walking frame, may be more relevant to this age group than expounding the role of specific nutrients.

The most effective nutritional messages are those geared to the desires for health, taste and convenience. The use of a variety of techniques is most likely to stimulate attention and to endorse the message for both short and long term memory. Visual aids, group discussion, quiz, questionnaire or lecture are best backed up by practical cooking demonstrations, taste sessions, reminder leaflets and specialised recipe books.

Involvement of the elderly meeting together in social groups for recipe demonstrations, tasting and discussion could stimulate their interest in the dietary guide-lines.

Practical difficulties (*Magdalena Krondl* Faculty of Medicine, University of Toronto, Canada). If elderly people are to be exhorted to eat more vegetables to increase dietary fibre and complex carbohydrates, it should be remembered that: (1) they will mostly only accept vegetables with taste already familiar to them or those which they perceive as 'healthy'; (2) they do not have a high tolerance of raw vegetables, irrespective of dietary fibre content; (3) acceptance of both cooked and raw vegetables is limited by digestive disturbances.

Barriers to the application of dietary guide-lines in institutional food services (*A. Stewart* The Flinders University of South Australia, Adelaide, Australia). Lack of authoritative, easy to follow guide-lines and suitable economical, nutritious, acceptable recipes; lack of conviction of the benefits of dietary changes, by both residents and staff; unimaginative presentation of food, with poor communication between reisdents, kitchen and nursing staff; lack of suitable in-service training courses.

Additional guide-lines for the elderly. Suggestions for additional guide-lines specifically for the elderly included the topics of fluid, sunlight/vitamin D, and calcium. In proposing a guide-line for the latter, *B.E.C. Nordin* agreed that the levels he suggested (so long as vitamin D levels were in the normal range) were compatible with normal dietary intakes from dairy products and other calcium foods.

In general discussion it was stressed that there is scope for dietary change and the introduction of new ideas for health benefits at any age. There is no question of a cut-off age at which guide-lines are not required. However, it is essential to recognize the wide range of life experience and physical and mental capacities of the elderly population. The question was raised: To whom should guide-lines be addressed? To the elderly themselves and or to those caring for them or both? Guide-lines need to be translated into terms of foods: practical, enjoyable and acceptable.

The organizer of this Workshop wishes to thank Alan Stewart for advice in the preparation of this summary and to express gratitude to all the speakers for making this a most exciting workshop. Our message to the next International Congress of Nutrition: we need to continue these stimulating discussions and present them in more detail in four years time.

XVI: Measuring food intake

Validation of food intake measurements

Wija A. VAN STAVEREN

Department of Human Nutrition, Agricultural University, De Dreijen 12, 6703 BC Wageningen, The Netherlands

Marr finished her famous review article 'Individual dietary surveys: purposes and methods' with the words 'The methods chosen must be known, or shown, to be reproducible and sufficiently valid for the purpose of the particular investigation'[7]. Since that time many studies have been carried out on the validity and reproducibility of methods assessing food consumption, but uncertainty still exists on the quality of these methods.

The *validity* of a method is defined as the demonstration that a method measures what it is intended to measure. This can only be assessed by comparing it with an independent method of indisputable accuracy. There is no such absolute method because of the nature of the data to be collected. Instead, either the relative validity or the concurrent validity may be established. The relative validity evaluates the method in terms of another generally accepted method, designed to measure the same concept. The concurrent validity compares the results of a method with a biological marker. Validity studies refer to information bias and systematic response errors.

A method is called *reliable* or *reproducible* if it gives the same results when used repeatedly in the same situation. The problem in food consumption surveys is that the situation is never absolutely identical. Reproducibility refers to the biological within-person variation (or true day-to-day variation) as well as to random response errors, because these two sources of variation can hardly be separated.

Accuracy incorporates elements of both validity and reproducibility. There are many sources of error in food consumption studies[8]. However, as Marr has pointed out[7] in judging the quality of research methods the differences in the purposes of different investigations should be appreciated. It is often said that for epidemiological studies it is not always necessary to produce accurate results for each individual, but methods yielding valid data on groups of individuals would be of great value[2]. To be able to obtain such valid data on a *group level* it is of the utmost importance to specify beforehand which kind of data the study should supply. In epidemiological studies data are required roughly on three different levels for various purposes[1,4]:

(A). Average energy and nutrient intake data for a group, in order to make group-group comparisons.

(B). The distribution of usual energy and nutrient intake data within a population, to detect groups of individuals at risk, if the risk is marked by a high or a low intake of a certain nutrient.

(C). The usual energy and nutrient intake of groups of individuals during a long period of time, to make correlation and regression analysis relating independent and dependent variables on an aggregate level.

In Wageningen, we have only used methods that produce quantitative estimates of energy and nutrient intake of Dutch adults. In all methods portion sizes have been checked by weighing and amounts of foods have been converted into energy and nutrients by the Dutch nutrient data base UCV.

Methods appropriate for purpose 'A'. The preferred approach for this purpose is to estimate the energy and nutrient intake of one day per person in a large representative sample with an adequate representation of all days of the week. A certain required precision for the mean intake (eg a standard error of 10 per cent or less of the mean value) does not necessarily fix the sample size and the number of days per person, but can be attained by a number of equivalent combinations[11]. A weighed record method has long been considered to be the gold standard and valid group estimates may be obtained with this method[6]. Based on studies comparing protein intake with urine nitrogen excretion we have concluded that valid group estimates on protein intake may also be obtained with the dietary history method estimating the usual food consumption of the previous month and with the 24-h recall method[9]. Study designs and interviews, however, should be made carefully, because it appears that systematic underestimates of energy and nutrient intake often occur with record as well as with recall methods. The importance of standardization and training of interviewers has been demonstrated recently[5].

Methods appropriate for purpose 'B' and 'C'. For these purposes it is necessary to assess the usual energy and nutrient intake of individuals, although the data are interpreted on an aggregate level. Sample size and number of observations required depend on the accuracy desired, and the ratio of within-person to between-person variation.

The dietary history method has been developed by Burke[3] to estimate the usual food consumption of individuals in one interview, sometimes completed with a 3-day record. The usual food consumption refer to the past year, six months, or season. According to Burke[3] this method can only be applied in groups of individuals with a rather constant dietary pattern, but since 1947, food consumption patterns have become much more complicated in industrialized countries and it is difficult now to interview individuals in industrialized countries about their usual food consumption over one year. Therefore, we have restricted the time of reference in our dietary history interviews to one month. Even then it is practically impossible to validate the results on an individual level.,

It has been suggested that recalls or records of a single day's food intake randomly selected to represent all days of the week and administered over an interval long enough to discover cyclic changes, will result in valid estimates of the usual intake of individuals. We have applied such a design with 14 monthly repeated 24-h recalls in 123 adult women[10]. This design should yield valid information for the purposes mentioned under B and C. Validity was examined firstly by comparing the mean daily energy intake with fluctuations in body weight. (The pattern of physical activity for all subjects was classified as light work.) Therefore the group was distributed in approximate quintiles of their energy intake. The results showed that subjects reporting a very low energy intake tend to under-estimate their energy intake and subjects reporting a very high energy intake tend to overreport their energy intake. Secondly, the validity was tested by comparing the mean daily protein intake assessed with the fourteen 24-h recalls with the mean protein intake as derived from the nitrogen excretion in at least 11 collections of 24-h urine per subject. With this test the same trend was found. In 20 subjects (16 per cent) the mean difference in daily protein intake between the two estimates exceeded 20 g. Sixteen of these 20 subjects reported either a very high ($n = 7$) or a very low ($n = 9$) energy intake.

In using 24-h urine nitrogen excretion as the reference method it should be recognized, that this method also has potential sources of error and variation which attenuate the relationship between protein intake as derived from the 24-h urine nitrogen excretion and from the estimated food consumption data. It is generally accepted that urine nitrogen excretion can hardly be used on an individual level as a biological marker to validate daily protein intake as estimated with food consumption data, even for an average of several days. Studies under controlled conditions have shown, however, that it is not very likely that these sources of error and variation would account for differences of more than 20 per cent from the protein intake derived from 24-h urine nitrogen excretion. In our study, this means that the difference between the two mean estimates for one person should not exceed the 20 g. Such a difference, however, is from a physiological point of view a large difference.

Thus, with not very strict criteria 16 per cent of the subjects were not able to provide valid 24-h food recalls. Most of these invalid recalls concerned participants who reported either an extremely high or an extremely low energy intake. This indicates that it is very difficult to determine within a group studied solely on the basis of food consumption the percentages of subjects with a high or a low health risk, if the risk is marked by a high or a low intake of a certain nutrient (purpose B). To relate intake data of certain nutrients with indicators of health status (purpose C) it has been suggested that oversampling should be practised, checking the data with an independent biochemical indicator. This makes it possible to discard data considered not to be trustworthy.

In conclusion: within an adequately formulated research design, the methods assessing food consumption described can be relatively valid for estimating intakes of energy and protein in groups (purpose A). If energy and nutrient intake data are to be related to health indicators (purpose C) repeated measures per person are necessary. Furthermore, oversampling and the checking of intake data with an independent biochemical or physiological indicator to discard data that are considered not to be trustworthy, are recommended. However, it is difficult to detect groups with a low or high intake of a certain nutrient within the study population (purpose B) if only data on food consumption are available. This is so, even if, based on the required accuracy and the ratio of the within-person to between-person variation, enough recalls are obtained per participant in a sample of sufficient size.

Further studies should be done to indicate whether the problems of overreporting and underreporting encountered in our study are especially associated with the 24-h recall method. It might be important to be able to characterize persons who either overreport or underreport their food consumption and why they do so.

1. Beaton, G.H. (1982): What do we think we are measuring? In *Symposium on dietary data collection, analysis and significance*, pp. 36–49 Boston: University of Massachusetts.
2. Block, G. (1982): A review of validations of dietary assessment methods. *Am. J. Epidemiol.* **115**, 492–505.
3. Burke, B.S. (1947): The dietary history as a tool in research. *J. Am. Diet. Ass.* **23**, 1041–46.
4. Callmer, E., Haraldsdottir, J., Løken, E.B., Seppänen, R. & Solvoll, K. (1985): Selecting a method for a dietary survey. *Näringsforskning* **29**, 43–52.
5. Frank, G.C., Hollatz, A.T., Webber, L.S. & Berenson, G.S. (1984): Effect of interviewer recording practices on nutrient intake — Bogalusa heart study. *J. Am. Diet. Ass.* **84**, 1432–1439.
6. Isaksson, B. (1980): Urinary nitrogen output as a validity test in dietary surveys. *Am. J. Clin. Nutr.* **33**, 4–12.
7. Marr, J.W. (1971): Individual dietary surveys: Purposes and methods. *World Rev. Nutr. Diet.* **13**, 105–164.
8. Van Staveren, W.A. & Burema, J. (1985): Food consumption surveys: frustrations and expectations. *Nähringsforskning* **29**, 38–42.
9. Van Staveren, W.A., De Boer, J.O. & Burema, J. (1985): Validity and reproducibility of a dietary history method estimating the usual food intake during one month. *Am. J. Clin. Nutr.* **42**, 554–559.
10. Van Staveren, W.A., Deurenberg, P., Burema, J., Hautvast, J.G.A.J. (In prep): Validity of a monthly 14 times repeated 24-h recall method.
11. Van Staveren, W.A., Hautvast, J.G.A.J. & Katan, M.B. (1982): Dietary fiber consumption in an adult Dutch population. A methodological study using a seven-day record. *J. Am. Diet. Ass.* **80**, 324–30.

National assessment of food intake studies in the Federal Republic of Germany

H. ROTTKA, Gabriele STRICKER and G. ZAUSCH
Institute for Social Medicine and Epidemiology, Federal Health Office, Postfach 33 00 13, D–1000 Berlin 33, Federal Republic of Germany.

No generally accepted method exists for measuring the dietary intake of people outside institutions despite a constant demand by nutritionists, epidemiologists, clinicians, the food industry and others for this kind of measurement. Accurate information is frequently needed on a few individuals, on representative groups, or on thousands of persons for prospective studies[2]. Such detailed information on food intake has to be collected directly from the individuals under study. This is costly of staff, time needed to record and evaluate the comprehensive data and in general.

For the purposes of the nutrition report of the Federal Republic of Germany (Ernährungsbericht der Bundesrepublik Deutschland) we developed an indirect method based on recording foods bought in the different types of household[1]. Records are based upon the so-called income and consumption sample (Einkommens- und Verbrauchs-Stichprobe; EVS) of household data collected every 5 years by the Federal Office of Statistics, Wiesbaden[4].

Individual household records of foods and drinks bought are available, classified by months and covering amounts and monetary values for one year. The sample comprises a total of 50 000 households and 4000 of these participate, on a monthly basis, in the detailed recordings of foods bought. Since representation of the individual population groups and seasons is not absolutely uniform, individual prognostication factors are used for standardization fixed by reference to the microcensus of the preceding year into size of household, income class, and occupation, allocating equal shares to the individual months. Data are available for each household on the monthly number of principal meals (lunch and dinner) taken by individual household members outside the home in cafeterias, restaurants, schools. By means of an estimation method, the results of an additional representative survey covering foods consumed in places outside the home especially cafeterias and restaurants, and included in the EVS.

It is impossible, however, to identify values for individuals from the data except for one-person households. For this reason, we tried to determine empirically a functional association between household and person-related values that meets this requirement. The model sets out with the assumption that, with increasing age, there will only be a gradual change in the amounts consumed. Thus the age-dependent amount of consumption of a particular food can be approximately described by the shape of a curve having various increase and decrease phases whose position and intensity are determined by the statistical material.

The estimate for each individual food depends on a regression of the average daily consumption (M) of a household predicted by age (T) and sex (m, w: men, women) of the persons within the household. The function of age was constructed, separately for each sex, as a polynomial of the third degree (Figure). Using values for decay and waste, it is possible to

$$\text{Figure.} \qquad M_1 = C_0 + \sum_j [\, f_m(T_j) + f_w(T_j)\,] + \mathcal{E}_1$$

$$M = \text{amount} \qquad\qquad f_m\,T\,/\,f_w\,T = \text{third} - \text{degree polynominal}$$

$$T = \text{age}$$
$$C_0 = \text{mean number persons / household}$$
$$m\,/\,w = \text{sex}$$

calculate the supply of energy, nutrients, vitamins and trace elements from individual foods and/or the whole diet for the different age and sex groups of the population. The data obtained on the basis of the computational steps outlined is quite close to the average consumption figures for foods and nutrients.

This 'Income and Consumption Sample' adopted for our purposes produced numerous tables which have been published in the Nutrition Report[1] published by the Federal Government (every 4 years). For example, separate tables show the amount of single food items consumed by males and females of different age groups, starting at 4 to 6 years and ending at 66 years and above. Each table contains 225 single food items. Other tables show the amounts of protein consumed by males and females of the same age groups, the protein coming from 21 food groups. The consumption of single food items in different parts of Germany ('Länder') are also shown together with the seasonal consumption figures for each month of a year. This procedure is a mixture of the direct and the indirect method. It is relatively easy and gives good results at relatively low cost.

The other method for measuring food intake on a national level is the National Food Survey using a direct method. This study was designed by a committee of our Federal Health Office and at the moment is conducted by GfK Marktforschung. It is based on a representative sample of

10 800 households, ie about 24 000 persons investigated in 20 administrative districts ('Regierungsbezirke') over a period of 3 years. For evaluating food intake a diary is used in which all foods, beverages and activities are recorded by each test person for her/himself, with the exception of children below 12 years of age, for whom the parents record. These recordings have to be done for 9 consecutive days. A preliminary period of 2 d is needed to eliminate possible effects of the survey on habits and to control the recordings of the test person and, perhaps, to improve recording. The following 7 d period serves to measure the average intake of energy and nutrients and to estimate energy expenditure. We also do a 24 h recall for validation purposes on beverages only. The test persons are instructed to take notes directly after each meal or during its preparation. This applies also to meals taken outside the home. Meals have to be recorded according to the individual ingredients and the way of cooking. To determine the amount of food consumed and its ingredients, the test person should use adequate scales. These are checked as to their degree of accuracy before using. It is also possible to define quantities in common household measuring units for bread, sausage, cheese, cakes and different sizes of dishes, cups and glasses. The status of each food (raw, cooked, amount of non-edible wastes etc.) is also noted.

Test persons are instructed by qualified nutritionists or specially trained staff. Intensive contact with test persons during the recording period is guaranteed by personal contacts or telephone calls. The first contact on the second day — personally or by telephone — serves to give additional instructions and to control the food protocols. The following calls on the 3rd and 5th day are necessary to stabilize motivation and to remove further difficulties. The extent of these contacts depends on the quality of recording of each member of the household.

The advantage of this method is that it permits the inclusion of differences in food intake which may occur from one day to the next. In comparison to the 24 h recall, the intra-individual variability of food intake is reduced because of a longer recording period. These average values obtained are very suitable to determine correlations.

The disadvantage of this method is the enormous amount of work for both the test persons and staff. Furthermore, recording of the consumed foods and beverages may result in an alteration of nutritional behaviour (mostly simplification) during the test period. This can be avoided if tape recorders are used.

Coding. For all direct methods coded on data sheets we use the Federal Food Coding System (Bundeslebensmittelschlüssel — BLS)[3]. The BLS has been developed as a standard uniform hierarchically structured code to meet the needs of research workers but also those of simple dietary assessments.

The code contains up to 7 digits, although for most uses 5 digits suffice and for less sophisticated studies, 3–4 digits are enough. For example when coding a meal with the BLS, red wine, strawberry, or ice cream need only 3 digits to describe them, but the pizza uses all 7 digits.

Data. The data bank based on this code contains 5000 food items, each with up to nine different methods of preparation. The 5000 items include 500 basic foods, 1300 industrially processed basic foods, 500 vegetarian and dietetic items — an additional 2700 industrially processed and prepared foods are required only for more extensive intake surveys. Up to now the Federal Food Code contains 1500 coded recipes of meals, from households, restaurants and food services. This will be extended in the near future to another 3000 recipes.

The constituents given, about 64 at the moment, are all macro nutrients and vitamins, 13 minerals and trace elements, 10 sugars, 5 dietary fibre components, 4 fatty acids and 3 risk substances: cholesterol, purine-nitrogen and oxalic acid.

We are trying to extend the constituents up to about 170, to include all 18 amino acids, 35 fatty acids, 18 organic acids and even 6 heavy metals.

In the Federal Food Coding System, losses are also determined in 9 selected cooking methods for each of the 64 nutrients. All the values have been selected from German, British, Dutch, American and other food tables or other published data. In cases where no analytic information is available, we developed special computer programs to calculate the missing values. This helps to avoid blanks which normally make it impossible to correct calculations of nutrients. These values determined by calculation will be marked to enable them to be replaced by analytical data. We plan to have user conferences on the BLS twice a year to make such replacements and to decide what other changes should be made, to keep the system alive and up to date.

1 Deutsche Gesellschaft für Ernährung (1976): *Ernährungsbericht 1976.* Frankfurt: Deutsche Gesellschaft für Ernährung
2 Marr, W. (1971): Individual dietary surveys. Purposes and methods. *Wld. Rev. Nutr. Diet.* **13**, 105–164.
3 Rottka, H., Polensky, W. and Scherz, H. (1985): Review of food composition tables and nutrient data banks in the Federal Republic of Germany. *Ann. Nutr. Metabol.* **29**, S1, 25–26.
4 Statistisches Bundesamt (1978): *Einkommens- und Verbrauchs stichprobe 1978.* Mainz: Kohlhammer.

Computer-assisted dietary assessment

Lenore ARAB
Klinisches Institut für Herzinfarktforschung, Universität Heidelberg, Bergheimer Str. 58, 6900 Heidelberg, Federal Republic of Germany.

Nutritional science, particularly when related to asessment of dietary intake is generally considered inaccurate, semiquantitative at best and largely unscientific. These prejudices (or truths) arise from severe methodological difficulties among other problems. Collection of information that is accurate and precise has been hindered by memory, bias, estimation difficulties, variation in intakes, communication problems, language, the extent of food offerings, time and expense. The current interest in dietary methodology is less one of scientific excitement about the methods than of a frustration with the status quo. As soon as an elegant, accurate and inexpensive method becomes available, it will be adopted and discussions of the pros and cons of the regular methods forgotten. This major breakthrough may be near, incorporating new applications and full automation from subject motivation and data capture to statistical analysis of the findings. This report is a projection on areas well suited to automation in which developments should be made to improve the scientific value of dietary methodologies, to simplify the process, reduce the costs, make dietary assessment available to more researchers and to speed the acquisition of results from months to minutes.

If a program is designed to be fun human beings will spend hours of time and lots of their own money in front of a terminal. The success of video games proves this. Application of such practical knowledge to diet assessment can help to attract the interest of our subjects and to motivate them. Direct input of the desired data into the computer saves time, trouble, and prevents many types of errors, and instant feedback, presenting information graphically is an extremely powerful method of information transfer. Evaluation of information entered can be transmitted in an informal, non-offensive but memorable fashion, by using computers.

The use of computers for interviewing is not new. In the medical area much pioneering work was done by Slack, first in proving that people will readily convey personal information to a computer[16]. Later he showed methods of feedback of subject responsiveness to the interview, such as responsiveness to heart beat rate, or the time lag in response to a question triggering a different line of questionning[15]. In 1972 they linked up a tape recorder to the computer to allow lengthy responses in a medical-psychological counselling situation[17].

The first reported computer dietary questionnaire was 12 years ago[9], a program inquiring about usual intake in a counselling situation has been in operation for 9 years[19].

A cornerstone study showed that computerized instruction could surpass written instruction or physicians' verbal explanations[10]; successful completion of a clean voided urine specimen by women was gauged by subjective opinion and objective testing. There was a significantly lower bacterial count in the computer-based explanation group of women. In Germany an automated 24-h recall has been successfully used in the field in a large epidemiological study, in which 20–40 persons per day were examined[4]. Dietary assessment generally involves collecting descriptive information on foods consumed by individuals (including parts eaten, parts discarded and preparation), quantifying the amount eaten, processing this information, often converting it to an estimate of nutrient intake and further statistical analysis, depending upon the hypothesis or purpose of the study. In Table 1 the probems in dietary assessment, and the degree to which they are currently being automated, are denoted.

Computer assistance: data collection. Data on intakes are currently and sporadically being collected with the assistance of computers, and will certainly be done increasingly in this manner in the future, in both small and large scale studies. This area of using computer support in standardizing questioning or easing the documentation of intakes is open to creative development. The automated 24-h recall mentioned earlier is one application in which the computer prompts questions about yesterday's intake (and activities). This method is divorced from interviewer bias and guarantees standardized question formulation, sequence and depth of probe, which is determined by the researcher and not the interviewer. An additional advantage is the elimination of coding steps, and the production of an immediate printout of intake of foods and nutrients consumed yesterday as well as the estimated energy expenditure (a sample segment is shown in Table 2). Another group has worked even longer with conversation-based computerized questionning of eating behaviour, particularly in patients with hyperlipidaemias[19], and reported a good level of acceptance. The system requires the subject to recall one typical day and record its composition in terms of foods usually eaten. Interesting graphics are used to motivate and stimulate the user while probing about the nutrient content of foods commonly eaten and to sum up total meals previously eaten in a commercially available program entitled the 'Eating machine'[18]. A Packman type character, with grins, grimaces and frowns lets you know how your behaviour compared with the recommended intake levels.

A new method of computerized assessment of eating behaviour is currently under development. Similar to a diet history, this is a quantitative assessment of regular intake structured by meals and day of the week. This program requires too much storage to be currently distributed widely on inexpensive microcomputers. It is being developed as a sensitive research tool for assessment and characterization of individual intakes over the last year. Space limitations

Table 1. *Areas of difficulty in dietary assessment*

	Current	Future automation		Current	Future automation
1. Time frame	−	−	5. Data processing	+ +	+ + +
2. Data collection	+	+ + +	6. Nutrient-to-food conversion	+ +	+ + +
3. Language and description	+	+ + +	7. Statistical analysis	+	+ + +
4. Quantification	+	+ +			

Table 2. *A sample of ESSEKAN questions (Q) and the responses (A) which in turn determine the next question from part of a 24-h recall from one subject.* The responses are the selections from a menu presented to the subject after each question. In response to their answer the next appropriate question is drawn from the program.

Q	A	Q*	A*
Did you eat or drink at mid-day?	Yes	Did you have something to drink?	Yes
Where did you eat it?	At home	What did you drink?	Wine
What did you have to eat?	Soup	What type of wine?	200 ml red
What type of soup was it?	150 ml clear broth	Can you think of anything else that you ate or drank at noon time?	No
Did you eat anything else?	Meat		
What type of meat?	Beef		
What was it exactly?	200 g fillet steak	What did you do between lunchtime and evening?	1.00 h of sleep
Did you eat anything else?	Vegetables		3.15 h of light work and some sports
What type of vegetables?	Cooked vegetables		
Which cooked vegetables?	120 g peas, 80 g carrots	What type of sport?	1.45 h swimming
Did you eat anything else?	Rice		
What type of rice?	150 g brown, cooked		
Did you eat anything else?	Dessert		
What type of dessert?	150 g apple	*Continued from left hand side of Table	
Raw, cooked or canned?	Raw		
Was there anything else?	No		

do not allow for complete description of the method. Dialogue begins with questions about how often per week breakfast is usually consumed and how many different sorts of breakfast are usually eaten. Detailed questionning of the sets of foods eaten and their amounts follow. The meal-organized questionning ends with an assessment of foods rarely or never eaten. The author predicts that all retrospective dietary intake information will be soon collected by standardized computerized programs.

Computer assistance: language and description. Language and terminology inexactness is a significant problem and yet a topic hardly dealt with in currently available software involved with dietary assessment. Many applications are imaginable and would be extremely useful. They include a system in which the input of any name prompts synonym lists or where this food relates to other foods in a thesaurus set up. When the item eaten represents a mixed dish, the recipe could be shown upon request in order to ensure that this name represents the combination of foods the subject is trying to describe. In 25 of the 69 data bases reviewed in the nutrient data base directory[11], ingredients are actually stored in the data base. This does not mean they are used for this type of identification, but they could be. In terms of cross-referencing among many different languages, experience has been gained through the development of an international multilingual agricultural thesaurus for the European Community use[1,12]. The European Community is increasingly solving its language problems through computerized language translations and this could help in the area of food tremendously. The problem of language and description can be expected to be eliminated by rapid access to extensive computer-stored memory of terms, synonyms, recipes and potentially images. These will in any case provide greater defense against incorrect, inexact terminology within and between languages. Taken further, the problem of identification would be greatly enhanced through full colour pictures of food items stored and recallable on the computer. This would lend the assurance to the researcher of a match based on vision instead of only verbal description. This approach could be also used for identification of parts of food actually analysed for nutrient content or parts of foods considered edible and inedible in different countries.

Computer assistance: quantification. Quantification of prior intakes will remain inaccurate, but simulation of reported intakes in two or three dimension can refine estimates and protect against gross errors. An existing two-dimensional fluid measure programme with interchangeable dimensions has been constructed (by Dr Ken Samonds, Director of the Massachusetts Nutrient Data Bank at the University of Massachusetts, Amherst) and includes typical beverage glass shapes, wine glasses, cups, mugs and short glasses. Visual filling and emptying of these images, after recreating the relevant size might enhance the effect. For prospective methods of dietary assessment, a kitchen scale linked to a recording device which understands natural language is available[7].

Another aspect of the quantification problems is the conversion of household units and common portion sizes to the gram amounts that most computerized data bases expect. Relief for the interviewer or dietician through computer-supported conversion of weight of items as purchased to weight of items as eaten (steak with bone, oranges, bananas) and prepared weight to dry weight (rice, noodles) and the differences due to peeling (carrots, potatoes) and coring (apples) is a task obviously suited to computerization thereby eliminating individual interviewer differences and miscalculations. It is however not as widely available in programs as might be expected: 44 of the 60 data bases summarized by Hoover report conversion capabilities. They are however rarely as wide reaching as to include all those mentioned above: 23 of those surveyed could not report the nutrient value of one serving of a given recipe. These conversions, the conversion of household measures to gram amounts (1 cup equals x grams of flour, sugar, salt, bran) and conversion of fluid measures into gram amounts would greatly relieve the tedium of thousands of dietary calculations confronting the dietician. Mass of weight conversions would free the subject to report food sizes in terms of height, width, depth without overwhelming the interviewer.

Computer assistance: data processing. Since it takes very long to clean up large data bases which do not have automated coding and entry procedures (12 man-years for the HANES II Study[13], 2 man-years for the Heidelberg Study[2]), advances are to be expected towards improving data processing. Data processing includes coding, entry, and validation of dietary information on nutrient content of foods. These are all expensive, time consuming and intellectually unstimulating tasks which could well and easily be automated. For example, coding and entry become internal tasks which are not visible to the interviewer or subject but conducted concurrently with the interview if the interview is computerized[6]. This will tremendously reduce error rates and save time.

Additionally, developments of automated coding systems with which prospective dietary assessments can be coded are possible[3] and new ones are under development[8].

A system for coding and entering food frequency information with options for seasonal behaviour, occasional consumption and consumption of specific foods being temperature (weather) dependent is described by Baghurst & Record[5]. Finally, a solution to the data processing involved with updating nutrient information would be possible through a centralized data resource and online access to the desired data similar to the information systems currently available for air line travel, stock reports and scientific literature. Some far-sighted individuals foresee the use of devices such as optic readers and bar-coded readers for nutritional assessment in the future[14]. The opinion of the author is that these will only be useful if apples and oranges received bar-codes as well as menu items in restaurants (which is not inconceivable).

Computer assistance: food to nutrient conversion. Independent from data base content is the influence of calculation of thousands of sets of information on the resulting products and sums. Automation would decrease the error rate, eliminate unnecessary calculation, and assure that the same algorithms are being undertaken.

Programs could also be designed to test and validate nutrient conversion programs in various systems, thereby enhancing the comparability of results between systems. Certainly the conversion of food amounts into a nutrient content estimation is the most widely advanced field of computerized dietary assessment.

Computer assistance: statistical analysis. The scientific goals of understanding the relationship between intakes and human health would be enhanced if the statistical analysis needed were more widely available and the programs providing statistical analysis for dietary information would allow or disallow the use of certain procedures for specific cases and would provide more explicit messages or warnings about the dependency of the results as a function of the study design, the sample size, and the dietary assessment method used, amongst other considerations.

Conclusions. There are many advantages to be foreseen from increased automation of dietary assessment in five basic areas — the *quality* (validity) of the information collected, the *time* and *effort* spared from tedious manual tasks, the *quality control* of data collected and data analyses, and the advantage of potentially better more lasting *behavioural change* through improved communication and stimulation. The dynamic quality of a computer session and the speed of results produced are strong potential motivators of interviewers, who see the results of their work immediatley; of subjects, who receive some information on the nutrient intake immediately; and of the scientists, who can much more rapidly begin to explore the interactions between nutrition and health which are currently prohibitively expensive and time-consuming. It should therefore be expected that enhanced activity in this area has a good chance of bearing fruit which could possibly have a terrific impact on nutritional research as well as the application of knowledge in our field.

1 Agrovoc. (1982): *A multilingual thesaurus of agricultural terminology.* Rome: Apimondia.
2 Arab, L., Schellenberg, B. & Schlierf, G. (1982): *Nutrition and health. A survey of young men and women in Heidelberg.* München: Karger.
3 Arab, L. (1983): Coding and entry of food intakes. In Proceedings of Eighth National Nutrient Data Bank Conference, ed R. Tobelman, pp. 13–22. Springfield, VA: National Technical Information Service.
4 Arab, L. & Bellin, O. (1983): Ein standardisiertes System für das 24-Stunden-Ernährungs- und Aktivitätsprotokoll, das die Befrager-Variabilität ausschließt. *Ernähr.-Umsch.* **30**, 249–258.
5 Baghurst, K. & Record, S. (1984): A computerized dietary analysis system for use with diet diaries or food frequency questionnaires. In *Community Health Studies*, **8**, 29–29a.
6 Bellin, O. & Arab, L. (1984): ESSEKAN. Ein standardisiertes 24-Stunden-Erinnerungsprotokoll über körperliche

Aktivität und Nahrungsmittelaufnahme. In *Entwicklung und Benutzung von Nährstoffdatenbanken in der Bundesrepublik Deutchsland*, ed L. Arab & G. Karg, pp.192–203.

7 Bingham, S.A., Cummings, J.H. & Murgatroyd, P.R. (1985): PETRA: a new device for weighed dietary intakes. XIII Int. Cong. Nutr. Abstr.

8 Buzzard, I.M. (1983): A microcomputer-based interactive model for collection and coding of dietary data. In *Proceedings of Eighth National Nutrient Data Bank Conference*, Springfield, VA: National Technical Information Service.

9 Evans, S.N., Gormican, A. (1973): The computer in retrieving dietary history data. 1. Designing and evaluating a computerized diabetic dietary history. *J. Am. Diet. Ass.* **63**, 397–402.

10 Fisher, L.A., Johnson, T.S., Porter, D., Bleich, H.L. & Slack, W.V. (1977): Collection of a clean voided urine specimen: a comparison among spoken, written, and computer-based instructions. *Am. J. Publ. Hlth* **76**, 640–644.

11 Hoover, L.W. (1984): *Nutrient data bank directory*, 4th Edn. The Curators of the University of Missouri.

12 Iljon, A. (1977): Development of a multilingual thesaurus for food science and technology. *Alimenta* **16**, 163–166.

13 National Center for Health Statistics (1981): *Plan and operation of the second National Health and Nutrition Examination Survey, 1976–1980. Vital and health statistics: series 1, programs and collection procedures, No 15*, Hyattsville: Department of Health and Human Services.

14 Sawicki, M. & Endres, J. (1983): Energy and nutrient calculations using an optical character reader system. *Continuing Education*, **82**, 135–141.

15 Slack, W. (1971): Computer-based interviewing system dealing with non-verbal behaviour as well as keyboard responses. *Science*, **171**, 84–87.

16 Slack, W.V. & van Cura, J.L. (1968): Patient reaction to computer-based medical interviewing. *Comput. Biomed. Res.* **1**, 527–531.

17 Slack, W.V. & Slack, C.W. (1972): Patient-computer dialogue. *New Engl. J. Med.* **286**, 1304–1309.

18 Thorne, B.S. (1982): *The eating machine*. Baltimore: Muse Software.

19 Witschi, J., Porter, D., Vogel, S., Buxbaum, R., Stare, F.J., Slack, W. (1976): A computer-based dietary counselling system. *J. Am. Diet. Ass.* **69**, 385–390.

Food intake studies in Australian aborigines: some methodological considerations

Ingrid H. E. COLES-RUTISHAUSER
Department of Human Nutrition, Deakin University, Geelong 3217, Australia.

Australian aborigines, today, live under a wide variety of climatic, geographic and socio-economic conditions. Places where aborigines live range from seasonal coastal and inland camp-sites, located mainly in the centre and the north of the continent, to conventional town housing in the large urban areas in the south of the continent. Between these extremes many aboriginal communities live under a variety of conditions in the vicinity of old government settlements, mission and cattle stations, or small mining and country towns.

Until recent years almost no quantitative information was available on the food intake of Australian aborigines living outside government settlements. This was because food intake data were usually collected in the course of anthropological rather than nutritional studies. The main exception to this was the food intake data collected by the American–Australian Scientific Expedition to Arnhem Land in 1948[6,7].

Conditions in the 1980s, however, are very different from those in 1948 particularly with respect to the availability of food. In 1948 rations were provided on a regular basis to aborigines living in settlements while to-day most food has to be purchased with the fortnightly pay or pension cheque except by those aborigines living at traditional bush camp-sites. Consequently for most aborigines the purchase of food now competes with other demands on a limited income and since the cost and availability of food vary with the location, as do the facilities for preparing food, there is no typical aboriginal diet. In this paper some of the methodological problems encountered in obtaining a valid assessment of food intake, under a variety of living conditions, are discussed by reference to a number of recent studies which have specifically attempted to obtain quantitative information on food intake in Australian aborigines.

Methodological problems associated with studies in the traditional environment. A number of problems are encountered in trying to assess food intake in a traditional bush

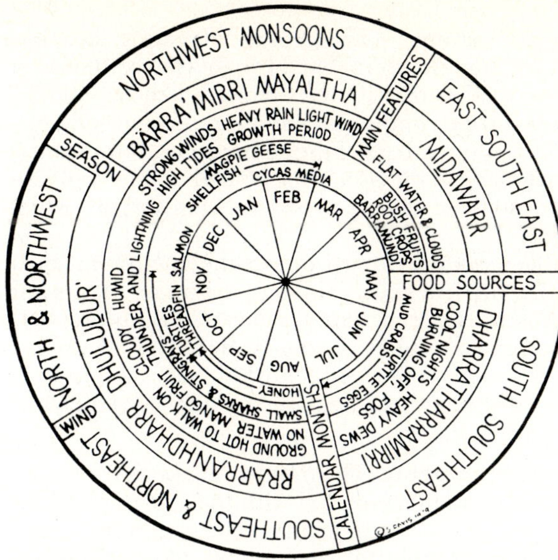

Figure 1. *A seasonal calendar of foods available in north east Arnhem Land*[10].

environment. These are well illustrated by a study undertaken by Meehan[8] to assess the role of shellfish in the diet of a group of Anbarra tribespeople living in out-station camps on the Arnhem Land coast of northern Australia.

Since season has a major influence on the availability of different types of animals and plants which are used for food (Fig. 1) an important requirement for this study was that observations should be made during all seasons. Moreover, to do this successfully meant living with the Anbarra for the whole year in order to be present whenever food collecting activities took place. Because of the division of food foraging activities between men and women, a study of the total diet also required not only constant observation but also the presence of both male and female observers. For example both traditionally and to-day the men in the community provide the fish, birds and larger mammals in the diet while the women provide the lizards, small mammals, shellfish and vegetable foods such as tubers, nuts and fruits.

To-day the main dietary sources of vegetable foods are purchased from the nearest store even by those living at bush camps so that traditional vegetable foods now make only a small contribution to the total diet (Fig. 2). Measuring the actual amounts of food available for consumption, however, presents difficulties in the traditional bush environment. Nuts and fruits, for example, are eaten whenever available, being swiftly taken from the tree and popped into the mouth.

Even foods not consumed as soon as collected present problems of quantification since a considerable amount of the food collected on foraging expeditions is not brought back to the

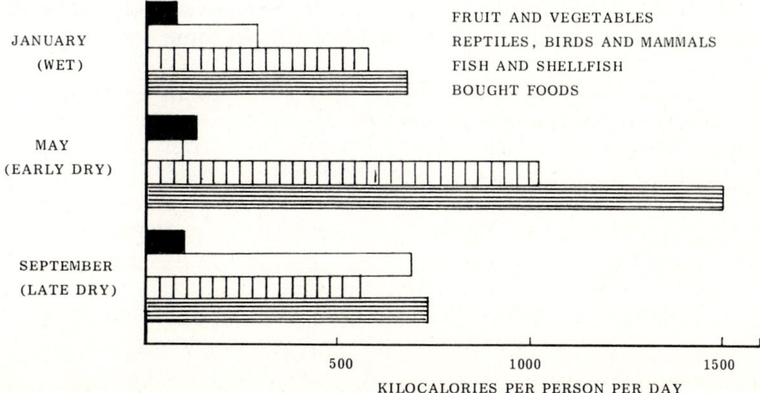

Figure 2. *Seasonal variations in major energy sources in the Anbarra diet. (Adapted from*[8]*).*

main camp-site but consumed at 'dinner-time' camps. This pattern of eating provides considerable incentive, not only to the dietary investigators but also to the Anbarra, to accompany food collecting expeditions because food is distributed among all those who are present. The practice of consuming food at dinner-time camps also has an important influence on the amount and type of food available to different members of the community. For example because of the different role that men and women have in the procuring of food, males probably not only consume considerably more meat but also have greater access to livers and fat, which are especially valued items of the diet, than females.

A further problem associated with food intake studies carried out in the traditional bush environment is the lack of information about the nutrient composition of the many plants and animals used for food. Several laboratories in Australia are currently engaged in analysing both traditional animal and plant foods used by aborigines[9], but as yet the available information is limited. Not infrequently the concentration of nutrients reported in 'bush' foods is found to be considerably higher than that in related cultivated species because of their higher content of dry matter.

Methodological problems in studies at rural settlements. The number of aborigines living in out-station camps in the bush and on the coast is small compared with those living at small permanent settlements in rural areas. One feature of such settlements is the community store which is often the only source of bought foods for perhaps 100 km or more. Consequently it provides a useful source of information about the food supply of the community particularly as in the permanent settlements little traditional food is now available in the immediate vicinity of the settlements, these areas having been gradually depleted of bush food by over-utilisation.

A number of investigators have utilised food store records to estimate per caput availability of foods and nutrients in these communities[1,4,11]. Care, however, needs to be exercised in interpreting data obtained in this way. For example, Meehan[8] writing about the foods purchased by the Anbarra reports that much of the food, especially flour and sugar, is never consumed. A sizeable quantity is ruined during periods of rain because people fail to protect it properly or because their houses leak. In addition some of the flour is fed to the family dogs, and both flour and sugar are wasted because of the way in which damper (a kind flat bread) and tea are prepared.

Another more obvious problem with food stores records is the fact that such records exclude foods not purchased at the store but available from the bush, from gardens or purchased elsewhere. The combined effect on the estimated daily nutrient availability of including meat available from hunting expeditions and allowing for a 20 per cent loss of all flour and sugar purchased is seen in Table 1. The overall effect of these adjustments is only a small increase in the energy available for consumption but a marked increase in the nutrient density of the available diet with respect to protein, iron and riboflavin. Clearly the nutrients most affected will vary according to the type of bush food which is available but since the energy density of most bush foods is relatively low, making the appropriate adjustments to food store records will generally increase the nutrient density of the available diet.

Although the majority of food in rural settlements is purchased, food intake studies indicate that there are marked seasonal differences in intake of at least some nutrients.

Table 1. *The effect of adjusting food store records for bush food and for a 20 per cent loss of flour and sugar. (Adapted from* [11]*)*.

	Basic records	Adjusted records	Per cent increase
	Nutrients per person per day		
Energy, MJ	9.6	9.8	3
Energy, kcal	(2280)	(2335)	–
Protein, g	72	106	47
Iron, mg	14	19	36
Thiamin, mg	0.92	0.94	2
Riboflavin, mg	0.37	0.67	81

Methodological problems in studies of urban populations. Very little information is available on the food intake of Australian aborigines living under urban conditions. The diet of two aboriginal families living in the town of Bourke in New South Wales[5] and similar data on eight households living in and around a country town in the south-west of Western Australia[3] have been described. In neither study were the families randomly selected and they may not have been representative of the local population. Dietary patterns and nutrient intakes were found to differ markedly between the reserve and town families. With the exception of energy (85 per cent) and thiamin (86 per cent) the diet of the town families provided on average at least 90 per cent of the recommended allowance for the major nutrients while that of the reserve families provided less than 70 per cent of the allowance for calcium (43 per cent), vitamin A (68 per cent), riboflavin (47 per cent) and vitamin C (39 per cent). An obvious difference in food consumption pattern between the two groups of households was that the reserve households generally only prepared two meals daily while the town households usually had three meals per day. The only notable difference between reserve and town households in food purchasing patterns, however, appeared to be that the town families purchased bread while the reserve families bought flour instead, and a smaller quantity and variety of fruit and vegetables than the town families. This would suggest that the two diets were not too different in terms of the major sources of energy in the diet. Figure 3 shows that this was clearly not the case with bread and flour apparently contributing 57 per cent of the total energy available in reserve households but only 33 per cent of that available in town households. It is not unlikely that the bulk purchase of flour (10 kg bags) as opposed to bread, as well as the losses of flour referred to earlier exaggerate the apparent difference between town and reserve households in this respect.

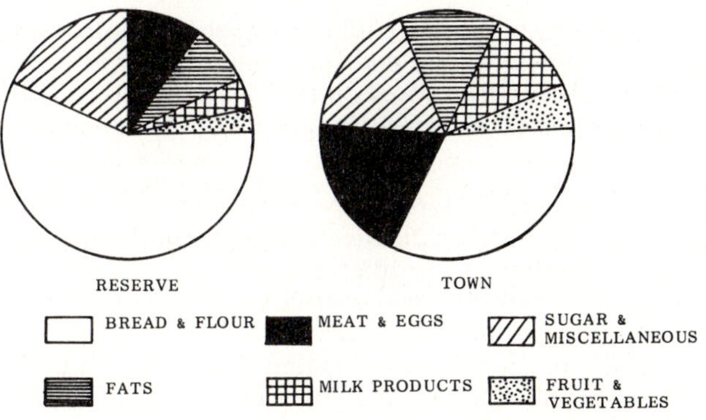

Figure 3. *Energy sources in the diets of reserve and town households. (Adapted from[3]).*

A further problem in food intake studies of aboriginal Australians is the close relationship between dietary quality and pay day[2]; immediately after pay day the diet usually contains meat, fruit and vegetables but these items are usually absent for some days before pay day. Clearly any studies of food intake in this population must also taken into account the usual pay cycle which is not necessarily a weekly one. The main conclusion from this review is that detailed information about the lifestyle and environment of the people being studied is an essential ingredient of all surveys seeking to provide valid data on food intake.

1 Coles-Rutishauser, I.H.E. (1979): Growing up in Western Australia: If you are Aboriginal. *Proc. Nutr. Soc. Aust.* **4**, 27–33.
2 Cutter, T. (1978): Nutrition and food habits of the Central Australian Aboriginal. In *The nutrition of Aborigines in relation to the ecosystem of Central Australia*, ed B.S. Hetzel & H.J. Frith, pp. 63–70. Melbourne: Commonwealth Scientific and Industrial Research Organization.
3 Hitchcock, N.E. & Gracey, M. (1975): Dietary patterns in a rural aboriginal community in South-West Australia. *Med. J. Aust.* **2**, 12–16, (Special Suppl.).
4 Kailis, D.G. (1979): Groote Eylandt Studies 3. The influence of diet on the prevalence of dental caries in aboriginal children at Groote Eylandt, N.T. Australia 1973. *Proc. Nutr. Soc. Aust.* **4**, 118.
5 Kamien, M., Woodhill, J.M., Nobile, S., Rosevear, P., Cameron, P. & Winston, J.M. (1975): Nutrition in the Australian aborigine. *Fd Technol. Aust.* **27**, 93–103.

6 McArthur, M. (1960): Food consumption and dietary levels of the aborigines at the settlements. In *Records of the American–Australian Scientific Expedition to Arnhem Land Vol. 2*, ed C.P. Mountford, pp. 14–26. Melbourne: Melbourne University Press.

7 McArthur, M. (1960): Food consumption and dietary levels of groups of aborigines living on naturally occurring foods. In *Records of the American–Australian Scientific Expedition to Arnhem Land Vol. 2*, ed C.P. Mountford, pp. 90–134. Melbourne: Melbourne University Press.

8 Meehan, B. (1982): The role of shellfish in the total diet. In *Shell bed to shell midden*, pp. 141–161. Canberra: Australian Institute of Aboriginal Studies.

9 O'Dea, K. (1983): Register of laboratories analysing bush foods. In *Proceedings aboriginal bush foods workshop Brisbane, November 1983*, ed K. O'Dea pp. 77–78. Heidelberg: Department of Medicine Repatriation General Hospital (Mimeographed).

10. Rae, C.J., Lamprell, V.J., Lion, R.J. & Rae, A.M. (1982): The role of bush foods in contemporary aboriginal diets. *Proc. Nutr. Soc. Aust.* **7**, 45–52.

11. White, I.M. (1977): Pitfalls to avoid: the Australian experience. In *Health and disease in tribal societies*, Ciba Foundation Symposium 49 pp. 269–301. Amsterdam: Elsevier.

Assessment of long-term intake

L. STOCKLEY
AFRC Food Research Institute, Norwich, Colney Lane, Norwich NR4 7UA, UK.

The measurement of long-term dietary intake is one of the most difficult problems confronting the research nutritionist. The amounts and types of food consumed change through the lifetime of an individual, and other fluctuations are superimposed on this overall pattern. The sources of this variation are examined below in terms of the type of long-term study which they affect.

Types of study for long-term dietary assessment. *Between group comparisons (cross-sectional studies).* This type of comparison may be carried out to examine the effect of long-term changes in a more rapid way than is possible with longitudinal studies. Some differences between groups may be due to biological changes, but difficulties in interpretation can arise because of socio-economic and cultural influences during the lifetime of the groups, and differences in survival rates. Despite these difficulties cross-sectional data can be invaluable, for example in monitoring changes in the national diet over a number of years, and in assessing changes in a population when, for some reason, it is not possible to carry out a longitudinal study.

Repeated studies on a group (longitudinal studies). There are particular problems in continuing a dietary investigation over a number of years. In addition to 'survival' effects there may be selective loss of participants through non-cooperation or migration, and it has been suggested that bias might be introduced into the results as a consequence of subjects changing their behaviour because they are in study[10].

Sources of variation which are additional to biological effects include changes in the environment; religious feasts and fasts; seasonal changes; and day of the week differences have also been reported. The extent of these effects varies between countries, and regional and socio-economic groups within the countries.

Classification of individuals within a group. There are a number of reasons why individuals may be incorrectly classified in relation to each other on the basis of a few days dietary study, even though all individuals are surveyed at the same time of year and on the same days of the week. Some people have very irregular dietary patterns, and episodes of illness and convalescence, short-term changes in activity, changes in body weight, and personal celebrations may all affect intake.

In recent years statistical techniques have emerged based on the ratio of intra- to inter-individual variances, which enable the calculation of the number of days a study should be carried out to correctly classify a predetermined percentage of individuals into certain percentiles of the distribution for the group[5,11]. The number of days needed varies with the particular group of people, for example civil servants or students, and with the nutrient to be estimated.

Methods of assessment. *Biochemical measures* which reflect long-term intake of a nutrient are an attractive alternative to repeated dietary surveys. Unfortunately there are few such methods available, and they may be unsuitable for community studies because of the intrusive nature of the tests. The other consideration is that a knowledge of the biochemical level of a nutrient without knowing the dietary source can raise more questions than it answers.

Retrospective dietary assessment. The most usual methods for retrospective diet assessment are the dietary history, originally developed by Burke[6], the 24-h recall and the food frequency questionnaire. These methods do not cause any interference with usual eating patterns, co-operation rates are usually high, and for the 24-h recall and the diet history the subject does not need any literary skills.

The history method demands intensive input from the interviewer and so is not as suited to cover large number of people as the other two methods. It has been used in several epidemiological studies, notably the 20-year studies carried out by Beal[2,3]. However, comparisons of mean intakes for a group estimated using both the diet history and a weighed method have usually found various degrees of overestimation with the history[13,18].

Although the 24-h recall is used extensively in epidemiological studies in the USA, the majority of studies in developed countries have found that 24-h recall underestimates mean intakes by as much as 25 per cent when compared with a weighed method[7,17]. James *et al.*[14] conclude that the 24-h recall should be abandoned as an epidemiological tool, and point out that although numerous tests of repeatability have been carried out these cannot disprove a bias in the method.

The use of self-administered food frequency questionnaires is seriously limited by the consistent underestimation obtained using these compared with weighed methods[1,23].

Prospective dietary assessment. The methods which are available to measure intake prospectively include the larder inventory, a food diary with weights estimated using household measures, a weighed inventory of food either before and after preparation, or before consumption only, and analysis of duplicate diets. All of these approaches have been discussed in extensive reviews[19,20]. The two main types of error associated with their use include error in the measurement of the diet at the time of the study, and changes in habitual dietary patterns.

It has been recognised for many years that subjects may eat atypically during a dietary survey period. James *et al.*[14] have suggested that 24-h urinary nitrogen can be used to detect changes in usual dietary patterns. When this approach was used in a study of 30 men in each of four Scandinavian countries there were no significant changes in the diet during and after a duplicate diet collection[4]. However, when 28 adults were persuaded to maintain detailed diet records for one year, and asked to collect duplicate diets, urine and faeces for 7 days on four occasions during the year, there was a significant decrease in energy intake during the collection periods of 17 per cent for the men and 13 per cent for the women[12]. The scientific evidence for or against changes in the diet is scanty. It seems that this source of error *may* be of as much or more importance than measurement error, at least for duplicate diet collections.

Study design. Data from long-term studies have been analysed to assess the usefulness of intermittent sampling during the study to estimate intake. Chappell[8] concluded that a good estimate of mean intake was obtained by subdividing the year into equal strata, with a decrease in the confidence of the estimate with reduction in the number of strata. Kim *et al.*[16] compared nutrient intakes calculated for 1 day/month, 3 days/month, 7 days/month and for 365 days. The differences were only 3 to 8 per cent between methods, and the authors conclude that the results from all methods were comparable.

The number of sampling periods in the year, and the number of days of study in each period, depend upon the objective of the study, and the relative importance of the different sources of variation in the groups to be surveyed. It was suggested[15] that a knowledge of the extent of seasonal and other variations might be important in relating diet to disease patterns. To quantify this it would be necessary to measure intake over more days in each study period than if the aim is to assess average intake over a year.

A last source of error which has not been discussed so far is investigator-related. This affects all dietary studies, but long-term assessments are particularly prone to it. Over a long period of time changes in staff, and hence in staff-subject interactions, are almost inevitable. Staff changes are also responsible for differences in the interpretation and coding of food items. Food composition tables may be updated and revised, and the analytical methods for the tables and for duplicate diet analysis will probably be modified in some way.

The future. Computer technology is advancing rapidly and is becoming increasingly important in the processing of dietary data. At present it is standard procedure to store food composition data and use programs to calculate dietary intakes. Further development of nutrient data bases should enable comparisons between composition data used over a number of years, and so reduce the investigator-related errors to some extent.

Alternative methods of intake measurement are also being developed which are less demanding for the subjects and so may be more suitable for long-term measurements. A photographic approach has been tested[9], and another recently developed method, based on the use of a microcomputer also eliminates the need for a subject to read a balance or use a notebook[21]. Trials of the method have been completed in 29 subjects, who also kept seven day weighed diaries[22].

1 Acheson, K.J., Campbell, I.T., Edholm, O.G., Miller, D.S. & Stock, M.J. (1980): The measurement of food and energy intake in man — an evaluation of some techniques. *Am J. Clin. Nutr.* **33**, 1147–1154.

2 Beal, V.A. (1971): Nutritional studies during pregnancy: changes in intakes of calories, carbohydrate, fat, protein and calcium. *J. Am. Diet. Ass.* **58**, 312–320.

3 Beal, V.A. (1971): Nutritional studies during pregnancy: dietary intake, maternal weight gain, and size of infant. *J. Am. Diet. Ass.* **58**, 312–320.

4 Bingham, S., Wiggins, H.S., Englyst, H., Sëppanen, R., Helms, P., Strand, R., Burton, R., Jørgensen, I.M., Poulsen, L., Paerregaard, A., Bjerrum, L. & James, W.P. (1982): Methods and validity of dietary assessments in four Scandinavian populations. *Nutr, Cancer* **4**, 23–33.

5 Black, A.E., Cole, T.J., Wiles, S.J. & White, F. (1983): Daily variation in food intake of infants from 2 to 18 months. *Hum. Nutr. Appl. Nutr.* **37A**, 448–458.

6 Burke, B.S. (1947): The dietary history as a tool in research. *J. Am. Diet. Ass.* **23**, 1041–1047.

7 Campbell, V.A. & Dodds, M.L. (1967): Collecting dietary information from groups of older people. *J. Am. Diet. Ass.* **51**, 29–33.

8 Chappell, G.M. (1955): Long-term individual dietary surveys. *Br. J. Nutr.* **9**, 323–339.

9 Elwood, P.C. & Bird, G. (1983): A photographic method of diet evaluation. *Hum. Nutr: Appl. Nutr.* **37A**, 474–477.

10 Exton-Smith, A.N. (1982): Epidemiological studies in the elderly: methodological considerations. *Am. J. Clin. Nutr.* **35**, 1273–1279.

11 Gardner, M.J. & Heady, J.A. (1973): Some effects of within person variability in epidemiological studies. *J. Chron. Dis.* **26**, 781–795.

12 Holbrook, J.T., Patterson, K.Y., Bodner, J.E., Douglas, L.W., Veillon, C., Kelsay, J.L., Mertz, W. & Smith, J.C. (1984): Sodium and potassium intake and balance in adults consuming self-selected diets. *Am. J. Clin. Nutr.* **40**, 786–793.

13 Jain, M., Howe, G.R., Johnson, K.C. & Miller, A.B. (1980): Evaluation of a diet history questionnaire for epidemiologic studies. *Am. J. Epidemiol.* **111**, 212–219.

14 James, W.P.T., Bingham, S.A. & Cole, T.J. (1981): Epidemiological assessment of dietary intake. *Nutr. Cancer* **2**, 203–212.

15 Keys, A. (1979): Dietary survey methods. On: *Nutrition, lipids and coronary heart disease*, ed R. Levy, B. Rifkind, B. Dennis and N. Ernst, pp.1–23. New York: Raven Press.

16 Kim, W.W., Kelsay, J.L., Judd, J.T., Marshall, M.W., Mertz, W. & Prather, E.S. (1984): Evaluation of long term dietary intakes of adults consuming self-selected diets. *Am. J. Clin. Nutr.* **40**, 1327–1332.

17 Linussen, E.E.I., Sanjur, D. & Erikson, E.C. (1974): Validating the 24 hour recall method as a dietary survey tool. *Archs. Latinoam. Nutr.* **24**, 227–294.

18 Lonergan, M.E., Milne, J.S., Maule, M.M. & Williamson, J. (1975): A dietary survey of older people in Edinburgh. *Br. J. Nutr.* **34**, 517–527.

19 Marr, J.W. (1971): Individual dietary surveys: purposes and methods. *Wld. Rev. Nutr. Diet.* **13**, 105–164.

20 Pekkarinen, M. (1970): Methodology in the collection of food consumption data. *Wld. Rev. Nutr. Diet.* **12**, 145–171.

21 Stockley, L., Chapman, R.I., Holley, M.L., Jones, F.A., Prescott, E.H.A. & Broadhurst, A.J. (1986): Description of a food recording electronic device for use in dietary surveys. *Hum. Nutr: Appl. Nutr.* **40A**, 13–18.

22 Stockley, L., Hurren, C.A., Chapman, R.I., Broadhurst, A.J. & Jones, F.A. (1986): Energy, protein and fat intake estimated using a Food Recording Electronic Device compared with a weighed diary. *Hum. Nutr.: Appl. Nutr.* **40A**, 19–23.

23 Yarnell, J.W.G., Fehily, A.M., Milbank, J.E., Sweetnam, P.M. & Walker, C.L. (1983): A short dietary questionnaire for use in an epidemiological survey: comparison with weighed dietary records. *Hum. Nutr.: Appl. Nutr.* **37A**, 103–112.

Changes in dietary patterns over a 4-year period in an elderly population

P.J. GARRY, W.C. HUNT and J.S. GOODWIN
*Departments of Pathology and Medicine, University of New Mexico School of Medicine, (P.J.G.: Surge
Building, Room 236), Albuquerque, New Mexico 87131, USA.*

In 1979 we recruited 304 healthy men ($n = 138$) and women ($n = 166$) from the Alberquerque, New Mexico area for a longitudinal study of nutrition. Participation in this 8-year study was entirely voluntary and was limited to men and women over 60 years of age who were free of major illnesses and receiving no prescription medication. A specific aim of this longitudinal project is to determine whether nutritional status, as measured by yearly dietary, biochemical, and clinical examinations, is a determinant for subsequent morbid events in an aged population.

The average age at entrance was 71 years and all were Caucasian, 3 per cent of whom were of Spanish/Hispanic descent. They were highly motivated, physically active, healthy and well educated and from the middle income group.

The dietary intake information collected during the 1st year of the study (1980) has been published[2]. In the present report dietary intakes during the 2nd (1981) and 5th year (1984) of the study are compared with the data for the first year. (Dietary information was not collected during the 3rd and 4th year). In addition, the influence of changing health status on diet is investigated by comparing those who have remained in a constant state of good health with those who have been diagnosed for new illnesses subsequent to entrance into the study.

Subjects and methods. All volunteers were seen as outpatients each year in the Clinical Research Center at the University of New Mexico Hospital. A dietitian instructed the volunteers on how to keep an accurate 3-d food record. All food items and portions were recorded on standard forms for three successive weekdays. At the end of the 3-day recording period, a dietitian visited their homes to collect the diet records and obtain information about physical activity. All food records were coded by food item and amount and analyzed for nutrient composition using a computerized nutrient data base (1980 edn.) obtained from Case Western Reserve University, Cleveland, Ohio. An activity score, modified from Cassel[1], was obtained at the same time.

At the end of 1984, there were 238 of the original 304 elderly remaining in the study. There have been 25 deaths at the time of this report. For this report we have only included those elderly men ($n = 91$) and women ($n = 116$) who completed the 3-d diet records for both years. Health status was determined by reviewing the medical records for each participant over the 4-year period. Participants were classified as unhealthy if they had been diagnosed as having cardiovascular disease, cancer (excluding skin cancer that had been removed without complications), diabetes, senile dementia or chronic obstructive pulmonary disease. Using these criteria for illness, there were 54 women and 41 men who no longer were considered healthy at the end of 1984. Sixty-two women and 50 men had no significant change in health status. The mean ages of healthy and unhealthy women in 1980 were 69.5 ± 4.3 years and 72.0 ± 5.2 years, respectively. For men, the mean ages were 71.2 ± 4.2 years and 71.9 ± 4.6 years, respectively.

The study was approved by the Human Research Review Committee of the University of Mexico School of Medicine. Informed consent was obtained from each participant.

Results. Total energy, protein, fat and carbohydrate intakes decreased between 1980 and 1984 (Table 1). With the exception of carbohydrate intake for men, all decreases were statistically significant ($P < 0.05$ by paired t-test). The composition of the diet, as per cent of energy from protein, fat and carbohydrate, did not show any significant change over the 4-year period. Body weights also failed to show any significant change.

The observed decreases in intake were very similar for those subjects who have remained in good health for the four years when compared to those who experienced significant health

Table 1. *Mean and standard deviation (in parenthesis) of daily dietary intake of total energy protein, fat and carbohydrate.*

	Women (n = 116)						Men (n = 91)					
	1980		1981		1984		1980		1981		1984	
Energy												
MJ	6.81	(1.45)	6.40	(1.36)	6.18	(1.50)	9.25	(2.14)	8.76	(2.07)	8.57	(2.08
kcal	1628	(347)	1530	(324)	1477	(358)	2212	(512)	2094	(494)	2050	(497
Protein												
g	66.5	(15.0)	61.9	(13.6)	61.9	(16.0)	84.6	(19.7)	82.4	(19.8)	79.6	(21.4
% of energy	16.8	(4.4)	16.6	(3.9)	17.1	(4.1)	15.6	(3.1)	16.1	(3.3)	15.8	(3.6
Fat												
g	67.7	(27.2)	63.5	(20.5)	58.8	(21.8)	92.0	(29.2)	84.7	(25.9)	82.8	(26.9
% of energy	36.9	(6.8)	36.9	(7.1)	35.2	(7.4)	37.1	(6.5)	36.2	(6.4)	36.1	(6.9
Carbohydrates												
g	184.6	(41.6)	172.0	(41.7)	173.4	(47.1)	248.6	(66.9)	239.6	(69.8)	239.1	(74.2
% of energy	45.8	(7.1)	45.3	(8.2)	47.5	(8.5)	45.1	(7.5)	45.7	(7.1)	46.6	(8.2
Body weights (kg)	60.4	(9.4)	60.5	(9.4)	60.0	(9.3)	74.0	(10.3)	73.9	(10.3)	74.0	(10.2

Table 2. *Changes in energy, protein, fat and carbohydrate intakes, weight and physical activity between 1980 and 1984 in healthy and unhealthy subjects.*

	Women		Men	
	Healthy (n = 62)	*Unhealthy* (n = 54)	*Healthy* (n = 50)	*Unhealthy* (n = 41)
Energy				
MJ	−0.54	−0.74	−0.73	−0.62
kcal	−129	−177	−175	−147
Protein				
g	−3.2	−6.3	−4.5	−5.6
% of total energy	0.4	0.3	0.4	0.1
Fat				
g	−10.2	−7.8	−8.1	−10.7
% of total energy	−1.7	−1.6	−0.2	−1.9
Carbohydrates				
g	−11.0	−11.3	−12.8	−5.5
% of total energy	1.1	2.4	1.1	1.9
Weight (kg)	0.0	−0.9	0.0	−0.3
Activity	0.24	−2.15	0.18	−2.37

problems ($P > 0.30$ by t-test for all nutrients). (Table 2). Weight changes were small and were not significantly different between the two groups. Activity levels, however, decreased for the unhealthy group while remaining stable for healthy subjects. This difference is only marginally significant ($P = 0.06$ by t-test).

Discussion. In our earlier report[2] we used the 1980 Recommended Dietary Allowances (RDA) as the standard to assess adequacy of intake for energy, protein, vitamins and minerals. In the present work we did not attempt to compare intakes with any standard. Instead we were primarily interested in examining changes in dietary intake with age midway through our 8-year longitudinal study in order to obtain an initial insight into factors that may influence dietary intakes in a free-living elderly population.

The decrease in energy intake with advancing age has been reported previously[4] and has been attributed to small reductions in basal energy metabolism paralleling the reduction in lean body mass. In addition there is a decrease in physical activity with age.

When we separated our population into two distinct health categories we could find no significant differences in energy intake between healthy and non healthy, possibly because health status of the non-healthy individuals was not serious enough or their condition had not deteriorated to a critical point where it affected their appetite.

We examined the energy intakes of our elderly on a cross-sectional basis, dividing our population into two groups, those who were less than 72 years of age in 1980, and those who were 72 or older; the median age difference between the groups was 7 years for both the males and females. Average differences in energy intake between these two groups for 1980, 1981 and 1984 were only 31 kcal (130 kJ) for females and 78 kcal (327 kJ) for males. The older group had the lower energy intake. These values are appreciably less that the 4-year longitudinal changes noted, ie −151 kcal (632 kJ) and −162 kcal (678 kJ) for females and males respectively. The lower cross-sectional change noted in energy intake, as compared to the longitudinal findings, supports the earlier report[3] that 'it is difficult to separate the effects of aging and secular trend in a cohort study, because changes in age and time take place at the same time in the same population'.

It is well recognized that a major disadvantage of cross-sectional studies is that they represent one-point in time measures; however, it is not always apparent in a longitudinal study what other changes, in addition to increasing age, may be occurring. For example, our elderly volunteers eating habits may have changed over time. This is particularly likely since they were keenly aware of their participation in a long-term nutritional study. A suggestion of this influence can be noted in the energy intake in 1981 compared to 1980 and 1984 (Table 1). For women there was a 98 kcal (410 kJ) decrease in energy intake from 1980 to 1981 and a much smaller difference between 1981 and 1984 , 53 kcal (180 kJ). In men there was also a large decrease in energy intake from 1980 to 1981, 118 kcal (494 kJ) with a smaller decrease from 1981 to 1984, 44 kcal (184 kJ). We can only speculate why the relatively large decrease in energy intake occurred between the 1st and 2nd year. One possible explanation is that repetition or increased instruction resulted in more accurate dietary records in the 2nd and 5th year compared to the 1st.

Another possibility is that the elderly may have changed their eating habits during the 3-d record keeping periods for 1981 and 1984 by eating simple foods and by avoiding eating out, to make recording easier. In other words, the 1st year may have been a learning experience which resulted in simplifying the task of keeping a 3-d diet record in subsequent years. At this time, it does not seem possible to separate these effects from true age related changes.

In conclusion, this preliminary report of our longitudinal dietary intake data in an elderly population confirms the statement[5] that, 'A better, more sensitive definition of age (ie functional rather than chronological) must be formulated before epidemiology can be of optimal use in nutrition and aging research.'

Acknowledgements. The authors thank Susan Frye and Jeanie Schwartz for their help in preparing this report which was supported by grants from the United States Public Health Serve, AG 02049 and RR-00997-05,06.

1 Cassel, J. (1971): Occupation and physical activity in coronary heart disease. *Archs. Intern. Med.* **128**, 920–926.

2 Garry, P.J., Goodwin, J.S., Hunt, W.C., Hooper, E.M. & Leonard, A.G. (1982): Nutritional status in a healthy elderly population: dietary and supplemental intakes. *Am. J. Clin. Nutr.* **36**, 319–331.

3 Krombout, D. (1983): Changes in energy and macronutrients in 871 middle-aged men during 10 years of follow-up (the Zutphen Study). *Am. J. Clin. Nutr.* **37**, 287–294.

4 McGandy, R.B., Barrows, C.H., Spanias, A., Meredith, A., Stone, J.L. & Norris, A.H. (1966): Nutrient intakes and energy expenditure in men of different ages. *J. Gerontol.* **21**, 581–587.

5 Munro, H.N. & Everitt, A.V. (1981): Introduction to mini-symposium on nutrition and aging. In *Nutrition in health and disease and international development. Symposia from the XII International Congress of Nutrition.* ed A.E. Harper & G.K. Davis. pp. 677–685. New York: Alan R. Liss.

Host defences against infection

J.L. TURK

Department of Pathology, The Royal College of Surgeons of England, 35–43 Lincoln's Inn Fields, London, WC2A 3PN, UK.

Lymphocytes control the specificity of the immune response whether they are B-lymphocytes involved in humoral antibody production or T-lymphocytes carrying specific antigen reactive sites involved in cell-mediated immunity. Moreover, they are also the primary agents in the regulation of the immune response. T-lymphocytes may be divided into subclasses depending on their function which correlates with certain membrane antigens that can be identified by the use of monoclonal antibodies. Thus, we have T_{DTH} for effector cells of delayed hypersensitivity; T_C cytotoxic T-cells; T_H helper cells; T_S suppressor cells. In addition, there is a separate group of lymphocytes NK (natural killer) cells that can be activated, particularly by interferon. Regulation of a cell-mediated response may be by B-lymphocytes and macrophages as well as by T_S cells.

Lymphocyte function in infection cannot be discussed in isolation. The lymphocytes and macrophages work together. Indeed it has been suggested that macrophages show the same genetic restriction as lymphocytes. Macrophages and the closely related dendritic cells such as the Langerhans cells in the epidermis are needed for antigen presentation. In addition, in cell-mediated immune reactions macrophages play an important role both in resistance to infection, elimination of infecting organisms and in delayed allergic reactions leading to granuloma formation. One of the important questions that still needs to be answered is to what extent are lymphocytes involved in delayed hypersensitivity infection also involved in host resistance. The present communication deals briefly with three aspects of lymphocyte-macrophage function in chronic infectious diseases: (1) regulation of the normal immune response (2) lymphocyte activation of macrophage function (3) the role of cell-mediated immunity in granuloma formation.

Regulation of the normal immune response. The study of immune regulation in experimental animals has been greatly facilitated by the use of the drug cyclophosphamide to eliminate certain classes of cells regulating the immune response. A single dose of 200 to 300 mg/kg cyclophosphamide (CY) given before immunization eliminates temporarily rapidly dividing lymphocytes. The cells affected are the precursors, particularly of B-lymphocytes and T_S cells. The precursors of T_{DTH} remain unaffected. Thus, by eliminating suppressor cells without effector cells one is able to study the action of the immune response unaffected by control mechanisms. It becomes straightaway clear that not all forms of immune responses are affected equally. In the first place, cell-mediated immune responses are more affected than B-lymphocytes responses, although a number of situations can be uncovered in which there is an increased antibody response in CY pretreated animals. Moreover, the strength of immunological control is related to the strength of the immune response itself. The stronger the antigen, and thus the response of the animal, the stronger the control and the greater the increase in response following CY pretreatment. In addition to releasing the immune response from normal regulation CY can reverse certain states of immunological tolerance, particularly those induced by a heavy load of antigen. This indicates a contributory role of suppressor cells to this form of tolerance. In both normal immunization and immunological tolerance, suppressor cells show immunological specificity equivalent to that of the antigen inducing the response. However, there are two phenomena in which CY-sensitive suppressor cells are induced that are non-specific in their action. One of these is antigenic competition and the other is desensitization. It is possible that the action of suppressor cells in controlling a normal response could result in the release of factors that might restrict the response to antigens to which the individual might be exposed at the same time.

Lymphocyte activation of macrophage function. It is the macrophage that is the final effector cell in cell-mediated immune reactions *in vivo*. This is particularly so in delayed hypersensitivity reactions. Specifically sensitized lymphocytes in the presence of specific antigen release lymphokines which act directly on the macrophage cell membrane. Activation is through cyclic nucleotides and effects tubulin function, as a result of which macrophages round up and are inhibited from migrating. They are also induced to aggregate. Following this, they become activated showing increased Krebs cycle and hexose monophosphate shunt enzyme activity. This activation of energy is associated with an increased phagocytic activity.

The role of cell-mediated immunity in granuloma formation. In many chronic infectious diseases host resistance to infection is associated with granuloma formation. These are usually infections that need cell-mediated immune mechanisms for their control. This is a particular feature of mycobacterial infections. Granuloma formation is a feature of the allergic response of the individual, although the walling off of the area of infection probably plays an important role in limiting the spread of the organism. A granuloma may be defined as a collection of cells of the mononuclear phagocyte system with or without the addition of other cell types. The particular feature of allergic granuloma formation in these conditions is that cells of the mononuclear phagocyte system take on the appearance of 'epithelioid cells', many of which contain a prominent Golgi apparatus and rough endoplasmic reticulum. In addition, these cells are poorly phagocytic. Epithelioid cell granulomas are also the site of increased fibroblast activity and evidence will be presented to show that there is increased collagen synthesis.

Experimental mycobacterial granulomas. The granuloma of tuberculoid leprosy is a typical epithelioid cell granuloma associated with the presence of a strong state of delayed hypersensitivity and the ability to develop epithelioid cell granulomas (Mitsuda reaction) when the individual is injected intradermally with heat-killed *M. leprae*. This indicates that this granuloma is also produced by a cell-mediated immune response. In contrast the granuloma of lepromatous leprosy consists solely of macrophages that have ingested 'globi' of *M. leprae*, there is an associated specific defect in cell-mediated immunity and patients are unable to develop an epithelioid cell granuloma when injected intradermally with the Mitsuda reagent.

Models of these two types of granuloma have been developed in the auricular lymph node of guinea pigs injected in the dorsum of the ear with *Mycobacteria*[6]. The intradermal injection of BCG vaccine, live or cobalt irradiated, produced typical epithelioid cell granulomas in which the epithelioid cells were shown by electron microscopy to contain rough endoplasmic reticulum. These cells were similar to those seen in the zirconium granulomas. There were also considerable numbers of fibroblasts and evidence of new collagen formation. In contrast, the granulomas produced by the injection of cobalt irradiated *M. leprae* consisted mainly of macrophages which still contained ingested *M. leprae*. There was little evidence of phagocytosed bacteria in the cells of the mononuclear phagocyte series in the BCG granulomas. Quantitative evaluation of these granulomas according to the weight of the lymph nodes and the area of granulomatous infiltration, as measured by planimetry, indicated that the BCG granulomas reached their peak 2 weeks after induction, whereas the *M. leprae* granulomas peaked at 5 weeks.

Table 1. *Properties of large cells infiltrating granulomas as compared with peritoneal exudate macrophages.*

	Peritoneal exudate cells 72 H oil-induced	BCG (epithelioid cells) (2 week granuloma)	M. leprae macrophages (5 week granuloma)
Glass or plastic adherence	++ (~60%)	± (~10%)	+++ (~70%)
FC receptors	+++ (83%)	−	± (~10%)
C3 receptors	+++ (73%)	−	± (~10%)
Peroxidase	+++	−	−
Non-specific esterase	+++	++	++
Fibronectin	++	++	++
Specific macrophage antigen	++ (75%)	+++ (100%)	++ (80%)
Ia antigen	+ (35%)	− (0%)	++ (80%)

Comparison was made of a number of parameters, between cells of the mononuclear phagocyte series in these two types of granuloma and oil-induced peritoneal macrophages (Table 1). Both peritoneal macrophages and *M. leprae* macrophages were glass adherent. However, the epithelioid cells of the BCG granulomas did not adhere to glass. This was consistent with their failure to phagocytose. EA and EAC rosetting on the peritoneal cells showed that a large proportion of these macrophages carried surface receptors for the Fc component of IgG and C3. A high percentage of these macrophages also exhibited peroxidase and non-specific esterase activity. Immunofluorescence using FITC-conjugated monoclonal antibody against human fibronectin on peritoneal exudate cells showed the presence of fibronectin in these macrophages. A high percentage of cells of the MPS infiltrating the granulomas induced by BCG and *M. leprae* were esterase positive and also showed the presence of fibronectin. However, these cells did not carry Fc or C3 surface receptors nor did they exhibit peroxidase activity.

Despite the general acceptance that epithelioid cells were related to mononuclear phagocytes[3], it was important to demonstrate a formal immunological relationship between these two cell types, as the term 'epithelioid cell' had been used originally to cover all non-lymphoid mononuclear cells in granulomas whether of an immunological or non-immunological nature. A monoclonal anti-guinea pig macrophage antibody was therefore prepared using guinea pig peritoneal macrophages as antigen. This was specific for macrophages and not just directed against the Ia antigen or the Fc receptor, as it did not stain LC2 leukaemia cells (a B-cell line with Fc receptors and Ia antigens) and did not block EA rosetting. This was compared with an anti-guinea pig Ia monoclonal antibody (kindly given by Dr Ethan Shevach of the NIAID, NIH, Bethesda, Md) in immunofluorescence and immunoperoxidase studies[2]. Both BCG epithelioid cells and *M. leprae* macrophages stained with this reagent as did peritoneal exudate macrophages and Kupffer cells. Langerhans cells in the skin failed to have the specific macrophage antigen. Peritoneal macrophages, Kupffer cells, Langerhans cells and the *M. leprae* granuloma macrophages were Ia positive. However, epithelioid cells were Ia negative. Thus, it would appear that epithelioid cells are related antigenically to other cells of the mononuclear phagocyte series, including peritoneal and other macrophages. They differ in that they are poorly phagocytic and thus not glass adherent, and lack Ia antigen, indicating that they do not possess an antigen presenting function. The presence of a rough endoplasmic reticulum would probably indicate that these cells have a secretory rather than phagocytic function.

In order to see whether there was a relationship between epithelioid cell formation and increased fibroblast activity, collagen synthesis was examined in explants of auricular lymph nodes from animals injected with BCG and *M. leprae*, and compared with that in auricular lymph nodes from animals painted on the dorsum of the ear with 2,4-dinitro-fluorobenzene (DNFB). Lymph nodes were cut into small pieces and incubated with [^{14}C] proline for 24 h at 37° C. They were then homogenized in Tris-buffered water and divided into two aliquots. One was solubilized directly in 10 per cent TCA for counting the total protein (T). The other was treated with collagenase at 34° C for 90 min and the TCA precipitate solubilized to give a hydrolysed fraction (H) that did not contain collagen. The total protein less the hydrolysed fraction would then give the ^{14}C incorporated into collagen. In these studies it was evident that

Table 2. *Accessory cell (A) function of BCG epithelioid cells and* M. leprae *macrophages in concanavalin-A (Con A)-induced lymphocyte (L) proliferation.* (Values represent mean counts/min ± s.d.).

	BCG	M. leprae		*BCG*	M. leprae
Granuloma cells			*Peritoneal macrophages (control)*		
L + 3 µg Con A	240 ± 200	62 ± 32	L + 3 µg Con A	175 ± 3	60 ± 51
L + A	170 ± 26	44 ± 11	L + A	594 ± 64	294 ± 8
L + A + 3 µg Con A	16 269 ±4029	44 ± 5	L + A + 3 µg Con A	16 318 ± 4542	15 092 ± 1605

the nodes from animals injected with BCG synthesize high levels of collagen as compared with the nodes from animals sensitized with DNFB or injected with cobalt-irradiated *M. leprae*[7]. There was, therefore, a direct association between the presence of secretory epithelioid cells and the subsequent development of fibrosis. One possible explanation for the association between epithelioid cell granulomas and fibrosis is that fibroblast activation results from a release of a specific activating factor from the epithelioid cells with rough endoplasmic reticulum. Further experiments were therefore performed to see whether such a factor was released by granuloma tissues in culture.

Supernatants from both BCG and *M. leprae* granulomas were found to release soluble non-dialysable factors *in vitro* which stimulated [^{14}C]-proline and [^{14}C]-leucine incorporation in fibroblasts in culture and depressed their [^{3}H]-thymidine uptake. These supernatants did not show any detectable macrophage migration inhibitory activity *in vitro*. On the other hand, supernatants from sensitized lymphocytes incubated with tuberculin-PPD had no effect on fibroblasts. Supernatants from DNFB-sensitized lymph nodes also showed stimulation of [^{14}C]-proline incorporation into total protein synthesized by fibroblasts and depressed [^{3}H]-thymidine incorporation. It would appear therefore that fibroblast activation in lymph nodes containing mycobacterial granulomas could result from the release of soluble factors of lymphocyte origin rather than from cells of the mononuclear phagocyte series. These factors appear to be independent of classical lymphokines that act on macrophages *in vitro*. The indentification of these factors has however not clarified the mechanism of fibroblast activation in BCG granulomas, as compared with *M. leprae* granulomas, nor has it added to our knowledge of the function of the secretory epithelioid cell[5].

Despite this, it is clear that epithelioid cells form a distinct subpopulation of cells of the mononuclear phagocyte function for a secretory role. They are therefore not glass adherent and lack Ia antigens. As they can be recognized in tissues mainly by their typical appearance under the electron microscope, their presence cannot be determined by light microscopy alone. The role these cells play in the formation of certain granulomas is intriguing and requires further study.

The accessory cell function of granuloma cells. In view of the fact that the epithelioid cells of BCG granulomas were found to be mainly Ia antigen positive and the macrophages of *M. leprae* granulomas were Ia negative, it was important to see whether these cells could act as 'accessory cells'. An 'accessory cell' may be defined as a cell of the mononuclear phagocyte series or a dendritic cell that plays a role in antigen presentation and whose presence is necessary for T-lymphocyte proliferation. In this study it was possible to show that the total epithelioid cell population of BCG granulomas was able to support a mitogen (Concanavalin-A) induced proliferative response of macrophage-depleted autologous T-lymphocytes (Table 2). However, *M. leprae* granuloma macrophages failed to enhance this response. Neither mononuclear cell populations were able to act as accessory cells for antigen (tuberculin) induced T-cell proliferation. In these studies both epithelioid cells and macrophages were prepared in a purified state on a fluorescent activated cell sorter using a specific monoclonal anti-guinea pig macrophage antibody. The failure of BCG induced epithelioid cells to support tuberculin-induced proliferation could be due to their lack of Ia antigens. However, it has been shown[1] that Ia-negative macrophages can act as accessory cells for Con A induced proliferation, despite Ia positivity being necessary for proliferative responses to antigen. The lack of response when *M.*

leprae granuloma macrophages, which are Ia-positive, are used could be due either to an inability to secrete interleukin 1 (IL-1) or to the secretion of macrophage suppressor factors that might inhibit the secretion of IL-2. A range of accessory cell lymphocyte ratios were used in this study to exclude the possibility that a failure of cell response was due to suboptimal or supraoptimal accessory cell:lymphocyte ratios.

1 Kammer, G.M. & Unanue, E.R. (1980): Accessory cell requirements in the proliferative response to T-lymphocytes to hemocyanin. *Clin. Immun. Immunopath.* **15**, 434–443.
2 Mathew, R.C., Katayama, I., Gupta, S.K., Curtis, J. & Turk, J.L. (1983): Analysis of cells of the mononuclear phagocyte series in experimental mycobacterial granuloma by monoclonal antibodies. *Infect. Immun.* **39**, 344–352.
3 Metchinkoff, E. (1983): *Lectures on the Comparative Pathology of Inflammation*. Kegan Paul, Trench, Trubner. London.
4 Nagao, S., Ota, F., Emorik, K., Inoue, K. & Tanaka, A. (1981): Epithelioid granuloma induced by muramyl dipeptide in immunologically deficient rats. *Infect. Immun.* **34**, 993–994.
5 Narayanan, R.B., Curtis, J. & Turk, J.L. (1981*a*): Release of soluble factors from lymph nodes containing mycobacterial granulomas and their effect on fibroblast function *in vitro*. *Cell. Immun.* **65**, 93–102.
6 Narayanan, R.B., Badenoch-Jones, P. & Turk, J.L. (1981*b*): Experimental mycobacterial granulomas in guinea pig lymph nodes: ultrastructural observations. *J. Path.* **134**, 253–265.
7 Narayanan, R.B., Badenoch-Jones, P., Curtis, J. & Turk, J.L. (1982): Comparison of mycobacterial granulomas in guinea pig lymph nodes. *J. Path.* **138**, 219–233.

Intrauterine growth retardation and immune responses

Charlotte G. NEUMANN
University of California (UCLA), Schools of Medicine & Public Health, Los Angeles, CA, USA.

Intrauterine growth retardation (IUGR) may occur in as many as 20 per cent of all new-borns particularly in developing countries and in disadvantaged families in industrialized countries. These intrauterine growth retarded infants may experience increased neonatal morbidity and mortality with short-term complications and long-term sequelae in a number of areas of function[28]. A number of aetiologic factors are associated with IUGR, but most important globally are maternal malnutrition during pregnancy and placental insufficiency due to a variety of causes including toxaemia, vascular disease, placental malaria, maternal and intrauterine infections and toxins such as alcohol and nicotine[28].

Maternal malnutrition, whether due to the early onset of frequent and closely spaced cycles of pregnancy and lactation and/or energy deficits due to poor basic diet, hard physical work, and the catabolic effects of repeated bouts of infection, can lead to various 'maternal depletion' syndromes. Not only are energy deficits involved but often deficiencies of protein, iron, calcium, folic acid and, occasionally, vitamin A, pyridoxine and thiamin[15,28]. Recently, trace metal deficiencies, especially zinc, have been noted. Pregnancy outcome in the above circumstances may be poor with low birth-weight due to IUGR. Prematurity is often superimposed on the above situation.

Animal studies. A limited number of studies in humans actually document a link between maternal malnutrition and defective immune function in the neonate. However, well-controlled animal studies support this hypothesis. Animal studies furnish useful clues to the human situation in terms of which nutritional deficiencies may be most detrimental. These include energy and protein deficits, zinc, pyridoxine, folic acid, B_{12}, and choline deficiencies and are summarized in Table 1.

Immune function in IUGR in humans. *The maternal situation.* For the most part, in studies of immunocompetence in IUGR infants, the mothers were not examined for nutritional status, but rather it was inferred that because the mothers came from poor socio-economic circumstances,

Table 1. *Maternal malnutrition and immune defects in intra-uterine growth-retarded (IUGR) animals.*

Nutrient deficieny	Effects on progeny
Protein	Thymolymphatic atrophy
Energy	Impaired AB response to T-cell-dependent antigen
Pyridoxine[24]	Thymic size reduction
Zinc[1]	Cellular immunity decreased
Lipotropes[11]	Impaired ontogenesis of IgA (intergenerational)
Choline	Thymolymphatic atrophy
Methionine	Increased deaths from infection
|B$_{12}$	
Folic acid	

they were probably receiving poor diets, had suboptimal pregnancy weight gains and an increased likelihood of infection. In a number of studies of immune function in IUGR infants which demonstrated decreased cell-mediated immunity (CMI) in the infants, little is described about nutritional status of the mother. In our own studies Kenyan mothers were shorter and lighter and had a higher incidence of anaemia[22]. Levels of serum transferrin and albumin were slightly decreased compared to mothers of healthy full-term normal weight infants. Maternal protein depletion has also been associated with fetal malnutrition[27].

Studies of IUGR infants of poor Indian women stated merely that women were of lower socio-economic status. It was presumed, but not documented, that problems of malnutrition in the mothers were linked to fetal growth retardation and decreased immunity in the offspring[2,27].

Maternal\|folic-acid deficiency in humans can result in IUGR with decreased lymphoid and thymic tissue[12] and folic acid supplementation during pregnancy increases birth-weight. Zinc deficiency is suspected but more work is needed. Maternal short stature is highly correlated with IUGR offspring and a vicious cycle of nutritional deficiency *in utero*, low birth-weight, impaired physical growth during childhood and short adult stature follow and the cycle is thus repeated in the 2nd generation[6]. The mechanism of maternal malnutrition and neonatal immunodeficiency can be seen as: (1) decreased growth and development of fetal lymphoid tissue, thymus and spleen, and a decrease in T-cells; (2) limitation of synthesis of nucleic acid, protein, DNA, cell division, etc.; (3) possible role of cortisol crossing placenta in response to maternal infection and stress.

The role of toxaemia, hypertension, placental malaria and the TORCH (toxoplasmosis, 'other', rubella, cytomegalic inclusion disease, herpes simplex) infections are well-known contributors to the incidence of IUGR and these have a higher incidence in low socio-economic groups, particularly in developing countries[28]. Viral infections and malaria can cause obliterative vasculitis. Studies of Costa Rican infants[17] have demonstrated that elevated IgM levels, a sign of intrauterine infection, were associated with IUGR.

Any condition which reduces the vascularity and blood flow to the placenta, or causes decreased placental size, results in a diminished supply of energy and nutrients to the fetus and a higher incidence of IUGR infants. Growth of fetal lymphoid organs is retarded especially the thymus and impairment of the developing immune system results, with DNA synthesis decreased and cell division and growth severely restricted[20]. Infection *per se* can depress CMI.

Immune function and infection in IUGR infants. *Humoral immunity.* Humoral immunity is generally normal in terms of percentage and number of B-cells in IUGR infants[22] except in some studies in which B-cell number was reduced[5]. Some of the infants may have been preterm. Immunoglobulins have been found to be normal or increased except in situations where the IUGR infant is also preterm. IUGR infants born as a result of placental dysfunction may have low IgG levels because of decreased transfer via the placenta[6]. In a study of rural Costa Rican infants, elevated IgM levels in cord blood of IUGR infants were presumably due to high prevalence of infection while *in utero*[17] although this is not always the case.

Antibody response to tetanus and typhoid immunizations has been observed to be at protective levels in IUGR infants. However, a greater percentage of IUGR infants were found to have lower post-immunization concentrations of tetanus and typhoid antibodies than normal infants[5]. Sero-conversion with trivalent oral polio was seen in low birth-weight infants, both preterm and full-term, but the mean antibody titre was lower in IUGR infants at 4 and 8 weeks post-immunization than in normal BW infants. Haemaglutination inhibition antibody (HAI) responses to measles and pertussis vaccine at 6 months were found to be comparable in IUGR and normal infants when CMI was normal at birth, but lower antibody levels were found when CMI responses were diminished at birth[22].

Granulocyte function. A significant decrease in granulocyte number has been seen in IUGR infants. Decreased intracellular killing and a marked diminution in the bacteriocidal effect of plasma has been noted[5,30].

The nitroblue tetrazolium test (NBT) in the unstimulated state has shown no difference between IUGR and AGA infants but after latex stimulation, a decrease in NBT reduction was found[18] in IUGR infants. Impaired mobilization and killing capacity of polymorphs (PMN) have been documented in IUGR infants and can lead to suboptimal tissue inflammatory response with diminished host protection. Also, macrophages have shown similar diminished function[3].

Leukocyte metabolism studies in the blood of mothers of IUGR infants and cord blood leukocytes of such infants have shown alterations indicative of energy deficits. However, leukocytes did not necessarily show severe functional impairment relevant to host resistance to infection[19]. In other studies of energy metabolism, leukocytes in IUGR infants have shown that all basal activities of the leukocyte were significantly lower than in normal infants. Glucose 6 P-D and leukocyte oxidase activity, oxygen uptake and glucose conversion were studied. The response of all these parameters during stimulation was also significantly lower in IUGR than control infants[13].

Complement levels. For the most part, all complement components and kinetics of the classical and alternative pathway are significantly higher in IUGR infants than in AGA weight-matched preterm infants. Low birth-weight preterm infants have important defects in complement activity[23], the levels correlating mainly with gestational age.

Studies of Indian and Kenyan infants with IUGR were found to have normal concentrations of complement components C_3 and C_4. Only complement component Clq was found to be lower in IUGR infants. It does not appear that IUGR appreciably effects the complement system[14,24].

Cell-mediated immunity (CMI). All studies of IUGR infants, whether term or preterm, show diminished CMI[2,5,9,24,26]. This is expressed by multiple parameters such as decreased total lymphocyte count, reduced T-lymphocytes (percentage and number) and enumerated by E-rosette forming cells (RFC), and diminished delayed cutaneous hypersensitivity. IUGR infants given BCG at birth have a high percentage of negative reactions to intradermal PPD (tuberculin) after BCG immunization. *In vitro* lymphocyte stimulation is normal or increased at birth as there is increased spontaneous blastogenic activity among low and normal birth-weight neonates. The range of depression of CMI is similar in all the studies, that of a moderate but significant degree of decreased function. Rather than a threshold effect, a spectral or progressive depression of CMI is seen, depending on the degree of IUGR as noted by birth-weight deficit. In a study that examined IUGR infants, not only below 2500 g, but also between 2500 to 2800 g, the latter BW group had decreased CMI intermediate between controls and the smallest IUGR infant group (Figure)[22]. Other studies examining very-low birth-weight groups of IUGR infants also found a diminishing degree of CMI function with decreasing birth-weight[2]. It appears that the degree of IUGR is the main determinant of CMI depression (Table 2).

Serum thymic hormone activity in conjunction with CMI was studied in healthy neonates and in preterm and IUGR infants at birth, and at 1, 3, and 12 months. In the IUGR infants, thymic hormone activity and T-cells were reduced in all low birth-weight groups. These values returned to normal in the preterm AGA infants. However, values for lymphocyte stimulation and T-cell number remained low for 12 months in the IUGR infants with low thymic hormone

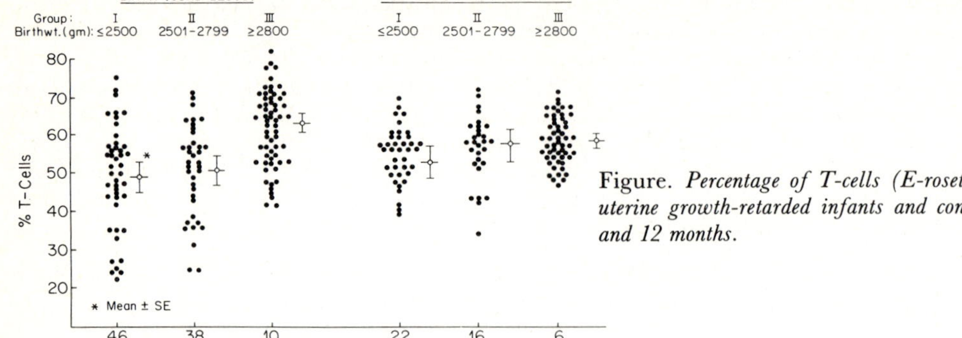

Figure. *Percentage of T-cells (E-rosettes) in intra-uterine growth-retarded infants and controls at birth and 12 months.*

Table 2. *Cell-mediated immunity in intra-uterine growth-retarded (IUGR) infants according to body weight in published studies expressed in terms of per cent rosette-forming cells (mean ± s.e.m.)*

Body weight (g)	Ferguson et al. (1974)[9]	Bhaskaram et al. (1977)[2]	Neumann et al. (1984)[22]	Singh et al. (1978)[26]
> 2800	65.1 ± 1.4	—	60.2 ± 1.1	—
2501–2800	—	56.8 ± 43[++]	56.5 ± 1.3	49.6 ± 6.7[+]
2250–2500	—	52.3 ± 3.26	52.5 ± 7.2	—
1801–2250	49.2 ± 2.0	36.3 ± 3.01	49.8 ± 5.2	54.4 ± 7.8
1501–1800	—	—	44.0 ± 8.3	23.9 ± 4.2

[+] BW groups 2600–3900 g; [++] BW group > 2500 g.

activity at one month of age[7]. Decreased thymic hormone activity has been suggested as being responsible for decreased CMI in IUGR infants and in older individuals[7,29].

Normal catch-up growth helps, only in part, to restore the impaired immune function. Unlike post-neonatally acquired PEM, where CMI shows recovery early in the course of nutritional rehabilitation (often by 10–14 d) the depressed CMI in IUGR infants is long term, lasting from 1 year to at least 5 years[4,8]. Also IUGR infants are at risk for superimposed post-natal PEM.

Functional outcomes. In regard to CMI status and immunization response, a group of nonresponders to pertussis and measles immunization were found to have a significantly higher percentage of infants with reduced T-cells than did vaccine responders[10,21]. BCG immunizations given at birth resulted in significantly lower percentages of positive tuberculin reactions at 6 months post-BCG in IUGR infants than in normal new-borns, another expression of depressed CMI[16,22]. Since depressed CMI is the main immunologic problem in IUGR, this may decrease the effectiveness of certain immunizations which are, at least in part, T-cell dependent such as for tuberculosis, measles and pertussis.

Clinical infections and cell-mediated immunity. In examining morbidity in IUGR infants in whom immune function had been studied, crude clinical infection rates from 0 to 6 months of life were higher than in normal BW infants. Episodes of lower respiratory infection, oral moniliasis and pertussis were higher in IUGR infants with decreased percentages of T-cells (50 per cent) compared to those with normal T-cells[22]. In the same study, over the entire 1st year of life, double the percentage of IUGR infants had ≥ 10 clinical infections compared to the normal BW infants (26 per cent vs 14 per cent). Forty-three per cent of the latter group had reduced T-cells compared to 13 per cent of the normal infants. Between 7 to 12 months of age, otitis media, clinically diagnosed tuberculosis and diarrhoea were more prevalent in the infants with decreased CMI than in infants with normal CMI.

A group of Indian IUGR infants followed for 6 months had a greater frequency and duration of skin sepsis, diarrhoeal disease, and septicaemia compared to normal infants[25].

In summary, the health implications of depressed cell-mediated immunity and of the opsonic and leukocyte abnormalities in the IUGR infant include increased susceptibility and lower resistance to infection and diminished response to certain immunizations.

1 Beach, R.S., Gershwin, M.E. & Hurley, L.S. (1982): Reversibility of development retardation following murine fetal zinc deprivation. *J. Nutr.* **112**, 1169–1181.

2 Bhaskaram, C., Ragharamulu, N. & Reddy, V. (1977): Cell-mediated immunity and immunoglobulin levels in light-for-date infants. *Acta Pediatr. Scand.* **66**, 617–619.

3 Blaese, M., Poplack, D.G. & Muchmore, A.V. (1979): The mononuclear phagocyte system role in expression of immunocompetence in neonatal and adult life. *Paediatrics* **64**, 829–833.

4 Chandra, R.K. (1974): Rosette forming T-lymphocytes and cell-mediated immunity in malnutrition. *Br. Med. J.* **3**, 60–69.

5 Chandra, R.K. (1975): Fetal malnutrition and postnatal immunocompetence. *J. Dis. Child.* **129**, 450–454.

6 Chandra, R.K. (1977): Biological Implications. In *Nutrition, immunity, and infection*, pp. 181–196. New York: Plenum Press.

7 Chandra, R.K. (1981): Serum thymic hormone activity and cell-mediated immunity in healthy neonates, preterm infants, and small-for gestational age infants. *Pediatrics* **67**, 407–411.

8 Ferguson, A.C. (1978): Prolonged impairment of cellular immunity in children with intrauterine growth retardation. *J. Pediatr.* **93**, 52–56.

9 Ferguson, A.C., Lawlor, G.J., Neumann, C.G., Oh, W. & Stiehm, E.R. (1974): Decreased rosette-forming lymphocytes in malnutrition and intrauterine growth retardation. *J. Pediatr.* **85**, 717–723.

10 Gallagher, M.R., Welliver, R., Yamanaka, T., Eisenberg, B., Sun, M. & Ogra, P.L. (1981): Cell-mediated immune responsiveness to measles. Its occurrence as a result of naturally acquired or vaccine-induced infection and in infants of immune mothers. *Am. J. Dis. Child.* **135**, 48–51.

11 Gebhardt, B.N. & Newberne, P.M. (1974): Nutrition and immunological responsiveness: T-cell function in the offspring of lipotrope and protein deficient rats. *Immunology* **26**, 489–495.

12 Gross, R.L., Reid, J.V.O. & Newberne, P.M. (1975): Depressed cell-mediated immunity in megaloblastic anemia due to folic deficiency. *Am. J. Clin. Nutr.* **28**, 225–232.

13 Hernandez, O., Frenk, S., Velasco-Candano, L., Urrusti, J., Yoshida, P., Bernel-Torres, A. & Rosado, A. (1980): Human fetal growth retardation. Metabolic response of leukocytes to phagocytosis. *Archs. Invest. Med.* **11**, 175–186.

14 Jagadeesan, V. & Reddy, V. (1978): Serum complement and lysozyme levels in light-for-date infants. *Acta Paediatr. Scand.* **67**, 237–238.

15 Jelliffe, D.B. (1966): *The Assessment of the nutritional status of the community.* WHO, 53 (Geneva).

16 Manerikaris, S., Malaviya, A.N. & Singh, M.B. (1976): Immune status and BCG vaccination in newborns with intrauterine growth retardation. *Clin. Exp. Immunol.* **26**, 173–175.

17 Mata, L.J. & Villatoro, E. (1977): Umbilical cord immunoglobulins. In *Malnutrition and the immune response*, ed R.M. Suskind. New York: Raven Press.

18 Merkiel, K., Kemona, H., Iwaszki-Krawczuk, W. & Prokopowicz, J. (1980): Nitroblue tetrazolium test in the term small-for-dates newborn. *Acta Paediatr. Acad. Sci. Hung.* **21**, 85–88.

19 Metcoff, J. (1974): Maternal leukocyte metabolism in fetal malnutrition. *Adv. Exp. Med. Biol.* **49**, 73–118.

20 Naeye, R.L., Blanc, W. & Paul, C. (1973): Effects of maternal malnutrition on the human fetus. *Pediatrics* **52**, 494–503.

21 Neumann, C.G., Stiehm, E.R. & Cherry, J. (1980): Immune function and infection in intrauterine malnourished infants. In *Procs. infections in the immunocompromised host-pathogenesis, prevention and therapy.* Amsterdam: Elsevier.

22 Neumann, C.G., Stiehm, E.R., Zahradnick, J., Newton, C., Weber, H., Swendseid, M.E., Cherry, J. & Carney, J. (1984): Immune function in intrauterine growth retardation. *Nutr. Res.* **4**, 399–419.

23 Notarangelo, L.D., Chirico, G., Chiara, A., Colombo, A., Rondini, G., Plebani, A., Martini, A. & Ugazio, A.G. (1984): Activity of classical and alternative pathways of complement in preterm and small-for gestational age infants. *Pediatr. Res.* **18**, 281–285.

24 Robson, L.C. & Schwartz, M.R. (1975): Vitamin B_6 deficiency and the lymphoid system 11. Effects of vitamin in utero on the immunological competence of the offspring. *Cell. Immunol.* **16**, 145–52.

25 Saha, K., Kaur, P., Srivastava, G. & Chaudhury, D.S. (1983): A six months follow-up study of growth morbidity and functional immunity in low birth weight neonates with special reference to intrauterine growth retardation in small-for-gestation age infants. *J. Trop. Paediatr.* **29**, 278–282.

26 Singh, M., Manerikar, S., Malaviya, A.N., Gopalan, R. & Kuman, R. (1978): Immune status of low birth weight babies. *Ind. Pediatr.* **4**, 563–566.

27 Stein, H. (1975): Maternal protein depletion and small-for-gestational age babies. *Archs. Dis. Childhood* **50**, 146–149.

28 Tafari, N. (1981): Low birthweight: an overview. *Adv. Int. Matern. Child Hlth* **1**, 105–127.

29 Wara, D.W. & Barrett, D.J. (1979): Cell-mediated immunity in the newborn: clinical apsects. *Pediatrics* **64**, 822–828.

30 Ziobro, J., Iwaszko-Krawczuk, W. & Prokopowicz, J. (1980): Bateriocidal capacity of plasma and granulocytes against *Escherichia coli* in the small-for-dates newborn. *Acta Paediatr. Hung.* **21**, 8–9.

Can dietary factors alter waning immunocompetence in old age?

R.K. CHANDRA
*Health Sciences Centre, Memorial University of Newfoundland, St. John's, Newfoundland
A1B 3V6, Canada.*

The question no longer is *whether* dietary factors and nutritional status effect immunocompetence and risk of disease, but *how* and *to what extent.* Nutritional deficiency is the most common cause of secondary immunodeficiency both in developing and industrialized countries.

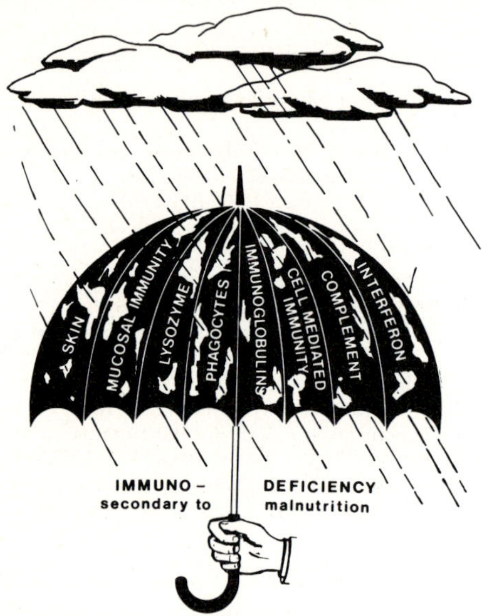

Figure. *The host-protective umbrella consists of anatomic barriers and non-specific and antigen-specific mechanisms.* Malnutrition produces defects in many of these factors.

Impaired immunologic and non-immunologic defense mechanisms (Figure) such as absent or reduced delayed cutaneous hypersensitivity response to common microbial antigens, decreased number of thymus-dependent T lymphocytes, reduced bactericidal capacity of neutrophils, lower mucosal secretory IgA antibody titre, and depressed complement system, have been consistently documented in several studies among undernourished children and adults[1,3].

The progressive increase in the proportion of elderly individuals has prompted a serious examination of the prevalence and causes of common illnesses affecting them. The frequent occurrence of infection, cancer and autoimmune disease suggests declining immunocompetence in old age. Indeed this has been amply confirmed in several recent studies in man and laboratory animals. However, immunological senescence is not universal and at least a proportion of the elderly maintain the ability to mount immune responses at levels comparable with those of the young. Obviously, both genetic and environmental factors are critical determinants of immunocompetence. Among the latter, nutrition is of prime importance.

Immunocompetence in the elderly. Many physiologic functions decline in old age. The immune system is no exception. Age-related changes in immune response have been studied extensively and have been reviewed[6]. The most dramatic effect is on cell-mediated immunity.

In individuals above the age of 65 years, delayed cutaneous hypersensitivity responses to ubiquitous recall antigens derived from bacterial and fungal products as well as to the strong chemical agent 2,4-dinitrochlorobenzene are reduced in frequency and size. The number of circulating rosette-forming T-cells is normal or slightly reduced. The recent availability of monoclonal antibodies to identify different subsets of lymphocytes has permitted analysis of T-cell subpopulations in the elderly. The number of T4+ helper cells is slightly reduced or normal whereas the proportion of T8+ suppressor/cytotoxic cells is often decreased. These changes could explain the functional alterations — reduced proliferation response to mitogens and antigens, decreased production of lymphokines such as the macrophage migration inhibition factor, impaired autologous mixed lymphocyte reaction, synthesis of T-cell growth factor, and natural killer-cell activity — observed by several investigators[12,14,16,18–20].

There are several hormonal, metabolic and regulatory changes observed in old age which may partly explain the above noted immunologic decline. T-cell maturation and differentiation is regulated by a number of inductive factors largely produced by the thymus. In individuals beyond 40 years of age, there is a sharp decline in the serum concentration and activity of these factors, including Facteur Thymique Serique. The activity is almost undetectable in those above 65 years. *In vitro*, thymic epithelium from young individuals permits the development and functional maturation of precursor cells derived from either young or old persons, whereas the thymic epithelial cultures from the elderly fail to achieve this. This emphasizes the critical role of thymus hormones in the development and maintenance of T-cell-dependent immune responses. There is growing evidence also for qualitative changes in T-cells, including the density of receptors on T-cells and the appearance of new receptors. A terminal differentiation antigen, the 'senescent cell antigen' appears on the membrane of cells as they age. Ultrastructurally, there is swelling of mitochondria and presence of myelin-like structures and reduced number of cristae in cells from old individuals. Metabolically, there is evidence of an imbalance in the level of cyclic AMP and GMP in resting and mitogen-stimulated T-cells.

Estimation of serum immunoglobulin concentrations has generally shown a reduction in serum IgG and increase in serum IgA levels in the elderly. The prevalence of autoantibodies increases, but this does not necessarily indicate the presence of underlying disease. Levels of circulating isoantibodies and natural heterophil antibodies decline with age. The proliferative response of B-lymphocytes to bacterial lipopolysaccharide, a B-cell mitogen, is normal or marginally reduced. In old animals, primary antibody response is decreased, but antibody titre after booster immunization is comparable in young and old animals. Moreover, there may be a delay in reaching the peak response. For many antigens, antibody production by B-cells requires the help of T-cell-generated helper factors. For such antigens, antibody titre in older individuals is decreased. Moreover, the affinity of antibody is reduced. In a small proportion of the elderly, monoclonal gammopathy is seen, and more rarely, there is development of multiple myeloma.

Neutrophils obtained from the elderly have reduced migration ability, both random and chemotactic. Phagocytosis, including the uptake of microorganisms and the ability to kill ingested bacteria, is largely intact. Killing of *Candida* is slightly decreased and the magnitude of metabolic burst associated with phagocytosis is limited.

Nutrition and immunity. Much of the data on nutritional regulation of immunity are derived from observations on young children, but there is good reason to expect that such information can be extended to other age groups including the elderly. At the same time, impaired immunocompetence in malnourished elderly is more difficult to repair, probably because there is an element of age-related irreversible decline in immunity.

Impairment of immune responses occurs both with generalized under-nutrition as well as with deficiencies or excesses of single nutrients[1–3,7]. The causal interaction between nutritional status and immunologic function is a complex one and depends upon a variety of factors, including the age of the subject, the type and duration of malnutrition, presence of specific nutrient deficiencies, nature of the underlying disease, and the presence of concurrent infection. The most prominent effects of nutritional deficiencies are observed on cell-mediated immunity, number of T-lymphocytes, helper T-cell function, complement system, mucosal IgA response, neutrophil bacterial killing capacity, and antibody affinity. Depression of host immune response in malnutrition is generally reversible. However, critical data about the rates of functional recovery of different components of the immune system, upon nutritional repletion, are only limited[8].

Influence of nutrition on immunity in old age. Recognizing the comprehensive observations on immunological changes in old age, on dietary intake and body composition of the elderly, and on the critical role of nutrition in regulation of immunocompetence, it is surprising that so little has been studied about nutritional regulation of immunity and disease in this age group[4,5]. Our study of the nutritional and immunological status of a group of elderly individuals who had no evidence of an underlying systemic disease showed that among those with clinical, haematologic and biochemical evidence of nutritional deficiency, there was a significant reduction in delayed cutaneous hypersensitivity, T-cell number and response to mitogen[10]. Nutritional advice and supplements given for 8 weeks resulted in improved skin test responses, increase in T-cell number and in lymphocyte proliferation response to phytohaemagglutinin. This improvement in immunologic function was associated with evidence of improved nutritional status, mainly in terms of levels of albumin, prealbumin, transferrin, retinol-binding protein, zinc and iron[11].

In another study, the administration of moderate amounts of zinc to subjects over 70 years of age for 1 month was associated with increase in the number of circulating T-cells, delayed cutaneous hypersensitivity to purified protein derivative, *Candida* and streptokinase-streptodornase, serum IgG antibody response to tetanus toxoid[13]. Vitamin C supplements of 500 mg per day for 1 month enhanced lymphocyte proliferative responses *in vitro* and skin reactivity to tuberculin *in vivo*[17]. There was no change in serum immunoglobulin levels or the proportion of rosetting T-cells. In a recent study, the elderly receiving megadose vitamin C supplements tended to respond better on skin testing, but the differences from non-supplemented controls were statistically non-significant[15] and there were no changes in lymphocyte responses to mitogens *in vitro*. Subjects taking megadoses of vitamin B complex or vitamin E had lower absolute lymphocyte counts than did controls. At the same time, we should recognize that large doses of 'essential' nutrients may produce deleterious effects[5].

Concluding remarks. In old age, there is a progressive decline in immunological vigour as well as in lean body mass. At the same time, many individuals above the age of 65 years have obvious or subclinical nutritional deficiencies. We suggest that such malnutrition contributes to immunologic senescence and that the correction of nutritional deficits and imbalances can reverse, in part, the impairment of cell-mediated immunity observed commonly in the elderly[4]. The provision of protein-energy supplement and correction of deficiencies of iron, zinc, vitamin C, E and B complex, is associated with improved immune responses[10]. Nutritional support also improves antibody response, and perhaps protection, following the administration of influenza pneumococcal, and tetanus immunization[9,11]. Preliminary data suggest that improved nutritional status not only results in enhanced immunocompetence but also reduces the burden of illness experienced by the elderly. These observations have considerable clinical and public health importance on a global scale.

Can dietary support improve waning immunocompetence in old age? The answer has to be in the affirmative.

 1 Beisel, W.R. (1983): Single nutrients and immunity. *Am. J. Clin. Nutr.* **35**, 417–468.
 2 Chandra, R.K. (1979): Nutritional deficiency and susceptibility to infection. *Bull. Wld Hlth Org.* **57**, 157–176.
 3 Chandra, R.K. (1983): Nutrition, immunity and infection: Present knowledge and future directions. *Lancet* **1**, 688–691.
 4 Chandra, R.K. (1984): Nutritional regulation of immune function at the extremes of life: in infants and in the elderly. In *Malnutrition: determinants and consequences*, ed P.L. White & N. Selvy, pp. 245–251. New York: Alan R. Liss.
 5 Chandra, R.K. (1984): Excessive intake of zinc impairs immune responses. *J. Am. Med. Ass.* **252**, 1443–1446.
 6 Chandra, R.K. (1985): *Nutrition, immunity and illness in the elderly* New York: Pergamon Press. (In press)
 7 Chandra, R.K. & Dayton, D. (1982): Trace element regulation of immunity and infection. *Nutr. Res.* **2**, 721–733.
 8 Chandra, R.K. & Puri, S. (1985): Nutritional regulation of host resistance and predictive value of immunologic tests in assessment outcome. *Pediat. Clin. N. Am.* **32**, 499–515.
 9 Chandra, R.K. & Puri, S. (1985): Nutritional support improved antibody response to influenza vaccine in the elderly. *Br. Med. J.* **291**, 705–706.
10 Chandra, R.K. *et al.* (1982): Nutrition and immunocompetence of the elderly. Effect of short-term supplementation on cell-mediated immunity and lymphocyte subsets. *Nutr. Res.* **2**, 223–232.
11 Chandra *et al*, (1985): Nutritional regulation of immunity and risk of disease in the elderly. *Abstr. Int. Congr. Gerontol.* New York, July 12–17.
12 Dworsky, R. *et al.* (1983): Immune responses of healthy humans 83–104 years of age. *J. Natl. Cancer Inst.* **71**, 265–268.

13 Duchateau, J. *et al.* (1981): Beneficial effects of oral zinc supplementation on the immune response of old people. *Am. J. Med.* **70**, 1001–1004.

14 Girard, J.P. *et al.* (1977): Cell-mediated immunity in an aging population. *Clin. Exp. Immunol.* **27**, 85–91.

15 Goodwin, J.S. & Garry, P.J. (1983): Relationship between megadose vitamin supplementation and immunological function in a healthy elderly population. *Clin. Exp. Immunol.* **51**, 647–653.

16 Hicks, M.J. *et al.* (1983): Age-related changes in mitogen-induced lymphocyte function from birth to old age. *Am. J. Clin. Path.* **80**, 159–163.

17 Kennes, B. *et al.* (1983): Effect of vitamin C supplements on cell-mediated immunity in old people. *Gerontology* **29**, 305–311.

18 Mascart-Lemone, F. *et al.* (1982): Characterization of immunoregulatory T lymphocytes during aging by monoclonal antibodies. *Clin. Exp. Immunol.* **48**, 148–154.

19 Rosenkoetter, M. *et al.* (1983): Modulation of T lymphocyte differentiation antigens: influence of aging. *Cell. Immunol.* **77**, 395–401.

20 Sohnle, P.G. *et al.* (1980): Failure of lymphokine producing lymphocytes from aging humans to undergo activation by recall antigens. *J. Immunol.* **124**, 2169–2174.

Trace elements and immunity

Gloria HERESI
Division of Human Nutrition and Medical Sciences, Institute of Nutrition and Food Technology (INTA), University of Chile, Santiago, Chile.

The effect of malnutrition on infection and function of the immune system is well established[7,34]. However, malnutrition is a complex syndrome with many nutrient deficiencies involved. How each one of these nutrients affects the immune status has been the focus of much research during the last decade, trace elements being the group most widely studied.

There are many trace elements but only zinc, copper, arsenic, chromium, cobalt, fluorine, iodine, iron, manganese, molybdenum, nickel, selenium, silicon, tin and vanadium fulfil the criteria for essentiality defined by Mertz[30]. For each nutrient there is a range of safe and adequate exposure, within which homoeostasis is able to maintain optimal tissue concentrations and functions. However, adverse deleterious effects may be expected when the range of safe and adequate exposure is violated either by excess or deficit. The biological importance of most trace elements stems primarily from their role in many vital enzymes or as components of biologically active molecules as hormones. There is considerable evidence that many individual trace elements influence the immune system in animals and man.

Iron. Infants, women and children are the groups most affected by iron deficiency[37]. Iron is essential for mammalian cells as well as for microorganisms, and conflicting data concerning iron deficiency and infection have been reported in the literature. Two main positions have emerged: some investigators have claimed that iron deficiency is associated with a high incidence of infection, while others point out that anaemia protects against infection. When the possible effect of an acidified iron-fortified formula upon infections was studied in a longitudinal field trial the incidence of gastrointestinal and respiratory infections was found to be similar to that of infants fed a non-acidified unfortified formula[24]. In another study, 654 infants with iron fortified milk and 585 with non-fortified milk were followed monthly. The number of episodes of diarrhoea per hundred infants was fewer in the group receiving the fortified formula during spring and summer[24].

Most of the studies done in this area can be criticized on methodological grounds, eg, lack of simultaneous controls or poorly defined criteria for the diagnosis of infection and in some studies infection rates were compiled retrospectively by questionnaire or recall[39]. There is need to make well-controlled field trials to obtain reliable information on this issue.

In relation to the immune system, most studies have shown impaired cell-mediated immune function and neutrophil activity in iron deficieny. Skin reactivity to a battery of recall antigens has been found to be decreased[6,26]. A low number of T-cells which return to normal after iron therapy has been described[3,6]. Lymphocyte transformation to mitogens and antigens is reduced[6,26]. Lymphokine production is similarly decreased in response to antigenic stimulation. Macrophage migration inhibitory factor, the only lymphokine to be studied, became normal after iron repletion[26]. Other investigators have not found alterations in cellular immune response in iron deficiency[22,29]. However, the small number of subjects studied, presence of associated infection and differences in techniques, are important variables to consider when interpreting the results of these studies[39]. Bactericidal activity against different bacteria was decreased when polymorphs from iron-deficient subjects were compared to control[5,40]. Bactericidal activity towards *E. coli* reverts to normal not sooner than 15 d after iron therapy, implying a need for iron during neutrophil maturation in the bone marrow[40]. Myeloperoxidase, a haem-containing enzyme which participates in bacterial killing, has been found decreased in iron deficiency[42].

Humoral immunity in humans is, apparently, unaffected by iron deficiency. A normal immunoglobulin level, secretory IgA and complement components have been described[6]. However, animal studies have shown that iron-deficient rats have decreased antibody titres to antigens[31]. Recently, it was demonstrated that iron deficiency during gestation and lactation resulted in decreased antibody formation to sheep red blood cells (SRBC) by offspring[27].

The mechanism involved in the immunological changes observed in iron deficiency may include: a decreased ribonucleotide reductase necessary for DNA synthesis and cell proliferation, a decrease in myeloperoxidase (an iron-dependent enzyme) and decreased formation of hydroxyl radicals within the phagocytic cell. However, the molecular defects involved have not yet been clearly established.

Zinc. Acrodermatitis enteropathica (AE), a genetic syndrome, and the animal model for this disease, the A-46 mutant cattle of the Dutch Friesian type have provided evidence that a normal zinc nutritional status is essential for the development and maintenance of a normal immune system. AE is a syndrome probably secondary to an inherited defect in zinc absorption[12]. Symptoms and signs appear during infancy, after weaning, and include mucocutaneous lesions, diarrhoea, anorexia, alopecia, growth retardation and a high susceptibility to infections. Children with AE manifest an abnormal immune response; the thymus is undersized, grossly absent or depleted of lymphocytes. Lymphocyte proliferation to phytohaemagglutinin (PHA) is decreased and delayed hypersensitivity response and monocyte chemotaxis are impaired[7,41].

Zinc deficiency has been reported in children with PEM. Thymic atrophy in malnourished children can be reversed with zinc supplements[19] and the local application of zinc sulphate ointment improves delayed cutaneous response to the candida antigen[20], though this has not been confirmed. In marasmic infants receiving zinc sulphate supplement for 3 months, a significant reduction in infectious episodes with normal delayed cutaneous response, as compared with a placebo group, has been reported[4]. No differences were found in lymphocyte proliferation to PHA.

Zinc deficiency in laboratory animals has helped to elucidate the role of this micronutrient on the immune system. Atrophy of the thymus, specially the cortical area, have been reported in mice and rats[8]. Zinc deprivation has an effect on the ontogeny of immunity. Moderate deprivation of zinc during prenatal life alone is associated with a depressed plaque-forming cell (PFC) response to SRBC inoculation and with impaired development of serum immunoglobulins[2]. These defects in immunological function persist into the 2nd and 3rd generation.

Marginal deficiencies in zinc during lactation greatly reduce the ability of suckling pups to mount antibody-mediated responses[17]. Low thymic hormone levels have been reported[9] and zinc administration restored normal hormone levels. It has been suggested that a nonactive zinc-deprived peptide is secreted in mice subjected long term to a diet marginally deficient in zinc[13]. The presence of a non-functional thymic hormone could explain some of the cellular impairments seen in zinc deficiency. A defective delayed-type hypersensitivity and lymphocyte proliferation to mitogen has been reported in mice and rats[18,21]. In one study the proliferative response restores to normal by adding levamisole to the culture[21]. Others have reported a normal lymphocyte proliferative response to mitogen in zinc-deficient animals[28].

A diminished natural killer-cell activity and an impaired generation of splenic cytotoxic T-lymphocyte response of tumour cells *in vivo*, but normal *in vitro*, have also been described[8,15]. The humoral immune response of animals deprived of zinc after weaning is better than when deprivation starts from the first day of life. A low antibody response to T-dependent and T-independent antigens, which returns to normal after zinc-supplementation, has also been reported[17]. Several studies have demonstrated a defective T-helper cell function[16].

Zinc excess *in vivo* was associated with reduction in lymphocyte stimulation to PHA and depressed chemotaxis and phagocytosis[11]. The underlying mechanisms are not clear. An increase in serum and membrane-associated low-density lipoprotein has been postulated to depress lymphocyte stimulation.

The mechanism by which zinc affects immunity is not clear. It is known that zinc is an essential factor for the activity of more than 100 metalloenzymes. Thus thymidine kinase, DNA polymerase and DNA-dependent RNA polymerase involved in RNA and DNA synthesis are zinc-dependent enzymes. The effect of these enzymes in nucleic acid synthesis could explain the effects of zinc on lymphoid cell proliferation. On the other hand, zinc is necessary for the activity of some immunity mediators like thymuline.

Copper. Menkes syndrome is a rare congenital disease with copper deficiency. These children die early in life usually from an infection such as pneumonia. Alteration of cell-mediated immunity has been described in some of these patients[32].

Studies in copper-deficient rehabilitated marasmic infants have shown impairment of phagocytic function which improves after 1 month of copper-supplementation[23]. A depressed blastic transformation to PHA has also been reported. Further studies have suggested that the depressed blastic transformation could be related to lack of copper or a copper dependent factor in the plasma or presence of a suppressor plasmatic factor induced by copper deficiency[23]. Copper deficiency prevented the reticulo-endothelial system from responding appropriately to infection with *S. typhimurium*.

A reduced PFC response to SRBC, decreased resistance to tumours and decreased response to mitogen in copper-deficient laboratory animals has been found[33]. However, one report shows normal lymphoproliferative response to PHA[38]. Granulocytes from copper-deficient cattle and lambs have a decreased microbicidal activity, but other reports have shown that copper enhances phagocytosis and oxygen transport in dog granulocytes[25]. Research is needed to clarify if copper acts upon the immune response through copper dependent enzymes or by other mechanisms as yet unknown.

Other trace elements. There is a scarcity of information on the influence of other trace elements on immunity. Dietary supplementation with selenium at levels above the nutritional requirements enhanced the primary immune responses. This was measured by the number of antibody-forming cells and levels of SRBC-agglutinating antibody[36]. Selenium promoted increased synthesis of IgM antibody. Dogs deficient in selenium and vitamin E developed low neutralizing antibody titres following vaccination[35]. The primary immune response to SRBC was not affected but secondary responses were reduced.

Magnesium deficiency in rats results in reduced levels of serum proteins and immunoglobulins G and M[1,14]. Little is known about other trace elements, and ultra trace elements, and immunity, but a summary of recent information from a workshop held at the National Institute of Health has been published[10].

Acknowledgements. I want to thank Dra Marta Colombo for her support and critical review of the paper and Miss Adriana Vargas for typing the manuscript. Part of these data was performed at the Division of Human Nutrition and Medical Sciences, INTA, University of Chile. This work was supported partially by Grant M 1321-8122 from University of Chile.

1 Alcok, N.W. & Shils, M.E. (1974): Serum immunoglobulin G in the magnesium depleted rat. *Proc. Soc. Exp. Biol. Med.* **145**, 855–858.

2 Beach, R.S., Gershwin, M.E. & Hurley, L.S. (1982): Gestational zinc deprivation in mice: persistence of immunodeficiency for three generations. *Science* **218**, 469–471.

3 Bhaskaram, C. & Reddy, V. (1975): Cell mediated immunity in iron and vitamin-deficient children. *Br. Med. J.* **3**, 522.

4 Castillo, C., Heresi, G., Fisberg, M. & Uauy, R. (1982): Zinc supplementation in marasmic infants under nutritional rehabilitation. *Rev. Chil. Nutr.* **10**, 21–33.

5 Chandra, R.K. (1973): Reduced bactericidal capacity of polymorphs in iron deficiency. *Archs. Dis. Child.* **48**, 864–866.

6 Chandra, R.K. (1975): Impaired immunocompetence associated with iron deficiency. *J. Pediatr.* **8**, 899–902.

7 Chandra, R.K. (1980): *Immunology of nutritional disorders*. London: Edward Arnold.

8 Chandra, R.K. & Au, B. (1980): Single nutrient deficiency and cell mediated immune responses 1. Zinc. *Am. J. Clin. Nutr.* **33**, 736–738.

9 Chandra, R.K., Heresi, G. & Au, B. (1981): Serum thymic factor activity in deficiencies of calories, zinc, vitamin A and pyridoxine. *Clin. Exp. Immunol.* **42**, 332–335.

10 Chandra, R.K. & Dayton, D.H. (1982): Trace element regulation of immunity and infection. *Nutr. Res.* **2**, 721–733.

11 Chandra, R.K. (1984): Excessive intake of zinc impairs immune responses. *J. Am. Med. Ass.* **252**, 1443–1446.

12 Danboet, N. & Closs, R. (1942): Acrodematitis enteropathica. *Acta Dermatol. Venereol.* **23**, 127–169.

13 Dardenne, M., Savino, W., Wade, S., Kaiserlian, D., Lemmonnier, D. & Bach, J.F. (1984): In vivo and in vitro studies of thymulin in marginally zinc-deficient mice. *Eur. J. Immunol.* **14**, 454–458.

14 Elin, R.J. (1975): The effect of magnesium deficiency in mice on serum immunoglobulin concentrations and antibody plaque-forming cells. *Proc. Soc. Exp. Biol. Med.* **148**, 620–624.

15 Fernandez, G., Nair, M., Once, K., Tanaka, T., Floyd, R. & Good, R.A. (1979): Impairment of cell mediated immunity functions by dietary zinc deficiency in mice. *Proc. Natl. Acad. Sci. USA.* **76**, 457–461.

16 Fraker, P.J., Depasquale-Jardieu, P., Zwickl, C.M., Lueke, R.W. (1978): Regeneration of T-cell helper function in zinc-deficient adult mice. *Proc. Natl. Acad. Sci. USA.* **75**, 5660–5664.

17 Fraker, P.J., Hildebrant, K., Lueke, R.W. (1984): Alteration of antibody-mediated responses of suckling mice to T-cell dependent and independent antigens by maternal marginal zinc deficiency: restoration of responsivity by nutritional repletion. *J. Nutr.* **114**, 170–179.

18 Fraker, P.J., Zwicki, C.M. & Luecke, R.W. (1982): Delayed type hypersensitivity in zinc-deficient adult mice: impairment and restoration of responsitivity to dinitro fluorobenzene. *J. Nutr.* **112**, 309–313.

19 Golden, M.H.N., Golden, B.E. & Jackson, A.A. (1977): Effect of zinc on thymus of recently malnourished children. *Lancet* **2**, 1057–1059.

20 Golden, M.H.N., Golden, B.E., Harland, P.S.E.G. & Jackson, A.A. (1978): Zinc and immunocompetence in protein-energy malnutrition. *Lancet* **1**, 1226–1228.

21 Gross, R.L., Osdin, N., Fong, L. & Newberne, P.M. (1979): Depressed immunological function in zinc deprived rats as measured by mitogen response of spleen, thymus and peripheral blood. *Am. J. Clin. Nutr.* **32**, 1260–1265.

22 Gross, R.L., Reid, J.V.O., Newberne, P.M., Burgess, B., Marston, R. & Hift, W. (1975): Depressed cell-mediated immunity in megaloblastic anemia due to folic acid deficiency. *Am. J. Clin. Nutr.* **28**, 225–232.

23 Heresi, G., Castillo-Duran, C., Muñoz, C., Arévalo, M. & Schlesinger, L. (1985): Phagocytosis and immunoglobulin levels in hypocupremic infants. *Nutr. Res.* (In press).

24 Heresi, G., Olivares, M., Pizarro, F. & Stekel, A. (1981): Incidence of gastrointestinal and respiratory infection in infants fed an iron fortified acidified milk. XIX Reunión Anual, SLAIP, Quito-Ecuador (Abstr. 9).

25 Jones, D.G. & Suttle, N.F. (1981): Some effect of copper deficiency on leucocyte function in sheep and cattle. *Res. Vet. Sci.* **31**, 151–156.

26 Joynson, D.H.M., Jacob, A., Murray, W.D. & Dolby, A.E. (1972): Defect of cell mediated immunity in patients with iron deficiency anemia. *Lancet* **2**, 1058–1059.

27 Kochanowski, B.A. & Sherman, A.R. (1985): Decreased antibody formation in iron-deficient rat pups — effect of iron repletion. *Am. J. Clin. Nutr.* **41**, 278–284.

28 Kramer, T.R. (1984): Reevaluation of zinc deficiency on cancanavalin-A-induced rat spleen lymphocyte proliferation. *J. Nutr.* **114**, 953–963.

29 Kulapongs, P., Vithayasai, V., Suskind, R. & Olson, R.E. (1974): Cell-mediated immunity and phagocytosis and killing function in children with severe iron-deficiency anemia. *Lancet* **2**, 689–691.

30 Mertz, W. (1981): The essential trace elements. *Science* **213**, 1332–1338.

31 Nalder, B.N., Mahoney, A.W., Ramakrishan, R. & Hendricks, D.C. (1972): Sensitivity of the immunological response to the nutritional status of rats. *J. Nutr.* **102**, 535–542.

32 Pedroni, E., Bianchi, E., Ugazio, G.A. & Burgio, R.G. (1975): Immunodeficiency steely hair. *Lancet* **1**, 1303–1304.

33 Prohaska, J.R. & Juka Sewycz, O.A. (1981): Copper deficiency suppresses the immune response of mice. *Science* **213**, 559–561.

34 Schlesinger, L., Muñoz, C. & Heresi, G. (1981): Impact of nutrition on host defense. In *Nutrition in health and disease and international development*, Symposium from the XII Int. Congr. Nutr., ed A.E. Harper & G.K. Davis, pp. 453–462. New York: Alan R. Liss.

35 Sheffy, B.E. & Schultz, R.D. (1979): Influence of Vitamin E and selenium on immune response mechanisms. *Fed. Proc.* **38**, 2139–2143.

36 Spallholz, J.E., Martin, J.L., Gerlach, M.L. & Heinzerling, R.H. (1973): Immunologic responses of mice fed diets supplemented with selenite selenium. *Proc. Soc. Exp. Biol. Med.* **143**, 685–689.

37 Stekel, A. (1984): *Iron nutrition in infancy and childhood*. New York: Raven Press.

38 Vyas, D. & Chandra, R.K. (1983): Thymic factor activity, lymphocyte stimulation response and antibody producing cell in copper deficiency. *Nutr. Res.* **3**, 343–349.

39 Vyas, D. & Chandra, R.K. (1984): Functional implication of iron deficiency. In *Iron nutrition in infancy and childhood*, ed A. Stekel. New York: Raven Press.

40 Walter, T., Arredondo, S., Arévalo, M. & Stekel, A. (1983): Effect of iron therapy on phagocitosis and bactericidal activity of iron deficient infants. Western Hemisphere Nutrition Congress VII, Miami Beach, Florida, U.S.A. (Abstr. 42).

41 Weston, W.L., Huff, J.C., Humbert, J.R., Hambidge, R.M., Nelder, K.H. & Walravens, P.A. (1977): Zinc correction of defective chemotaxis in acrodermatitis enteropathica. *Archs. Dermatol.* **113**, 422–425.

42 Yetgin, S., Altay, C., Aliv, G. & Yahja, L. (1979): Myeloperoxidase activity and bactericidal function of PMN in iron deficiency. *Acta Haemat.* **61**, 10–14.

Mechanisms for immune function modification by unsaturated fatty acids

V. UTERMOHLEN, S. KILBURN, I. KISELIS and D. MAO
Division of Nutritional Sciences, Cornell University, Ithaca, New York 14853, USA.

Sweeping changes in the fat consumption patterns have been urged on peoples consuming 'Western' diets, in order to decrease the risk of cardiovascular disease. Prominent among these changes is a decrease in the consumption of saturated fats and an increase in the ratio of polyunsaturated to saturated fats in the diet. This paper explores how changes in dietary fat types may, at least in theory, result in changes in immune function.

The mechanisms whereby dietary fatty acids may affect immune function fall into two broad categories: (1) effects secondary to changes in membrane composition and state; and (2) effects secondary to metabolism of the fatty acids.

Effects secondary to changes in membrane composition and state. Using a fluid-mosaic model it has been proposed that the cell membrane consists of a phospholipid bilayer in which proteins are embedded. It has been suggested[4] that some portions of the lipid bilayer are in a gel state, in which mobility of molecules is limited, while other portions are in a sol state, in which lateral mobility of molecules is relatively free (Fig. 1). The state of the membrane depends on the 'ordering' of acyl chains. The greater the number of *cis* double bonds, the less ordered are the acyl chains, and the more sol-like the membrane. According to this model, free fatty acids can be divided into two groups: Group A, consisting of oleic, linoleic and arachidonic acids, which partition preferentially into the sol phase; and Group B, consisting of elaidic, stearic and nona-decanoic acids which partition preferentially into the gel phase.

Experimentally, FFA can be added to cells, where they are incorporated either as FFA ($\simeq 95$ per cent of added fatty acid) or into phospholipids ($\simeq 5$ per cent)[4,9]. This addition results in at least four types of changes in the cell: (1) in antigen and receptor presentation and aggregation; (2) in transport protein function; (3) in cytoskeletal organization, and (4) in the cell cycle.

Antigen and receptor presentation and aggregation. A change in the sol-gel state of a plasma membrane will change the ability of macromolecules to move in the plane of that membrane. This type of movement may be extremely important to immune function, where receptor aggregation and cross-linking appear to be essential first steps in many immune responses. We have found that sodium linoleate, but not sodium oleate, significantly increases the diffusion coefficients of both labelled proteins and a lipid probe, 3,3′-dioctadecylindocarbocyanin, on lymphocytes[9]. By contrast, Karnovsky[4] found, in measuring 1,6-diphenyl-1,3,5-hexatriene (DPH) fluorescence decay, that oleate as well as linoleate increased the area of cell membrane in the sol state. It may be that lateral movement of membrane components requires changes in the underlying cytoskeleton (see below); or linoleate, but not oleate, may make sol domains contiguous, allowing flow of molecules from one domain to another. A third possibility, discussed below, is that each fatty acid is incorporated preferentially into one or another leaflet of the membrane,

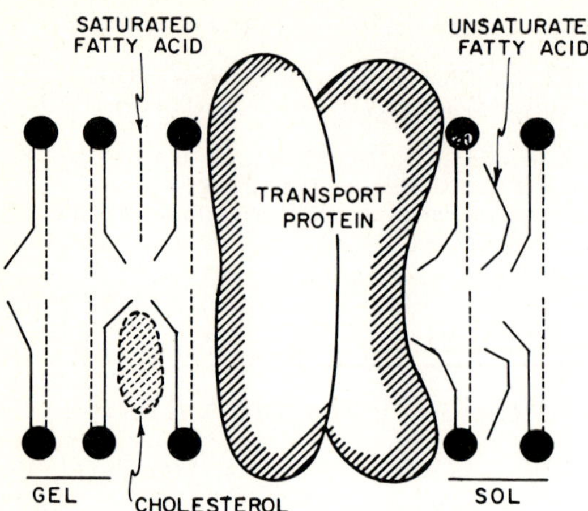

Fig. 1. *The sol-gel state of the membrane as determined by fatty acid and cholesterol composition, according to the model proposed by Karnovsky et al.*[4].

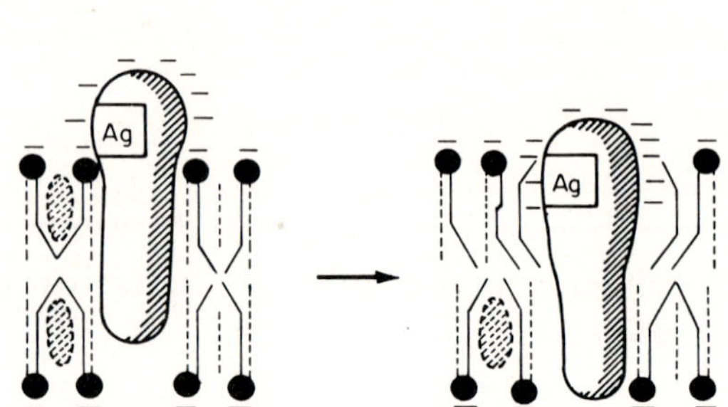

Fig. 2. *Modification of the vertical 'solubility' of membrane antigenic proteins by changes in the fatty acid composition of the membrane (Ag = antigenic site).*

with the result that some Group A fatty acids may increase lateral movement of membrane components while others may not.

Vertical mobility of proteins may also be important. An increase in the number of *cis*-unsaturated fatty acids may render the interior of the membrane less hydrophobic. Therefore we can expect, on thermodynamic grounds, that polar moieties of proteins will readily 'sink' into the plane of the membrane when the membrane is in the sol state, and rise out of the membrane in the gel state (Fig. 2). It has been shown that[7] vertical 'solubility' of proteins can be decreased by preincubating cells with cholesterol. In similar experiments, we have found that preincubation of sheep erythrocytes with oleate causes a decrease in their susceptibility to haemolysin plus complement (Kilburn & Utermohlen, unpublished data). Linoleate and arachidonate had no effect, though an effect might have been surmised from their structure. However, we found that more oleate than linoleate could be recovered from phosphatidyl ethanolamine (PE). If PE in sheep erythrocytes is in the outer leaflet of the membrane, as it is in the erythrocytes of other species, then we can expect that haemolysin susceptibility would correspond to changes in oleate levels, but not to changes in linoleate levels. Similar differential distribution may be expected in lymphocytes as well, with resulting changes in membrane receptor and antigen presentation.

Changes in transport function induced by incorporation of unsaturated fatty acids have been studied in many different cell types[6]. In cells of the lymphoid system transport of methotrexate into L1210 murine leukemia cells increased when the cells were grown in animals on high corn-oil diets, this finding being attributed to increased membrane fluidity as measured by spin-label probe[1]. By contrast, we have found that incubation of L1210 cells *in vitro* with either oleate (10 mM) or linoleate (10 mM) significantly *decreased* ^{14}C-methotrexate incorporation, while arachidonate (10 mM) had no effect (Kiselis & Utermohlen, unpublished). The effect of linoleate was dose-dependent between 10 and 40 mM. Indomethacin had no effect. In sum, there is strong evidence that transport protein function may be altered by changing the fatty acid composition of membranes, possibly through changes in protein conformation induced by the sol/gel and hydrophilic/hydrophobic milieu created by these fatty acids.

Changes in cytoskeletal organization. It has been demonstrated that lymphocyte (B-cell) cytoskeletal organization (tubulin, actin) is exquisitely sensitive to group A but not group B fatty acids[4]. Thus 10 mM linoleate causes a margination of cellular tubulin, which otherwise exists in a spoke-and-wheel pattern. This cytoskeletal reorganization is associated with failure of immunoglobulin-anti-immunoglobulin complexes on the cell surface to cap. Because the changes can be readily reversed with high levels (5 mM) of extracellular calcium, it was argued that the fatty acids displace calcium from cell surface glycoproteins to phospholipid head groups, where it becomes unavailable for transport into the cell[4]. Such a change in cytoskeletal organization may, then, be expected to alter both membrane function and the ability of cells to divide.

Control of the cell cycles. There is to date little evidence that exogenous fatty acids can alter cell cycle. However, in experiments using L1210 cells, we have found that linoleate at 20 mM and oleate at 10 mM may slightly but significantly shorten calculated cell cycle time in L1210 cells (Kiselis & Utermohlen, unpublished).

Are these experiments realistic? Insofar as cells of the immune system are constantly bathed in environments (plasma, lymph) containing large amounts of free fatty acids, and insofar as the exchange of fatty acids between the cells and the environment is rapid, the fatty acid composition of the mononuclear cell membrane reflects that of the environment[10]. In turn plasma and lymph fatty acid levels reflect diet levels, particularly with respect to essential fatty acids. Thus the changes we see *in vitro* may well be seen *in vivo*. However, from the *in vitro* experiments alone it is impossible to tell how important these changes are in the overall function of the immune system.

Effects secondary to metabolism of the fatty acids. Fatty acids of the n-6 and n-3 series (linoleic, arachidonic and α-linolenic acids), both in the membrane and within the cell, can serve as precursors for a variety of metabolically active molecules. Figure 3 summarizes the data concerning the roles of linoleate metabolites in T-cell and natural killer-cell activation. These metabolites can be ordered from immune-suppressive to immune enhancing as follows:

$$PGI_2 — PGE_2 — PGD_2 — PGF_{2\alpha} — TXA_2 — LT\text{'s.}$$

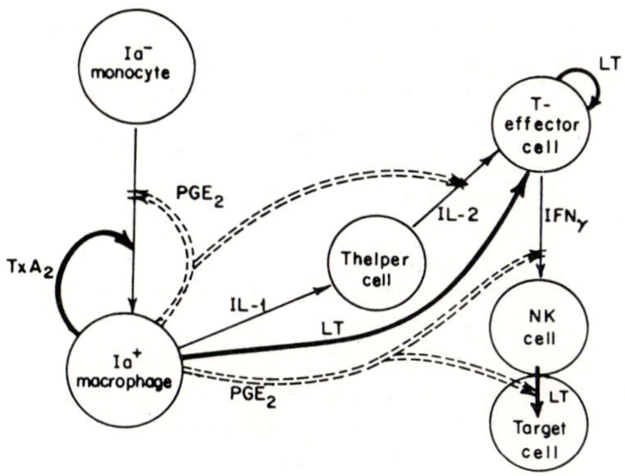

Fig. 3. *Some of the known effects of prostaglandins and leukotrienes on interactions of immunologically active cells.* TxA_2 = Thromboxane A_2; PGI_2 = Prostacyclin; PGE_2 = Prostaglandin E_2; IL-1 = Interleukin 1; IL-2 = Interleukin 2; LT = Leukotrienes; IFN_γ = Interferon γ; NK = natural killer. Solid lines indicate enhancing effects; dotted lines indicate inhibitory effects.

Immune-enhancing eicosanoids tend to increase intracellular calcium and decrease cAMP levels, while immunosuppressive eicosanoids tend to do the opposite.

In vivo, the results of the administration of dietary fat or prostaglandins depend strongly on the doses involved. For example, workers using anti-PGE_1 antibody could completely suppress immune function when PGE_1 production is completely blocked[5]. Provision of small amounts of PGE_1 restored immune function, while larger amounts were again suppressive. Similar results have been obtained with oral administration of polyunsaturated fatty acids: restoration of function at low doses, and suppression at high doses. The best interpretation of these and other data concerning eicosanoids and essential fatty acids[2,3] is that the dose response is bell-shaped, with one effect at both low and high levels and the opposite effect at intermediate levels.

In sum, there are many different mechanisms whereby essential fatty acids may affect immune function. The result of dietary administration of these fatty acids will depend in the very least on dose, on the relative levels of other fatty acids consumed, and on the immune function being studied. In any given situation, then, it may be difficult to predict whether the fatty acids will cause immune suppression or enhancement.

1 Burns, C.P., Lutteneger, D.G., Dudley, D.T., Buettner, G.R. & Spector, A.A. (1979): Effect of modification of plasma membrane fatty acid composition on fluidity and methotrexate transport in L1210 murine leukemia cells. *Cancer Res.* **39**, 1726–1732.
2 Gurr, M.I. (1983): The role of lipids in the regulation of the immune system. *Prog. Lipid Res.* **22**, 257–289.
3 Johnston, D.V. & Marshall, L.A. (1984): Dietary fat, prostaglandins and the immune response. *Prog. Food Nutr. Sci.* **8**, 3–25.
4 Karnovsky, M.J., Kleinfeld, A.M., Hoover, R.L., Davidowicz, E.A., McIntyre, D.E., Salzman, E.A. & Klausner, R.D. (1982): Lipid domains in membranes. *Ann. NY Acad. Sci.* **401**, 61–75.
5 Mertin, J. & Stackpoole, A. (1981): Anti-PGE antibodies inhibit *in vivo* development of cell-mediated immunity. *Nature* **294**, 456–458.
6 Poon, R., Richards, J.M. & Clark, W.R. (1981): The relationship between plasma membrane lipid composition and physical-chemical properties. II. Effect of phospholipid fatty acid modulation on plasma membrane physical properties and enzymatic activities. *Biochem. Biophys. Acta* **649**, 58–66.
7 Shinitzky, M. & Souroujon, M. (1979): Passive modulation of blood-group antigens. *Proc. Natl. Acad. Sci. (USA)* **76**, 4438–4440.
8 Singer, S.J. & Nicholson, G.L. (1972): The fluid mosaic model of the structure of cell membranes. *Science* **175**, 720–731.
9 Utermohlen, V., Coniglio, J., Mao, D., Sierra, J., Smith, R., Besner, G., Hutchins, S., Spitzer, K., Tomasso, J. & Boyar, A. (1982): Unsaturated fatty acids and human mononuclear cell function. *Prog. Lipid Res.* **20**, 739–741.
10 Wahle, K.W.J. (1983): Fatty acid modification and membrane lipids. *Proc. Nutr. Soc.* **42**, 273–296.

Nutritional and immunological consequences of infection

H.M. COOVADIA
Department of Paediatrics and Child Health, Faculty of Medicine, University of Natal, PO Box 17039, Congella 4013, Republic of South Africa.

Interaction between infection and nutrition. Infections of childhood usually have a detrimental effect on nutritional status. While this is of marginal importance in the richer countries of the north it is a significant contributory factor in the development and persistence of malnutrition in developing countries. The nutritional consequences of measles illustrates this best of all. It has been observed that about 5 per cent of children in Guatemala, and 13 per cent in West Africa develop overt kwashiorkor after an episode of measles.

The other side of the coin is the well-established predisposition of malnourished children to frequent, severe and often fatal infection. In developing countries infection occurs even before birth. Maternal disease is transmitted to the fetus and causes intrauterine growth retardation, embryopathy and loss of life. Growth retardation, occurring during the intrauterine stage and early infancy, may have lasting effects on eventual size. The postnatal infectious diseases of infancy and childhood result in weight loss, height arrest, sickness and occasionally death. Profound malnutrition is generally seen among adults in industrialized countries and is secondary to hospitalization, chronic debilitating diseases and alcohol abuse.

Immunological consequences of infection. Immunity and infectious organisms have evolved in parallel. As parasites expanded and refined their repertoire of devices to evade the immune responses in man, the latter increased the range, complexity and sophistication of protective mechanisms to contain or eliminate invading microbes. There is a dynamic interaction between man and microbe which most often leads to a relationship of easy or uneasy compromise between the two. However, on occasion, the intervention of changed circumstances alters the balance in favour of one to the detriment or destruction of the other.

Nutritional consequences of infection. *'Macro' level.* Anorexia, nausea and vomiting often accompany febrile illnesses causing a reduced food intake. Measles, herpes and candidiasis can cause a sore mouth and a resulting refusal to feed. In children with diarrhoea the protein and energy intake was 0.96 g and 75 kcal (314 kJ)/kg, respectively, compared to 1.89 g and 129.9 kcal (544 kJ)/kg among healthy controls[11]. Loss of nutrients may occur in stools, vomitus, sweat, sputum and urine. The nutritional consequences of infectious diarrhoea due to rotavirus, cholera, enterotoxigenic *E. coli* and shigella have shown that protein absorption is more seriously affected than that of carbohydrate and the most severe effect on both these nutrients is produced by shigella[14]. In addition diarrhoea may result in malabsorption of amino acids, fats, vitamins (A, B_{12}, folate), minerals and trace elements[17].

'Micro' level. Infections cause alterations in the metabolism of protein, carbohydrates, lipids, vitamins, minerals, trace elements and electrolytes. Infections raise the resting metabolic expenditure and produce a negative nitrogen balance. The metabolic consequences of fever include increased oxygen consumption and heat production; electrolytes are lost in the sweat and there is a negative balance of nitrogen, potassium, magnesium and phosphate. Hormonal changes accompany febrile episodes; these include increases in glucocorticoids, mineralocorticoids and thyroxine. Hepatic glycogen is rapidly depleted by these changes. Severe changes occur in the production and breakdown of proteins[3]. The wasting of tissues detected clinically as growth retardation is a direct result of this deviation in protein metabolism. There is a diversion of amino acids and proteins away from peripheral tissues, principally skeletal muscle, towards the provision of building blocks for an amplifying immune response, for production of energy and to continue maintenance of essential organs such as the brain and heart. Proteins are degraded in muscle and skin and the amino acids released into the circulation, particularly phenylalanine, alanine, tryptophan and glutamine, are taken up by the liver for two special reasons: the synthesis and release of acute phase reactants to facilitate protection against the invading organism (Table 1) and the acceleration of gluconeogenesis for energy. Branched chain amino acids derived from protein catabolism in skeletal muscle are retained in muscle to serve as a source of energy or to synthesize alanine or glutamine.

Table 1. *Utilization of proteins during infections.*

Phagocytes	Lymphokine production
Acute phase reactants	Immunoglobulins
Inflammation	Complement
Lymphocyte proliferation	

Table 2. *Effects of leucocyte endogenous mediators.*

Granulocyte release from bone marrow	Increased hepatic production of acute phase proteins
Increased hepatic uptake of Fe, Zn and amino acids	Increased secretion of insulin and glucagon
Increased hepatic synthesis of nucleic acids	

In brief, the effects of infection on protein nutrition include anorexia, impaired absorption, altered metabolism and increased loss in urine, stools, sweat and sputum.

Despite an accelerated synthesis and release of glucose through hepatic gluconeogenesis, glycogenolysis and the effect of increased output of glucagon, adrenocortical and growth hormones, there is glucose intolerance and occasionally hypoglycaemia develops[12].

Lipid metabolism is affected by Gram negative sepsis[8]. There is an elevation of serum triglycerides, FFA and very-low-density lipoproteins. Despite the need for extra energy there is defective ketogenesis and this may account for accumulation of lipid within the hepatocytes.

The effect of infection on vitamins (especially A, C, thiamin, folic acid and B_{12}), electrolytes (especially in diarrhoea) and trace elements (in particular Fe, Zn and Cu) is often determined by the microbial agent causing disease[15,19]. Iron and zinc levels fall while serum copper rises. Large quantities of iron can be lost in malaria, hookworm, schistosomiasis and trichuris trichiura. Intracellular electrolytes (potassium, magnesium, zinc, sulphur and phosphorus) are lost during infection. Sodium and chloride are lost through diarrhoea, vomiting and sweating, and there may be a dilutional hyponatraemia.

Infections may precipitate overt signs of xerophthalmia, beriberi, megaloblastic anaemia and other vitamin deficiencies.

Some mechanisms responsible for these metabolic rearrangements have been identified. Particular attention has been given to endogenous mediators released by leucocyte activity[15] (Table 2).

Immunological consequences of infection. *Immunological maturation and infections among children in poor communities.* Soon after delivery the exposed and easily accessible surfaces of the body, such as the gut and the skin, are rapidly colonised by microbial organisms derived from the mother and the immediate surroundings. This interaction between host and an expanding army of parasites persists throughout life. Nearly all children are subject to this general pattern of development, but some major differences exist between those growing up in a prosperous industrialized country and those living in poorer communities in the third world. With very few exceptions, the former are endowed with and maintain an intact immune system which deals adequately with the relatively limited challenges from infectious agents in the environment. In striking contrast to this, the growing child in developing countries is often immunologically compromised and is frequently bombarded with a vast array of germs. These frequent infections often undermine immune mechanisms of children and provide a suitable environment for the unchecked proliferation of infectious organisms. The growth and development of the immunological apparatus and response are governed, not only by genetic endowment, but also by the nature and amount of antigenic challenge. It is therefore not surprising that immunological indices of normal children in the third world who spend a lifetime swimming in a sea of antigens will be different from their counterparts in developed countries[9]. Healthy children living in the tropics have higher levels of serum IgG, IgM and IgA and marked increases in serum IgE; apparently normal new-borns have relatively high concentrations of cord blood IgM and IgA and there may be an absence of the physiological hypogammaglobuli-naemia which occurs in early infancy. There is an earlier development of adult levels of IgA and IgM in Black children eg the IgM level of a Black infant could be within the normal White adult range within 2 weeks of birth. Auto-antibodies, especially rheumatoid factor, are detected more often. Immune complexes which are due to the combination of excess antigen with antibody, are often positive in normal sera from African children. B lymphocytes have been reported to be higher and T lymphocytes and neutrophils lower in adult Africans[4]. In comparison with Dutch children, normal African children between the ages of 6 months and 6 years have higher total lymphocyte counts[7]. This increase is accounted for mainly by more B cells and other mononuclear cells which cannot easily be classified as either T cells or B cells (ie NULL cells and cells with markers of both T and B lymphocytes).

Effect of infections on different components of the immune response: non-specific immunity. (1) Neutrophils. Bacterial superinfection is known to occur during the course of other infections. This may be due to transient defective bacterial killing ability by neutrophils during septicaemia and sluggish chemotaxis in measles[1] and influenza[13].

(2). Macrophages. The function of macrophages can be enhanced or diminished by a number of infections common in tropical countries. BCG, listeria, malaria and bacterial and T-cell products activate macrophages to improve their killing function. Such activated macrophages kill not only the stimulating organism but also other bacteria, protozoa and tumour cells. Infection of macrophages by viruses such as polio[20] and influenza[16] causes defective processing of antigens and results in impaired cell-mediated immunity (CMI). An abnormal CMI decreases defences against viruses, fungi and intracellular organisms.

(3). Natural antibodies. The extensive exposure to antigens among poor children results in antibodies to one organism which protect against another. Infection by *E. coli*, which may be asymptomatic, results in antibodies against some strains of meningococcus, pneumococcus and *Haemophilus influenzae*[18].

(4). Complement. The level of serum C3 done on admission is useful in management of certain tropical renal diseases. It is markedly reduced in post-streptococcal glomerulonephritis (PSGN), moderately decreased in typhoid glomerulonephritis and almost normal in post-streptococcal nephrotic syndrome[6].

Specific immunity. Infecting organisms possess variable numbers of antigens ranging from a few in the case of viruses to more than 50–100 in bacteria and helminths. These elicit immune responses in the host specific to each antigen. These responses may be antibodies and cell-mediated immunity (CMI). Most infectious agents stimulate both.

Antibody works in the following ways: opsonisation, neutralisation, lysis, and prevention of attachment to mucosal surfaces.

CMI is necessary for intracellular organisms, against which antibody has little effect; these are viruses, protozoa and intracellular bacteria such as mycobacteria, salmonella and brucella.

Sensitized T cells react with specific antigens on these organisms and produce at least two effects: T killer lymphocytes emerge and damage the cell membrane of the microorganism causing cell death and T cells release a number of substances called lymphokines which attract macrophages to the site of inflammation, concentrate them to the site and enhance their killing capacity.

Antibody can work in concert with mononuclear cells (K cells) to kill viruses, bacteria, yeasts or trypanosomes. This is known as antibody-dependent cell mediated cytotoxicity (ADCC).

Immunoclinical consequences of infection. Infection can therefore lead to a number of different effects in man and these are determined primarily, though not entirely, by the nature of the immune response elicited, as follows: (1) Nothing apparent may happen in the infected individual. This is due to innate immunity which is absolute and of which little is known. (2) There may be transient, long-lasting or permanent immunity after a brief period of clinical or subclinical disease. (3) Immune responses directed against the invading microbe may, paradoxically, harm the host. This results in immunopathological disease. (4) Immune responses, either specific or non-specific, may be suppressed. This allows the development of severe disease by the infecting agent, lowers the barriers against other organisms and opens the way to superinfection. Measles, which remains a major killer of children in the third world, is particularly damaging in this respect[5]. Immunoparesis caused by measles virus affects almost all components of the immune response and when immunological attrition is profound there is superinfection with other viruses (herpes simplex, adenovirus) and bacteria. Immune responses may also be weakened by other viruses and schistosomiasis, malaria and trypanosomiasis. (5) There may be 'immunological priming' analogous to that caused by allergens. Antibody elicited during an initial infection or transmitted placentally, combines with similar microbial antigens during a second infection with disastrous results, eg dengue haemorrhagic fever[10], respiratory syncitial virus[2]. (6) Tolerance may be induced. (7) Infection may be co-carcinogenic.

1 Anderson, R., Rabson, A.R., Sher, R. & Koornhof, H.F. (1976): Defective neutrophil motility in children with measles. *J. Paed.* **89**, 27–32.

2 Anon (1970): A puzzling respiratory virus. *Br. Med. J.* **1**, 317.

3 Beisel, W.R. (1977): Metabolic and nutritional consequences of infection. In *Advances in nutritional research*, ed Harold H. Draper, pp. 125–166. London: Plenum Press.

4 Brain, P., Cox, J., Duursma, J. & Pudifin, D.J. (1976): T and B lymphocytes in three population groups. *Clin. Exp. Immunol.* **23**, 248–251.

5 Coovadia, H.M. (1980): Recent advances in the understanding of measles. *S. Afr. J. Hosp. Med.* **6**, 141–148.

6 Coovadia, H.M. (1983): Glomerulonephritis in childhood. *S. Afr. J. Hosp. Med.* **9**, 7–11.

7 Coovadia, H.M. (1985): Immunological factors in childhood disease: a third world challenge. *S. Afr. J. Cont. Med. Educ.* In press.

8 Gallin, J.I., Kaye, D. & O'Leary, W.M. (1969): Serum lipids in infection. *New. Engl. J. Med.* **281**, 1081–1083.

9 Greenwood, B.M. & Whittle, H.C. (1981): *Immunology of medicine in the tropics*, pp. 1–20. London: Edward Arnold.

10 Halstead, S.B., Marchette, N.J. & O'Rourke, E. (1978): Immunologically enhanced dengue virus infection of mononuclear phagocytes. A mechanism which may regulate disease severity. *Asian J. Infect. Dis.* **2**, 55–93.

11 Hoyle, B., Yunus, Md. & Chen, L.C. (1980): Breast-feeding and food intake among children with acute diarrheal disease. *Am. J. Clin. Nutr.* **33**, 2365–2371.

12 Kinney, J.M. (1966): Energy deficits in acute illness and injury. In Proc Conf. 'Energy metabolism and body fuel utilization', ed A.P. Morgan, p. 173. Cambridge, Mass.: Howard University.

13 Larsen, H.E. & Blades, R. (1976): Impairment of polymorphonuclear leucocyte function by influenza virus. *Lancet* **1**, 283.

14 Molla, A.M., Molla, A. & Khatoon, M. (1983): Nutritional consequences of infectious diarrhoea. *XVII Int. Cong. Pediatr.* Abstracts **2**, 576. (Philippines).

15 Powanda, M.C. (1977): Changes in the body balances of nitrogen and other key nutrients: description and underlying mechanisms. *Am. J. Clin. Nutr.* **30**, 1254–1268.

16 Roberts, N.J. & Steigbigel, R.T. (1978): Effect of in vitro virus infection on response of human monocytes and lymphocytes to mitogen stimulation. *J. Immunol.* **121**, 1052–1058.

17 Rosenberg, Irwin, H., Solomons, N.W. & Schneider, R.E. (1977): Malabsorption associated with diarrhea and intestinal infections. *Am. J. Clin. Nutr.* **30**, 1248–1253.

18 Schneerson, R. & Robbins, J.B. (1975): Induction of serum *Haemophilus influenzae* type b capsular antibodies in adult volunteers fed cross-reaching *Escherichia coli* 075:K100:H5. *New. Engl. J. Med.* **292**, 1093–1096.

19 Scrimshaw, N.S., Taylor, C.E. & Gordon, J.E. (1968): *Interactions of nutrition and infection.* Monograph 57. Geneva: WHO.

20 Soontiens, F.C.J. & Van der Veen, J. (1973): Evidence for a macrophage mediated effect of poliovirus on the lymphocyte response to phytohaemagglutinin. *J. Immunol.* **111**, 1411–1419.

Nutrition and immunity: a workshop report

R.K. CHANDRA (Organizer) and R.R. WATSON (Co-chairman)
Memorial University of Newfoundland, St. John's, Newfoundland, Canada; University of Arizona, Tucson, Arizona, USA.

The Workshop was held under the joint auspices of the International Nutritional Immunology Group. Epidemiological studies have shown a correlation between severity of malnutrition and mortality, particularly due to diarrhoeal disease and infections. The several factors that increase susceptibility to infection in malnutrition are recognized and include poor sanitation, overcrowding, poor personal hygiene and impaired immunocompetence. Early studies have confirmed the consistent impairment of cell-mediated immunity, bactericidal capacity of phagocytes, complement system, secretory IgA antibody response and antibody affinity. Recent work has emphasized the role of specific nutrients, viz trace elements, vitamins and lipids. It has also become clear that excessive intake of 'essential' nutrients may also suppress immune responses.

Coovadia (Durban, South Africa) reviewed the influence of malnutrition on infection and of infection on immunity. Post-streptococcal glomerulonephritis rarely occurs in malnourished patients and it is possible that malnutrition reduces the deposition of immune complexes. Alterations in the production of lymphokines and in the inflammatory response may influence the expression of immune complex disease. Bacterial meningitis is uncommon in malnourished children but mortality is increased in *Haemophilus influenzae* infections. The South African experience with measles differs considerably from the West African. Children with measles who died had comparable nutritional status with that of non-infected controls. The duration of hospitalization and of the infectious period was also similar in malnourished and healthy children. Overcrowding, with consequential larger dose of the virus, was an adverse prognostic factor. Post-measles immunosuppression can induce disseminated herpes infection.

Heatley (Leeds, UK) examined the role of nutritional factors in the immunological profile of patients with Crohn's disease. Emaciation is a major problem in this condition and anthropometric assessment of nutritional status often reveals the presence of malnutrition. Oral polymeric diet given for 2 months produced a significant improvement in anthropometric measurements and number of T-cells. The T4/T8 ratio was unchanged. The production of immunoglobulins *in vitro* was decreased initially and improved on nutritional support.

Chandra (St. John's, Canada) assessed the impact of malnutrition on respiratory mucosal immunity. Chest infection is a major cause of morbidity and mortality in malnourished children and elderly subjects. Secretory immunoglobulin A (sIgA) concentration in nasopharyngeal secretions and specific sIgA-antibody responses to attenuated measles virus vaccine are decreased. This may be the result in part of a reduced number of IgA-producing plasma cells in submucosal location. Alveolar fluid cell count is high in malnourished individuals, a reflection of more frequent infection. The T4 helper/T8 suppressor cell ratio is decreased. There is increased binding of bacteria to respiratory epithelial cells and the local delayed hypersensitivity reaction is blunted. Ciliary activity is slow and gets almost totally knocked off in the presence of infection. These changes in the local non-specific and antigen-specific responses could enhance the risk of respiratory infectious disease in the malnourished.

Bhaskaram (Hyderabad, India) studied macrophage function in malnutrition. Spontaneous bactericidal capacity was slightly high, due perhaps to bacterial stimulation *in vivo*. Mobilization of macrophages was delayed whereas opsonic activity and migration inhibition factor production were normal. *Sakamoto* (Tokyo, Japan) examined the restoration of immunological function following parenteral nutrition of malnourished rats. Complement C3 level and macrophage function returned promptly to normal but skin reactivity to purified protein derivative was unchanged in many animals. The contributing factors that influence immunological recovery during nasogastric tube feeding were not clear.

Several presentations highlighted the critical role of certain nutrients in modulating immunity. *Watson* (Tucson, U.S.A.) found that increasing dietary retinyl palmitate given to mice enhanced macrophage activity whereas the natural killer (NK) cells were unaffected. Dietary retinyl palmitate given together with selenium enhanced phagocytosis and inhibited the growth of papilloma tumour. Selenium alone tended not to enhance immune responses. High doses both of selenium and retinoids suppressed cellular immunity *in vitro*. *Bendich* (Nutley, USA) created vitamin E deficiency of varying severity in rats and found depressed T-cell and B-cell proliferation responses to mitogens. Mitogenesis correlated with vitamin E content of diet. Polyunsaturated fatty acids (PUFA) produced immunosuppression and the addition of moderate amounts of vitamin E did not overcome this depression. Plasma vitamin E concentrations were lower in animals fed PUFA-supplemented diets. T-helper and T-suppressor-cell numbers were not affected by vitamin E deficiency or by PUFA. *Sherman* (Urbana, USA) confirmed the adverse influence of iron deficiency on T-cell-dependent antibody production in rats. The effect was more pronounced and difficult to correct when iron deficiency was induced during gestation or neonatal period. Iron excess had little effect on immunoglobulin production, whereas NK activity was unchanged or slightly suppressed. *Malave* (Caracas, Venezuela) observed improved responses to mitogens in a low-responder strain of mice when cells were cultured in the presence of a moderate excess of zinc. The effect was not seen in a high responder strain, indicating a threshold phenomenon. The presence of 2-mercaptoethanol influenced the effects of zinc on mitogen responses. *Kramer* (Grand Forks, USA) found depressed NK cell activity and increase in null cells in zinc deficient animals. BCG vaccine suppressed T-cell mitogenesis and phagocytosis measured by chemiluminescence. The latter was also depressed in zinc deficiency and T-cell response to mitogens was decreased also in copper deficiency. *Mark* (New York, USA) examined the modulation of autoimmune disease by dietary cholesterol. Immunosuppression produced by PUFA may be the result of altered prostaglandin production by T-cells or macrophages or both. Cholesterol also suppressed immune responses, whereas vitamin E supplementation may counter the effects on prostaglandin production.

The discussion highlighted the importance of several confounding variables that influence immune responses in nutritional deficiencies. Among others, the nature and extent of nutrient deficit or excess, the dose of mitogen, choice of animal species, T-cell dependent nature of antigen, organism chosen to test susceptibility to infection, presence of latent infection, can influence the results. It was also recognized that *in vitro* experiments are a poor representation of events *in vivo*. Finally, we must attempt to separate epiphenomena from those changes in immunocompetence that are of biological and clinical relevance.

XVIII: Food intolerance

Classification and mechanisms of food intolerance

M.H. LESSOF

Department of Medicine, Guy's Hospital Medical School, London, SE1 9RT, UK.

Food intolerance has been defined as a reproducible, unpleasant (ie adverse) reaction to a specific food or food ingredient which is not psychologically based[24]. *Food allergy* is a form of food intolerance caused by an abnormal immunological reaction to the food. *Food aversion* is either an avoidance of food for psychological reasons or an unpleasant bodily reaction caused by emotional mechanisms rather than by the food itself.

Leaving aside the psychological problems of food aversion, intolerance may be due to a number of causes. It can result from irritant, toxic, pharmacological and metabolic effects of food. It can also be the result of enzyme deficiencies, an untoward immune response, or the release of substances produced by the fermentation of food residues in the bowel. The susceptibility of particular individuals varies enormously, as can be seen when foods which are normally well-tolerated upset patients with peptic ulceration or fatty foods cause nausea in patients with gall bladder disease. A similar variation in individual susceptibility is found throughout the whole range of food intolerant symptoms, whether they are toxic effects, immunologically based, or due to quite different causes.

Potentially toxic foods are too numerous to review in anything less than a textbook.

Pharmacological effects. Caffeine is the most widely used stimulant drug in the world and two cups of coffee or three of tea contain a highly effective dose of about 200 mg. Over-stimulation of the nervous system, cardiovascular effects, oesophageal reflux and the secondary consequences of caffeine-induced diuresis can all lead to problems[11,13,27].

Pharmacological effects may also be apparent after the ingestion of foods which contain vasoactive amines, including the tyramine present in cheeses and pickled fish; it has been claimed (but also disputed) that enough may be absorbed to provoke migraine in susceptible subjects[14].

Indirect pharmacological effects have also aroused interest. Since histamine and other amines cannot readily penetrate the mucosal barrier, and high levels in the portal venous blood may not reach the systemic circulation[23], strawberry and other foods which stimulate the release of histamine and other mediators in the body may provoke symptoms more readily than those which have a high amine content.

Enzyme defects. Many people throughout the world have primary lactase deficiency[12]. For these individuals the lactose present in cow's milk remains unabsorbed, is fermented to lactic acid, and can lead to osmotic effects, diarrhoea and malabsorption[25]. Furthermore, recurrent infectious diarrhoea or other bowel disorders can denude the intestinal mucosa and give rise to a secondary deficiency of lactase and, in some cases, of other disaccharidases[12].

Few other enzyme deficiencies are sufficiently common to affect substantial numbers of people. These include aldehyde dehydrogenase deficiency, which affects 40 per cent or more of many Asian communities and is associated with intolerance to alcohol[15]. Haemolytic anaemia due to glucose-6-phosphate dehydrogenase deficiency is also seen in 1 per cent or more of some populations and predisposes to the development of haemolytic anaemia after eating such foods as fava beans or foods which are coloured by the dye orange-RN[1].

Immunological reactions. A number of patients with food intolerance have evidence of an allergic reaction to the food concerned, as shown by a positive immunoglobulin E (IgE) radioallergosorbent test (RAST) or a positive skin-prick test to the food concerned[18]. Positive tests are frequently seen in patients with food-provoked asthma or eczema, are not uncommon in those who develop urticaria or angioedema, and are least frequent in those whose food-intolerant reactions are confined to the gastrointestinal tract or associated with rhinorrhoea.

More insidious immunological reactions also occur, possibly including the villous atrophy of gluten enteropathy. In this case, however, despite the evidence of immunoglobulin G antibody production and the formation of immune complexes, the precise mechanism is not fully understood.

Gastrointestinal stimulation. Recent studies of the irritable bowel syndrome[16] have suggested that patients who have no evidence of an enzyme defect or an immunological abnormality may nevertheless develop gastrointestinal symptoms several hours after taking specific foods, sometimes accompanied by objective evidence of an increased rectal release of prostaglandins. The most common foods to be involved are wheat products and other cereal foods. Many of the symptoms may depend on the release of intestinal gas through bacterial fermentation of food residues[19], and it is known that colonic bacteria can both produce and consume hydrogen[20]. Changes in bacterial flora might therefore be a factor in some cases, and it is of interest that many patients date the onset of their symptoms to a gastrointestinal infection or to antibiotic treatment.

Mechanisms. When reactions are confined to the gastrointestinal tract there is evidence that increased peristalsis of the bowel is associated with a release of prostaglandins[16]. Drugs which inhibit prostaglandin synthesis can prevent such reactions[6] and it therefore seems likely that prostaglandin release plays an important part in mediating the increased gut motility which is the main manifestation of this reaction. Not all of these reactions are accompanied by the presence of IgE antibodies or evidence of an immediate allergic response outside the gastrointestinal tract.

As a wider range of mediators have come to be studied, it has become apparent that inflammatory mediators are released from mast cells, basophils, platelets and other cells, in a wide variety of circumstances. Immediate allergic reactions are not unique in being able to stimulate mediator release, and non-immunological reactions are being recognized in increasing numbers. As in pseudo-allergic drug reactions, including those provoked by aspirin[2,3] abnormal patterns of mediator release appear to be provoked by pharmacological mechanisms.

Patients who react to aspirin have also implicated azo dyes and preservatives (eg benzoates) as substances which are capable of triggering asthma[8] and it is possible that a pharmacological mechanism rather than an allergic mechanism is involved in such cases. Asthma, wheezing, and in some cases flushing and hypotension have also been reported after food or drinks which contain sodium metabisulphite added as a preservative. There is evidence that such foods can release sulphur dioxide at a concentration of 1–3 mg/kg or more which is sufficient to provoke bronchospasm in susceptible asthmatics[5]. Direct irritant effects on the bronchial mucosa thus appear to be capable of triggering a similar sequence of events to those which are seen in allergy.

In a number of other cases the evidence is less clearcut. In children who have chronic urticaria of obscure origin, it has been claimed that a diet that is free of azo dyes and preservatives can lead to a remission of symptoms in something like 50 per cent of cases[26]. Of those who lose their symptoms, however, fewer than half react to colouring matter or benzoate when a double-blind challenge is arranged.

Childhood hyperactivity and disruptive behaviour have also been blamed on food intolerance[9] but this remains controversial. Although mood alterations may accompany reactions to food which involve migraine, urticaria, eczema and diarrhoea[10], behaviour disorders which are unaccompanied by these symptoms are seldom seen as the sole expression of food intolerance. Indeed a recent study of 17 healthy children presenting at an allergy clinic[28] showed the frequency with which mothers can mistakenly restrict their children's diet to an unsafe degree, encouraged by organizations which claim to have special techniques for the diagnosis of food intolerance. In at least ten of these cases, a more appropriate diagnosis was that of 'food intolerance by proxy'[22].

Even in well-documented anaphylactic reactions a number of conditioning factors may also operate. For example, it has been reported that a patient with anaphylactic reactions to shellfish, who had clearly demonstrable IgE antibodies, developed his anaphylactic responses only when a meal of the appropriate food was followed by exercise[21]. A similar relationship has also been described in three patients with an allergy to celery who developed symptoms only when exercise was taken after eating this food[17]. A similar complexity may also apply to food-induced migraine — whether provoked by allergy as proposed by Egger and his colleagues[10] or by a pharmacological response to amines[14]. Regardless of any relationship to food, many migraineurs report that the most common precipitating factor appears to be stress, while lack of food can also precipitate migraine in those who are predisposed[7].

Reactions to food do not only develop after a single exposure. Eczema provides an insidious form of rash which, although complex in its origin, is increasingly found to be associated with food intolerance or allergy[4].

1 Akinyanju, O.O. & Odusote, K.A. (1983): Cause of red suya syndrome in food dye organge-RN. *Lancet* **2**, 1314.
2 Asad, S.I., Kemeny, D.M., Youlten, L.J.F., Frankland, A.W. & Lessof, M.H. (1984): Effect of aspirin in 'aspirin-sensitive' patients. *Br. Med. J.* **288**, 745–748.
3 Asad, S.I., Youlten, L.J.F., Lessof, M.H. & Holgate, S.T. (1984): Mediators of inflammation in aspirin intolerant patients. Abstract of Proceedings of the Fifth Charles Blackley Symposium. Midlands Asthma Research Association, Nottingham.
4 Atherton, D.J. (1982): Atopic eczema. *Clins. Immunol. Allerg.* **2**, 77–100.
5 Baker, G.J., Collett, P. & Allen, D.H. (1981): Bronchospasm induced by metabisulphite-containing foods and drugs. *Med. J. Aust.* **71**, 487–489.
6 Buisseret, P. (1978): Common manifestations of cow's milk allergy in children. *Lancet* **1**, 304–305.
7 Blau, J.N. & Pyke, D.A. (1970): Effect of diabetes on migraine. *Lancet* **2**, 241–243.
8 Committee on Adverse Reactions to Foods (1984): In *Adverse reactions to foods, US Department of Health and Human Services*. NIH Publication No. 84–2442. Joint Report of American Academy of Allergy and Immunology and of National Institute of Allergy and Infectious Diseases.
9 Egger, J., Carter, C.M., Graham, P.J., Gumley, D. & Soothill, J.F. (1985): Controlled trial of oligoantigenic treatment in the hyperkinetic syndrome. *Lancet* **1**, 540–544.
10 Egger, J., Carter, C.M., Wilson, J., Turner, M.W. & Soothill, J.F. (1983): Is migraine food allergy? A double-blind controlled trial of oligoantigenic diet treatment. *Lancet* **2**, 865–869.
11 Finn, R. & Cohen, H.N. (1978): 'Food allergy': fact or fiction? *Lancet* **1**, 426–428.
12 Gray, G.M. (1980): Absorption and malabsorption of dietary carbohydrate. In *Nutrition and gastroenterology*, ed M. Winick, pp. 45–53. New York: Wiley.
13 Greden, J.F. (1974): Anxiety or caffeinism; a diagnostic dilemma. *Am. J. Psychiat.* **131**, 1089–1092.
14 Hanington, E. (1983): Migraine. In *Clinical reactions to food*, ed M.H. Lessof, pp. 155–180. Chichester: Wiley.
15 Harada, S., Agarwal, D.P., Goedde, H.W., Tagaki, S. & Ishikawa, B. (1982): Possible protective role against alcoholism for aldehyde dehydrogenase isoenzyme deficiency in Japan. *Lancet* **2**, 827.
16 Jones, V.A., McLaughlan, P., Shorthouse, M., Workman, E. & Hunter, J.O. (1982): Food intolerance: a major factor in the pathogenesis of irritable bowel syndrome. *Lancet* **2**, 1115–1117.
17 Kidd III, J.M., Cohen, S.H., Sosman, A.J. & Fink, J.N. (1983): Food-dependent exercise-induced anaphylaxis. *J. Allerg. Clin. Immunol.* **71**, 407–411.
18 Lessof, M.H., Wraith, D.G., Merrett, T.G., Merrett, J. & Buisseret, P.D. (1980): Food allergy and intolerance in 100 patients in local and systemic effects. *Quart. J. Med.* **49**, 259–271.
19 Levitt, M.D., Lasser, R.B., Schwartz, J.S. & Bond, J.H. (1976): Studies of a flatulent patient. *New Engl. J. Med.* **295**, 260–262.
20 Levitt, M.D., Berggren, T., Hastings, J. & Bond, J.H. (1974): Hydrogen (H^2) catabolism in the colon of the rat. *J. Lab. Clin. Med.* **84**, 163–167.
21 Maulitz, R.M., Pratt, D.S. & Schocket, A.L. (1979): Exercise induced anaphylactic reaction to shellfish. *J. Allerg. Clin. Immunol.* **63**, 633–634.
22 Meadow, R. (1982): Munchausen syndrome by proxy. *Archs. Dis. Child.* **57**, 92–98.
23 Moneret-Vautrin, D.S. (1983): False food allergies: non-specific reactions to foodstuffs. In *Clinical reactions to food*, ed M.H. Lessof, pp. 135–153. Chichester, Wiley.
24 Report of Joint Committee of the Royal College of Physicians and British Nutrition Foundation (1984): M.H. Lessof, Chairman. *J. R. Col. Physns* **18**, 83–123.
25 Sandine, W.C. & Daly, M. (1979): Milk intolerance. *J. Fd Protect.* **42**, 435–437.
26 Supramanium, G. & Warner, J.O. (1983): Abstract from meeting International Paediatric Association, Manila.

27 Turnberg, L.A. (1978): Coffee and gastrointestinal tract. *Gastroenterology* **75**, 529–530.
28 Warner, J.O. & Hathaway, M.A. (1984): The allergic basis of Meadow's Syndrome. *Archs. Dis. Child.* **59**, 151–156.

Intolerance of amines and additives

D. Anne MONERET-VAUTRIN
Service de Medecine D, Immuno-allergologie, C.H.U. de Brabois, 54500 Vandoeuvre-les-Nancy, France.

Evidence is accumulating that adverse reactions to foods are of considerable importance. Excluding metabolic food reactions and toxic reactions (food poisoning), there are two distinct categories: the first is food allergy, or hypersensitivity, the mechanism of which is immunological, usually IgE-dependant. The second is variously described as food sensitivity, food idiosyncrasy, food intolerance, pharmacological food reactions, etc. Those non-specific reactions to foods are usually termed food intolerance or, when the symptoms mimic those of true hypersensitivity, false food allergies (FFA). The clinical symptoms of FFA are mainly chronic urticaria and angioneurotic oedema, vasomotor headaches, intestinal functional disorders, attacks of rhinitis, or asthma and histaminic shock. Subjective complaints, eg, fatigue, depression, are troublesome and need serious consideration about the tests to be used to confirm their reality.

Mechanisms. These may be classified in three types, from the best-documented to the speculative.

(1) The excessive intake of biogenic amines was first illustrated with histamine, contained in fermented food. Biogenic amines are formed by decarboxylation of amino acids: even in small quantities, they induce different physiological actions, such as vaso-active effects. They exist pre-formed in different foodstuffs, or are produced in the intestine, from the amino acids, by microorganisms[15]. At present, cooked pork, sauerkraut, fermented cheeses, tuna fish in cans, red wines, spinach, are the common causes of this syndrome (Table 1), but an excessive production of endogenous histamine may be the consequence of increased microbial synthesis in the intestines. This is due, in turn, to an excessive intake of starchy foods, containing cellulose, which increase the processes of fermentation.

Table 1. *Foods rich in histamine (µg/g)*

Fermented cheeses	up to 1330	Meats	10
Fermented drinks (wine)	20	Vegetables	traces
Fermented foods		Tomato	22
sauerkraut	160mg/kg	Spinach	37.5
	(a portion of 250g=40mg)	Deep-frozen fish	1
Dry pork and beef sausage	225	Fish, fresh shellfish	0.2
Pig's liver	25	Fish:	
Tinned tuna	20	tuna	5.4
Tinned anchovy fillets	33	sardine	15.8
Tinned smoked herring's	350	salmon	7.35
eggs		anchovy fillets	44
Tinned foods	from 10 to 350		

Normal protective mechanisms are involved at the intestinal level, the hepatic level and the blood level. At the intestinal level, gut mucoproteins, secreted locally by the intestinal epithelium, fix and inactivate histamine. That which is unfixed passes into the mucosa and is subject to enzymatic destruction by mono-amine oxidase in the eosinophils. Portal histamine is

Table 2. *Effects on blood pressure and pulse rate of infusing histamine (1.75 mg/kg) or placebo into the duodenum of 13 healthy volunteers in a double-blind study*

Substance	n	Pulse rate (per min)		Blood pressure (mm Hg)			
				Systolic		Diastolic	
		b	a	b	a	b	a
Placebo	6	81	73	128	113*	69	64
Histamine	7	78	105*	132	116*	72	58*

b = before; a = 3 min after. *Significantly different from initial value ($P < 0.05$).

Table 3. *Foods rich in tyramine (µg/g)*

French cheeses:	
Camembert	20–86
Brie	180
Gruyère	516
Cheddar	1466
Roquefort, hung game	High but variable
Brewer's yeast	1500
Soused herrings	3030
Chianti	25

Chocolate contains methyltyramine

degraded by the liver. Post-hepatic free histamine is adsorbed on platelets, or fixed on glycoproteins. Plasma free histamine is low, less than 2 ng/ml. In man, the instillation of histamine by duodenal tube confirms the harmlessness of large doses in the healthy subjects, in amounts up to 2.75 mg/kg.

We carried out a study in volunteers who were undergoing surgery for gall-stones. For a dose of 1.75 mg/kg, there is no significant rise in portal vein histamine level: the gut mucosa acts as a barrier. For higher doses of histamine, the portal level is increased, but the peripheral level is unchanged, demonstrating the role of the liver[9].

In healthy subjects, a double-blind study shows that significant symptoms due to histamine are a slight tachycardia, and a lowered diastolic blood pressure lasting for 5 minutes or less. (Table 2). The same symptoms are observed in patients with FFA, but other reactions are quoted: facial flush, pruritus, urticaria, headaches. The main point seems to be their duration, lasting more than ten minutes. This fact points to the possibility of an impaired permeability of the gut mucosa, as well as an impaired hepatic enzyme function. In 77 patients whose clinical troubles were related to foodstuffs, without immunological findings, the response to a duodenal bolus of histamine was abnormal in 58 per cent of cases, when evaluated 10 minutes after the instillation: headaches occurred in 64 per cent of cases, then tachycardia (40 per cent), urticaria (28 per cent), abdominal pain (8.8 per cent), hypotension (6.6 per cent) and, rarely, bronchospasm (2.2 per cent).

Another biogenic amine is tyramine, which is found in different foods such as fermented foods, (Table 3), or which may arise from an excessive endogenous synthesis by bacterial decarboxylation of tyrosine in the intestines.

Tyramine elicits headaches[3] and urticaria[7]. Other amines, such as phenylethylamine, should be taken into consideration in cases of vasomotor headaches[12]. Vaso-active amines may act as 'starting-blocks', precipitating spontaneous platelet aggregation and adhesion. Platelets might release 5-hydroxy-tryptamine. A deficiency in platelet mono-amine oxidase has also been reported.

(2) The mechanisms related to the degranulation of mucosal mast cells (MMC) are gaining more and more interest. They are very numerous in the lamina propria: $20\,000/mm^3$, and predominate in the stomach, duodenum and ileum lining the surface of the gastrointestinal tract[1]. They are normally unresponsive to histamine releasers, such as bee venom peptide 401, or compound 48/80[11]. Their number could be increased by magnesium-deficiency, which might also increase their releasability. There are substantial data to support their involvement in food allergy, but few studies on mucosal mast cells and pseudo-allergic reactions are available. We studied six patients with FFA and observed a considerable degranulation of the MMC in the duodenal mucosa. Incubation of duodenal biopsy material with various histamine-releasing substances (compound 48/80, concanavalin A, the calcium ionophore A 23 187) confirmed the susceptibility of duodenal mast cells to non-specific release of histamine[8].

Non-specific histamine release reactions may occur with various foods: egg ovomucoid[14], shellfish, strawberries, tomatoes[13], chocolate, fish, pork, pineapple and ethanol. This type of disorder is often observed in young children less than 8 years old, who have an atopic disease: they show a tendency to release histamine easily. Apart from the common symptoms (urticaria, angioneurotic oedema), there may be an exacerbation of atopic dermatitis, because the eczematous skin is very rich in mast cells. Histamine is then released in greater quantities than elsewhere and pruritus causes a scratching which accentuates the lesions. Those foods act like histamine-releasers, directly on the membrane of mast cells. A similar effect is postulated for other foods by two other mechanisms: the degranulating effect of lectins, contained in leguminous plants, peanuts and cereals[4], or of anaphylatoxins generated by food contaminants, such as bacterial endotoxins and fungal products[16].

Chemical mediators other than histamine might be liberated by the mast cells. The activation of the metabolism of arachidonic acid either towards prostaglandins, or leukotrienes, or oxygen-free radicals[2,5,6] must also be considered. Intolerance to food additives might be related to the interference of these substances with the metabolism of arachidonic acid, leading to an excessive production of oxygen-free radicals.

(3) The third group of mechanisms includes the possible activation of lymphokines[16] and the interference of food additives with the autonomic nervous system. The multiplicity of the mechanisms, as well as our lack of knowledge, raises obstacles to the diagnosis of food intolerance, more especially as several mechanisms may be triggered by a single food.

FFA does not only originate from an unbalanced diet, with an excessive intake of certain food categories, but it is probably favoured by irritative and inflammatory events acting on the gut mucosa, either of viral, parasitic, or chemical origin. A noxious exposure could stimulate neuro-peptide-containing C fibres in the mucosa, which would release substance P and somatostatin from the peripheral terminals. Complex interactions between the sensory neuropeptides and mucosal mast cells could account for an abnormal release of the chemical mediators from those cells[10].

Whatever the mediators which are predominantly liberated, it must be emphasized that the same effects could be observed: hyperpermeability of the intestinal epithelium and of the small vessels, increased muscle contraction, stimulation of pain fibres and recruitment of inflammatory cells. An increased passage of macromolecules across the intestinal barrier then ensues, and may be considered as an enhancing factor of sensitization, creating food allergy. It may also be feared that this phenomenon could trigger the connective tissue mast cells in the submucosa, and induce an amplification of the liberation of mediators. Undoubtedly most clinical reactions to foods are non-immunological. Subtle alterations of the gut mucosa, which may underlie the symptoms of FFA are not clearly identified, but MMC appear to play a major part. This fact may support the hypothesis that interrelationships do exist between FFA and food allergy.

1 Barrett, K.E. & Metcalfe, D.D. (1984): The mucosal mast cell and its role in gastrointestinal allergic diseases. *Clin. Rev. Allergy.* **2**, 39–53.

2 Buisseret, P.D., Youlten, J.F., Heinzelmann, D.I. & Lessof, M.H. (1978): Prostaglandin synthetase inhibitors in prophylaxis of food intolerance. *Lancet* **1**, 906–907.

3 Hanington, E. (1983): Migraine. In *Clinical reactions to food*, ed M.H. Lessof, pp. 155–175. Chichester: John Wiley.

4 Helm, R.M. & Froese, A. (1981): Binding of the receptors for IgE by various lectins. *Int. Archs. Allergy Appl. Immunol.* **65**, 81–84.

5 Larsen, J.C. (1983): Absorption and transformation: intolerance to certain foreign chemicals. In *Allergy and hypersensitivity to chemicals.* (Proc. WHO/CEE Workshop, Frankfurt, pp. 162–214). Copenhagen: WHO.

6 Lessof, M.H. & Anderson, J.B. (1984): Prostaglandins and other mediators in food intolerance. *Clin. Rev. Allergy* **2**, 79–93.

7 Moneret-Vautrin, D.A. (1983): False food allergies — non-specific reactions to foodstuffs. In *Clinical reactions to food*, ed M.H. Lessof, pp. 135–154. Chichester: John Wiley.

8 Moneret-Vautrin, D.A., de Korwin, J.D. & Tisserant *et al.* (1984): Ultrastructural study of the mast cells of the human duodenal mucosa. *Clin. Allergy* **14**, 471–481.

9 Moneret-Vautrin, D.A., Viniaker, J., Boissel, P., Noel, M. & Kim, K. (1981): Effets de l'instillation d'histamine dans l'intestin grêle chez l'homme. 1. Variations de l'histiminémie portale et périphérique. *Ann. Gastro-Entérol. Hépatol.* **17**, 395–400.

10 Payan, D.G., Levine, J.D. & Goetzl, E.J. (1984): Modulations of immunity and hypersensitivity by sensory neuropeptides. *J. Immunol.* **132**, 1601–1604.

11 Pearce, F.L., Befus, A.D., Gauldie, J. & Bienenstock, J. (1982): Effects of anti-allergic compounds on histamine secretion by isolated intestinal mast cells. *J. Immunol.* **128**, 2481–2486.

12 Sandler, M., Youdim, M.B.H. & Hanington, E. (1974): A phenylethylamine oxidising defect in migraine. *Nature* **250**, 335–337.

13 Schachter, M. (1956): Histamine release and the angiooedema type of reaction. In *Histamine*. Ciba Fdn. Symp. London: J. & A. Churchill.

14 Schachter, M. & Talesnik, J. (1952): The release of histamine by egg-white in non-sensitized animal. *J. Physiol.* **118**, 258–263.

15 Tarjan, V. & Janossy, G. (1978): The role of biogenic amines in foods. *Die Nahrung* **22**, 281–285.

16 Weck de, A.L. (1984): Pathophysiological mechanisms of allergic and pseudo-allergic reactions to foods, food additives and drugs. *Ann. Allergy* **53**, 583–586.

Lactose intolerance

V.I. MATHAN
The Wellcome Research Unit, Christian Medical College Hospital, Vellore 632 044, India.

Lactose intolerance is a clinical entity, individuals developing otherwise unexplained gastrointestinal symptoms of bloating, flatulence, abdominal cramps and sometimes diarrhoea, associated with eating lactose containing foods[11]. This clinical manifestation is the result of a deficiency of the disaccharidase, lactase (β-galactosidase), in the enterocyte brush border membrane[2,10]. Dietary lactose is then not hydrolysed to the constituent monosaccharides, glucose and galactose and cannot be absorbed. The accumulation of unhydrolysed lactose in the lumen of the intestinal tract leads to osmotic diarrhoea and to gas production due to bacterial fermentation, especially in the colon[3,4,6,16]. Milk and milk-derived foods are the most important source of dietary lactose, but many prepared articles of food in the developed world may contain sufficient added lactose to produce symptoms in a susceptible individual. All individuals with low lactase concentration in the intestinal mucosa do not develop symptoms and therefore hypo-or a-lactasia is not synonymous with lactose intolerance.

Epidemiology. Lactase is usually present in adequate quantities in healthy infants and toddlers and congenital absence of the enzyme is rare. Intestinal lactase concentrations start to decrease by 4 or 5 years of age and become very low in early adulthood[5]. In certain geographic areas and ethnic groups, this decline of intestinal lactase starts earlier and is more complete and many adults may be alactasic. The majority of the world's population — most of tropical Africa, Asia and Central and South Amercia — appear to be genetically programmed to develop primary adult onset hypolactasia. Significantly low lactase concentrations are found in about 15 per cent of the population of adults in the USA while a prevalence of over 60 per cent is present in other areas such as southern India[14]. Striking regional differences are shown by a much lower prevalence (28 per cent) in northern India. The precise genetics of the prevalence of adult onset hypolactasia is not fully understood. The observed patterns suggest that descendants of ethnic groups who were predominantly herders are less likely to develop hypolactasia[13]. It is important to emphasize that clinically-significant lactose intolerance is seldom encountered in these areas probably related to the low consumption of milk and milk products.

Secondary hypolactasia especially as a transient phenomenon is more widely encountered in clinical situations. Viral gastroenteritis, Crohn's disease, coeliac disease, tropical sprue, drugs, irradiation and other such conditions which damage the small intestinal enterocyte can reduce intestinal lactase and lead to intolerance. The clinical syndrome is often provoked by such patients being given large amounts of milk during convalescence. It can lead to a potentially fatal situation in young children in developing countries who are recovering especially from viral gastroenteritis[16].

Clinical presentation. The manifestation of symptoms of lactose intolerance in adults is related to the amount of lactose taken in the diet. In a group of healthy southern Indian adults diarrhoea occurred consistently when 20 g lactose was given in the fasting state, but 10 g was tolerated by over 90 per cent and 15 g by over 50 per cent. 100 ml of milk will contain about 4 g of lactose and is well-tolerated by most such people.

Secondary hypolactasia must be kept in mind in devising diets for most patients with malabsorption syndromes. It is not necessary to completely omit milk and milk products. A small quantity of milk may be well-tolerated and a variety of fermented milks including yogurt or curds may not give rise to any problems. It has been suggested that a β-galactosidase of bacterial origin in yogurt is able to hydrolyse lactose in the alkaline pH of the upper small intestine and may prevent the occurrence of symptoms of lactose intolerance and make lactose available for nutrition.

The syndrome of lactose intolerance in the post-enteritis state is particularly important. This problem is prevalent worldwide and is one of the commonest causes of persistent diarrhoea in young children. Milk is the preferred food in this age group and additional milk is likely to be given to such children to improve their nutritional status. The problem is complicated since some of these children especially infants may also develop cow's milk protein allergy in addition to hypolactasia. Milk withdrawal from the diet will not distinguish between these two conditions, but an enteropathy can be demonstrated in jejunal biopsies from infants with milk protein intolerance. In isolated lactase-deficiency the jejunal mucosa is morphologically normal.

Diagnosis. Clinically lactose intolerance can be diagnosed if the patient's symptoms improve on excluding lactose completely from the diet and relapses on the reintroduction of lactose. In addition to milk and milk-derived foods it is important to remember that a variety of prepared foods contain lactose and that it is used in many pharmaceuticals. Symptomatic lactose intolerance appears to be dose related and a small amount of lactose may not produce any gastrointestinal problems.

Estimation of lactase concentration in jejunal mucosal samples[15] obtained by peroral biopsy is necessary to confirm the diagnosis of hypo-or a-lactasia. Several other tests have been devised which are particularly useful in population studies and can diagnose low lactase levels by non-invasive means.

Lactose tolerance test. The determination of peak blood glucose concentration after an oral dose, usually 50 g lactose, and comparing it with the response to 25 g of glucose is the classical way of determining the ability of the intestine to hydrolyse lactose. Variables which might influence the test include rate of gastric emptying and diabetes[4].

Breath hydrogen estimation. The fermentation of unhydrolysed carbohydrates by the bacterial flora of the gastrointestinal tract releases hydrogen which is absorbed into the blood stream and can be estimated in expired air[1,9]. Since the fermentative activity is maximal in the colon, significantly elevated breath hydrogen estimation several hours after an oral dose of lactose would suggest lactase deficiency. If the dose of lactose initiates a severe osmotic diarrhoea the breath hydrogen estimation may not be accurate. In a small proportion of individuals, hydrogen producing organisms may be absent in the gastrointestinal tract and in others bacterial colonization in the small intestine may produce an early peak of breath hydrogen or a high background level making the test unsuccessful.

Differential urinary excretion of sugars. A large number of variables affect the urinary excretion of a substance given by mouth. These include rate of gastric emptying, intestinal transit, hydrolysis, absorption, permeation of the mucosa, metabolism and rate of urinary excretion. In order to study lactose hydrolysis it is possible to find another disaccharide of similar molecular weight and size which is handled similarly by all variables except intestinal hydrolysis. Lactulose has been found to be suitable for this and if a mixture of lactose and lactulose is given by mouth all the variables except intestinal hydrolysis will act on both the sugars in the same fashion. Since both the sugars are excreted in the urine if they permeate the intestinal mucosa any difference in urinary excretion will reflect the extent to which the lactose is hydrolysed by the intestinal epithelium. This noninvasive test which involves a 5 h urine collection has now been evaluated and preliminary results suggest that it is a valid test especially for field studies[8,11,12].

Nutritional significance of lactose intolerance. In the clinical situation where a patient presents with symptoms, the diagnosis of a-lactasia and lactose intolerance and appropriate dietary advice to exclude dietary lactose can solve the problem. However, since it has now been established that large segments of the world's population are hypo-or a-lactasic, there may be wider nutritional implications. In many of the third-world countries, one of the efforts to improve nutrition is to promote animal husbandry so that milk and milk-products are more widely available. As an example, in India, a major operation — 'Operation flood' — has been undertaken at a national level and preliminary results suggest that the milk intake of the population will significantly increase. Is the increased milk consumption likely to make symptomatic lactose intolerance a major problem in areas like southern India with high prevalence of adult onset hypolactasia? If this situation does arise, it would have serious implications on the success of the programme. Our preliminary results suggest that up to 10 g of lactose (250 ml milk) can be tolerated as a single dose and indicates that hypolactasia may not be a major problem in the success of milk based nutritional programmes. The suggestion that lactose intake in fermented milk is better tolerated also indicates an alternative way to overcome the problems of prevalence of hypolactasia[7].

1 Bond, J.H. Jr. & Levitt, M.D. (1972): Use of pulmonary hydrogen measurements to quantitate carbohydrate absorption: study of partially gastrectomized patients. *J. Clin. Invest.* **51**, 1219–25.

2 Crane, R.K., Menard, D., Preiser, H. & Eerda, J.J. (1976): The molecular basis of brush border membrane disease. In *Membranes and diseases*: International Conference on Biological Membranes, ed L. Botz, J.F. Hoffman & A. Leaf, pp. 229–241. New York: Raven Press.

3 Cuatrecasas, P., Lockwood, D.H. & Caldwell, J.R. (1965): Lactase deficiency in the adult. *Lancet* **1**, 14–18.

4 Dawson, A.M. (1970): *Modern trends in gastroenterology*, ed W.I. Card & B. Creamer. London: Butterworths.

5 Gray, G.M. (1978): Intestinal disaccharide deficiencies and glucose-galactose malabsorption. In *The metabolic basis of inherited diseases*, 4th edn. ed J.B. Stanbury, J.B. Wyngaarden & D.S. Fredrickson, pp. 1526–1536. New York: McGraw-Hill.

6 Gray, G.M. (1981): Carbohydrate absorption and malabsorption. In *Physiology of the gastrointestinal tract*, ed L.R. Johnson, pp. 1063–1072. New York: Raven Press.

7 Kolars, J.C., Levitt, M.D., Mostafa Aouji & Savaino, D.A. (1984): Yogurt — an autodigesting source of lactose. *New. Engl. J. Med.* **310**, 1–3.

8 Laker, M.F. & Menzies, I.S. (1977): Increase in human intestinal permeability following ingestion of hypertonic solution. *J. Physiol.* **265**, 881–894.

9 Levitt, M.D. (1969): Production and excretion of hydrogen gas in man. *New. Engl. J. Med.* **281**, 122–7.

10 Malathi, P., Ramaswamy, K., Caspary, W.F. & Crane, R.K. (1973): Studies on the transport of glucose from disaccharides by hamster small intestine in vitro. I. Evidence for a disaccharidase-related transport system. *Biochim. Biophys. Acta.* **307**, 613–626.

11 Menzies, I.S. (1982): Medical importance of sugars in the alimentary tract. In *Developments of sweetners*, 2, ed T.H. Grenby, K.J. Parker & M.G. Lindley, pp. 89–117. London: Applied Science Publishers.

12 Menzies, I.S., Mount, J.N. & Wheeler, M.J. (1978): Quantitative estimation of clinically important monosaccharides in plasma by rapid thin layer chromatography. *Am. J. Clin. Biochem.* **15**, 65–76.

13 Simoons, F.J. (1969): Primary adult lactose intolerance and the milking habit: a problem in biological and cultural interrelations. I. Review of the medical research. *Am. J. Dig. Dis.* **14**, 819–36.

14 Swaminathan, K., Mathan, V.I., Baker, S.J. & Radhakrishnan, A.N. (1970): Disaccharide levels in jejunal biopsy specimens from American and south Indian control subjects and patient with tropical sprue. *Clin. Chim. Acta* **30**, 702–712.

15 Walter, W.M. & Gray, G.M. (1968): Enzyme assay of peroral biopsies. Storage conditions and basis of expression. *Gastroenterology* **54**, 56–59.

16 Weijers, H.A., Van De Kamer, J.H., Mossel, D.A. & Ijsseling, J. (1960): Diarrhoea caused by a deficiency of sugar splitting enzymes. *Acta Paediatrica* **50**, 55–71.

Coeliac disease (gluten enteropathy)

B. McNICHOLL, Bridie EGAN-MITCHELL, Fiona M. STEVENS, P.F. FOTTRELL and C.F. McCARTHY
Department of Paediatrics, Medicine and Biochemistry, University College Galway, Republic of Ireland.

Samuel Gee's description of 'the coeliac affection' in 1888[10] is regarded as the classical one of this disease, which had probably been described as early as the 2nd century AD by Arataeus of Cappodocia. Coeliac disease is the term used in most English-speaking countries and indicates a condition related to dietary gluten, hence the synonym 'gluten enteropathy'. Although Gee and others recognized the adverse effects of farinaceous foods in the acute stages of the disease, it remained for Dicke[6] to identify wheat and rye as the primary cause, confirmed later by himself and his colleagues[7]. The first demonstration of the intestinal mucosal pathology[16] was followed by the introduction of the Crosby capsule[5] and later fibre-optic endoscopy[18] enabling per-oral biopsy of the intestinal mucosa, to allow definitive histological diagnosis and surveillance as well as immunological and biochemical studies. Typical changes are shown in the Figure.

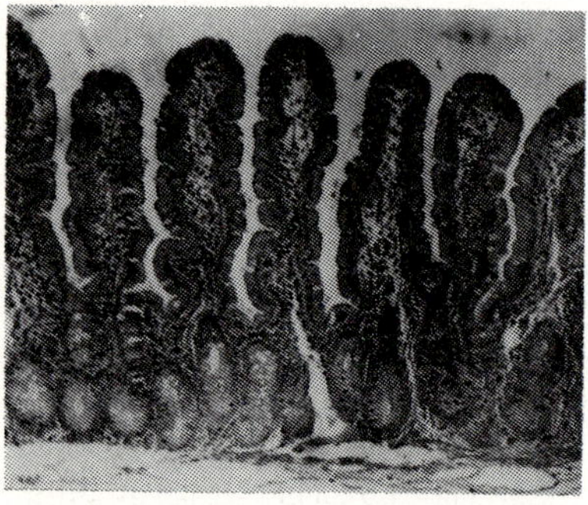

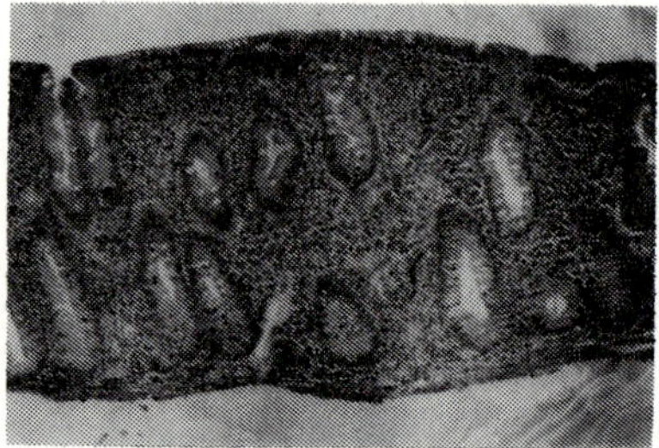

(b) Section of jejunum from 15-month-old child with active coeliac disease. Note the absence of villi, reduced height of the columnar surface epithelium, which is infiltrated with lymphocytes, and the increased cellularity of the lamina propria, mainly due to plasma cells.

Fig. 1. *(a) Histological section of normal jejunum from a child.* Note slender villi, with tall columnar epithelium and a minimum of cells in the lamina propria.

In children the disease usually appears in the first 2 years; the interval between first gluten feeding and the appearance of symptoms is rarely less than about 2 months, but can vary from that to several years. The classical picture is of diarrhoea, weight loss, growth retardation, loss of appetite, irritability and abdominal distention. In mild cases, there may be no intestinal symptoms and growth retardation may be the only notable finding. We have emphasized that in some children constipation may be a presenting sign[8]. In the adult, diarrhoea and weight loss, anaemia of iron or folate deficiency (particularly during pregnancy) and bone decalcification may present. In established cases, in both children and adults, nutritional deficiencies arise from malabsorption of iron, folate, fats, fat-soluble vitamins, proteins and calcium. Excess faecal fat (steatorrhoea), once thought to be an invariable feature, is variable and often absent in the early stages of the disease in childhood. The extensive literature on clinical and aetiological aspects of the disease has been well summarized[2,4].

Incidence and genetics. Biopsy studies of families have shown an incidence of between 5 per cent[17] and 10 per cent[15] of first-degree relatives. Incidence has varied from close to 1/300 births in the west of Ireland[14] to a virtual absence in black and Asiatic peoples. Other areas of high incidence are Austria, Sweden and Switzerland, and some parts of the UK, Canada and Chile. Coeliac disease has been described in Punjabis and Pakistanis, in Israel, Iraq, Lebanon, Kuwait, Sudan, and in North Africans in Paris, but there are no estimates of incidence. (References available on request).

Genetic markers are HLA B_8[9] and HLA DR_3[11]. In our patients, another marker on chromosome 6, is complement 4 S, found in 23 per cent of our patients but in no controls. Present theories require two genes acting together, one on chromosome 6 and another (unidentified) on the same or another chromosome, to interact with dietary gluten. The HLA B_8 on DR_3 haplotypes have their highest prevalence in the west of Ireland, HLA B_8 being 45 per cent[19], and the prevalence of the latter decreases as one moves south-eastwards across Europe, falling to 5 per cent in Israel. The spread of wheat farming north-eastwards from the Middle-East from 5000BC onwards has been mapped[1], and contrasted with HLA B_8 prevalence, suggesting that as wheat eating spread north-westwards, people with HLA B_8 haplotypes would have tended to be eliminated by natural selection, resulting in the higher prevalence of these haplotypes in north-west Europe. In keeping with this theory is the study of cereal consumption in England, Scotland and Wales in 1801, which showed a striking predominance of oats and barley in the Celtic fringes of Scotland and Wales[3]. Oats and barley were also the staple cereal of the Irish until the potato famine of 1847, when wheat was established as the staple cereal in a population hitherto little exposed to it and with a high prevalence of the susceptible haplotypes. The scene for the high incidence of coeliac disease in the Irish was thus set.

Aetiology. The precise mechanism of mucosal damage is still uncertain. Alpha gliadin is thought to be or to contain the toxic fraction which interacts in a pathological manner with the intestinal mucosa of people with the susceptible genotype. Earliest theories presumed an immune defect, which would allow binding of gliadin to the cell membrane, either causing direct damage to the cell, or altering its antigenic expression to one foreign to the body's immune system. It is probable that most of the immunological abnormalities, such as elevated serum IgA levels, circulating immune complexes, relative deficiency of T lymphocytes and abnormal behaviour of lymphocytes when stimulated with different substances are epiphenomena, as they tend to return to normal with withdrawal of gluten from the diet. Reduced splenic hypofunction in our adult coeliacs has been shown to reverse with strict gluten withdrawal. Although most patients exhibit a high serum IgA level, we have shown that a selective deficiency of IgA makes an individual 15 times more likely to develop coeliac disease than those with normal IgA levels.

Absence of a mucosal enzyme which would allow accumulation of toxic peptides was one of the earlier theories, not yet fully excluded, but lacking firm evidence. Increased intestinal permeability to probe molecules has been shown in the untreated coeliac but there is conflicting evidence concerning the reversion of this abnormality with treatment. It has also been suggested that an abnormality of the glyco-protein structure of the cell membrane may allow damaging binding by gluten lectins.

Management. A strict gluten-free diet leads to clinical and mucosal remission in children, but not in all adults, although it nearly always leads to improved health. Whereas absorption soon normalizes with treatment, specific deficiencies of iron, folic acid and vitamins should be speedily treated. In prolonged or extensive disease, vitamin B_{12} and trace elements such as zinc, copper and selenium will also need to be restored. Depression of the epithelial surface disaccharidases and peptidases leads to digestive difficulties, and low lactase levels can lead to temporary lactose intolerance. Strict adherence to a gluten-free diet (GFD) seems to be the best guarantee of normal health, and in particular, of normal growth in the child. Re-introduction of a normal diet leads to mucosal relapse in 95 per cent of children, but there is evidence that this may take some years, during which the child seems well, this leading to a false impression of gluten tolerance[13]. A new assay for gliadin developed in this centre[12] (Table 1) for the first time allows us to be precise about dietary management.

Table 1. *Mean concentration of gliadin in some foods (g/kg ± s.d.). From* McKillop *et al.* (1985).

Wheat flour	57 ± 8.0
Oatmeal flour	2.40 ± 0.5
Cornflour	0.47 ± 0.25
Rice	0.46 ± 0.23
Soya flour	0.70 ± 0.23
'Gluten-free' flour 'a'	0.35 ± 0.27
'Gluten-free' flour 'b'	0.50 ± 0.18

Table 2. *Incidence of coeliac disease related to total births in County Galway for 22 years (1960–1981)*

	1.1.60–30.1.65	1.7.65–31.12.70	1.1.71–30.6.76.	1.7.76–31.12.81
Coeliacs/births	1/604	1/590	1/514	1/1376
Coeliacs/10^5 births	165	169	194	73

Malignancy. A disquieting feature is the increased risk of malignancy, commonly malignant histiocytosis, less commonly carcinoma of the intestine. In Galway, of 41 deaths in coeliacs, 24 have been due to malignancy, at a mean age of 58 years (McCarthy & Stevens, personal communications). We have some evidence that adherence to a GFD will defer this risk, but whether adherence to a GFD from childhood will prevent or defer the tendency to malignancy, will require surveillance for 50 to 60 years from diagnosis, or 30 to 40 years in our patients diagnosed by the earliest biopsies of 25 years ago. The present registration of almost all known coeliacs in Ireland, North and South, in a computer in Galway, should help to answer these vital questions, but in the meanwhile we recommend a permanent GFD on grounds of general health as well as reducing the risk of malignancy.

Decreasing incidence in children. Most European countries have noticed a decrease in the incidence of CD in children over the last 10 years. Table 2 shows our experience over 22 years, with a 60 per cent reduction since 1975. Of the possible factors, we believe that the most important is the general trend to defer wheat feeding to infants until the 4th or 5th month, in comparison with the practice in the 60s and 70s of frequently introducing wheat in the early weeks and almost always by 2 months or so. When wheat feeding is deferred until close to 6 months of age, important maturational changes have occurred in the infant gut, particularly a decrease in permeability[21] and an increase in IgA[20] from the low levels of early infancy, rendering the gut more competent to handle the potentially toxic gliadin. Recalling the 15-fold increased risk of coeliac disease in older subjects with IgA deficiency, it is not surprising that the young infant, with low IgA levels, is at risk. Other factors which may contribute are the increase in breast-feeding (in the area from virtually none in the 50s to about 30 per cent now at 6 weeks of age), and the decrease in protein content and osmolarity of cow's-milk based infant formulae from around 1976. Breast-milk, as well as being immunologically neutral for the infant, also contains IgA as well as some trophic factors for the gut. Lowering the protein levels in infant formulae, even if more β-lactoglobulin is being used, has probably led to decreased antigenicity, as processing tends to lessen the antigenicity of all the proteins, including β-lactoglobulin. Passage of time will again be needed to tell us whether the reduced incidence of CD we are now experiencing will be permanent, or only a postponement until later in life.

1 Ammerman, A.J. & Cavalli-Sforza, L.L. (1971): Measuring the spread of early farming in Europe. *Man.* **6**, 674–688.
2 Cluysenaer, O.J.J. & Van Tongeren, J.H.M. (1977): Malabsorption in coeliac sprue. The Hague: Martinus Nijhoff.
3 Collins, E.J.T. (1975): Dietary change and cereal consumption in Britain in the nineteenth century. *Agric. Hist. Rev.* **23** (2), 97–115.
4 Cooke, W.T. & Holmes, G.K.T. (1984): *Coeliac disease.* Edinburgh: Churchill Livingstone.
5 Crosby, W.H. & Kugler, H.W. (1957): Intraluminal biopsy of the small intestine. *Am. J. Dig. Dis.* **2**, 236–241.
6 Dicke, W.K. (1950): Coeliakie. Een onderzoek naar de nagelige invloed van sommige graansoorten op de lijder aan coeliakie. MD thesis, Utrecht.
7 Dicke, W.K., Weijers, H.A., Kamer, J.H. & Van de (1953): Coeliac disease: presence in wheat of a factor having deleterious effect in cases of coeliac disease. *Acta Paediatr. Scand.* **42**, 34–42.
8 Egan-Mitchell, B. & McNicholl, B. (1972): Constipation in childhood coeliac disease. *Archs. Dis. Child.* **47**, 238–240.
9 Falchuk, Z.M., Rogentine, G.N. & Strober, W. (1972): Predominance of histocompatibility antigen HLA 8 in patients with gluten-sensitive enteropathy. *J. Clin. Invest.* **51**, 1602–1605.
10 Gee, S.J. (1888): On the coeliac affection. *St. Bartholomew's Hosp. Rep. Lond.* **24**, 17–20.

11 Keuning, J.J., Pena, A.S., van Leeuwen, A., van Hooff, J.P. & van Rood, J.A. (1976): HLA-Dw3 associated with coeliac disease. *Lancet* **1**, 506–508.
12 McKillop, O.F., Gosling, J.P., Stevens, Fiona M. & Fottrell, P.F. (1985): Enzyme immunoassay of gliadin in food. *Biochem. Soc. Trans.* **13**, 486–487.
13 McNicholl, B., Egan-Mitchell, B. & Fottrell, P.F. (1979): The variability of gluten tolerance in treated childhood coeliac disease. *Gut* **20**, 126–132.
14 Mylotte, M., Egan-Mitchell, B., McCarthy, C.F. & McNicholl, B. (1973): Incidence of coeliac disease in West of Ireland. *Br. Med. J.* **1**, 703–705.
15 Mylotte, M., Egan-Mitchell, B., Fottrell, P.F., McNicholl, B. & McCarthy, C.F. (1974): Family studies in coeliac disease. *Quart. J. Med.* **43**, 359–369.
16 Paulley, J.W. (1954): Observations of the aetiology of idiopathic steatorrhoea; jejunal and lymph-node biopsies. *Br. Med. J.* **4**, 1318–1321.
17 Rolles, C.J., Kyaw-Myint To & Sin, W.K. (1974): Family studies of coeliac disease. In *Coeliac disease*, ed W.T.J.M. Hekkens & A.S. Pena. Leiden: Stenfert Kroese.
18 Stevens, Fiona M. & McCarthy, C.F. (1976): The endoscopic demonstration of coeliac disease. *Endoscopy* **8**, 177–180.
19 Stevens, Fiona M., Egan-Mitchell, B., Watt, D.W., Baker, S.H., McNicholl, B. & McCarthy, C.F. (1978): HLA antigens in coeliac disease and in control population in the west of Ireland. In *Perspectives in coeliac disease*, ed B. McNicholl, C.F. McCarthy & P.F. Fottrell, pp. 137–143. Lancaster: MTP.
20 Tomasi, T.B. (1975): The development of the secretory system. In *The immune system of secretions*, ed A.G. Olster, L. Weiss, pp. 41–56. Englewood, NJ: Prentice Hall.
21 Udall, J. & Walker, W.A. (1982): The physiologic and pathologic basis for the transport of the macromolecules across the intestinal tract. *J. Pediatr. Gastroenterol. Nutr.* **1**, 295–301.

XIX: Food processing

The social responsibility of the food industry

C.L. ANGST
Nestlé SA, 1800 Vevey, Switzerland.

When Professor Waterlow asked me quite some time ago to talk about corporate responsibility, I accepted without hesitation, appreciating the opportunity to address this conference. It occurred to me recently that I neglected to ask why the subject was chosen; a subject which is rather controversial, ill-defined and frequently misunderstood. I then assumed that this is simply a reflection of our time where it has become fashionable to talk about corporate responsibility or corporate conscience, not infrequently with an implicit or even explicit assumption of guilt. If so, Nestlé might be considered an ideal partner for discussion or confrontation, being one of the leading consumer product companies and, as quite a few among you know, having been the object of criticism related to what is sometimes called the 'infant formula issue'.

Being sure that you are not interested in generalizations and banalities, I shall draw on Nestlé's experiences during these last 10 years, but, where appropriate, I shall not hesitate to extrapolate this experience to multinational companies in general. I would also hope to have your agreement when I stray on occasion beyond the food industry's specific interest and particularities without, of course, losing sight of the fact that this Congress is all about nutrition. I doubt, however, that you wish to hear about the ABC of the food industry and its main objective of transforming perishable food and raw material into nutritionally high quality products, with guaranteed shelflife, at reasonable prices.

Hence, I take it that I shall have your attention with a discussion of not only how the food industry but industry in general and multinational corporations in particular fit into today's society and environment and whether they meet their obligations towards this society.

Assuming now that I have more or less zeroed in on what the organizers intended, let me start with the obvious statement that industry has come a long way since the era of Taylorism. This was characterized by putting millions of untrained, and often illiterate, men and women into factories, creating a system of a privileged class which thinks and gives orders, and of the large masses who, unthinkingly, execute their highly limited and segmented jobs.

We should perhaps not be too surprised if the entrepreneur of that time, spanning the second half of the last and the beginning of this century, is frequently portrayed as a ruthless and exploiting capitalist. Undoubtedly, this image reflects to some extent a reality of that time, but is today nothing but a caricature, even if some people still enjoy using it if it suits their purpose. Furthermore, to be fair to the industrialists of that era, there were some quite enlightened ones around as demonstrated by Julius Maggi who founded the company which, today, is part of the Nestlé Group. In the 1870s he was already preoccupied with the consequences of having more and more women working in factories who no longer had time to prepare meals in the time-consuming fashion of that period. To avoid the negative effects on the family diet, Julius Maggi developed a nutritious, powdered pea soup for easy preparation, thus combining the prospects of a promising business venture with a contribution to improving the health of the population.

Taylorism is now a thing of the past and industry has long since entered a phase of what might indeed be called social responsibility, reflected in the respect for the individual and offering the best possible working conditions. So what is then the explanation for the fact that industry, and above all multinational companies, have been exposed to so much criticism? That the phenomenal growth of multinational companies after the Second World War provoked fears of too much concentration of power and risk of abuse, is to some extent understandable. But this perceived power belongs, more often than not, to the realm of fiction. Industry itself is partly to blame for this image, having failed to explain its activities as well as to act and react in good time, to enter into candid dialogue and to correct errors where they exist. Of course, errors did occur. In fact, I would find it rather inconceivable that somebody might go through life without committing errors, be it an enterprise or even an individual, unless he never gets out of bed. As we all know, infallability is a quality reserved to a very few exalted positions in this world. On the other hand, just as important, is the extent to which widely varying concepts of corporate responsibility, seen from different social, religious, and political perspectives, have been promoted over the past two decades. These concepts, together with a frightening amount of misinformation, have combined to form the public image of multinational corporations. This, of course, was also helped by some over-eager media. As a foreigner speaking in the UK, I am of course not thinking of the BBC, but, as a Swiss, I dare say that Swiss television has every so often proven to be a champion in slanting information to turn it into dramatized misinformation. I do not think that any representative of Swiss Television is here, but, if so, I do not mind being quoted.

Private enterprise often shies away from raising publicly political and ideological aspects and yet, why should we remain silent in the face of statements emanating, for instance, from such morally-authoritative sources as the 1983 Vancouver Congress of the World Council of Churches, to the effect that 'Capitalism is incompatible with Christianity', and that 'Profit and transnational companies are inherently evil'?

In some people's mind, corporate responsibility appears to be equated with philanthropy. Corporations are regarded by some as having responsibilities which go well beyond the traditional concepts of producing guaranteed quality goods or services at a fair price; beyond providing decent wages and working conditions; even beyond being a good corporate citizen, participating in the economic development of the country. Some go as far as to demand — and here I am citing a declaration published last year by American bishops — that every economic decision be judged by the effect it will have on human beings. Such a declaration, at first sight as unattackable as motherhood, completely ignores the fact that social justice will not necessarily lead to economic justice and progress, as sadly demonstrated by countries which put welfare before economic progress with disastrous results.

When it comes to the specific problems of the third world, we are not infrequently asked what we are doing to alleviate hunger in those countries. I hardly need to emphasize that we are all equally distressed by this sad situation and we are also all equally anxious to help in finding a solution. Where we often differ from certainly well-meaning philanthropic organizations, however, is how best to achieve this objective. Our approach is businesslike — I intentionally and emphatically use this expression — creating agricultural and industrial activities.

Let me cite a practical example, demonstrating corporate responsibility the way we see it with regard to developing countries. I am thinking of Brazil where our first milk factory, put into operation of 1921, marked the beginning of a vast undertaking consisting of teaching farmers the raising and care of livestock, providing free veterinary advice and opening roads to permit an efficient milk collection, thus enabling the farmers in remote areas to have a regular and guaranteed outlet for their surplus milk. Today, we operate in Brazil eight milk factories and each one helps to raise the living standard in the area. In the State of Minas Gerais, for instance, through the impact of our plant inaugurated in 1964, milk production increased from 75 000 t to 320 000 t in 1980. What is most important is the fact that close to 80 per cent of the milk received in the factory is provided by small producers, delivering less than 100 litres/day. Many of those small producers had no regular source of income before the advent of the factory and, contrary to frequently heard statements, this development has not resulted in monoculture, but rather permitted the farmers to diversify. Thus one factory, in itself not of tremendous size, provides direct and indirect income to more than 80 000 people and, counting also family members, it certainly can be said that the living standard of some 30 000 people has been raised. This one example, extrapolated to some hundred Nestlé factories in developing countries or, why not, to thousands of other multinational companies' factories, demonstrates the contribution multinational corporations can make and how, through their normal activity, they fulfil their social obligations.

Economic development is in the interest of any country, be it in the North or the South. Industry cannot live up to its social responsibilities, as some kindhearted souls continue to proclaim, by doling out money left and right, and by indulging in a proliferation of welfare programmes. The purpose of business is still business, and only the generation of profits by business makes it possible to render services to a community, a region and a country. Ideological schemes demanded by those who cry the loudest against multinational activities would actually retard economic growth. These people would be well advised to set aside their preoccupation with imagined evils and look objectively at the positive consequences of free-enterprise activities. If I insist now on the term 'free enterprise', I might as well add that they should also look at the living standard in countries which adopted and encouraged the free enterprise concept and compare it with those who do not.

Let us not forget either that the multinational corporation in a developing country cannot afford many mistakes. Its arrangements with the host country must be equitable if it wants to survive — which is in the interest of both, the company and the host country.

Addressing this Congress without mentioning the famine ravaging some African countries might be considered negligence or skirting the most urgent issue. What we are witnessing is tragic beyond comprehension, but just as tragic is the fact that it is caused as much by men as by nature. Natural disasters are exacerbated by the neglect of agriculture, priorities accorded to armaments, tribal warfare, the clash of political ideologies helped or even triggered from the outside, mishandling and misappropriations of funds and plain corruption. Adding to all of this the continuing population growth, outpacing food production, health and education facilities, the immensity of the problem seems to be beyond the grasp of any organization or institution. We can nevertheless all agree that a long-term solution can only be found through the patient development of local agriculture. This, fortunately, was publicly recognized at the July meeting of the Organization for African Unity which had the courage and wisdom to accept their share of responsibility for the calamity.

Of course, charitable food aid is sometimes an urgent necessity, but, long term, philanthropy is entirely misplaced. As I have tried to demonstrate, only a pragmatic approach, profitable to all parties concerned, can achieve success. Multinational corporations therefore have a role to play, which, I am glad to say, is now being more and more recognized.

Corporate responsbility, as far as Nestlé is concerned, has undoubtedly passed through its most sensitive and most controversial phase with the infant formula issue. Henri Nestlé, the founder of our Company and of the modern infant food industry, wrote as long ago as 1869 that 'every mother able to do so should herself breast-feed her children'. His successors have been saying the same ever since, although — I must now, and do, admit with hindsight — not always loudly enough. Nobody has really ever questioned that breast-feeding is best for babies and we can also all agree that the feeding of substitutes or supplements is hazardous if the necessary hygienic conditions are absent, if the utensils are dirty and the water is contaminated. It is exactly in recognition of these risks that great emphasis has always been put on information and education. The infant food industry has, since its beginnings, accepted the responsibility to assist health services in educating mothers, not only regarding the superiority of breast-feeding and the correct preparation of substitutes and supplements where necessary, but also of general maternal and child health care.

Much of this consumer education was greatly appreciated by the health services, hence you may understand our perplexity and dismay when, all of a sudden, the company became the focus of violent attacks by critics, who, in addition to drawing attention to some admittedly inappropriate marketing methods, questioned how commercial interests could ever provide disinterested and objective advice to mothers. Management was at fault in reacting too slowly to these attacks although this was perhaps understandable in view of the distortions and mud-slinging which exaggerated beyond all recognition the extent of the errors and the supposed conflict of interest between industry's educational and promotional activities.

The adoption of the WHO Code finally provided general guidance to governments and industry on these questions, even if the ambiguity of some important provisions resulted in widely differing interpretations. By adopting a very candid and open approach to these problems, resulting in the company's unequivocal adoption of the WHO Code throughout the developing world — where the problems of malnutrition which the Code seeks to address, are widespread — Nestlé finally put this disagreeable conflict behind it. This does not mean that the issue itself is really over, since quite a few activists continue to question the role of industry, and continue to claim that even the basic provision of instructions, through the health services, for the correct use of infant formula, is no more than a disguised form of promotion. Such ill-founded propositions simply cloud the issue because the root of the problem is poverty, and the need to improve child health among deprived populations requires concerted action by all interested parties — above all WHO, governmental health services and industry. Since manufacturers are prevented by the WHO Code, as well as by pressure groups, from providing direct assistance to mothers, this basic task falls now entirely on the shoulders of the authorities. Unfortunately, governmental health services are frequently overstretched or plainly inadequate for the task. It may also be useful to point out that, although the WHO Code was approved by 118 member states, only 13 developing countries have enacted voluntary or mandatory measures closely following the WHO model. The infant formula issue therefore is far from being solved and progress will certainly not be achieved through continuing discord and uncoordinated actions.

In spite of this, one of the more positive consequences for Nestlé of the infant formula issue, which lasted over some 10 years, is that the participants — adversaries and concerned people in general — got to know each other. I am glad to say that a spirit of cooperation exists today between industry, WHO, UNICEF and church groups; a fruitful dialogue with the World Council of Churches has started. I can even add with a degree of satisfaction that we are on speaking terms with some of the most aggressive of our former foes. I also had the privilege to meet a number of personalities, in the other camp so to speak, for whom I have great respect and whom I consider today as friends. Inevitably, there were others whose ambition in life seems to be to search and search for errors, closing their eyes to the tremendous progress which has been achieved so that they may continue once they think they identified an error, to judge and to condemn. These people are often wrong, but they are never in doubt. They make poor partners for a concerted effort which is so badly needed.

The need to inform and, indeed, to educate the consumer is of course not limited to infant nutrition. WHO has identified food safety as a worldwide public health problem. Illness caused by contaminated food is a leading cause of sickness in the developing world, affecting untold millions. While it is clearly a government responsibility to enforce food safety standards and encourage appropriate educational measures, I am happy to state that WHO also seeks the assistance of the food industry in promoting positive health messages. All responsible manufacturers will welcome the opportunity for such cooperation with the United Nations systems and with governments.

In the Western world, excessive consumption of fats, sugar, salt and whatever other components happen to hit the headlines, has become a daily topic. While the diseases of the affluent society are an undeniable fact, it is likewise true that the science of nutrition has a long way to go to clear up a great deal of conflicting evidence. It would be rather presumptious on my part to treat this subject in front of an audience so much more knowledgeable than I, but I do wish to point out that the food industry, has the responsibility to inform. This can only be done by acquiring first the underlying knowledge. Hence, research is certainly one the the basic responsibilities of the food industry and, in my view, considerable progress has been made by the largest food manufacturers in cooperation with leading academic institutes. As some of you may know, Nestlé devotes a great deal of effort and money to increase its knowledge in food science and nutrition and, as a concrete manifestation of our endeavours, a new nutrition research centre designed to further our basic knowledge will be opened in about one year's time.

While we attempt on one hand to better understand malnutrition in all its forms, we also tackle on the other hand specific problems in developing countries and to this effect two new R & D centres have been put into operation, one in Latin America and one in South-East Asia. Their main task is the development of moderate cost food, to meet the needs of the indigenous populations, based on locally available raw material, of high nutritional value and good eating qualities.

It is self-evident that it is not altruism which motivates this research, but it is likewise self-evident that the results of this research will ultimately benefit not only the corporation, but society as a whole. Discussions on whether the first obligation of a corporation is towards its shareholders, or its employees, or its customers, or whether it should be extended beyond these groups to the environment and society at large, are really quite academic. No enterprise, and certainly no consumer product company, can succeed long term if it does not take care of all these aspects. I therefore maintain that a well-managed company which has moved along with the rapid evolution in every sphere of human life through these last few decades, takes good care of its social responsibilities.

If you need further convincing, let me add that, in today's age, all the men and women working for a corporation are very much aware of its image and they would want it to be such that they can be proud of it. Each corporation has its own identity, often rooted in its founder's personality and concepts, adopted by subsequent generations. This is fashionably called 'corporate culture', reflected in the contacts with the community, consumers and in its respect for the employees. Their loyalty, so important to an enterprise, is assured when they find personal satisfaction, when they can put their potential to good use and when they know that their company honours its social obligations. It is thus that the corporation remains strong in a changing environment, and its lasting success is proof that its coporate culture is in harmony with society.

I am conscious of having made quite a few statements in my address to you which would have caused angry protests only a few years ago. Of course, there are probably still some, even among you, who are inclined to manifest their objections. By and large, however, a change has fortunately taken place and emotions and fanaticism have been replaced, at least to some extent, by rational thinking and good sense. Multinational corporations are being recognized for their positive impact on progress in developing countries.. The free enterprise concept seems to be gaining. This must not now be a cause for smug satisfaction, but, quite on the contrary, it encourages us to live up to this newly emerging image and to continue to carry out our social responsibilities. If I succeeded to convince at least some of you of what we have achieved and can achieve, then I shall be happy and grateful for having had this opportunity to talk to you.

FOOD PROCESSING AND NUTRITION

Food processing and nutrition: an overview

O. FENNEMA
Department of Food Science, 1605 Linden Drive, University of Wisconsin-Madison, Madison, WI 53706, USA.

Chemical, enzymatic and physical changes can and do occur during the processing, handling and storage of foods (hereafter simply called food processing) and some of these changes influence nutritive value. When physical factors affect nutritive value they do so by causing selective separation of nutrients (eg leaching, milling) or by indirectly influencing chemical reactions, eg ice formation can alter the pH and concentration of oxygen in the unfrozen phase of a frozen food and these changes will in turn affect rates of chemical reactions. In this presentation major emphasis will be on chemical and enzymatic reactions that cause damage to the nutritive value of foods since these reactions are far more complex and less well understood than damage caused by physical factors.

The primary purpose of many food processes is to inactivate or retard the growth of microorganisms. This is achieved by thermal processing, chilling, freezing, drying, irradiation or chemical treatments. Other purposes of processing are to improve the convenience, and stabilize or improve the sensory properties of foods or food ingredients. Retention or improvement of nutritive value during food processing has received comparatively little attention at the commercial level until recently.

Chemical changes during food processing can be desirable or undesirable. Desirable changes generally involve sensory properties (eg intentional browning of cereal products, hydrogenation or interesterfication of lipids, isomerization of glucose, chemical modification of starch, or firming of plant tissue), although nutritional properties can be improved if nutrients are added. Occasionally, desirable nutritive changes occur incidentally. Soy proteins, for example, are often heated to alter their functional properties, but this heat treatment also inactivates some antinutritive substances, thus rendering the proteins more digestible.

Unfortunately, many chemical changes occur during food processing that are undesirable from the standpoint of both sensory properties and nutritive value. These undesirable changes are accepted as an unavoidable penalty that must be paid to achieve the primary goal of lessening or stopping microbial spoilage. Since the advantages of microbiological stability are generally considered to more than counterbalance any detrimental effects on sensory properties and nutritive value, processed foods have come to represent a prominent (greater than half) and increasing proportion of the average diet of individuals in developed countries. This should not be a cause for alarm, but food processors and government regulatory agencies should feel an increasing responsibility to assure that those processed foods representing major components of the average diet should also be fair-share contributors to fulfilment of recommended dietary allowances.

Major factors governing chemical changes during food processing. These factors are enumerated in Table 1 and their relative importance depends on the type of food and the kind of conditions to which the food is exposed. Indicated in Table 2 is the relative importance of these factors in influencing loss or inactivation of nutrients during various kinds of food processing, and the seriousness of nutrient reductions as a function of process type.

Effect of food processing on major classes of nutrients. It is appropriate now to consider the effects of food processing on major classes of nutrients and on interactions between nutrients. Primary attention will be given to heat processes since, unfortunately, they cause the greater nutrient damage in processed foods. However, other degradation factors will also be mentioned where appropriate.

Proteins. The nutritive value of proteins can be modified by heating, oxidation, exposure to

Table 1. *Factors governing kinds and rates of chemical reactions that occur in food processing.*

I. Product composition
　—Kinds of components
　—pH, a_w, catalysts, $[O_2]$
II. Process and storage factors
　—Time and temperature
　—Composition of the atmosphere
　—Chemical or biological treatments
　—Exposure to radiant energy (light, x-rays, gamma rays)
　—Exposure to high energy electrons
　—Unintentional events (contamination, physical abuse)

Table 2. *Nutrient stability during food processing: factors influencing and degree of damage*

Process	Factors normally of major importance	Normal degree of damage
Heat sterilization	Time-temperature, product composition	Moderate
Freezing	Product composition	Insignificant
Dehydration	Time-temperature, product composition	Insignificant to moderate
Irradiation (sterilization)	Dose, product composition	Moderate
Fat and oil processing	Time-temperature, product composition	Slight
Protein processing	Time-temperature, product composition	Slight
Milling of wheat	Separation (altered product composition)	Substantial
Storage:		
Canned or irradiated	Time-temperature, product composition	Moderate
Frozen	Time-temperature, product composition, atmospheric composition	Moderate
Dry	Time-temperature, product composition, atmospheric composition	Moderate
Fresh	Time-temperature, product composition, atmospheric composition	Insignificant to moderate

alkaline conditions and by reaction with nonprotein constitutents in food. Extensive information on these reactions has accumulated in recent years[8,13–15,18,22,24,26,27,29,32,37,44,47].

Heating of moist, acidic proteins in the absence of both oxygen and active non-protein carbonyl groups can result in unfolding of the molecule (denaturation) some crosslinking and, if heating is severe, some destruction of component amino acids[22,29]. Denaturation usually results in inactivation of enzymes (desirable with regard to stability of some vitamins) and inactivation of proteinaceous antinutritional substances[9,38,46]. Heat treatments administered under these conditions and in accord with good manufacturing practices usually have either positive effects or negligible negative effects on protein nutritive value.

Heating of moist proteins in the presence of active carbonyl groups (eg reducing sugars and products of lipid oxidation) will favour the Maillard reaction, Strecker degradation (when discarbonyls are present) sugar crosslinks and protein-lipid complexes. Browning-type reactions can have a substantial negative effect on protein nutritive value. Whether toxic substances develop to a level of significance during browning is still a matter of investigation and debate[14,15,22,26,37,44,47].

Heating of moist proteins in the presence of alkali results in two important changes that influence nutritive value: racemization and formation of crosslinks (compounds of the lysinoalanine type)[13,18,27,29,37]. Both occurrences have negative effects on protein nutritive value, but appear to have no toxicological effects of significance.

Oxidation of proteins, whether or not accompanied by heat, can result in thiol-disulfide interchange reactions, crosslinking (eg, S-S, dityrosine) and the formation of protein degradation products. Among these, dityrosine linkages and oxidative degradation products are known to detract from protein nutritive value[13,15,29,32,37]. Toxic constituents can form during protein oxidation, but it seems likely under mild oxidizing conditions that the kinds and concentrations do not pose a significant threat to health.

Lipids. Especially when unsaturated, lipids undergo many kinds of chemical changes during processing and some of these changes can affect their nutritional value and wholesomeness[1,6,7,16,28,30,31,36,47]. Unsaturated lipids are susceptible to oxidation when exposed to oxygen, radiant energy and/or a variety of organic and inorganic catalysts. When this occurs, several chemical changes can be observed that are of importance nutritionally and perhaps toxicologically.

Formation of hydroperoxides. These are more toxic than the unoxidized parent compounds and some believe them to be carcinogenic[11].

Partial conjugation of the double-bond system in lipids. Conjugated fatty acids apparently are more likely to covert to the *trans* configuration and are also more likely to engage in dimerization and polymerization reactions than the nonconjugated *cis* counterparts. Fatty acid dimers and polymers when fed to rats have no nutritive value and cause growth suppression and poor reproduction[28,33,47].

Partial conversion of natural cis fatty acids to trans fatty acids. Formation of *trans* fatty acids can occur during hydrogenation or oxidation of lipids. Studies with animals have indicated that *trans* fatty acids have no essential fatty acid properties, however they are calorically available. When *trans* monoenes are incorporated in the diets of animals at levels normally encountered in human foods, the effects approximate those obtained by feeding saturated fats[3,12,40,41]. *Trans* dienes are of greater concern from the standpoint of wholesomeness, but these types of fatty acids occur only at very low levels in foods[1].

Peroxidizing lipids also exert negative effects on the nutritive value and perhaps wholesomeness of foods by their interaction with proteins and vitamins. Peroxidizing lipids in the presence of proteins can cause protein crosslinking, formation of oxidative degradation products of proteins and, most importantly, can cause the Maillard reaction with its detrimental effects on the nutritive value of proteins. In the presence of vitamins, peroxidizing lipids reduce the activity of vitamins A, C, D, E and folate[42].

Heating of lipids can cause the formation of many new compounds including ketones, cyclic fatty acid monomers, dimers and polymers. These changes cause a reduction in caloric value, and cyclic fatty acid monomers are of some concern because of their toxic potency[2,16,17,47].

Carbohydrates are generally less susceptible than proteins and lipids to processing-induced chemical changes that impair nutritive value or increase toxicity. Carbohydrates with active carbonyl groups do, of course, participate readily in Maillard reactions and Strecker degradation of proteins and thereby have an adverse effect on protein nutritive value and perhaps toxicity. Other types of carbohydrate reactions that would have a negative effect on nutritive value and perhaps wholesomeness of foods are caramelization of sugars, and thermal degradation of carbohydrates in an aqueous environment (eg formation of furfural, hydroxymethylfurfural)[5,20,21,26,35,39,45].

Vitamins. Some of the vitamins are labile and therefore losses are incurred during certain kinds of food processing[4,19,42]. Vitamins C, D, E, A and folate are especially prone to inactivation by oxidation, and vitamins C, folate, thiamin and B_6 are subject to degradation during heating in the presence of water. Riboflavin is especially susceptible to light-catalyzed degradation. Product composition (pH, water-activity (a_w), catalysts, binding agents, oxidized lipids, $[O_2]$ and added chemicals such as sulfites, nitrites and ethylene oxide) has a profound effect on vitamin stability. Water soluble vitamins also can be lost during exposure of foods to water (eg blanching) and the concentration of all vitamins can be significantly reduced by separation processes (eg milling of wheat, peeling of potatoes). When foods are exposed to long-term methods of preservation (heat sterilization, freezing, dehydration, irradiation) plus lengthy storage, losses of the more labile vitamins can be substantial.

In a few instances, moderate heat treatments can have beneficial effects on vitamin (eg biotin, niacin) bioavailability or stability by inactivating binding agents[9,10,23,34] or by inactivating enzymes.

Minerals. Losses of minerals from foods during processing can be substantial especially if the food is exposed to an abundance of water (eg blanching of vegetables in water) or if separation processes are utilized (eg milling of wheat, peeling of potatoes)[43]. The bioavailability of a mineral can be influenced by factors such as chemical form, particle size, composition of the food and processing. Iron is a good example since its bioavailability is influenced by all of these factors. The bioavailability of ferrous gluconate is very good, whereas that of ferric sodium pyrophosphate is poor; a small particle size for elemental iron favours bioavailability; ascorbate and fructose increase iron bioavailability, whereas phytates (di and tetra-ferric phytates) decrease it; and thermal processing of spinach in the presence of abundant water increases bioavailability of iron[25].

Processing can also increase the mineral content of food. This, in a sense, is a form of contamination since the added minerals come from water, utensils or machinery used for processing, or from packaging materials, especially metal cans[43].

Conclusions. It must be acknowledged that nutrient loss or inactivation often does accompany food processing, handling and storage and this reduction in nutrient value of the food can be substantial in some situations. It is therefore a desirable goal of the food industry to minimize any reduction in the nutritive value of food. Much is known about the means by which nutrients are inactivated during food processing, but like most complicated subjects, much also remains to be learned, especially with regard to chemical mechanisms of nutrient inactivation. This information is of great importance since it will enable development of practical methods for inhibiting some of these reactions. In the mean time, the food industry can justifiably argue that most foods currently processed and handled in accord with good manufacturing practices are valuable wholesome components of the diet and that processed foods of the future will, in all probability, exhibit improved nutritional qualities because of improvements in processing and handling techniques and because addition of nutrients to foods will become more common.

1 Applewhite, T.H. (1981): Nutritional effects of hydrogenated soya oil. *J. Am. Oil Chem. Soc.* **58**, 260–269.

2 Artman, N.R. & Smith, D.E. (1972): Systematic isolation and identification of minor components in heated and unheated fat. *J. Am. Oil Chem. Soc.* **49**, 318–326.

3 Beare-Rogers, J.L. (1983): *Trans-* and positional isomers of common fatty acids. *Adv. Nutr. Res.* **5**, 171–200.

4 Bender, A.E., ed (1978): *Food processing and nutrition.* London: Academic Press.

5 Birch, G.G. (1977): Chemical, physical and biological changes in carbohydrates induced by thermal processing. In *Physical, chemical and biological changes in food caused by thermal processing*, ed T. Høyem & O. Kvåle, pp. 152–167. London: Applied Science Publishers.

6 Bollard, J.L. & Koch, H.P. (1945): The course of autoxidation in polyisoprenes and allied compounds. Part IX. The primary thermal oxidation of ethyl linoleate. *J. Chem. Soc.* 1945, 455–447.

7 Carpenter, D.L. & Slover, H.T. (1973): Lipid composition of selected margarines. *J. Am. Oil Chem. Soc.* **50**, 272–276.

8 Cheftel, J.C., Cuq, J.L. & Lorient, D. (1985): Amino acids, peptides and proteins. In *Food chemistry*, 2nd edn., ed O. Fennema, pp. 246–369. New York: Marcel Dekker.

9 Chichester, C.O. & Lee, T.C. (1981): Effect of food processing in the formation and destruction of toxic constituents in food. In *Impact of toxicology on food processing*, ed J.C. Ayres & J.C. Kirschman, pp. 35–56. Westport, CT: AVI.

10 Clegg, K.M. (1963): Bound nicotinic acid in dietary wheaten products. *Br. J. Nutr.* **17**, 325–329.

11 Cutler, M.G. & Schneider, R. (1973): Sensitivity of feeding tests in detecting carcinogenic properties in chemicals: examination of 7, 12-diethylbenz[a]-anthracene and oxidized linoleate. *Fd Cosmet. Tox.* **11**, 443–457.

12 Emken, E.A. (1984): Nutrition and biochemistry of *trans* and positional fatty acid isomers in hydrogenated oils. *Ann. Rev. Nutr.* **4**, 339–376.

13 Feeney, R.E. (1980): Overview on the chemical deteriorative changes of proteins and their consequences. In *Chemical deterioration of proteins*, ed J.R. Whitaker & M. Fujimaki, pp. 1–47. Washington, DC: American Chemical Society.

14 Feeney, R.E. & Whitaker, J.R. (1982): The Maillard reaction and its prevention. In *Food deterioration — mechanisms and functionality*, ed J.P. Cherry, pp. 201–229. Washington, DC: American Chemical Society.

15 Finot, P.A. (1982): Nutritional and metabolic aspects of protein modification during food processing. In *Modification of proteins: food, nutritional and pharmacological aspects*, ed R.E. Feeney & J.R. Whitaker, pp. 91–124. Washington, DC: American Chemical Society.

16 Firestone, D., Horwitz, W., Friedman, L. & Shue, G.M. (1961): Heated fats I. Studies on the effects of heating on the chemical nature of cottonseed oil. *J. Am. Oil Chem. Soc.* **38**, 253–257.

17 Frankel, E.N., Smith, L.M., Hamblin, C.L., Creveling, R.K. & Clifford, A.J. (1984): Occurrence of cyclic fatty acid monomers in frying oils used for fast foods. *J. Am. Oil Chem. Soc.* **61**, 87–90.

18 Gould, D.H. & McGregor, J.T. (1977): Biological effects of alkali-treated protein and lysinoalanine: an overview. In *Protein crosslinking: nutritional and medical consequences, Part B*, ed M. Friedman, pp. 29–48. New York: Plenum Press.

19 Harris, R.S. & Karmas, E, eds (1975): *Nutritional evaluation of food processing, 2nd edn.* Westport, CT: AVI.

20 Hodge, J.E. & Osman, E.M. (1976): Carbohydrates. In *Principles of food science, Part 1, food chemistry*, ed O. Fennema, pp. 41–138. New York: Marcel Dekker.

21 Houminer, Y. (1973): Thermal degradation of carbohydrates. In *Molecular structure and function of food carbohydrates*, ed G.G. Birch & L.F. Green, pp. 133–155. London: Applied Science Publishers.

22 Hurrell, R.F. & Carpenter, K.J. (1977): Nutritional significance of crosslink formation during food processing. In *Protein crosslinking: nutritional and medical consequences, part B*, ed M. Friedman, pp. 225–258. New York: Plenum Press.

23 Koetz, R. & Neukom, H. (1977): Nature of bound nicotinic acid in cereals and its release by thermal and chemical treatment. In *Physical, chemical and biological changes in food caused by thermal processing*, ed T. Høyem & O. Kvåle, pp. 305–310. London: Applied Publishers.

24 Lea, C.H. & Hannan, R.S. (1949): Studies of the reaction between protein and reducing sugars in the 'dry' state. I. The effect of activity of water, of pH and of temperature on the primary reaction between casein and glucose. *Biochim. Biophys. Acta* **3**, 313–325.

25 Lee, K. (1982): Iron chemistry and bioavailability in food processing. In *Nutritional bioavailability of iron*, ed C. Kies, pp. 27–54. Washington, DC: American Chemical Society.

26 Lee, C.M., Lee, T.-C. & Chichester, C.O. (1975): Physiological consequences of browned food products. *Proc. IV Int. Congr. Fd Sci. and Technol.* **1**, 587–603.

27 Masters, P.H. & Friedman, M. (1980): Amino acid racemization in alkali-treated food proteins — chemistry, toxicology and nutritional consequence. In *Chemical deterioration of proteins*, ed J.R. Whitaker & M. Fujimaki, pp. 165–194. Washington, DC: American Chemical Society.

28 Matsuo, N. (1962): Nutritional effects of oxidized and thermally polymerized fish oils. In *Lipids and their oxidation*, ed H.W. Schultz, E.A. Day & R.O. Sinnhuber, pp. 321–359. Westport, CT: AVI.

29 Mauron, J. (1977): General principles involved in measuring specific damage of food components during thermal processes. In *Physical, chemical and biological changes in food caused by thermal processing*, ed T. Høyem and O. Kvåle, pp. 328–359. London: Applied Science Publishers.

30 Morton, I.D. (1977): Physical, chemical and biological changes related to different time-temperature combinations — changes in fat. In *Physical, chemical and biological changes in food caused by thermal processing*, ed T. Høyem & O. Kvåle, pp. 135–151. London: Applied Science Publishers.

31 Nawar, W.W. (1985): Lipids. In *Food chemistry, 2nd edn.* ed O. Fennema. pp. 140–244. New York: Marcel Dekker.

32 Neukom, H. (1980): Oxidative crosslinking of proteins and other biopolymers. In *Autoxidation in food and biological systems*, ed M.G. Simic & M. Karel, pp. 249–259. New York: Plenum Press.

33 Perkins, E.G. (1967): Formation of non-volatile decomposition products in heated fats and oils. *Fd Technol.* **21**, 611–616.

34 Rajalakshmi, R., Nanavaty, K. & Gumashta, A. (1964): Effect of cooking procedures on the free and total niacin content of certain foodstuffs. *J. Nutr. Diet.* (India) **1**, 276–280.

35 Rice, E.W. (1972): Furfural: Exogenous precursor of certain urinary furans and possible toxicological agent in humans. *Clin. Chem.* **18**, 1550–1551.

36 Richardson, T. & Korycka-Dahl, M. (1984): Lipid oxidation. In *Developments in dairy chemistry, 2nd edn.* ed P.F. Fox, pp. 241–363. Barking, England: Applied Science Publishers.

37 Satterlee, L.D. & Chang, K.C. (1982): Nutritional quality of deteriorated proteins. In *Food protein denaturation — mechanisms and functionality*, ed J.P. Cherry, pp. 409–431. Washington, DC: American Chemical Society.

38 Schwimmer, S. (1981): *Source book of food enzymology.* Westport, CT: AVI.

39 Simonyan, T.A. (1969): Toxico-hygienic characteristics of oxymethylfurfural. *Voprosy Pitomiya* **28**, 54-58.

40 Sommerfeld, M. (1983): *Trans* unsaturated fatty acids in natural products and processed foods. *Prog. Lipid Res.* **22**, 221–233.

41 Spence, M., Davignon, J., Holub, B., Little, J.A. & McDonald, B.E. (1980): *Report of the ad hoc committee on the composition of special margarines.* Ottawa, Canada: Ministry of Supply and Services.

42 Tannenbaum, S.R., Archer, M.C. & Young, V.R. (1985): Vitamins and minerals. In *Food chemistry*, 2nd edn. ed O. Fennema, pp. 447–544. New York: Marcel Dekker.

43 Tannenbaum, S.R. & Young, R. (1979): Minerals. In *Nutritional and safety aspects of food processing*, ed S.R. Tannenbaum, pp. 139–152. New York: Marcel Dekker.

44 Waller, G.R. & Feather, M.S., eds. (1983): *The Maillard reaction in foods and nutrition.* Washington, DC: American Chemical Society.

45 Whistler, R.L. & Daniel, J.R. (1985): Carbohydrates. In *Food chemistry*, 2nd edn, ed O. Fennema, pp. 70–137. New York: Marcel Dekker.

46 Whitaker, J.R. (1981): Naturally occurring peptide and protein inhibitors of enzymes. In *Impact of toxicology on food processing*, ed J.C. Ayres & J.C. Kirshman, pp. 57–104. Westport, CT: AVI.

47 Yannai, S. (1980): Toxic factors influenced by processing. In *Toxic constituents of plant foodstuffs*, 2nd edn. ed I.E. Liener, pp. 371–427. New York: Academic Press.

Significance of food processing in developing countries

R. ORRACA-TETTEH
Department of Nutrition and Food Science, University of Ghana, Legon, Ghana.

Famine and starvation are stalking the continent of Africa more than ever before. The toll in deaths may be counted in thousands, but the toll in impaired and impoverished lives will be in millions. Various factors from drought, civil wars, underproduction of food, economic recession, rapid and unprecedented growth in populations have been invoked as immediate or short term causes.

The food production potentials of most of these developing countries have not been utilized to the full. This is because of poor farming technology, unavailability of inputs such as machinery, fertilizers, improved seeds and planting materials, and lack of good extension services. Where food is produced in abundant quantities, these occur only during certain seasons of the year with a glut on the market. The abundance of food during these harvest periods leads to food waste, because of the perishable nature of food materials. Food and the associated processes, such as storage, processing, preparation and cooking have always been regarded as the domain of women in Africa and in most developing countries. Thus the science and technology of food has not developed much beyond the art of indigenous preparation.

Food science has been defined as 'an integrated body of scientific knowledge on the chemical, physical, structural, nutritional, toxicological, microbiological and organoleptical properties of food systems and on the changes occurring during handling, conversion, fabrication preservation and storage'. Thus defined, the vast scope of food science and its application in food processing, storage and manufacture in relation to the food needs of developing countries is of prime concern. The science of food, important for understanding the basic foods and their products used in many developing countries, has not advanced very much.

Maize and its products. Maize and maize foods illustrate this lack of knowledge of foods of developing countries. In Ghana, maize is an important staple food. The maize is generally used as whole meal and only occasionally as polished grain. The maize is soaked in water for 2 days and the water discarded. The grain is then ground in the corn mill of the attrition type into a fine flour. The flour is mixed with water and kneaded to form a dough, which is allowed to ferment for 2 days and then used in making various traditional foods. The chemical and microbiological changes which occur in these foods have been studied only to a very limited extent. The preparation of these foods is still carried out by laborious small-scale methods. Maize porridge (Akassa) is the traditional infant weaning food. The consistency of this porridge affects the amount of porridge the infant can consume. It is usually in a thin gruel form, which affects the nutrient and energy concentration of the porridge and consequently the nutrient intakes of the infant. The viscosity of the porridge has a relationship to the amount of maize meal used and the energy content. Fermented maize meal has lower viscosity than unfermented maize meal, and thus larger amounts of fermented meal can be utilized for making porridge with lower viscosity. Addition of a small amount of germinated maize meal to a porridge of unfermented maize can also reduce appreciably the viscosity of the porridge.

Rice processing. The processing of rice has been a classical example of the influence of processing on nutrition in developing countries. In Ghana, rice processing by traditional pounding and winnowing was the rule until machine milling was introduced on a large scale in the late 50s. This led to the production of white polished rice, evidently with the loss of most of the B complex vitamins. When such rice was used in feeding pigeons, avain beriberi (polyneuritis) was produced. Those fed the polished rice plus the rice bran and polish, and those fed the unpolished rice did not develop the disease. Chemical analyses for thiamin showed, however, that the amount of thiamin, though low, was enough for the requirements of man. The implication of this is that if some consumers use exclusively polished rice without other sources of thiamin there could be a possibility of thiamin-deficiency in the diet.

Cassava processing. Cassava (*Manihot utilissima*) is a main staple food in many tropical developing countries. The root contains the cyanogenic glucosides, linamarin, and lotaustralin, which are concentrated in the peel and outer layers, with varying concentration in the pulpy inner part. The root is peeled, cut into pieces and boiled in water for about 20 to 30 min until cooked. The cooking of the root inactivates the enzyme linamarase, which is needed to liberate the cyanide from the cyanogenic glucoside.

The fresh cassava roots after peeling may be cut into chips and dried in the sun for several days. The dried chips are then pounded in a mortar to reduce their sizes and then ground in a mill into flour. The drying of the chips in the sun helps to inactivate the enzyme linamarase and this prevents the release of the cyanide. The drying of the cassava chips is most often not done under controlled conditions, and this leads to mould growth on the chips. The fungus *Aspergillus flavus* has been found to grow on the chips and aflatoxin contamination thus occurs under such conditions. Because of the possible carcinogenic implication of aflatoxin, the need for good processing of cassava chips is important.

The cassava roots can also be used in making a farina like product, Gari. For this product, the fresh cassava roots are peeled, and grated into a pulp. The pulp is put into cloth or jute sacks or sometimes into baskets and the water pressed out of it. During this period of 3 to 5 days some fermentation of the pulp takes place in addition to the loss of the sap. The sap which can be collected contains some amount of starch. The pressed pulp is dried in the sun and then roasted in a large iron pan, over a firewood fire, with constant stirring until very dry. This is Gari, a farinaceous products, which stores very well. A similar product farinhade mandioca is made in central and south America, particularly in north-east Brazil.

The fresh cassava root when uprooted does not store for long. It rots within 3 to 4 d, due to its high moisture contents and from growth of various microorganisms. Thus as a high-energy yielding crop in developing countries of the tropical region, its preservation through good processing is important for the nutrition of large population groups.

The consumption of cassava has been associated with the development of goitre in the Bauchi Plateau region of Nigeria[1] and also the development of ataxic neuropathy, in some consumers in Nigeria. In all these areas it is found that proper processing of the cassava, by the traditional method which destroys the cyanide and some goitrogenic factors, does not lead to the incidence of the diseases.

Fish processing. In most developing countries with coastal boundaries, or which have rivers and lakes, fishing is an important activity. There is abundance of fish at certain seasons of the year, whilst in the lean season, there is a scarcity of fish. In Ghana as in most developing countries processing of fresh fish is by smoking, salting and pickling, drying, frying and canning.

Smoke-curing of fish as practised in many countries aims at reducing the moisture content of fish and imparting to it a characteristic flavour. In Ghana the fish is first dried for a few hours in the sun, and then packed on perforated metal or mesh based trays. These are then placed in the smoking ovens which are fired for a day or two by firewood and smoke producing materials such as bagasse, sawdust and wood shavings. When the heating is properly controlled a dark brown product is produced. But when this is not done, a black and sometimes charred product is obtained. This tends to affect the quality of the protein, which can be drastically reduced, (Table)[2]. The smoke-curing of fish is carried out by artisan processors, almost entirely women, since there is no large-scale smoke-curing of fish.

Some relationship is considered to exist between smoked food products and cancer, but this needs more investigation, particularly in developing countries where traditional smoking of fish is the foremost method of fish processing, and since most consumers prefer smoked fish[3]. In Africa sun drying of both fresh and salted fish is carried out. The fish are spread out on mats or sometimes on the bare cement or tarred floors for several days. The drying is effected by the heat of the sun which is, in most tropical areas, very intense. Because of the method of drying, the microbiological quality of the fish is not as good as it should be. It is therefore necessary that because of abundance of sunshine in most developing countries, proper design of solar dryers for

Table *Protein value of fish processed by modern and traditional methods*

Types of fish	Origin	Net protein utilization
Fresh fish (marine)	UK	0.90
Kippers	UK	0.81
Stock fish	Norway	0.91
Cod (salted)	Norway	0.69
Catfish (smoked)	Ghana	0.65
Tilapia (salted, sun dried)	Ghana	0.57

fish and other food materials should be investigated. Because of the environmental conditions of high humidity and high temperatures coupled with presence of many microbial agents there is quick spoilage of foods. Thus proper processing of fish and meat, both domestic and game, is essential for much needed protein-rich foods for the populations.

Legume processing. Legumes are important protein-rich foods for most low income groups in developing countries since the price of fish and meat almost invariably is beyond their purchasing power. Groundnuts (*Arachis hypogea*), cowpeas (*Vigna sp*), soya bean (*Glycine max*), pigeon peas (*Cajanus cajan*), Bambara groundnut (*Voandzeia subterranea*), winged bean (*Psophocarpus tetragonolobus*), locust bean (*Parkia sp*) and various peas are grown and widely used. Apart from canning, which is used more in developing countries, these legumes undergo very little processing except drying by the sun. Some of these legumes can be processed into flours which then when properly packaged will provide readily available products. Legumes are susceptible to attack by insects and fungus which cause great damage to them and thus affect their potential as low cost protein rich foods. Legumes are difficult to cook and the use of a lot of fuel to cook them tends to discourage their increased use by populations in rural areas where fuel resources such as firewood are diminishing. The processing of legumes by soaking them in solutions of sodium tripolyphosphate, sodium carbonate for about 24 h before cooking reduced considerably the cooking time sometimes to about one-third the normal cooking time — Figure[4].

Groundnuts have for a long time been processed into paste which is used on a wide scale as spreads and in making soups and stews. Because of aflatoxin contamination there is need for good drying of the groundnuts so that fungal growth is prevented.

Fruits and vegetables. The easily perishable nature of fruits and vegetables necessitates their good processing to preserve them for use. Unfortunately the canning and frozen storage which are the best means for preservation of vegetables are methods which demand high outlays for necessary equipment and these are generally not available in developing countries. Though some canning of various foods including fruits and vegetables takes place in developing countries the processing costs involved tend to form about 50 per cent of the cost of the final product. Thus appropriate technology is needed to enable low-cost processing of fruits and vegetables. Bottling of fruits and fruit juice and some vegetables is also practised.

Drying of fruits and vegetables helps in preserving them, but this leads to the loss of one of their important contributions to the diet, vitamin C. Since fruits and vegetables are important articles of diet providing vitamins including vitamin A in the yellow and green varieties, minerals and fibre in the diet, their proper processing is vital in developing countries.

Sugar, alcohol and soft drinks. These adjuncts to the diet have assumed an important position in the diets of the world out of all proportions to their value in the diet. Their processing and easy availability have increased tremendously over the past few years. Though various traditional soft drinks can be made through fermentation of cereals, such as maize for cornwine (Nmeda), millets for Pito and Brukutu and others, these seem to be overshadowed by the Coca cola, Pepsi cola, Fanta, Sprite, Mirinda. Processing and preservation with greater use of traditional soft drinks needs to be encouraged.

Spices, condiments and salts. Most developing countries — because of the tropical climate — produce various spices such as pepper, curry, nutmeg, ginger. When properly processed, and exported, these are important foreign exchange commodities. In addition developing countries with coastal boundaries can process the important trade commodity, salt, for both home consumption and export. There is, however, the need to improve the processing and possible iodization of salt for some of the countries where endemic goitre is a problem.

Quick-cooking winged beans

STEP   Dry winged bean seeds

I   BLANCH
                       ↓
            2 min in boiling water
                       ↓
II   SOAK
            24 h in solution of
            2% sodium chloride
         1% sodium tripolyphosphate
         0.75% sodium bicarbonate
          0.25% sodium carbonate
                 at 20 °C
                       ↓
III   DRAIN
                       ↓
IV   COOK
        15 to 20 min in boiling water

Figure. *Procedure for preparing quick-cooking salt-soaked beans from whole, raw dry beans.*

Research and training. Most developing countries have several traditional food processing methods, including fermentation which need to be studied and adopted. This demands good training of a cadre of food scientists, food technologists and nutritionists oriented to work in their environment of villages, rural areas and towns. Research costs money and particularly in many developing countries this is an obstacle to research work by nutritionists, food scientists and technologists. Obviously research scientists see in applied research instead of pure research some way out of this difficulty. But more importantly scientists in developing countries have the urgent task of involving themselves in applied research which is necessary for dealing with the immediate problems of food and nutrition in their environment.

There is need for developed countries, and particularly their scientific associations, to assist their counterparts in developing countries with some of their research needs of equipment, chemicals, journals and experts. The International Union of Nutritional Science, the International Union of Food Science and Technology, and their constituent members could provide such assistance.

Appropriate technology in food processing, in combination with modern food technology, can help in providing abundant, safe and nutritious food for the people of the developing world.

Dedication. This paper is dedicated to the memory of the late Professor Benjamin Stanley Platt CMG, father, teacher and friend of nutrition workers from developing countries.

1 Ekpechi, O.L. (1967): Pathogenesis of endemic goitre in Eastern Nigeria. *Br. J. Nutr.* **21**, 537–545.

2 Orraca-Tetteh, R. (1961): The place of food science and technology in the campaign against malnutrition. Problems and some Solutions: Ghana. *Proc. Nutr. Soc.* **20**, 109–112.

3 Orraca-Tetteh, R. & Nyanteng, V.K. (1977): Consumer attitudes to cured fish. Consultancy report to FAO. Rome: FAO.

4 Rockland, L.B., Zaragosa, E.M. & Orraca-Tetteh, R. (1979): Quick cooking winged beans (*Psophocarpus tetranoglobus*). *J. Fd Sci.* **44**, 1004–117.

Significance of processing in industrialized countries. Searches for the diverse roles of foods

H. NAITO
Laboratory of Nutritional Biochemistry and Animal Nutrition, Department of Agricultural Chemistry, University of Tokyo, Yayoi, 1-1-1, Bunkyo-ku, Tokyo 113, Japan.

While the shortage of food is still a matter of great concern as a global problem, it is also true that special attention should be paid to some social strata suffering from diseases caused by a daily intake of an excess amount of food. In addition, there are a number of symptoms caused by mineral deficiency even under conditions of apparently normal supply.

Ingestion of a food causes a variety of biological responses other than the nutritional effects of supplying the constituent materials to the body. In this regard, foods possess several functions part of which are latent and are revealed only after ingestion or during metabolism.

Function of food. Basically, a food exhibits primary and secondary functions; the former are manifested in the use of the constituent nutrients, and the latter relate to sensory properties, such as palatability, olfactory quality or masticatory characteristics. Furthermore, many foods also have a third function, which produces various physiological responses on food ingestion, eg wakefulness, calmness, allergies. Thus, food function can be classified into following three categories[2]: (1) nutritional, (2) sensory, (3) physiologically conditioned.

Food processing should be planned so as to enhance the merits or to remove the demerits of a food, taking these functions into account. Many kinds of processed food have been exploited in this respect. For example the preparation of Tofu, soyabean curds, was devised almost a thousand years ago in Japan and this food is now valued as a health food by many nations. Here I shall describe examples of food proteins which produce novel effects on mineral utilization.

The formation of physiologically active peptides during intestinal digestion of food proteins. Although ingested protein is normally rapidly digested, and the free amino acids and oligopeptides are absorbed and utilized for body needs, there seems to be a possibility that a small amount of peptide fragments escape further proteolysis and remains free within the intestinal lumen. This phenomenon is essentially due to the properties of the amino acid sequence in a protein molecule, which causes a block to the limited proteolysis of intestinal peptidases.

Recently, several studies have reported that proteolytic cleavage *in vitro* of cereal proteins and of caseins gives rise to peptide fragments having an opioid-like activity[1,10] or an inhibitory action on renin-angiotensin conversion[6].

This aspect of the field of nutrition seems to be attractive, since ingestion and the subsequent varying extent of alimentary digestive proteolysis of proteins results in the formation of widely diverse species of peptide fragment. If some of these peptides possess a biological activity, the overall effect must be altered if the process of digestion is changed, provided that the above mentioned *in vitro* events also occur within the intestinal tract.

In this respect, we have attempted to investigate whether the ingestion of different protein sources could directly affect mineral absorption. Most of the studies so far reported refer to the effect of dietary protein quality on mineral absorption, revealed by feeding trials of varying length. This kind of experiment discloses nutritional effects of protein quality which indirectly affect nutrient absorption through an alteration in the metabolism of the intestinal tissues.

In our experiments, rats were fed an experimental diet containing 200 g test protein/kg for only 1 or 2 days. Shortly after food intake, rats were killed, the small intestinal contents were flushed out and the amount of soluble or insoluble mineral was measured. Such an experiment ensures direct interactions between protein and minerals so we can assume some specific effects on mineral availability. Figure 1 shows that most of the minerals tested are very soluble in the

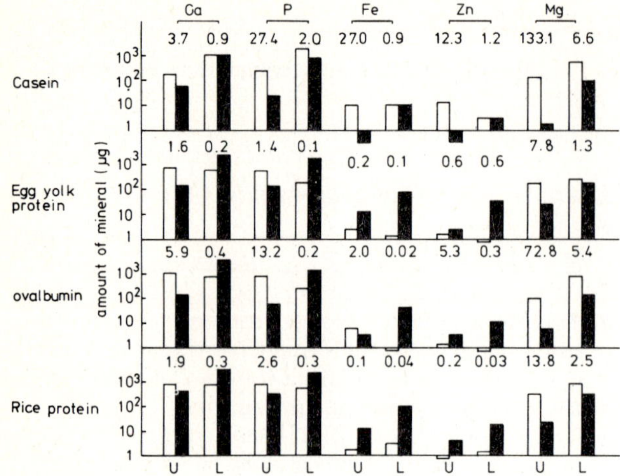

Fig. 1 *Distribution of soluble (□) and insoluble (■) forms of minerals in the upper (U) and lower (L) halves of small intestine of rats shortly after giving various protein diets (200 g protein/kg).* Figures on top of columns represent soluble/insoluble ratios.

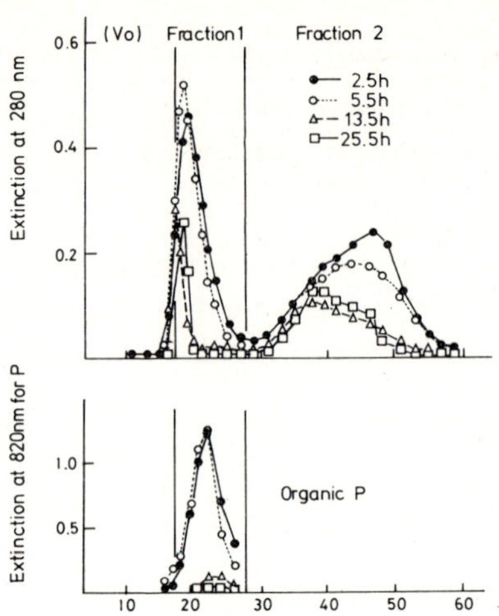

Fig. 2 *Changes in the elution patterns with period after meal for intestinal contents after ingestion of 200 g casein/kg diet.* V0, void volume; Fraction 1, macrophosphopeptides. (Lee *et al.*, 1980)

proximal portion of the small intestine, but tend to be insoluble in the distal portion where the pH shifts to become slightly alkaline. Among the dietary proteins tested, the effect of casein revealed most markedly the highest soluble/insoluble ratios of all five minerals. On the contrary, rice protein and egg yolk protein tended to increase the precipitation of minerals. These results suggest that the difference in the protein source might be a principal cause of altered solubility of minerals, though influences from some minor inclusions in protein materials cannot be neglected. Our attention was, at first, focused on the high solubility of Ca and Fe of the intestinal contents of rats fed casein diet.

Caseinphosphopeptides (CPP) and intestinal calcium absorption. When a semi-synthetic diet containing 200 g casein/kg was fed to rats, the small intestinal digesta appeared to contain a larger amount of soluble Ca and a small amount of macrophosphopeptides. The latter were separated by gel-filtration after precipitation of protein with trichloroacetic acid[3] Fig. 2. The administration of a diet containing β-casein gave rise to a phosphopeptide which was characteristically comprised of a major portion of the amino acid sequence of that obtained by trypsin digestion *in vitro*. This CPP, as well as tryptic CPP, exhibits a peculiar property of preventing the precipitation of calcium phosphate at physiological pH and temperature. Since, this inhibitory activity much diminished when CPP was previously dephosphorylated[7], the cost portion of CPP molecule, where adjacent sequenced phosphoserine residues are located (Fig. 3), seems to be essential for the onset of the inhibitory action.

The estimated amount of CPP in distal small intestine of rats shortly after feeding a casein diet, was less than 5 mg or 10^{-4} mol/l, which is enough to inhibit the precipitation of Ca. The increasing amount of soluble Ca in the distal small intestine raises the gradient concentration of Ca between lumen and blood plasma, which may lead to the stimulation of a passive type of Ca transport[4].

This enhancement in Ca absorption by CPP could be demonstrated *in situ* by the tied-loop method. The results (Table) are shown in comparison with rats fed soyabean protein isolate. Thus, it is assumed that milk and other dairy products contain at least two kinds of factor stimulating Ca absorption. Lactose is the one which has been known from earlier times, although the mechanism of its action on Ca transport is still unclear. CPP is another agent whose action is latent in the casein molecule but manifests during the intestinal digestion of casein. In this respect, surveys on cheese products are a matter of interest, because they contain

H₂N–Arg–Glu–Leu–Glu–Glu–Leu–Asn–Val–Pro–Gly–Glu–
(positions 1 ... 10)

Ile–Val–Glu–Ser–Leu–Ser–Ser–Ser–Glu–Glu–Ser–Ile–
(positions 15 ... 20, with P under Ser residues)

Thr–ArgOH
(position 25)

Fig. 3 *Primary structure of caseinphosphopeptide obtained by trypsin digestion of bovine β-casein. Arrows represent possible splitting positions in vivo within the small intestine.*

Table. *The absorption of Ca, observed by subtracting the amount of* ^{40}*Ca or* ^{45}*Ca in the ileal contents of rats killed 3.5 h (60 min after ligation) from those killed 2.5 h (0 min after ligation) after ingestion of a diet containing 200 g/kg of casein or soyaprotein isolate (SPI): Mean values ± s.e. for four rats. (Sato et al., unpublished)*

Diet	Casein	SPI
Absorption of ^{40}Ca(g)	81.5	36.3
Absorption of ^{45}Ca[a](dpm × 10⁶)	4.17 ± 0.55	1.35 ± 0.13**
Femur uptake of ^{40}Ca[b]	1.96 ± 0.37	0.58 ± 0.08*

[a] ^{45}CaCl₂ was injected into ileal loops (8 cm) at 0 min.
[b] Total radioactivity of femur/(sum of initial and final specific radioactivity of luminal contents/2). Difference between casein and SPI group was significant: **$P < 0.01$, *$P < 0.05$.

little lactose, but the beneficial effect of these foods on Ca utilization has been noted. Feeding cheese to rats led to an increase in the amount of soluble Ca in the luminal contents, suggesting the formation of CPP from cheese. Some sorts of phosphopeptide are also formed by microbial proteases during the ripening process of cheese.

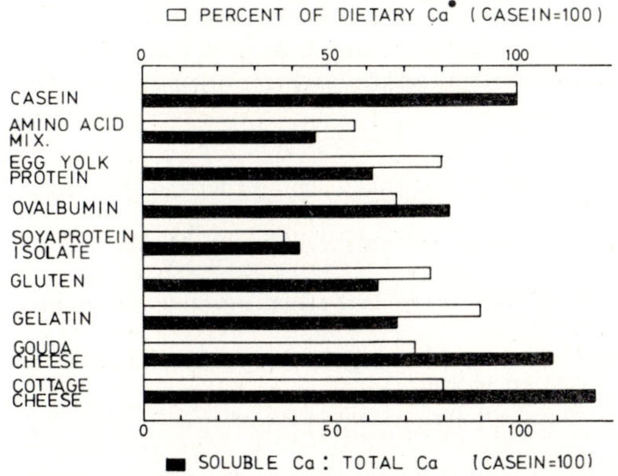

Fig. 4. *The amount of soluble Ca in whole small intestinal contents of rats given 200 g/kg protein diets.*

$$\text{*} \frac{\text{Soluble Ca/PEG in the contents}}{\text{Total Ca/PEG in the diet}} \times 100$$

PEG = polyethylene glycol.

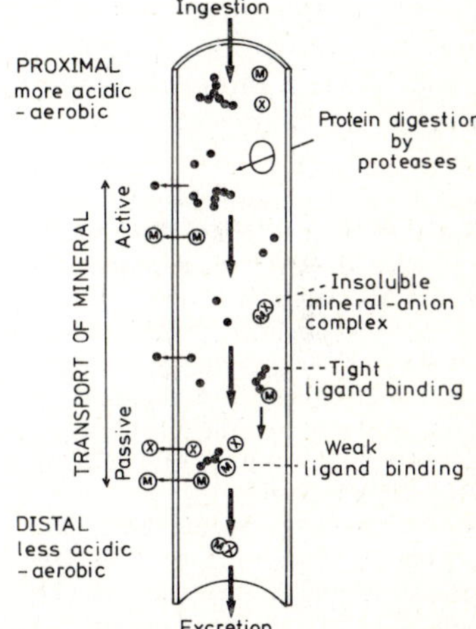

Fig. 5. *Schematic diagram showing the relationship between protein digestion and mineral absorption in the small intestine.*

These preformed CPPs seem to be equally effective on Ca utilization as those formed during luminal digestion. Because the quality of Ca solubilized by CPP was much larger than that of CPP, some ten- to 100-fold on a molar basis, these phosphopeptides may act simply as an inhibitor of hydroxyapatite crystal formation, and not as a carrier of ions.

Phosphopeptides and the utilization of iron. Although, the mechanism of the absorption of iron is far more complicated than that of Ca, its soluble form must be favourable to absorption, and the amount of soluble iron is also variable with the kind of dietary protein.

Feeding a casein diet increased the amount of soluble Fe compared with other protein sources (Fig. 1). On the contrary, feeding another type of phosphoprotein, phosvitin from hen egg yolk, strongly accelerated the precipitation of Fe within the intestinal lumen[9]. The interactions between CPP and Ca, and between phosvitin phosphopeptides and Fe, are the respective causes of enhancement and of deterioration in mineral absorption processes.

However, the mechanisms of these interactions between minerals and peptide substances affecting mineral absorption processes have not yet been well elucidated. Experimental results on the solubility of Ca and Fe in the presence of phosphopeptides *in vivo*, for example, seem to be quite different from those obtained from *in vitro* studies.

In *in vitro* systems, CPP plays a role as a catalytic agent of the oxidation of Fe^{2+} to Fe^{3+}, and the subsequent precipitation of iron[5].

However, the presence of CPP in the intestinal lumen seems to slow down the precipitation of iron. This is in contrast to the action of phosvitin phosphopeptides in accelerating the oxidation and precipitation of iron, both *in vivo* and *in vitro*[8,9]. These results suggest that the availability of minerals seems to be greatly influenced by the presence of peptides originated from dietary protein digests (Fig. 5). Food processing may also affect the availability of minerals by altering their solubility, although the latter may not always match the extent of absorption.

Conclusion. From the nutritional viewpoint, food protein is primarily utilized as a source of amino acids, and the availability of dietary minerals may be indirectly affected by the quality of protein which alters the efficiencies of nutrient absorption through changes in the metabolism of alimentary tissues. On the other hand, the absorption of minerals may be directly influenced by ingested proteins, because most minerals are more or less bound to proteins or peptides, and the strength of the binding is variable depending on the property of the ligands and on physiological environment.

In this paper, the author described a mineral-peptide interaction occurring within intestinal lumen after protein digestion, which causes the promotion or antagonism of mineral absorption.

It is very important to investigate the mechanism and effects of peptide-mineral interactions on mineral absorption, in order to improve the availability and to remove factors inhibitory to the absorption of minerals. Food processing should also be directed toward the improvement of mineral availability and other desirable food characteristics.

1 Brantle, V., Teschemachen, H., Henscham, A. & Lottsperch, F. (1980): Novel opioid peptides derived from casein (β-casomorphins). *Hoppe-Seyler's Z. Physiol. Chem.* **360**, 1211–1216.

2 Fujimaki, M. (1983): Systematic analyses of food functionalities and their development (in Japanese). *Jpn. Scientific Monthly* **36**, 690–694.

3 Lee, Y.S., Noguchi, T. & Naito, H. (1980): Phosphopeptides and soluble calcium in the small intestine of rats given a casein diet. *Br. J. Nutr.* **43**, 457–467.

4 Lee, Y.S., Noguchi, T. & Naito, H. (1983): Intestinal absorption of calcium in rats given diets containing casein or amino acid mixture: the role of casein phosphopeptides. *Br. J. Nutr.* **49**, 67–76.

5 Manson, W. & Cannon, H. (1978): The reaction of α_{s1} and β-casein with ferrous ions in the presence of oxygen. *J. Dairy Res.* **45**, 59–67.

6 Maruyama, S. & Suzuki, H. (1982): A peptide inhibitor of angiotensin I converting enzyme in the tryptic hydrolysate of casein. *Agric. Biol. Chem.* **46**, 1393–1394.

7 Sato, R., Noguchi, T. & Naito, H. (1983): The necessity for the phosphate portion of casein molecules to enhance Ca absorption from the small intestine. *Agric. Biol. Chem.* **47**, 2415–2417.

8 Sato, R., Lee, Y.S., Noguchi, T. & Naito, H. (1984): Iron solubility in the small intestine of rats fed egg yolk protein. *Nutr. Rep. Int.* **30**, 1319–1326.

9 Sato, R., Noguchi, T. & Naito, H. (1985): The formation and iron binding property of phosphopeptides in the small intestinal contents of rats fed egg yolk diet. *Nutr. Rep. Int.* **31**, 245–252.

10 Zioudrou, C., Streaty, R.A. & Klee, W.A. (1979): Opioid peptides derived from food proteins. The exorphins. *J. Biol. Chem.* **254**, 2446–2449.

Effects of processing of fats

M.H. GORDON
Food Science Department, University of Reading, Whiteknights, PO Box 226, Reading RG6 2AP, UK.

Fats are amongst the most heavily processed of all food components (Fig. 1). When extracted from plants, animals or fish, edible fats may be highly coloured, unpleasant tasting materials of poor quality. The food manufacturer aims to refine these fats into pale yellow materials with a bland flavour and high chemical stability such that the material is stable under normal processing conditions. Modification of the physical properties of the fat may also be required. These processes involve deliberate changes in the chemical composition of the fat, which may have nutritional consequences. Also, the use of fats in food products or food processes introduces the possibility of deterioration of the fat which may lead to loss of nutrients or formation of toxic components

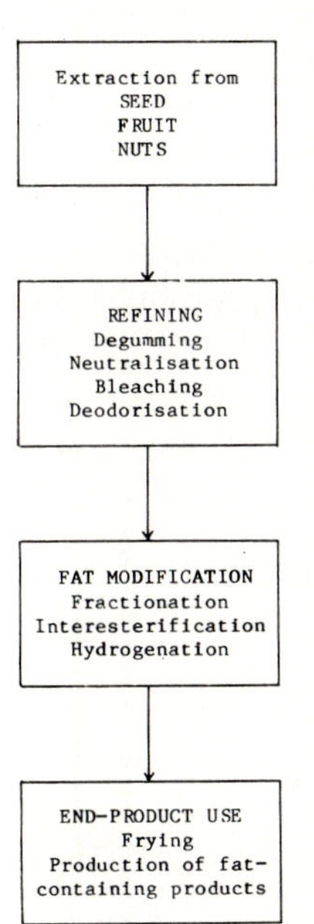

Fig. 1. *The processing of fats.*

Refining. The main aim of refining is the removal of small concentrations of components, which contribute strongly to the colour or odour of a fat. The first stage of the refining process is degumming. This involves the addition of hot water or hot phosphoric acid to precipitate gums which contain high concentrations of phospholipids. The next stage involves the addition of caustic alkali to neutralize the free fatty acids, which are removed by treatment with a bleaching earth. This is followed by the deodorization step, which involves passing superheated steam through the fat under high vacuum (typically 250 °C at 6 mm Hg pressure for 30 min) to remove volatile impurities.

The main changes of nutritional consequences during the refining of fats are the loss of some vitamin E and β-carotene. There is no change in composition of the triacylglycerols. In order to compensate for the loss of vitamin E, which serves as an antioxidant in the fat, synthetic antioxidants are added at the end of the refining process. Synthetic antioxidants are allowed in fats at levels up to 200 ppm, but research on the safety of these additives has intensified in recent years. It has been shown that butylated hydroxyanisole may induce cancer in the forestomach of rats, and both butylated hydroxyanisole and butylated hydroxytoluene may promote carcinogenesis in the bladder initiated by other carcinogens[14]. These studies have led to the banning of butylated hydroxyanisole as an additive in Japan.

Fat modification. Major changes in the composition of fats are caused by the fat modification techniques of fractionation, interesterification and hydrogenation. These techniques are mainly used in order to change the melting range and crystallization properties, and increase the stability of edible fats for use in food products.

Fractionation involves the physical separation of triacylglycerols into high melting and low melting fractions. There is no chemical change in the triacylglycerols, and the only nutritional consequences arise from the increased saturated and reduced polyunsaturated fatty acid content of the high melting fraction. Typical changes during fractionation are given in Table 1.

Interesterification is a chemical process which causes the randomization of fatty acids across all the triacylglycerols of the fat (Fig. 2). There have been reports that interesterification can affect the atherogenicity of edible oils. Studies on peanut oil showed that interesterification reduces the atherogenicity for cholesterol-fed rabbits and monkeys. The changes in the composition of the oil are shown in Table 2. Detailed studies indicated that the effects of interesterification were due to events subsequent to the release of cholesterol-containing chylomicrons and very-low-density lipoproteins by the small intestinal epithelial cells into the

Table 1. *Fractionation of palm kernel oil.* Data from Thomas & Paulicka (1976).

	Oil	Stearin	Olein
Melting pt (°C)	28.5	31	22.5
Yield		50%	50%
Fatty acid composition (%)			
Saturated	84.2	94.5	74.5
18:1	13.7	4.8	21.4
18:2	1.9	0.6	4.0

Table 2. *Changes in the major fatty acids at the 2-position of peanut oil (PNO) triacylglycerols after interesterification.* Data from Myher et al., (1977).

Fatty acid	PNO	Interesterified PNO
16:0	2.2	11.5
18:1	50.8	50.9
18:2	46.2	27.9

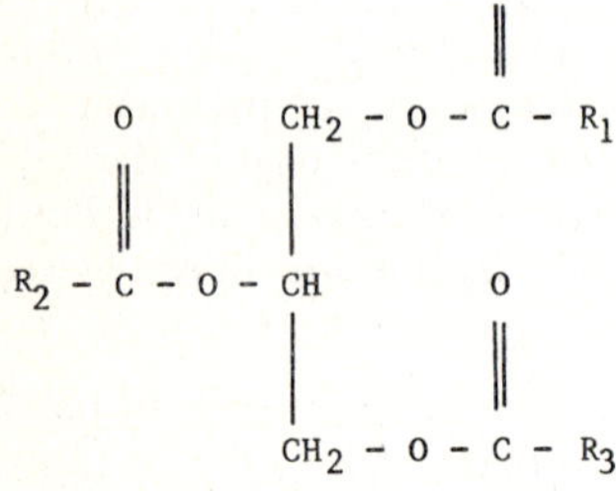

Fig. 2. *Changes in triacylglycerols during interesterification.*

plasma[25]. Pancreatic lipase which plays a key role in the conversion of triacylglycerols to monoacylglycerols in the duodenum is specific for fatty acids at the 1 and the 3 positions of the triacylglycerols, and therefore the fatty acid in the 2-position is retained in this position to a large extent during the biosynthesis of triacylglycerols and phospholipids.

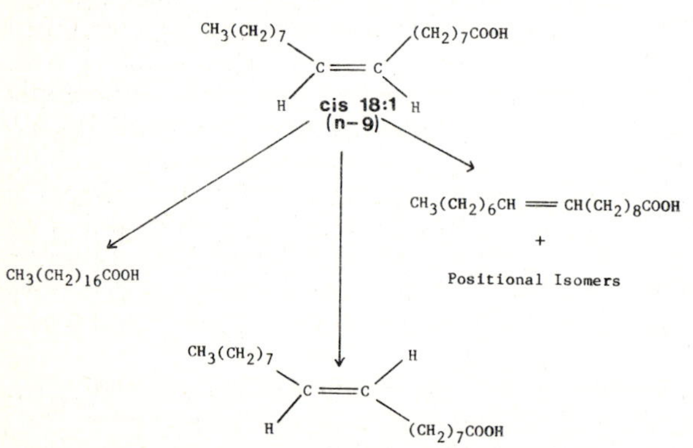

Fig. 3. *Changes in fatty acids during hydrogenation.*

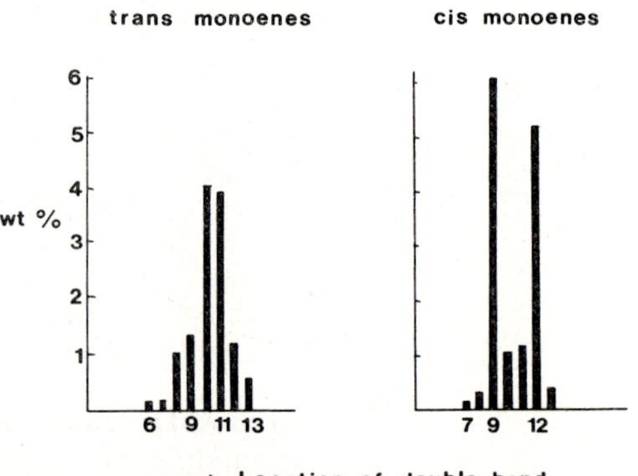

Fig. 4. *Formation of positional isomers during hydrogenation of linoleate.*

The hydrogenation of a fat causes major changes in the fatty acid composition. The degree of saturation of the fatty acids is increased, and isomerisation of unsaturated fatty acids also occurs with the conversion of the naturally occurring cis-unsaturated double bonds to trans-unsaturated double bonds (Fig. 3). A large number of positional isomers are formed (Fig. 4). These changes in composition are controlled by the manufacturer by the use of different catalysts and hydrogenation conditions, in order to achieve a fat with the desired physical properties and stability. About 24 per cent of the vegetable oils used in food products in the UK are hydrogenated. These hydrogenated fats are used in margarines, shortenings, chocolate-flavoured couvertures, and frying fats. Many margarines contain 20–40 per cent trans fatty acids, although samples with levels in excess of 60 per cent have been reported[3].

Table 3. *Fatty acid composition of soybean oil (SBO) and partially hardened soybean oil (HSBO).* HSBO(1), HSBO(2) and HSBO(3) were hydrogenated to iodine values of 110, 105, and 76 respectively. Data from Applewhite (1981).

Fatty acid	SBO	HSBO(1)	HSBO(2)	HSBO(3)
16:0	11	11	11	11
18:0	4.1	4.3	7	10
Cis - 18:1	22	29	33	18
Trans - 18:1	–	12	12	51
Cis-9, cis-12 - 18:2	54	31	22	–
Non-conjugated cis, trans - 18:2	– ⎰	6	10	9
Non-conjugated trans, trans - 18:2	–	–	–	–
Conjugated - 18:2	–	2	0.5	–
18:3	7.5	2.3	2.0	–

A complex mixture of trans fatty acids are formed during the hydrogenation of fats (Table 3). The fatty acids formed differ from natural fatty acids not only in the stereochemistry of the double bonds but also in the position of the double bonds along the fatty acid chain. There have been many studies relating to the absorption and metabolism of hydrogenated fats, and the effect of trans fatty acids on the metabolism of other fatty acids (reviews[2,4,16]).

Several studies have concentrated on the relationship between consumption of trans fatty acids and coronary heart disease (CHD). Alarming results were obtained from a swine-feeding study at the University of Illinois which appeared to demonstrate a relationship between consumption of trans fatty acids and atherosclerosis[17]. However, this interpretation has been strongly challenged, since allowance was not made for the high fat:protein ratio, and borderline essential fatty acid deficiency. Subsequent studies of young swine using higher protein:fat ratios and increased EFA levels failed to confirm any deleterious effects of trans fatty acids on swine atherosclerosis[15].

In experimental animals, trans, monounsaturated fatty acids tend to be similar to saturated fatty acids in their effect on serum lipids, but trials on man have produced divergent results[10]. Like saturated fatty acids, trans, monounsaturated fatty acids occur mainly in position 1 of phospholipids, whilst cis unsaturated fatty acids occupy position 2[22]. The similarity in the incorporation of trans, monounsaturated and saturated fatty acids into phospholipids is not surprising in view of the shapes of the fatty acids (Fig. 5), since this affects the packing of the molecules in membranes, which is relevant to the fluidity and permeability of the membrane. The phospholipids in membranes can influence the levels of activity of the constituent enzymes. Thus in one study, the red blood cells of animals fed hardened olive oil with a high trans content suffered haemolysis five times more rapidly than normal controls, and the liver mitochondria swelled two to three times faster than the controls[9]. These effects are similar to those observed in animals suffering essential fatty acid deficiency.

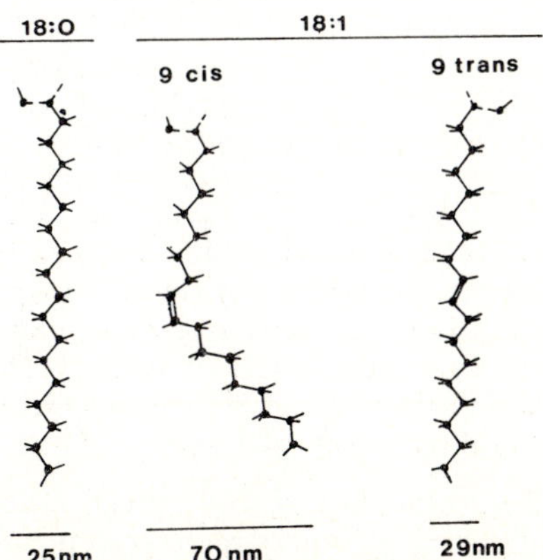

Fig. 5. *Shapes of fatty acids.*

In recent years there has been considerable research on the nutritional effects of specific trans fatty acids in the diet, since it is clear that polyunsaturated trans fatty acids have very different effects from monounsaturated trans acids, and there are also significant differences between positional isomers. Trans, trans-octadecadienoic acid has been shown to inhibit arachidonic acid synthesis in rats, resulting in low serum levels of prostaglandins[13]. As shown in Table 4, the synthesis of both PGE$_1$ from 20:3 (n-6) and PGE$_2$ from 20:4 (n-6) was reduced. It does appear, however, that trans, trans octadecadienoic acid is only present in food products based on hydrogenated fats in trace amounts[6]. The cis, trans isomers of linoleic acid occur in margarines in large amounts than the trans, trans isomer. However, research on the nutritional effects of the cis, trans isomer is limited due to the difficulty of synthesizing the fatty acid. It has been shown that cis-9, trans-12 but not cis-12, trans-9-octadecadienoic acid can be converted to an eicosatetraenoic acid[1].

Table 4. *Effect of dietary fatty acids on key platelet fatty acids and serum concentrations of prostaglandins.* Data from Hwang & Kinsella (1979).

Dietary fatty acids	20:3 (n-6) (%)	PGE$_1$ (ng/ml)	20:4 (n-6) (%)	PGE$_2$ (ng/ml)
Hydrogenated coconut oil	Trace	1.1	1.9	2.2
Trans, trans-18:2	Trace	0.2	1.4	0.2
Mixture of trans, trans-18:2				
+ cis, cis-18:2 (1:1)	0.1	3.5	14.1	11.6
Cis, cis-18:2	0.3	5.7	17.6	24.9

Table 5. *Effect of dietary cis-18:1 and trans-18:1 concentrates on PUFA in rat liver phosphatidylcholine (PC) (Lawson* et al. *1985).* Diets contained 23 per cent fat and their fat composition is shown at the foot of the table.

PUFA	Control	PHSO	Trans	Cis	1.5 Cis
18:2	10.1	13.3	16.0	8.8	8.9
20:3 n-9	0.67	0.45	0.39	1.9	2.6
20:4 n-6	20.5	12.0	10.9	17.1	14.4
20:5 n-3	1.0	1.6	2.0	0.8	0.7
Composition of fat (%)	21.2 beef tallow, 1.0 corn oil, 0.84 linseed oil	17.9 partially hardened soybean oil, 2.53 beef tallow, 1.61 corn oil, 0.99 linseed oil	20.02 trans concentrate*, 1.99 corn oil, 0.99 linseed oil	10.3 cis concentrate**, 10.9 beef tallow, 0.9 corn oil, 0.93 linseed oil	15.42 cis concentrate**, 5.75 beef tallow, 0.86 corn oil, 0.97 linseed oil

*Trans concentrate contained 5.8% Cis-18:1 and 41% trans-18:1
**Cis concentrate contained 28%-18:1 and 56% Cis-18:1

Significant differences in the metabolism of positional isomers of cis and trans monounsaturated fatty acids have been observed[12]. Differences in the rates of lipolysis, oxidative catabolism and incorporation into phospholipids have been observed for various positional isomers of oleic and elaidic acids. There have also been reports demonstrating that the rates of desaturation of these fatty acids, and their effect on the rates of desaturation and chain elongation of essential fatty acids show considerable variations. Table 5 summarizes the effect of unusual cis-18:1 and trans-18:1 isomers on the concentrations of n-6 and n-3 polyunsaturated fatty acids (PUFA) in liver phosphatidylcholine[19]. The data clearly show a suppression of the PUFA in the phospholipids.

Thus it is clear that the nutritional effects of hydrogenated fats can only be fully understood if further research on the effects of specific trans fatty acids is pursued. However, on the basis of the available information, the Committee on Medical Aspects of Food Policy (1984)[7] report recommended that trans fatty acids should be regarded as equivalent to saturated fatty acids for the purpose of recommendations on saturated fat intake and P/S ratios. Otherwise it made no specific recommendation about the dietary intake of trans fatty acids.

Heating of fats. Major changes occur in edible fats during their exposure to elevated temperatures. This is particularly important during commercial deep fat frying, where oils may be kept at temperatures of about 180 °C for several hours. High concentrations of oxidized and polymerized products are formed under these conditions. The nutritional implications of this deterioration have caused concern for many years[5]. It has been shown that if fats and oils are heated for very long periods at extremely high temperatures, the samples can become toxic. It was found that the feeding of heated fats to animals caused irritation of the gastrointestinal tract, diarrhoea and growth retardation[8]. In some cases the animals died. These dramatic results have been ascribed to uncommon compounds formed under the particularly extreme heating conditions used, and in some cases to the complete destruction of essential nutrients including linoleic acid.

A detailed study was performed of the nutritional effects of fats heated under normal frying conditions, containing 10–20 per cent oxidized and polymerized components[18]. Soybean oil and hardened groundnut oil, heated for 96 h at 175 °C, in the presence and absence of frying foods were fed to three generations of rats forming 10 per cent of the diet.

No deleterious effects were observed during this study, and it was concluded that heated fats were not harmful if they were not heated above normal frying temperatures.

This conclusion has been confirmed by several other studies in which edible fats were heated under normal food processing conditions. When the non-triacylglycerol fraction was isolated from fats heated under normal conditions[21], the heated fats themselves containing normal quantities of these oxidized and polymerized components produced no ill-effects on animals, although this fraction proved somewhat toxic when fed to animals in big doses.

There has been some interest in the extent to which oxidized and polymerized components of heated oils accumulate in body tissues. The tissues of rats which were fed heated soybean oil at a concentration of 20 per cent in their food for 2 months were investigated and the kidney fat, subcutaneous fat and fat extracted from the liver, were analysed[23]. The fat from the tissues contained less than 3 per cent of the degradation products, whereas the original heated fats contained up to 31 per cent of these compounds.

It was concluded that oxidized and polymerized triacylglycerols do not accumulate in body tissues. In particular, dimeric triacylglycerols were shown to be almost totally absent from the tissues although present at quite high levels in the heated fat. In the light of these studies, the German Society for Fat research has recommended[11] that a used frying fat should be discarded when the concentration of polar components reaches 27 per cent. Normally fats are discarded before they deteriorate to this extent because the flavour deteriorates and the colour darkens. Thus, it does not appear that used frying fats present a danger to health in practice.

Conclusions. Major changes in edible fats occur during food processing operations, with changes during hydrogenation and deep fat frying being the most significant. The physiological effects of fats subjected to these processes require further investigation. However, in the light of present knowledge it does appear that trans fatty acids can be considered as equivalent to saturated fatty acids in the diet, whilst fats used in deep fat frying can be consumed without ill effects as long as the fat has not been allowed to deteriorate excessively.

1 Anderson, R.L., Fullmer, C.S. Jr, & Hollenbach, E.J. (1975): Effects of the transisomers of linoleic acid on the metabolism of linoleic acid in rats. *J. Nutr.* **105**, 393–400.
2 Applewhite, T.H (1981): Nutritional effects of hydrogenated soya oil. *J. Am. Oil Chem. Soc.* **58**, 260–269.
3 Beare-Rogers, J.L., Gray, L.M. & Hollywood, R. (1979): The linoleic acid and trans fatty acids of margarines. *Am. J. Clin. Nutr.* **32**, 1805–1809.
4 Beare-Rogers, J.L. (1983): Trans and positional isomers of common fatty acids. In *Advances in nutritional research*, Vol. 5, ed H.H. Draper, pp. 171–200. New York: Plenum Press.
5 Billek, G. (1985): Heated fats in the diet. In *The role of fats in human nutrition*, ed F.B. Padley & J. Podmore, pp. 163–172, Chichester: Ellis Horwood.
6 Carpenter, D.L. & Slover, H.T. (1973): Lipid composition of selected margarines. *J. Am. Oil Chem. Soc.* **50**, 372–376.
7 Committee on Medical Aspects of Food Policy (1984): *Diet and cardiovascular disease.* London: HMSO.
8 Crampton, E.W., Common, R.H., Harmer, F.A., Berryhill, F.M. & Wiseblatt, L. (1951): *J. Nutr.* **44**, 177–189.
9 Decker, W.J. & W. Mertz. (1967): Effects of dietary elaidic acid on membrane function in rat mitochondria and erythrocytes. *J. Nutr,* **91**, 324–330.
10 Emken, E.A. & Dutton, H.J. (1979): *Geometrical and positional fatty acid isomers.* Champaign, Illinois: American Oil Chemists Society.

11 German Society for Fat Research (1979): Symposium Brat und Siedefette. *Fette Seifen Anstrichm.* **81**, 572–574.

12 Holman, R.T. (1985): Influence of hydrogenated fats on the metabolism of polyunsaturated fatty acids. In *The role of fats in human nutrition*, ed F.B. Padley & J. Podmore, pp. 48–61. Chichester: Ellis Horwood.

13 Hwang, D.L. & Kinsella, J.E. (1979): The effects of trans, trans methyl linoleate on the concentration of prostaglandins and their precursors in rats. *Prostaglandins* **17**, 543.

14 Imaida, K., Fukushima, S., Shirai, T., Ohtani, M., Nakanishi, K. & Ito, N. (1983): *Carcinogenesis* **4**, 895–899.

15 Jackson, R.L., Morrisett, J.D., Pownall, H.J., Gotto, A.M. Jr., Kamio, A., Imai, H., Tracy, R. & Kummerow, F.A. (1977): Influence of dietary trans-fatty acids on swine lipoprotein composition and structure. *J. Lipid Res.* **18**, 182–190.

16 Kinsella, J.E., Bruckner, G., Mai, J. & Shimp, J. (1981): Metabolism of trans fatty acids with emphasis on the effects of trans, trans-octadecadienoate on lipid composition, essential fatty acids, and prostaglandins: An overview. *Am. J. Clin. Nutr.* **34**, 2307–2318.

17 Kummerow, F.A., Mizuguchi, T., Arima, T., Cho, B.H.S., Huang, W.Y. & Tracy, R.E. (1978): *Artery* **4**, 360.

18 Lang, R. (1978): *Z. Ernährungswiss.* Suppl. 21.

19 Lawson, L.D., Hill, E.G. & Holman, R.T. (1985): Dietary fats containing concentrates of cis or trans octadecenoates and the patterns of polunsaturated fatty acids of liver phosphatidylcholine and phosphatidylethanolamine. *Lipids* **20**, 262–267.

20 Myler, J.J., Marai, L., Kuksis, A. & Kritchevsky, D. (1977): Acylglycerol structure of peanut oil of different atherogenic potential. *Lipids.* **12**, 775–785.

21 Nolen, G.A., Alexander, J.C., Artman, N.R. (1967): Long-term feeding study with used frying fats. *J. Nutr.* **93**, 337–348.

22 Reichwald-Hacker, I., Grosse-Oetringhaus, S., Kiewitt, I. & Mukherjee, K.D. (1980): Molecular structure of glycerolipids in rats fed partially hydrogenated triacylglycerols. *J. Nutr.* **110**, 1122–1129.

23 Strauss, H.J. & Billek, G. (1974): Nutritional and physiological properties of frying fats V. *Z. Ernährungswiss.* **13**, 81–88.

24 Thomas, A.E. & Paulicka, F.R. (1976): Solvent fractionated fats. *Chem. Ind.* 774–779.

25 Tso, P., Pinkston, G., Klurfeld, D. & Kritchevsky, D. (1984): The absorption and transport of dietary cholesterol in the presence of peanut oil or randomised peanut oil. *Lipids* **19**, 11–16.

Effects of processing on proteins

J. MAURON
Nestlé Ltd, Research Department, Avenue Nestlé 55, CH-1800 Vevey, Switzerland.

Protein reactions and interactions. *Formation of iso-peptides.* Severe heating of relatively pure proteins leads to the formation of internal peptide links between the ε-amino group of lysine and amide groups in the protein (asparagine, glutamine)[3]. These internal peptide links represent a steric hindrance for the digestive enzymes and can make parts of the protein nutritionally unavailable.

It should be noted that the free iso-peptide ε-(γ-glutamyl)-lysine is fully available as source of lysine for both rats and chicks since it is hydrolyzed in the kidneys[6]. The free ε-(β-aspartyl)-lysine is, on the other hand, nutritionally unavailable.

Lysinoalanine formation. Lysinoalanine (LAL) can be formed in proteins by reaction of lysine with dehydroalanine produced by cysteine and serine degradation. It can be formed in considerable amounts during alkaline treatments of protein-containing foods but can also be present in heated foodstuffs, including milk products[9]. LAL is absent from spray-dried milk powders. UHT treatment followed by aseptic filling gives much less LAL than HTST or conventional in-can sterilization (300; 540; 710 mg/kg protein). LAL formation in food proteins has been reviewed extensively[7]; in general, one may state that LAL is possibly a toxicological problem, not a nutritional one. Indeed, it has been shown to produce renal cytomegaly in rats. The latter has, however, never been found in any other species, and even in rats it is reversible. The LD-isomer of LAL is about ten times more active at provoking cytomegaly than the LL-form[5]. Since the kidney lesions were observed only in the rat and are reversible, there is no need to fix limits for the presence of lysinoalanine in foods (Codex Alimentarius, document CX/VP 82/5).

In infant formulas, however, it would still be wise to limit the lysinoalanine formation in using the least severe sterilization process possible.

Racemization. Alkaline treatments are today a classic processing operation for plant proteins. There have been several reports of the racemization of amino acids during food processing by alkaline treatments[18], as well as in protein-sugar and protein-fat reactions[12]. The racemization of amino acids in differently processed proteins has been studied in our laboratory (Table 1)[17]. When five commercially prepared products containing soya protein or sodium caseinate were analysed, including a soya-based infant formula, it was reported that 9 to 17 per cent of the aspartic acid was in the D-form[8]. Racemization does not play an important role in food processing but, with the increased use of alkaline treatments, the danger of racemization increases and should be kept under control.

Table 1. *Percentage of D-amino acids in food proteins after varying treatments.* 50% D-amino acid = 100% Racemization.

Amino acid	Chicken muscle (2 h at 121°C)	Milk powder (20 min at 230°C)	Casein solution (1 h at 80°C) 0.2M NaOH	1M NaOH
Ala	0	3	20	42
Val	0	0	4	18
Leu	0	2	9	34
Ileu	1	0	4	30
Cys	0	0	–	–
Met	0	0	30	43
Phe	0	1	31	44
Lys	0	0	13	41
Asp	15	31	37	51
Glu	0	9	28	42
Ser	1	0	44	54
Thr	0	0	28	34
Tyr	1	0	14	49
Hist	–	–	36	49

Protein-carbohydrate interactions. *The Maillard reaction.* The reaction of proteins with reducing sugars is the major source of nutritional damage to food proteins during processing and storage[19].

Early Maillard reactions. The first step involves the condensation reaction between the carbonyl group of the reducing sugar and the amino-group of lysine. The reaction rapidly proceeds via the Schiff base to the deoxy-ketose compound or Amadori rearrangement product. This is a relatively stable derivative and is the major form of blocked lysine after early Maillard reactions. At this stage, there is no colour formation. The main consequence of the early Maillard reactions is the loss of nutritive value since lysine blocked with its ε-amino group in the form of the Amadori compound (fructose-lysine) was shown to be biologically unavailable in the rat. Upon acid hydrolysis fructose-lysine yields furosine (32 per cent in milk products), that can be used to determine the percentage of lysine residues blocked as lactulosyl lysine during the processing of milk (Table 2), using the formula[19]:

$$\% \text{ blocked lysine} = \frac{3.1 \text{ furosine} \times 100}{\text{total lysine} + 1.87 \text{ furosine}}$$

Advanced Maillard reactions. Under more severe heating conditions, the Maillard reaction proceeds further to the different advanced steps; they lead to the formation of literally thousands of compounds which are responsible for the numerous flavours and odours in heated foods. Recently it has been shown that fructose-lysine can be degraded in an advanced Maillard reaction to N^{ε}-carboxymethyl-lysine[24]. The later stage of the advanced Maillard reaction

Table 2. *Blockage of lysine as Amadori product in milk products.*
UHT = Ultra high temperature; HTST = high temperature short
time.

Heat process	% Blocked lysine
Freeze-drying	0
Pasteurization	0
UHT sterilization	0–2
Spray-drying	0–2
Spray-drying infant formula	5–10
HTST sterilization	5–10
Conventional sterilization	10–15
Roller drying	20–50
Spray-drying lactose-hydrolysed milks or casein-glucose mixtures	15–70

results in the formation of a great number of heterocyclic compounds involving oxygen, nitrogen and sulphur.

Final Maillard reactions. The final phase of the Maillard reaction produces the brown melanoidin pigments. It appears that they have a molecular weight above 1000 and are chemically and biologically relatively inert substances.

Experimental separation of early and advanced Maillard damage in storage experiments. Whole milk powders containing 2.5 per cent moisture were stored for several weeks at 60 °C and 70 °C and the fate of lysine, methionine and tryptophan was investigated[15]. Storage at 60 °C is an example of early Maillard damage. After 9 weeks storage, the product still retained its natural colour, even though about 40 per cent of the lysine was blocked as lactulosyl lysine. Methionine, cystine, tryptophan and leucine were stable. At 70 °C, 50 per cent of the lysine units were blocked as lactulosyl lysine after only 2 weeks storage; from 3 weeks onwards the product became a deep red brown colour as lactulosyl lysine degraded and advanced Maillard reactions took place. Lysine was destroyed and available methionine and tryptophan, as measured by *Streptococcus zymogenes*, were progressively reduced, due to an impairment of protein digestibility (cross-link formation). It is interesting to note that at 60 °C storage temperature, the Maillard reactions stops at the early stage, whereas at 70 °C, the advanced Maillard reactions takes place. The high lysine losses at 70 °C are somewhat academic since the brown products are organoleptically unacceptable. Of greater practical importance is the fact that at 60 °C there is a great reduction of available lysine without any significant change in product colour.

Protein-oxidized lipid interactions. The oxidation of unsaturated lipids proceeds in three steps, ie the formation of (a) primary products (hydroperoxides); (b) secondary products (aldehydes, ketones, etc.); (c) stable compounds (carboxylic acids and polymerization products).

A study of the interaction between protein and lipid oxidation products has been made in our laboratory[21], incubating whey protein with methyllinolenate under varying conditions of temperature, water activity and oxygen tension. There were important losses of lysine and moderate of tryptophan. Separate determination of methionine and methionine sulphoxide showed extensive oxidation of methionine to its sulphoxide. All amino acid losses showed the same pattern: degradation was highest at high water activity, excess oxygen and high temperature. Methionine reacted most rapidly followed by lysine and, after a time, tryptophan. This is in accordance with the proposed mechanisms, namely that methionine is oxidized by the hydroperoxides, whereas lysine reacts with the carbonyls formed on hydroperoxide degradation. The low reactivity of tryptophan would indicate that it reacts only with some very active secondary degradation products.

Growth trials and N-balance studies on rats confirmed the results concerning amino acid losses obtained chemically; with increasing water activity and temperature, the values of protein efficiency ratio, true digestibility and biological value fell. The losses in bioavailability (slope ratio rat assay) were least for tryptophan, intermediate for sulphur amino acids and highest for lysine.

Protein-polyphenol interactions. In modern plant processing, protein extraction with alkali is a frequent operation during which browning reaction with polyphenols can occur.

The quinones (oxidation products of polyphenols) can react with the free amino group of lysine. The mechanism of this reaction is not yet completely understood. Two initial reactions can be envisaged: lysine reacts with its ε-amino group at the position 6 of the quinone molecule forming a substituted quinone or the ε-amino group of lysine could form a Schiff base with the keto group of the quinone (alkaline conditions). Further reactions lead then to complexes between the lysine substituted and ordinary quinones. In our laboratory the polyphenol-protein reaction has been studied using a model system containing casein and caffeic acid[14]. They found that the *in vivo* loss of availability was greatest for lysine, moderate for methionine and smaller for tryptophan. It was greater in the sample treated at pH 10.0 than in that treated with tyrosinase at pH 7.0. The loss of *in vivo* availability was due in part to reduced protein digestibility and in part to specific reactions of the amino acid side-chains. Lysine appeared to form covalent lysine-caffeoquinine complexes.

Pyrolysis. Heating foodstuffs at temperatures above 300 °C leads to so-called pyrolysis reactions. Since pyrolysis compounds can be formed from pure proteins, they must be distinguished from the Maillard reaction.

Health aspects of processing damage to proteins. For many decades, processing damage to proteins has been almost synonymous with loss in nutritive value or in amino acid availability. It was only in the 60s that the possibility of the formation of anti-nutritive or even toxic substances during processing was envisaged. The toxicological aspects of Maillard reaction products have been discussed[16,19].

Fructose-lysine (FL) in heated protein-glucose mixtures induces a renal lesion in rats which is similar to that induced by LAL[25]. It has been suggested that chelation of zinc ions may be involved in the development of the lesion[13] and it has been shown that casein-glucose mixtures fed to rats increased the urinary zinc in proportion to the FL content[10]. The effect was only partly due to lysine-deficiency.

A more recent development is the detection of the formation of mutagenic compounds during food processing. In 1978, it was reported that mutagens are found in commercial beef extract, as well as in ground beef hamburgers when they are cooked at temperatures around 200 °C[4]. Although the heating conditions in beef extract and grilled hamburgers are quite different (100 °C for a day against ∼ 200 °C for a minute), the mutagens formed are similar in both cases and were found to be imidazo-derivatives of quinoxaline and quinoline (IQx; IQ)[11]. These mutagens must be considered as the product of an advanced Maillard reaction which is known to produce nitrogen heterocyclics. They are also highly carcinogenic[23].

Another kind of mutagen is found in the charred part of fish and beef. This mutagenic activity is due to pyrolysis. Indeed, pyrolysates of proteins, peptides and amino acids can be highly mutagenic[22]. It is important to note that mutagenic activity appeared only at pyrolysis temperatures above 400 °C. These mutagens are therefore different from those found in beef extract and grilled hamburgers which are of the very advanced Maillard type.

Still another group of completely different mutagens is found in moderately heated or carbohydrate rich foods, such as bakery products, coffee and tea. These compounds are relatively weak mutagens and they are generally metabolically deactivated by microsomes[2]. These products correspond to the moderately advanced Maillard compounds, formed under not too severe conditions in food relatively rich in carbohydrates.

The influence of the different parameters in the Maillard reaction on mutagenicity has been studied systematically in our laboratory using reaction models (glucose-amino acid mixtures)[1]. The most interesting result of these model assays is that mutagenicity increases in parallel with the formation of brown pigments, but only up to a certain point, after which increased browning did not increase mutagenicity any more, on the contrary (Table 3). It should also be noted that the Amadori product of ε-N-lysine with fructose was not mutagenic in the Ames test.

Table 3. *Correlation between mutagenicity and browning* (S-9 = microsomal activation mix).

Coefficient of browning (ext 480 nm, 1% DM)	Mutation frequency of Ames tester strain TA 100 250 mg reaction product per plate	
	−S-9	+S-9
0.15	1.5	1.1
0.30	19	1.3
0.50	2.2	1.6
0.80	2.8	1.7
1.00	1.8[a]	1.6
1.50	1.7[a]	1.5
3.00	1.7[a]	1.4

[a] 125 mg reaction product per plate.

The sequence of events during the progression of the Maillard reaction seems therefore to be the following: during the initial, colourless stage of the Maillard reaction, the products formed are not mutagenic; then, with the appearance of the first brown products, mutagenicity increases in parallel to browning, but diminishes again in the final stage of the Maillard reaction. In addition, in protein rich foods such as meat and fish, the advanced Maillard reaction can take a particular pathway to yield strongly mutagenic substances. For all Maillard reactions, mutagenicity increases with pH, temperature and reaction time — except for the final stage.

I would like to propose a coherent but tentative scheme in order to try to clarify the situation as regards the relationship between mutagenicity and heat damage to proteins (Table 4). This is certainly an over-simplified generalization but may help to order the great number of findings in this field.

Table 4. *Heat damage and mutagenicity — a simplified overview.* TA = tester strains, S-9 = microsomal activation mix.

Type of damage	Compound	Mutagenicity			
		TA-100		TA-98	
		+S-9	−S-9	+S-9	−S-9
I. Early Maillard	Amadori	0			
II. 1 Advanced Maillard	Enediols				
Mild conditions	Reductones	0	++		
(early browning)	1,2-dicarbonyls				
or carbohydrate-rich food	Maltol	++	0	0	0
2 Advanced Maillard	Quinolines			++++	0
Severe conditions	Quinoxalines				
(late browning)					
protein-rich food					
III. Final Maillard	Melanoidins	0			
IV. Pyrolysis	α,γ-Carbolines			+++	0
	Pyrido-imidazoles				

Conclusions. Millions of tons of foods are saved every year through processing and proper storage. Interactions between food constituents are the price we have to pay for it.

Although the precise chemical mechanisms of the different interactions is not yet fully elucidated, we can state that we have most of them under control and can now orient with processing operations in the desired way to obtain a maximal benefit with a minimum of draw-back (for a review see also: Mauron, 1985[20]).

1 Aeschbacher, H.U. (1982): The significance of mutagens in food. In *Mutagens in our environment*, ed M. Sorsa & M. Vainio, pp. 349–362. New York: Liss.

2 Aeschbacher, H.U., Chappuis, Ch., Manganel, M. & Aeschbach, R. (1981): Investigation of Maillard products in bacterial mutagenicity test systems; in *Progress in food and nutrition science*, Vol. 5: *Maillard reactions in food*, ed C. Eriksson, pp. 291. Oxford: Pergamon.

3 Bjarnason, J. & Carpenter, K.J. (1970): Mechanisms of heat damage in proteins. *Br. J. Nutr.* **24**, 313–329.

4 Commoner, B., Vithayathil, A. & Dolara, P. (1978): Mutagenic analysis as a means of detecting carcinogens in foods. *J. Fd Prot.* **41**, 996–1003.

5 Feron, V.J., van Beek, V.S., Slump, L. & Beems, R.B. (1978): Toxicological aspects of alkali treatment of food protein. Biochemical aspects of protein food. *FEBS Lett.* **44**, 139–147.

6 Finot, P.A., Mottu, F., Bujard, E. & Mauron, J. (1978): N-substituted lysines as sources of lysine in nutrition; in *Nutritional improvement of food and feed proteins*, ed M. Friedman. pp. 549–570. New York: Plenum Press.

7 Finot, P.A. (1983): Lysinoalanine in food proteins. *Nutr. Abstr. Rev. Clin. Nutr.* A **53**, 67–80.

8 Friedman, M., Zahnley, J.C. & Masters, P.M. (1981): Relationship between in vitro digestibility of casein and its content of lysinoalanine and D-amino acids. *J. Fd Sci.* **46**, 127–134.

9 Fritsch, R.J. & Klostermeyer, H. (1981): Bestandesaufnahme zum Vorkommen von Lysinoalanin in milcheiweis- shaltigen Lebensmitteln. *Z. Lebensmittelunters. -Forsch.* **172**, 440–445.

10 Furniss, D.E., Hurrell, R.F. & Finot, P.A. (1985): Excessive urinary zinc excretion in the rat associated with the feeding of Maillard reaction products. Nordic Symp. Loen (Norway) on Metabolism of trace elements related to human diseases.

11 Hargraves, W.A. & Pariza, M.W. (1983): Purification and mass spectral characterization of bacterial mutagens from commercial beef extract. *Cancer Res.* **43**, 1467–1472.

12 Hayase, F., Kato, H. & Fujimaki, M. (1979): Racemization of amino acid residues in proteins during roasting. *Agric. Biol. Chem.* **37**, 191–192.

13 Hayashi, R. (1982): Lysinoalanine as a metal chelator. *J. Biol. Chem.* **257**, 13896–13898.

14 Hurrell, R.F., Finot, P.A. & Cuq, J.L. (1982): Protein-polyphenol reactions. 1. Nutritional and metabolic consequences of the reaction between oxidized caffeic acid and lysine residues of casein. *Br. J. Nutr.* **47**, 191–211.

15 Hurrell, R.F., Finot, P.A. & Ford, J.E. (1983): Storage of milk powders under adverse conditions. 1. Losses of lysine and other essential amino acids. *Br. J. Nutr.* **49**, 343–354.

16 Lee, T.C., Kimiagar, M., Pintauro, S.J. & Chichester, C.O. (1981): Physiological and safety aspects of Maillard browning of foods; in *Progress in food and nutrition science, Vol. 5: Maillard reactions in food*, ed C. Eriksson, pp. 243–256. Oxford: Pergamon Press.

17 Liardon, R. & Hurrell, R.F. (1983): Amino acid racemization in heated and alkali-treated proteins. *J. Agric. Fd Chem.* **31**, 432–437.

18 Masters, P.M. & Friedman, M. (1979): Racemization of amino acids in alkali treated food proteins. *J. Agric. Fd Chem.* **27**, 507–511.

19 Mauron, J. (1981): The Maillard reaction in food: a critical review from the nutritional standpoint: in *Progress in food and nutrition science. Vol. 5: Maillard reactions in food*, ed C. Eriksson, pp. 5–35. Oxford: Pergamon Press.

20 Mauron, J. (1985): Influence of processing on protein quality. *Bibl. Nutr. Dieta* **34**, 56–81.

21 Nielsen, H.K. (1984): Nutritional aspects of reactions between oxidizing lipid and protein with emphasis on tryptophan. Thesis No 865, University of Fribourg, Switzerland.

22 Sugimura, T. (1978): Let's be scientific about the problem of mutagens in cooked food. *Mut. Res.* **55**, 149–152.

23 Sugimura, T. (1985): Carcinogenicity of mutagenic heterocyclic amines formed during the cooking processing. *Mut. Res.* **150**, 33–41.

24 Thorpe, S.R., Baynes, J.M. & Ahmed, M.V. (1985): Commun. 3rd Int. Symp. on the Maillard Reaction, Tokyo (July 1985).

25 von Wangenheim, B., Hänichen, T. & Erbersdobler, H. (1984): Histopathologische Untersuchungen an Rattennieren nach Fütterung hitzegeschädigter Proteine. *Z. Ernährungswiss.* **23**, 219–229.

Effects of food processing on vitamins

A.E. BENDER
2, Willow Vale, Fetcham, Leatherhead, Surrey, KT22 9TE, UK.

It seems to be accepted generally that processing damages vitamins (and other nutrients) so that manufactured foods are regarded as being nutritionally inferior to the domestic equivalent. For example the policy statement of the American Medical Association (1982) states, *inter alia*, that nutrient losses can occur in storage, processing or handling of foods and that restoration helps to assure that the levels of nutrients in the food are similar to those originally present. Such restoration would almost inevitably bring the levels of nutrients above those in the domestic equivalent. The statement continues by emphasizing that good processing techniques should be employed to conserve nutrients.

However, the passage of foodstuffs through the factory does not necessarily produce nutritionally inferior products and there is no simple statement that can summarize the effect of processing on the vitamin and nutrient content of processed foods.

Over the past century and a half a range of processes — canning, oven and vacuum drying, various chemical treatments and freezing — were introduced before much was known about nutrients and nutrition, but there is no evidence that such processes have had any detrimental effects although any conclusions are clouded by the simultaneous increase in variety and availability of foods.

However, any novel foods or processes that are expected to replace traditional foods to any extent will, in the light of our present knowledge, require detailed investigation.

Prediction of losses. Nutritional labelling makes it increasingly necessary to be able to predict the stability of the vitamins in a processed food. This is fraught with difficulties. Vitamin C, for example, would appear to present a relatively simple system but there are conflicting reports that the destruction of vitamin C follows a first order reaction or a second order reaction[7,9,20]. It has been pointed out that the destruction of vitamin C occurs through varying mechanisms including oxidation and non-enzymic browning[11]. In the latter reaction, activation energy increases with decreasing moisture content, while the reverse is true for vitamin-enriched cereal mixtures.

Even greater complexity was revealed when 15 cultivars of green beans grown under the same conditions were examined[13]. These cultivars were found to differ in: (1) their vitamin C content; (2) the proportions of ascorbic to dehydroascorbic acid; (3) the amounts of these extracted into the canning brine, and (4) the amounts destroyed in canning under two sets of conditions.

Benefits of processing. When discussing the effects of processing on nutrients the benefits are often ignored. The principal benefit, of course, is the preservation of the food itself but processing has a marked effect on preserving vitamins despite any immediate loss.

There can be extremely rapid loss of vitamin C from freshly harvested foods. It was reported that there was 5–18 per cent loss of vitamin C within 2 h of harvesting green leaves, increasing to 38–66 per cent after 10 h, the time at which they were locally purchased[8].

Folate appears to be similarly unstable with the added complication of some apparent conversion of the complex derivatives, thought to be largely unavailable, into the free, available form (Table 1)[4,15]. Endive lost 10 per cent of the total folate in 6 h after harvesting when stored at 23 °C, increasing to 20 per cent after 24 h.

An additional benefit of processing is the liberation of bound, unavailable, niacin from cereals on heat and/or alkaline treatment, and the synthesis of niacin from trigonelline on roasting coffee. Sprouting and fermentation can increase the vitamin content.

Table 1. *Loss of folate after harvesting (µg/100g dry wt).* Nik-Daud (1983).

| Time (h) | Endive stored at 23°C | | | | Time (d) | Brussels sprouts stored at 18°C | | | |
| | Free folate | | Total folate | | | Free folate | | Total folate | |
	content	% loss	content	% loss		content	% loss	content	% loss
0	390		1845		0	280		2220	
6	345	−12	1660	−10	4	320	+15	1740	−20
24	315	−20	1450	−20	7	340	+20	1300	−40
48	420	+ 7	1160	−40					

Perspective. There are numerous papers describing losses of vitamins during manufacture but before drawing any conclusions it is essential to view these findings in perspective[2].

Some losses are intentional. Where a process involves a selection of the more attractive part of a food — such as milling to produce white flour or rice, and evisceration of fish, and selection of the more palatable parts of fruits and vegetables — the concomitant discard is a loss of vitamins and, of course, all nutrients. Such a loss is not inherent in processing as such but presumably a response to consumer demand and so the loss, if it is so regarded, is intentional.

Some losses are inevitable. Under the most carefully controlled laboratory conditions some loss of vitamins is inevitable, especially water-soluble vitamins and those more sensitive to heat.

Table 2. *Vitamin C content of garden peas (mg/100 g).* Robertson & Sissons (1966).

Process	Freshly cooked		Frozen	Freeze-dried	Air-dried	Canned
Cooking time (min)	10	10	3.5	2	15	'boil'
Vitamin C content	16.4[a]	18.5[b]	14	15.8	11.3	9.2

[a] and [b] are duplicate samples.

Table 2 shows the losses of vitamin C from green peas that have been freshly cooked — presumably the standard comparison for processing — which, is virtually the same as the loss in several established factory processes.

Some losses are in place of those incurred domestically, not additional. Many manufactured foods are partly or completely cooked so that the consumer cooks them for a shorter time than would be needed for the raw food; or they can be consumed without any further treatment. Table 3 indicates some of the stages of losses in various processes including the final reheating by the consumer.

Table 3. *Cumulative loss (per cent) of vitamin C.* Mapson (1956).

Processing procedure	Fresh	Frozen	Canned	Air-dried	Freeze-dried
Successive	—	Blanch 25	Blanch 30	Blanch 25	Blanch 25
stages in	—	Freeze 25	Can 37	Drying 55	Drying 30
the processing	—	Thaw 29			
Final processing	Cook 56	Cook 61	Heat 64	Cook 75	Cook 65
by consumer					

Comparisons must be made 'on the plate'. Errors arise from comparisons of the food before and after treatment when the storage period is not taken into account. Many foods, especially dried and canned foods are stored for long periods, up to several years, before consumption and need to be examined at the time of consumption — 'on the plate' — rather than at the end of the factory production line.

Table 4. *Percentage loss of vitamins from canned meals after canning and storage at 22 ± 2°C. Hellendoorn et al. (1971).*

| | | | Percentage loss after | | |
| | Initial | | | Storage | |
Vitamin	value[a]	Canning	1.5 years	3 years	5 years
Vitamin A	16.5 µg	50	100	—	—
Vitamin E	80 mg	0	0	50	50
Thiamin	9 mg	50	75	75	75
Riboflavin	6 mg	0	0	0	0
Pyridoxine	5 mg	0	0	0	0
Vitamin B_{12}	18 µg	0	0	0	0
Niacin	110 mg	10	20	20	20
Pantothenate	21 mg	25	50	50	50
Folic acid	14 µg	0	0	0	0
Inositol	26 mg	0	0	0	0
Choline	27 mg	0	0	0	0

[a]Total per can (ie meal).

Few reports include such storage; Table 4 reveals the storage losses as well as the initial processing loss.

Treatment with sulphite not only caused some immediate loss of thiamin but enhanced the subsequent loss on frying (Table 5).

Table 5. *Loss of thiamin from half potatoes soaked for 16 h in water or metabisulphite solution and subsequently fried (thiamin content in 2 mm slices, µg/100 g). Oguntona & Bender (1976).*

| | Soaked in water | | | Soaked in sulphite | | |
	Raw	Fried	Loss %	Raw	Fried	Loss %
1st layer	39.2	35.2	10.2	20.6	16.5	19.9
2nd layer	42.5	38.2	10.1	30.3	23.6	22.1
3rd layer	41.7	37.3	10.6	32.0	25.2	21.2

The role of the food in the whole diet must be taken into account. Some of the losses of nutrients in processing are unimportant in the diet as a whole. The loss of vitamin A appears to be considerable, but the amount initially present was so small that it is of no significance if all had been preserved or all had been destroyed (Table 4). The reverse is true of the thiamin since the content was so high that even after 75 per cent loss the food was still a rich source of this vitamin.

However, there are sections of the population who may be relying more heavily than the average on individual foods so that losses of vitamins that are insignificant in the average diet might be important to them.

Losses must be balanced against advantages. Apart from the beneficial effects discussed earlier, processing confers certain advantages even where there is an accompanying loss of nutrients. When milk is pasteurized there is a loss of about 25 per cent of the vitamin C and 10 per cent of some of the other vitamins but this would generally be regarded as a price worth paying for microbiological safety.

Outstanding problems. *Analytical methods.* Some reports on vitamin C suffer from the wrong selection of method of analysis. The simple titration with dichlorophenol indophenol does not measure the biologically active dehydroascorbic acid (DHA) unless this is reduced back to ascorbic acid (AA).

Raw fruits and vegetables vary enormously in their proportions of AA and DHA[6,14] and in the proportion of AA converted into DHA on processing.

Before 1971 it was accepted practice to determine provitamin A activity as total carotenoids but it was then shown that wet heat processing, as in canning, causes partial isomerization of all-trans isomers into neo-isomers of lower potency[19]. Green vegetables contain mainly β-carotene and the authors calculated a loss of 15–20 per cent potency through canning, while yellow vegetables, mainly α-carotene, lose 30–35 per cent.

It is noteworthy that at this late date in the history of vitamins — as recently as 1985 — it was possible for an international committee to recommend reliable methods for vitamin A, β-carotene, B_1, C and E; to quote tentative methods for B_2, B_6 and D, to give only references for niacin and folate, and not even to give references for B_{12}, K, pantothenate and biotin[5].

There is some difficulty in extracting fat-soluble vitamins from foods. Several workers have uncritically reported an increase in carotene after heating a food, which was due to the incomplete extraction from the raw food compared with the heated food where the cell walls were degraded.

The problem was clearly demonstrated when water-dispersible carotene beadlets were added to a low-fat starchy slurry and the mixture dried on a roller dryer. Saponification followed by standard extraction with solvent yielded only 70 per cent recovery, and complete recovery required enzymic hydrolysis or prolonged solvent extraction treatment[3].

Bioavailability. We cannot usually measure the bioavailability of the vitamins and are forced to use chemical or physical indices of the amount present.

In the early days of investigating human requirements, such as the Medical Research Council's (MRC) work of 1942–44 for vitamin A and vitamin C, the bioavailability for human subjects was revealed at the same time. With modern techniques for assessing requirements, such as the changes in a labelled pool of the vitamin, such information is not revealed.

So if a novel food were to replace a traditional food to any considerable extent in the diet of the community there may be a need to determine the true, ie human, bioavailability of the vitamins. The same would be true of a novel process — such as irradiation and extrusion.

The whole topic is submerged beneath the finding in the MRC experiments that the physical form of the food controls the availability of the vitamin to a greater extent than any other factor. The availability of carotene from carrots was increased three-fold as the particles of carrot were subdivided — homogenized carrot was better than finely minced, which was, in turn, better than coarsely minced carrot.

A recent investigation of vitamin A in foods using HPLC methods reported the various isomers of retinol and their relative stabilities. The findings that there was no loss of vitamin A from lamb kidney on frying, a fall to half when ox kidney was stewed and to a quarter when pig kidney was stewed, illustrate the difficulty of quoting average figures for loss of vitamins and the need for specific analyses when reliable information is required[18].

Conclusions. We have little relevant knowledge of the effects on vitamins of large-scale production of foods — model systems and laboratory-scale preparations do not provide a very useful basis for factory production of complex mixtures. Consequently, there is often a considerable difference between what should happen, as predicted from the laboratory, and what, in practice, does happen, and the difference can rarely be explained.

1 American Medical Association (1982): The nutritive quality of processed foods; general policies for nutrient additions. *Nutr. Rev.* **40**, 93–96.

2 Bender, A.E. (1978): Food processing and nutrition. London, New York: Academic Press.

3 Bender, A.E. & Macfarlane, A. (1965): Determination of β-carotene in a roller-dried food. *Analyst* **90**, 536–540.

4 Bender, A.E. & Nik-Daud, N.I. (1984): Folic acid, assay and stability. In *Thermal processing and quality of foods* ed P. Zeuthen, J.C. Cheftel, C. Eriksson, M. Jul, H. Leninger, P. Linko, G. Varela, & G. Vos. pp. 880–884. London and New York: Elsevier Applied Science Publishers.

5 Brubacher, G., Muller-Mulot, W. & Southgate, D.A.T. (1985): Methods for the determination of vitamins in food. Recommended by COST. London and New York: Elsevier Applied Science Publishers.

6 Clegg, K.M. (1974): Frozen vegetables. *Nutr. Fd Sci.* **36**, 6–8.

7 Eison-Perchonok, M.H. & Downes, T.W. (1982): Kinetics of ascorbic acid autoxidation as a function of dissolved oxygen concentration and temperature. *J. Fd Sci.* **47**, 765–767.

8 Fafunso, M. & Bassir, O. (1976): Effect of cooking on the vitamin C content of fresh leaves and wilted leaves. *J. Agric. Fd Chem.* **24**, 354–355.

9 Freed, M., Brenner, S. & Wodicka, V.C. (1949): Prediction of thiamin and ascorbic acid stability in stored and canned foods. *Fd Technol.* **3**, 148–151.

10 Hellendoorn, E.W., Groot, A.P., de Mijlldekker, L.P., Van der Slump, P. & Willems, J.J.L. (1971): Effects of heat sterilisation and prolonged storage. *J. Am. Diet. Ass.* **58**, 434–441.
11 Labuza, T.P. (1972): Nutrient losses during drying and storage of dehydrated foods. *CRC Critical Rev. Fd Technol.* **3**, 217–240.
12 Mapson, L.W. (1956): Effect of processing on the vitamin content of foods. *Br. Med. Bull.* **12**, 73–77.
13 Marchesini, A., Majorino, G., Montuori, F. & Cagna, D. (1975): Changes in the ascorbic acid and dehydroascorbic acid content of fresh and canned beans. *J. Fd Sci.* **40**, 665–668.
14 Mokady, S., Cogan, U. & Lieberman, L. (1984): Stability of vitamin C in fruits and fruit blends. *J. Sci. Fd Agric.* **35**, 452–456.
15 Nik-Daud, N.I. (1983): An assay of folates in foods. Ph. D. Thesis. University of London.
16 Oguntona, T.E. & Bender, A.E. (1976): Loss of thiamin from potatoes. *J. Fd Technol.* **11**, 374–352.
17 Robertson, J. & Sissons, D.J. (1966): The effects of maturity, processing and storage in the pod and cooking on the vitamin C content of fresh peas. *Nutrition* **20**, 21–27.
18 Sivell, L.M., Bull, N.L., Buss, D.H., Wiggins, R.A., Scuffam, D. & Jackson, P.A. (1984): Vitamin A activity in foods of animal origin. *J. Sci. Fd Agric.* **35**, 931–939.
19 Sweeney, J.P. & Marsh, A.C. (1971): Effect of processing on provitamin A in vegetables. *J. Am. Diet. Ass.* **59**, 238–243.
20 Wanninger, L.A. (1972): Mathematical model predicts stability of ascorbic acid in food products. *Fd Technol.* **26**, 42–45.

★ ★ ★

PROCESSING TECHNIQUES AND NUTRIENT COMPOSITION

The effect of irradiation on the nutrient composition of food

A.W. HOLMES and V.M. WILKINSON
Leatherhead Food Research Association, Randalls Road, Leatherhead, Surrey KT22 7RY, UK.

Recent developments in the legal position of food irradiation are the result of a report of the Joint FAO/WHO/IAEA Committee on 'Wholesomeness of irradiated food' (the JECFI report), published in 1981, which was based on the results of a 10 year, internationally-funded project[9]. It concluded that irradiation of any food commodity up to an overall average radiation dose of 10 kGy presents no toxicological hazard and, furthermore, introduced no special microbiological or nutritional problems.

Ionizing radiation can be used to treat food for the purposes listed in the Table. In view of the number of applications, treatment of a wide range of foodstuffs can be envisaged and these will include some of our key dietary constituents.

Table. *Food irradiation applications*

Objective	Radiation dose range (kGy)
Inhibition of sprouting, eg onions, potatoes	0.05–0.15
Control of insect infestation, eg fruit, cereals	0.25–0.75
Control of maturation and senescence of fruit and vegetables	0.25–1
Increase shelf-life by controlling spoilage micro-organisms, eg meat, fish, fruit	1–3
Control of pathogenic organisms, eg poultry, (shell-fish)	3–7
Disinfestation of food ingredients, eg spices, herbs	7–10

Nutrient composition of irradiated food. The radiostability of the major food components in the pure state, in solution and in model systems has been extensively studied but foods, which are complex systems, may not react as predicted, the effect depending on many factors, eg (1) radiation dose; (2) food composition; (3) environment during- and post-irradiation.

Proteins. Reviews of the radiation chemistry of proteins have been published[5,21]. The principal radiolytic changes occurring in aqueous solutions of amino acids are deamination and decarboxylation. However, at the radiation doses employed for food irradiation, there are no significant changes in the amino acid composition of food and no measurable nutritional loss of protein value.

Enzymes in foods are well-protected and the radiation requirements for inactivation are large (> 10 kGy). Autolytic changes in high-protein foods are therefore not inhibited.

Fats. The radiation chemistry of fats has been reviewed[17,18]. The effects of ionizing radiation on lipids are similar to those produced by oxidative and heat processes. The main reactions involve oxidation, polymerization, decarboxylation and dehydration. Non-oxidative reactions can also occur. The overall digestibility of fats is unaffected by irradiation[10].

Unsaturated fats are more readily oxidized than saturated fats. Rancidity off-flavours are characteristic of irradiated foods with a high unsaturated fat content and such foods may be unsuitable for irradiation, unless nitrogen- or vacuum-packed.

Carbohydrates. Reviews of the radiation chemistry of carbohydrates are available[1,4]. The main effects of ionizing radiation on carbohydrates are hydrolysis and oxidative degradation. For lower saccharides, oxidation at the ends of the molecule produces acids. Ring scission forms aldehydes. For higher saccharides cleavage of the glycosidic link results in fragmentation into smaller units. Changes in irradiated carbohydrates increase with increased radiation dose.

Solubilization of pectins, cellulose, hemicellulose and starch in response to radiation doses exceeding 0.6 kGy is observed and results in softening of fresh fruits and vegetables[11]. The extent of softening depends on the commodity irradiated; for example, strawberries can be successfully treated at 2 kGy. However, the above have been shown to be of no nutritional significance.

In some cases, irradition may have a beneficial effect. Radiation-induced textural changes have been considered as a means to reduce the cooking time of dehydrated soup vegetables and pulses. As prolonged heating is known to destroy B-vitamins, a reduction in cooking time may result in better retention of vitamins in irradiated pulses[19].

Vitamins. Radiation-induced changes in vitamins have been reviewed[2,16,20]. Losses of vitamin A are very variable and depend not only on radiation dose but also on the complexity of the food product. Radiation doses at which significant losses occur, eg milk at 4.8 kGy, are very likely to cause undesirable organoleptic changes. Some apparent loss is due to *cis trans* isomerization rather than degradation. Retention of carotene in irradiated mangoes and papayas was high[3] and, in the case of papayas, was greater than when fruit was processed by freezing and canning.

Thiamin (vitamin B_1) is the most radiolabile of the B-vitamins. Losses of thiamin in irradiated food are well documented. A 15 per cent loss of thiamin has been reported in fish treated with 3 kGy[9], and a 47 per cent loss in cod treated with 6 kGy[12]. Thiamin losses depend not only on radiation dose but also on the particular food product, the method of preparation for processing and storage conditions. Losses of thiamin in foods are reduced by irradiation at sub-freezing temperatures and storage losses are reduced by packing in the absence of air[6]. The JECFI report concluded that a partial loss of thiamin in fish would be of concern only if that was the key source of thiamin in a particular population[9].

Nicotinic acid (niacin) and riboflavin (vitamin B_2) are generally more resistant to ionizing radiation than is thiamin. Minor losses of niacin have been observed in irradiated wheat flour treated with radiation doses between 0.3 and 0.5 kGy. However, the levels of niacin were shown to be higher in bread baked from the irradiated wheat flour[8]. This suggests that radiation plus heat treatment released some niacin from a bound form[7].

There have been fewer studies on the radiation stability of other B-vitamins (folic acid, vitamin B_6 (pyridoxine), vitamin B_{12}, pantothenic acid and biotin). In irradiated fish, 25 per cent pyridoxine may be lost and pyridoxine appears to be relatively sensitive to irradiation[9]. No significant losses have been demonstrated in other B-complex vitamins. A radiation dose of 0.2–0.5 kGy, which is recommended for disinfection of cereal grains, will not cause a destruction of B-complex vitamins. This is of particular importance if irradiation is to be applied on a large scale in countries where cereals are the staple diet[14]. Vitamin C is one of the more radiation-sensitive vitamins and conflicting results on losses have been reported in the radiation dose range 1–10 kGy. However, there is evidence for the conversion of ascorbic acid into dehydro-ascorbic acid, which is also biologically active[9].

The effect on vitamin C content of foods has been studied extensively, mostly at doses below 5 kGy. In general, losses rarely exceed 20–30 per cent and are of no direct nutritional consequence[20]. Losses may well be less if the dehydro-ascorbic acid content were taken into account.

Retention of ascorbic acid in irradiated mangoes and papayas has been shown to compare well with that in fruit processed by other methods[3]. The differences between control and irradiated Bing cherries is so small as to be meaningless from a nutritional point of view[15]. A study of the effect of storage on vitamin C in strawberries[13] showed that directly following irradiation there was a reduction in total ascorbic acid which increased with increased dose to a maximum loss of 12 per cent at 3 kGy. Decrease during storage was similar for both control and irradiated samples. It must be borne in mind that irradiated samples will potentially store for two or three times longer than control samples and therefore full-scale storage tests of this nature are required.

Vitamin D is more stable to irradiation than vitamin A. It is stable to radiation doses above 10 kGy.

Vitamin E is considered to be the most radio-sensitive among the fat-soluble vitamins; the highest losses induced by irradiation occur in food products having a high fat content. A protective effect is exerted by low temperatures and exclusion of oxygen by vacuum-packaging or packing under nitrogen[6]. This type of packaging is likely for food products with a high fat content.

The stability of vitamin K in irradiated plant products is reported to be very high[20].

Minerals. There are few specific reports on the effects of irradiation on food mineral composition, absorption and utlization but there is no reason to believe there will be any change.

Conclusion. Radiation doses used to treat food will be selected on the basis of objective and on retention of sensory quality of the food. At low radiation doses (< 1 kGy), appropriate for the disinfection treatment, vitamin losses are negligible compared with the large variations between cultivars and changes caused by growth conditions, storage, transport. In the medium-dose range (1–10 kGy), used to control microbial growth, the lowest possible dose will be selected because of the importance of retaining sensory quality and on economic grounds. Losses of vitamins, particularly B_1, C and E, will therefore be minimised. In the low or medium-dose range, nutritional changes in proteins, fats and carbohydrates are negligible.

Under commercial conditions, the effect of irradiation on the nutrient composition of food will be similar in degree or less than that observed with other food preservation methods and no special nutritional problems are associated with the technique.

1 Adam, S. (1983): Recent developments in radiation chemistry of carbohydrates. In *Recent advances in food irradiation*, ed P.S. Elias & A.J. Cohen, pp. 149–170. Amsterdam: Elsevier Biomedical.

2 Basson, R.A. (1983): Recent advances in radiation chemistry of vitamins. In *Recent advances in food irradiation*, ed P.S. Elias & A.J. Cohen. pp. 59–77. Amsterdam: Elsevier Biomedical.

3 Beyers, M. & Thomas, A.C. (1979): Irradiation of Subtropical fruits. 4. Changes in certain nutrients present in mangoes, papayas, and litchis during canning, freezing and α-irradiation. *J. Agric. Fd Chem.* **27**, 48–51.

4 Dauphin, J.F. & Saint-Lebe, L.R. (1977): Radiation chemistry of carbohydrates. In *Radiation chemistry of major food components*, ed P.S. Elias & A.J. Cohen. pp. 131–186, Amsterdam: Elsevier.

5 Delincée, H. (1983): Recent advances in radiation chemistry of proteins. In *Recent advances in food irradiation*, ed P.S. Elias & A.J. Cohen, pp. 129–147. Amsterdam: Elsevier Biomedical.

6 Diehl, J.F. (1979): Verminderung von strahleninduzierten Vitamin-E-und-B_1-Verlusten durch bestrahlung von lebensmitteln bei tiefen temperaturen und durch ausschluss von luftsauerstoff. *Z. Lebensm. Unters. Forsch* **169**, 276–280.

7 Diehl, J.F. (1981): Effects of combination processes on the nutritive value of food. In *Combination processes in food irradiation*, Proc. Symp. Colombo, pp. 349–366. Vienna: IAEA.

8 Heiligman, F., Rice, L.J., Smith, L.W. Jr., Thomas, M.H., Kelley, N.J. & Wierbicki, E. (1973): Irradiation disinfection of flour. II. Storage studies of irradiated flour. Presented at 33rd Ann Meeting, Inst. Food Technol.

9 Joint FAO/IAEA/WHO Expert Committee report (1981): *Wholesomeness of irradiated food*. Tech. Rep. Ser. No. 659. Geneva: WHO.

10 Josephson, E.S., Thomas, M.H. & Calhoun, W.K. (1978): Nutritional aspects of food irradiation: an overview. *J. Fd Proc. Preserv.* **2**, 299–313.

11 Kader, A.A, Lipton, W.J., Reitz, H.J., Smith, D.W. & Tilton, E.W. (1984): Irradiation of plant products. In Comments from CAST, April 1984 (ISSN 0194–4096).

12 Kennedy, T.S. & Ley, F.J. (1971): Studies on the combined effect of gamma radiation and cooking on the nutritional value of food. *J. Sci. Fd Agric.* **22**, 146–148.

13 Kim, H.S., Kim, Y.S. & Park, K.T. (1969): Studies on the storage of fruits by irradiation. II. On the storage of strawberry. *J. Nucl. Sci (Seoul)* **9**, 111–118.

14 Lorenz, K. (1975): Irradiation of cereal grains and cereal grain products. *CRC Critical Rev. Fd Sci. Nutr.* **6**, pp. 317–382.

15 Maxie, E.C., Sommer, N.F. & Brown, D.S. (1964): Cherries. In *Radiation technology in conjunction with post-harvested procedures as a means of extending the shelf-life of fruits and vegetables*, pp. 105–108. Annual Report Feb 1, 1963–Jan 30, 1964. UCD-34P80-2.

16 Murray, T.K. (1981): Nutritional aspects of food irradiation. *Fd Irradiation Information* **II**, 21–32.

17 Nawar, W.W. (1977): Radiation chemistry of lipids. In *Radiation chemistry of major food components*, ed P.S. Elias & A.J. Cohen, pp. 21–61. Amsterdam: Elsevier.

18 Nawar, W.W. (1983): Comparison of chemical consequences of heat and irradiation treatment of lipids. In *Recent advances in food irradiation*, ed P.S. Elias & A.J. Cohen, pp. 115–127. Amsterdam: Elsevier Biomedical.

19 Sreenivasan, A. (1974): Compositional and quality changes in some irradiated foods. In *Improvement of food quality by irradiation*. Panel Proceedings Series, pp. 129–155. Vienna: IAEA.

20 Tobback, P.P. (1977): Radiation chemistry of vitamins. In *Radiation chemistry of major food components*, ed P.S. Elias & A.J. Cohen. pp. 187–220. Amsterdam: Elsevier.

21 Urbain, W.M. (1977): Radiation chemistry of proteins. In *Radiation chemistry of major food components*, ed P.S. Elias & A.J. Cohen. pp. 63–130. Amsterdam: Elsevier.

Frying

G. VARELA
Institute of Nutrition (CSIC), Faculty of Pharmacy, 28040 Madrid, Spain.

Deep frying (DF), one of the oldest culinary methods in existence, originated and developed in countries where the olive was grown. It was not a popular method in areas where olive oil was not produced and a 'black legend' even grew up around frying. For instance, until recently it was held that fried foods were indigestible and there was even talk of their possibly being toxic. However, these ideas have begun to change owing, amongst other things, to the studies carried out in several laboratories, including our own, to bring to the fore the positive aspects of this process. It can, in fact, be asserted that DF is gaining ground in countries where it has hitherto been unpopular. The different facets of DF have been studied in our laboratory for many years now[5,6].

When talking about DF we should establish a few facts clearly: (a) we are referring to deep frying, not to sautéeing, (b) any changes indicated refer to when the food is actually being fried in the fat, not to overheating, (c) whether the food is breaded or not.

The process of frying. The number of factors make this an extraordinarily complex process. This very complexity was what prompted researchers working in this subject area[1–3] to employ 'models' that were sufficiently representative of the process and in which the different variables involved in the process could be isolated.

We embarked on our study with a very simple model[4]. We diced potatoes into cubes of different surface/volume ratios and then, in a laboratory deep fryer or a household frying pan, studied the changes in temperature both inside the food itself and in the container, as well as the penetration kinetics of the fat. The temperature within the food was determined by a thermometer, whereas fat penetration was studied in two ways: by determining the total fat absorbed or the area penetrated by the fat using a fluorescent method devised by us. Employing this model, we examined the influence of a number of factors: temperature, time, water content/fat penetration ratio, physical and chemical changes in the fat and the food, the material the container was made of, antioxidants and acceptance by a panel of tasters testing the palatability of the fried food. We tested virtually all the cooking fats available on three foods to start with: potatoes, bananas and hake.

We discovered that the temperature of the fat in which the food is fried has relatively little bearing on the thermal damage to the food, provided the latter has a high water content. Within the range of frying temperatures, the temperature inside potatoes does not rise above approximately 100 °C while the water is evaporating and the fat does not start to penetrate into the food until a very substantial portion of the water has evaporated. As the fat acts on the inside of the food for a short time, DF does no more harm than other culinary methods. We have also demonstrated that the penetration kinetics of cooking fats differs; for instance, when potatoes are fried in olive oil, the oil remains on the outside, whereas other fats penetrate deeply into the food, making the fried food greasy and unacceptable.

Changes occurring in the nutritional value of the food. Changes may occur in the three parameters that determine the nutritional utlization of food: palatability, digestibility and metabolic utlization. One of the most positive aspects of frying is that it makes fried food extremely palatable since it has been enriched by the fat. As the actual time during which the fat acts on the food is short, it is to be expected that any alterations produced on digestive and metabolic utlization would be of little significance, as we later confirmed in trials on rats and, in some cases, on humans.

Changes occurring in the cooking fats. These may be greater than the changes in the nutritional value of the fried foods and depend on numerous factors that are particularly relevant in repeated fryings (RF). To supply an example of this complexity, in our work we point out the difficulty in maintaining the necessary food/cooking fat proportion in RF, as well as the errors in the calculation of the changes in the fatty acids when expressed as percentages instead of as absolute values.

What exactly are the practical repercussions of these changes? (1) *Length of time fats can be used*. We ran tests on various types of oils in 36 RF of potatoes and 22 of hake, finding no important changes in any of them throughout, except for the smoking point[7]. When precautions are not taken to keep the food/oil ratio constant, the oil is practically used up in repeated fryings. These conclusions are valid for our experimental conditions only and should not be considered as applying generally. (2) *Digestibility*. Literature abounds on the digestibility of raw oils, whereas we know nothing about fats used in RF. We recently studied the digestibility of a number of fats used in 10 RF of potatoes, meat and sardines. We discovered that the process did not affect their digestibility and that in every case digestibility was greater with olive oil than with the other fats. (3) *Metabolic utilization*. Great interest has arisen lately in ascertaining how changes in fats can affect their metabolism. Amongst other things, this marked interest has grown up because the proportion of PUFA in the diet is related to cholesterol levels and cardiovascular diseases and the PUFA are the first to alter in RF.

Working on rats, we investigated the influence diets of olive oil or margarine used in 30 RF of potatoes have on lipid levels. We found no significant differences, compared with raw oils, as regards total cholesterol or lipoprotein distribution. However, these findings obtained with rats cannot be extrapolated to human beings because the cholesterol metabolism and lipoprotein pattern of rats are different. It would therefore be worthwhile extending these studies to human beings, which is precisely one of the objectives pursued in our laboratory.

New opportunities for frying. DF has great scope in fast-food establishments where, in fact, deep fryers and grill plates are used exclusively. Perhaps from a nutritional point of view, the most interesting problem posed by modern life-styles is the increase in the number of people who eat lunch out five times a week. One of the greatest drawbacks lies in the losses that occur in the nutritional value of the food when it is kept hot until ready to be consumed (warm holding), which is when the greatest amount of thermolabile nutrients are lost. We believe that DF can substantially cut these losses since it is technically possible to design a fryer outfit equipped with a belt that conveys the food into the fat at a speed which is automatically regulated, depending on demand.

Among the different systems employed in catering, the one that seems to offer the best advantages is Cooking-Freezing-Reheating. We have studied how DF in olive oil affects the protein quality of different types of foods of animal origin (meats, fish and eggs).

The food was first fried in olive oil at 180 °C, then frozen at −18 °C for 30 d and finally reheated in a micro-wave oven; we discovered that the system overall did not affect either the digestive or metabolic utilization of the protein in the different foods studied.

1 Dagerskog, M. (1977): Time-temperature relationships in industrial cooking and frying. In *Physical, chemical and biological changes in food caused by thermal processing*, ed T. Hoyem & O. Kvále, pp. 77–100. London: Applied Science.
2 Morton, I.D. (1977): Physical, chemical and biological changes related to different time-temperature combinations. In *Physical, chemical and biological changes in food caused by thermal processing*, ed T. Hoyem & O. Kvále, pp. 135–151. London: Applied Science Publishers Limited.
3 Paulus, K.O. (1984): Modelling in industrial cooking. In *Thermal processing and quality of foods*, ed P. Zeuthen *et al.*, pp. 304–312. London: Elsevier Applied Science Publishers.
4 Varela, G. (1977): Les graisses chauffées: contribution à l'étude des processus de la friture des aliments. *Biblio. Nutr. Dieta* **25**, 112–121.
5 Varela, G. (1980): Nutritive aspects of olive oil in the frying process. *Proc. IIIrd Int. Cong. Biological value of olive oil*, Crete (Greece), pp. 385–402.
6 Varela, G. (1982): Nutritional aspects of home frying. In *Home cooking nutrient changes and emerging problems*. Proceedings of workshop. Rome: EEC, COST-91.
7 Varela, G., Moreiras-Varela, O. & Ruiz-Roso, B. (1983): Utilización de algunos aceites en frituras repetidas. Cambios en las grasas y análisis sensorial de los alimentos fritos. *Grasas y Aceites* **34**, 101–107.

Nutritional effects of extrusion-cooking

J.C. CHEFTEL
Laboratoire de Biochimie et Technologie Alimentaires, Université des Sciences et Techniques, 34060 Montpellier, France.

The extruder is viewed as a continuous chemical reactor processing food mixes at high temperatures (up to 250 °C) for relatively short residence times (usually 1–2 min), at high pressures (up to 25 mPa), under high shear forces, and in most cases at relatively low water contents (below 30 per cent), although some recent applications are carried out in twin-screw extruders at 40–80 per cent moisture[11,15].

While nutritional changes are of little concern in some extruded foods, prevention or reduction of nutrient destruction, together with improvements in starch or protein digestibility are of importance in most other applications. Extrusion also permits the inactivation of several anti-nutritional or toxic factors, of deterioration enzymes and of microorganisms. Detailed surveys of the nutritional effects of extrusion-cooking have been published[2,9].

Protein. *Physico-chemical modifications.* Soyabeans and many legume-or oil-seeds provide a good example of improved protein digestibility and bioavailability of (limiting) sulphur amino acids through (1) thermal unfolding of the major seed globulins and (2) thermal inactivation of trypsin inhibitors and other growth-retarding factors[10].

Improved nutritional value of the protein is consistently obtained, as shown by protein efficiency ratio determinations on rats (from 1 to 2.15 after extrusion of raw soyabeans).

In the texturation of vegetable proteins by extrusion-cooking, advantage is taken of unfolding and aggregation reactions to promote the formation of insoluble dry expanded and fibrous structures that readily rehydrate into chewy meat extenders or analogues. Specific conditions are necessary to obtain satisfactory texturation. The exact texturation mechanisms are not known, although protein insolubilization clearly results from new hydrogen, hydrophobic and disulfide bonding. Other covalent cross-links such as lysinoalanine and lanthionine are not formed in appreciable amounts.

The protein nutritional value of experimental and commercial extruded texturized vegetable protein has been assessed in human adolescents and adults, and with rats[8,14].

Extrusion-cooking usually brings about complete enzyme inactivation in spite of the HTST process conditions[11].

Chemical changes. Extensive lysine loss and nutritional damage can take place when cereal flours or cereal/legume blends are extruded into biscuits, crispbread, breakfast cereals or instant flours under severe conditions of temperature or shear forces at low moisture, especially in the presence of reducing sugars (≥ 3 per cent glucose, fructose, maltose, lactose)[4,6,13]. Decreases in total and FDNB-reactive lysine contents and in the bioavailability of lysine were respectively equal to 37, 37 and 50 per cent when a biscuit mix containing starch, protein and sucrose was extruded under excessive conditions[13].

With food mixes of low initial dextrose equivalent ($DE \leq 1$) containing starch but no sucrose, no nutritional damage is observed under mild processing. Under more severe conditions, however serious decreases in the lysine content and in the protein biological value were noted[4].

It is not fully understood whether the damaging effects at low water contents are due to local temperature increases through intense shear forces, to specific mechanical effects (splitting of the glycosidic bonds of starch, decrease in the diffusion barrier existing at low water content), to an enhancing effect of low moisture on the Maillard condensation, or to a combination of these effects. Reducing sugars can be formed from starch or oligosaccharides under severe extrusion conditions[11]. Model studies in rheometers permitting high shear at low moistures are needed to determine reaction kinetics, activation energies, effect of mix composition and comparison of various time-temperature conditions.

In order to keep lysine losses within the 10–15 per cent limit accepted in bread baking, it is necessary: (1) to avoid extrusion above 180 °C at water contents below 15 per cent (even if a subsequent oven-drying step is then necessary), and (2) to avoid the presence of reducing sugars during extrusion.

New applications include: (1) manufacture of gelatin gel confectionery; (2) transformation of acid casein into sodium caseinate, at 100 °C and 20 per cent moisture; (3) destruction of aflatoxin in peanut meal with 2 per cent NH_3; (4) chemical modification of protein such as covalent attachment of fatty acids, etc.; (5) improvement in the functional properties of protein through mild mechanical/thermal processing; (6) pasteurization or sterilization (baby foods, animal blood, etc.); (7) moist solubilization of collagen or keratin; (8) acid/mechanical hydrolysis of vegetable protein or fish mince as an initial step in sauce preparation, and (9) wet-state texturization. Continuous gelation of soy proteins, continuous restructuring of mechanically-deboned meat, continuous emulsification of dairy products into process cheese can all be achieved in a twin-screw extruder. Wet-state extrusion (40–85 per cent water) does not induce high pressure, intense shear or expansion. Severe chemical changes and nutritional damage are therefore unlikely.

Starch. *Physicochemical and chemical modifications.* Extrusion-cooking, depending on process conditions and food mix composition, causes swelling and rupture of starch granules, cold water solubility and reduced viscosity of starch, and partial to complete release of amylose and amylopectin[11].

Viscosity and molecular-weight determinations clearly indicate that amylose and amylopectin are partly hydrolysed to maltodextrins as a result of high shear extrusion of wheat starch but not of drum-cooking[7]. Starch constituents in cereal or legume flours may be more readily hydrolysed than in purified starches, probably because endogenous amylases are active during the initial extrusion steps.

Crystalline complexes are known to form between amylose and polar lipids during the extrusion of cereal starches.

Increased in vitro *enzymatic digestibility of starch.* Mildly or severely extruded wheat flours are as available *in vitro* to α-amylase as autoclaved controls, and more available than boiled, and especially raw, controls. Extrusion probably increases the enzymatic availability of starch by way of gelatinization, inactivation of endogenous α-amylase inhibitor, disruption of cellular structure and size reduction.

The same extruded flours, when suspended in water and used for mouth rinse, were readily fermented to organic acids by microorganisms in the dental plaque, with resulting decreases in pH. Judging from this, extruded flours must be considered as more cariogenic than boiled or drum-cooked flours.

Increased in vivo *digestibility of starch*. Rat balance experiments showed that both raw wheat starch and extruded wheat starch (or starch from extruded wheat flours) were completely digested *in vivo*. However, these experiments cannot discriminate between digestion plus absorption, and bacterial fermentation in the colon[3].

The wheat flours that had been subjected to *in vitro* α-amylolysis were also investigated for *in vivo* starch absorption, as judged by plasma glucose levels within a 2 h period after gastric intubation of young rats. The plasma glucose responses varied in the following order of intensity: severe extrusion > mild extrusion (flat crispbread type) = boiling = soft bread-baking > regular mild drum-cooking and drying[3]. Slowly absorbed carbohydrates are considered as beneficial.

Dietary fibres. Severe extrusion-cooking of wheat flours cause a 1 to 6 per cent apparent increase in dietary fibres due to the formation of amylase-resistant starch fractions.

Extrusion-cooking of white wheat flour was found to cause an alteration in the ratio of insoluble to soluble dietary fibre[5] when 50–75 per cent of total fibre was soluble in the extruded flour, compared with 40 per cent in the raw flour.

Rat balance experiments showed that dietary fibre in raw white wheat flour was highly available to bacterial degradation since the faecal recovery of arabinose, xylose and glucose averaged a low 22 per cent. After mild extrusion, the faecal recovery further decreased to 12 per cent. The higher solubility is probably responsible for this increased fermentability. The faecal recovery of fibre constituents from raw whole grain wheat flour was higher ($\simeq$ 42 per cent) and remained unchanged after extrusion. Some chemical structures are therefore resistant to bacterial degradation *in vivo*, in spite of the intense shear treatment during extrusion.

Lipids. Most extruded cereal foods contain less than 6 to 7 per cent lipids immediately after extrusion, because high lipid concentrations prevent expansion. Preliminary investigations indicate that the extent of hydrogenation and cis→trans isomerization of fatty acids that take place during extrusion is too small to be nutritionally significant.

Vitamins and minerals. The retention of B-group vitamins has been investigated during crispbread production. A linear relationship has been established between the destruction of the most thermolabile B-vitamins (folic acid, B_1, B_{12} and B_6) and the energy input[12].

Data on the stability of carotenoid pigments were obtained during extrusion and subsequent storage of corn starch[1]. Carotenoids resisted extrusion fairly well but some were further oxidized during storage.

Twenty to 40 per cent losses of vitamin C are consistently observed during extrusion.

It is advisable to carry out vitamin fortification after extrusion, whenever possible.

The digestibility and bioavailability of Fe, Cu, Zn, Mg is usually low in plant foods since these elements may be present as insoluble complexes with dietary fibres, phytate or proteins. Data concerning minerals in extruded foods are scarce and partly contradictory, and additional research is needed.

1 Berset, C., Debontridder, J. & Marty, C. (1984): Stabilité de quelques pigments caroténoïdes en cuisson-extrusion. In *Thermal processing and quality of foods*, ed P. Zeuthen *et al.*, pp. 168–174. Barking, Essex: Elsevier Applied Science.

2 Björck, I. & Asp, N.G. (1983): The effects of extrusion-cooking on nutritional value. A literature review. *J. Fd Eng.* **2**, 281–308.

3 Björck, I., Asp, N.G., Birkhed, D. & Lundqvist, J. (1984): Effects of processing on starch availability *in vitro* and *in vivo*. Extrusion-cooking of wheat flours and starch. *J. Cereal Sci.* **2**, 91–103.

4 Björck, I., Asp, N.G. & Dahlqvist, A. (1984): Protein nutritional value of extrusion-cooked wheat flours. *Fd Chem.* **15**, 203–214.

5 Björck, I., Nyman, M. & Asp, N.G. (1984): Extrusion-cooking and dietary fiber: effects on dietary fiber content and on degradation in the rat intestinal tract. *Cereal Chem.* **61**, 174–179.

6 Björck, I., Noguchi, A., Asp, N.G., Cheftel, J.C. & Dahlqvist, A. (1983): Protein nutritional value of a biscuit processed by extrusion-cooking: effects on available lysine. *J. Agric. Fd Chem.* **31**, 488–492.

7 Colonna, P., Doublier, J.L., Melcion, J.P., de Montredon, F. & Mercier, C. (1984): Extrusion-cooking and drum-drying of wheat starch. I. Physical and macromolecular modifications. *Cereal Chem.* **61**, 538–543.

8 Elias, L.G., Braham, J.E., Navarrete, D.A. & Bressani, R. (1984): Calidad proteinica de productos comerciales de proteina texturizada de soya y de mezclas con carne. *Archiv. Latinoam. Nutr.* **34**, 355–364.

9 de la Guerivière, J.F., Mercier, C. & Baudet, L. (1985): Incidences de la cuisson-extrusion sur certains paramètres nutritionnels de produits alimentaires notamment céréaliers. *Cashiers Nutr. Diet.* **20**, 201–210.

10 Harper, J.M. & Jansen, G.R. (1985): Production of nutritious precooked foods in developing countries by low-cost extrusion technology. *Fd Rev. Int.* **1**, 27–97.

11 Linko, P., Colonna, P., & Mercier, C. (1981): High temperature, short time extrusion-cooking. *Adv. Cereal Sci. Tech.* **4**, 145–235.

12 Millauer, C., Wiedmann, W.M. & Killeit, U. (1984): Influence of different extrusion parameters on vitamin stability. In *Thermal processing and quality of foods*, ed P. Zeuthen *et al.*, pp. 208–216. Barking, Essex: Elsevier Applied Science.

13 Noguchi, A., Mosso, K., Aymard, C., Jeunink, J. & Cheftel, J.C. (1982): Maillard reactions during extrusion-cooking of protein-enriched biscuits. *Lebensm. Wiss. Technol.* **15**, 105–110.

14 Vemury, M.K.D., Kies, C. & Fox, H.M. (1976): Comparative protein value of several vegetable protein products fed at equal nitrogen levels to human adults. *J. Fd Sci.* **41**, 1086–1091.

15 Zeuthen, P., Cheftel, J.C., Eriksson, C., Jul, M., Leniger, H., Linko, P., Varela, G. & Vos, C. eds (1984): *Thermal processing and quality of foods*. Barking, Essex: Elsevier Applied Science.

Microwave cooking

C.E. ERIKSSON
SIK — The Swedish Food Institute, Box 5401, S-402 29 Göteborg, Sweden.

Radiation can be defined in terms of ionizing radiation produced by gamma-rays and x-rays, optical radiation where we find ultra-violet, visible and infrared light and finally radio-frequency radiation such as microwaves, and ordinary radiowaves. By international agreement two microwave frequencies are allowed for our purpose, 915 MHz (320 mm) and 2450 MHz (120 mm) are mostly used. Microwaves can be reflected and absorbed like light.

The first commercial microwave ovens for home use appeared on the market 1955. In 1980 four million ovens were sold in US which means that one in five US households owned a microwave oven. The estimated number in 1985 is six million units or every second household having a microwave oven. US and Japan are the prime manufacturers of microwave ovens. In fast-food establishments microwave heating is used for thawing precooked frozen meals and in reheating catered foods. In food processing microwaves can be used in, for instance, freeze-drying, to improve rehydration properties, in dough proofing, and in cooking bacon and chicken.

Microwaves are absorbed unevenly in the food depending on the chemical composition in different parts of the food and this can lead to an uneven temperature profile in the food. Through evaporative cooling the surface reaches a lower temperature than the inner parts. Fatty parts can sometimes be overheated. Since microwaves behave as light, refraction and focusing can lead to heat concentration at corners, peaks and edges. Thawing of frozen food can be very rapid; however there is a much larger absorption of microwave energy in water than in ice.

Since 1982, four reviews on the nutritional consequences of microwave heating of food have been published[5–7,15]. While the latter[15] deals primarily with the nutrition in food items such as fish, meat, vegetables, the others[5–7] report on the effects on individual nutrients such as protein, fat, vitamins, the last two primarily in animal foods. All these surveys conclude that, in general, little or no differences exist between the effects of microwave and conventional cooking. This is to be expected as the heat effect at the same 'doneness' should theoretically be the same, irrespective of the heating method used. There are, however, some differences in microwave heating as compared with other methods which makes a comparison difficult. This often depends on the initial temperature unevenness in microwave-heated foods, to the fact that temperature measurements were difficult until microwave-safe thermometers were used more widely and to the moisture content of the food.

The data presented here are selected from studies where proper comparisons can be made. Since the sensory quality of cooked food also has an implication on its nutrition a few examples of flavour and colour effects have been included.

Meat. Meat is not browned when applying microwave cooking which has an appreciable influence on flavour and appearance. When cooking of minced beef to the same degree of 'doneness' in microwave and conventional ovens was studied judges noted more blood-like and less meaty roasted aroma in the microwave-cooked beef[13]. Untrained judges could not differentiate the samples.

An attempt was made to establish the optimum cooking time both for flavour (F) and for over-all acceptability (A), for conventional and microwave-cooking of beef[3]. There are very large differences in cooking time due to the more rapid and direct heating brought about by microwaves, viz. the relevant times were, for conventional cooking 88 min (F) and 84 min (A) and for microwave 2.8 min (F) and 3.4 min (A). Sensory properties of beef heated to 70 °C internal temperature at two microwave effects, 500 W and 1050 W, were compared with those at conventional heating[17]. The flavour of beef cooked at 1050 W had more intense, and at 500 W less intense, flavour than beef cooked in the conventional oven. No differences in flavour were noted for beef cooked dry or moist in microwave ovens.

Less warmed-over-flavour in microwave reheated beef slices than in conventionally reheated samples was reported[9]. No differences in juiciness were found between top round steaks cooked with microwaves or conventionally provided that the microwave heating was properly controlled and that a reduced effect was used.

When beef roast-cooked conventionally was compared with beef cooked by microwaves, to the same internal temperature (58–60 °C), little difference in thiamin retention was found: the percentage retention for conventional cooking was 88 at 95 °C, 88 at 149 °C and 67 at 204 °C, while for microwave it was 86[11]. In another study[2] cooking of beef, pork and lamb by conventional methods (C) was compared with microwave 1054 W (M1) and microwave 492 W (M2), for thiamin retention. The results (percentages) were: beef C 69, M1 61 and M2 49; pork C 72, M1 73 and M2 67; lamb C 52, M1 52 and M2 49 showing that low-microwave effect gave less thiamin retention, but this was not confirmed for beef in a subsequent study[18]. Significantly higher riboflavin retention was found in microwave-cooked beef roasts as compared with conventional cooking — 90 per cent vs 81 per cent — but the difference in niacin was not significant — 52 per cent vs 50 per cent[10]. The sodium content in lamb cooked in a conventional oven was higher than after microwave cooking[2].

Vegetables. Peas cooked in a microwave oven scored higher for flavour, greenness and colour uniformity compared with conventional heating if the microwave-cooking was made at reduced power[12]. Addition of some water had a positive influence on all characteristics. The same authors also found significally higher scores for colour of peas cooked in a home microwave oven than in an institutional microwave and conventional oven. No differences were found for carrots.

No differences in flavour of frozen spinach cooked in microwave and conventional oven were found[8]. Depending on the evaporative cooking of the surface, broccoli and carrots develop tougher outer parts and softer inner parts in microwave than conventional cooking[16].

Microwave-baked potato were judged by trained panels to be inferior in appearance and flavour as compared with conventionally baked, while a consumer panel could not differentiate between them[14].

In general, microwave cooking results in a retention of vitamins and pigments equal to or higher than that in conventionally cooked vegetables. A number of research groups have found a significantly better retention of vitamin C in microwave-cooked vegetables (M) vs conventionally-cooked vegetables. Reported results (mg/100 g AA) include: 117 M vs 73 C, cabbage 43 M vs 25 C, cauliflower 85 M vs 48 C, green beans 6 M vs 5 C and spinach 24 M vs 15 C. (From G. Armbruster, Thermador/Waste King pamphlet MHS-1). However, the cooking time seems to have the greatest influence.

Significantly greater amounts of thiamin were found in microwave-baked potatoes as compared with other cooking methods[1]. A number of studies have revealed that the cooking time and amount of water are important factors in the retention of riboflavin in microwave-cooked vegetables. For folic acid no differences have been found.

Carotene seems to be completely stable in microwave cooking of carrots[4,8]. Chlorophyll retention has also been reported to be significantly higher in microwave cooked peas.

Bread. No crust is formed in microwave baking which gives microwave-baked bread less flavour. The consistency has been reported to be rubber-like and moist. The water content of the dough seems to be of utmost importance. Depending on the no-crust formation the loss of lysine is less than in conventionally baked bread. Bread fermentation can be performed in a microwave oven more rapidly than when using conventional technique due to the fact that the temperature of the bread interior can be brought very rapidly to the optimal fermentation temperature around 38 °C. This might however result in a lesser degradation of phytate and reduced availability of minerals, eg iron and zinc.

Conclusions. Microwave cooking is for most people a novel way of preparing food. One must know how to place the food in a correct geometrical manner to avoid the special corner and edge effects so that the food is evenly heated. One should allow some after-cooking time to equilibrate the temperature.

There are no special effects produced by the microwaves *per se*. Basically the events in the food when microwave-cooked are introduced are influenced by the same parameters as in conventional cooking, that is to say by the choice and composition of the raw materials, temperature, time and water relationships. Because of evaporative cooling and high moisture in the surface no searing or browning occur unless a special device is used. Low power setting should be used, if possible, for thawing since water absorbs microwave energy far better than ice, for tenderization of tough meat and vegetables and for fermentation of bread.

The main advantages with microwave cooking are convenience and short cooking time and addition of little water, which has an advantageous influence on nutrients, especially vitamins, of which smaller quantities are destroyed and minerals which are leached out to a lesser extent.

1 Augustin, J., Johnson, S.R., Teitzel, C., True, R.H., Hogan, J.M., Toma, R.B., Shawn, R.L. & Deutsch, R.M. (1978): Changes in nutrient composition of potatoes during home preparation: II. Vitamins. *American Potato J.* **55**, 653–662.

2 Baldwin, R.E., Korschgen, B.M., Russel, M.S. & Mabesa, L. (1976): Proximate analysis, free amino acid, vitamin and mineral content of microwave cooked meat. *J. Fd Sci.* **41**, 762–765.

3 Bodrero, K.O., Pearson, A.M. & Magee, W.T. (1980): Optimum cooking times for flavor development and evaluation of flavor quality of beef cooked by microwaves and conventional methods. *J. Fd Sci.* **45**, 613–616.

4 Chung, S.Y., Morr, C.V. & Jen, J.J. (1981): Effect of microwave and conventional cooking on the nutritive value of Colossus Peas. *J. Fd Sci.* **46**, 272–273.

5 Cross, G.A. & Fung, D.Y.C. (1982): The effect of microwaves on nutrient value of foods. *CRC Crit. Rev. Fd Sci. Nutr.* **16**, 355–381.

6 Dehne, L., Bögl, W. & Grossklaus, B. (1983): *Fleischwirtschaft* **63**, 231–237.

7 Dehne, L. & Bögl, W. (1983): *Fleischwirtschaft* **63**, 1206–1211.

8 Eheart, M.S. & Gott, C. (1964): Conventional and microwave cooking of vegetables. Ascorbic acid, carotene retention and palatability. *J. Am. Diet. Ass.* **44**, 116–119.

9 Johnston, M.B. & Baldwin, R.E. (1980): Influence of microwave reheating on selected quality factors of roast beef. *J. Fd Sci.* **45**, 1460–1462.

10 Korschgen, B.M. & Baldwin, R.E. (1978): Moist-heat microwave and conventional cooking of round roasts of beef. *J. Microwave Power* **13**, 257–262.

11 Lushbough, C.H., Heller, B.S., Weir, E. & Schweigert, B.S. (1962): Thiamin retention in meats after various heat treatments. *J. Am. Diet. Ass.* **40**, 35–38.

12 Mabesa, L.B. & Baldwin, R.E. (1978): Flavor and color of peas and carrots cooked by microwaves. *J. Microwave Power* **13**, 321–326.

13 MacLeod, G. & Coppoch, B.M. (1978): Sensory properties of the aroma of beef cooked conventionally and by microwave radiation. *J. Fd Sci.* **43**, 145–151.

14 Maga, J.A. & Twomey, J.A. (1977): Sensory comparison of four potato varieties baked conventionally and by microwaves. *J. Fd Sci.* **42**, 541–542.

15 Ohlsson, T. & Åström, A. (1982): Sensory and nutritional quality in microwave cooking. *Microwave Wld.* **3**, 15–16.

16 Schrumpf, E. & Charley, H. (1975): Texture of broccoli and carrots cooked by microwave energy. *J. Fd Sci.* **40**, 1025–1029.

17 Snider, S. & Baldwin, R.E. (1981): Flavor intensity as related to the creatine and creatinine content of microwave and conventionally cooked beef. *J. Fd Sci.* **46**, 1801–1804.

18 Voris, H.H. & van Duyne, F.O. (1979): Low voltage microwave cooking of top round roasts: Energy consumption, thiamine content and palatability. *J. Fd Sci.* **44**, 1447–1450, 1454.

Nutritional changes in food processing: fermentation

R.F. McFEETERS
Food Fermentation Laboratory, US Department of Agriculture, Agricultural Research Service, and North Carolina Agricultural Research Service, Department of Food Science, North Carolina State University, Raleigh, NC 27695, USA.

The greatest nutritional significance of food fermentations is that these processes allow for improved utilization of foods either by preservation of perishable commodities or by improving the organoleptic qualities of foods to increase acceptability. Pickles, sauerkraut and cheese, for example, were undoubtedly used as foods because they could be stored safely much longer than cucumbers, cabbage or milk. Products such as tempeh, a fungal fermentation of cooked soybeans by *Rhizopus oligosporus*, or idli, a heterolactic acid fermentation of rice and blackgram, are brief fermentations which have as their primary goal improvement of the flavour and texture of the food. Certainly the most important source of nutrients in all fermented foods is the nutrient content of the starting ingredients. However, it is clear that the fermentation process can often cause changes in nutrient concentrations which, in special instances, could be of significant benefit. It is clear that rapid development of techniques to modify microorganisms genetically offers many possibilities for improvement of both the nutritional and functional qualities of fermented products. The purpose of this presentation is to review some of the direct nutritional effects of fermentation and to consider what types of research are needed if we are to successfully improve the nutrient content of these products.

Changes in energy content. Data have not been published on changes in the energy content of fermented foods. As a general rule, large changes in energy values would not be expected. In the case of a product like tempeh, with about a 24 h aerobic growth period for a mould, the fermentation period would appear to be too short to allow large losses in the lipids or proteins, which are the major constituents of the soyabean. On a theoretical basis, lactic acid or alcoholic fermentations, which use glycolysis as the major energy pathway, should only cause about a 5 per cent energy loss since only 2 mol of ATP/mol of glucose are generated compared to a potential of 38 mol of ATP for aerobic metabolism of glucose.

Changes in proteins. *Protein content.* Fermentations have not been found to cause large changes in protein content. No significant change in protein concentration was observed in idli[16] or khaman[12]. Small increases in protein concentration attributed to loss of other components have been found in tempeh[8,23] and fermented milks[3]. Small decreases in fermented milk products have also been found[15]. An exception to this general pattern is a case in which *Candida tropicalis* was grown on cassava flour to produce yeast biomass. This resulted in an increase in protein from 3.1 per cent in the starting material to 18 per cent after fermentation[4].

Protein quality changes. The protein efficiency ratio (PER) change as a result of fermentation has generally ranged from slightly negative to about + 0.5 (Table). There have been differences in reported PER changes in idli fermentations by different workers. An increase of up to 60 per cent in methionine during idli fermentations was reported[11] — although, in other studies, no change was observed[21] the different results being attributed by the authors to variations in preparation techniques and different microflora in the natural fermentations.

Table. *Changes in protein efficiency ratio (PER) in fermented foods.*

Product	Change in PER	References	Product	Change in PER	References
Idli 4:1 blackgram/rice	0.27	Rao, 1961	Soybean tempeh	0.10	Wang *et al.*, 1968
Idli 1:1 blackgram/rice	−0.15	Van Veen *et al.*, 1967	Soybean tempeh	0.26	Kao & Robinson, 1978
Idli 1:2 blackgram/rice	0.50	Rajalkshimi & Vanaja, 1967	Wheat/soybean tempeh 1:1	0.30	Wang *et al.*, 1968
Soybean tempeh	−0.07	Hackler *et al.*, 1964	Wheat tempeh	0.50	Wang *et al.*, 1968

In one of only a few attempts intentionally aimed to improve the nutritional quality of fermented foods, lysine-excreting lactobacilli variants were selected from natural microbial populations[19,20]. Efforts are being made to introduce these organisms into traditional fermentation processes to improve the quality of low-lysine cereal ingredients[9].

There appear to be possibilities of significantly improving protein quality by fermentation processes. However, the fermentations must be better understood before consistent improvements can reasonably be expected. There would also be many difficulties in changing traditional fermentations to incorporate technical advances.

Changes in vitamins. The concentrations of most vitamins which have been investigated have been found to increase substantially in some fermentations — riboflavin[22], niacin[10], folic acid[17], thiamin[2], and vitamin B_{12}[22]. In most instances, it has not been clearly defined which organisms are responsible for vitamin production and under what conditions the vitamin increases will consistently occur. There is some evidence that *Aerobacter cloacae* and *Lactobacillus delbrueckii* may be responsible for riboflavin increases in ogi[1], and idli[13], respectively. *Aerobacter cloacae* was also implicated with niacin increases in ogi[1]. In addition to riboflavin, *L. delbrueckii* also appeared to be responsible for thiamin increases in idli fermentations[13].

Some particularly interesting observations have been made with regard to vitamin B_{12} synthesis: an increase of over 30-fold in vitamin B_{12} concentration in tempeh fermentations[22]; an increase in B_{12} in traditional tempeh fermentations, but not in pure culture fermentations with inoculated *Rhizopus oligosporus*[7]. This indicated that the vitamin was produced by a contaminating unidentified organism in the natural fermentation. Vitamin B_{12} was intentionally increased in kimchi fermentations[18] by the addition of a *Propionibacterium freudenreichii* culture to the natural fermentation.

As in the case of protein quality changes, vitamin increases associated with fermentations have been commonly observed, but they are by no means consistent. However, there does appear to be a potential for producing significant amounts of vitamins with a number of different fermentations provided appropriate organisms are selected and fermentation conditions are defined.

Conclusions. There appear to be a number of opportunities to improve substantially the nutritional attributes of fermented foods. However, concerted long-term efforts to increase nutrients have not been made. For many traditional fermentation processes, it is particularly critical to identify which microorganisms cause nutrient changes. Once this step has been taken and procedures to get a consistent increase in a nutrient are defined, it should then become possible to make use of modern genetic techniques to engineer improved strains. In this area, the approach taken by Sands & Hankin[19,20] looks to be particularly promising.

Many additional opportunities to improve nutritional quality will almost certainly emerge as techniques are developed to carry out genetic transfers in important food fermentation microorganisms.

1 Akinrele, I.A. (1970): Fermentation studies on maize during the preparation of a traditional African starch-cake food. *J. Sci. Fd Agric.* **21**, 619–625.
2 Aliya, S. & Geervani, P. (1981): An assessment of the protein quality and vitamin B content of commonly used fermented products of legumes and millets. *J. Sci. Fd Agric.* **32**, 837–842.
3 Alm, L. (1982): Effect of fermentation on proteins of Swedish fermented milk products. *J. Dairy Sci.* **65**, 1696–1704.
4 Azoulay, E., Jouanneau, F., Bertrand, J.C., Raphael, A., Janssens, J. & Lebeault, J.M. (1980): Fermentation methods for protein enrichment of cassava and corn with *Candidi tropicalis. Appl. Environ. Microbiol.* **39**, 41–47.
5 Hackler, L.R., Steinkraus, K.H., Van Buren, J.P. & Hand, D.B. (1964): Studies on the utilization of tempeh protein by weanling rats. *J. Nutr.* **82**, 452–456.
6 Kao, C. & Robinson, R.J. (1978): Nutritional aspects of fermented foods from chickpea, horsebean, and soybean. *Cer. Chem.* **55**, 512–517.
7 Liem, I.T.H., Steinkraus, K.H. & Cronk, T.C. (1977): Production of vitamin B_{12} in tempeh, a fermented soybean food. *Appl. Environ. Microbiol.* **34**, 773–776.
8 Murata, K., Ikehata, H. & Miyamoto, T. (1967): Studies on the nutritional value of tempeh. *J. Fd Sci.* **32**, 580–585.
9 Newman, R.K., Sands, D.C. & Scott, K. (1984): A microbiological approach to nutrition. *J. Am. Diet. Ass.* **84**, 820–821.
10 Nilson, K.M., Vakil, J.R. & Shahani, K.M. (1965): B complex vitamin content of cheddar cheese. *J. Nutr.* **86**, 362–368.
11 Padhye, V.W. & Salunkhe, D.K. (1978): Biochemical studies on black gram (*Phaseolus mungo* L.). III. Fermentation of the black gram and rice blend and its influence on the *in vitro* digestibility of the proteins. *J. Fd Biochem.* **2**, 327–347.
12 Rajalakshmi, R. & Vanaja, K. (1967): Chemical and biological evaluation of the effects of fermentation on the nutritive value of foods prepared from rice and grams. *Br. J. Nutr.* **21**, 467–473.
13 Ramakrishnan, C.V., Parekh, L.J., Akolkar, P.N., Rao, G.S. & Bhandari, S.D. (1976): Studies on soy idli fermentation. *Plant Foods for Man* **2**, 15–33.
14 Rao, M.V.R. (1961): Some observations on fermented foods. In *Progress in meeting protein needs of infants and pre-school children*. National Academy of Science, National Research Council, Washington, DC, Publ. no. 843.
15 Rao, D.R., Pulvsani, S.R. & Rao, T.K. (1982): Amino acid composition and nutritional implications of milk fermented by various lactic cultures. *J. Fd Quality* **5**, 235–243.
16 Reddy, N.R., Sathe, S.K., Pierson, M.D. & Salunkhe, D.K. (1981): Idli, an Indian fermented food: a review. *J. Fd Quality* **5**, 89–101.
17 Reif, G.D., Shahani, K.M., Vakil, J.R. & Crowe, L.K. (1976): Factors affecting B-complex vitamin content of cottage cheese. *J. Dairy Sci.* **59**, 410–415.
18 Ro, S.L., Woodburn, M. & Sandine, W.E. (1979): Vitamin B_{12} and ascorbic acid in kimchi inoculated with *Propionibacterium freudenreichii* ss. *shermanii. J. Fd Sci.* **44**, 873–877.
19 Sands, D.C. & Hankin, L. (1974): Selecting lysine-excreting mutants of lactobacilli for use in food and feed enrichment. *Appl. Microbiol.* **28**, 523–524.
20 Sands, D.C. & Hankin, L. (1976): Fortification of foods by fermentation with lysine-excreting mutants of lactobacilli. *J. Agr. Fd Chem.* **24**, 1104–1106.
21 Van Veen, A.G., Hackler, L.R., Steinkraus, K.H. & Mukherjee, S.K. (1967): Nutritive quality of idli, a fermented food of India. *J. Fd Sci.* **32**, 339–341.
22 Van Veen, A.G. & Steinkraus, K.H. (1970): Nutritive value and wholesomeness of fermented foods. *J. Agr. Fd Chem.* **18**, 576–578.
23 Wang, H.L., Ruttle, D.I. & Hesseltine, C.W. (1968): Protein quality of wheat and soybeans after *Rhizopus oligosporus* fermentation. *J. Nutr.* **96**, 109–114.

XX: Food safety and health

Food safety and health

Workshop

Nutrition and toxicology

Workshop

FOOD SAFETY AND HEALTH

Food-borne infections and malnutrition

L. MATA
Instituto de Investigaciones en Salud (INISA), University of Costa Rica, Ciudad Universitaria Rodrigo Facio, Costa Rica.

Until recently, public health practice in the less developed countries did not consider food-borne infection in the complex web of sources of diarrhoeal diseases and malnutrition. This omission rested on the belief that cooked foods, eaten in the home or in the street, generally do not carry the agents of diarrhoeal diseases. Food-borne infections were thought of as resulting from massive contamination of food in restaurants and from caterers.

The frequent occurrence of diarrhoea in families in tropical countries during the warmer and rainy months, and the occurrence of outbreaks after family or community festivities makes food and water an important suspect in the epidemiology of diarrhoea. Prior to 1970, the study of aetiologic agents of diarrhoea included shigellae, salmonellae and enteropathogenic *Escherichia coli*[6] (FAO/WHO, 1984). Enterotoxigenic and enteroinvasive *Escherichia coli*, rotaviruses, *Campylobacter* and *Cryptosporidium* have become better known in recent times[13]. Intrafamilial person-to-person spread was considered the most important mechanism, coupled with water transmission, but more recently, food has been suspected for the following reasons: (a) some foods, well-cooked before being eaten, are often stored at room temperature and become heavily contaminated; (b) some foods are often kept warm favouring replication of bacteria; (c) heating does not have an effect of many toxins of microbial origin[6].

Village food as a source of infectious diarrhoea. Field observations in Guatemala showed that 'tortillas' (flat cooked pancakes of lime-treated corn), generally considered free of pathogens, become contaminated with faecal bacteria during preparation[5]. Tortillas are the main food for many villages in Middle America, and are among the first foods given to weanlings. Tortillas are often stored in small baskets covered with a wet cloth to keep them soft which then favours proliferation of *Bacillus cereus* and of species of *Staphylococcus*, *Streptococcus* and *Clostridium*, all agents of diarrhoea (Table 1). Heating and reheating of tortillas significantly

Table 1. *Faecal bacteria and other potential enteric pathogens in village weaning foods*

Community	Food	Bacteria, $\log_{10}$/g food	Reference
Cauqué, Guatemala	Tortilla	*Escherichia coli*, 3–7 *Staphylococcus aureus*, 7–8 *Bacillus cereus*, 9 *Clostridium* sp., 1–2	Capparelli & Mata (1975)
Kenneba, The Gambia	Cereal gruels, milk	*Escherichia coli*, >5 *Staphylococcus aureus*, 2–6 *Bacillus cereus*, 4–6 *Clostridium welchii*, 3–5	Barrell & Rowland (1979)
Metlab, Bangladesh	Rice, milk	*Escherichia coli*, 2–7	Black *et al.* (1982)

reduce the levels of bacteria, but these proliferate again upon overnight storage. The sources of contamination are water used in their preparation and soiled hands of village women. Survival of microorganism after heating of tortillas suggests that other village foods also become contaminated in a similar fashion. This was recently demonstrated in The Gambia and Bangladesh[3,4]. The studies in Bangladesh showed that food contamination was more frequent and intense during the warm and humid months of the year, coinciding with the increase in community diarrhoea during the monsoon.

Transmission of enteric infection. Possible modes of transmission of diarrhoea involve human-to-human and animal-to-human contact. *Campylobacter fetus jejuni*, enterotoxigenic *Escherichia coli*, rotaviruses, and *Cryptosporidium* are harboured by humans and animals; the latter may be more important than initially suspected, particularly in rural settings where children often cohabitate with animals. Transmission is primarily determined by cultural, religious, social and economic factors. The contrast of two typical villages in Guatemala and Bangladesh revealed strikingly similar determinants of spread of diarrhoea agents, Table 2[11]. In both settings, the common source of contamination is faeces which reach the hands, food, water and utensils, and eventually the mouth[2,8].

Enteric infection and malnutrition. Food-borne diarrhoea results in diminished food consumption, reduced nutrient absorption, increased secretion, protein-losing enteropathy, and metabolic alterations. Diarrhoea interferes with food consumption as a result of anorexia, vomiting, dehydration, fever, discomfort and anxiety[12]. Anorexia and vomiting are common findings. Severe restriction of food intake for days or weeks is common and as much as 20 to 50 per cent of the total home diet is lost due to diarrhoea alone[9,14].

Adhesion of bacteria to the mucosa, release of toxins, direct damage to the enterocyte and crypt cells, bacterial hydrolysis of bile acids and carbohydrates, and other pathogenic actions result in a diminished capacity of the mucosa to absorb macro- and micronutrients. A decreased absorption of nitrogen, energy, fat, and carbohydrate in children with specific diarrhoeas was found in Bengali children[14].

Augmented secretion results from damage and lysis of villous tips of absorptive enterocytes and replacement by immature crypt-like cells. Other causes of hypersecretion are stimulation of cyclic AMP and cyclic GMP by bacterial heat-labile and heat-stable toxins, or by increased bile and fatty acids from bacterial metabolism, or by hormones and neurotransmitters. Hypersecretion results in deficits in sodium, potassium, chloride, water, vitamins and trace elements[12].

Alterations of mucosal epithelium by *Shigella*, rotaviruses and probably *Campylobacter*, lead to a protein-losing enteropathy syndrome. An increased ratio of α_1-antitrypsin (stool over serum values) was observed in many diarrhoeas due to rotavirus and *Shigella*[16]. There are losses of plasma and epithelial and blood cells. The consequences are more serious for malnourished children. The protein-losing enteropathy could explain the occurrence of kwashiorkor after epidemics of diarrhoea.

Recurrent diarrhoeas lead to malnutrition, especially if rehydration and alimentation are not promptly instituted. Metabolic alterations such as negative balances of nitrogen, magnesium,

Table 2. *Food contamination and opportunities for exposure in two villages with low socioeconomic development.* (After Mata, 1983[11]).

Faecal contamination of	Cauqué, Guatemala (Mata)	Teknaf, Bangladesh (Aziz)
Hands	Cleaning children	Cleaning children
	Handling animal faeces	Handling animal faeces
Mouth	Touching nipple	Touching nipple
	Handling foods, feeding with fingers	Handling foods, feeding with fingers
	Play with children	Play with children
Foods	Making mashes, purees	Making mashes, purees
	Peeling and serving fruits	Peeling and serving fruits
	Incubating in environment	Incubating in environment
	Exposure to insects	Exposure to insects
Water	Contamination with faeces	Contamination with faeces
	Touching with hands	Touching with hands
	Serving water	Serving water
Utensils	Touching with fingers	Touching with fingers
		Ablution
Feet	Cleaning site soiled with faeces	Cleaning site soiled with faeces
		Touching foot with hand during prayer
Ground	Outdoor, indoor	Indoor, outdoor

potassium, and phosphorus; mobilization of amino acids from muscle for gluconeogenesis; augmented synthesis of acute-phase reactant proteins; and sequestration of trace elements, are to be expected. Diarrhoea induces acute weight loss and arrest in linear growth[8]. Inspection of individual growth curves of cohort children shows weight faltering following diarrhoea attacks. Progressive weight deterioration (wastage) and marked growth retardation (stunting), are already evident in many children at the end of the first year of age. Stunting was more marked in children who had experienced fetal growth retardation[12].

It can be concluded that diarrhoeas are a major cause of chronic malnutrition and stunting of village children, especially when there is fetal growth retardation and borderline dietaries. Wasted and/or stunted children, on the other hand, tend to suffer from more severe diarrhoea and also have an increased risk of death.

Control of food-borne infections. Any attempt to control and prevent food-borne enteric infection must take into account their transmission cycle, which is dependent on human behaviour and environmental conditions. The approach must be holistic with emphasis on improving personal hygiene and environmental sanitation. Control must capitalize on 'maternal technologies'[9] and health education[12]. Personal hygiene (one of the maternal technologies) is an endowment that promotes child nutrition and health; often they are independent of schooling and economic condition. Women living in poverty and deprivation may possess maternal technologies that protect infants from diarrhoea and malnutrition. For instance, they may know how to cook and mix local village foods to produce nutritious and safe weaning mixtures; they may know how to handle food without contaminating it with faeces; they may wash their hands frequently and may protect drinking water from contamination[9,11].

Health education technique has been passive in the past because it aimed at diffusing knowledge through the radio, posters, and other audiovisual aids, often utilizing the infrastructure of the elementary school system. It was not until the concept of primary health care developed that health education reached the home to involve the family in the process[7,17]. More recently, the child-to-child concept was developed in recognition that older children in traditional societies are responsible — along with mothers — for the care and rearing of younger siblings[1]. Mothers can become part of the health team, contributing to growth monitoring, oral rehydration and promotion of child nutrition and health[10].

Current packages of health education have given little consideration to food safety[15], probably as a result of the slow pace of incorporation of new knowledge on etiology and epidemiology of diarrhoeal disease; another is the unawareness of the importance of food as a source of diarrhoea and poisoning under rural condition. On the other hand, there is still lack of information on the role of food in transmission of several important agents of diarrhoeal disease.

1 Aarons, A. & Hawes, H. (1979): *Child-to-child*. The Macmillan Press, London.

2 Aziz, K.M.A., Hasan, K.Z. & Datwarg, Y. (1981): A study of interpersonal spread of human feces in rural Teknaf of Bangladesh. Manuscript ICDDR,B., Dhaka, Bangladesh.

3 Barrell, R.A.E. & Rowland, M.G.M. (1979): Infant foods as a potential source of diarrhoeal illness in rural West Africa. *Trans Roy. Soc. Trop. Med. Hyg.* **73**, 85–90.

4 Black, R.E., Brown, K.H., Becker, S., Alim, A.R.M.A. & Merson, M.M. (1982): Contamination of weaning foods and transmission of enterotoxigenic *Escherichia coli* diarrhoea in children in rural Bangladesh. *Trans Roy. Soc. Trop. Med. Hyg.*, **76**, 259–264.

5 Capparelli, E. & Mata, L. (1975): Microflora of maize prepared as tortillas. *Appl. Microbiol.*, **29**, 802–806.

6 FOA/WHO (1984): *The Role of food safety in health and development*. Tech. Rep. Ser. 705. Geneva: WHO.

7 King, M. & King, F. (1979): *Primary child care. A guide for the community leader, manager, and teacher*. Book Two. Oxford: Oxford University Press.

8 Mata, L.J. (1978): *The children of Santa Maria Cauqué. A prospective field study of health and growth*. Cambridge, Mass.: The MIT Press.

9 Mata, L. (1979): The malnutrition-infection complex and its environment factors. *Proc. Nutr. Soc.* **38**, 29–40.

10 Mata, L., Allen, M.A., Jimenez, P., Garcia, M.E., Vargas, W., Rodriguez, M.E. & Valerin, C. (1982): Promotion of breast-feeding, health, and growth among hospital-born neonates, and among infants of a rural area of Costa Rica. In *Diarrhea and malnutrition, interactions, mechanisms and interventions*, ed L. Chen & N.S.S. Scrimshaw, pp. 177–202. New York: Plenum.

11 Mata. L. (1983): Food-borne enteric infections: health education and training aspects in less developed countries. EFP/FOS/EC/WP, Geneva, 30 May-6 June.

12 Mata, L. (1983): Influence on the growth parameters of children. Comments. In *Acute diarrhea: its nutritional consequences in children*, ed J.A. Bellanti, pp. 85–94, New York: Nestlé, Vevey/Raven Press.

13 Mata, L, Urrutia, J.J. & Simhon, A. (1984): Infectious agents in acute and chronic diarrhea of childhood. In *Chronic diarrhea in children*, ed E. Lebenthal, pp. 237–252. New York: Nestlé Vevey/Raven Press.

14 Molla, A., Molla, A.M., Rahim, A., Sarker, S.A., Mozaffar, Z. & Rahaman, M.M. (1982): Intake and absorption of nutrients in children with cholera and rotavirus infection during acute diarrhea and after recovery. *Nutr. Res.* **2**, 233–242.

15 Pan American Health Organization (1982): *Health for all by the Year 2000. Plan of action for the implementation of regional strategies*. PAHO Document No. 1979, Washington, DC.

16 Rahaman, M.M. & Wahed, A. (1983): Direct nutrient loss and diarrhea. In *Diarrhea and malnutrition. Interactions, mechanisms, and interactions*, ed L.C. Chen & N.S. Scrimshaw, pp. 155–160, New York: Plenum Press.

17 World Health Organization (1980): *The primary health worker*. Geneva: WHO.

Interventions to promote microbiological food safety

F.K. KÄFERSTEIN
World Health Organization, 1211 Geneva 27, Switzerland.

Nature and extent of the problem of food safety. The attention of the public is always drawn to the problem of food-borne illness if something spectacular happens. The suffering of some 20 000 people of whom as many as 350 died and which might have been caused by the consumption of contaminated cooking oil in Spain in 1981 and 1982 has caused a lot of concern[8] and has made many headlines in the national and international press. The same is certainly true for the recent 'Illinois-outbreak' for which *Salmonellae* in dairy products seemed to be responsible[3]. However, headlines seldom dwell on the suffering and death of millions of people from diarrhoea.

According the available data 1000 million episodes of diarrhoea occur in developing countries of Asia (except China), Africa and Latin America in children under the age of 5 years alone. Of these, about 5 million children die[4] which is equivalent to ten diarrhoeal deaths every minute of each single day of the year.

A substantial number of cases of acute diarrhoea is caused by microbiologically contaminated food[2,7] and the resulting malabsorption reduces the nutritional status, a specially serious consequence in the case of marginally-nourished or already mal-nourished persons. When one adds to this total other food-borne diseases such as botulism, typhoid fever, and parasitism, as well as the mainly chronic effects of chemical contamination of food, the number of people affected and the impact of food contamination on function and well-being is appalling.

Equally important is the effect of such widespread acute and chronic debilitation on the economic and financial situation of the world community. It is therefore not surprising that an Expert Committee on Food Safety, which met in 1983 in Geneva, came to the conclusion that 'illness due to contaminated food is perhaps the most widespread health problem in the contemporary world and an important cause of reduced economic productivity'[7]. This conclusion is certainly not only true for developing countries, for although food-borne mortality rates in industrialized countries are statistically insignificant, the morbidity rates are appalling as well.

It is an undisputed fact that in many developing countries, food production does not keep pace with population growth. According to FAO and the World Bank, 450 million — others even say up to one billion — people do not have enough food[6]. Food safety may seem insignificant *vis-à-vis* this food shortage and famine. However, under these conditions, the situation becomes even more disastrous if the little food available is unsafe, especially through microbiological contamination, which leads to diarrhoea and nutrient loss, thus initiating or aggravating malnutrition. Thus, there is no conflict between the effort to provide *enough* food and the effort to provide *safe* food; a programme to ensure food safety will help to increase the availability of food by decreasing losses attributable to spoilage and contamination[7]. The control of microbiological food contamination will help to reduce diarrhoea and other mainly acute food-borne diseases. In view of the potential long-term impact on human health of chemicals in food, the control of chemical food contamination and the use of only safe food additives under good manufacturing practice are of equal public health significance.

Factors affecting the safety of food. The aforementioned Expert Committee on Food Safety has devoted an entire chapter of its report[7] to discussing the various factors affecting food safety. In this paper, however, it is only possible to highlight some of those, which in my view, are not yet universally appreciated. In every society, the nutritional items identified as food, their mode of preparation, the conditions under which they are eaten, the proscriptions and prescriptions relating to ritual and other occasions, all reflect basic cultural values, premises about life, religious convictions and often, national pride. Food practices have, from the standpoint of health, both positive and negative aspects. Some of these practices appear to be universal; others are culture-specific in that they characterize one or several societies.

Widespread customs conducive to food safety include the thorough cooking of food, the peeling of fruits, the boiling of milk and the preservation of meats and fruits through salting and/or sun or air drying. Culture-specific food practices that promote food safety include, for instance, the oriental custom of cutting meat into small pieces, thus permitting effective heat penetration during the cooking, and the fermenting of milk to make yogurt.

Unfortunately, negative factors in food handling are also widespread. Many of these factors naturally stem from the poor environmental sanitation prevailing in much of the world. But many negative factors are largely or entirely cultural and improvement can be effected with correct information and the willingness to give up traditional ways that are detrimental to health.

Strategies for the prevention and control of food-borne diseases of microbiological origin. Having reviewed the nature and extent of the problem, as well as some of the factors affecting it, it is not surprising that the World Health Organization considers food safety as one of its priorities. This concern is reflected in the so-called essential components of primary health care[5] through which WHO and its member states approach the target of 'Health for all by the year 2000'.

Primary health care emphasizes the need for action at the level of the individual, the family and the community. At the same time, it stresses the need for governmental and non-governmental support to the community through a system of decentralization and referral.

The above mentioned Expert Committee on Food Safety in its report on *The role of food safety in health and development*[7] drew attention to the fact that the Declaration on primary health care of Alma-Ata[5] only implicitly covered food safety as an essential component of primary health care. The Expert Committee emphasized that food safety and adequate nutrition were basic to the reduction and prevention of disease and to the promotion of health. It recommended that 'food safety should be considered an integral part of the primary health care delivery system' since the consumption of safe and nutritious food was vital for health. This recommendation has to be seen in light of the following facts: (1) epidemiological data from industrialized countries indicate that food safety programmes, as commonly carried out (eg through official control of production, processing and marketing of food and food establishments), have failed to reduce the incidence of food-borne disease; (2) in the developing countries, only a very small proportion of food is subject to inspection, the extent and quality of which varies from country to country, but is generally inadequate.

In these seemingly discouraging circumstances, the only rational approach to bring about improved levels of food safety would be appropriate action taken by individuals, families and/or communities themselves which need to be encouraged and supported by the health team and helped further through a coordinated effort by all sectors with responsibility for food safety. All efforts should be aimed at enabling individuals, families and communities to be intelligently involved in maintaining or obtaining safe food and in this way, in preventing food-borne illness and food losses.

However, the preceding three paragraphs have not been included in order to suggest that in the future, the responsibility for food safety, especially for microbiological food safety, should rest solely on the shoulders of consumers. What is suggested is a concerted effort of the three parties involved, namely governments, food industry and trade, and consumers.

For this reason, the Expert Committee on Food Safety[7] recommended that a national strategy for the prevention and control of food-borne diseases by the improvement of food safety should start with the *identification of the prevailing problems*. Many developing and industrialized countries have not as yet formulated mechanisms for the assessment of the true extent of morbidity and mortality from food-borne disease. Thus, the responsible technical staff are often not fully acquainted with the reality of the problem. Consequently, they are frequently unable to express actual health situations in concrete terms to policy makers. In addition, it is often not precisely known which of the many factors that may influence the safety of food are of particular concern to one specific culture or society. This, however, is one of the pre-conditions for cost-effective interventions to reduce food contamination.

As already mentioned, improvements in food safety cannot be expected without the involvement of the consumer. For this reason, the Export Committee on Food Safety believed that it was also very important to *identify target groups* within a society on which attention should be focused. In selecting target groups for the prevention of diarrhoeal disease and malnutrition, attention should be focused mainly on mothers of pre-school children since weaning children in particular are the most vulnerable group in terms of morbidity and mortality in many parts of the developing world. In industrialized countries on the other hand, mothers of pre-school children would not necessarily be a special target group.

Having sufficient data on the prevailing problems of food safety and on specific target groups would allow the formulation of interventions. In general, the Expert Committee on

Food Safety proposed several direct and supportive interventions for consideration by member states.

Direct interventions for ensuring food safety. These may basically be approached in three ways: (a) regulatory food control as being the governmental responsibility for food safety; (b) voluntary food control as being the responsibility of industry, trade, food premises, etc. for food safety; and (c) community participation through public education since the consumers themselves must be able to assume responsibility for food safety.

The objectives of national *food control* systems are varied but they all play an equally critical role in ensuring food safety for the population. In order to be effective, there must be a legislative framework and the necessary infrastructure for its implementation and enforcement.

The *commercial sector*, in turn, has the responsibility for ensuring, as far as practicable, that every unit of food is safe. Food control authorities should encourage the establishment by the food industry of quality assurance programmes which, in turn, should result in less frequent need for inspection and sampling by the authorities.

Probably the greatest need, however, is for the *education of the public*. The most effective incentive for the commercial sector to improve hygiene is consumer response, ie the unwillingness of the consumer to buy food from unhygienic premises and those that have a bad reputation for safety. Furthermore, it should be recognized that good commercial food safety practices can be nullified if the food is mishandled at home[1]. Therefore, governments and industry should be encouraged to play a role in educating the public in the safe handling of food at the domestic level. For rural populations living to a large extent on food not moving in trade and therefore not usually subject to any form of control, education on proper food handling is probably the single most important measure for preventing food-borne diseases and unnecessary food losses.

These direct interventions for the improvement of food safety can and must be backed up by several *supportive interventions*, over which, however, governmental authorities having responsibility for food safety and control, often have no direct control.

The following supportive interventions have been identified: (1) environmental protective measures; (2) zoonose control; (3) medical care and patient education, and (4) improvement of the nutritional quality of food. Addressing nutritionists, it is certainly appropriate briefly to discuss (3) and (4) in more detail. It is recognized that, in the short-and medium-term, there will be a need for treatment of acute diarrhoeal diseases. The treatment of institutionalized cases and out-patients should be seen as an opportunity for educating patients and their families on why food-borne diseases occur and how they can be prevented. In formulating strategies to prevent food-borne diseases by improvement of food safety, they should be linked to the health delivery system based on primary health care. This is turn implies that more attention should be given to ascertaining local needs, resources, and attitudes, and the development of appropriate health education and information.

In considering food quality it is important to remember that it comprises two, perhaps even three different aspects. The food hygienist usually limits quality to microbiological safety, avoidance of filth, minimising chemical contaminants, such as heavy metals and pesticide residues, and refraining from the use of unsafe food additives. On the other hand, in the eyes of nutritionists, food quality refers mainly to matters such as proteins, dietary energy, amino acids, minerals, vitamins and others. Finally, the third — the aesthetic aspect, relates to appearance, smell, freshness.

In the view of the Expert Committee on Food Safety, any strategy to interrupt the diarrhoeal disease/malnutrition cycle should, however, emphasize both the hygienic and the nutritional aspects of food quality. Accordingly, in the strategic matrix for the prevention and control of diarrhoeal diseases and malnutrition, it is essential to incorporate the concept of nutritional quality of individual foods and total diets from the perspectives of both prevention and therapy. It is for this very reason that WHO proposed to the Organizing Committee for the XIII International Congress of Nutrition the holding of a colloquium on Food Safety and Health in order to underline the need for nutritionists and food hygienists to join forces and to work together for the prevention and control of the food-borne diarrhoeal disease/malnutrition cycle.

1 Allen, R.J.L. & Käferstein, F.K. (1983): Foodborne disease, food hygiene and consumer education. *Arch. Lebensmittelhyg.* **34**, 86–89.
2 Barua, D. & Käferstein, F.K. (1983): The role of food in the epidemiology of acute enteric infections and intoxications. WHO offset document EFP/FOS/83.48.
3 MMWR (1985): Milk-borne salmonellosis in Illinois. *MMWR* **34**, (15), 215.
4 Snyder, J.D. & Merson, M.H. (1982): The magnitude of the global problem of acute diarrhoeal diseases. *Bull. Wld Hlth Org.* **60**, 605–613.
5 WHO (1978): *Primary health care.* Report of the International Conference on Primary Health Care, Alma-Ata, USSR, 1978. WHO 'Health for all' Series No. 1. Geneva: World Health Organization.
6 WHO (1980): *Sixth report on the world health situation* (1973–77). *I. Global analysis.* Geneva: World Health Organization.
7 WHO (1984): *The role of food safety in health and development.* Report of a Joint FAO/WHO Expert Committee on Food Safety, Geneva 1983. WHO Tech. Rep. Ser. No. 705. Geneva: World Health Organization.
8 WHO/EURO (1984): Toxic oil syndrome. Mass food poisoning in Spain. Report on a WHO meeting, Madrid, 21–25 March 1983, WHO/EURO.

Food preparation — the faults that lead to food-borne disease

Diane ROBERTS
Food Hygiene Laboratory, Central Public Health Laboratory, 61 Colindale Avenue, London NW9 5HT, UK.

There is some indication from the reports received by the disease surveillance centres in most countries that food-borne illness, rather than abating or remaining static, is on the increase. In England and Wales for example, 15 168 cases of bacterial food-poisoning and salmonella infection were reported in 1983, a 20 per cent increase over the 1982 figure (12 684), which was a 19 per cent increase over the numbers reported in 1981 (10 665)[7–9]. These values exclude symptomless involvement of salmonellas.

Improvement of food preparation processes and education of those responsible for provision of food, particularly in mass catering, would undoubtedly reduce the incidence of food-poisoning. In order that this can be brought about it is essential to know the factors which have contributed to the incidents.

The various characteristics of food that may play a part in allowing bacterial multiplication include pH, water activity (a_w), redox potential and levels of other organisms which may compete with, or inhibit, the growth of potential pathogens, or both. Certain characteristics of food-poisoning bacteria, such as production of heat resistant spores, ability to grow at relatively high temperatures, and tolerance of high salt and sugar levels, also contribute to incidents of food-poisoning.

In the sequence of events which occurs when persons succumb to bacterial food-poisoning the dose of organisms in a food must usually increase from an initial harmless level to a harmful one, of the order of 10^6 organisms/g or more. Many malpractices take place in food preparation which permit contamination, survival and growth of food-poisoning agents. A number of studies of these factors have been carried out in the USA[1], UK[10,11] and Canada[12].

Analysis of contributory factors. The study made recently of 1044 outbreaks of food-poisoning which occurred from 1970 to 1979 in England and Wales[10] has been extended to include the years 1980–1982. The results of this extended analysis of contributing factors is presented to illustrate the faults in food preparation that lead to food-borne disease. The data have been extracted from routine reports of general and family outbreaks made to the PHLS

(Public Health Laboratory Service) Communicable Disease Surveillance Centre, supplemented by published reports, and by information from correspondence and questionnaires accompanying cultures of *Clostridium perfringens*, *Staphylococcus aureus*, *Bacillus cereus* and other *Bacillus* spp. and food samples, sent to the Food Hygiene Laboratory for further testing.

Table 1. *Distribution of 1479 general and family outbreaks of food-poisoning analysed (1970–1982).*

Causal agent	Number of outbreaks	Causal agent	Number of outbreaks	Causal agent	Number of outbreaks
Salmonella spp.	566	Other — bacterial		Other — non-bacterial	
C.perfringens	525	*V.parahaemolyticus*	9	Scrombrotoxin	124
S.aureus	166	*E.coli*	3	Red kidney beans	8
B.cereus and	63	*C.botulinum*	1	Virus	3
other *Bacillus* spp.		*Y.enterocolitica*	1	Not known	10

The outbreaks studied were mostly due to bacteria, but some episodes due to scombrotoxic fish-poisoning, red kidney bean poisoning and viral gastroenteritis are included (Table 1). The reports analysed varied in the amount of detail furnished, in some as many as five or six contributory factors being recorded whereas in others there was only one. In the latter instance it is likely that other factors were involved, but as they were not recorded they could not be included. The total of 1479 represents only about 20 per cent of such outbreaks reported to the PHLS during that period. This figure is low and includes only a fraction of the reported incidents of salmonella food-poisoning, because in only a small proportion of these outbreaks is the food vehicle ever traced. In the period 1969 to 1982 the vehicle of infection was determined in only 10 per cent of incidents of salmonella food-poisoning, while for other types of bacterial food-poisoning this figure exceeded 80 per cent and often approached 100 per cent. Thus the proportion of salmonella outbreaks included in this analysis does not bear any relationship to the number reported. The foods implicated in the outbreaks studied are summarized in Table 2. Cold cooked meats and poultry and desserts were the foods involved in incidents of staphylococcal food-poisoning.

Table 2. *Foods implicated in 1479 outbreaks of food poisoning, England and Wales (1970–82)*

Food	Number of outbreaks (%)					Total
	Salmonella	C.perfringens	S.aureus	B.cereus	Other[a]	
Meat	141 (25)	367 (70)	89 (53)	2 (3)	3 (2)	602 (40)
Poultry	324 (56)	136 (26)	43 (26)	—	2 (1)	505 (34)
Milk	75 (13)	—	—	—	—	75 (5)
Seafood	6 (1)	2 (<1)	10 (6)	1 (2)	138 (87)	157 (11)
Rice	—	—	—	52 (83)	—	52 (3)
Other	30 (5)	20 (4)	25 (15)	8 (13)	16 (10)	99 (7)
Total	576[b]	525	167[c]	63	159	1490

[a]See Table 1 [b]In ten outbreaks two foods were involved [c]In one outbreak two foods were involved.

Table 3 gives data on the places where food was prepared in the 1479 outbreaks. This shows that it is in situations where food is prepared in quantity for a large number of people that most problems arise.

The factors which contributed to the 1479 outbreaks of food-poisoning in England and Wales are summarized in Table 4.

Discussion. In the domestic kitchen it is fairly easy to time preparation and cooking of food so that a meal can be served hot immediately; in mass catering this is not as straight-forward. When large numbers of people require feeding in a short space of time or a meal service is required outside the normal working day, as is the case with shift workers, it is often necessary to prepare food hours before it is needed and to hold until required, either under refrigeration or in a hot-holding apparatus. If this procedure is strictly controlled and the storage temperatures are

Table 3. *Place where food prepared in 1479 outbreaks of food poisoning, England and Wales (1970–82)*

Place	Salmonella	C.perfringens	S.aureus	B.cereus	Other[1]	Total (%)
Mass catering						
Restaurants, hotels, clubs	126	90	17	32	9	274 (19)
Banquets, dinners, receptions, parties	77	19	23	1	3	123 (8)
Hospitals, old people's and other homes	19	180	15	2	1	217 (15)
Schools, canteens	19	156	23	1	3	202 (14)
Colleges, Institutions	12	16	6	—	1	35 (2)
Sub total						851 (58)
Home catering	14	—	—	—	2	16 (1)
Other	14	30	5	—	7	56 (4)
Retail						
Shops, bakeries, takeaways, milk rounds	179	2	22	23	2	228 (15)
Family homes	106	32	55	4	5	202 (14)
Non recorded	—	—	—	—	2	2 (0.1)
Scombrotoxin incidents[2]	—	—	—	—	124	124 (8)
Total	566	525	166	63	159	1479

[1]'Other' outbreaks listed in Table 1 [2]Full data not analysed.

Table 4. *Factors contributing to 1479 outbreaks of food poisoning, England and Wales (1970–82)*

Contributing factors	Salmonella	C.perfringens	S.aureus	B.cereus	Other	Total
Total	566	525	166	63	159	1479
Preparation too far in advance	240 (42)	464 (88)	80 (48)	54 (86)	6 (4)	844 (57)
Storage at ambient temperature	172 (30)	276 (53)	75 (45)	39 (62)	4 (3)	566 (38)
Inadequate cooling	125 (22)	313 (60)	12 (7)	17 (27)	1 (1)	468 (32)
Inadequate reheating	76 (13)	275 (52)	5 (3)	33 (52)	2 (1)	391 (26)
Contaminated processed food	110 (19)	19 (4)	27 (16)	4 (6)	86 (54)	246 (17)
Undercooking	139 (25)	74 (14)	2 (1)	1 (2)	7 (4)	223 (15)
Contaminated canned food	2 (<1)	4 (1)	42 (25)	1 (2)	55 (35)	104 (7)
Inadequate thawing	61 (11)	34 (6)	—	—	—	95 (6)
Cross contamination	84 (15)	8 (2)	2 (1)	—	—	94 (6)
Raw food consumed	84 (15)	—	1 (1)	—	8 (5)	93 (6)
Improper warm holding	15 (3)	52 (10)	—	8 (13)	2 (1)	77 (5)
Infected food handlers	13 (2)	—	50 (30)	—	2 (1)	65 (4)
Use of left overs	25 (4)	25 (5)	11 (7)	1 (2)	—	62 (4)
Extra-large quantities prepared	29 (5)	17 (3)	2 (1)	—	—	48 (3)

at levels which will not permit bacterial multiplication then there need not be any hazard. Food to be held hot must be placed immediately after cooking into a hot holding apparatus already at a temperature of at least 145 °F/62.8 °C (UK) or 140 °F/60 °C (USA) and maintained at that level until required. In many incidents, however, food has been left for long periods at ambient temperatures, placed in hot holding equipment which has not been preheated — or is set at too low a temperature, or has been 'reheated' by the addition of hot gravy or sauce. All these practices produce ideal conditions for, and growth of, any organisms which have survived the cooking procedure or may have been picked up after cooking.

When foods are undercooked, such as can occur when large joints of meat or poultry, especially large frozen turkeys, are cooked for too short a time — or at too low a temperature, or from an improperly thawed state — then there is a greater chance of survival of organisms such as *Salmonella* and subsequent poor storage will permit multiplication.

During cooking oxygen will be driven out of food thus creating an anaerobic environment. Heat-resistant spores of *C.perfringens* that survive most conventional cooking procedures will be heat-activated and during a long slow cooling process there will be germination and rapid multiplication. *C.perfringens* has a high optimum temperature for growth (43–47 °C) and a short generation time of about 12 min. The organism is widespread in the environment, is usually present in the animal intestine and will therefore be present naturally in most foods, particularly those of animal origin. Rapid cooling of large bulks of food prior to refrigeration is therefore essential. Foods which are to be stored cold should be refrigerated within 90 min of cooking so that surviving organisms do not have the opportunity to begin multiplying rapidly.

Poultry is a particular problem in relation to *Salmonella* food-poisoning. Many oven-ready chickens and turkeys enter the kitchen already contaminated with salmonellae. A recent survey in London[3] showed that 79 of 100 frozen chickens from retail outlets were contaminated. The procedures carried out during the preparation of poultry for the table offer many opportunities for the spread of contamination. In poultry-associated outbreaks factors such as adequate thawing, undercooking and cross contamination are important contributory factors. The larger the bird the greater the problem in ensuring adequate thawing, cooking, cooling and storage.

Although cross contamination appears quite low in the list of contributory factors (Table 4) it probably plays a much greater part than is indicated. If raw and cooked foods are prepared on the same surfaces, by the same personnel, and using the same equipment, or are stored in close proximity, there are great opportunities for spread of organisms to foods which will receive no further heat-treatment before consumption. Separate surfaces, equipment and personnel for raw and cooked foods, regular hand-washing, particularly after handling raw foods, and good cleaning schedules regularly enforced are essential in keeping cross contamination to a minimum.

Infected food handlers do not play a significant role except in instances of *S.aureus* food-poisoning. The organism is frequently carried in the anterior nares, less commonly on the skin and most importantly in septic lesions on the hands. In many incidents the same phage and exterotoxin producing type of *S.aureus* was isolated from both food handler and food. Foods which act as vehicles of intoxication are usually those which have received much handling during preparation, such as cold meats and desserts which are consumed without further heat-treatment. In a small proportion of salmonella outbreaks infected food handlers may have been the source of the contaminating organisms; however, more often the food handlers are victims, not sources, who become infected either from frequent contact with contaminated raw food, from tasting during preparation, or from eating left over contaminated food.

Of the non-bacterial food-poisonings, scombrotoxic fish-poisoning is probably beyond the control of the food handler and the consumer. The fault lies at the processing stage when scombroid fish (tuna, mackerel, bonito), rich in histidine, are stored at warm temperatures. The normal fish flora decarboxylate the histidine to histamine, is the toxic factor or closely associated with it[4]. The toxin is very stable and cannot be destroyed by curing or heating, so outbreaks can occur from canned fish[5].

Outbreaks associated with red beans are due to consumption of the food in an uncooked or undercooked state. The toxin which is a natural constituent of the red kidney bean (*Phaseolus vulgaris*) and some other beans is inactivated by cooking the beans until soft[6].

Conclusion. The final line of defence in the prevention of most types of bacterial food-poisoning is good kitchen hygiene.

A recent publication from the WHO[2] is aimed at drawing the attention of catering and health officials to the relationship between mass catering and public health. WHO also have a surveillance programme for the control of food-borne infections and intoxications in Europe, its third report deals with food-borne diseases in 21 European countries in 1982[13].

1 Bryan, F.L. (1978): Factors that contribute to outbreaks of foodborne disease. *J. Fd Protect.* **41**, 816–827.
2 Charles, R.H.G. (1983): *Mass catering*. WHO Regional Publications, European Series No. 15. Copenhagen: World Health Organization.
3 Gilbert, R.J. (1983): Food-borne infections and intoxications — recent trends and prospects for the future. In *Food microbiology: advances and prospects*, ed T.A. Roberts & F.A. Skinner. Society for Applied Bacteriology Symposium Series No. 11, pp. 47–66. London & New York: Academic Press.
4 Gilbert, R.J., Hobbs, G., Murray, C.K., Cruickshank, J.G. & Young, S.E.J. (1980): Scombrotoxic fish poisoning: features of the first 50 incidents to be reported in Britain (1976–9). *Br. Med. J.* **281**, 71–72.
5 Murray, C.K., Hobbs, G. & Gilbert, R.J. (1982): Scombrotoxin and 'Scombrotoxin-like' poisoning from canned fish. *J. Hyg., Camb.* **88**, 215–220.
6 Noah, N.D., Bender, A.E., Reiaidi, G.B. & Gilbert, R.J. (1980): Food poisoning from raw red kidney beans. *Br. Med. J.* **281**, 236–237.
7 Public Health Laboratory Service (1982): Food poisoning and salmonellosis surveillance in England and Wales: 1981. *Br. Med. J.* **285**, 1127–1128.
8 Public Health Laboratory Service (1984): Food poisoning and salmonella surveillance in England and Wales: 1982. *Br. Med. J.* **288**, 306–308.
9 Public Health Laboratory Service (1985): Food poisoning and salmonella surveillance in England and Wales: 1983. (In press).
10 Roberts, D. (1982): Factors contributing to outbreaks of food poisoning in England and Wales 1970–1979. *J. Hyg., Camb.* **89**, 491–498.
11 Roberts, D. (1985): Good food handling — the final line of defence against foodborne Salmonella infection. In *Proc. Int. Symp. Salmonella*, ed G.H. Snoeyenbos, pp. 289–295. University of Pennsylvania: American Association of Avian Pathologists.
12 Todd, E.C.D. (1983): Factors that contributed to foodborne disease in Canada. 1973–1977. *J. Fd Protect.* **46**, 737–747.
13 World Health Organization (1984): *WHO surveillance programme for control of foodborne infections and intoxications in Europe. Third report, 1982.* Berlin: FAO/WHO Collaborating Centre for Research and Training in Food Hygiene and Zoonoses.

Food composition and safety: an industrial perspective

R.L. HALL
McCormick and Company, Inc., 11350 McCormick Road, Hunt Valley, Maryland 21031, USA.

Safety is not an absolute, and absolute safety is absolutely unattainable. Safety is a relative term, and it is relative freedom from risk or hazard. While many categorizations of food hazards are possible, a useful and familiar one is[1]:
Microbiological contamination
Nutritional hazards

Natural toxicants
Environmental contaminants

Pesticide residues
Food additives
This is not an equally spaced ranking; there are large gaps between the first two and the middle two, and between the middle and the last two. And while the ranking remains everywhere generally the same, the magnitude of these hazards varies enormously in different countries, depending on the general level of sanitation and other personal and public health practices, the effectiveness of the infrastructure for food control, and the training and sophistication of the agricultural and food processing industries. Even though popular concern and media attention frequently reflect a virtually inverted perception, all available data support this ranking.

The impact of food processing. When, about 12 000 years ago, our distant ancestors changed from hunting and gathering to herding and farming — the Neolithic Revolution — they accomplished two significant changes. They enormously increased the supply of available food, and they made necessary what we now know as food processing — doing something to food so it could be kept in edible condition for later consumption.

Many of the most serious sources of food risks, some of the microbiological contaminations and mycotoxins, for example, first arose then. That set a pattern that continues to this day. We now process food for many reasons beyond mere preservation. Improved nutritive value, acceptability, convenience, and waste reduction all are important. There are many variations on food processing the better to serve these purposes, but there are only six basic processes. They are:

Physical (washing, peeling, sorting, cutting, etc.)
Thermal (pasteurizing, heating, cooking, retorting, etc.)
Refrigeration (cooling, freezing)
Chemical (fermentation, fumigation, preservatives, etc.)
Dehydration (concentration, drying, evaporation, etc.)
Radiation (by gamma radiation, electron beams)

The history of food processing and food control is the history of extending the benefits and reducing the risks.

The 'newer' hazards in our initial tabulation are the last three — those from environmental contaminants, pesticide residues, and food additives. These three have lent themselves — in part logically, in part by historical accident — to evaluation by toxicological methods and to regulatory control. Partly for that reason, as we have begun to consider the safety of 'novel foods', we have, usually without much thought, assumed that toxicological evaluation and regulatory control should work here as well. It is the purpose of this paper to argue that more thought and ingenuity are needed.

Toxicology — benefits and limitations. Toxicology is the study of poisons — of chemical disruption of living systems. It grew out of pharmacognosy, pharmacology, and nutrition, usually from the study of low levels of physiologically active materials. The use of animals as experimental models began early. Toxicology has recently been applied to many substances in our environment, including some showing only moderate or little physiological activity.

In order to elicit a response with a necessarily limited number of test animals, it has frequently become the practice to feed very high doses to increase the likelihood of observing a response. This likelihood is purchased at the price of possible irrelevance. Metabolic pathways may become saturated as the dose rises, and spill over into pathways little used, or not used at all at normal exposure levels. This will frequently produce effects not relevant to human exposures.

The use of an experimental animal model is based on broad and unquestionable similarities between species. It has frequently been our only window of insight into safety, and has served us very well.

But it has become a highly developed technology that has exceeded its base of fundamental understanding. The most elaborate toxicological test, the two-species, two-year chronic study, is a tool that deals very well with strong and clear-cut effects. But as one moves toward effects that are less clear-cut, or are weak, or uncertain, or merely hypothetical, the weaknesses of the model loom larger. Opportunities for false positives, insensitivity, error-proneness and 'noise' – random effects – abound. Increasing the cost and complexity, the more sophisticated statistical techniques should not – and must not be allowed to – conceal the biological uncertainty.

These are the problems of toxicology applied to trace ingredients and contaminants. Even more daunting are the problems posed by new foods and new processes.

Problems raised by novel foods — lessons from irradiation. This topic is now receiving increasing attention, most recently in the MAFF/DHSS 'Memorandum on the testing of novel foods'[3]. This thoughtful set of guide-lines is a considerable advance over previous efforts. It would be even more valuable had it recognized that safety testing of novel foods, unfortunately, is likely to present exactly the situation in which conventional animal-feeding tests are most insensitive. If one recognizes this explicitly, one can then devise strategies to avoid or reduce this insentivity by sharpening the focus of such tests, or at least not expect more of them than they can reveal.

Of our six basic food processes, only irradiation post-dates toxicology. Irradiated foods have been examined in toxicological studies over the past 30 years. The results have been consistently negative, but unimpressive.

This conclusion emerges from the report on the 'Wholesomeness of irradiated food'[4], a report covering approximately 142 tests on eight foods or food categories. Of these, 68 were animal-feeding tests for toxicity or reproductive effects. Of the 68, 15 did not involve feeding the unirradiated food as a control diet, so possible adverse effects from feeding the test food itself at elevated levels could not be determined. In the remaining 53, one-half, or 27 tests, showed adverse effects from the *un*irradiated diet as compared with standard laboratory chow controls. Of the total 68, only five reported any adverse effects possibly attributable to irradiation. In all of these five, the effects were slight and questionable, and in the one test repeated, not reproducible.

There can now be no reasonable doubt that irradiation processing is safe under the conditions of intended use. But also there can be no doubt that in retrospect, most of this testing effort was well intended, but without value. The intent of the testing far exceeded the capability of the test system[2].

We cannot evaluate traditional foods and their natural components by toxicological methods. As the MAFF/DHSS memorandum[3] points out, we cannot cram enough of them into the diet of animals to support a conventional safety factor. They may be nutritionally inappropriate. Many of the unavoidable minor components are far too toxic to meet customary criteria. Specifications useful for toxicological purposes often are difficult or impossible to devise. Earlier toxic manifestations from one constituent may overshadow or preclude later consequences from another.

These are the reasons why 30 years of testing of irradiated foods in various countries yielded uniformly negative results. It is clear in the light of what we have discussed here that this was inevitably to be the case. Unless irradiation had created potent toxicants, which would have been analytically determinable, the problems and insensitivities of toxicological testing dictated that very little, other than random variation from negative results, could have been expected.

Gradually attention shifted to efforts to determine the nature and extent of the chemical changes resulting from irradiation. The focus became the 'unique radiolytic products' (URPs). After much study, there remains very little concern about the safety of the URPs. We should also remember that just as there are URPs so are there 'unique canning and cooking products' (UCCPs), and indeed, unique products of any process, including — worst of all — natural spoilage.

Potential improvements. Looking forward, then, in dealing with novel foods, we should focus our attention on the analytically determinable results of the new or changed process and the extent to which the result of the process differs, not from the unprocessed material, but from the same material processed by other methods whose results we readily — if usually uncritically —accept.

We should use conventional and long-accepted processes as benchmarks for acceptable risks. We should use analytical techniques to measure how far and in what directions a new process departs from these benchmarks. If the sum of the departures is in the direction of net risk reduction, then the conclusion on safety should be favourable.

This approach will require that we pay more attention than we have to the level of risk from natural toxicants in food and to the risk consequences of traditional processes.

The advantage of this approach is that it avoids the need to try to measure risks in the absolute terms now favoured by practitioners of 'risk analysis'. Risk analysis attempts to use various mathematical models to extrapolate risk from the experimentally observed range in animal-feeding studies to the range of human exposure — usually several orders of magnitude less. Typically, the results of different models disagree widely, and we know too little biology to choose the right model — if there is one. After such risky extrapolation, one must then generalize from the animal model to man. How much better simply to compare analytical results against an acceptable benchmark!

It will not be necessary to subject to formal toxicological evaluation every analytically detectable change. The trivial can be ignored. Others can be prioritized by available systems for predictive toxicology. Only rarely will actual toxicological testing be required.

Toxicology must continue to play an important supporting role in establishing the possible risk of the benchmark components in conventional foods and the 'unique processing products' in new foods. But for the reasons outlined previously, it cannot measure the risk of the foods in which these substances are found nor the processes, natural or human, that produce them. To apply toxicology as we have in the case of food irradiation, or as is sometimes urged in the case of new food components and new processes, is simply to use a tool because it is familiar even though it is likely to be irrelevant or useless. It is time we drew upon the experience of the experimental species with which we are most concerned – man – and used as our criteria for acceptable safety the processes we have come to value over the years. If something new appears safer than those, then it should be accepted in order that human experience, that final arbiter of safety, can be brought to bear on it as well.

1 Anonymous (1971): Wodicka rates food additive hazard as low. *Fd Chem. News* **12**, March 1, 11–12.
2 Hall, R.L.: Food irradiation-safety aspects. Proceedings of Foodanza 85 (Convention of Australian Institute of Food Science and Technology and New Zealand Institute of Food Science and Technology), Christchurch, New Zealand, May 20–23, 1985. (In press).
3 Ministry of Agriculture, Fisheries, and Food Department of Health and Social Security (1984): *Memorandum on the testing of novel foods incorporating guidelines for testing by the Advisory Committee on Irradiated and Novel Foods.* London, England: MAFF.
4 World Health Organization Joint FAO/IAEA/WHO Expert Committee (1981): *Wholesomeness of irradiated food,* technical report series No 659. Geneva, Switzerland: WHO.

Standards for pesticide residues in foods: a workshop report

J.N. HATHCOCK and A. ZARBA-VARY (Organizers)
Food and Nutrition Department, Iowa State University, Ames, Iowa, USA.

Participants. *I. Akinyele* (Faculty of Medicine, University of Ibadan, Ibadan, Nigeria); *S. Berger* (Human Nutrition Institute, Warsaw Agricultural University, Warsaw, Poland); *N. Librojo* (Institute of Chemistry, University of the Philippines at Los Banos, College, Laguna, Philippines).

There are at least three aspects of the nutritional importance of pesticides that may be important in setting standards: (1) protecting raw agricultural commodities (RACs) from various pests and therefore contributing to food production needed for the increasing, undernourished world population; (2) alteration of the nutritive values of various food products; and (3) possible modification of several physiological functions of nutrients after the pesticide is consumed.

The contribution of pesticides to food production and economic availability is difficult to estimate on a world-wide basis because of multiple agricultural variables and geographic differences in pesticide use. It is widely recognized, however, that in many locations production would be drastically curtailed if pesticides were not available. This high utility of chemical pesticides does not imply that other methods such as integrated pest management should not be used to decrease the economic and environmental costs of pesticide use.

The application of pesticides, substances of high biological activity, causes several disturbances in plant metabolism that lead to alterations in nutrient composition of plants and perhaps their flavour. For example, various pesticides have been found to cause about a 30 per cent decrease in ascorbic acid levels in several different crops. This aspect, as well as the possible adverse effects of pesticides on animals and humans, is a major concern in assessing the safety of pesticide use. Therefore, studies to eliminate or diminish any negative effect of pesticides on human nutrition and health are very important. Examples of such research include the effect of integrated pest management (IPM) on residue levels in RACs, as well as determination of pesticide residue levels in processed foods[2]. Not only the choice of pesticide, its dosage, formulation, and methods and time of application but also home and industrial food processing seem to play important roles in this regard[7].

Although results of most surveys indicate that no one pesticide is present at or above the maximum permitted intake in the daily diet, it is important to remember that exposure to multiple pesticides can occur and that other foreign substances are also present in our food and water. The interaction between pesticide and foreign substance has not been well-studied nor is such a study completely feasible, given the number of known harmful substances and possible combinations. In evaluating nutritional implications of pesticide residues in consumed food, food consumption patterns may be of great importance, and therefore maximum residue limit (MRL) values must be adjusted accordingly.

Estimating or predicting the exposure of consumers to pesticide residues is important to those in environmental health work and in regulatory agencies. Although reproducible scientific data are the only completely acceptable basis for pesticide regulation, estimates of exposure most often represent informed judgments, even when they are based on finite numbers such as the MRLs. The MRL is defined as the maximum permissible concentration of a pesticide residue resulting from the use of good agricultural practice (GAP). These values are recommended by the FAO/WHO Codex Alimentarius Commission as acceptable in or on a food, agricultural commodity or animal feed. The concentration is expressed in mg pesticide residue/kg RAC[5].

The MRL is set at the maximum level that is 'safe' or the level resulting from GAP, whichever is less[8]. In most cases the MRL is based on GAP data provided from supervised field trials. These, however, may not adequately account for the wide variety of climate and soil conditions. Nevertheless, the outcome of this approach tends to leave a wide margin of safety between the MRL and the concentration that is toxicologically considered acceptable.

The NOEL (no observed effect level) process is used to determine the level of pesticide residue considered 'safe'. This level is based on the following toxicological animal data: short-term (90 d) animal feeding studies; metabolic studies; teratology studies; carcinogenicity studies; reproduction studies and special studies (eg behavioural studies; potentiation studies).

The NOEL, which assumes that a threshold exists for all toxic effects, is used to calculate the acceptable daily intake (ADI). The ADI is the daily exposure level giving no appreciable risk during the entire life span and is expressed as mg pesticide residue/kg body weight per d.

Presently, the ADIs for many pesticides are based on incomplete data and/or data derived from studies performed utilizing protocols which are no longer considered valid. The NOEL process raises the following problems. (1) There are no guide-lines for defining effect, which may include induction of the mixed-function oxidase. (2) There is difficulty in establishing a negative, ie, that no effect occurred. (3) Sometimes wide intervals between dose levels in animal studies can affect the magnitude of the ADI identified.

To account for the uncertainty in extrapolation from animals to humans and the wide variability in exposure of the human population to a particular pesticide, the NOEL is divided by a safety factor (usually 100) to calculate the ADI. Ariens & Simonis[1] cite examples of the application of different safety factors to different environmental contaminants, with the selection of safety factor being influenced by reserve functional capacity in the affected physiological system and other factors.

In setting MRLs, the FAO/WHO uses estimated actual residue intakes derived from supervised field studies using GAP and 9th-decile level of food consumption reflecting typical dietary patterns. The United States uses mean intake of food items and theoretical maximum residue intakes (TMRI) to set a tolerance level for a pesticide residue in a particular food. The TMRI is calculated by multiplying tolerance or MRL for each commodity by a food factor (F) or the average daily per caput consumption of the food commodity and the average daily dietary weight (D) of RACs: TMRI (mg/d) = Σ(MRL $\times$ F $\times$ D). The calculation assures that, for a given pesticide, the maximum residue level is present in the food at the time of consumption and the residue is present in the total production of every approved commodity.

The FOA/WHO Codex Alimentarius Commission has published a guide to Codex maximum limits for pesticide residues[4] which gives values for both acceptable daily intakes (ADI) and maximum residue limit (MRL) for many pesticides in raw agricultural commodities (RACs) for crops on which their use is approved. Specific MRL values are calculated from the ADI and F, which is the decimal fraction of that RAC in a typical diet. Other techniques include examining the variability of the field trial residue levels, the distribution of the residue between edible and non-edible portions of the commodity, and the fate of the residues upon cooking or processing to help define the intake. One of the difficulties with these procedures is that dietary patterns differ substantially between countries and ethnic groups within countries. Whatever pattern is used in the calculation may be inappropriate for a particular country.

FAO/WHO pesticide standards were evaluated by calculating TMRIs (used in the USA assessment system) for Polish and Honduran dietary patterns, as follows: $\text{TMRI} = \Sigma\text{MRL} \times F \times D$ where D is the daily individual weight (kg) of RACs for that particular country. In the US assessment system, the TMRI should not exceed the maximum permitted intake (MPI). The MPI is calculated as $\text{MPI} = \text{ADI} \times W$, where W is the arbitrary human body weight (kg). Data reported indicate that the TMRI exceed the MPI for 16 of 33 pesticides commonly used in Poland and for 10 of 20 pesticides commonly used in Honduras, indicating that many MRL values are not completely appropriate for either dietary pattern[6]. The mean of the TMRI/MPI ratio values for pesticides is 3.09 for Poland and 1.73 for Honduras, indicating that many TMRI values are too high with that combination of MRL and particular dietary pattern. The mean for Poland includes two exceptionally high values, 19.5 for aldrin-dieldrin and 18.1 for fenethion.

Despite the fact that FAO/WHO considers the TMRIs inappropriate for deriving realistic estimates of pesticide intakes[5], several points are worth mentioning: when the Polish and Honduran dietary patterns are related to Codex MRLs through TMRI calculations the potential becomes apparent for over consumption of certain pesticides, especially aldrin-dieldrin, fenethion, carbaryl and malathion. Whether over-consumption actually occurs has to be determined by surveys at the local level and these have not been done in many locations. The potential appears to exist for over-consumption of aldrin-dieldrin in some locations regardless of GAP.

Estimating the daily intake of pesticide residue is a difficult way of evaluating the safety of specific pesticide registrations in agricultural commodities. The best method is to determine the actual daily residue intakes by total diet studies on ready-to-eat foods consumed by the public. It is in this direction that the US Environmental Protection Agency is moving[3]. FAO/WHO uses estimated actual levels of pesticide residues in food, ie, estimated actual residue intakes, and not the theoretical maximum intake (TMRI). The real levels must be known in order to assess exposure of populations to specific pesticides.

In many countries, obtaining appropriate human samples to verify the degrees of exposure is often extremely difficult. Because widespread food sampling in remote localities is not economically or practically feasible and analyses are difficult and expensive, the 'real' residue levels in food and the exposure to pesticides are unknown for most locations. Data described for malathion in human urine in two localities in the Philippines revealed higher malathion concentrations in an easily accessible lowland location (Cabuyao) with good exposure to local government extension service information than in a remote location (Loo Valley) in which the education level is much lower. Yet in interviews massive overuse of pesticides (including malathion) is commonly reported to occur in the Loo Valley. Possible reasons for these contradictory results include unaccounted differences in soil composition, different dietary consumption patterns and less rain water runoff from the lowland location.

The provision of an adequate and safe food supply for consumers requires a high degree of government involvement in setting and enforcing pesticide standards. High standards, however, may act as a barrier to other countries. In an effort to bring about international uniformity in terms of import requirements for food. FAO and WHO established the Joint FAO/WHO Food Standards Programme in 1962. Its objective is to avoid or eliminate non-tariff trade barriers through the development of food standards that will gain international acceptance. The greatest advance by the Commission has been in the area of standards for food additives and pesticide residues.

Data available indicate that Nigeria typifies a developing country that has invested heavily over the years in different pesticides in an effort to boost agricultural production. It is interesting to contemplate how much money could be saved in a developing country's budget if techniques of integrated pest management were better developed. Local standards might give better fit between MRL values and particular dietary patterns but there would be a lack of uniformity from one country to another which would impede trade. Standards adopted locally might be based mostly on political considerations, rather than scientific data. A commitment by both industry and government to provide safe and nutritious food must always be supported by a regulatory framework with appropriate preventive measures and penalty systems. This will foster confidence in the system by importers from non-industrialized nations.

Conclusions. Expansion and enforcement of uniform standards internationally will ensure safer and wholesome products. These efforts should involve the following. (1) Continued establishment of MRLs that are based on better determination of actual residue intakes. (2) Development of pre-shipment inspections of exports in each country. (3) Monitoring of residue levels in commodities imported into countries within a designated area. (4) Further determination of pesticide effects on the nutrient composition of foods.

1 Ariens, E.J. & Simonis, A.M. (1982): In *Nutritional toxicology, Vol. 1*, ed J.N. Hathcock, pp. 17–80. New York: Academic Press.
2 Berger, S., Pardo, B. & Skorkowska-Zieleniewska, J. (1980): Nutritional implications of pesticides in food. *Biblio. Nutr. Diet.* **29**, 1–10.
3 Chaisson, C.F., Peterson, B., White, S.B., Clayton, A., Brassard, D. & Johnson, P. (1984): *The tolerance assessment system: background information*. Washington DC: United States Environmental Protection Agency.
4 FAO/WHO Codex Alimentarius Commission (1978): *Guide to Codex maximum limits for pesticide residues*. Rome: Joint FAO/WHO Food Standards Programme.
5 FAO/WHO Codex Alimentarius Commission (1984): *Recommended national regulatory practices to facilitate acceptance and use of Codex limits for pesticide residues in foods*. Rome: Joint FAO/WHO Food Standards Programme.
6 Hathcock, J.N., Vary, A.Z., Berger, S. & Brzozowska, A. (1983): Evaluation of FAO/WHO pesticide standards in relation to Polish and Honduran diets. *Regul. Toxic. Pharmac.* **3**, 216–223.
7 Kubacki, S.J. & Lipowska, T. (1980): In *Food and health: science and technology*, pp. 215–226, ed G.G. Birch & K.J. Parker. London: Applied Science Publishers.
8 Turtle, E.E. (1980): In *Food and health: science and technology*, pp. 201–214, ed G.G. Birch & K.J. Parker. London: Applied Science Publishers.

★ ★ ★

NUTRITION AND TOXICOLOGY

Diet as a source of natural toxicants

R.F. CURTIS
AFRC Food Research Institute, Norwich, Colney Lane, Norwich NR4 7UA, UK.

There are several distinuished texts[13,19,23] which very adequately catalogue the vast number of natural toxicants, predominantly of plant origin, which may arise in human food. Fungal and fish toxins should not be excluded from consideration.

To constrain this paper to a reasonable length only plant products are considered and natural toxicants are defined as 'compounds present in food plants, or their products, which elicit a deleterious physiological or pharmacological effect when ingested by man'. The conceptual problems which underlie any attempts to define rational research programmes in this area will be discussed and illustrated with reference to the glycoalkaloids, a group of acutely toxic compounds occurring at significant concentration in the potato — the most important vegetable in the Western world. These compounds were, until recently, generally ignored by plant breeders, food scientists and toxicologists. They are heat-stable and little affected by cooking although somewhat reduced by the peeling process.

It must be evident that any really deleterious effects are likely to be chronic, because over the years of human development acute effects would have been readily detected. It might, of course, be argued that low-level consumption of toxicants is one of the normal hazards of life and since this low level of ingestion of active principles cannot be directly associated with human disadvantage the matter can be safely left to one side. However, the safety of any national food supply is of serious political, economic and social importance and current attitudes toward natural foods (and natural toxicants) contrast strongly with the continued attention which is applied to the criticism and evaluation of synthetic additives to food. In the longer run, questions comparable to those raised about synthetic additives must surely be raised about natural constituents as well.

Health hazards associated with the consumption of food may originate from a variety of sources. Natural toxicants are but one of the health hazards which potentially endanger the food supply. They can be conveniently grouped into order of decreasing risks as follows: (1) microbial contamination; (2) nutritional imbalance; (3) environmental contamination; (4) natural toxicants — (3 and 4 are 1000-fold less than 1 and 2); (5) pesticide residues, and (6) food additives — (5 and 6 are 100-fold less than 3 and 4). While this assessment is generally accepted[19,25], Hall[9] has drawn attention to the fact that this order is far removed from the public perception of food-related problems and from the concerns of regulatory authorities, the food industry, the quality press and what has been described as the 'fringe hysteria' element. In every category of interest, natural toxicants are regarded as the least important and while pointing out that this is based on US data, it has been suggested, nevertheless, that the situation is similar in most Western countries[8]. It is this perception which is so puzzling — that natural toxicants are relatively unimportant *vis-à-vis* other hazards, that they are not 'chemicals' in the same sense as food additives and that because they occur 'naturally' they must therefore be non-hazardous, or might even be beneficial (= natural).

If natural products are to be treated on a par with other chemicals then integrated toxicological studies are required. Reliable data on the biological potency of the compounds of interest are essential, to define an appropriate level of concern before analytical methods can be specified. However, one feature which is unique about natural toxicants among potential deleterious compounds is that the biological data are generally *not* available; moreover, there is little incentive to collect such data because there is not usually an immediately apparent economic advantage to do so. This is particularly true of chronic long-term effects.

Research on natural toxicants needs to be directed towards identification and isolation, coupled with examination of long-term effects in animals and preferably humans, together with rational methods for reduction of these compounds where they appear potentially hazardous for man. However, because of the general absence of overt effects, the approach to this area is very difficult but any programme should contain the following elements: (1) isolation of toxic principles and criteria needed; (2) acute and chronic toxicity studies; (3) analytical methodology; (4) estimates of intake, and (5) techniques for reduction or control.

The critical issue is the identification of criteria for proceeding with isolation studies. Some factors which might be considered relevant are: (1) epidemiological relationships; (2) physiological and diet-related disturbances in man; (3) performance data from farm animals; (4) extent of use of wild types in breeding programmes; (5) physico-chemical/chemical effects in non-food systems, and (6) serendipity.

Epidemiological relationships are the most difficult to identify, especially as diets become more and more internationalized. Useful examples generally relate to diets of particular groups of people in particular societies and would include haemolytic syndromes associated with legume consumption (related to vicine content) in certain individuals of Mediterranean origin[2], cancer related to bracken-shoot consumption in Japan which has recently been associated with the presence of a potent mutagen[10] and 'vomiting sickness' in Jamaica associated with hypoglycaemia following the consumption of the fruit of the ackee tree, *Blighia sapida*[12,13].

In the context of the average Western diet the other factors noted above are likely to be more important. For example, the acute physiological disturbances in man associated with ingestion of potatoes containing high levels of glycoalkaloids are well documented[11] and there is long-standing but clear cut evidence of hypnotic and opiate effects due to lettuce which have never been fully explained[4]. Performance data in farm animals are particularly useful, for example: the clear evidence of 'kale anaemia' in cattle associated with S-methyl cysteine sulphoxide; disturbed metabolism in poultry, cattle and pigs due to glucosinolates[6]; pulmonary disease in cattle associated with furano-terpenes[24], and reproductive malfunction in cattle and sheep due to plant oestrogens[22] are all due to compounds normally present in plant foods for humans.

The extent of use of wild types in plant-breeding programmes has never been fully assessed and little is known about the effect of such breeding programmes on the chemical composition of the plants. It is, however, certain that present day cultivars of many of our common vegetables have changed dramatically in a comparatively short historical time span, mainly due to crossing with wild types. Potatoes are a particularly good example. Carrots have changed from white to yellow and then to orange in a period of less than 500 years, as a perusal of old masters will reveal.

The recognition of the physico-chemical effects of plant extracts in non-food systems should also be a useful pointer to potential problems in food plants. For example, saponins are widely distributed in the plant kingdom and the effects of those compounds as potent surface-active agents is well known. What is missing is information about the qualitative and quantitative nature of saponins in food plants for man[17].

Finally, serendipity. The recent observation[1] of enhanced oestrogenic activity in urine from humans as a consequence of the microbial conversion of isoflavone precursors obtained by feeding an increased amount of soya protein in the diet is a salutary reminder of the importance of serendipity and the prepared mind. This observation stemmed from routine examinations of urine using HPL/MS techniques rather than the establishment of observed oestrogenic effects. It is, however, a very clear illustration of a wholly unexpected consequence of increased ingestion of vegetable protein — a thoroughly 'healthy' objective.

Some of the above points can be well illustrated by work on glycoalkaloids which has been carried out over the past 10 or so years. The potato is a staple crop in many parts of the world — at about 300 million tonnes per annum it is the third most important crop after wheat and rice. For over a century there have been recorded instances of human illness and, occasionally, death following consumption of low grade or 'greened' potatoes[14,18] and these effects were associated with the presence of glycoalkaloids, which have been shown to be potent cholinesterase inhibitors[11]. There is considerable species variation in sensitivity to these compounds[15] and the lethal dose in man is not known, although it is known that the compounds are not readily excreted. Outbreaks of human poisoning are not now common but do still occur. There was a quite well documented case in Lewisham, UK in 1979 where 78 school children were affected, with three seriously ill, following a school dinner based upon potatoes containing glycoalkaloids at the 33 mg/100 g level[14]. Most cases, however, relate to abused potatoes since normal cultivated varieties contain typically 3–8 mg/100 g fresh weight. There is, unlike food additives, no statutory control but a generally recognized limit is 20 mg/100 g — primarily derived from the observation that above this level the potato becomes increasingly bitter and toxic[21]. If it were seriously to be suggested that compounds with the biological activity of glycoalkaloids should be added to any food, let alone a staple food, there would be the most outraged response. There are double standards in these things.

The factors which influence glycoalkaloid content are: (1) cultivar; (2) environment; (3) exposure to light; (4) storage conditions — time/temperature; (5) maturity, and (6) stress. The significance of these factors and the potential importance of the problem became clear in 1972 when the new cultivar Lenape with excellent processing and agronomic characteristics, introduced in the USA after all the appropriate trials, had to be removed very suddenly[26]. This followed the realization that when grown under particular combinations of day-length and temperature in the north-eastern states of the USA the cultivar produced very high levels of glycoalkaloids — up to 65 mg/100 g. This resulted in bitterness and physiological effects in consumers on a scale previously unrecognized. The cultivar was hastily withdrawn and investigation quickly showed that the problem was directly attributable to a grandparent cross with the wild potato *Solanum chacoense*, which had been used for its desirable characteristics of disease resistance. In the case of potatoes some wild species have high levels of glycoalkaloid (up tp 150 mg/100 g) and it was then shown[20] that this characteristic is highly heritable. A rather similar situation arose in the UK, but because of the American experience it was identified before it could have commercial consequences. The Scottish Plant Breeding Station in Pentlandfield, Edinburgh, has an outstanding reputation for its Pentland varieties and their research programme had the important objective of attempting to enhance resistance of their cultivars to eelworm attack by the use of wild species *Solanum vernei* which has excellent resistance characteristics. The Institute sought to assure itself in the light of the American experience that it did not have a similar problem. Unfortumately, it did and a large number of potentially successful new clones about to go for final trial and selected for yield, shape, size, disease resistance, cooking quality etc, as well as eelworm resistance, had to be withdrawn at a late stage.

As a result of these problems new analytical techniques for chemical analysis of glycoalkaloids were developed[3] but these were extremely laborious for large scale screening of a breeding programme and a simple much more rapid ELISA method has now been described[16]. New cultivars are now routinely screened for glycoalkaloid content with a guide-line that material with greater than 20 mg/100 g should be rejected by plant breeders. A retrospective study of potatoes in the retail market in the UK has also been carried out to cover varieties introduced over the past 20 years and this has provided reassurance on current levels[5]. There are, however, still unanswered questions about the long-term effects of ingesting these pharmacologically active compounds.

Notwithstanding the problems outlined, some encouragement may be taken from a number of recent events. In the USA, the USDA have made available $9 million in support of studies on naturally occurring food toxicants and work at the Northern Regional Research Centre, Peoria has concentrated on such compounds in brassicas[7]. In Switzerland, the Institute of Toxicology of the ETH and University of Zurich under the leadership of Professor Schlatter is an excellent example of the utilization of a multidisciplinary approach (involving amongst others, chemists, nutritionists and biochemists) in the complex area of food toxicology. Finally the International Union of Pure and Applied Chemistry (IUPAC) have recognized the importance of dietary toxicants and have set up a working party, with experts drawn from various continents, to identify specific areas where research is needed. It is to be hoped that developments such as these will help to point the way forward and that some of the ideas presented here may be useful in advancing an understanding of this very difficult area.

Acknowledgement. I am grateful for the very great assistance I have received from Dr G.R. Fenwick of this Institute in preparing this paper.

1 Axelson, M., Sjövall, J., Gustafsson, B.E. & Setchell, K.D.R. (1984): Soya — a dietary source of the non-steroidal oestrogen equol in man and animals. *J. Endocr.* **102**, 49–56.
2 Chevion, M., Mager, J. & Glaser, G. (1983): Naturally occurring food toxicants, favism-producing agents. In *Handbook of naturally occurring food toxicants*, ed M. Rechcigl, jr., pp. 63–79. Boca Raton Florida: CRC Press.
3 Coxon, D.T. (1984): Methodology for glycoalkaloid analysis. *Am. Pot. J.* **61**, 169–184.
4 Crosby, D.G. (1963): The organic constituents of food. 1. Lettuce. *J. Fd Sci.* **28**, 347–355.
5 Davies, A.M.C. & Blincow, P.J. (1984): Glycoalkaloid content of potatoes and potato products sold in the UK. *J. Sci. Fd Agric.*, **35**, 553–557.
6 Fenwick, G.R., Heaney, R.K. & Mullin, W.J. (1983): Glucosinolates and their breakdown products in foods and food plants. *CRC Crit. Rev. Food Sci. Nutr.* **18**, 123–201.
7 Gould, D.H., Fettman, M.J., Daxenbichler, M.E. & Bartuska, B.M. (1985): Functional and structural alterations of the rat kidney induced by the naturally occurring organonitrile, 2S-1-cyano-2-hydroxy-3,4-epithiobutane. *Tox. Appl. Pharmocol.* **78**, 190–201.
8 Gray, J. (1985): How safe is your diet: general review. *Chemy Ind.* 146–148.
9 Hall, R.L. (1971): Information, confidence, and sanity in the food sciences. *Flav. Ind.* Aug. 2, 455–9.
10 Hirono, I., Aiso, S., Yamaji, T., Mori, H., Yamada, K., Niwa, H., Ojika, M., Wakamatsu, K., Kigoshi, H., Niiyama, K. & Uosaki, Y. (1984): Carcinogenecity in rats of ptaquiloside isolated from bracken. *Gann* **75**, 833–836.
11 Jadhav, S.J., Sharma, R.P. & Salunkhe, D.K. (1981): Naturally occurring toxic alkaloids in foods. *CRC Crit. Rev. Toxicol.* **11**, 21–104.
12 Kean, E.A. (ed) (1976): *Hypoglycin.* New York: Academic Press.
13 Liener, I.E. (1980): *Toxic constituents of plant foodstuffs.* New York: Academic Press.

14 McMillan, M. & Thompson, J.G. (1979): An outbreak of suspected solanine poisoning in schoolboys. *Q. J. Med.* **48**, 227–243.

15 Maga, J.A. (1980): Potato glycoalkaloids. *CRC Crit. Rev. Food Sci. Nutr.* **12**, 371–405.

16 Morgan, M.R.A., McNerney, R., Matthew, J.A., Coxon, D.T. & Chan, H.W-S. (1983): An enzyme-linked immunosorbent assay for total glycoalkaloids in potato tubers. *J. Sci. Fd Agric.* **34**, 593–598.

17 Oakenfull, D. (1981): Saponins in food — a review. *Food Chem.* **7**, 19–40.

18 Oslage, H.F. (1956): Über das Solanin in der Kartoffel und seine Wirkung auf das Tier. *Kartoffelbau* **7**, 204–11.

19 Roberts, H.R. (1981): *Food safety*. New York: John Wiley.

20 Sinden, S.L. & Webb, R.E. (1974): Effect of environment on glycoalkaloid content of six potato varieties at 39 locations. *Tech. Bull. No. 1472, Agr. Res. Sci. USDA*, 1–30.

21 Sinden, S.L., Deahl, K.L. & Aulenbach, B.B. (1976): Effect of glycoalkaloids and phenolics on potato flavour. *J. Fd Sci.* **41**, 520–531.

22 Stob, M. (1983): Naturally occurring food toxicants: estrogens. In *Handbook of naturally occurring food toxicants*, ed M. Rechcigl, jr., pp. 81–100. Boca Raton, Florida: CRC Press.

23 Strong, F.M. (ed) (1973): *Toxicants occurring naturally in foods*. Washington DC: National Academy of Sciences.

24 Uritani, I., Oba, K., Takeuchi, A., Sato, K., Inoue, H., Ito, R. & Ito, I. (1981): Biochemistry of furanoterpenes produced in mold-damaged sweet potatoes. In *Antinutrients and natural toxicants in foods*, ed R.L. Ory, pp. 1–16. Westport, Connecticut: Food and Nutrition Press.

25 Wodicka, V.O. (1971): Remarks before the National Agricultural Outlooks Conference sponsored by the USDA Feb. 23, *Fd Chem. News*, 1st March, 130–2.

26 Zitnak, A. & Johnson, G.R. (1970): Glycoalkaloid content of B5 141–6 potatoes. *Am. Pot. J.* **47**, 256–260.

Nutritional effects of toxicants

L. HAMBRAEUS
Institute of Nutrition, University of Uppsala, Uppsala, Sweden.

Every healthy individual consumes a multitude of toxic substances in his normal diet every day, without, in most cases any obvious signs of intoxication. This might be due to the fact that the toxicants usually exert their effects only when they are consumed under special conditions, ie malnutrition, metabolic disorders or when there are other potentiating substances present. Furthermore, the concentration of toxicants *per se* in the food is often so low that the food item must be consumed in large amounts for a number of days for intoxication to occur. Finally, it should be remembered that the organism is suited to handle small amounts of various toxicants and most of the toxic effects of various chemicals that are potentially hazardous do not show an additive effect.

Potential toxic compounds in food can be separated into the following groups. *(1) Natural or inherent toxins* which occur naturally as a result of the endogenous metabolism of the animal or plant. Most of the naturally occurring antinutritive factors or toxins are of vegetable origin. They are concentrated along the food chain and those natural toxins which are found in animal products are usually derived directly or indirectly from vegetable sources, which have been consumed by the animal and which they have not been able to detoxify. *(2) Acquired toxicants* are those which emanate from *microbial action* on foodstuffs, due to poor food hygiene, or from *enzymatic degradation* during storage, ie goitrogenic compounds which occur from the action of myrosinase on glycosinolates. *(3) Environmental toxins* are accumulated in the food components from the environment, or unintentionally introduced during processing, handling and storage. They may be of microbial as well as of chemical origin. These *man-made toxicants* include such components as residues from the use of biocides, herbicides, pesticides and fertilizers. Other examples are residues from pharmaceutical treatment of animals before slaughter, or chemical substances that are produced during the processing of food or various food additives and preservatives used in food technology, as well as components which may be derived from the packing material. *(4)* A fourth group of antinutrients or potentially toxic components are the *allergens* or components that may act as allergens. However, this is best considered as a problem of *food allergy* and not of food toxicology.

Effect of antinutrients. The effect of the antinutrients can be manifold. In one situation the antinutrient or toxicant may interfere with the uptake of certain nutrients, in another situation with their metabolism. The antinutritive effect will also depend on the specific metabolic situation of the individual. Furthermore there are also antagonistic interactions leading to the fact that some ingredients interfere and reduce the toxic effect of other components, ie fat-soluble vitamins.

Although there are a number of inborn errors of metabolism where the consumption of various normal constituents can lead to deleterious effects, sometimes even fatal[13], ie galactosaemia, fructose intolerance, hypercholesterolaemia, Refsum's disease, phenylketonuria, urea cycle disorders, the specific nutritional effects reported in these patients are more related to the practical problems of furnishing the patients with adequate amounts of the nutrients on a restricted, often synthetic , diet, than to any specific nutrient deficiency.

The toxic effects can be due to an abundance in the diet of various compounds which then exert their effect. Sometimes there is an absolute excess as a result of a deviation in the food habits. The increase in the fat energy percentage of the diet of the population of affluent societies and its relation to the observed increase of cardiovascular diseases as well as of certain forms of cancer, ie breast cancer, colon cancer, could also be considered as a toxic effect and has thus led to various epidemiological studies. The high intake of sucrose in the Western diet has been discussed as cause of the high frequency of caries as well as a trigger for cardiovascular disease, obesity and diabetes, and is still disputed. An increased intake of polyunsaturated fatty acids is reported to lead to some potentially toxic or antinutritional effects, ie an increased requirement for vitamin E.

In another case it could be due to an *unbalanced intake* of certain components, ie the pellagra-like disease reported in leucine-isoleucine amino acid imbalance[5].

There may also be a relative excess due to a change in the metabolic capacity. Thus a genetic disturbance can increase the susceptibility for a normal constituent which due to the metabolic disturbance is converted to a toxicant, ie phenylalanine toxicity in phenylketonuria, favism in glucose-6-phosphate dehydrogenase deficiency. Some components have a potential as antinutrients although they constitute natural components of a healthy diet. The dietary intake of lactose through dietary products can lead to gastrointestinal problems due to a low lactose intolerance resulting from a decreased lactase activity in the intestinal mucosa which occurs in adults in the majority of the human race.

During the last decade the belief in megadoses of vitamins has increased as a component of the increased interest in food faddism[4]. This makes the potential risk of vitamin intoxication, especially of the fat-soluble vitamins, a reality. Furthermore there is a tendency to use fortification and enrichment of various food items with vitamin and mineral supplements to a greater extent in fabricated food products. This may secondarily lead to a potential risk of overconsumption of some vitamins, and calls for some guide-lines[3]. Although excessive amounts of the water-soluble vitamins can be excreted in the urine the increased use of megavitamin doses have shown that this does not necessarily mean that they can be considered as non-toxic. A direct toxic effect of megadoses of the vitamin or its metabolites has been reported for ascorbic acid, niacin, pyridoxine, thiamin and folic acid, and withdrawal symptoms may occur when megadoses of ascorbic acid, pyridoxine and pantothenic acid are abruptly discontinued[1].

Antivitamins. A number of substances have been reported to reduce the availability of vitamins and are consequently referred to as antivitamins. They can be structurally divided into two major groups[12]: (a) those who compete with the vitamins due to their similar chemical structure, and (b) those that destroy or decrease the effect of a vitamin by modifying its molecule or by forming a complex. Most of the antivitamins occurring in food, ie thiaminase, avidin, pyridoxine antagonists, seem to belong to the latter group.

Enzyme inhibitors. The legumes contain a number of antinutritional factors, many of them in the form of enzyme inhibitors[8]. As these inhibitors seem to be protein in nature, they lose their activity at denaturation by heat. However, the temperature of the treatment must be sufficiently high and the increasing use of 'slow cookers' or 'crock pots' seem to increase the risk of toxicity problems due to insufficient inactivation.

An enzyme inhibitor can affect the binding and transformation of substances or make the substrate unavailable to the enzyme. It can also interfere with the biosynthesis of the enzyme or affect the turnover of the enzyme or influence the regulator of activity. The most common way seems to be to exert the effect as substrate or cofactor analogue. They also form strong bindings to the active sites of the enzyme resulting in enzymatically inactive compounds.

There are also non-protein inhibitors, which may not be inactivated by heat treatment and still represent a potential hazard in the diet. The best example seems to be solanine, an inhibitor of cholinesterase which occurs in potatoes, tomatoes, eggplants, sugar beets and apples. Moderate and even severe poisoning including gastrointestinal disturbances and neurological symptoms are regularly reported as a result of the intake of solanine-containing potatoes.

Organ-specific toxins and toxins with specific nutritional effect. The goitrogens comprise some of the most common toxicants in human food. There is, however, little evidence that endemic goitre could be related to the consumption of goitrogenous food in man. However, leaf protein concentrates which are produced from various cabbage species may contain considerable amounts of glucosinolates and consequently give rise to goitrogenous effects[7].

Lectins comprise a number of antinutrients, usually of glucoprotein origin, which have a very selective impact on the intestines and their absorption of various nutrients. This has been postulated to be due to a specific combination with the cells in the intestinal wall thereby blocking absorption[6]. Lectins are usually inactivated by heat treatment. However, the ingestion of raw or partially cooked bean products, using slow cookers, has been reported to result in intoxication in humans probably due to their lectin content[2].

Interference with mineral metabolism. Oxalic acid and phytic acid represent compounds that interfere with mineral metabolism as they form chelates with calcium, iron and zinc, to mention a few examples. Phytic acid plays a more dominant role as chelator as it forms phytates with a number of minerals which are then almost unsoluble. The role of phytic acid has been of special concern throughout the last decades because of the increased interest in the use of dietary fibre, such as wheat bran, as well as of meat analogues based on vegetable proteins, which all contain phytic acid.

Antinutrients and malnutrition. Cyanogenetic glucosides occur in a number of plants, ie cassava, and can give rise to hydrogen cyanide, a very potent cytochrome oxidase inhibitor. However, only a few of those plants are really used as human food, cassava and almond being the commonest examples. Cyanide intoxication has recently been discussed as an important cause of epidemic outbreak of spastic paraplegia (Mantakassa disease) in Mozambique during drought conditions when cassava was harvested as the only food available[9]. It is assumed that the usual detoxification of ingested cyanide to thiocyanate is dependant on the availability of sulphur containing amino acids and vitamin B_{12} and that this detoxification was inadequate due to malnutrition[11]. Likewise, outbreaks of *lathyrism* have been described associated with famine, when large quantities of lathyrus meal have been consumed.

Carcinogens. During the last few years an increased interest has been devoted to the occurrence of various compounds in food that may have a carcinogenic effect. The committee on diet, nutrition and cancer of the National Academy of Sciences[10] recently evaluated the risk of dietary-induced cancer.

Effect of irradiation. From the nutritional point of view it seems that irradiation represents one of the least disturbing preservation techniques available. An oxidation of polyunsaturated fatty acids may occur and vitamin B_1, A, C, and E seem to be somewhat sensitive. However, no effects are to be expected at the low doses presently recommended. Although it cannot be excluded that some minor amounts of radiolysis products may occur after irradiation, such components also occur naturally. It should be stressed that irradiation does NOT result in the production of any radioactive isotopes in the food, a very common misinterpretation.

Microbial toxins. Naturally occurring toxicants in food, due to microbial actions, refer essentially to toxins which are produced prior to ingestion of the contaminated food, where the microorganisms have proliferated under suitable conditions. It is obvious that most microbial toxins exert their nutritional effects by inducing dehydration and electrolyte disturbances secondarily to the diarrhoea which may be intensive, or to malnutrition as result of nausea and vomiting.

Trace elements. The daily intake of various trace minerals such as lead, mercury, and cadmium may be low. However, as there is very limited capacity in the body to excrete them, even low intakes may result in the accumulation of toxic levels of minerals and trace elements in the body. The increased use of copper pipelines in the water systems in housing may lead to rather high dietary intake of copper through the water used in food preparation and interfere with the metabolism of other minerals, eg iron, zinc. This has especially been discussed with regard to formula feeding of infants.

Conclusion. Exposure to toxic compounds in the food is by no means a problem confined to the last decades. It seems to be a valid statement that more people to date have died because of naturally occurring toxicants of chemical or microbiological origin in food or to starvation due to food shortage secondary to the extensive loss of food during storage than due to the use of preservatives in food technology. The use of certain additives and preservatives in food technology is essentially based on the assumption that they will maintain, prolong, or even enhance the nutritional quality of the products throughout storage, as well as reduce microbial contamination or growth of microorganisms during handling and storage. Obviously man has a capacity to handle these toxic components to some degree through the detoxifying capacity of the liver. Thus the nutritional effects of the various toxicants is limited. Nevertheless specific legislation regarding the use of additives and preservatives in food is extremely rigorous.

1　Alkadeff, L., Gualtieri, C.T. & Lipton, M. (1984): Toxic effects of water-soluble vitamins. *Nutr. Rev.* **42**, 33–40.
2　Bender, A.E. & Reaidi, G.B. (1982): Toxicity of kidney beans (Phaseolus vulgaris) with particular reference to lectins. *J. Plant Foods* **4**, 15–22.
3　Darby, W.J. & Hambraeus, L. (1978): Proposed nutritional guidelines for utilization of industrially produced nutrients. *Nutr. Rev.* **36**, 65–71.
4　Dubick, M.A. & Rucker, R.B. (1983): Dietary supplements and health aids. A critical evaluation. Part 1 — Vitamins and minerals. *J. Nutr. Educ.* **15**, 47–53.
5　Gopalan, C. & Rao, K.S.J. (1975): Pellagra and amino acid imbalance. *Vitam. Horm.* **33**, 505–528.
6　Jaffé, W.G. (1983): Nutritional significance of lectins. In *CRC Handbook of naturally occurring food toxicants*, ed M. Reichcigl Jr, pp. 31–38. Boca Raton, Florida: CRC Press.
7　Langer, P. (1983): Naturally occurring food toxicants: goitrogens. In *CRC Handbook of Naturally occurring food toxicants*, ed M. Reichcigl Jr, pp. 101–129. Boca Raton, Florida: CRC Press.
8　Liener, I.R. (1980): *Toxic constituents of plant foodstuffs.* 2nd edn. New York: Academic Press.
9　Ministry of Health, Mozambique (1984): An epidemic of spastic paraparesis associated with chronic cyanide intoxication in a cassava staple area of Mozambique. 2. Nutritional factors and hydrocyanic acid content of cassava products. *Bull WHO* **62**, 485–492.
10　National Academy of Science. (1982): *Diet, nutrition and cancer.* Washington: National Research Council. National Academy Press.
11　Osuntokun, B.O. (1981): Cassava diet, chronic cyanide intoxication and neuropathy in the Nigerian Africans. *Wd Rev. Nutr. Diet.* **36**, 141–173.
12　Somogyi, J.C. (1978): Natural toxic substances in food. In *Foreign substances and nutrition*, ed J.C. Somogyi & R. Tarjan, *Wld Rev. Nutr. Diet.* **29**, 42–59.
13　Stanbury, J.B., Wyngaarden, J.B., Fredrickson, D.S., Goldstein, J.L. & Brown, M.S. (1983): *The metabolic basis of inherited disease*, 5th edn, New York: McGrawHill.

Cooperative research in food safety and nutrition

A. MALASPINA
International Life Sciences Institute, 1126 Sixteenth Street, NW, Washington, DC 20036, USA.

The interactions between two sciences, nutrition and toxicology, are involved in many of today's scientific and regulatory issues and many reports have emphasized that the composition of the diets used in toxicological studies may affect the results. For example, a high protein intake decreases the sensitivity of rats to pesticides, while energy restriction reduces the incidence of spontaneous or chemically-induced tumours.

As these complexities continue to emerge, it has become apparent that interdisciplinary approaches are needed to resolve nutrition and food safety questions. Furthermore, the issues are so complex that more sophisticated research, utilizing modern methods of molecular biology, is necessary for their resolution.

Unfortunately, in the last decade or so, research needs have not been met, since funding from government agencies has decreased significantly. Many governments have channelled relatively larger percentages of their budgets into social programmes, energy research, and defence spending. And in some countries, including the USA, large budgets have been approved for routine chemical testing, while funds to support more basic research in nutrition and toxicology have been inadequate. As a consequence, alternative funding sources must be identified. In addition, the current situation has led to the recognition of the benefits of cooperative research programmes in government, industry and academia. Such efforts can maximize efficiency by pooling financial resources and technical expertise. They can also minimise unnecessary and wasteful duplication of effort.

The International Life Sciences Institute-Nutrition Foundation, or ILSI-NF, is a model of the collaborative approach to resolving scientific issues. ILSI-NF is the consolidation of the US Nutrition Foundation with ILSIs US branch. Prior to the merger, ILSIs main emphasis had been on toxicology and food safety, while the Nutrition Foundation's programmes stressed nutrition.

Throughout its 43-year history, the Nutrition Foundation sponsored a wide variety of activities in nutrition and food science. The Foundation provided much-needed money for research in the 1940s, and promoted cooperation between the food industry and the academic community. It began publishing *Nutrition Reviews* in 1943 to communicate the results of nutrition research to the scientific community. For 20 years of so, many young scientists who made significant discoveries, particularly in the areas of amino acids, vitamins and minerals, received support from the Foundation.

Since the mid 1970s, the Nutrition Foundation has served as the Secretariat for the International Consultative Groups on vitamin A and nutritional anaemia. Through these projects, which are financed primarily by the US Agency for International Development, guide-lines and recommendations are prepared to assess the regional magnitude of vitamin-A-deficiency and nutritional anaemia, and to develop intervention strategies. Recently, the Foundation sponsored research on dental caries, and a review of diet and hyperactivity.

ILSI was established in 1978. Its goals are to expand the scientific data base through research on specific ingredients and food components, to promote the international harmonization of toxicological testing, and to advance the science of nutrition.

During the past few years, the activities of ILSI and the Nutrition Foundation began to duplicate one another, because of the increasing overlap between nutrition and toxicology. In order to maximize resources and promote collaboration, the two organizations merged in January 1985. New activities are being developed, while the major programmes of both organizations have continued.

Many of ILSI-NFs programmes are conducted through Technical Committees. In the US, 12 committees have been organized. Scientists from member companies volunteer their time to direct each technical committee, with the guidance of scientific advisors, who are usually from the academic sector. These committees support research, hold workshops and symposia, and publish scientific papers and monographs.

For example, the Caffeine Committee sponsored a carcinogenicity bioassay, and research on the effects of caffeine on the cardiovascular and endocrine systems. The Committee also supported a project on the effect of caffeine on brain neurotransmitter levels in rats, as well as behavioural studies in children. The Caffeine Committee has held five international workshops, and has recently published a monograph which is a comprehensive review of current research findings.

The value of ILSIs international network of scientists was evident in 1982 when Japan proposed a ban on BHA, one of the most important food antioxidants. ILSI was instrumental in organizing a group of government and university scientists who worked with industry to review the data upon which the Japanese based their proposed action. This dialogue resulted in a postponement of the ban, and led to further research to characterize the nature of the BHA risk. The Antioxidant Committee is continuing to sponsor research, and has prepared scientific monographs on five food antioxidants.

The Saccharin Committee has initiated a research programme which focuses on explaining the mechanism of saccharin's effects in male rats. We are discovering that various salt forms of saccharin have different effects on the bladder. Sodium saccharin causes a higher rate of bladder cell proliferation than either acid saccharin or calcium saccharin. We are also learning that the composition of the diet fed to experimental animals can modify their carcinogenic response to saccharin. This finding is another example of the need to combine the disciplines of nutrition and toxicology in safety evaluation.

ILSI-NF is also examining the questions about residues in foods. We will prepare monographs on specific pesticides and identify areas which need additional information. The scope of activity will be expanded to include environmental contaminants and package migrants.

Other specific educational activities are coordinated by ILSI's Expert Committees. The Nutrition Expert Committee is currently preparing a monograph on calcium, and is planning additional ones on zinc and dietary fibre. The Pathology/Toxicology Expert Committee is developing a series of ten monographs on the Pathology of Laboratory Animals. Each reviews one organ system. Monographs on the Endocrine and Respiratory Systems have already been published. The Committee also sponsors seminars to train pathologists in the diagnosis of neoplastic and non-neoplastic diseases. These seminars are held annually at medical schools in West Germany, Japan, and the USA. More than 400 pathologists attend these seminars every year.

In addition, this Expert Committee has issued two monographs on current issues in toxicology. In the first volume, the Committee addressed the issues in selecting doses in toxicity testing and the effect of the ageing process on toxicological results. The second volume reviewed the factors that must be considered when extrapolating animal data to humans, and discussed the validity of mutagenicity testing. A third volume on reproductive toxicity is in preparation. Criteria for assessing the adequacy of animal teratology data for subsequent extrapolation to humans are the major topics considered in this monograph.

ILSI has also recognized the need to sponsor basic research that will help to define the mechanism of toxicity in experimental animals. In 1984, ILSI established a Research Foundation, which is guided by nine Scientific Directors, five of whom are Nobel Laureates. The aim of the Foundation is to support the research of young scientists who are involved in fields such as molecular biology, immunology, nutrition and genetics. This year ILSI will award four $100 000 grants.

The most recent development within the ILSI international structure is the establishment of a Risk Science Institute. The idea originated at a symposium ILSI held in 1983 together with the US FDA and the Canadian HPB, entitled 'Safety Assessment: The Interface between Science, Law and Regulation'. At this symposium, many questions were raised about the scientific validity of the assumptions used in quantitative risk assessment. Therefore, it became evident that a major research effort would be required to improve the methodology used in risk assessment.

Many of the questions and uncertainties involve the extrapolation of animal data to estimate potential risk to humans. For instance, the high dose levels required under current regulatory procedures may result in abnormal physiological changes. These changes may themselves cause adverse effects which are unrelated to the inherent toxicological properties of the compound. Data are needed at the lower end of the dose-response curve to more closely approximate human exposure. The Risk Science Institute will study how new methods can best be incorporated into safety assessment protocols.

Also, when a chemical is treated in several species but found to be carcinogenic in only one, as a matter of policy, the regulatory agencies often rely on the single positive result, whether or not it may be relevant to human health. To address this particular problem, we must generate data on the mechanism of the toxic response in the sensitive species. We must then find out whether the same mechanism exists in humans, in order to determine what role the findings from the sensitive species should play in regulatory decisions.

Interpretation and evaluation are further complicated by the expanding amount of information available from new, highly sensitive analytical techniques. In addition, in recent years, regulatory agencies have required more and more routine animal data. However, the ability to estimate risk does not necessarily increase by using larger numbers of animals, examining more tissues, increasing the numbers of doses and dose levels, and extending the duration of tests. We need to streamline the process. Data from comparative metabolism and pharmacokinetic studies would be very valuable.

The further development and validation of *in vitro* tests using tissue cultures and bacteria are critical. If these tests can predict *in vivo* responses to chemicals, not only will time and money be saved, but the controversial use of increasing numbers of laboratory animals will be addressed.

Recently, new scientific fields have been developed such as behavioural toxicology and immunotoxicology. They have raised interesting questions. For instance, if a substance causes changes in the behaviour or the immune system of test animals, it is necessary to find ways to determine whether or in what manner it might affect humans, given the ethical constraints of human testing.

In addition, we have to examine the many environmental and physiological factors which potentially confound the results of epidemiological studies, both in terms of exposure estimates and the end-point being measured. The Risk Science Institute will work to decrease the uncertainties associated with epidemiological research and to correlate epidemiological studies with toxicologic research to answer critical questions in safety assessment.

We have also begun exploring opportunities for collaborative research programmes between government laboratories and universities. We will develop a small grants programme to stimulate interest among academic investigators in risk-assessment research, and to support the development of projects that can later attract major funding from Federal agencies. Through funding from the Risk Science Institute, scientists in various research settings will be able to investigate new and interdisciplinary approaches to risk assessment.

We are excited about this institute, because it has the potential to address creatively a significant scientific and public health need. The scientific community has a mandate to improve the methodologies used in risk assessment, and the advantages of collaborative research should be encouraged and stimulated.

The formation of mutagens and carcinogens during food processing

T. SUGIMURA
National Cancer Center, Chuo-ku, Tokyo, Japan.

Dietary factors play an important role in the development of some human diseases. Cancer development is also thought to be closely related to the diet[3]. Trials to detect carcinogens in food have been made and the presence of carcinogenic polycyclic hydrocarbons in cooked foods confirmed[17,18]. These earlier investigations relied on chemical methods, which cannot easily detect new carcinogens. In this context, the introduction of a mutation assay system using bacteria to detect probable carcinogens[1] has been most valuable and has been used by us to investigate the presence of carcinogens in broiled fish and fried meat[29].

Formation of mutagenic and carcinogenic heterocyclic amines during heating of foodstuffs. Mutagens formed during broiling fish and frying beef were purified by monitoring their mutagenicity to *S. typhimurium* TA98 with metabolic activation. From broiled sun-dried sardines two mutagenic principles were isolated and identified as 2-amino-3-methylimidazo-[4,5-*f*]quinoline (IQ) and 2-amino-3,4-dimethylimidazo[4,5-*f*]quinoline (MeIQ)[14,15]. From fried beef, 2-amino-3,8-dimethylimidazo[4,5-*f*]quinoxaline (MeIQx) was isolated[13]. Their chemical structures suggested that the imidazole moiety may be derived from creatinine and the pyridine or pyrazine moiety from the Maillard reaction between amino acids and sugars[10]. When a mixture of creatinine, glucose and glycine or threonine was heated at around 130 °C for 2 h in diethylene glycol/water, the formation of MeIQx was confirmed[11]. Together with MeIQx, two isomers of the methyl derivative of MeIQx, ie, 2-amino-3,4,8-trimethyl-imidazo[4,5-*f*]quinoxaline (4,8-DiMeIQx) and 2-amino-3,7,8-trimethylimidazo[4,5-*f*]quino-xaline (7,8-DiMeIQx) were formed from the glycine and threonine mixtures, respectively[22,23]. Recently we found the actual presence of 4,8-DiMeIQx in beef extract[32].

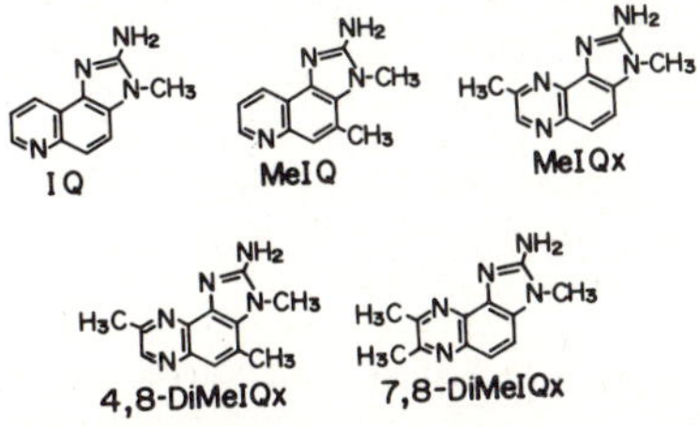

Fig. 1. *Structures of mutagenic amino-methylimidazoquinolines and amino-methylimidazoquinoxalines (see text for full chemical names).*

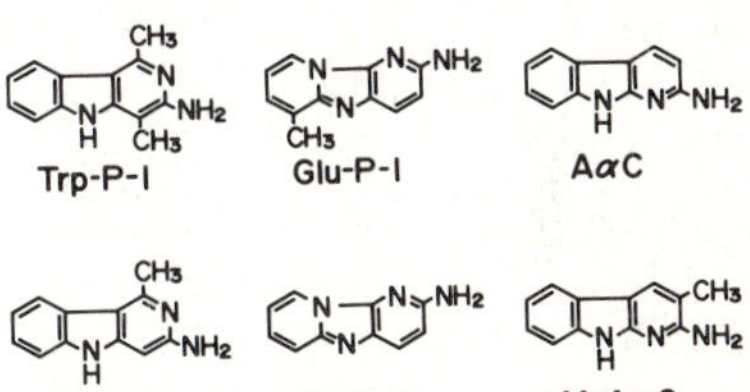

Fig. 2. *Structures of mutagenic hetero-cyclic amines isolated from amino acid and protein pyrolysates (see text for full chemical names).*

All these aminomethylimidazoquinoline and aminomethylimidazoquinoxaline compounds (Fig. 1) exert marked mutagenicities toward *S. typhimurium* TA98 with S9 mix, which range from 150 000 to 660 000 revertants per µg[30,31]

Chemically synthesized IQ, MeIQ and MeIQx, were mixed in the diet and given continuously to mice and/or rats. IQ, when fed to CDF mice at 0.3 g/kg diet, induced hepatocellular carcinomas, squamous cell carcinomas in the forestomach and lung adenocarci-nomas[26]. In the F344 rats the same dose of IQ in the diet also showed multipotent carcinogenicity, inducing hepatocellular carcinomas, adenocarcinomas in the small and large intestines and squamous cell carcinomas in the Zymbal gland, skin and oral cavity[36]. Induction of adenocarcinomas in the mammary gland was also shown when IQ was administered by gavage into female SD rats[37]. MeIQ at 0.4 g/kg diet induced squamous cell carcinomas in the forestomach and hepatocellular carcinomas in mice[25]. MeIQx was also recently shown to be hepatocarcinogenic in mice (unpublished observation).

Mutagenic heterocyclic amines are isolated also from the pyrolysates of amino acids and proteins. They are formed at higher temperatures and in this process the radical reaction may be involved. Chemical structures of these heterocyclic amines are shown in Fig. 2. 3-Amino-1,4-dimethyl-5H-pyrido[4,3-b]indole (Trp-P-1) and 3-amino-1-methyl-5H-pyrido-[4,3-b]indole (Trp-P-2) were first isolated from a tryptophan pyrolysate[28] and 2-amino-6-methyldipyrido[1,2-a:3′,2′-d]imidazole (Glu-P-1) and 2-amino-dipyrido[1,2-a:3′,2′-d]imidazole (Glu-P-2) were from a glutamic acid pyrolysate[42]. The specific mutagenic activities of these compounds are 2 000 to 100 000 with S9 mix[30,31]. 2-Amino-9H-pyrido[2,3-b]indole (AαC) and 2-amino-3-methyl-9H-pyrido[2,3-b]-indole (MeAαC) were isolated from a soybean globulin pyrolysate[43] and their specific mutagenic activities are 300 and 200 revertants/μg, respectively in the same bacterial strain with S9 mix[30,31]. The target organ for all these carcinogens in mice was the liver, where hepatocarcinomas developed[19,27]. Haemangioendothelial sarcomas in the brown adipose tissue of the interscapular region and some other parts were also induced by Glu-P-1, Glu-P-2, AαC and MeAαC[27]. In rats also, hepatocarcinomas were induced by all these heterocyclic amines. Additionally, tumours in the small and large intestines, the Zymbal gland and the clitoral gland were also induced by Glu-P-1 and Glu-P-2[7,34,35].

The presence of some of the above heterocyclic amines has been confirmed in cooked foods[30]. We have developed a simple method, with good recoveries, for the quantification of heterocyclic amines in food. It depends on an initial partial purification by adsorption to and elution from blue cotton, followed by acid-base partition and fractionation with a SEP-PAX cartridge and a final quantification step using HPLC with electrochemistry[33]. By using this method precise data on the amounts of heterocyclic amines in various cooked foods are being accumulated.

Oncogene activation in experimental tumours induced by heterocyclic amines. To investigate the possible activation of oncogenes in tumours by these heterocyclic amines, DNAs were extracted from hepatomas induced by IQ in rats and transferred to NIH3T3 cells. Southern blot analysis of DNAs isolated from primary and secondary transformants showed the presence of rat repetitive sequences. Moreover, in transformants obtained by the DNA isolated from one hepatoma (IQ4), the presence of rat H-*ras* was detected[8]. In another transformant obtained by transfection of DNA from another hepatoma (IQ7), the activation of rat *raf* oncogene was found[9]. The same line of study has so far revealed the activation of N-*ras* in a small intestinal adenocarcinoma induced in a rat by Glu-P-2 (unpublished observation). These studies should elucidate the molecular mechanisms of carcinogenesis by heterocyclic amines and they may also help to clarify the role of these environmental agents in human cancer development.

Mutagens in coffee. The mutagenicity of coffee has been well documented with freshly brewed, instant and also with caffeine-free coffees[16,21]: the mutagens are formed during the roasting process. Dicarbonyl compounds have been identified in coffee and among them methylglyoxal is a major mutagen[12]. It was found that the generation of hydrogen peroxide started right after making the coffee and increased with time. When hydrogen peroxide was added to methylglyoxal, the mutagenicity increased markedly over that due to hydrogen peroxide or methylglyoxal alone[20]. Accordingly the total mutagenicity of coffee can be fully explained by the presence of methylglyoxal and hydrogen peroxide together in a coffee solution. When methylglyoxal was injected subcutaneously into rats, the induction of subcutaneous sarcomas at the injection sites was observed. The effect of oral administration of this compound is being studied.

Precursors of mutagens formed during food processing. The correlation between the incidence of gastric cancer and the amount of nitrate ingested has been demonstrated[4]. Soya sauce developed marked mutagenicity after treatment with nitrite under acidic conditions. These mutagen precursors are (-)-(1S,3S)- and (-)-(1R,3S)-1-methyl-1,2,3,4-tetrahydro-β-carboline-3-carboxylic acids (MTCAs) and tyramine (Fig. 3)[24,41]. MTCAs are formed by the

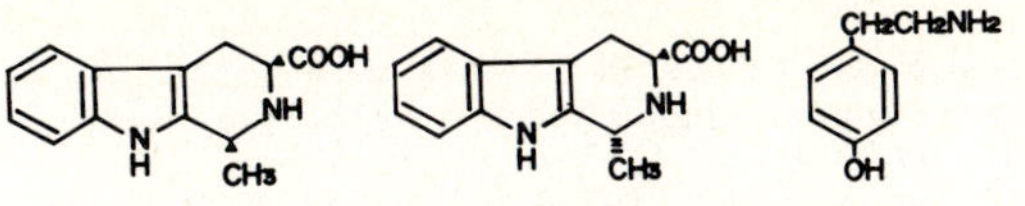

Fig. 3. *Mutagen precursors in soya sauce which are converted into active mutagens by nitrous acid (see text for full chemical names).*

(−)−(1S,3S)form   (−)−(1R,3S)form   Tyramine

1−Methyl−1,2,3,4−tetrahydro−β−carboline−
3−carboxylic acid (MTCA)

condensation of tryptophan and acetaldehyde and tyramine from tyrosine through decarboxylation by a bacterial enzyme during the processing of soyabeans. The direct-acting mutagen formed from tyramine by the nitrite treatment was identified as 4-(2-amino-ethyl)-6-diazo-2,4-cyclohexadienone[24]. When this mutagen was administered to rats in the drinking water, the induction of squamous cell carcinomas in the oral cavity was observed.

Indole derivatives from the Chinese cabbage have also been identified as mutagen precursors. They are indole-3-acetonitrile, 4-methyoxy-indole-3-acetonitrile and 4-methyoxy-indole-3-aldehyde. The direct mutagen formed by nitrite treatment of indole-3-acetonitrile was 1-nitrosoindole-3-acetonitrile[39,40].

Conclusion. During food processing and cooking, many new types of mutagens and carcinogens and their precursors are formed, which induce tumours in animals. Data on their exact amounts in foods are being obtained, which may help in evaluating the risk of these mutagens and carcinogens for human cancer development.

Carcinogenesis is a complex process. Chemicals which induce mutation can potentially activate oncogenes by point mutation, translocation or amplification. These cells are susceptible to the action of tumour promoters, which promote the process of carcinogenesis. Some tumour promoters like phorbol esters and newly discovered promoters such as teleocidin and aplysiatoxin[5] exert their action at very minute concentrations by activating protein kinase C, which is regarded as their receptor on the cell membrane, in the presence of calcium ions and phospholipid[2,6]. However, other types of tumour promoters whose biological action is not well defined are present in relatively larger quantities in our environment and in our bodies. They are alcohol, sodium chloride, fat, various amino acids and various hormones and bile acids[30]. These common tumour promoters, as well as some pathological conditions of the human body[38], may play a major role in human carcinogenesis initiated by mutagens and carcinogens. Qualitative and quantitative studies on all modifying factors in food, working positively but sometimes negatively on carcinogenesis and present along with mutagens and carcinogens in food, may eventually lead to a better understanding of the mechanisms of human cancer development and point the way to its prevention.

Acknowledgements. Our studies cited in this article were supported by Grants-in-Aid for Cancer Research from the Ministry of Health and Welfare, and the Ministry of Education, Science and Culture, Japan.

1 Ames, B.N., McCann, J. & Yamasaki, E. (1975): Methods for detecting carcinogens and mutagens with the Salmonella/mammalian-microsome mutagenicity test. *Mutation Res.* **31**, 347–364.
2 Castagna, M., Takai, Y., Kaibuchi, K., Sano, K., Kikkawa, V. & Nishizuka, Y. (1982): Direct activation of calcium-activated, phospholipid-dependent protein kinase by tumour-promoting phorbol esters. *J. Biol. Chem.* **257**, 7847–7851.
3 Doll, R. & Peto, R. (1981): The causes of cancer: Quantitative estimates of avoidable risks of cancer in the United States today. *J. Natl. Cancer Inst.* **66**, 1193–1308.
4 Fine, D.H., Challis, B.C., Hartman, P. & Van Ryzin, J. (1982): Endogenous synthesis of volatile nitrosamines: model calculations and risk assessment. In *N-Nitroso compounds: occurrence and biological effects*, IARC Sci. Publ. No. 41, ed H. Bartsch, I.K. O'Neill, M. Castegnaro, M. Okada & W. Davis, pp. 379–396. Lyon: IARC.
5 Fujiki, H. & Sugimura, T. (1983): New potent tumor promoters: teleocidin, lyngbyatoxin A and aplysiatoxin. *Cancer Surveys* **2**, 539–556.
6 Fujiki, H., Tanaka, Y., Miyake, R., Kikkawa, V., Nishizuka, Y. & Sugimura, T. (1984): Activation of calcium-activated phospholipid-dependent protein kinase (protein kinase C) by new classes of tumor promoters: teleocidin and debromoaplysiatoxin. *Biochem. Biophys. Res. Commun.* **120**, 339–343.
7 Hosaka, S., Matsushima, T., Hirono, I & Sugimura, T. (1981): Carcinogenic activity of 3-amino-1-methyl-5H-pyrido[4,3-b]indole (Trp-P-2), a pyrolysis product of tryptophan. *Cancer Lett.* **13**, 23–28.
8 Ishikawa, F., Takaku, F., Nagao, M., Ochiai, M., Hayashi, K., Takayama, S. & Sugimura, T. (1985): Activated oncogenes in a rat hepatocellular carcinoma induced by 2-amino-3-methylimidazo[4,5-f]quinoline (IQ). *Jpn. J. Cancer Res.* **76**, 425–428.

9 Ishikawa, F., Takaku, F., Ochiai, M., Hayashi, K., Hirohashi, S., Terada, M., Takayama, S., Negao, M. & Sugimura, T. (1985): Activated c-*raf* gene in a rat hepatocellular carcinoma induced by 2-amino-3-methylimidazo[4,5-*f*]quinoline. *Biochem. Biophys. Res. Commun.* **132**, 186–192.

10 Jägerstad, M., Laser Reuterswärd, A., Öste, R. & Dahlqvist, A. (1983): Creatinine and Maillard reaction products as precursors of mutagenic compounds formed in fried beef. In *The Maillard reaction in foods and nutrition*, ACS Symposium Series 215, ed G.R. Waller & M.S. Feather, pp. 507–519. Washington, DC: American Chemical Society.

11 Jägerstad, M., Olsson, K., Grivas, S., Negishi, C., Wakabayashi, K., Tsuda, M., Sato, S. & Sugimura, T. (1984): Formation of 2-amino-3,8-dimethylimidazo[4,5-*f*]quinoxaline in a model system by heating creatinine, glycine and glucose. *Mutation Res.* **126**, 239–244.

12 Kasai, H., Kumeno, K., Yamaizumi, Z., Nishimura, S., Nagao, M., Fujita, Y., Sugimura, T., Nukaya, H. & Kosuge, T. (1982): Mutagenicity of methylglyoxal in coffee. *Gann* **73**, 681–683.

13 Kasai, H., Yamaizumi, Z., Shiomi, T., Yokoyama, S., Miyazawa, T., Wakabayashi, K., Nagao, M., Sugimura, T. & Nishimura, S. (1981): Structure of a potent mutagen isolated from fried beef. *Chem. Lett.* 485–488.

14 Kasai, H., Yamaizumi, Z., Wakabayashi, K., Nagao, M., Sugimura, T., Yokoyama, S., Miyazawa, T. & Nishimura, S. (1980): Structure and chemical synthesis of Me-IQ, a potent mutagen isolated from broiled fish. *Chem. Lett.* 1391–1394.

15 Kasai, H., Yamaizumi, Z., Wakabayashi, K., Nagao, M., Sugimura, T., Yokoyama, S., Miyazawa, T., Spingarn, N.E., Weisburger, J.H. & Nishimura, S. (1980): Potent novel mutagens produced by broiling fish under normal conditions. *Proc. Jpn Acad.* **56B**, 278–283.

16 Kosugi, A., Nagao, M., Suwa, Y., Wakabayashi, K. & Sugimura, T. (1983): Roasting coffee beans produces compounds that induce prophage in *E. coli* and are mutagenic in *E. coli* and *S. typhimurium*. *Mutation Res.* **116**, 179–184.

17 Kuratsune, M. (1956): benzo[a]pyrene content of certain pyrogenic materials. *J. Natl. Cancer Inst.* **16**, 1485–1496.

18 Lijinsky, W. & Shubik, P. (1964): Benzo[a]pyrene and other poly-nuclear hydrocarbons in charcoal-broiled meat. *Science* **145**, 53–54.

19 Matsukura, N., Kawachi, T., Morino, K., Ohgaki, H., Sugimura, T. & Takayama, S. (1981): Carcinogenicity in mice of mutagenic compounds from a tryptophan pyrolyzate. *Science* **213**, 346–347.

20 Nagao, M., Suwa, Y., Yoshizumi, H. & Sugimura, T. (1984): Mutagens in coffee. In *Coffee and health*, Banbury Report 17, ed B. MacMahon & T. Sugimura, pp. 69–77. Cold Spring Harbor, New York: Cold Spring Harbor Lab.

21 Nagao, M., Takahashi, Y., Yamanaka, H. & Sugimura, T. (1979): Mutagens in coffee and tea. *Mutation Res.* **68**, 101–106.

22 Negishi, C., Wakabayashi, K., Tsuda, M., Sato, S., Sugimura, T., Saitô, H., Maeda, M. & Jägerstad, M. (1984): Formation of 2-amino-3,7,8-trimethylimidazo[4,5-*f*]quinoxaline, a new mutagen, by heating a mixture of creatinine, glucose and glycine. *Mutation Res.* **140**, 55–59.

23 Negishi, C., Wakabayashi, K. *et al.* (1986): Identification of 4,8-diMEIQX, a new mutagen. *Mutation Res.* **147**, 267–268.

24 Ochiai, M., Wakabayashi, K., Nagao, M. & Sugimura, T. (1984): Tyramine is a major mutagen precursor in soy sauce, being convertible to a mutagen by nitrite. *Gann* **75**, 1–3.

25 Ohgaki, H., Hasegawa, H., Kato, T., Suenaga, M., Ubukata, M., Sato, S., Takayama, S. & Sugimura, T. (1985): Induction of tumors in the forestomach and liver of mice by feeding 2-amino-3,4-dimethylimidazo[4,5-*f*]quinoline (MeIQ). *Proc. Jpn Acad.* **61B**, 137–139.

26 Ohgaki, H., Kusama, K., Matsukura, N., Morino, K., Hasegawa, H., Sato, S., Sugimura, T. & Takayama, S. (1984): Carcinogenicity in mice of mutagenic compound, 2-amino-3-methylimidazo[4,5-*f*]quinoline, from broiled sardine, cooked beef and beef extract. *Carcinogenesis* **5**, 921–924.

27 Ohgaki, H., Matsukura, N., Morino, K., Kawachi, T., Sugimura, T. & Takayama, S. (1984): Carcinogenicity in mice of mutagenic compounds from glutamic acid and soybean globulin pyrolysates. *Carcinogenesis* **5**, 815–819.

28 Sugimura, T., Kawachi, T., Nagao, M., Yahagi, T., Seino, Y., Okamoto, T., Shudo, K., Kosuge, T., Tsuji, K., Wakabayashi, K., Iitaka, Y. & Itai, A. (1977): Mutagenic principle(s) in tryptophan and phenylalanine pyrolysis products. *Proc. Jpn Acad.* **53**, 58–61.

29 Sugimura, T., Nagao, M., Kawachi, T., Honda, M., Yahagi, T., Seino, Y., Sato, S., Matsukura, N., Matsushima, T., Shirai, A., Sawamura, M. & Matsumoto, H. (1977): Mutagen-carcinogens in food with special reference to highly mutagenic pyrolytic products in broiled foods. In *Origins of human cancer*, Book C, ed H.H. Hiatt, J.D. Watson & J.A. Winsten, pp. 1561–1576. Cold Spring Harbor, New York: Cold Spring Harbor Lab.

30 Sugimura, T. & Sato, S. (1983): Mutagens-carcinogens in foods. *Cancer Res. (Suppl.)* **43**, 2415s–2421s.

31 Sugimura, T. & Sato, S. (1983): Bacterial mutagenicity of natural materials, pyrolysis products and additives in foodstuffs and their association with genotoxic effects in mammals. In *Developments in the science and practice of toxicology*, ed A.W. Hayes, R.C. Schnell & T.S. Miya, pp. 115–133. Amsterdam: Elsevier.

32 Takahashi, M., Wakabayashi, K., Nagao, M., Yamaizumi, Z., Sato, S., Kinae, N., Tomita, I. & Sugimura, T. (1985): Identification and quantification of 2-amino-3,4,8-trimethylimidazo[4,5-*f*]quinoxaline (4,8-DiMeIQx) in beef extract. *Carcinogenesis* **6**, 1195–1199.

33 Takahashi, M., Wakabayashi, K., Nagao, M., Yamamoto, M., Matsui, T., Goto, T., Kinae, N., Tomita, I. & Sugimura, T. (1985): Quantification of 2-amino-3-methylimidazo[4,51-*f*]quinoxaline (MeIQx) in beef extracts by liquid chromatography with electro-chemical detection (LCEC). *Carcinogenesis* **6**, 1195–1199.

34 Takayama, S., Ishikawa, T., Nakatsuru, Y., Sato, S. & Sugimura, T. (1985): Carcinogenicity in rats of a mutagenic compound from tryptophan pyrolysate. *Jpn J. Cancer Res. (Gann)* **76**, 815–817.

35 Takayama, S., Masuda, M., Mogami, M., Ohgaki, H., Sato, S. & Sugimura, T. (1984): Induction of cancers in the intestine, liver and various other organs of rats by feeding mutagens from glutamic acid pyrolysate. *Gann* **75**, 207–213.

36 Takayama, S., Nakatsuru, Y., Masuda, M., Ohgaki, H., Sato, S. & Sugimura, T. (1984): Demonstration of carcinogenicity in F344 rats of 2-amino-3-methylimidazo[4,5-*f*]quinoline from broiled sardine, fried beef and extract. *Gann* **75**, 467–470.

37 Tanaka, T., Barnes, W.S., Weisburger, J.H. & Williams, G.M. (1985): The fried food mutagen 2-amino-3-methyli-midazo[4,5-*f*]quinoline (IQ) is a powerful carcinogen for rat mammary gland. *Jpn J. Cancer Res. (Gann)* **76**, 570–576.

38 Templeton, A.C. (1975): Acquired diseases. In *Persons at high risk of cancer. An approach to cancer etiology and control*, ed J.F. Fraumeni Jr., pp. 69–84. New York: Academic Press.

39 Wakabayashi, K., Nagao, M., Ochiai, M., Tahira, T., Yamaizumi, Z. & Sugimura, T. (1985): A mutagen precursor in Chinese cabbage, indole-3-acetonitrile, which becomes mutagenic on nitrite treatment. *Mutation Res. Lett.* **143**, 17–21.

40 Wakabayashi, K., Nagao, M., Tahira, T., Saito, H., Katayama, M., Marumo, S. & Sugimura, T. (1985): 1-Nitroso-indole-3-acetonitrile, a mutagen produced by nitrite treatment of indole-3-acetonitrile. *Proc. Jpn Acad.* **61B**, 190–192.

41 Wakabayashi, K., Ochiai, M., Saito, H., Tsuda, M., Suwa, Y., Nagao, M. & Sugimura, T. (1983): Presence of 1-methyl-1,2,3,4-tetrahydro-β-carboline-3-carboxylic acid, a precursor of a mutagenic nitroso compound, in soy sauce. *Proc. Natl. Acad. Sci. USA* **80**, 2912–2916.

42 Yamamoto, T., Tsuji, K., Kosuge, T., Okamoto, T., Shudo, K., Takeda, K., Iitaka, Y., Yamaguchi, K., Seino, Y., Yahagi, T., Nagao, M. & Sugimura, T. (1978): Isolation and structure determination of mutagenic substances in L-glutamic acid pyrolysate. *Proc. Jpn Acad.* **54B**, 248–250.

43 Yoshida, D., Matsumoto, T., Yoshimura, R. & Matsuzaki, T. (1978): Mutagenicity of amino-α-carbolines in pyrolysis products of soybean globulin. *Biochem. Biophys. Res. Commun.* **83**, 915–920.

What laboratory diets should be used in the study of response to xenobiotes? a workshop report

D.L. FRAPE (Organizer)
CANTAB Group of ICLAS, Cambridge, UK.

Contributors. *J.J. Knapka* (National Institute of Health, Bethesda, Maryland); *A.C. Beynen* (State University, Utrecht, Netherlands); *A. Wise* (Robert Gordon's Institute of Technology, Aberdeen); *I.R. Rowland* and *A.K. Mallett* (BIBRA, Carshalton, UK); *M.R. Spivey Fox* and *J.I. Rader* (Food and Drug Administration, Washington, DC, USA); *M.A. Bieber, B. Scott Appleton* and *R.E. Landers* (Best Foods, Union, New Jersey, USA).

This workshop had the objectives of discussing critical issues in laboratory diet composition for animals on experiment and of making recommendations in succession to those formulated at the 12th International Congress of Nutrition held at San Diego, California in 1981.

The diet AIN-76 is a purified diet, the origin and purpose of which are short-term experimentation. No published work is available that has established the most suitable purified diet for lifetime studies, or that indicates whether similar life spans are possible with purified diets to those achieved with natural diets. As distinct from animals in feeding studies of short duration, those subjected to lifetime studies and receiving purified diets are likely to require a dietary source of all trace elements established to be nutrients for that species. For instance, the absence of nickel from diet AIN-76 may only jeopardize the growth and health of rats in feeding studies of long duration.

As distinct from the influence of nutrients on animal responses, dietary sources of fat and carbohydrate and organic structural elements of plant cells can have a remarkable effect on health in life span studies. The high concentration of sucrose in diet AIN-76 is not only unrepresentative of human diets, but is a cause of pathological changes during extended feeding. The inclusion of purified sources of indigestible carbohydrate in these diets may extend life-expectancy, but the effect on microbial enzyme activity in the large intestine is unlikely to be the same as that observed with similar indigestible substances forming normal constituents of natural diets. In particular, the addition of cellulose to a purified diet reduces the microbial flora in the rat's caecum and makes its metabolic profile even more unlike that in rats fed stock diet than they are in rats given fibre-free purified diet. Experiments have shown that the activities of hind gut microbial nitro and nitrate reductases not only differ amongst rodent species and man, but also differ between natural and purified diets given to those animals. The flora that are preferentially selected are likely to be those which most effectively metabolize the fermentable substrate. Interestingly, rodents given purified diets evince activities for these two enzymes closer to those expressed by human gut flora. The reason for this is unknown, but it may rely upon the physical relationships amongst the structural components of plant cells signifying that the modelling of the human predicament should take into consideration both the chemical and the physical characteristic of food.

The simulation of metabolic events in the human is an important objective of animal modelling, but an alternative and perhaps equally justifiable objective of experimentation in this field that should yield valuable information would be to measure the consequences of changes in the activities of key microbial enzymes under defined and reproducible conditions rather than attempt to mimic the human situation.

Evidence has demonstrated a higher incidence of metabolic disorders in rodents receiving purified diets over extended periods than in controls receiving natural, or stock, diets of similar chemical composition. Nevertheless the frequency of spontaneous tumours and some metabolic disorders is still too high in rodents receiving many stock diets during life span studies. There has therefore been widespread interest in the formulation of diets and of feeding regimes that reduce this background incidence which is considered to make more difficult the detection of adverse events simultaneously caused by xenobiotes administered in safety bioassays. However, the experimental efficiency of such assays is a function of a ratio, the magnitude of the response per unit dose of the test substance divided by the residual variance. Many diets that are designed to reduce the incidence of spontaneous metabolic disorders, including for example renal, hepatic, cardiac and peripheral vascular lesions, hypertension and oncogenesis may also suppress the toxicity of test substances and the incidence of test substance-induced lesions, decreasing the coefficient of regression of response to test dose.

Although much work remains to be done in this area and although the mechanisms by which spontaneous disorders occur may be poorly understood a rational approach can still be taken in the recommendation of diets for testing the various classes of xenobiotes An understanding of the mechanisms of action and dietary interaction of a test substance would nevertheless assist in the rational selection of the preferred dietary characteristics and nutrient contents yielding the most sensitive response to test substance. This implies that dietary analysis for the critical nutrients should be undertaken on each batch of feed and the uniformity of distribution established at concentrations that without good reason should be of minimum adequacy. A conclusion to this discussion is that no one basal diet would be suitable for testing all types of xenobiote.

A full understanding of diet x xenobiote interaction will yield invaluable information on potency and the likely minimum effective and toxic doses for man when, subsequently, clinical tests are undertaken in individuals of differing ethnic origins distributed across a variety of environments. An understanding of any interactive metabolism may also point the way to dietary means of combatting clinical toxicity or side-effects of drugs in the target species without diminishing efficacy.

A number of metabolic disorders are correlated with fat consumption in both laboratory animals and man. Longevity can be increased by reducing the fat content of diets where this is excessive. However, high dietary fat concentrations may be desirable for research into many drugs and other test substances. Some evidence suggests that the critical characteristic of diet in the induction or promotion of certain disorders, including oncogenesis and some other types of metabolic derangement, is metabolizable or net energy intake. Energy consumption can be reduced by restricting daily intake, rather than by reducing the energy density of diets most commonly achieved through lowering the fat content and increasing the dietary concentration of structural carbohydrates. A number of studies have already been reported where rodents have been managed with the restriction of daily dry matter intake. This concept suggests that a more appropriate model of man for many functions might be obtained from use of meal eaters, such as pigs rather than by use of nibblers, such as rodents. Although much work is required to resolve the issues involved the scheduled and limited access of rodents to feed may provide a better model than that in which rodents are given unlimited access.

More information is needed on the nutrient requirements of adults. Nevertheless it is well established that the adult animal requires lower concentrations of many nutrients in its diets than do growing animals and it may for that reason display fewer diet x drug interactions. Diets for adults should be capable of preventing fat deposition unless such deposition forms part of the model. Whether high concentrations of indigestible carbohydrates would be counterproductive must depend on the mode of action of the substance under test.

Adult DNA is more sensitive to chemical lesions and any influence diet may have in protecting DNA from the disruptive influence of some xenobiotics would seem to imply that the adult is the more appropriate model for discerning drug x diet oncogenic influences. It is likely that previous dietary history has an influence on the susceptibility of the adult to oncogenesis. Therefore the adult would be a reliable model only if that history was constant and known. Where the diet has been purified rather than stock, subsequent sensitivity is likely to be enhanced.

The chemical characteristics of the structural and other carbohydrates and lignin should be described as the various forms act differently. Information about many other characteristics of diet not routinely determined at present may be required by the investigator. These include phytates, digestible protein, available dietary indispensible and dispensible amino acids, digestible energy or net energy for various functions, lipid composition, including the concentrations of various sterols and a complete fatty acid analysis. Most currently used diets are analysed for a range of vitamins, minerals and trace elements, although where purified diets are under scrutiny the number of trace elements monitored, amino acid, lipid, etc. may not be necessary for each study but those of particular relevance must be carried out and carefully controlled from batch to batch. Water composition should be constant and should also be known in many cases.

More rapid progress in the understanding of diet x xenobiotic interaction and the definition of the most appropriate diet for a particular field of research would be fostered by detailed and intelligent dietary description in many specific journals. It was proposed that these goals could be attained with greater expedition by the formulation of a 'critical path' procedure for diet formulation in which the most appropriate characteristics of each component of the diet for a specified objective would be decided by the investigator following a plan. Such a plan could be adapted for computer programming.

It is accepted that purified diets are more expensive than natural diets. Nevertheless the additional cost is small in comparison to other costs and the addition investment in diet is likely to be outweighed by the improvement in definition of dietary composition, experimental efficiency, and reproducibility between laboratories, saving time, facilities and animals, especially in studies evaluating the safety, or effect, of long-term low level exposure to various compounds. The reasons for differences in response between purified and natural diets must be clarified as the objective is to model man, whose nutriture would seem to span a spectrum from entirely natural ingredient diets in the case of rural populations of Africa and those diets of other undeveloped communities to those ingested by some Western societies for which any natural origin may be difficult to discern.

Conclusions and recommendations. (1) Information is urgently required to establish the characteristics and desirable nutrient contents of purified diets for life-span studies. (2) The reasons for many differences in response of animals to purified and natural diets are not adequately understood, due in part to a failure to analyse natural ingredient diets thoroughly, or to the use of closed formula diets the composition of which may not be reproducible. (3) Comparison of effects obtained with purified vs natural diets may provide information on nutrient-xenobiotic interactions, and lead to the development of better (ie, more sensitive) test diets. (4) Knowledge of the function, toxicity and mechanism of action of a particular xenobiote can be extremely useful for the formulation of an appropriate test diet. It follows that no one standard purified diet could be conceived. Use of well-designed and reproducible test diets can contribute significantly to knowledge of the function, toxicity, and mechanism of action of particular xenobiotics. (5) Diets that reduce the incidence of metabolic disorders may also decrease the sensitivity of response to test substances and so fail to improve experimental efficiency if the denominator of the F ratio is not also decreased adequately. The number of animals required to achieve a given probability level will be affected accordingly. (6) Restriction of daily food consumption and use of 'meal eaters' may improve the modelling of man. (7) More appropriate chemical analyses and description of diets is essential for interpretation of animal response. Greater cooperation from scientific journal editors is required. (8) Guide-lines to those formulating diets with specific objectives in mind are required. (9) Unless there is a specific reason for doing otherwise, diets should be balanced with respect to nutrient requirements and should not contain excessive concentrations of nutrients that could mask adverse effects of a xenobiotic.

INTERACTIONS THAT AFFECT NUTRITIONAL VALUE OF THE DIET

Interactions between the individual and food choice

Barbara J. ROLLS
The Johns Hopkins University School of Medicine, Department of Psychiatry and Behavioral Sciences, 600 N. Wolfe Street, Meyer 4–119, Baltimore, MD 21205, USA.

Every interaction an individual has with food is a potentially significant influence on later food choices. Because of the complexity of factors that can affect food habits, a number of recent studies of human food selection have concentrated on defining the general principles by which foods come to be considered as palatable. Palatability, or the hedonic response to food, is dependent on the taste, smell, texture and appearance of the food, and can be influenced by social, cultural and economic factors as well as by the internal physiological state and previous experiences with the food.

Effects of palatability on food intake. Palatability can affect meal size and pattern of eating. Increasing palatability leads to an increase in meal size and duration, and a decrease in chewing time and the number of chews per piece of food[1,6]. During and two hours after a meal of palatable foods, hunger and the desire to eat have been found to be higher than with a less preferred meal. Consumption of more palatable foods may also lead to more positive moods and feelings[5].

Palatability is not a fixed property of foods, but can change from meal to meal and within a meal (see below). The changing palatability of foods is illustrated by dietary selection in newly weaned infants[4]. These children, who had no preconceived ideas about how many foods they should eat or what was appropriate, showed themselves to be omnivorous by consuming most of the wide variety of foods presented. Although they demonstrated preferences within a meal in that they would consume significant quantities of two or three foods, these preferences were not predictable from meal to meal. Thus the overall pattern of consumption was one of variety. Palatability, as judged by the amount of particular foods eaten, tended to change from meal to meal.

Sensory-specific satiety. Palatability also changes during a meal. As an individual becomes satiated on a food its palatability changes so that the sensory properties, including taste, smell, appearance and texture, are significantly less pleasant than they were at the start of eating. Cabanac[3] suggested that the liking for particular foods depends on the internal physiological state. In support of this he found that, as a sweet solution was ingested, subjective measurements of its pleasantness decreased progressively over 45 to 60 minutes. Because of this slow time course, and because changes also occurred following intragastric preloads of glucose, it was thought that sensory stimulation by the preloads at the oropharyngeal level had little influence on these changes, which were presumed to be due to an alteration in the physiological need for particular substances. Our recent experiments challenge the suggestion that the pleasantness or palatability of food depends upon its physiological usefulness.

In a series of experiments we have investigated the role of sensory properties in the changing hedonic response to foods. The aim of the first experiment[8] was to determine whether the liking for the taste of a food which was eaten until the subjects were satisfied declined more than the liking for foods which were not consumed. To assess this, subjects were asked to rate their subjective liking for the taste of eight foods. After this initial rating they were given the opportunity to eat as much as they liked of one of these foods which had been tasted (either cheese on crackers or sausages). Two minutes after eating had stopped, the subjects again tasted and rated the eight foods they had sampled at the start of the test. When the changes in the response to the foods over the course of the meal were analysed, there was a significantly greater decrease in the ratings of the liking for the taste of the food which had been eaten to satiety than for the foods which had been tasted but not eaten.

Satiety appeared to be specific to the food that had been consumed, and it was of interest to know whether such changes in the hedonic response to foods would be related to the amount eaten subsequently. To test this, subjects were given an unexpected second course just after they completed the second series of ratings. If the subjects were given the same food in the second course that they had consumed in the first course, their intake fell to half that eaten in the first course, whereas if they were given a different food, intake was the same in the second course as in the first course. The changes in liking over the first course were found to be significantly correlated with the amount eaten in the second course. Thus, as a food is consumed, its taste is liked less and this change in hedonic response is related to the amount of food that will be consumed during the rest of the meal. A selective change in the palatability of food, or sensory-specific satiety, favours switching from one food to another during a meal, and thus promotes intake of a balance of nutrients. Sensory-specific satiety therefore provides a means of ensuring good nutrition.

We have also looked at the changes in the hedonic response to foods over a four-course meal which consisted of two savory courses followed by dessert and fruit[10]. The purpose of this experiment was to see if the specific changes in the pleasantness of foods already eaten give way to a more general satiety after several courses, so all foods become unpleasant. Forty-eight subjects of normal weight were tested twice at lunch time. On one occasion they were given a varied meal consisting of four successive courses which were sausages, bread and butter, chocolate whipped dessert and bananas. On the other occasion they were given a plain meal which consisted of just one of the four foods offered repeatedly in the four courses. Energy intake was elevated 60 per cent in the varied meal. The pleasantness of the taste of the eaten foods decreased rapidly, whereas the pleasantness of foods which had not been eaten remained relatively unchanged. The change in the pleasantness of a food correlated well with the subsequent intake of that food. Therefore sensory specific satiety was still found after eating four different courses in a meal, and general satiety did not result.

Variety in the sensory properties of foods. Thus offering a succession of foods which differed in a number of ways, ie flavour, appearance, texture and composition, greatly enhanced intake. In a series of experiments we have investigated whether varying just the sensory properties of foods, or just one sensory property, while keeping the nutrient composition constant, can enhance intake.

Variations in the flavour of food can enhance intake. We found that successive courses of three different flavours of cream cheese sandwiches (salt, curry, and combined lemon and saccharin) enhanced intake by 15 per cent compared to the successive presentation of the favourite food[9]. Variations in the shape of food which change both the appearance and mouth feel can also affect intake. Thus we found that successive courses of three different shapes of pasta enhanced intake by 14 per cent compared with the successive presentation of the favourite shape[9]. We have also looked at the effect of varying appearance by offering candy-coated chocolates of different colours both successively and simultaneously, and comparing intake to that of the favourite colour presented alone. We found no effect of the variety of colours on intake, although we did find that when just one colour was available, the pleasantness of that colour decreased significantly more than that of the uneaten colours[9].

Time course of the changing palatability of foods. The change in the hedonic response to the food which had been eaten was seen 2 minutes after the termination of the meal, ie before there would have been time for absorption of most of the food. This indicates that the sensory properties of the food were probably a major factor in this response. This was examined further in a study in which the time course of the changes in the pleasantness of a number of sensory properties of foods was tracked over the hour after the meal[7]. The rationale was that if the hedonic changes that occur with eating are due to sensory stimulation by the foods, they should occur rapidly and then decline with time after eating. On the other hand if the changes are primarily due to post-absorptive effects of foods they should increase in magnitude over the hour after eating. The changes in the pleasantness of the taste, texture, appearance, and smell of cheese on crackers after a meal of cheese on crackers are shown in the Figure. The changes in the pleasantness of the sensory properties of eight uneaten foods arc meaned together for

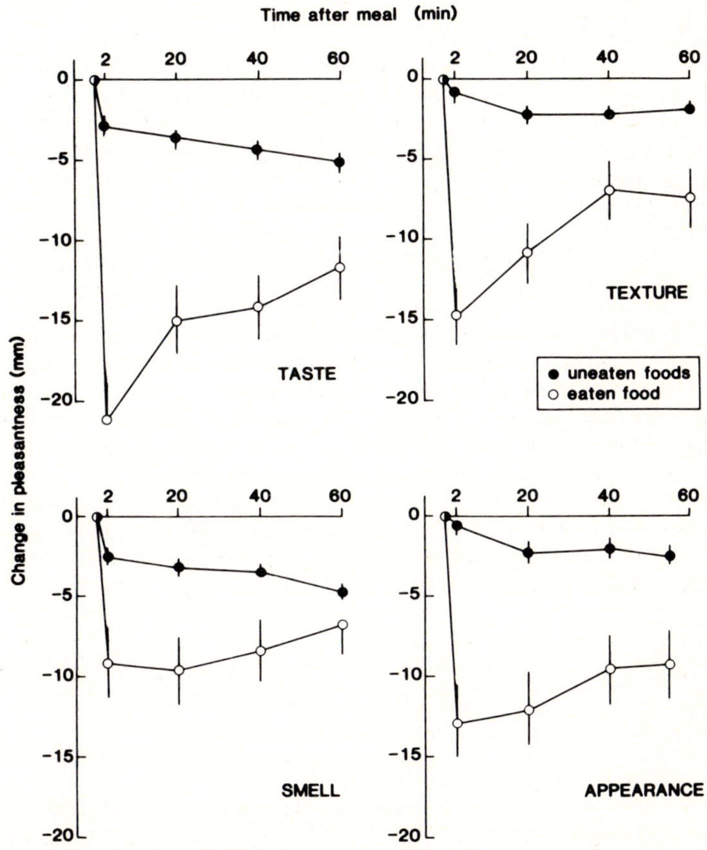

Figure. *Mean (± SEM) changes in the taste, texture, smell and appearance of the eaten food and the uneaten foods following a meal of cheese on crackers at 2, 20, 40 and 60 min after the meal. For all sensory variables except smell the most significant decline in the pleasantness of the eaten food occurred 2 min. after the meal.*

comparison with the eaten food. For all of the sensory properties there was a bigger decrease in the pleasantness of the eaten food than the uneaten foods. The changes tended to be greatest at 2 minutes after the meal, with a gradual recovery in pleasantness over the hour after eating. Since the largest changes were seen before most of the food would have been absorbed, a major influence on the hedonic response to foods comes from the sensory properties of the foods.

Energy density and sensory-specific satiety. In order to further clarify the relative importance of sensory stimulation and energy value, we conducted an experiment using foods which had similar sensory qualities (appearance, smell, texture, and taste) but which differed in energy density[7]. We tested 24 normal-weight non-dieting females, 12 of which were assigned to a soup condition and 12 of which were assigned to a jello condition. Half of the subjects in each group received the high-calorie version (0.49–0.54 kcal/g) of the test meal on the first test day and half received the low calorie version (0.07–0.09 kcal/g) on the first test day. Before the meal subjects were asked to rate hunger, stomach fullness and the pleasantness of nine sample foods on visual analogue scales and then to eat as much of the test meal as they liked. At 2, 20, 40 and 60 minutes after consumption subjects were asked to make these judgements again. After this period subjects were offered a second course of cheese on crackers to test whether there would be a compensation for differences in energy uptake in the first course.

Subjects consumed similar weights of the high and low energy foods. This meant there were highly significant differences in energy intake between the two versions of the same food. Despite these differences in intake, ratings of hunger and stomach fullness did not differ following the high and low energy foods. For both versions of the soup and jello test meals the greatest decline in pleasantness occurred at 2 minutes after consumption for the eaten food. The differences in energy value of the test meals had no differential effect upon the development, time course or magnitude of sensory-specific satiety. That subjects were unable to detect differences in energy density was supported by the finding that there was no energy compensation in the second course following the low energy test meals. This experiment clearly demonstrates that the sensory properties of foods are a major determinant of the changing response to foods. Also, when subjects are unaware of the energy contents of foods, intake during a meal appears to be controlled primarily by cognitive factors, perhaps related to portions previously learned to be satisfying, rather than by regulation of energy.

Conclusions. Interactions with food influence food choices from an early age. Infants show the capacity to consume appropriate amounts of food and to eat a varied diet. The consumption of a varied diet is likely to be due at least in part to sensory specific satiety since young children show a decrease in preference for a food following consumption[2]. We propose that sensory-specific satiety, or the change in the hedonic response to foods, is inborn and from the start of mixed feeding will help to ensure that a variety of nutrients is ingested.

Studies in which a variety of foods offered in a meal is changed or in which the energy content of foods is disguised indicate that food intake is not under precise physiological control. If we are to understand abnormalities of eating behaviour or body weight regulation, there must be more studies which clarify how an individual's interactions with foods affect food intake and selection.

1 Bellisle, F. & Le Magnen, J. (1980): The analysis of human feeding patterns: the edogram. *Appetite* **1**, 141–50.

2 Birch, L.L. (in press): The acquisition of food acceptance patterns in children. In *Food habits*, ed R. Boakes, D. Popplewell & M. Burton. Cambridge: Cambridge University Press.

3 Cabanac, M. (1971): Physiological role of pleasure. *Science* **173**, 1103–1107.

4 Davis, C.M. (1928): Self selection of diet by newly weaned infants. An experimental study. *Am. J. Dis. Child.* **36**, 651–679.

5 Hill, A.J., Magson, L.D. & Blundell, J.E. (1984): Hunger and palatability: tracking ratings of subjective experience before, during and after the consumption of preferred and less preferred food. *Appetite* **5**, 361–371.

6 Hill, S.W. & McCutcheson, N.B. (1975): Eating responses of obese and nonobese humans during dinner meals. *Psychosom. Med.* **37**, 395–401.

7 Rolls, B.J., Hetherington, M., Burley, V.J. & van Duijvenvoorde, P.M. (in press): Changing hedonic responses to foods during and after a meal. In *The chemical senses and nutrition*, eds M.R. Kare & J.G. Brand. New York: Academic Press.

8 Rolls, B.J., Rolls, E.T. & Sweeney, K. (1981): Sensory specific satiety in man. *Physiol. Behav.* **27**, 137–142.

9 Rolls, B.J., Rowe, E.A. & Rolls, E.T. (1982): How sensory properties of foods affect human feeding behavior. *Physiol. Behav.* **29**, 409–417.

10 Rolls, B.J., van Duijvenvoorde, P. & Rolls, E.T. (1984): Pleasantness changes and food intake in a varied four course meal. *Appetite* **5**, 337–348.

Meal composition, gastric emptying and the control of food intake

H.R. KISSILEFF and T.B. VAN ITALLIE
From the Departments of Medicine (TBVI) and Psychiatry (HRK), College of Physicians & Surgeons, Columbia University at St. Luke's-Roosevelt Hospital Center, Amsterdam Ave. at 114th Street, New York, NY 10025, USA.

In this discussion of the effect of meal composition on ingestive behaviour, we have made the basic assumption that stomach fullness is an important contributor to meal termination. If this assumption is correct, gastric emptying rate and quantity of food consumed may be interrelated via the following sequence: (1) the composition of the meal modulates gastric emptying; (2) gastric emptying influences gastric fullness; (3) food intake is inversely proportional to gastric fullness at the onset of a meal.

Recent studies using separate isotopic markers for emptying of solids and liquids have confirmed earlier work using primarily serial test liquid meals removed from the stomach at intervals[11], showing that gastric emptying is slowed by various nutrient-related influences on the duodenum. Primary among these influences are the effects of increasing osmotic concentration, increasing acid content, increasing fat content, and increasing fibre content.

Energy density. The resultant of these mechanisms has been carefully examined in the rhesus monkey. Over a narrow range of energy concentrations in food (which is probably wide in relation to gastric chyme), macronutrients empty from the simian stomach at between 0.4 and 0.5 kcal (1.7–2.1 kJ)/min. Therefore, inhibition of gastric emptying occurs in direct proportion to energy concentration. However, when the concentration of energy was doubled from 0.7 to 1.4 kcal (5.8 kJ)/ml in a liquid meal, the rate of transfer was only increased by 50 per cent[9]. Thus, at concentrations above 0.7 kcal (2.9 kJ)/ml, gastric emptying is increasingly slowed. Nevertheless, this slowing is not sufficient to maintain delivery to the duodenum at the low rate of 0.4 kcal (1.7 kJ)/min. It has been suggested that, as result of this failure of gastric emptying to slow sufficiently to offset the increases in diet concentration, food intake is less inhibited and overconsumption of food energy can occur.

Exceptions across food groups. Although gastric emptying appears to be related to energy density, within limits, there appear to be some exceptions. First, when alcohol is added to a beverage, emptying rate is not necessarily reduced; for example, wine, when compared with low-alcohol wine, did not significantly alter gastric emptying of either solid or liquid food components[22]. Kaufman & Kaye[12] similarly found no relation between energy density and gastric emptying when alcohol was substituted for glucose in a liquid test meal. In fact, the test meal emptied more slowly when its glucose content was greater. These results also confirmed earlier work showing that glucose added to ethanol would delay emptying and ethanol absorption[15].

The addition of soluble fibre is another factor that slows gastric emptying. A study that found that the addition of guar to a meal, increasing its viscosity, inhibited gastric transit time assessed by ^{24}Na also shows a significant correlation between mean gastric emptying time and subjective measure of satiety[29]. Further, ^{131}I-labelled cellulose emptied very slowly from the stomach as compared with water-soluble fibres[18]. In contrast, it has been reported[25] that gastric emptying time was prolonged approximately twofold after a week on a diet supplemented with 20 g/d of apple pectin. The same amount of cellulose was ineffective.

Exceptions within nutrient groupings. In addition to the exceptions to the relationship between emptying and energy content across nutrient groupings, there are notable exceptions within them. First, among the sugars, fructose empties twice as fast as glucose[23], but they inhibit food intake equally in a 4-h test, thereby giving emphasis to the fact that receptors beyond the stomach are involved in the relationship between nutrient interaction and the control of food intake.

Among the products of protein digestion, phenylalanine and tryptophan appear to play a special role. Several studies[3,7,27,28] have shown that these two amino acids are more potent on a molar basis or acid basis than other amino acids in inhibiting gastric emptying. Cooke & Ward[3] suggest further that the effect of tryptophan is mediated by a receptor in the gut, not by a systemic effect on the stomach, or the brain, or by its metabolites. This conclusion was reached because only its gastric administration, neither its intravenous infusion nor infusion of its metabolites, had this effect.

As regards the fats, earlier work in man showed that increasing the chain length of the contituent fatty acids could influence inhibition of gastric emptying, increasing the inhibition at first and then decreasing it[10]. Recent studies in the rat[17], have not demonstrated an effect of chain length on emptying rate; however, it seems clear that emptying of the oil phase of a meal is dependent upon its hydrolytic products, since sucrose polyester, a non-digestible fat, has been shown to empty at the same rate as water. When water and fats were administered in a mixture, water emptied first, indicating the ability of the stomach to control emptying of individual components[4,5]. It is interesting to note that inhibition of emptying of organic acids, such as citrate, acetate, and lactate, rose with increases in the number of carboxyl groups and the molecular weight of the acid[1].

Solids vs liquid emptying. The nutrient effects on gastric emptying described above were obtained from experiments using liquids. It is reasonable to study effects of liquids on gastric emptying, because even solid food is liquified by digestion and admixture with saliva and gastric juices. However, it is now well known that solid particles empty from the stomach as well. To empty under normal conditions, such particles must be no larger than 0.5 mm in diameter[21]. In addition, the rate of emptying of solids from the stomach follows a linear mathematical function, while the emptying of liquids is either negatively accelerated, or linear after an initial rush[20], depending on the nature of the food consumed. The physical form of a food as well as its nutrient composition, therefore, plays an important role in determining the rate of gastric emptying.

Relationship of gastric emptying to food intake. There is now sufficient evidence from the study of the effects of preloads on gastric emptying and food consumption to support the hypothesis that fullness of the stomach, as assessed by its reciprocal, emptying of the stomach, is an important contributor to satiety, the inhibition of consumption and, thereby, the control of food intake. McHugh has shown by elegant studies that a precise relationship can be demonstrated between the rate at which energy empties from the stomach and inhibition of 4-h food intake in the monkey. When preloads were given over a range which maintained emptying at 0.4 kcal (1,7 kJ)/min, intake was suppressed by precisely the amount of energy that was loaded[19]. It is likely that this precise one-to-one relationship between preload, emptying and intake breaks down as the nutrient density increases, because in most studies on the relationship between intake and preloads, the preload suppresses subsequent intake by less than 1 kcal for each kcal of preload[13], while under some circumstances, for example, when the preload was a warm broth, intake was reduced by more than the energy content of the load[11].

Mechanisms. Several recent studies have shed light on the possible mechanisms by which preloads could slow gastric emptying and thereby reduce further intake. Some of these mechanisms may help to explain the interactions, ie nonadditive effects that apparently occur. One of the best studied and most likely contributors to such interactions is the gut hormone cholecystokinin (CCK), which has been shown to reduce food intake in man[14] and to slow gastric emptying in monkeys[24] and dogs[6]. Indeed, McHugh has demonstrated that the satiety effect of CCK, with doses in the physiological range, fails to occur unless the stomach is partly filled[24]. Furthermore, both the satiety effects[26] and the slowing of gastric emptying[30] disappear after vagotomy. Another possible type of interaction is the systemic effect of nutrient absorption on gastric emptying. For example, experimentally induced hyperglycaemia retards gastric emptying[16] while a decrease in glucose availability to cells, as in experimental diabetes, enhances it[8]. The locus of action for this effect is unknown. Finally, the role of adrenergic receptors has been suggested as playing a role in the control of gastric emptying because the reduction in emptying rate induced by acid-containing test meals is eliminated if intramuscular reserpine is given[2].

1 Blum, A.L., Hegglin, J., Krejs, G.J., Largiarder, F., Sauberli, H., & Schmid, P. (1976): Gastric emptying of organic acids in the dog. *J. Physiol. (Lond)*. **26**, 285–299.

2 Cooke, A.R. & Clark, E.D. (1976): Effect of first part of duodenum on gastric emptying in dogs: response to acid, fat, glucose, and natural blockade. *Gastroenterology*. **70**, 550–555.

3 Cooke, A.R. & Ward, W.O. (1976): Effect of tryptophan and its metabolites on gastric emptying of liquid meals in dogs. *Proc. Soc. Exp. Biol. Med.* **152**, 656–658.

4 Cortot, A., Phillips, S.F. & Malagelada, J.R. (1981): Gastric emptying of lipids after ingestion of a solid-liquid meal in humans. *Gastroenterology* **80**, 922–927.

5 Cortot, A., Phillips, S.F. & Malagelada, J.R. (1982): Parallel gastric emptying of nonhydrolyzable fat and water after a solid-liquid meal in humans. *Gastroenterology* **82**, 877–881.

6 Debas, H.T., Farooq, O. & Grossman, M.I. (1975): Inhibition of gastric emptying is a physiological action of cholecystokinin. *Gastroenterology* **68**, 1211–1217.

7 Fisher, M. & Hunt, J.N. (1977): Effects of hydrochlorides of amino acids in test meals on gastric emptying. *Digestion* **16**, 18–22.

8 Granneman, J.G. & Stricker, E.M. (1984): Food intake and gastric emptying in rats with streptozotocin-induced diabetes. *Am. J. Physiol.* **247**, R1054–R1061.

9 Hunt, J.N. (1980): A possible relation between the regulation of gastric emptying and food intake. *Am. J. Physiol.* **239**, G1-G4.

10 Hunt, J.N. & Knox, M.T. (1968): A relation between the chain length of fatty acids and the slowing of gastric emptying. *J. Physiol., London* **194**, 327–336.

11 Hunt, J.N. & Knox, M.T. (1968): Regulation of gastric emptying. In *Handbook of physiology, Section 6: Volume IV. Motility*, ed C.F. Code. Washington, DC: American Physiological Society.

12 Kaufman, S.E. & Kaye, M.D. (1979): The effect of ethanol upon gastric emptying. *Gut* **20**, 688–692.

13 Kissileff, H.R. (1984): Satiating efficiency and a strategy for conducting food loading experiments. *Neurosci. Biobehav. Rev.* **8**, 129–135.

14 Kissileff, H.R., Pi-Sunyer, F.X., Thornton, J. & Smith, G.P. (1981): C-terminal octapeptide of cholecystokinin decreases food intake in man. *Am. J. Clin. Nutr.* **34**: 154–160.

15 Klotz, H., Hahn, S., Priesnitz, E. & Stefanelli, N. (1977): The extent to which ethanol absorption is influenced by an alteration of gastric emptying (auth. trans.). *Wien. Klin. Wochenschr.* **89**, 161–164.

16 MacGregor, I.L., Gueller, R., Watts, H.D., Meyer, J.H. (1976): The effect of acute hyperglycemia on gastric emptying in man. *Gastroenterology* **70**, 190–196.

17 Maggio, C.A. & Koopmans, H.S. (1980): The satiety effects of triglycerides with different chain length. *Alim. Nutr. Metab.* **1**, 312, (Abstr.)

18 Malagelada, J.R., Carter, S.E., Brown, M.L. & Carlson, G.L. (1980): Radiolabeled fiber: a physiologic marker for emptying and intestinal transit of solids. *Dig. Dis. Sci.* **25**, 81–87.

19 McHugh, P.R. & Moran, T.H. (1978): Accuracy of the regulation of caloric ingestion in the rhesus monkey. *Am. J. Physiol.* **235**, R29–34.

20 McHugh, P., Moran, T., Wirth, J. (1982): Postpyloric regulation of gastric emptying in rhesus monkeys. *Am. J. Physiol.* **243**, R408–R415.

21 Meyer, J.H. (1980): Gastric emptying of ordinary food: effect of antrum on particle size. *Am. J. Physiol.* **239**, G133–135.

22 Moore, J.G., Christian, P.E., Datz, F.L. & Coleman, R.E. (1981): Effect of wine on gastric emptying in humans. *Gastroenterology* **8**, 1072–1075.

23 Moran, T.H. & McHugh, P.R. (1981): Distinctions among three sugars in their effects on gastric emptying and satiety. *Am. J. Physiol.* **241**, R25–R30.

24 Moran T.H. & McHugh, P.R. (1982): Cholecystokinin suppresses food intake by inhibiting gastric emptying. *Am. J. Physiol.* **242**, R491–497.

25 Schwartz, S.E., Levine, R.A., Singh, A., Scheidecker, J.R. & Track, N.S. (1982): Sustained pectin ingestion delays gastric emptying. *Gastroenterology* **83**, 812–817.

26 Smith, G.P., Jerome, C., Cushin, B.J., Eterno, R. & Simanksy, K.J. (1981): Abdominal vagotomy blocks the satiety effect of cholecystokinin in the rat. *Science* **213**, 1036–1037.

27 Stephens, J.R., Woolson, R.F. & Cooke, A.R. (1975): Effects of essential and nonessential amino acids on gastric emptying in the dog. *Gastroenterology* **69**, 920–927.

28 Stephens, J.R., Woolson, R.F. & Cooke, A.R. (1976): Osmolyte and tryptophan receptors controlling gastric emptying in the dog. *Am. J. Physiol.* **231**, 848–853.

29 Wilmshurst, P. & Crawley, J.C.W. (1980): The measurement of gastric transit time in obese subjects using 24Na and the effects of energy content and guar gum on gastric emptying and satiety. *Br. J. Nutr.* **44**, 1–6.

30 Yamagichi, T. & Debas, H.T. (1978): Cholecystokinin inhibits gastric emptying by acting on both proximal stomach and pylorus. *Am. J. Physiol.* **234**, E375–E378.

Nutrition, neurotransmission and behaviour

Harris R. LIEBERMAN and Richard J. WURTMAN
Departments of Psychology (HRL) and Nutrition (HRL, RJW) Massachusetts Institute of Technology, Cambridge, MA 02139, USA.

Over the last 15 years it has become apparent that certain foods and food constituents can affect the brain and behaviour. The effects of these foods on the brain are mediated by changes in the plasma concentrations of certain neurotransmitter precursors. The concentrations of most plasma constituents are, by and large, independent of the amounts of these compounds that happen to be present in the diet. Homoeostatic mechanisms exist which keep, for example, plasma calcium from rising when milk is consumed, or plasma osmolarity from increasing by more than a few percent after a meal rich in salt or potassium. However, plasma levels of a few constituents apparently are unregulated, rising and falling substantially depending on the composition of the food currently being digested, and the rates at which the food constituents leave the blood stream (by being taken up into tissues, catabolized, or excreted into the urine). Examples of unregulated plasma constituents are the neurotransmitter precursors, amino acids and choline. Plasma levels of an amino acid like leucine or valine can quite normally vary over a six-fold range, depending on the amounts of protein and carbohydrate in the foods currently being ingested. A high-protein meal elevates their plasma levels substantially (because both are relatively abundant in protein), while a high-carbohydrate, protein-free meal depresses them (compared with those seen in the fasting state, because insulin facilitates their uptake into and catabolism by skeletal muscle)[13].

The changes in plasma choline and amino acid concentrations which follow eating can have important effects on the nervous system, modulating the rates at which particular neurons convert these nutrients to neurotransmitters, and the quantities of transmitter subsequently released when the neurones fire. Moreover their effect on the brain can be amplified by administering them in pure form, as though there were drugs, and, in the case of amino acids, by giving them along with carbohydrates, which potentiate their brain uptake by causing an insulin-mediated fall in plasma levels of other amino acids that would otherwise compete with them for transport across the blood-brain barrier.

Dietary constituents which affect the brain. One neurotransmitter precursor which can, under certain conditions affect the brain, is choline. The most common dietary precursor of acetylcholine found in food is phosphatidylcholine (PC) — also known as lecithin although commercial lecithins may contain as little as 10 per cent, and rarely more than 30 per cent, PC.

The sequence of events that couples the consumption of, for example, a choline-rich meal to an increase, somewhere within the body, in cholinergic transmission can be described as follows (for a detailed review[2]). (*1.*) The individual consumes a meal, for example, one containing lecithin-rich foods like eggs or liver; the lecithin is broken down to free choline within the mucosal cells that line the gut; this choline passes into the plasma, causing blood choline levels to rise (as much as three-fold after a breakfast and lunch of omelettes). (*2.*) The rise in plasma choline causes a concurrent increase in brain choline levels. This is because a specialized macromolecule exists within the endothelial cells lining the brain capillaries which facilitates the bi-directional diffusion of choline across the blood-brain barrier[10]. Moreover the kinetic characteristics of this transport system are such that it is unsaturated with its ligand (choline) at normal plasma choline concentrations; thus an increase in plasma choline can cause an immediate increase in the transport molecule's saturation, and in the passage of choline into the brain. (*3.*) Once in the extracellular fluid, the choline can be taken up into all brain cells by a low-affinity transport system, and into cholinergic terminals by an additional high-affinity system. Once within the terminals of a cholinergic neurone, part of the choline is acetylated by the enzyme choline acetyltransferase (CAT) to form acetylcholine (ACh); another part is phosphorylated (by choline kinase) to form phosphocholine. Both of the enzymes involved also have low affinities (high Kms) for choline, and are highly unsaturated with their substrates. Hence a rise in intracellular free choline can rapidly increase the formation of both ACh and phosphocholine. (Apparently CAT is not subject to end-product inhibition, which might otherwise shut off the acceleration in ACh synthesis.) (*4.*) The responsiveness of a particular cholinergic neurone to additional choline depends upon its level of physiological activity: neurones that have been firing frequently for prolonged periods are highly responsive to supplemental choline, so that administration of choline (or lecithin) markedly amplifies their output of ACh. Because most cholinergic neurones are not physiologically active at any moment, the physiological consequences of choline administration will be quite selective. These effects might be expected to be greatest when the continued firing of a particular cholinergic tract or nerve is important for maintaining some key bodily function, or when most of the neurones in that tract or nucleus have been damaged by a disease or injury.

The mechanism that couples tyrosine availability to catecholamine synthesis is similar to the one coupling choline to ACh, in that tyrosine levels are very important in neurones that are firing frequently, but relatively ineffective in affecting catecholamine output from quiescent neurones. The mechanisms that couple the firing of a catecholaminergic neurone to its precursor-responsiveness involve: (a) the phosphorylation (and consequent activation), of the enzyme tyrosine hydroxylase when the neurone is depolarized; and (b) a transient depletion of tyrosine that probably occurs within nerve terminals when they have been converting relatively large amounts of the amino acid, irreversibly, to a catecholamine. Real foods probably have too small an effect on brain tyrosine to bring about useful changes in catecholamine synthesis and release; it is necessary to give tyrosine itself, alone or with a carbohydrate, for this purpose. The reason that dietary proteins have little effect on brain tyrosine is that they also contain even larger quantities of the other large neutral amino acids (LNAA), eg leucine, valine, which compete with tyrosine for transport across the blood-brain barrier. Brain tyrosine levels depend not on plasma tyrosine alone, but on the plasma tyrosine ratio, ie the ratio of the tyrosine concentration to the summed concentrations of the other five or six LNAA that compete most strongly with tyrosine for brain uptake. Choline, unlike the neutral amino acids, appears to have no important circulating competitors for blood-brain barrier transport; hence brain choline levels vary directly with plasma choline concentrations.

The effects of dietary amino acids, and of protein and carbohydrate foods, on brain neurotransmitters probably underlie the behavioural effects, discussed below, of these nutrients and foods. It is also true that other food constituents besides proteins, carbohydrates, and lecithin can affect the brain, for example, caffeine, and the vitamins and trace minerals that may be deficient in malnutrition. Moreover, other neurotransmitters besides the ones discussed above probably are affected by nutrient (precursor) availability, but, for a claim that a certain food constituent affects a particular behaviour to be taken seriously, some evidence must be available that the food does indeed produce neurochemical effects, and that those effects are consistent with the behavioural change (ie, that it be compatible with other data, derived from studies on drugs or diseases, that associate the transmitter with behaviour).

Behavioural studies with foods. Behavioural research conducted on the acute responses of normal adults to various foods and nutrients makes it now appear virtually certain that such responses occur. These effects are subtle and not necessarily those predicted by traditional folk wisdom, nor by advocates of particular dietary regimens.

Amino acid neurotransmitter precursors. At noted above, certain LNAA, which are found in protein-containing foods and the blood stream, are the precursors of brain neurotransmitters underlying important behaviours. One such LNAA is tryptophan, the precursor of the

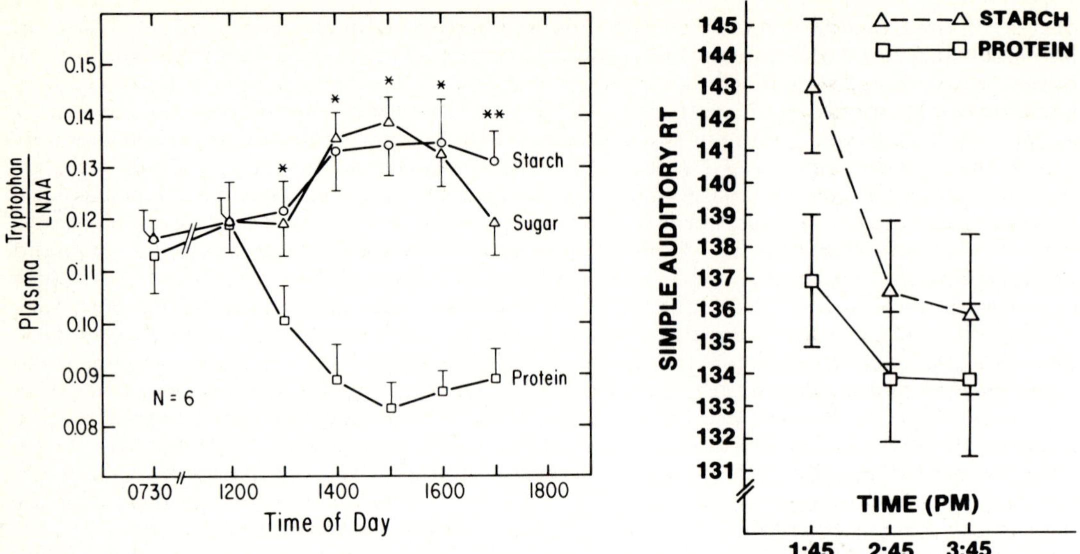

Fig 1 (above left). *The effects of isoenergetic lunch meals on the ratio tryptophan : other large neutral amino acids (LNAA) in the plasma of human subjects.* Changes in plasma tryptophan ratios predict brain tryptophan concentration. The meals contained either 120 g of starch (circles), 120 g of sucrose (triangles) or 80 g animal protein (squares) and were administered at noon. *indicates a P < 0.01 difference between protein and the other meals; **indicates a difference of P < 0.05 between all meals. Bars indicate s.e.m.

Fig 2 (Above, right). *Mean simple reaction time (RT in ms) at three different intervals following administration of an isoenergetic protein or carbohydrate (starch) meal at noon[8].* Forty young males participated in this cross-over study. The protein and starch meals were the same as those used for the amino acid study illustrated in Fig. 1. Reaction times were significantly slower (P < 0.05) at 1:45 pm on the day the subjects consumed the carbohydrate meal. Bars indicate s.e.m.

neurotransmitter serotonin. When tryptophan is administered systemically in pure form, it increases brain tryptophan and serotonin levels, concurrently affecting mood, sleep, and pain sensitivity in normal subjects[5,9,11]. Levels of L-tyrosine, the LNAA precursor for the neurotransmitters dopamine and norepinephrine can affect the synthesis of these important transmitters, and tyrosine administration can thereby affect certain behaviours associated with neurones releasing these neurotransmitters (such as motor activity, mood-state, and behavioural responses to acute stress)[1,3,4,7].

There is little doubt that L-tryptophan, when administered in sufficient quantities, has sedative-hypnotic properties. Numerous investigators have demonstrated effects of tryptophan on human alertness as measured by self-report mood questionnaires[9] and on latency to fall asleep as measured by EEG recordings[5]. The hypnotic-like effects observed in humans after tryptophan administration are consistent with reports implicating brain serotonin neurones in the regulation of sleep[6], since tryptophan has been shown to increase brain serotonin in animals. Although tryptophan does not appear to be as potent as prescription hypnotic drugs, it may have some clinical utility as a treatment for mild insomnia. It should be noted that the doses of tryptophan that have, to date, been shown to be psychopharmacologically active, probably produce changes in brain tryptophan larger than those produced by dietary carbohydrates. Therefore, it may be necessary to give the tryptophan in pure form, preferably along with carbohydrates which increase its brain uptake, in order to obtain substantial hypnotic-like effects.

Few studies have been conducted on the behavioural effects of giving tyrosine to normal humans; however, animal experiments and clinical studies with patients suffering from depression suggest that under certain conditions (such as stress), tyrosine could have positive behavioural effects[1,7].

Protein and carbohydrate foods. Studies on the behavioural responses of adults to protein and carbohydrate foods have been largely inspired by the demonstration that high protein and high carbohydrate meals have opposite effects on the brain concentration of tryptophan and its neurotransmitter product serotonin[13]. Because tryptophan is present in protein, but not in carbohydrate foods, one might assume ingestion of protein would elevate plasma and therefore brain concentration of tryptophan. However, this is not the case. Protein meals do elevate plasma levels of tryptophan, but this amino acid competes with all other LNAAs at the blood-brain barrier for access to the brain. Therefore, the parameter determining the access of tryptophan into the brain is the ratio of its plasma concentration to the other LNAAs, not its absolute plasma concentration. Since tryptophan is the rarest of the LNAAs with regard to its concentration in most protein foods, its plasma *ratio* (as opposed to concentration) *declines* after such foods are ingested (Fig. 1). Protein meals therefore decrease plasma tryptophan ratio so that less tryptophan enters the brain and is available for serotonin synthesis.

It might also be anticipated that a pure carbohydrate meal would have little effect on either plasma tryptophan or tyrosine concentration, since these amino acids are not present in such foods. However, carbohydrate meals do significantly affect the ratio of plasma tryptophan to the other LNAAs as a result of the secretion of insulin elicited by such meals. Insulin lowers the plasma levels of other LNAAs relative to tryptophan. Carbohydrate meals, therefore, have an effect opposite to that of protein meals on plasma tryptophan ratios. Such meals increase the tryptophan/LNAA ratio regardless of the type of carbohydrate tested, as shown in Fig. 1. Since more tryptophan is available for transport into the brain, carbohydrate meals can increase brain serotonin. The effects of a carbohydrate meal thus should resemble those following the administration of pure tryptophan, which provides a similar rise in the plasma tryptophan ratio.

Since carbohydrate meals increase brain serotonin and protein meals have the opposite effect, behavioural studies have been conducted with these foods to determine if they have opposite effects on behaviour. Since serotonin neurones are known to participate in the onset and maintenance of sleep, one would predict that carbohydrate foods, relative to protein foods, would increase sleepiness. Results suggest that from approximately 1–3 h after ingestion of high carbohydrate (as opposed to high protein) meals, performance is somewhat impaired (Fig. 2) and sleepiness increases, especially in older subjects[8,12].

1 Brady, K., Brown, J.W. & Thurmond, J.B. (1981): Behavioral and neurochemical effects of dietary tyrosine in young and aged mice following cold swim stress. *Pharmacol. Biochem. Behav.* **12**, 667–674.

2 Blusztajn, J.K. & Wurtman, R.J. (1983): Choline and cholinergic neurons. *Science* **221**, 614–620.

3 Gelenberg, A.J., Wojcik, J.D., Gibson, C.J. & Wurtman, R.J. (1983): Tyrosine for depression. *J. Psychiat. Res.* **17**, 175–180.

4 Gibson, C.J., Deikel, S.M., Young, S.N. & Binik, Y.M. (1982): Behavioral and biochemical effects of tryptophan, tyrosine and phenylalanine in mice. *Psychopharmacology* **76**, 118–121.

5 Hartmann, E. (1983): Effects of L-Tryptophan on sleepiness and on sleep. *J. Psychiat. Res.* **17**, 107–113.

6 Jouvet, M. (1973): Serotonin and sleep in the cat. In *Serotonin and behavior*, ed J. Barchas & E. Usdin, pp. 385–400. New York: Academic Press.

7 Lehnert, H., Reinstein, D.K., Strowbridge, B.W. & Wurtman, R.J. (1984): Neurochemical and behavioral consequences of acute, uncontrollable stress: effects of dietary tyrosine. *Brain Res.* **303**, 215–223.

8 Lieberman, H.R., Spring, B.J. & Garfield, G.S. (In Press): The behavioral effects of food constituents: strategies used in studies of amino acids, proteins, carbohydrate and caffeine. In *Diet and behavior: a multidisciplinary evaluation*, ed G.H. Anderson, W. Lovenberg, A.H. Lubin & D.H. Morris. Washington DC: Nutrition Foundation.

9 Lieberman, H.R., Corkin, B.J., Growdon, J.H. & Wurtman, R.J. (1983): Mood, performance, and pain sensitivity: changes induced by food constituents. *J. Psychiat. Res.* **17**, 135–145.

10 Pardridge, W.M., Cornford, E.M., Braun, L.D. & Oldendorf, W.H. (1979): Transport of choline and choline analogues through the blood-brain barrier. In *Nutrition and the brain, V. 5*, pp. 25–34, ed A. Barbeau, J.H. Growdon & R.J. Wurtman. New York: Raven Press.

11 Seltzer, S., Stoch, R., Marcus, R. & Jackson, E. (1982): Alteration of human pain thresholds by nutritional manipulation and L-tryptophan supplementation. *Pain* **13**, 385–393.

12 Spring, B., Maller, O., Wurtman, J.J., Digman, L. & Cozolino, L. (1983): Effects of protein and carbohydrate meals on mood and performance: interactions with sex and age. *J. Psychiat. Res.* **17**, 155–167.

13 Wurtman, R.J., Hefti, F. & Melamed, E. (1981): Precursor control of neurotransmitter synthesis. *Pharmac. Rev.* **32**, 315–335.

Interactions of nutrients, foods and drugs

A. Stewart TRUSWELL
Biochemistry Department, University of Sydney, NSW 2006, Australia.

In earlier reviews[15,16] six different types of interactions were distinguished (*1.*) *Foods can affect drugs*, for example by affecting absorption, an acute effect of single meals. (*2.*) *Nutrition can affect drugs*: either the nutritional state or particular foods regularly eaten can affect drug metabolism and hence dosage and toxicity. (*3.*) *Drugs can affect nutrition*: appetite, nutrient absorption, metabolism of macronutrients, vitamins and nutrient elements can each be affected, positively or negatively, by different drugs. (*4.*) *Drugs can affect foods*, causing unpleasant reactions to minor components in some foods, whose metabolism we normally take for granted, eg, hypertension from tyramine in cheese in patients taking monoamine oxidase inhibitors. (*5.*) *A few drugs are used as food*, as part of the usual diet: alcoholic drinks, coffee, tea and carbonated cola beverages. (*6.*) *Nutrients are used as drugs*: the nutrients are all obtainable now in pure form. Some have established, others suggested, effects in pharmacological dosage.

But these six categories do not cover all the interactions between food and drugs. In 1985 I suggest we have to consider another three. (*7.*) *Drugs and breast feeding*: can a drug, indicated for a lactating mother, affect the volume of her milk or its nutrients? Will the drug be excreted in the milk in sufficient amount to affect the baby? (*8.*) *'Health foods' overlap with herbal medicines*: in health food stores pharmacological actions are claimed for ordinary foods like rice or honey. Alongside these foods whose nutrients appear in our food tables are herbal medicines — camomile tea, raspberry leaves, aloe vera, ginseng, and many others whose nutrient composition and pharmacological properties (if any) are *terra incognita* for most nutritional scientists. (*9.*) *In-vitro incompatibilities between nutrients for parenteral nutrition* are primarily the concern of manufacturers and hospital pharmacists but need to be appreciated by nutritionists working in that field.

The following is a brief review of seven of these interactions.

1. 'Should I take the medicine before or after meals, Doctor?'[11]. To prescribe a drug with meals is one of the best ways of reminding people to take their nutrition regularly. Forgetting a dose means a lower blood level than any interfering effect of a meal. *Antibiotics* which are acid-labile should be taken *½ hour before meals*: ampicillin, penicillin G, cloxacillin, erythromycin, lincomycin, tetracycline, rifampicin and isoniazid. *Some antidiabetic* drugs, glibenclamide and glipizide, should also be taken before meals and so of course should *appetite-suppressants*.

Most drugs and medicines are best taken with or just after meals, either for convenience or because they are *gastric irritants* (salicylates, indomethacin, phenylbutazone, prednisone, chlorpropamide, phenformin, metronidazole, phenothiazines, haloperidol, thiazides, theophylline, nicotinic acid, iron compounds, potassium supplements, reserpine, etc.). Absorption of some of these may be a little delayed but this is preferable to an increased chance of gastric irritation.

When taken with food, blood levels of digoxin do not peak as high but persist for longer. This moderating effect makes it preferable to prescribe cardiac glycosides with meals.

A few drugs are *better absorbed* when taken with meals. Griseofulvin absorption is enhanced by fatty meals and the bioavailability of some drugs that are subjected to extensive pre-systemic metabolism is increased by food: hydralazine, alprenolol, metoprolol and labetalol.

Plenty of water should be taken with uricosurics (to prevent renal precipitation), cholestyramine and bulk formers like methyl cellulose.

2. The nutritional state or dietary components taken regularly can affect metabolism of some drugs. In rats underfeeding affects the rate of metabolism of some but not all drugs and foreign compounds. There are differences between males and females in mature animals.

Starvation impairs drug-metabolizing enzymes that are androgen-dependent (eg, hexobarbital hydroxylase and aminopyrine N-demethylase) but does not decrease enzymes that are not sex-dependent (p-nitroanisole O-demethylase, zoxazolamine hydroxylase and aniline hydroxylase). Effects are greater, therefore, in male animals. Starvation also reduces glucuronide conjugation of drugs[12].

Protein depletion decreases metabolism of some drugs, along with reduction of cytochrome P-450 per unit of liver weight. However, deficient animals have still shown induction of cytochrome P-450 when given multiple doses of inducing drugs like phenobarbitone[10]. Activity of nitro reductase was reduced in immature rats fed a low protein diet but aromatic hydroxylation (substrate biphenyl) was not. Glucuronide conjugation is less affected by protein depletion than phase 1 metabolism[6].

In human protein-energy malnutrition, fasting for obesity for 7 d had no effect on antipyrine or tolbutamide metabolism. Dosages for malnourished people should at least be adjusted for body weight. Is this enough correction? In malnutrition, digestion of drugs given in ester form might be reduced by pancreatic atrophy or absorption of drugs might be affected by gut atrophy; liver metabolism or renal clearance might be reduced or the activity of drugs carried mostly protein-bound in plasma might be increased by hypoalbuminaemia. Research on this aspect of childhood protein-energy malnutrition has come late but a series of studies mostly by Buchanan[3] and also by workers in India, Uganda and Chile and Sudan now give information about the handling of most of the major drugs likely to be needed for malnourished children. To summarize, slowed clearances are reported of antipyrine, acetanilide, chloramphenicol, chloroquine, gentamicin, penicillin and sulphadiazine. In some cases this is attributed to impaired liver, in other cases renal function. The dosage should be reduced.

Several drugs show decreased *in-vitro* binding to plasma proteins in serum from kwashiorkor patients: cloxacillin, flucloxacillin, digoxin, salicylate, PAS, phenobarbitone, thiopentone, phenylbutazone, streptomycin and tetracycline. This is particularly important for digoxin and thiopentone. Doses of these drugs should therefore be reduced in kwashiorkor.

Other components of the diet can affect liver microsomal activity. Fats, especially those rich in polyunsaturated fats are required for normal function in rats. Some foods contain appreciable amounts of natural xenobiotics (safrole, flavones, certain xanthines and indoles) which are known to be strong inducers of liver microsomal drug oxidizing system. Charcoal-broiled beef (which contains aromatic polycyclic hydrocarbons, inducing agents) stimulates hepatic and intestinal drug metabolism in rats and humans[8]. By different mechanisms the nutritional state can affect drug metabolism in four additional specific ways: (a) Extra vitamin B-6 reduces the effectiveness of L-Dopa[9]. (b) Leafy vegetables, such as spinach and kale are high in vitamin K. Patients stabilized on oral anticoagulants should therefore avoid excessive consumption of these and any other foods containing significant amounts of vitamin K for this will reduce the anticoagulant effect. (c) Ascorbic acid supplements enhance the antiamphetamine and cataleptogenic effects of haloperidol. The vitamin seems to act by blocking forebrain dopamine receptors[13]. (d) On a strict low sodium diet the dose of anti-hypertensive drugs to achieve a given blood pressure is less than in patients taking their usual diet.

3. Particular drugs can affect the nutritional state[14], altering biochemical tests or even leading on occasions to clinical under-, over- or mal-nutrition (general or specific). The following are examples.

Appetite may be decreased by anorectic drugs, bulking agents, dexamphetamine, phenformin, cardiac glycosides, glucagon, morphine, phenylbutazone, indomethacin, cyclophosphamide, 5-fluorouracil, methylphenidate, salbutamol, levodopa, etc., and by drugs that alter taste (griseofulvin, penicillamine and lincomycin).

Appetite may be increased by sulphonylureas, oral contraceptives, cyproheptidine, chlorpromazine, androgens, anabolic steroids, corticosteroids, insulin, lithium, amitryptyline, pizotifen, clomipramine, benzodiazepines, metoclopramide.

Malabsorption for more than one nutrient may be induced by neomycin, kanamycin, paromomycin, colchicine, phenindione, PAS, chlortetracycline, cholestyramine, colestipol, cyclophosphamide, indomethacin, liquid paraffin (fat soluble vitamins), methotrexate, methyldopa.

Energy metabolism may be stimulated by caffeine, smoking, some sympathomimetic drugs.

Carbohydrates. Increased blood glucose may be produced by corticosteroids, thiazide diuretics, diazoxide, oral contraceptives and phenytoin.   Hypoglycaemia may be produced (as well as sulphonyl-ureas, biguanides and insulin) by propranolol and by alcohol.

Lipids. Plasma total cholesterol may be raised by chlorpromazine and large intakes of coffee and some oral contraceptives. As well as specific cholesterol-lowering drugs, aspirin, PAS, colchicine, trifluperidol, phenformin and sulphinpyrazone may lower total cholesterol. *Plasma HDL cholesterol* may be raised by phenytoin, ethanol, cimetidine, terbutaline and prazosin. It may be lowered by propranolol and oxprenalol. *Plasma triglycerides* may be raised by propranolol, ethanol and (oestrogenic) oral contraceptives. They may be lowered by norethidrone (norethisterone). *Protein. Nitrogen balance* may be made negative by cortico-steroids, vaccines and tetracyclines. It may be made positive by insulin or anabolic steroids. *Plasma aminoacids* may be increased by tranyl-cypromine and lowered by oral contraceptives. Plasma phenylalanine may be raised by trimethoprim and methotrexate.

Thiamin absorption can be reduced by ethanol or by antacids.

Riboflavin status may be lowered by oral contraceptives and by chlorpromazine.

Niacin may be antagonized by isoniazid.

Vitamin B-6 may be antagonized by isoniazid, hydralazine, thiosemicarbazide, cycloserine, ethionamide, penicillamine, oral contraceptives, oestrogens, hydrocortisone, imipramine, levodopa, piperazine and pyrazinamide.

Folate may be antagonized by ethanol, phenytoin, oral contraceptives (uncommonly), cycloserine, triamterene and cholestyramine. In addition several drugs owe their antibacterial action to antagonism of folate metabolism — more in microbial than mammalian cells pyrimethamine, trimethoprim and pentamidine. Then methotrexate, aminopterin and amethopterin are potent folate antagonists which have more effect on rapidy dividing cells, eg, cancer cells.

Vitamin B-12 absorption may be impaired by Slow K, PAS, metformin, colchicine, trifluoperazine by high doses of vitamin C, cholestyramine and methotrexate. Prolonged nitrous oxide anaesthesia antagonizes vitamin B-12 (can oxidize the vitamin *in vivo*). Smoking and oral contraceptives reduce the plasma level.

Vitamin C. Plasma concentrations are lowered by oral contraceptives, smoking, aspirin and tetracycline. Ascorbate excretion is increased by corticosteroids, phenylbutazone, sulphinpyrazone and chlorcyclizine.

Vitamin A plasma concentration is increased by oral contraceptives. Absorption may be reduced by liquid paraffin and cholestyramine.

Vitamin D status is lowered by anticonvulsants, eg, phenytoin, phenobarbitone, glutethimide and when taken in high dose for long periods rickets can occur.

Vitamin E. Iron antagonizes in premature newborns.

Vitamin K. Coumarin drugs are antimetabolites. Purgatives and intestinal antibiotics (eg, neomycin, tetracyclines, sulphonamides) may remove the contribution from colonic bacteria). Salicylates and cholestyramine may reduce absorption and cefoperazone antagonizes the vitamin K-expoxide cycle.

Potassium. Drugs are important causes of potassium depletion: purgatives and laxatives increase faecal loss; thiazide diuretics and furosemide and ethacrynic acid increase renal loss. Other drugs that may increase urinary potassium are carbenicillin, penicillin, glucocorticoids, licorice, outdated tetracycline, gentamicin and alcohol.

Calcium. Absorption may be increased by aluminium hydroxide or by cholestyramine and decreased by phosphates and corticosteroids. Thiazide diuretics decrease urinary calcium. Gentamicin, mithramycin, actinomycin D and ethacrynic acid increase it.

Iron. Allopurinol, fructose and ascorbic acid increase absorption. Antacids, phosphates and tetracycline decrease it. Oral contraceptives tend to increase serum iron.

Iodine. Sulphonylureas, phenylbutazone, PAS, cobalt and lithium can cause goitre; they interfere with iodine uptake in the gland. Serum protein-bound iodine is increased by oral contraceptives, X-ray contrast media and potassium iodide, and decreased by phenytoin.

Phosphate absorption is decreased by aluminium and calcium.

Zinc depletion from increased urinary excretion may be produced by thiazide diuretics and furosemide, by cisplatin, penicillamine and alcohol.

Magnesium depletion from increased urinary loss may be produced by thiazides and furosemide, cisplatin, alcohol, aminoglycosides, amphotericin, cyclosporin and gentamicin.

4. Drugs can affect foods. The most important example is that drugs which inhibit monoamine oxidase prevent the normal metabolism of amines like tyramine, present in fermented protein-rich foods like cheese and other foods containing amines, pickled fish, chocolate, some wines, hung game, broad beans, yoghurt, stored liver, Bovril, Marmite and Vegemite. A dangerous rise of blood pressure can occur when these foods are eaten by people taking phenelzine or tranylcypromine, iproniazid, isocarboxizid, nialamide, mebanazine and furoxone.

A different reaction is caused by drugs which inhibit ethanol metabolism at the acetaldehyde stage so that there are symptoms of flushing, nausea, etc., after an alcoholic beverage. Disulfiram (Antabuse) is used deliberately for this effect. It is a side effect of some other drugs, particularly metronidazole and chlorpropamide, also less often furazolidine and nifuratel.

5. Some drugs are used as part of the daily diet by most people. Coffee, tea and cola beverages (in that order) are taken at least partly because they contain caffeine. We found 58–168 mg/cup of coffee and 43 to 92 mg/cup of tea as made and consumed in British homes, cafes and restaurants[1]. A considerable amount of work has now been done on the pharmacokinetics, metabolism and toxicology of caffeine[5].

Alcohol is the other psychotropic agent taken as a normal part of the diet by most people. Alcohol itself can affect metabolism of other drugs if taken in large amounts. It acutely potentiates the CNS depressant effect of tranquillizers. Chronic alcoholics may show increased metabolism of (and so tolerance to) barbiturates, warfarin, sulphonylureas and phenytoin[7].

6. Some nutrients are used as drugs. Nicotinic acid (but not nicotinamide) is a standard plasma lipid-lowering agent, used in amounts 150 times or more the nutrient requirement. Tryptophan may be useful as anti-depressant or hypnotic. Magnesium sulphate is used both by mouth as a purgative and by injection as a sedative. Iodides have several uses, eg, as an expectorant.

As to the claim that pharmacological doses of ascorbic acid prevent upper respiratory infections, over 30 controlled trials have found negative results on the prevention of episodes in the majority of cases, including all the best designed and analysed trials.

7. Can drugs cause trouble in lactation? Before describing a drug for a lactating woman, three questions must be asked: can it affect the volume of milk? can it affect the nutrient composition of the milk? can the drug be excreted in the milk in sufficient amount to affect the infant?

The most frequently indicated drugs for lactating women are oral contraceptives. Oestrogen-progestin pills tend over time to suppress the milk volume; progestin-only pills do not[2]. So far no effect of oral contraceptives on vitamins in human milk has been found[4].

Most drugs only reach the milk in tiny amounts; their concentration in milk is about the same as in mothers' plasma. The infant would receive 1 per cent or less of the maternal dose. But a minority of drugs are concentrated in the mammary gland[17]. The milk/plasma ratio is 12/1 for propylthiouracil and 25 for iodine-131. Other drugs are contraindicated in lactation if they are radioactive, or can cause allergy, agranulocytosis or bleeding disorders or are poorly metabolised in the newborn. Examples are chloramphenicol, indomethacin, diazepam, reserpine, anti-cancer drugs, lithium and some others. Tetrahydrocannabinol is concentrated in the milk of cannabis smokers, as are opiate narcotics in the milk of those taking them.

One final point. Interactions of drugs and nutrition are likely to cause more trouble in the elderly than in younger people. Old people take more drugs; their dose is not always adjusted for body weight, let alone for lean body mass or functioning liver mass. Because they eat less their liver microsomes are likely to be less induced by substances in food and they are more susceptible to micro-nutrional deficiency.

1 Al Samarrae, W., Ma, M.C.F. & Truswell, A.S. (1975): Methylxanthine consumption from coffee and tea. *Proc. Nutr. Soc.* **34**, 18A.
2 American Academy of Pediatrics Committee on Drugs (1981): Breast feeding and contraception. *Pediatrics* **68**, 138–140.
3 Buchanan, N. (1984): Effect of protein-energy malnutrition on drug metabolism in man. *Wld. Rev. Nutr. Diet.* **43**, 129–139.
4 Cumming, F.J. (1985): Lactation in Australian women: the effect of oral contraceptives on the vitamin and trace element content of breast milk. PhD Thesis, Deakin University, Victoria, Australia.
5 Dews, P., Grice, H.C., Neims, A., Wilson, J. & Wurtman, R. (1984): Report of 4th International Caffeine Workshop, Athens, 1982. *Fd Chem. Toxic.* **22**, 163–169.
6 Dickerson, J.W.T., Basu, T.K. & Parke, D.V. (1976): Effect of protein-energy nutrition on the activity of hepatic microsomal drug-metabolizing enzymes in growing rats. *J. Nutr.* **106**, 258–264.
7 Griffin, J.P. (1974): Drug interactions: 3. With alcohol. *Prescribers' Journal* **14**, 55–58.
8 Kappas, A., Alvares, A.P., Anderson, K.E., Pantuck, E.J., Pantuck, C.B., Chang, R. & Conney, A.H. (1978): Effect of charcoal-broiled beef on antipyrine and theophylline metabolism. *Clin. Pharmac. Ther.* **23**, 445–450.
9 Mars, H. (1974): Levodopa, Carbidopa and pyridoxine in Parkinson disease. Metabolic interactions. *Arch Neurol.* **30**, 444–447.
10 McLean, A.E.M. & Day, P.A. (1975): The effect of diet on the toxicity of paracetamol and the safety of paracetamol-methionine mixtures. *Biochemical Pharmac.* **24**, 37–42.
11 McLean, A.K. & Melander, A. (1983): The influence of food on oral drug usage. *Curr. Ther.* September, pp. 51–58.
12 Parke, D.V. & Ionnides, C. (1981): The role of nutrition in toxicology. *Ann. Rev. Nutr.* **1**, 207–234.
13 Rebec, G.V., Centore, J.M., White, L.K. & Alloway, K.D. (1985): Ascorbic acid and the behavioural response to haloperidol: implications for the action of anti-psychotic drugs. *Science* **227**, 438–441.
14 Roe, D. (1984): Nutrient and drug interactions. *Nutr. Rev.* **42**, 141–154.
15 Truswell, A.S., (1977): Interactions of nutrition, food and drugs. *Pharmaceutic. J.* March 12, p. 127.
16 Truswell, A.S. (1978): Interactions of nutrition, food and drugs. In *Early nutrition and later development*, ed A.W. Wilkinson, pp. 206–218. London: Pitman Medical.
17 Wilson, J.T. (1981): *Drugs in breast milk*. New York, Sydney: Adis Press.

★ ★ ★

FOOD ACCEPTABILITY AND NUTRITION

Taste preference of the newborn: what the perinatal human infant can report on his food-likes and dislikes

J.E. STEINER
Department of Oral Biology, The Hebrew University Hadassah Faculty of Dental Medicine, Jerusalem 91010, Israel.

Psychometrics, or cognitive psychophysical scaling, ranking or rating are among the main tools introduced by the discipline of psychology for sensory analysis of food items. Psychophysical rating and ranking or estimation provide a semi-quantitative dimension for the assessment of perceived sensations. Quality intensity and hedonics (pleasantness) are the most widely used parameters in the assessment of tase-, odour-, and texture-induced feelings related to food items[5].

The application and use of such tests in sensory analysis depends on several major factors, such as: (a) the questioned consumer (the testee) should have the proper ability to understand the questions directed to him, (b) there should be no language and cultural barrier between the experimenter (or his questionnaire) and the testee, (c) the testee should have the abstractive ability to express his sensory experience reflecting this on a relative verbal, numerical or spatial scale.

The above mentioned, and many more conditions on which psychophysical testing is dependent, restrict the use of this important and widely used most valid tool to the intelligent collaborative adult testee.

The pre-verbal human infant cannot, therefore, be tested in a psychophysical, consumer-survey even for baby-food items. Nonetheless, the young infant does have his own food preferences and aversions. Whether certain food items, though considered rich in nutritive value and safe from the point of view of health, are acceptable, palatable or aversive to the young infant, presents not only an academic problem, but has practical interest too. The sick child with appetite problems or those sick young infants who are restricted to a specific diet deserve special attention.

The process of sensory experience, the elicitation of feelings, takes place in the living organism's most private domain. The cognitive processes on which psychometrics and psychophysical estimates are based, are not the only indicative mechanisms which can be used to assess quality, intensity and hedonics of taste, odour and texture sensations induced by food items. Behavioural manifestations can be considered as equally valid indicators to assess food acceptability or aversion. The observation, recording and quantitative analysis of stimulus-dependent motor or secretory responses can reflect the quality, intensity and the hedonics of sensations. Behavioural research on food-preference has, in fact, a rather long history. The Roman physician Galenus is known to have carried out food-preference experiments, with most proper, almost modern, design[6].

Man — as compared to many animal species — is known to have a rather limited repertoire of endogenous (instinctive) stereotyped behavioural displays. Many of these endogenous instinctive motor and secretory coordinations are closely related to food-intake and are elicitable in peri-natal age. Nonhuman primates, both adult and juvenile, were found to respond to gustatory stimulation with differential and oral-facial behaviour reactions. These responses were found to be similar to and comparable with the human gustofacial response[13,14].

Experimental. In previous studies we have described the *gustofacial reflex* and the *nasofacial response*[6–11]. Stimulation of the neonate infant's peripheral gustatory or olfactory apparatus with delicate amounts of tastants or with food-related odorants, activate stereotype fixed distinct motor patterns in the oral, perioral and facial areas.

Stimulation with a 12.5 per cent sucrose solution, or with a 2.5 per cent citric-acid solution or with an 0.25 per cent quinine hydrochloric (bitter) solution (all presented in volumes of 0.2–0.3 ml) elicit different sets of motion features. These result in a differential facial play. The neonate infant's resting face, the sequences of the orofacial motor reactions to distilled water and to the gustatory stimulants are video-recorded and the recordings, in which the stimulus conditions are identified by a code only, can be subjected to an assessment by one or more evaluators. Based on a large number of observations, a special notational system, encompassing all of the taste-induced-facial-expressive motion features, could be composed. Using this notational system it was possible not only to distinguish between motor action patterns induced by each of the taste qualities, but the responses were found to vary in frequency and intensity of their appearance with the intensity (concentration) of the stimulant[3]. A further study revealed that the sweet-induced motion response can be classically conditioned already at the age of 2–48 hours of life in the human neonate[1]. Some of the most characteristic facial expressive features are shown in Fig. 1.

The differential fixed facial action patterns elicited by gustatory stimuli carry a non-verbal communicational message indicating the hedonic note of a specific taste sensation. The semi-quantitative evaluation of such motor behaviours in adolescents is an equally reliable indicator of the sensory experience of gustation, as are the psychometric indicators[16]. In the same study we could show that changes in heart rate of human examinees may also be used to indicate taste quality and hedonics. The neonate was also found to display changes, both in cardiac activity and in the performance of nutritive sucking encountering different gustatory

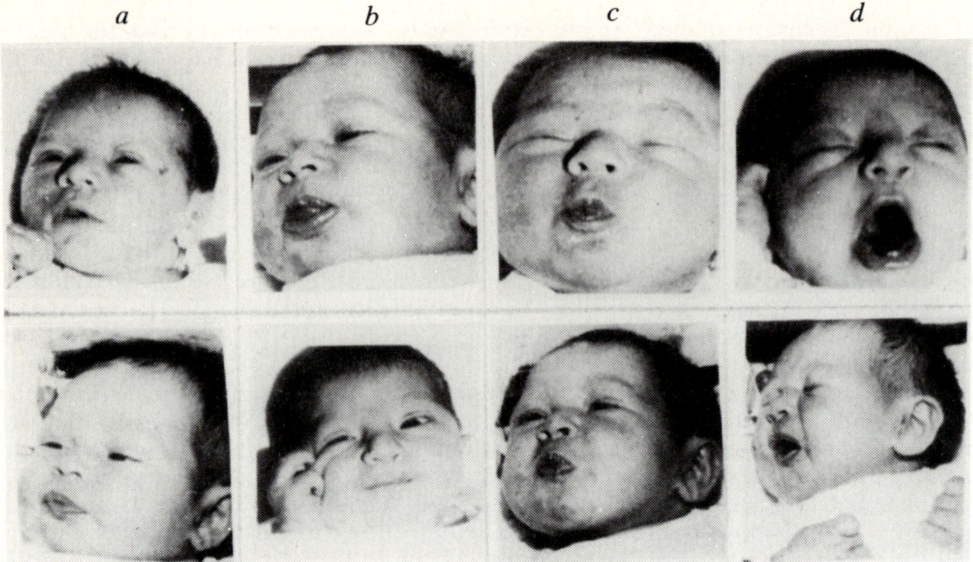

Fig. 1. *Facial expressions of perinatal infants in response to intraoral stimulation: (a) with distilled water, (b) with sweet taste, (c) with sour taste, (d) with bitter taste (stimuli were presented between birth and first contact with food).*

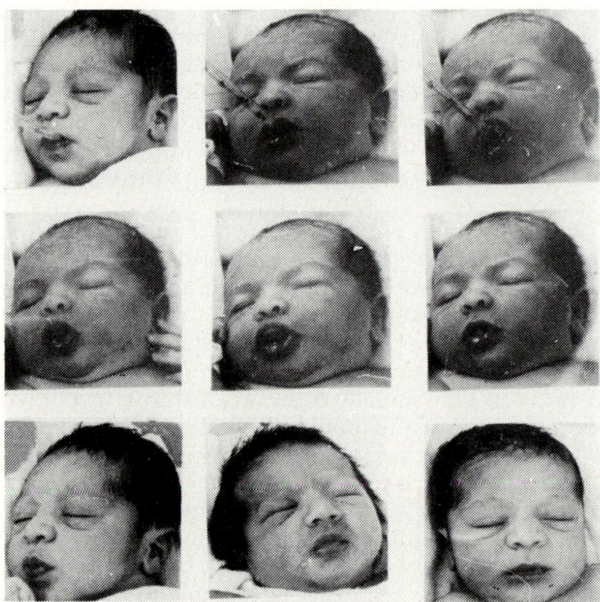

Fig. 2. *Some facial expressions in response to intraoral stimulation with a vegetable broth seasoned with 0.5 per cent mono-sodium glutamate (MSG).* Note the resemblance of the orofacial expressions in these pictures to those shown in Fig. 1(b) (sweet response).

stimuli[2,4]. Furthermore, it was shown that electro-encephalographic arousal reaction can also reliably reflect taste hedonics, both in animal and man[15,16].

It is evident that consumatory behaviour can also be used even in very young human infants as a valid aid for the assessment of taste preference and aversion respectively. It seems that the assessment of taste preference and taste aversion by the aid of stimulus-induced behavioural events and by the semiquantitative analysis of these is superior to the consumatory studies, since the latter involve the ingestion of relatively large volumes of liquids by the infant, while the former techniques require the intraoral application of minute amounts of taste solutions only.

In a more recent large scale study the behavioural assessment method was utilized to investigate the palatability of a clear vegetable broth seasoned with different concentrations of two glutamate salts: monosodium glutamate (MSG) and potassium glutamate (PG). Samples of the unseasoned broth and samples seasoned with 0.1, 0.25 and 0.5 per cent of the glutamic salts were presented to 110 normal healthy perinatal infants in the age range of 3–96 hours of both sexes[12].

This study was carried out in two different stages, first, with the MSG-seasoned, then with the PG-seasoned broth. For the sake of comparison, reactions to bitter (0.25 per cent quinine HCl) and to sweet (12.5 per cent sucrose) stimuli were also elicited. All the responses were video-recorded and the obtained tapes were submitted to independent evaluators. Some samples of the facial expressive features elicited by the 0.5 per cent MSG-seasoned broth are shown in Fig. 2.

The findings of this study revealed that: (a) Sweet and bitter stimuli induced the typical acceptance and aversion reactions respectively; (b) the *unseasoned* soup induced a clear aversion response, and (c) Most of the glutamate-seasoned samples induced features of acceptance response. The behavioural features characteristic of the orofacial response induced by the 0.5 per cent MSG seasoned samples are almost identical with those composing the sweet reaction.

The findings of this study were strongly supported by the results of a psychophysical study carried out on young mothers within 4 d after child birth. These rather finicky and choosy testees rated those glutamate-seasoned samples as palatable ones which also induced acceptance responses in the neonates. Furthermore, the majority of the tested mothers declared their willingness to use that broth sample, which they found most palatable, as a baby-food item to their own infants.

Finally, in a pilot study, the orofacial behaviours induced by a 1 mg/ml aspartame solution was compared with the acceptance response induced by a 12.5 per cent sucrose solution. Twenty healthy neonate infants (ten baby boys and ten girls) were tested. The motion features comparing the behavioural response to aspartame were found to be overlapping with those of the sweet response. The evaluators' hedonic score (in a double-blind setting) showed an almost identical distribution for the two types of sweet response. It was, therefore, possible to conclude that the natural and the tested artificial sweeteners are equally palatable and acceptable to the neonate.

1 Blass, E.M., Ganchrow, J.R. & Steiner, J.E. (1984): Classical conditioning in newborn humans 2–48 hours of age. *Infant Behav. Dev.* **7**, 223–235.

2 Crook, C.K. (1982): Modulation of the sucking reflex by olfaction and taste. In *Determination of behaviour of chemical stimuli*, ed J.E. Steiner & J.R. Ganchrow, pp. 117–126. London: Information Retrieval.

3 Ganchrow, J.R., Steiner, J.E. & Daher, M. (1983): Neonatal facial expressions in response to different qualities and intensities of gustatory stimuli. *Inf. Behav. Dev.* **6**, 473–484.

4 Lipsitt, L.P. (1977): Taste in human neonates: its effects on sucking and heart-rate. In *Taste and development — the gensis of sweet preference*, ed J.M. Weiffenbach, pp. 125–142. Bethesda, MD: NIH-DHEW.

5 Moskowitz, H.R. (1975): Application of sensory measurement to food evaluations. I. Threshold, category and discrimination scales. (Review article) *Lebensm. -Wiss. u. -Technol.* **8**, 245–248.

6 Siegel, R.E. (1973): *Galen on psychology, psychopathology and function and diseases of the nervous system. An analysis of his doctrines, observations and experiments.* Basel, Karger.

7 Steiner, J.E. (1973): The gustofacial response: observations on normal and anencephalic newborn infants. In *Symposium on oral sensation & perception — IV*, ed, J.F. Bosma pp. 254–278. Bethesda MD: NIH-DHEW.

8 Steiner, J.E. (1974): Innate discriminative human facial expression to taste and smell stimulation. (Discussion paper). *Ann. NY Acad. Sci.* **237**, 229–233.

9 Steiner, J.E. (1977): Facial expressions of the neonate infant indicating the hedonics of food-related chemical stimuli. In *Taste and development — the genesis of sweet preference*, ed J.M. Weiffenbach, pp. 173–188. Bethesda, MD, NIH-DHEW.

10 Steiner, J.E. (1979): Human facial expressions in response to taste and smell stimulation. In *Advances in child development and behaviour*, ed H.W. Reese & L.P. Lipsitt, pp. 257–295. New York: Academic Press.

11 Steiner, J.E. (1979): Oral and facial innate motor responses to gustatory and to some olfactory stimuli. In *Preference behavior and chemoreception*, ed. J.H.A. Kroeze, pp. 247–262. London, Information Retrieval Ltd.

12 Steiner, J.E. (1985/6): Palatability of a glutamate-seasoned vegetable broth to the perinatal infant. (An observational study, using a behavioral assay). In prep.

13 Steiner, J.E. & Glaser, D. (1984): Differential behavioral responses to taste stimuli in nonhuman primates. *J. Hum. Evol.* **13**, 709–723.

14 Steiner, J.E. & Glaser, D. In press: Orofacial motor patterns induced by gustatory stimuli in apes. Procs VII Annual Mtg. Ass. Chemoreception Sciences, Sarasota. *Chemical Senses* **10**(3).

15 Steiner, J.E. & Reuveni, J. (1979): Differential arousal response to gustatory stimuli in the awake rabbit. *EEG & Clin. Neurophysiol.* **47**, 1–11.

16 Steiner, J.E., Reuveni, J. & Beja, Y. (1982): Simultaneous multidisciplinary measures of taste-hedonics in *Determination of behavior by chemical stimuli*, ed J.E. Steiner & J.R. Ganchrow, pp. 149–160. London: Information Retrieval Ltd.

Changing needs and life-styles in developing countries

A. OMOLOLU
Department of Human Nutrition, University of Ibadan, Ibadan, Nigeria.

Twenty-five years ago, very few mothers in developing countries, apart from a few of the elite, fed their infants artificial milk. Due to the increasing affluence in most of these countries, the mass importation and availability of breast-milk substitutes and the all-pervading mass media advertisement of the baby food manufacturers the picture has changed radically. Whereas breast-milk used to be the main food for babies up to 2 to 3 years, with local weaning and other foods serving as supplements, breast-milk is now being supplemented in most areas of the developing world with breast-milk substitutes and other commercial foods by the 2nd or 3rd month. Due to the poor environmental sanitation, inadequate potable water, high cost of imported foods and ignorance of the proper use and care of utensils, more and more cases of infective diarrhoea and marasmus are now being seen in these countries. The impact of the WHO Code on Breast-milk substitutes (1981) is still to be felt in most countries of the developing world, as most have not passed the necessary laws that will give effect to the code.

There is a very important point about taste in the introduction of artificial milk to a baby during the first 2 or 3 months of life. Working mothers in developing countries need to get back to work by the second month of delivery. Most of these mothers try to introduce artificial feeding by the end of the first month with the idea of giving breast-milk in the mornings and evenings on return to work.

These mothers report that within a month of starting this form of 'mixed up feeding' — breast-milk in the mornings and evenings and bottles of artificial milk during the day — the infants refuse the breast. This is shown by biting the nipple and screaming until the bottle of artificial milk is offered. Many reasons have been adduced for this refusal of breast-milk, including the difference between sucking from the breast and sucking from the teat. However, the use of sucrose in the making up of artificial milk must play a part. Lactose, the main sugar of breast-milk, is not as sweet as sucrose and one gets the feeling that the infant at this early age, must be influenced and fascinated by the difference in taste. It is important for the future of breast feeding in the developing countries that a proper study be carried out to find out if the sweetness of sucrose is a deciding factor in this common refusal of the breast by infants.

Fermented foods are common in the dietary of most developing countries of the world. In West and Central Africa, fermented cassava 'manihot' is widely used. In Ethiopia, the cereal teff is usually eaten fermented as 'injera'. In the Far East, fermented soya beans in many forms and shapes abound. The taste of fermented foods is slightly sour and this sourness is highly desired. It is an acquired taste that one learns to appreciate. Fermented foods like soya sauce, tempeh and gari have spread all over the world, though they are still mostly eaten in their areas of origin.

The traditional processing methods of producing these fermented foods depend upon the use of mixtures of 'wild' organisms. As these wild organisms cannot be used for commercial processing due to standardisation and toxicity, these fermented foods cannot be produced on a commercial scale and in large enough quantities; thus, they are becoming expensive. In some areas, they are now delicacies to be taken on special occasions; in other areas, production is limited to the villages and rural areas.

Bland foods that are not fermented are taking over in most areas of the developing countries. Rice is an important cereal in this respect. Though produced in the poorest parts of the developing world, the amounts produced have increased to satisfy the needs of the world. Once parboiled or polished, rice has a long shelf-life and can be easily transported. Thus, it can be readily made available all over the world at a very competitive price. Fortunately too, rice has a high prestige status. It has therefore become an acceptable food not only in the developing world but also in most parts of the developed countries.

Condiments, side-plates or soups have always been important in the dietary of developing countries. Foods were eaten from two plates or bowls. One bowl contained the main carbohydrate food — rice, injera, foofoo, yam, taro — whilst the other bowl contained the condiment or soup. The condiment/soup was made up of spices, onions, tomatoes, oil, dark green leafy vegetables, meat/fish/shrimps. Nutritionally, this second bowl was the main source of the protein, fat, and minerals of the diet. It also supplied the pepper. Pepper was highly desired and the amounts used were very high. Pepper in large doses was a very important ingredient of all foods. In most developing countries, there are sayings and proverbs showing the importance of peppers in the dietary — 'a soul without pepper is a very weak soul'. 'Pepper is the medicine for long life' etc. The mainstay of the dietary of any seriously ill person or of someone recuperating from an illness was the 'pepper soup', a watery soup of fish, shrimps or meat lavishly garnished with pepper. It was normally taken with slices of bread. After a few sips or spoonfuls, the patient perspired profusely and was drenched in sweat. This was thought to be a good sign. The patient's clothing was changed and he had a good sleep.

This reverence for and love of peppers is now fast becoming a thing of the past. The younger generation has objected to the 'torture' of getting conditioned to peppers. The conditioning to pepper starts in infancy and during the weaning process the younger child has to get used to the hotness of pepper. Some nutritionists are sure that, during weaning, many children refuse to eat the adult diet with the hot pepper thereby laying the foundation for malnutrition.

The above are examples of the changing needs and life styles of the developing countries. In these countries, there can be said to be three main groups — the urban elite and middle class; the urban poor and slum dwellers; and the rural group.

Members of the first group, made up of the elite and urban middle class, are comparable with their counterparts in developing countries. The young working mothers are faced with the problems of the care of their infants and young children, how to continue breastfeeding with early return to work after parturition, the problems of artificial feeding and weaning of children. The elite wives and their families are moving to fast foods and away from traditional heavy breakfast, lunch and dinners. The busy executive husbands have to wrestle with obesity and hypertension arising from too many official parties, lack of exercise and the stress of traffic hold-ups. For this group, 'fast foods' are in — television snacks, small portions quickly cooked; no formalities.

The problems of the urban poor and slum dwellers are the lack of money, poor services and infrastructure — houses, roads, water, toilets, food and social services. Living in an environment 'which is more conducive to the multiplying of pests and insects than for human survival', the people here will eat anything, anywhere and in whatever form as long as it is food. Due to their constant contact with hunger and starvation, they learn not to give a high priority to food. Whenever they get some money, good food is never a priority — any food goes. They would rather have alcohol, cigarettes and cars than good food.

The rural group has a monotonous diet which is prescribed by tradition and availability. Their dietary is based on what they grow and what is available. They are afraid of new foods yet they see the changes all around them. Their children go to school and bring back new habits and new foods. They see the doctor's wife feeding her baby artificially and wonder why she does not breastfeed. They listen to the radio and sometimes watch television from where they learn of new food fashions.

Thus, the developing countries are changing, but changing at different rates and under different stresses. The elite and literate learn of new foods and because they understand, accept them. The slum dwellers accept the foods because they see the elite eating them, because the mass media advertise them or because they are cheap and available. The rural dwellers who form the bulk of the population are in the middle, pulled and pushed by the mass media and the actions of their offsprings and masters.

Governments, due to lack of foreign exchange and expertise stall, 'In doubt to act or rest'. The small but vociferous elite has to be heard, whilst the silent majority of rural dwellers are bypassed or left untouched. Nutritionally, the future is not rosy. The rising population growth, decreasing agricultural production and the depressing North-South divide, all call for urgent action. Life styles in the developing countries are changing. The nutritional needs of most of their populations are not being met. There is a need for national and international action to avert the impending chaos.

Changing needs and life-styles in developed countries

H.G. SCHUTZ and Debra S. JUDGE
Department of Consumer Sciences, University of California, Davis, California 95616 USA.

Changes in the larger conditions in and around society can result in changes in individual or household behaviour. Individual perceptions of self, society and the world also induce individual or household behaviours that affect other aspects of life-style and the structure of society. Thus, a model with macro-economics, demographic parameters, and personal values influences life-style from one direction while societal variables (production to meet demand, distribution, public education, attention from the popular media) influence life-style (including food habits and acceptance) from another. Food habits determine nutrient intake and influence health, both of which influence general life-style.

Life-style changes. The increased employment of women has impelled widespread life-style changes in the developed countries. In the USA, between 48 and 52 per cent of women participate in the paid labour force. Increased time spent for education and in work outside of the home has resulted in smaller average household size, changes in family incomes and changes in the relative importance of constraints on food habits. Time is now a more important consideration in food purchase and preparation choices for many. With more time-demands outside and fewer members in the household, family eating patterns are apt to fragment (members eating at different times, at home or away, full meals or snacks). These changes encourage the use of convenience foods and time saving methods of preparation. The food industry responded to time concerns with the development of prepared meals, new technology for expedient preparation (eg microwave ovens) and the availability of fast food away from home.

From 1976 to 1985, the percentage of households with an employed female head of household increased from 35 to 46 per cent. Concomitantly, household size decreased by 2.1 per cent *per annum* from 1980 to 1985 from a mean of 3.1 to 2.8 persons[8]. Single-headed households have increased; one in four households is headed solely by an adult female. In households with two employed heads of household there is a decrease in time available for household management and an increase in household income. In single-headed households, there is a decrease in time and most often a decrease in household income. In both cases, family activities outside the home and fewer members for whom meals may be prepared result in more meals either skipped or eaten away from home.

In a study of food purchasing practices in a southern urban locale, *per capita* income explained 55 per cent of the variability on grocery expenditures[15]. If food purchases away from home were included, the variability explained by *per capita* income would increase. Households with annual incomes less than \$5000 (13 per cent of 1977–78 sample) averaged \$1.93 *per* person *per* week spent on food away from home whereas those with incomes over \$25 000 (10 per cent of sample) averaged \$8.94[13]. Frequency of meals away from home continues to increase; in 1973, 12 per cent of all potential dinners were eaten away from home versus 22 per cent of all dinners in 1985[8]. Young adults (18 to 24 years) eat approximately 40 per cent of all their meals away from home. *Per capita* income is positively associated with meals away from home for all age groups, except school-age children, but household size is not associated with frequency of eating out[9]. More meals were eaten away from home when the female head of household was employed or in single-headed households (either male or female) than when the female head did not work outside the home or the family had two household heads present[9]. A household production model predicts that as female wages increase, the number of meals eaten away from home increases due to higher valuation of the preparation labour for the home meal[13].

Snacking (eating items between or around regular meal times) declined between 1973 and 1981, but has increased more recently. Current levels of snacking are greater than in 1981 but still less than in 1973[8]. Smaller household size was associated with higher snacking rates[9]. Income is positively associated with increased snacking for all age/sex classes. Female-headed households exhibit less snacking behaviour than do dual or male-headed households. Snacking is more frequent in suburban than in urban or non-metropolitan households. Foods used as snacks include the commonly envisioned sweets (40 per cent of reported snacks), beverages (53 per cent), fruits and vegetables (22 per cent), nuts and crackers, and yoghurt[8]. Ten per cent of all meals also are being skipped entirely by Americans (versus 8 per cent in 1973)[8].

There is increased attention to the relationship of diet and health. Government and private agencies have released information linking diet to health issues (eg, the relationship of coronary disease to diets high in saturated fats, of breast cancer to high fat diets, and the increased risk of certain forms of cancer to low-fibre diets[16]. Publicity about the negative effects of high sodium/salt intake on blood pressure and of cholesterol on the cardiovascular system have resulted in demand for, and introduction of, formulations of familiar products with lower sodium and/or less cholesterol. A recent survey indicated that approximately 60 per cent of Americans are on some kind of diet and 90 per cent of the dieters are on a reduced energy diet (Vance Research Services, *pers. comm.*); interest in such items has been sufficient to support the growth of new publications emphasizing diet and health.

Segments of the population are eating more nutritious foods due to increased emphases on health and nutrition. However, responses to consumer surveys indicate a wide disparity in the degree to which consumers are incorporating health/nutrition information into their everyday habits. In 1977–78, the average *per* person expenditure for food prepared at home was \$15.38 for households with *per annum* incomes of less than \$5000 and \$19.66 for households with incomes greater than \$25 000[13]. Average *per* person, weekly expenditures for foods prepared at home had increased to \$24.00 by 1985[4]. Seventy-eight per cent of the women responding to a survey in 1980 indicated that budgetary constraints were a major barrier to good nutrition for their families and 71 per cent said that they were giving up more expensive foods[7]. A consumer survey in 1980 indicated that cost and nutritional value were equivalent in importance to food purchase and consumption; both were less important than sensory attributes (Schutz, Judge & Gentry, unpubl.). It was later reported[2] that nutritional concerns among consumers had stabilized and that food cost was a major concern. Five per cent of 200 metropolitan women cited price as most important in deciding on food purchases; 35 per cent were primarily interested in 'quality' ('fresh', 'without preservatives')[14]. FMI reported that 59 per cent of the consumers interviewed in 1985 reported being at least somewhat concerned with nutrition, down 4 per cent from their 1984 sample[4]. Personal values also influence the importance of various factors in food purchases; the importance of nutrition and of taste has been reported as being correlated with a set of personal values in exactly opposite directions[12].

Nutritional implications of life-style changes. Small proportions of the population do have severely substandard diets[13]. In the USA these occur primarily in areas of extreme poverty such as American Indian reservations, among migrant workers, and the urban homeless. Population segments following certain restrictive diets may show nutritional problems (eg pre-school children on vegetarian diets[3]). However, over-consumption of fats and refined carbohydrates is more common, an average increase of 50–80 kcal (210–335 kJ) for non-dieters being reported between 1965 and 1977[11]. Over all subjects there was an energy *decrease* reflecting lower consumption of protein, fats, and carbohydrates. Higher levels of vitamin C, thiamin, riboflavin, and vitamin B_6 were calculated for the 1977 sample of adults; however, lower levels of riboflavin, magnesium, and B_6 were found in some age groups of children. All groups were below the RDA for magnesium. Teenage girls were deficient in iron and calcium. Calcium and vitamin D malnutrition are commonly cited as prevalent nutritional problems in industrialized countries[5]. Non-animal products have increased in importance in providing magnesium and riboflavin and the increased adult consumption of fruits and vegetables has resulted in higher intakes of vitamin A, vitamin C, and fibre[11].

Snacks generally provided 20 per cent of the energy, 15 per cent of the vitamins, 16 per cent of the fat, and 25 per cent of the carbohydrates *per* day in most age groups[10]. In 1979, approximately 11 per cent of the total food service industry was 'fast food'[1]. Increased fast food consumption implies a decreased ratio of polyunsaturated to saturated fats (from 1.45 to 0.78)[1]. Approximately 20 per cent of energy, protein, and fats and 15 per cent to 18 per cent of vitamins and minerals are obtained away from home[6]. Increasing away from home consumption may exacerbate current dietary problems and/or create demand for more nutritionally sound restaurant food. The impact of fast food marketing on the nutritional status of individuals in many developed countries is increasing with expansion of many American burger outlets to Japan, continental Europe, and Britain. As faster, simpler meals become more popular (expedient) both at home and away, potential for the food variety recommended to ensure a balanced diet declines. MRCA[8] reports that over the past several years there has been a 12 per cent decline in the number of main dishes served during at home meals along with a 19 per cent decrease in side dishes and a 22 per cent decline in desserts. Dishes that include a variety of items (often meat with vegetables or starches) are increasing in frequency in the American home. Decreased numbers of separate dishes and increased use of combination dishes may tend to cancel each other out in terms of nutrient components; however, the trend towards reduced preparation meals requires that the ingredients be carefully balanced when such meals are formulated for convenience packaging and preparation as they constitute a larger proportion of the overall energy and nutrient intake.

1 Chang, C.M. & Livingston, G.E. (1979): Eating at home vs away from home: problems in following a prudent diet. In *American Health Foundation — Food and Nutrition Committee Activities Report No. 2*. pp. 41–52.

2 Chou, M. (1983): The impact of the economy on food habits. *Fd. Agric. Rural Affairs Intelligence Rep.* January, 1983.

3 Dwyer, J.T., Palombo, R., Thorne, H., Valadian, I. & Reed, R. (1978): Preschoolers on alternate life-style diets. *J. Am. Diet. Ass.* **72**, 264–270.

4 Food Marketing Institute (1985): *Trends: consumer attitudes and the supermarket*. Washington DC: Research Division, Food Marketing Institute.

5 Foulkes, E. & Katz, S. (1977): Nutrition, behavior, and culture. In *Malnutrition, behavior, and social organization*, ed Lawrence Greene, pp. 219–231. New York: Academic Press.

6 Guenthe, P.M. & Chandler, C.A. (1980): Nutrients in foods at home and away. In *Outlook 1981*. USDA Agricultural Outlook Conference 1980, Washington DC.

7 Maracom Research Corporation (1980): *A summary report on US consumers' knowledge, attitudes, and practices about nutrition — 1980*. Minneapolis, MN: Maracom Research Corporation.

8 Market Research Corporation of America (1985): The changing shares of America's stomach. MRCA Information Services.

9 Morgan, K.J. & Goungetas, B. (1984): Snacking and eating away from home. Paper presented at the National Research Council's "What is America Eating?" Annual Symposium, December 1984, Washington, DC.

10 Pao, E.M. & Mickle, S.J. (1981): Nutrients from meals and snacks. In *Outlook 1981*. USDA Agriculture Outlook Conference 1980, Washington, DC.

11 Rizek, R.L. & Jackson, E.M. (1980): Current food consumption practices and nutrient sources in the American Diet. Paper presented (in part) at the International Symposium on Animal Products in Human Nutrition, Iowa State University, Ames, Iowa, 1980.

12 Rudell, F. (1979): *Consumer food selection and nutrition information*. New York: Praeger.

13 Senauer, B. (1984): Eating patterns: an economic/nutritional perspective. Paper presented at the National Research Council's 'What is America eating' symposium, December 1984, Washington, DC.

14 Sloan, A.E., Leone, L.C., Powers, M. & McNutt, K.W. (1984): Changing consumer life-styles. *Fd. Technol.* **38**, (11), 99–103.

15 Technical Committee SM–35 (1972): Food purchasing practices related to behavioural and socioeconomic characteristics. USDA Southern Cooperative Series Bulletin 172.
16 Weisburger, J.H. & Arnold, C. (1979): Dietary Risk Factors in Cardiovascular Disease and Cancer. In *American Health Foundation Food and Nutrition Committee Activities Report No. 2.* pp. 6–25.

Relating objective sensory analysis to consumer acceptability

D.H. LYON
Campden Food Preservation Research Association, Chipping Campden, Gloucestershire GL55 6LD, UK.

Sensory evaluation of foods can be defined as the examination and measurement of the attributes of the food which can be perceived by sight, sound, smell, taste and touch.

The findings reported here are those of a joint project between a research association and a leading manufacturer of orange juice who wished to find out how their standard blend compared to their main competitors, both objectively by trained sensory panels using quantitative descriptive analysis and subjectively by consumer testing. The manufacturers also wished to find out how a modified blend of their own product compared to their competitors product and whether this was seen by consumers as an improvement on their standard blend. Nine varieties of orange juice were supplied by our sponsor for this investigation.

Method. *(a) Objective sensory analysis.* In consultation with our client, the trained sensory panel at Campden developed a profile for orange juice to cover flavour, mouthfeel and after-flavour characteristics. The descriptive vocabulary was generated by the panel during informal discussion sessions when samples of the type to be profiled were presented to the panel. Each of the terms used by the panel was also defined to enable the sponsors of the research to understand the interpretation the panel placed on each attribute (Table 1). The Campden panel uses an unstructured line scale for each attribute anchored only at the ends either by 'Not at all' at one end to 'Very' at the other end. For each sample, the panellists record a vertical mark across the line at the point related to the intensity of that attribute. This mark is subsequently converted to a numerical score from 0–50 as the data are entered onto a computer using a graphics tablet and a pen-like stylus to record the position of the mark on the line. Each sample is assessed on six occasions by a panel of six trained assessors and the samples are presented randomised and

Table 1. *Orange juice descriptors and definitions.*

Flavour		*Mouthfeel*	
Sweet	One of the basic flavours of which sucrose is a typical example	Thick	Has body; not thin and watery
Sharp/acid	One of the basic flavour of which citric acid is a typical example.	Dry/astringent	Causes a drying of the mouth.
Bitter	One of the basic flavours of which quinine and caffeine are typical examples	*Aftertaste*	
		Sweet	Leaves a sweet taste in the mouth after swallowing.
Saccharin	Has a chemical sweet/bitter taste typical of saccharin.	Acid	Leaves a sharp/acid taste in the mouth after swallowing
Orange	'Natural' orange juice	Bitter	Leaves a bitter taste in the mouth after swallowing.
Artificial orange	Reminiscent of orange squash or powdered orange drink.	Saccharin	Leaves a chemical sweet/bitter taste in the mouth, typical of saccharin, after swallowing.
Processed	Cooked, caramelized.		
Perfumy	Floral, scented.		
Pithy/peely	Reminiscent of orange pith/peel.		
Smooth, rounded	Well balanced flavour, lacking harshness.		
Overall Strength	Strength of the overall flavour.		

coded so that the panel members are unaware which sample is being assessed. All samples are assessed independently by the panel members and there is no discussion of the sample until the trial is complete.

(b) Consumer Acceptability. A consumer study was carried out by our sponsor simultaneously to the trained panel assessments. The survey was conducted nationwide using a panel of housewives of all age groups and covering all social classes. The methodology used for the tests was blind comparisons.

Results. *Objective sensory analysis.* The results of profile assessments at Campden are usually presented in graphic form to give a clear and easy to understand comparison between samples. The attributes determined by the panel are plotted on a linear scale with each scale forming a radius of a circle. The conventional radial diagram, or star profile diagram, has been modified by reversing the usual scale so that the low scores are peripheral and the high scores are central as this gives a clearer representation of the flavour attributes. Panel means are plotted for each attribute and the 95 per cent confidence limits of the mean applied. If the diagram is drawn on a clear acetate sheet then it is simple to make direct comparisons between products by superimposing one diagram on top of another (Fig. 1). If the lines diverge, this represents a difference between the samples which becomes significant once the lines no longer overlap.

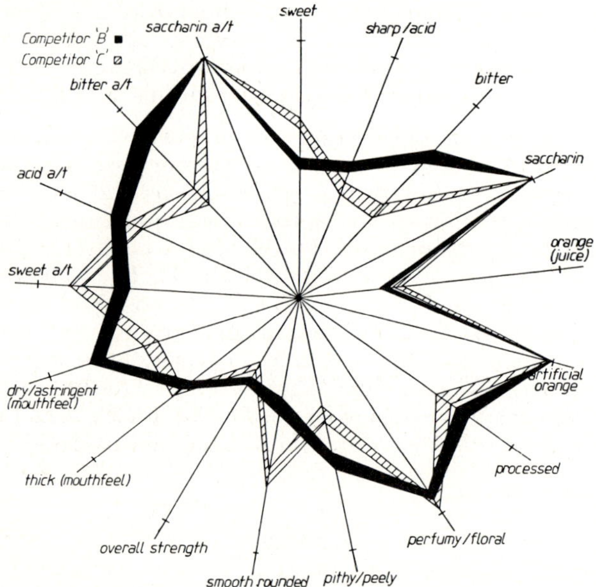

Fig. 1.

The mean scores and 95 per cent confidence interval of the means for each attribute are listed in Table 2 and Table 3.

The data have also been summarised using principal component analysis or mapping. If the first two principal components contain a high percentage of the total original variances, a scatter diagram of the attributes and samples can be plotted on axes of the principal components which then shows most of the differences in two diagrams, (Figs 2, 3).

This method is most useful where a large number of samples have been assessed making comparison of all star profile diagrams confusing.

Consumer test. Full details of the results of the consumer tests is beyond the scope of this paper. Table 4 is a summary of the consumers likes and dislikes of a juice compared with the standard product against the trained panel information on differences between the products. It is apparent from the table that there is a close relationship between both sets of information.

Table 2. *Mean score and 95 per cent confidence interval (95% CI) of the mean* (Std = standard, Mod B = modified blend).

Juice code	Sweet	Sharp	Bitter	Saccharin	Orange	Artificial Orange	Processed	Perfumy	Pithy/ peely	Smooth/ rounded	Overall strength
Std	24.7	30.6	23.7	–	41.1	–	19.1	1.7	27.9	28.0	41.0
Mod B	25.6	28.5	19.6	–	40.4	–	16.9	3.2	24.5	31.9	38.9
A	25.9	31.5	23.5	–	41.7	–	18.7	3.3	27.7	29.9	40.7
B	28.7	27.1	16.1	–	39.9	–	13.8	4.7	20.9	34.6	37.5
C	19.3	32.5	33.3	–	37.2	–	18.8	2.5	31.9	17.3	41.4
D	25.5	30.1	25.1	–	40.4	1.4	18.3	5.7	28.5	28.0	40.1
E	21.9	31.6	29.0	–	38.8	–	17.6	1.7	29.2	24.1	39.9
F	30.4	27.2	10.2	–	45.7	–	1.1	6.4	19.3	42.1	39.4
G	27.9	30.9	36.3	34.6	1.4	50.1	2.9	20.3	43.0	9.2	46.8
95% CI	2.7	2.6	4.0	0.8	2.1	1.0	3.9	2.9	3.9	4.2	1.8

Table 3. *Mouthfeel and aftertaste: mean score and 95 per cent confidence interval of the mean.*

Juice code	Thick	Dry/astringent	Sweet	Acid	Bitter	Saccharin
Std	28.4	18.4	14.3	17.7	16.9	–
Mod B	29.2	13.9	18.4	16.0	10.1	–
A	27.8	17.8	16.0	19.7	15.0	–
B	27.7	11.9	19.9	14.7	8.4	–
C	25.1	24.9	9.1	19.2	27.9	–
D	27.6	18.0	14.2	18.4	18.6	–
E	26.1	20.8	10.5	17.8	21.8	–
F	26.3	7.7	22.0	15.4	4.1	–
G	11.5	29.7	20.0	12.4	29.8	31.7
95% CI	2.9	3.7	3.7	3.3	5.2	0.6

Fig. 2.

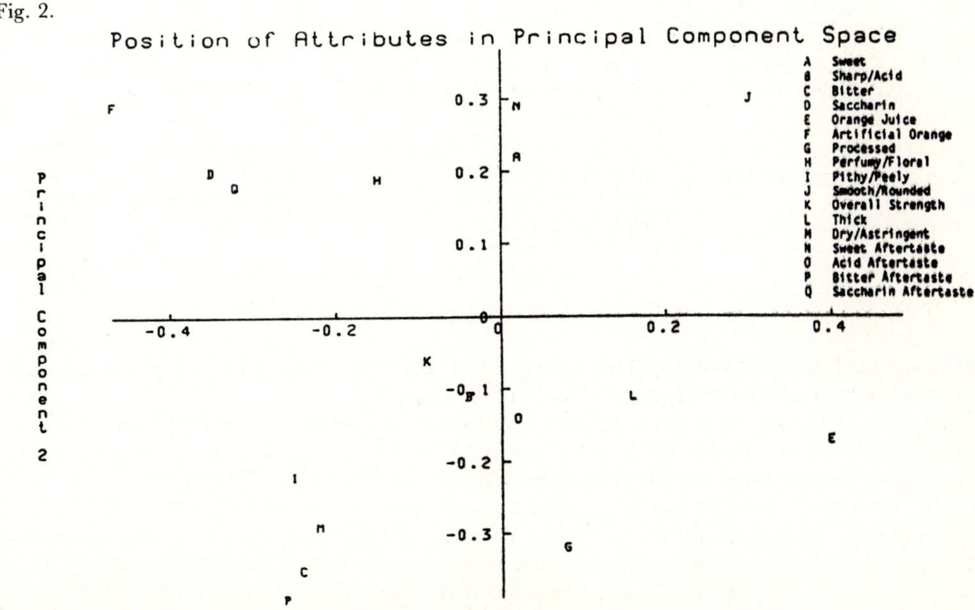

Fig. 3.

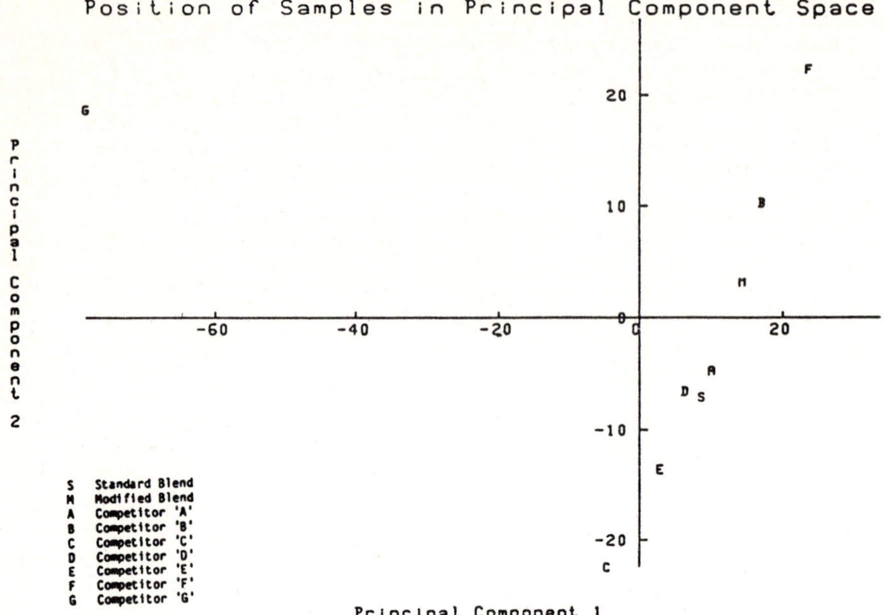

Table 4. *Comparison of reasons for consumer preferences and profile differences.*

Standard vs	Consumer reason	Profile	Standard vs	Consumer reason	Profile
Modified blend	More fresh taste, more bitter, not so sweet.	Less bitter, less strong, less dry.			
Competitor A	No outstanding reasons.	Similar.	Competitor D	Less strong orange flavour, more fruity, less sweet, thinner.	Less processed, more perfumy, slightly artificial.
Competitor B	Less strong, more fresh taste, not so bitter, smoother.	Less processed, less acid less pithy/peely, more round flavour.	Competitor E	More bitter, less sweet, not so thick.	Less sweet, more bitter.
Competitor C	More bitter, less sweet, less taste.	Taint. Less sweet, more pithy, less smooth, more astringent.	Competitor F	Not so bitter, thinner, better fresh, orange taste	Much less processed, more orange flavour, more perfumy, more smooth, sweeter, less bitter, less dry.

Conclusions. The results of this joint approach between objective and subjective panels helped our sponsors draw some conclusions about their products.

In particular, Competitor 'B' was considered worthy of further investigation. Trained panel assessments can now be carried out to 'predict' the likely response of the consumer and to narrow down the products to put forward for full consumer testing. This will obviously have cost and time advantages for the manufacturer.

In summary, therefore, the use of trained sensory panels alongside consumer testing can assist manufacturers to understand the quality attributes of their products, can give guidance on how product modifications can be made and used correctly and has been shown to be helpful as a tool to predict likely consumer responses to formulation changes.

The composition and properties of rice in relation to acceptability

B.O. JULIANO
Cereal Chemistry Department, The International Rice Research Institute, Los Baños, Laguna, P.O. Box 933, Manila, Philippines

Rice (*Oryza sativa* L.) is the staple food in tropical Asia. It is consumed mainly as surface-abraded milled or polished rice after dehulling of rough rice and abrasive milling of the resulting brown rice. Consumer acceptability of rice grain is determined both by composition and physicochemical properties[6].

Compositional factors. *Brown rice vs milled rice.* Comparison of the nutritional value of brown and milled rice in rats and preschool children confirmed similar nitrogen balance, but slightly lower energy digestibility, in brown rice[4,15]. Thus, the major nutritional advantage of brown rice over milled rice is its high content of vitamins of the B group. Rice is seldom stored as brown rice in tropical Asia because stone dehullers predominate which bruise the bran layers during dehulling of rough rice resulting in hydrolytic rancidity of the fat due to lipase activity. The use of rubber rollers for dehulling in Japan improves the storage quality of brown rice.

Degree of milling affects whiteness and keeping quality of milled rice. The higher crude fat content of the surface of undermilled rice reduces its shelf life compared to well-milled rice due to oxidative and hydrolytic rancidity.

Protein content. Within a variety, a high protein content (>9 per cent) improves grain translucency, head-rice yield, and hardness[1,3]. The milled rice, however, takes longer to cook[5].

Lipids and aroma. Total lipids of milled rice are about 1.5–1.7 per cent, but waxy rices have highest level (1.3 per cent) of nonstarch lipids which are subject to rancidity, in contrast to starch lipids. The popcorn-like aroma principle in cooked rice of various highly-priced aromatic rices was identified to be 2-acetyl-1- pyrroline[2].

Physicochemical factors. *Grain appearance.* A recent survey of price and quality characteristics of market samples of raw milled rice in three Southeast Asian countries verified that consumers give premium to whole-grain or head rice over brokens and to whiteness and translucency[16]. Consumer preference survey also verified the preference for whole, translucent non-waxy grains[11]. Waxy or glutinous rice has an opaque endosperm. Consumers also use the characteristic grain size and shape for variety identification.

Starch properties. Extensive studies have demonstrated that the texture of cooked rice prepared in a similar manner is mainly determined by amylose (linear): amylopectin (branched) ratio of starch[6]. The preferred amylose type varies greatly among countries and even within a country. Three starch properties are measured routinely in the IRRI rice breeding programme, amylose content by iodine colorimetry[7] (waxy 1–2 per cent, low 10–20 per cent, intermediate 20–25 per cent, high 25–33 per cent); gelatinization temperature (GT) by alkali spreading value[10] (low 6–7, intermediate 4–5, intermediate-high 3, high 2), and gel consistency[3] (soft 61–100 mm, medium 41–60 mm, hard 25–40 mm). An increase in ambient temperature during ripening may reduce amylose content and, independently, increase starch GT[14].

The three-country survey also confirmed consumer preference for low- to intermediate-amylose rices over high-amylose rices in Southeast Asia[10]. Among high-amylose rices, the softer cooked rice of soft gel consistency rices is preferred by consumers over that of hard gel consistency rices. Steamed waxy rice is the staple food in north and northeast Thailand and in Laos. Instrument methods for measuring hardness (softness) and stickiness of cooked rice are at least as sensitive as sensory evaluation in ranking cooked rices according to hardness or stickiness[8,9]. With rices cooked to optimum softness, glossiness and colour of cooked rice were negatively correlated with amylose content[6]. However, varietal differences in texture of samples of cooked rice with similar amylose contents have also been documented, which require further study.

Basmati-type rices show extreme elongation during cooking of presoaked grain whereas most varieties expand girthwise[6]. These varieties tend to have intermediate amylose content, low GT, and medium gel consistency, but the exact nature of this property is not well understood.

Ageing and parboiling. Ageing or storage changes occur in rice grain, particularly during the first 3–4 months after harvest[12,17]. Aged rice is commonly used for milling and cooking tests because it has improved total and head milled rice yields during milling and the milled rice has higher volume expansion and water absorption during cooking and less solids in cooking gruel than freshly harvested rice. The nature of these changes is not well understood but occurs regardless of whether the grain is stored as rough, brown, or milled rice.

Rice parboiling in India probably evolved from efforts to reduce the pastiness of freshly harvested rice. The process consists of steeping the rough rice in water below the starch GT, followed by steaming with minimal volume expansion, and drying[13]. The starch gelatinization results in a hard, translucent milled rice with higher head rice yield. Parboiled rice, mostly high amylose rice, is the main staple in Sri Lanka and Bangladesh and about 50 per cent of rice is parboiled in India and Pakistan. Parboiled rice takes longer to cook particularly when not presoaked. Although traditional parboiled rices are dark coloured and may have off-odours and mycotoxins, modern parboiling processes have minimized the differences between raw and parboiled rices.

1 Blakeney, A.B. (1979): Rice grain quality evaluation in Australia. In *Proceedings of the Workshop on Chemical Aspects of Rice Grain Quality*, Los Baños, 1978, pp. 115–121. International Rice Research Institute, Los Baños, Laguna, Philippines.

2 Buttery, R.G., Ling, L.C., Juliano, B.O. & Turnbaugh, J.G. (1983): Cooked rice aroma and 2-acetyl-1- pyrroline. *J. Agric. Fd. Chem.* **31**, 823–826.

3 Cagampang, G.B., Perez, C.M. & Juliano, B.O. (1973): A gel consistency test for eating quality of rice. *J. Sci. Fd. Agric.* **24**, 1589–1594.

4 Eggum, B.O., Juliano, B.O. & Maningat, C.C. (1982): Protein and energy utilization of rice milling fractions in rats. *Qual. Plant. Plant Foods Hum. Nutr.* **31**, 371–374.

5 Juliano, B.O. (1972): Physicochemical properties of starch and protein in relation to grain quality and nutritional value of rice. In *Rice beeding*, pp. 389–405. International Rice Research Institute, Los Baños, Laguna, Philippines.

6 Juliano, B.O. (1979): The chemical basis of rice grain quality. In *Proceedings of the Workshop on Chemical Aspects of Rice Grain Quality*, Los Baños, 1978, pp. 69–90. International Rice Research Institute, Los Baños, Laguna, Philippines.

7 Juliano, B.O., Perez, C.M., Blakeney, A.B., Castillo, D.T., Kongseree, N., Laignelet, B., Lapis, E.T., Murty, V.V.S., Paule, C.M. & Webb, B.D. (1981): International cooperative testing on the amylose content of milled rice. *Starch* **33**, 157–162.

8 Juliano, B.O., Perez, C.M., Barber, S., Blakeney, A.B., Iwasaki, T., Shibuya, N., Keneaster, K.K., Chung, S., Laignelet, B., Launay, B., del Mundo, A.M., Suzuki, H., Shiki, J., Tsuji, S., Tokoyama, J., Tatsumi, K. & Webb, B.D. (1981): International cooperative comparison of instrument methods for cooked rice texture. *J. Texture Studies* **12**, 17–38.

9 Juliano, B.O., Perez, C.M., Alyoshin, E.P., Romanov, V.B., Blakeney, A.B., Welsh, L.A., Choudhury, N.H., Delgado, L.L., Iwasaki, T., Shibuya, N., Mossman, A.P., Siwi, B., Damardjati, D.S., Suzuki, H. & Kimura, H. (1984): International cooperative test on texture of cooked rice. *J. Texture studies* **15**, 357–376.

10 Little, R.R., Hilder, G.B. & Dawson, E.H. (1958): Differential effect of dilute alkali on 25 varieties of milled white rice. *Cereal Chem.* **35**, 111–126.

11 Del Mundo, A.M. & Juliano, B.O. (1981): Consumer preference and properties of raw and cooked milled rice. *J. Texture Studies* **12**, 107–120.

12 Perez, C.M. & Juliano, B.O. (1981): Texture changes and storage of rice. *J. Texture Studies* **12**, 321–333.

13 Raghavendra Rao, S.N. & Juliano, B.O. (1970): Effect of parboiling on some physicochemical properties of rice. *J. Agric. Fd. Chem.* **18**, 289–294.

14 Resurreccion, A.P., Hara, T., Juliano, B.O. & Yoshida, S. (1977): Effect of temperature during ripening on grain quality of rice. *Soil Sci. Plant Nutr.* **23**, 109–112.

15 Santiago, M.I.C., Roxas, B.V., Intengan, C.Ll. & Juliano, B.O. (1984): Protein and energy utilization of brown, undermilled and milled rices by preschool children. *Qual. Plant. Plant Foods Hum. Nutr.* **34**, 15–25.

16 Unnevehr, L.J., Juliano, B.O., Perez, C.M. & Marciano, E.B. (1985): Consumer demand for rice grain quality in Thailand, Indonesia and the Philippines. *IRRI (International Rice Research Institute, Los Baños, Laguna, Philippines) Res. Paper Ser. No. 118.*

17 Villareal, R.M., Resurreccion, A.P., Suziki, L.B. & Juliano, B.O. (1976): Changes in physicochemical properties of rice during storage. *Starch* **28,** 88–94.

XXII: Animal production

Matching livestock systems with available feed resources in tropical countries

T.R. PRESTON
International Livestock Centre for Africa, PO Box 5689, Addis Ababa, Ethiopia.

It is frequently claimed that there would be no shortage of food in developing countries if only they could emulate the rates of agricultural productivity that have been achieved in the industrialized world. In terms of output per unit of land, labour and feed there is no doubt that there are enormous disparities in rates of livestock production between the developed and the developing regions of the world. For example, beef production per head of cattle per annum averages 93 kg in the industrialized world and 25 kg in the third world[7]. It is equally true that the high rates of animal productivity in the industrialized countries have been achieved through a disproportionate use of the world's resources[2] especially fossil fuels, marine fisheries and the protein-rich cakes and meals.

Developing countries are important producers of oilseed cakes (the third world exports 10.8 million tonnes protein oilcakes p.a. and imports 1.7 million tonnes — balance -9.1 million tonnes[2]) but most are consumed by European livestock (industrialized countries import 18.7 million tonnes and export 9.4 million tonnes — annual balance $+9.3$ million tonnes[2]), adding to the milk and meat mountains, which cause despair to the tax payer and finally serve to restrict the market of third-world countries which need to export in order to earn foreign currency to pay their debts. Even worse, the surpluses become 'gifts' which further restrict the possibilities for developing indigenous livestock industries in developing countries.

The disparity in energy use is equally great. While the energy consumed in the form of food is 50 per cent higher per person in industrialized as compared with developing countries, the total energy used (eg in manufactured goods, infrastructure, machinery and other services), is six times higher. The 'efficient' animal industries of the industrialized countries would be much less efficient if their access to fossil-fuel-derived inputs was limited to that presently imposed on the poorest countries.

It is relevant to this discussion to pose the question: why do we need efficient animal production systems? An argument used frequently by animal scientists is that biological efficiency is a direct function of rate of animal productivity. Almost unlimited goals have been set by animal geneticists for more milk per cow and more weight per day of age. The cost has been an increasing sophistication in nutrition to the point that only the most digestible feeds of high protein content (largely cereal grains and oilseed meals) are selected in the least-cost formulations.

For the industrialized countries, mostly situated in regions with temperate climates, it has not been too difficult to secure the required feed resources since cereals and highly nutritious forages can readily be grown. Countries without available land to grow these feeds (eg Japan, Taiwan, Israel, Arabian countries), because of their industrial base or wealth from oil, were able to import these feeds at relatively low cost and release them to farmers at prices often highly subsidised.

Developing countries by definition do not have these assets. Most developing countries are situated in the tropics. Their economies do not generate the necessary foreign exchange to import the 'quality' feeds used in intensive animal production systems. Moreover, one can generalize and conclude that there are not the world resources available — even if there was the wealth — for the poor countries to aspire to the degree of resource use now enjoyed by the industrialized world.

The challenge that faces the planners in the developing countries is thus formidable: how to raise the standard of living by the rational use of their own 'national' resources, with only minimal help from resources from other parts of the world.

Technology transfer. Early development strategy assumed that technology transfer not research was the key to progress. But it has been proved that, at least in the field of animal production, the direct transfer of technologies from developed to developing countries has rarely been successful by any standard, either technical or economic. Livestock production systems in the developed countries have a high degree of specialization and high rates of animal productivity, usually approaching the genetic potential of the animals. These systems have developed because of the advantages to profitability conferred by a large enterprise which permits optimal use of inputs of capital, labour and feed.

The transfer of specialized animal production technologies from developed to developing countries, occasionally led to short-term gains in production of animal protein (eg establishment of milk production colonies and intensive poultry enterprises on the outskirts of cities). However, the longer-term consequences have been a 'dependency' on imported feeds and the 'superior' animals to take maximum advantage of the transferred systems. Such imports are becoming increasingly difficult to sustain in the light of the shortages of foreign exchange in almost all developing countries, and the higher priority attached to imports of oil and other more basic needs of a country's economy. Another negative side-effect of 'imported technologies' has been the serious neglect of indigenous breeds and feed resources.

A specific example of a failure of technology transfer is that of tropical legumes. For the last 20 years, this has been a favourite topic for livestock planners, who extolled the role of legume-rich pastures in countries with profitable livestock industries such as New Zealand and the success of Australian scientists in developing tropical counterparts. But the technology has yet to provide the predicted breakthrough in tropical animal production. The reason is primarily because the legume/grass system promoted by the grassland experts did not match the livestock systems promoted by their livestock counterparts. Tropical legume/grass pastures are not sufficiently nutritious for dairy cows of high genetic merit which need high-quality feeds such as cereal grains and maize silage; and they are too expensive for specialized beef production (even in Australia) which because of low productivity requires minimum inputs. Strangely, tropical legumes are likely to find their role in the development of the one cattle production system (dual purpose milk-beef) which, although the system of choice of tropical farmers, has been almost completely ignored by tropical scientists.

A third example of transfer failure is the case of livestock feeding standards and nutrient requirements. From the economic standpoint, the fundamental flaw is the inherent concept of maximising livestock productivity, which results in attempts to find (usually by importing) the feeds to match the livestock. But there are also technical difficulties, especially with tropical foods, where non-additive-associated effects and interactions result in predictions of performance from feed analysis being a poorer guide than the rule of thumb method of the practising farmer.

Food versus energy. The increase in the price of fossil fuel has focused attention on the need to investigate alternative sources of energy especially those which are renewable. If it is assumed that the additional energy which will be needed in the future by developing countries must come mainly from renewable sources, then it is relevant to make some projections for a future world population which is expected to reach 16 billion. It has been estimated[14] that if the efficiency of solar-energy capture remains at the existing level (0.2 per cent) then the cultivated land area must be almost doubled (from 1400 to 2500 million hectares). Conversely the efficiency of solar-energy capture must be increased. Thus, either a considerably greater proportion of the earth's surface must be used for solar-energy capture or the efficiency of conversion of solar energy into biomass must be dramatically increased. It is therefore disappointing to learn that despite the dramatic increases in cereal grain production, resulting from the 'green revolution', there has been no commensurate increase in the efficiency with which the new cereal crops capture solar energy; apparently, grain yields have risen primarily because of changes in partitioning of energy within the plant, and not by overall increases in total plant productivity[6].

Socio-economic constraints to livestock production. It is not easy to introduce technological innovations in livestock production at the level of the smallholder. Without adequate knowledge of religious or other taboos, customs and the sociology of village communities, the researcher has little hope of establishing methods to improve traditional systems. Subsistence-farmers must first ensure their family's food supply. Only then can they think of improving the condition of their livestock. Thus, technical innovations, if they are to be successful, must be introduced within a framework which takes into account the following considerations: an immediate financial return from application; relative simplicity and lack of interference with normal farm activities, such as planting or harvesting; minimum risk; hazardous and arduous features to be ruled out unless returns are exceptionally high, and avoidance of any threat to religious or cultural activities.

Even with the right technology or innovation, the constraints to improving livestock production in developing countries are considerable. The application of scientific knowledge to the poorest people in the third world does not seem to lie solely in the realm of the extensionist. The reasons for this are that there are too many livestock owners, often remote from highways and often there is a language barrier. The answers seen to lie more in action by the community itself, by, for instance, increasing the degree of self-reliance. This topic is discussed in detail by Dolberg[3,4] on the basis of experience with the introduction of livestock technologies in India and Bangladesh. His analytical framework for a livestock development strategy illustrates the complex factors that interact to affect the success or otherwise of development.

Education and research as tools of development. There is an increasing awareness of the probability that direct technology transfer from the industrialized to the third world may have led to more problems than progress. Many mistakes arose because of the original definition of the objectives of agricultural development, which tended to be simplistic (eg increased food production).

The critical role of food supplies in developing countries became apparent with increasing urbanization. This was often a product of the development strategy promoted during the last two decades. Provided people remain in rural areas, food supplies are only a problem in time of natural or man-made disasters. It is the growth of cities which has distorted development. Employment opportunities in cities tempt people to leave the village and at the same time reduce the capability to produce food. The solution was believed to be 'the introduction of the so-called advanced technologies which would increase productivity'. Unfortunately, the technologies were mostly highly energy-dependent.

The concept of technology transfer was feasible when fossil fuel was inexpensive, but now it is relatively expensive. Pressure to procure fuel in order to promote or accelerate development has been mainly responsible for the present crisis, and the serious financial and sociological problems that have resulted in the poorer countries. Technology alone is not enough; in fact, applied indiscriminately, and out of the context of the local situation, technology is harmful.

What are the alternatives? Goals must be set and aims must be defined if there are to be sustainable solutions to these problems. The realization that the poorest people in the developing world were those who had benefited least from the aid process is leading to a redefinition of the target groups. The world's poor mostly live in the rural areas and these are the major producers of the nation's staples. Therefore, efforts to aid the rural poor, on the farm and in the village, will yield dividends both in food supply and in countering the migration to urban slums which are serious problems for the economies of emerging nations.

The objective of a rural-oriented development strategy can be defined as: increasing the income and the well-being of the rural poor, which is synonomous with both 'small farmers' and landless labourers, as almost all rural dwellers are involved in one way or another with farming.

The role of agricultural education and research in this development strategy is not easy to define. It was much simpler in the 'technological era'. To increase animal productivity can be a simple exercise (eg feeding high-concentrate diets). However, when the technology has to fit into the socio-economic framework of a village, interactions and associated effects limit its application. It is certain that not only the implementation but also the design of technologies require the involvement of multidisciplinary teams of scientists.

Measuring the impact of a proposed innovation becomes more difficult as the goals broaden. How does one measure 'well-being' of a family? What is the role of livestock as a means of improving the standard of living or the quality of life? It is certain that increasing fuel resources at the village level will be as important as generating more food. In many ways 'household' fuel is becoming an important constraint to development since, as it becomes scarcer, a greater effort is required to collect it. As a result a considerable amount of available family labour is diverted to this activity[8,9].

The technique of measuring the impact of technology in terms of energy transfer is an appropriate way to assess change[11]. Innovations which lead to increased fixation of solar energy and atmospheric nitrogen as biomass, and reduction of wastes through recycling, have important ecological advantages as well as contributing to greater self-reliance in village societies. The scientists who participate in the evolution of these strategies must have, in addition to their particular specialization, a broad experience and understanding of development issues. This is only likely to come about if the future architects of agricultural development strategies are trained in the environment where these same strategies are to be applied[22].

The long-term training of agricultural students from developing countries in advanced institutions overseas has also created special difficulties of identifying priorities for research and development.

A strategy for livestock development. The challenge to agricultural scientists is thus equally formidable as that facing the sociologists and economists; the task must be to maximize energy production from biomass while maintaining food supplies. And to do this in the framework of an overall strategy which rates socio-economic issues of employment creation more important than technical yardsticks; and where self-reliance is to be prized over self-sufficiency.

The identification of needs and a careful study of existing resources — feeds, livestock and farmers — are essential first steps. And resources must be examined in the broadest sense of soils and climate and crops which might be grown. Livestock systems must then be matched with the resources in a way that aims for economic optimization rather than biological maximization. New technologies have to be developed; but it may be more important to start with the improvement of existing ones. The present passion for 'farming systems research' is a result of the belated recognition of the obvious — that third-world farmers are much wiser and more knowledgable than planners or livestock specialists when it comes to utilization of resources.

Appropriate livestock technologies. Four examples may be chosen of technologies which appear to merit more widespread promotion: the dual-purpose system of milk and beef production, calf-rearing by restricted suckling, production of feed and fuel from dual purpose high-biomass-producing crops, integrated farming systems and urea/molasses supplements.

Dual-purpose milk-beef systems. Such systems have been, and still are practised by almost all traditional livestock farmers in developing countries; the motivation being as strongly economic (to pay the wages of the herd attendant) as nutritional (eg in the Borana tribe in East Africa where human comp004tition for the cow's milk is to the economic detriment of calf growth). There are sound reasons for believing that the most economic way of meeting an increasing demand for milk and meat in developing countries is through improvement of the existing livestock production systems based on the multipurpose animal, rather than by development of specialized milk and meat production[15]. The bases for the argument are: the relative consumption pattern of meat and milk in non-vegetarian communities; intensive milk production (more than 3000 litres/animal) competing for the same food resource as monogastric animals and man; the preference for high-fat milk from buffalo, particularly in the Indian subcontinent; the increasing role of draught animals, and the need to produce suitable animals for this purpose from animals kept for milk, and in most countries, the need for flexibility because of inadequate marketing.

The consumption ratio for milk relative to beef appears to be maintained at a fairly constant level of about 3–5 litres of milk for every kilogram of carcass meat which seems to be independent of the expendable income. This demand-ratio has been largely ignored by livestock planners whose recommendations invariably have been to establish separate and independent milk and beef production systems.

The disadvantages of such strategies are that the output from a specialized milking herd is between 10 and 25 litres milk/kg of meat (assuming that an intensively fed dairy cow will produce 3000 to 6000 litres of milk annually and that the beef from her offspring and from the cow when slaughtered represents 250 kg per year). If the male calves are slaughtered at birth (which frequently happens in the highly specialized dairy enterprises) then the production ratio of milk and meat widens to 50:1. Thus to satisfy the consumption ratio of 3–5 litres milk per kg meat will require four to five additional beef cows to balance the milk and meat outputs from one high-yielding dairy cow. The net result of specialization is a decline in numbers of dairy cows in national herds. Specialized dairy cows are highly efficient biologically. In contrast, specialized beef cows are inefficient, since their productivity is governed by their reproductive rate. This is always less than one offspring per year, which is considerably inferior to other meat-producing species such as pigs, poultry, sheep, goats and rabbits.

Specialized beef herds have largely developed in countries where grazing land is readily available (eg in parts of North and South America, Africa and Australia). In Europe, beef herds are highly specialized to guarantee an adeqaute income to farmers who are not diversified. In developing countries the increasing pressure on land implies that future priorities may favour sheep and goat production (because of their higher reproductive rate and multi-purpose traits of meat, milk, wool and hair production). The growing of biomass for fuel in traditional grazing areas is another alternative that is of increasing importance. A major advantage of multi-purpose meat/milk systems is that diverting milk to the young animal by using restricted suckling throughout lactation provides a 'catalytic' supplement so that the basal feed resource is used more efficiently. Better protein/energy nutrition in early life should ensure a higher mature bodyweight which could be important for draught oxen. A multipurpose animal and production system offers other advantages in those tropical countries where the native cattle are inherently low milk producers. Even when nutritional and environmental constraints are removed their productivity is much less than other breeds and crossbreeds[18].

A further consideration is that, as population pressure for increased feed production increases, it may be necessary to decrease populations of oxen in favour of cows that produce milk and offspring as well as work.

Dual-purpose cattle are easily produced by inseminating native (adapted) animals with semen from exotic bulls that have been proven for milk production. Such bulls should preferably be from breeds or strains with good meat characteristics as this will help to confer multi-purpose traits (milk, meat and traction) on their offspring.

Restricted suckling. Unselected crossbred cattle with more than 50 per cent of *Bos indicus* genes are reluctant to 'let down' their milk without the presence of the calf. This has led scientists to stress the advantages of developing breeds with proportions of genes from European dairy breeds exceeding 5/8. This appears to be the minimum level of exotic blood necessary to ensure adequate milk 'let-down' without stimulation from the calf[1].

But milk 'let-down' is only a problem in intensive milk production units with the need for high-throughput, low-labour milking sheds such as the 'herringbone' and 'rotary' designs. Such management systems are inappropriate in the majority of situations in developing countries where herd size is one to five animals, where family labour is readily available and the maintenance of machinery is difficult. The major advantage of combined milking and restricted suckling, is that both cow and calf benefit in the following ways: the system matches production with demand (5 kg milk: 1 kg beef); moderate lactation yield (2000 kg) and high beef potential (1.2 kg/d) can be met from available feed and genetic resources; simple management (once-a-day milking); better herd health, and faster and more efficient calf growth.

Feed and fuel from dual-purpose crops. The importance of developing fuel supplies from renewable resources cannot be stressed too highly. It seems logical that the humid tropics will be the focus of many such programmes. They offer much more potential (see Table) than temperate regions, first because of the possibility of growing crops all the year round and secondly because of the higher efficiency of photosynthesis in tropical plants.

Table. *Comparison of biomass production from annual temperate crops and perennial tropical crops grown for energy (E) or protein (P)*

Type	Species	Harvests /year	Carbohydrate: protein ratio	Biomass (tonnes DM/ ha/year)
Temperate	Sorghum (E)	2.5	10	20
	Soyabean (P)	3	2	9
Tropical	Sugar cane (E)	1	13	34
	Gliricidia *(P)	5	4	25

*A tree legume

A consequence of the rise in oil prices is that the difference in the value of carbohydrate as a source of fuel or food has narrowed. This encourages the growing of crops which can be used for fuel as well as food production, and is to the long term advantage of high-biomass-producing tropical plants such as sugar cane and leguminous trees. A previous disadvantage of these plants, as conventional feeds, was the high proportion of the crop in the form of lignified cell wall. With the new 'fuel' option, the fibre becomes an asset instead of a liability.

The effective utilization of these dual-purpose crops requires the application of fractionation technologies to permit optimum use of the end-products[16]. The logic behind this is that the contents of plant cells (largely sugars) and the leaves (which are high in protein) are most appropriately used for feed; while, the structural carbohydrates of plant cell walls are best directed into fuel. Sugar cane and legume trees are particularly suited for this purpose, the former providing the energy and the latter the protein; fuel is a byproduct (or primary product) of both (Fig. 1).

This development has opened up exciting new possibilites from tropical animal-production systems, which promise extremely high rates of animal and unit area productivity based on

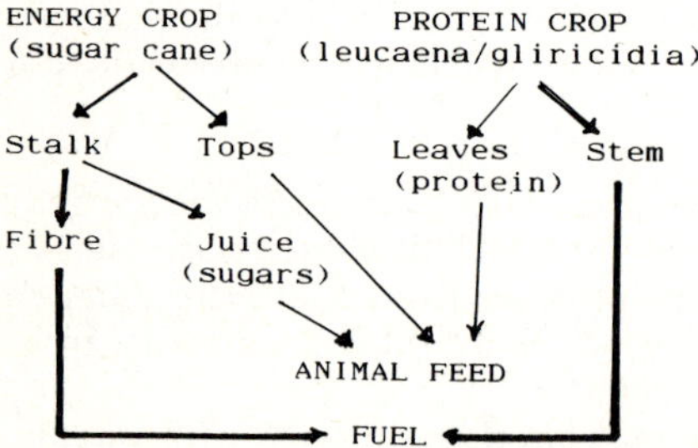

Fig. 1 *Fractionation of energy (eg sugar cane) and protein (eg Leucaena or Gliricidia) crops into energy and food.*

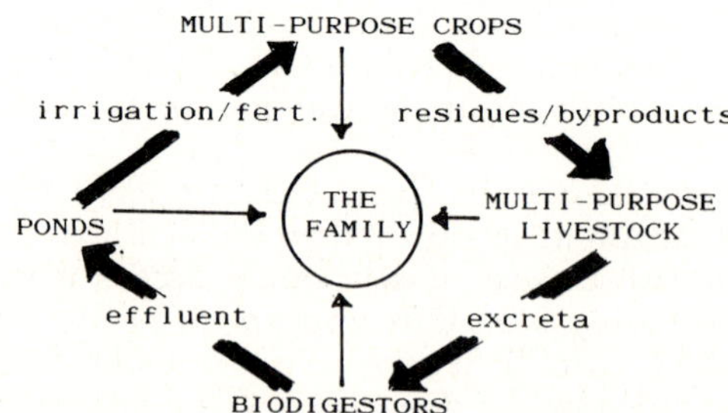

Fig. 2 *Flow diagram for integrated farming systems.*

truly indigenous crops and technologies. Thus there are reports that the rate of productivity in pigs and cattle fed sugar-cane juice equals, and may even exceed, that recorded on grain based diets[5,16,21]. The residual fibre following partial juice extraction has been a satisfactory fuel for producer gas generation (A. Lindgren personal communication). Leaves of the gliricidia tree, already widely used throughout tropical America as a 'live'post in fence lines are collected, sun-dried and incorporated in poultry diets as a substitute for imported synthetic pigments for egg yolk coloration in Colombia[13]. As a protein-supplement in ruminant diets it may be more appropriate than the herbaceous legumes, if for no other reason that it already exists as a weed in much of the tropics.

Integrated farming systems. Integrated systems aim to optimise overall agricultural and livestock productivity from available resources through the growing of multipurpose crops, with recycling of residues and byproducts both as nutrients for animals and plants and also for fuel. Figure 2 illustrates how the basic natural resources of solar energy, rainfall, atmospheric nitrogen, soil and farm management can be combined in an integrated production system, which aims to optimize resource use with minimum waste.

Urea-molasses supplements. All crop residues, which form the bulk of the diet of ruminants in many tropical countries, and natural grazings during the dry season of the year, contain insufficient nitrogen to provide the ammonia needed by rumen microorganisms for the efficient fermentative digestion of such feeds. In these situations, supplementing ruminant animals with urea can bring about marked improvements in performance or increase survival rates when droughts occur.

The main limitation of this technology is the difficulty of adding urea to the diet in a convenient way, and the toxicity hazard of doing this incorrectly. Incorporating urea in solid molasses-based blocks has overcome these difficulties and has been widely accepted by village livestock owners and by pastoralists[10,20].

The choice of livestock production systems. The argument for developing intensive pig and poultry production is based on the high feed-conversion efficiency of these species and their high reproductive capacity. Ruminants by contrast have the capacity to convert refractory carbohydrate resources, when properly supplemented, into protein of high biological value.

The important issues, especially in terms of resource utlization in most developing countries, are that the superiority of pigs and poultry is only apparent when grain-based feeds are available at low cost. Additionally, these industries need high management skills and controlled environments (good housing with control of temperature and humidity, and adequate disease prevention). Without these safeguards, the improved genotypes — an essential component of the superior performance — have difficulty in surviving let alone producing under village conditions. These represent major constraints, and as they are tied to fossil-fuel prices, will become increasingly difficult to resolve.

Efficiency in ruminants is not simply total feed use per unit of production since the basal component of their diet is frequently a residue or byproduct which has little value — other than for feeding to ruminants. In this situation, efficiency may be regarded as the utilization of the supplement component — which has alternative uses (eg for export, feeding to monogastric animals or even in the human diet). The comparison is, then, between conversion rates of 2 to 4 kg grain per kg liveweight for poultry and pigs respectively; and the conversion of supplement in a diet based on crop residues or byproducts fed to ruminants which can sometimes be less than 1:1 (eg use of fish meal in molasses and ammoniated straw-based diets) and is usually in the range of 1 to 2 kg supplement per kg liveweight gain[19].

Although the arguments in favour of ruminant-based livestock industries are complex, the major differences are in the relative needs for fossil-fuel-based inputs which are much higher for intensive pig and poultry enterprises and may be almost zero in village-based ruminant systems. When valuable supplements are scarce, then ruminants certainly should have priority.

1 Alvarez, F.J., Saucedo, G., Arriaga, A. & Preston, T.R. (1980): Effect on milk production and calf performance of milking crossbred European/Zebu cattle in the absence or presence of the calf, and of rearing their calves artificially. *Trop. Animal Prod.* **5**, 25–37.

2 Borgstrom, G. (1980): The need for appropriate animal production systems for the tropics. In *Animal production systems for the tropics*. Publ. No. 8 International Foundation for Science: Stockholm.

3 Dolberg, F. (1982): An analytical framework for livestock strategy in Bangladesh. In *Maximum livestock production from minimum land*, ed C.H. Davis, T.R. Preston, M. Haque & M. Saadullah, pp. 144–152. Mymensingh: Bangladesh Agricultural University.

4 Dolberg, F. (1982): Political influences on the formation of livestock policies in India. In *Maximum livestock production from minimum land*, ed T.R. Preston, C.H. Davis, F. Dolberg, M. Haque & M. Saadullah, pp. 236–258. Mymensingh: Bangladesh Agricultural University.

5 Duarte, F., Elliott, R. & Preston, T.R. (1982): Fattening cattle with sugar cane juice: effect of the conservation of the juice with ammonia and the use of Leucaena leucocephala as a source of protein and forage. *Trop. Animal Prod.* **7**, 169–173.

6 Evans, L.T. (1983): Photosynthetic activity and partitioning. In *Chemistry and world food supplies: the new frontiers* (Chemrawn II) ed L.W. Shemilt, pp. 621–631. Oxford: Pergamon Press.

7 FAO (1980): *Production yearbook*. Rome: FAO.

8 Gill, G.C. & Sultana, W. (1982): Women's role in small farm resource management: a case study in Joydebpur, Bangladesh. In *Maximum livestock production from minimum land*, ed T.R. Preston, C.H. Davis, F. Dolberg, M. Hague & M. Saadullah, pp. 236–258. Mymensingh: Bangladesh Agricultural University.

9 Laumark, S. (1982): Women's contribution to intensive household production in Bangladesh. In *Maximum livestock production from minimum land*, ed T.R. Preston, C.H. Davis, F. Dolberg, M. Haque & M. Saadullah, pp. 79–104. Mymensingh: Bangladesh Agricultural University.

10 Leng, R.A. & Preston, T.R. (1984): Nutritional strategies for the utilization of agroindustrial byproducts by ruminants and extension of the principles and technologies to the small farmer in Asia. In *Proc. 5th Wld. Conf. animal production*, pp. 310–318, (Tokyo).

11 Lewis, C. & Slessor, M. (1982): *Bio-energy resources*. London: Chapman and Hall.

12 Mena, A., Elliott, R. & Preston, T.R. (1981): Sugar cane juice as an energy source for fattening pigs. *Trop. Animal Prod.* **6**, 338–344.

13 Llano, A. (1985): A case study: Colombia. In *Expert consultation on the substitution of imported concentrate feeds in animal feeding systems in developing countries*. Bankok: FAO.

14 Porter, G. (1983): Food and energy: interdependent world needs. In *Chemistry and world food supplies — the new frontiers*, ed G. Bixler & L.W. Shemilt. Manila: IRRI.

15 Preston, T.R. (1977): Strategy for cattle production in the tropics. *Wld Animal Rev.* **21**, 11–17.

16 Preston, T.R. (1980): A model for converting biomass (sugar cane) in animal feed and fuel. In *Animal production systems for the tropics*. Publ. No. 8. International Foundation for Science: Stockholm.

17 Preston, T.R. (1983): Restricted suckling: effects on cow and calf performance. In. *Maximum livestock production from minimum land*, ed C.H. Davis, T.R. Preston, M. Haque & M. Saadullah, pp. 54–66. Mymensingh :Bangladesh Agricultural University.

18 Preston, T.R. and Willis, M.B. (1974): *Intensive beef production*, 2 edn. Oxford: Pergamon Press.

19 Preston, T.R. & Leng, R.A. (1984): Supplementation of diets based on fibrous residues and byproducts. In *Straw and other fibrous byproducts as feed*, ed F. Sundstol & E. Owen, pp. 373–413. Amsterdam: Elsevier Press.

20 Preston, T.R & Leng, R.A. (1985): *Matching livestock systems with available feed resources*. International Livestock Centre for Africa (ILCA) Publishing Unit, in press.

21 Sanchez, M. & Preston, T.R. (1980): Sugar cane juice as cattle feed: comparisons with molasses in the absence or presence of protein supplement. *Trop. Animal Prod.* **5**, 117–124.

22 Tarte, R. (1984): Lineamientos de una estrategia para fortalecer la cooperacion regionalen materia de investigacion y desarrollo agropecuario. In *Seminario-Taller sobre politica de investigacion y desarrollo*. Turrialba: CATIE.

Prospects of food production from animals in semi-arid areas

J.G. CLOETE
Animal and Dairy Science Research Institute, Private Bag X2, Irene 1675, Republic of South Africa.

Semi-arid areas are normally characterized by a vegetative period of 90–180 days, precipitation of $\simeq$ 500 mm p.a. and limited crop husbandry. Hence, farming practices are invariably directed at the natural range. A fairly permanent vegetation cover is possible, but land use has been described as 'backward' due to simple and out-dated management practices and a precariously slow application of technology[13].

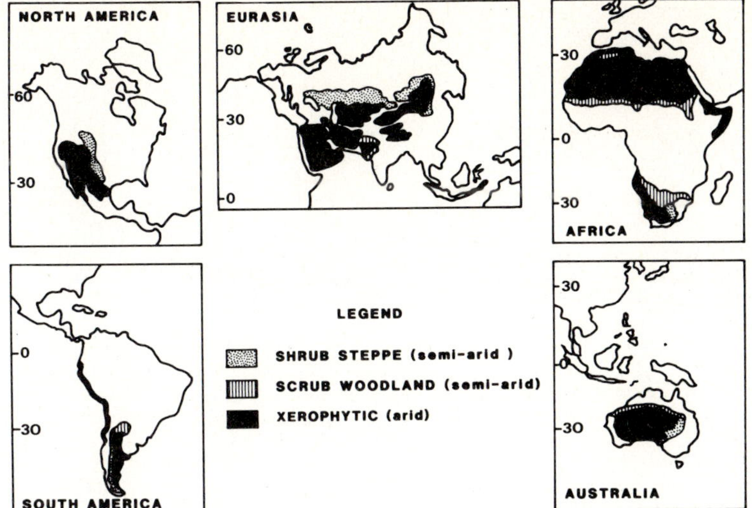

Figure. *Distribution of arid and semi-arid lands in each continent.*

A disturbing lack of data on the status and potential of animal production in the truly arid global grazing regions (rainfall $\simeq$ 250 mm p.a. and vegetative period restricted to 90 days) prompted their inclusion in this assessment.

Status and constraints of animal productivity in dry areas. Grazing in these areas, shown in the Figure may be grouped broadly into three zones, viz shrub-steppe and scrub-woodland (semi-arid) and xerophytic (arid) areas, and comprising roughly 2010 million ha or 63 per cent of global permanent pastures[4,12].

Nineteen major grazing regions were identified comprising: shrub-steppe (W. USA, S. America, Southern USSR, N.W. China, Southern Africa, E. Australia — 706 million ha), scrub-woodland (Sahel, Southern Africa, N.W. India, N. Australia, N. Africa — 464 million ha) and arid areas (S.W. USA, N. Africa, Near East, Middle East, S.W. China, S.E. USSR, S. America — 841 million ha).

These grazings are characterized by seasonal dry periods of up to 9 months resulting in significant changes in chemical composition (DM digestibility, crude protein and P may be reduced by 50 per cent) which lead to animal mass losses of up to 40 per cent in S. Africa, low calf and lamb crops (10–50 per cent in the Middle East and N. Africa) and mortality of up to 60 per cent (N.W. India) according to various reports.

The chancy nature of animal productivity is, furthermore, accentuated by various socio-economic and cultural (literacy) constraints, eg communal tenure, in which livestock is privately owned and the range nationalized, is the basis of 90 per cent of production and 78 per cent of the 369 million large stock units (LSU), or 25 per cent of global cattle, sheep and goats, are managed under migratory systems[3].

The increase in the human population is 2.9 per cent per annum compared with 0.63 per cent for developed economies while GDP (per caput) is \$US 565 compared to \$US 5289[8].

Variability in rainfall (CV > 35 per cent) and regular droughts (once every 2 to 4 years[2]), further reduce meat production/LSU to low levels (16.6 vs 36.5 kg per LSU) or 46 per cent of the global mean.

Various reports indicate overstocking and grazing destruction in these dry areas to be rife. Although open to criticism, the following is an attempt to quantify overstocking in the three zones by superimposing long-term effective grazing norms as calculated for Southern Africa (Table[2]).

The semi-arid scrub-woodland (10.4 million LSU) and xerophytic arid areas (16.6 million LSU) thus exhibited the largest increases in LSU during the last 7 years and also the most

Table. *Livestock numbers and grazing pressure in dry areas (1975–1982)*

Grazing[a] zone	Area (million ha)	Cattle (million)	Camels (million)	Sheep (million)	Goats (million)	LSU[b] (million)	Change in LSU (million)	Grazing pressure (ha/LSU)	Overgrazing (%)
Shrub-steppe (semi-arid):									
W. USA	128	28.7	0	12.0	1.4	30.4	− 2.2	4.21	0
S. America	28	5.2	0	1.8	0	5.5	+ 1.4	5.09	0
N.W. China	174	57.4	0	96.0	0	72.0	− 0.3	2.42	72
USSR	188	58.4	0	71.0	0	68.0	+ 4.0	2.76	51
S. Africa	15	3.5	0	11.4	0.4	5.1	− 0.3	2.94	41
Australia	173	1.3	0	20.0	0	4.3	− 0.3	–	0
Total	706	154.5	0	212.2	1.8	185.3	+ 2.3	3.81	9
Scrub-woodland (semi-arid):									
Sahel	200	52.0	10.5	62.0	69.0	81	+10.0	2.47	183
S. Africa	63	6.6	0	0	0	6.6	− 0.2	9.56	0
N.W. India	40	5.9	1.1	10.3	25.0	12.0	+ 0.2	3.33	110
Australia	113	0.5	0	0	0	0.5	–	–	0
N. Africa	48	4.3	0.4	28.6	9.0	10.1	+ 0.4	4.75	47
Total	464	69.3	12.0	100.9	103.0	110.2	+10.4	4.22	65
Xerophytic (arid):									
S.W. USA	90	12.6	0	11.7	8.6	15.5	+ 2.4	5.81	138
S. Africa	88	1.5	0	16.6	4.2	4.5	+ 0.2	19.6	0
N. Africa	23	3.1	0.4	11.8	3.8	5.8	0	3.97	249
Near East	145	31.5	1.5	117.0	39.5	53.7	+ 6.0	2.70	411
Middle East	108	11.1	1.3	35.7	31.8	22.0	+ 5.0	4.91	181
N.W. China	235	0	1.2	27.0	83.0	17.1	+ 2.6	13.74	181
USSR	94	0	0.2	57.0	6.1	9.2	+ 0.1	10.2	1
S. America	58	0.7	0	17.4	1.0	4.6	+ 0.3	12.6	35
Total	841	60.5	4.6	294.2	178.0	132.0	+16.6	6.37	117

[a]Distribution of livestock in USSR and N.W. China is estimated; [b]LSU–large stock unit; SSU–small stock unit; 1LSU = 7SSU taking cattle, camels, sheep and goats into account[9].

severe overstocking particularly in the Sahel, N.W. India, N. Africa, the Near and Middle East, which illustrates their greater vulnerability to increased desertification.

Notwithstanding increases in ruminant meat production in the scrub-woodland and arid areas of 14.5 and 20.2 per cent respectively during the past 7 years, daily per (human) caput animal protein production still amounts to only 71 per cent of the global mean of 23.8 g. The short-fall must be examined in conjunction with: the importation of live animals from eg Australia to OPEC countries (11.7 million sheep during 1980/81), meat exports from Sahel countries (70 000 tonne beef and 80 000 tonne (metric) mutton during 1975–82) and a significant increase in dairy cows (35 per cent) in N. Africa and the Near and Middle East — although yield/cow is only 59 per cent of the global mean and, through corn and soya imports, a spectacular (73 per cent) increase in poultry meat production in OPEC countries.

The contribution of milk and poultry meat in OPEC countries to per caput protein supply, however, still only amounts to seven and 25 per cent respectively. Likewise, per caput energy supply is only 91 per cent of the global mean.

Even though animal protein is not directly necessary in the human diet[7] the contribution to global animal production from these dry grazing lands has distinct value. Despite low off-takes from grazing (8 per cent in the Sahel to 22 per cent in the W. USA); these areas produce 17 per cent of estimated global beef, mutton and goat meat (4.2, 1.5 and 1.8 million tonne in the shrub-steppe, scrub-woodland and arid areas respectively), 43 per cent of its wool and > 90 per cent of its pelts, with energetically more efficient conversion ratios than those of the intensive systems[1]. Limited planted pastures and cropping (50 per cent of global mean), however, indicate that productivity increases were mainly achieved to the detriment of rangelands.

Future prospects. Global population pressure (1.7 per cent p.a.) to 2000 A.D. may jeopardise future intensive animal-production systems since anticipated shortages of 240 million tonne feed grains and 22 million tonne feed protein are anticipated[8], which will increasingly direct their use to human consumption[10]. A strong positive relationship (r = 0.91), however, appears to exist between expected GDP growth rate to 2000 A.D. and human preference for animal over plant protein[8]. Hence, it was established that, as personal incomes rise above $US 250/caput/ annum, the demand for animal protein becomes increasingly important[5].

While animal products generally contribute only 22.5 per cent to mean daily per caput global energy supply (17 per cent in the dry areas) and the production potential of the dry areas appears limited, animal productivity may yet be considerably improved despite formidable constraints.

Correction of the complex food problem in the most severely overgrazed regions, in which the peasant farmer should be fully involved[3], should be directed at alleviating poverty and a more even distribution of cultural and economic resources[7]. Despite the magnitude of foreign development programmes, the first essential should be to stabilise grazing through the following severe destocking goals: the Sahel by two-thirds, N.W. India by half, the arid S.W. USA by half, N. Africa by two-thirds, the Near East by three-quarters and the Middle East by two-thirds, subject to rigid statutory control. Efforts should involve: deferred grazing (including reseeding), refinements to migratory systems (cooperative grazing societies), sub-division of grazing into smaller units, resettlement of grazing communities to allow greater stratification of productive stock to adjacent cropping areas for finishing, continuing introduction of drought resistant fodder crops *(Antemisia, Atriplex, Salsola, Kochia, Agave, Opuntia)*, rotational grazing where fencing is practised, adequate watering points and remote sensing to monitor stock numbers and their movement, migration routes and vegetation cover directed at optimum carrying-capacity. The imposition of grazing and marketing subsidies by authorities may, in addition, arrest reluctance to dispose of stock[2]. In view of a general paucity of means to disseminate quantitative information, limited efforts in all these areas should be substantiated by multi-disciplinary national and even international action to avoid the creation of vast eroded bare areas and their possible detrimental influence in modifying global climate[11].

The fragmentary grasp of efficient management is, apart from overstocking, the most glaring constraint which restricts animal productivity in these areas. Even under fenced conditions in S. Africa, off-take may be doubled by merely raising management standards to acceptable levels[6].

Proposed destocking implies that 129 million LSU (or 27 per cent of the total) harboured by the three zones, should be withdrawn. A doubling in off-take by acceptable management of the remaining 73 per cent may increase red meat production by 44 per cent or 4.4 million tonne p.a. (virtually 50 per cent of present production), certainly a lucrative incentive associated with improved grazing and animal management.

Further prerequisites are: due to weak heterosis response, selection in these harsh environments should aim at exploiting the most productive indigenous animals[6]; more judicious mating and rearing practices geared to optimal nutrition levels; adequate disease control and the introduction of strategic supplementary and drought feeding once smaller grazing units have been established, ie conserved forage, by-products, NPN, molasses, by-pass (undegradable) protein and P[2].

Since possible hazards associated with diets high in saturated fats to human health still appear to be inconclusive, and substitutes for animal products still at low (but increasing) levels, an enhanced demand for animal protein, particularly in these mainly developing areas, is undoubtedly a future reality.

Conclusions. An assessment of the potential of animal production in 19 major dry grazing regions of the globe (2010 million ha), indicates that even after severe destocking in particularly the Sahel, N.W. India, the Near and Middle East and arid S.W. USA, animal protein production may be substantially increased (ruminant meat production by 44 per cent) by introducing acceptable management standards. A significant correlation ($r = 0.91$) between anticipated GDP growth rate to 2000 A.D. and human animal protein demand, particularly in these mainly developing economies, appears to be a reality.

1 Belyea, J. & Tribe, D.E. (1983): Animal production and energy resources. In *World animal science A1*, ed L. Peel & D.E. Tribe, pp. 235–254. Oxford: Elsevier.
2 Cloete, J.G. (1980): *Evaluation of drought feeding practices in Southern Africa*, pp. 1–21. Pretoria: Dept. of Agriculture.
3 Demirüren, A. (1982): Migratory (transhumance) systems. In *World animal science C1*, ed I.E. Coop, pp. 425–440. Oxford: Elsevier.
4 Food and Agriculture Organisation (1983): *FAO production yearbook*, *Vol. 37*. Stat. Ser. No. 48. Rome:FAO.
5 Henzell, E.F. (1981): Contribution of forages to world-wide food production [Citing Schrimshaw & Taylor, 1980]. In *Proc. 14th Int. Grassl. Congr.* (Lexington), ed J.A. Smith & V.W. Hays, pp. 42–46. Boulder, Colorado: Westview Press.
6 Hofmeyr, J.H. (1968): An evaluation of the status and potential of animal production on the African continent. *Proc. S. Afr. Soc. Anim. Prod.* **7**, 77–95.
7 Holmes, J.H.G. (1983): Animal production and the world food situation. In *World animal science A1*, ed L. Peel & D.E. Tribe, pp. 255–284. Oxford: Elsevier.
8 Hoshiai, K. (1981): Present and future protein demand for animal feeding. *Int. Symp. on Single Cell Proteins* (Paris) ed J.C. Senez, pp. 34–63.
9 Meissner, H.H. (1982): Substitution values of various classes of farm and game animals in terms of a biologically defined large stock unit. In *Farming in South Africa, beef cattle*. Leaflet C3, Pretoria: Government Printer.
10 Morley, F.W.A. (1983): Grazing animals in the next few decades. In *World animal science A1*, ed L. Peel & D.E. Tribe, pp. 331–345. Oxford: Elsevier.
11 Munn, R.E. & Machta, L. (1979): Human activities that affect climate. In *Proc. Wld Climate Conf.* (Geneva), pp. 170–229. Geneva: World Meteorological Organisation.
12 Rumney, G.R. (1968): *Climatology and the world's climates* ed G.R. Rumney, pp. 108–109. New York: Macmillan.
13 Walker, B.H. (1979): *Management of semi arid ecosystems*, ed B.H. Walker, p. 3. Oxford: Elsevier.

Cattle production in the tropics

R.A. LENG and P. BRUMBY
Department of Biochemistry, Microbiology and Nutrition, University of New England, Armidale NSW 2351, Australia and the International Livestock Centre for Africa, Addis Ababa, Ethiopia.

Much of the world's tropics are in 'developing countries' where cattle are often largely owned by subsistence farmers and have multipurpose roles. They provide draught power and milk, meat, hides and manure for fuel and fertiliser. They are often the most important source of cash income to the small-holder, and they provide financial security. Institutional credit for small farmers is a rarity, particularly in Africa, and livestock are the key source of any critical increase in the cash flow of most subsistence farmers. The sale of livestock products often provides the only available source of funds for agricultural development (eg purchase of improved seeds and fertilisers) and the first step in increasing the standard of living of subsistence farmers is frequently through an increase in animal productivity.

Limitation to cattle and buffalo productivity in developing countries. Cattle account for about 70 per cent of the domestic livestock in Africa. In India 86 million dairy buffalo produce some 60 per cent of the total milk supplies. On both continents the primary limitation to ruminant productivity is the imbalanced nature of the available forages and not their low digestibility[9]. Forage availability fluctuates widely during the year. A major stress period occurs during the crop-planting season when grazing is curtailed and cattle depend on crop residues, usually straw stored from the previous crop. In the rangelands or communal grazing areas the available forages during the dry season(s) are mature, low in N and are of low digestibility. In India the major feed resources, year round, for buffalo and cattle are cereal crop residues.

The principles underlying the efficient use of these mature forage resources by large ruminants have been discussed previously[8]. They focus on 'creating an efficient rumen ecosystem for fermentation of fibre in the rumen' and also 'balancing the products of fermentative digestion with dietary *escape* or *bypass* nutrients (largely protein) to optimise productivity'. The forages available are deficient in fermentable-N and bypass protein, and once these have been corrected mineral deficiencies may become important.

Balancing low digestibility forages to increase ruminant productivity. The key roles of urea (to supply fermentable-N) and of bypass protein (which supplies amino acids directly to the animal) in promoting productivity of ruminants fed on low digestibility forages may be summarized: (a) urea supplementation assists in ensuring the birth of a viable calf or lamb; (b) production of protein and urea helps to increase live weight gain in pregnant ruminants and milk yield in lactating animals[4]; (c) supplements of urea and protein stimulate intake and growth of young animals; (d) cows supplemented with protein during dry seasons have higher body weight at maturity, and (e) supplements of protein during dry seasons increase live weight and conception rate of cows[1,2,5,6,10].

Improving productivity of cattle and buffalo in small holdings in developing countries. The application of techniques which achieve these changes has major implications for increasing productivity of small-holder cattle in developing countries, but these changes are difficult to implement. One important reason for this is the reluctance of small-holder farmers to feed urea, where it is available, because its misapplication can easily lead to death of a cow from ammonia toxicity and such a loss is disastrous.

A second problem is the widely held concept that increases in productivity on straw based diets can only be achieved by feeding 'balanced concentrate'. The specific use of bypass nutrients, although now well documented[8] is rarely put into practice and there is an urgent need to find methods for applying these new concepts of feeding livestock under management systems pertaining to the small-holder farmer.

Research (and often therefore foreign aid) often finds its initial focus in application on large farms with the subsistence farmer only later receiving the benefits of research. A lack of appropriate technologies, logistical difficulties in communication to the large numbers of farmers with only one to five animals, and the very limited available resources on small farms are key reasons for this situation.

The use of molasses/urea nutrient blocks in India. Recent developments in India and elsewhere amply confirm that small farmers accept innovations if appropriate technologies are introduced. The National Dairy Development Board of India recently introduced the use of nutrient blocks for lactating buffalo under village conditions to meet the need of these animals for fermentable-N (urea), and other rumen microbial growth factors[3].

Multi-nutrient block-licks, based on molasses, have increased intake and growth of cattle on straw-based diets (Table) under village conditions and have led to large increases in milk-yield

Table. *Intake of rice straw by Jersey bulls (300 kg live weight) given 1 kg of concentrate with or without access to a urea/molasses block* (Kunju, G., Tripathi, A. & Leng, R.A., unpublished observations).

	Straw intake (kg/d)	Intake of block (g/d)	Live wt. change (g/d)	Total feed costs (rupees*/d)	Feed costs per kg gain (rupees*/kg)
Straw plus 1 kg concentrate	6.4	0	220	2.0	9.3
Straw plus 1 kg concentrate + block	6.8	530	700	2.6	3.7

*Indian rupees.

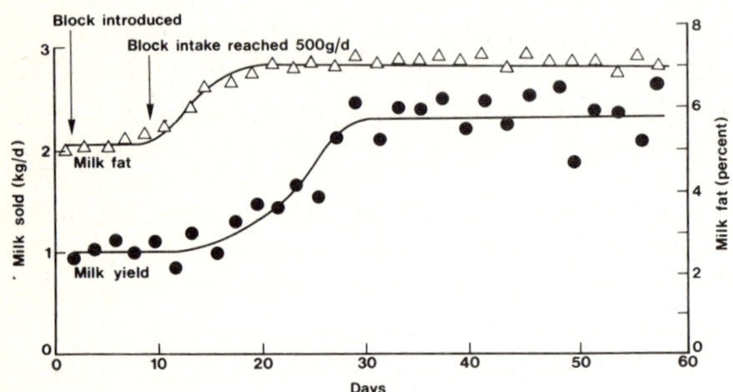

Figure. *The effects of introducing a molasses/ urea block (20 per cent urea) to a milking buffalo in a village in Mehsana, Gujarat, India.* It took approximately 8 d before the buffalo consumed significant amounts of the block (500 g/d). Milk sold on its fat content (from records of milk sales) increased after a time lag of 7–10 d. The basal diet was millet straw with a handful of green forage (Kunju, G., Dave, A. & Leng, R.A. 1985, unpublished observations).

and milk-fat percentages (Fig.) thereby reducing a dependence of milk production on concentrate feeding[7]. The implications of the successful introduction of the same technology into Africa are enormous.

Feeding bypass protein. The use of bypass proteins to supplement cattle under small-holders management are hindered by the lack of availability of high-protein meals specifically targeted at the ruminant industries.

Potential application of strategies aimed at maximising ruminant productivity in Africa. Imports of meat and milk into Africa have risen seven fold on a *per caput* basis and in 1979 cost close to $US5 billion per year. Widespread effective supplementation of the prevailing roughage diets on which ruminants depend could dramatically improve the efficiency of ruminant production and in this way reduce dairy or meat inputs, increase the output of draught animals and stimulate food grain production.

Body size is a primary constraint to the work load that draught animal can sustain. The use of a single animal as against two for cultivation of land can be facilitated if its mature weight is increased by strategic supplementation with urea and bypass protein during its lifetime as demonstrated by Hennessy[1]. The consequent use of a single draught animal for work reduces competition for available feed resources and enables an overall increase in livestock productivity to occur.

The more obvious effects of low-protein undernutrition in cattle, are low calving percentages, low birth-weights of calves, high calf death rates, low weaning weights, stunted mature body size and late sexual maturity. Animals raised in the traditional pastoral systems are smaller at all ages, the big difference being in weaning weight. The demand for milk for human use in pastoral areas severely restricts calf growth and sets in chain the spiral of events that reduces overall body size of cattle in developing countries.

The key to increasing the productivity of these cattle is to supplement them with fermentable-N and protein meals at critical periods. The calf begins life at a disadvantage with a low-birth-weight which can be corrected apparently by making sure the dam is not deficient in rumen fermentable-N. Subsequent supplementation of the calf with an oil seed cake, or leguminous forage, can substantially replace the milk needed for human use. One practical way of achieving this is to supplement calves and breeding cows directly with urea/molasses in small quantities preferably in association with small amounts of high quality bypass protein. In the pastoral areas protein can also be provided from small areas sown down to forage and/or tree legumes.

1 Hennessy, D.W. (1984): PhD thesis, University of New England, Armidale, NSW, 2351, Australia.
2 Hennessy, D.W. (1986): Lactational anoestrus in first-calf heifers grazing native pastures in the subtropics. (Submitted for publication — pers. comm.).
3 Leng, R.A. (1984): The potential of solidified molasses-based blocks for the correction of multinutritional deficiencies in buffaloes and other ruminants, fed low-quality agro-industrial byproducts. In *The use of nuclear techniques to improve domestic buffalo production in Asia*, pp. 135–150. Vienna: IAEA.
4 Leng, R.A. & Preston, T.R. (1984): Nutritional strategies for the utlization of agro-industrial byproducts by ruminants and extension of the principles and technologies to the small farmer in Asia, pp. 310–318. In *Proc. 5th Wld Conf. Animal Prod.* (Tokyo).
5 Lindsay, J.A. & Loxton, I.D. (1981): Supplementation of tropical forage diets with protected proteins. In *Recent advances in animal nutrition in Australia, 1981*, ed D.J. Farrell, pp. 1A. Armidale: University of New England.
6 Lindsay, J.A., Mason, G.W.J. & Thomas, M.A. (1982): Supplementation of pregnant cows with protected proteins when fed tropical forage diets. *Proc. Aust. Soc. Anim. Prod.* **14**, 67–78.
7 National Dairy Development Board of India (1984): Annual report.
8 Preston, T.R. & Leng, R.A. (1984): Supplementation of diets based on fibrous residues and byproducts. In *Straw and other fibrous byproducts as feeds*, ed F. Sundstol & E. Owen, pp. 373–413. Amsterdam: Elsevier Press.
9 Preston, T.R. & Leng, R.A. (1985): *Matching livestock production to available feed resources*. Addis Ababa, Ethiopia: ILCA.
10 Stephenson, R.G.A., Cobon, D., McGuigon, K.R. & Hopkins, P.S. (1981): The measurement of rumen ammonia concentrations as an indicator of the nitrogen status of lambing ewes. *Proc. Aust. Soc. Anim. Prod.* **15**, 601–603.

Food production from goats

C. DEVENDRA
Malaysian Agricultural Research and Development Institute, Serdang, Selangor, Malaysia;
Present address: Division of Agriculture, Food and Nutrition Sciences, International Development Research Centre (IDRC), Tanglin PO Box 101, Singapore 9124.

The main thesis of this paper is that goats can contribute to increased food production. Improvements can come from four main areas: better use of existing breeds and improved breeding, increased efficiency of feeding, improved health and the formulation of priorities that focus specifically on goats. Table 1 shows the distribution of the world population of goats. The economic contribution of goats in developing countries is reflected in the main products from them: meat, milk, skins and mohair. (Table 2).

Meat. Three types of goat meat are produced[3]: meat from kids (cabrito, 8–12 weeks of age); meat from young goats (1–2 years of age) and meat from old goats (2–6 years of age). The first type of meat is very popular in Latin America and the Caribbean. The second category is possibly the most widely produced meat, while the third group generally produces tougher meat. A large proportion of the meat produced in the tropics comes from this group.

At present, the demand for goat meat is in excess of supply and this has resulted in very high prices for the meat as well as live animals. In many countries, eg in South-East Asia, the West Indies and parts of Africa, goat meat is the highest-priced relative to all other meats sold in the market. This has resulted in three notable developments. First, there has been an increased import of feral goat meat from Australia and New Zealand to lucrative markets in the Near East region. Secondly, there has also been considerable substitution of goat meat by poor quality mutton to take advantage of the high price differential between the meats. The third development, and a continuing one, is increased slaughter especially of breeding animals, which

Table 1. *The world population of goats by region*[9]

Region	Population (10⁶)	Distribution (per cent)	Av. growth rate/yr (1961–1965 to 1980–1982) (%)	Ratio goat:sheep
Africa	152.2	32.2	1.9	1: 1.2
N.C. America & Caribbean	10.9	2.3	−1.6	1: 2.1
S. America	19.6	4.1	−1.5	1: 5.5
Asia and the Pacific	271.3	57.4	1.8	1: 1.3
Europe	12.3	2.6	−1.0	1: 11.6
Oceania	0.4	0.1	6.4	1:530
USSR	6.1	1.3	−0.4	1: 23.3
World	472.8	100.0	1.3	1: 2.5
Developed	25.7	5.4	−1.0	1: 21.1
Developing	447.1	94.6	1.3	1: 1.4

Table 2. *The economic contribution of goats in the developing countries*[9]

Product	Production (10³ m tons)	Av. growth rate/yr (1961–1965 to 1980–1982) (%)
Meat	1 950 (92.5%)[a]	1.1
Milk	5 619 (73.0%)[a]	2.7
Fresh skins	368.7 (94.3%)[a]	2.0
Mohair[b]	14 550	−

[a]As per cent of total world population; [b]From the main mohair producing countries: South Africa, Turkey, Texas (USA), Lesotho and Argentina.

has had the effect of reducing the rate of growth of the base population. A case in point is Central America and the Caribbean where increased demand for goat has resulted in this situation (Table 1.).

The quantitative and qualitative aspects of meat production from goats has been recently reviewed[7]. It is generally believed that goat meat has more lean than mutton[6], and this is associated with less subcutaneous and intermuscular fat than in sheep[13,17–19]. The total edible and commercially valuable portions of the carcass are important aspects of economic goat production. These values are high in many countries in the tropics. In temperate countries, a recent development has been the use of goat meat in the sausage industry. Up to 20 per cent goat meat has been used in frankfurters[8,15]. The addition of up to 40 per cent had little effect on processing characteristics or palatability.

Milk. Goat milk is widely consumed wherever it is produced. It is usually consumed fresh, but is also used for making other products. In view of the impact in recent years to promote increased milk production from cows and/or buffaloes, especially for the urban areas in many developing countries, the value of goats producing milk for the rural areas has become especially important.

The nutritive value of goat milk is of special interest[12]. Although goat, cow and human milks are approximately isocaloric and supply about 3.10 MJ/litre of energy, there are differences in the proportions of the energy derived from lactose and protein. In goat and cow milk, fat, protein and lactose account for about 50, 25 and 25 per cent of the energy, but in human milk they furnish 55, 7 and 38 per cent. Calculations of the nutritional adequacy of goat milk for human infants[12] demonstrated that the supply of protein, calcium, phosphorus, vitamin A, thiamin, riboflavin, and pantothenate were in excess. On the other hand, it was deficient in iron and vitamin A, B_{12} and C. Goat milk, like cow milk, had a satisfactory balance of essential amino acids equalling or exceeding the WHO (1973) requirements[20].

Three special attributes of goat milk are worthy of mention. (1) The fat globules are small in size. While the range of size of the fat globules is the same as the cow (1–10 μm in diameter), the content of smaller globules is greater[10]. Up to 4.5 μm in diameter, the percentage distribution of fat globules was 85.7 per cent in sheep, 82.7 per cent in goats, 62.4 per cent in cow and 40.9 per cent in buffalo milks. (2) The fat and protein contents are more easily digestible. Tubercle bacillus is rare and there are also anti-allergy properties. Thus goat milk can replace cow milk for those allergic to the latter. (3) The vitamin A is carried intact.

In addition to the use of goat milk for consumption, other products include cheese, butter and yogurt. Cheeses are particularly popular and several hundred cheeses have been described[11]. Either pure goat milk or goat milk combined with cow, buffalo or sheep milks may be used[2]. Fresh cheese ('Queso Blanco' in Latin America), soft cheeses (Greek 'feta') or hard cheeses ('Chevrotin' in France) can be produced.

In Cyprus 'halloumi', a semi-hard cheese is produced and is widely consumed. Other goat milk products include low-fat, fortified, flavoured or condensed milks, buttermilk, butter and ice-cream; the data on these however, are very limited[14].

The goat genetic resources. It is estimated that there are approximately 300 breeds and types of goats in the world, the majority of which are found in the tropics and sub-tropics[6]. Of these, 70 breeds are found in Africa and 22 in South-East Asia.

Table 3 lists the important improver indigenous breeds in the tropics and sub-tropics according to speciality, excluding the improved dairy breeds from the temperate regions. At least 23 breeds are identified in terms of above-average productivity with respect of meat, milk, prolificacy, mohair, pashmina and skin production.

There appear to be only two examples of breeds which have been selected and improved through well-planned breeding programmes. One concerns the Boer goat in South Africa and the other is the Damascus in Cyprus. These however represent only two out of a total of 23 potentially valuable improver breeds.

Considerable opportunities exist however to select within existing breeds for particular traits and to assess their potential thoroughly in the environment to which they are adapted. Further improvements can be achieved through genetic upgrading using improved breeds from the temperate environment.

Efficient use of the feed resources. Efficient utilization of forages, agro-industrial byproducts and non-conventional feeds is a definite means of increasing performance per animal, and therefore, output per unit area of land. In many situations, dietary protein rather than energy is the main limiting factor. Thus, supplementary protein ensures that requirements are met and there is high animal performance. Good quality protein sources such as groundnut cake and soybean meal are generally expensive and in short supply, which means that these are best retained for non-ruminant feeding. A realistic alternative approach is to use good quality leguminous forages as sources of supplementary protein.

There exist several good examples of forages mainly green leaves, which include leucane (*Leucaena leucocephala*), gliricidia (*Gliricidia maculata*), sesbania (*Sesbania grandiflora*), pigeon pea (*Cajanu cajan*) and cassava (*Manihot esculenta* Crantz). *Leucaena* for example, provides a source of supplementary energy, protein and sulphur and is an economical way of improving feeding systems which use crop residues and agro-industrial byproducts. When included in diets with Napier grass (*Pennisetum purpureum*), up to 75 per cent *Leucaena* enabled a higher uptake of metabolizable energy (ME) and it stimulated live weight gain (Table 4). ME was correlated to live weight gain ($r = 0.970$, $P < 0.01$) and gave the relationship $Y = 4.492 + 10.470X$ where Y is the live weight gain (g) and X is ME intake (MJ/day)[4]. Similarly, Abilay & Arinto[1] also fed up to 75 per cent *Leucaena* and reported that this level did not affect reproductive performance in goats.

Aside from forages, there also exist an abundant variety of crop residues, agro-industrial byproducts and non-conventional feeds. The latter for example, constitute approximately 45

Table 3. *Improver indigenous breeds in the tropics and sub-tropics*

Breed	Speciality	Country of origin
Angora	Mohair	Turkey; subtropical dry
Barbari	Meat, prolificacy	India; tropical, dry
Beetal	Milk	India; tropical, dry
Black Bedouin	Milk, meat (dessert)	Israel; Egypt, tropical, dry
Black Bengal	Prolificacy, skin	India; tropical, dry
Boer	Meat, prolificacy	S. Africa; tropical, dry
Criollo	Prolificacy	S. America; tropical, subtropical
Damani	Milk	Pakistan; tropical, dry
Damascus*	Milk, prolificacy	Syria, Lebanon; subtropical, dry
Dera Din Panah	Milk	Pakistan; tropical, dry
Jamnapari	Milk, meat	India; tropical, subtropical, dry
Kamori	Milk	Pakistan; subtropical, dry
Kilis	Milk	Turkey; subtropical, dry
Katjang	Meat, prolificacy	Indonesia; Malaysia; tropical, humid
Malabar	Milk, prolificacy	India; tropical, humid
Maradi	Skin	Niger; Nigeria; tropical, dry
Marwari	Milk	India; tropical, dry
Ma T'ou*	Meat, prolificacy	China; subtropical, humid
Mubende	Skin	Uganda; tropical, dry
Sudanese Nubian	Milk	Egypt; Sudan; tropical, dry
Sudanese Desert	Meat, prolificacy	Sudan; tropical, dry
West African Dwarf	Prolificacy	West Africa; tropical, dry
Zaraiby*	Milk	Egypt; tropical, dry

*Indicates breed is polled

Table 4. *The effect of supplementation with leucaena forage on the intake and utilization of rice straw[5].*

Treatment	DMI as % of body weight	OM digestibility	ME intake (MJ/kg)	N retention as % of intake
100% Rice straw (RS, chopped)	2.9 a*	50.9 a	3.63 a	0.1 a
90 : 10, RS : leucaena[†‡]	2.6 a	51.3 a	4.22 b	20.2 b
80 : 20, RS : leucaena[†]	2.6 a	49.5 a	4.39 b	16.4 b
70 : 30, RS : leucaena[†]	2.7 a	52.5 b	5.17 c	23.6 b
60 : 40, RS : leucaena[†]	3.1 a	53.3 b	6.04 d	31.5 c
50 : 50, RS : leucaena[†]	2.7 a	55.5 b	6.76 e	27.5 c
40 : 60, RS : leucaena[†]	2.6 a	52.4 b	4.74 b	30.8 c

*Means on the same line with different superscripts differ significantly ($P < 0.05$)

[†]In the total dry matter intake; [‡]leucaena forage : 22% crude protein and 22.18 MJ/kg gross energy content.

per cent of the total availability of byproducts from both types of crops in Asia and the Pacific. Many of these are valuable for feeding goats.

Two types of feeding strategy are possible in the utilization of crop residues, agro-industrial byproducts and non-conventional feedstuffs in the tropics. One option is to utilise the feeds intact, in suitable combinations and dietary mixtures which are palatable and provide the necessary nutritional requirements. Untreated rice straw for example supplemented with *Leucaena* increased both ME and N intakes.

The second alternative is to use some form of processing techniques (physical, biological or chemical) on the crop residues or agro-industrial byproducts. However, the case for processing and/or chemical treatment will need to consider the availability of reliable and proven techniques, practicability, applicability to real farm situations, and more particularly whether it can be economically justified. The latter can only be justified if these are significantly lower than the added benefits in terms of animal response. It is important to use the recommended nutrient levels according to NRC 1981[16].

Acknowledgement. The author appreciates the support of IDRC for participation in the Congress.

1 Abilay, T.A. & Arinto (1981): The influence of ipil-ipil *Leucaena leucocephala* (Lam) de Wit leaves feeding on the reproductive performance of goats in the tropics. *Int. Symp. on Nutrition and Systems of Goat Feeding*, 12–15th May, 1981, Tours, France, *Vol 2*: 623–634.

2 Delforno, G. (1977): Some cheeses of the Piedmontesealps. *Mondo del Lattle*, 31:13.

3 Devendra, C. (1981): Meat production from goats in developing countries. *Occ. Publ., Br. Soc. Anim. Prod.* **4**, 395–406.

4 Devendra, C. (1982): The nutritive value of *Leucaena leucocephala* cv. Peru in balance and growth studies with goats and sheep. *MARDI Res. Bull.*, **2**, 138–150.

5 Devendra, C (1983): Physical treatment of rice straw for goat and sheep and response to substitution with variable levels of cassava (*Manihot esculenta* Crantz), leucaena (*Leucaena leucocephala*), gliricidia (*Gliricidia maculata*) forages. *MARDI Res. Bull.*, **11**, 272–290.

6 Devendra, C. & Burns, M. (1983): *Goat Production in the Tropics. Tech. Commun. Common. Bur. Anim. Breed. Genet.* Farnham Royal: Commonwealth Agricultural Bureaux.

7 Devendra, C. & Owen, J.E. (1983): Quantitative and qualitative aspects of meat production from goats. *Wrld. Anim. Rev.* (FAO), **47**, 19–29.

8 Eggen, N.R., Smith, G.C., Carpenter, Z.L., Berry, B.W. & Shelton, M. (1973): Composition of Angora goat carcases. *J. Anim. Sci.* **37**, 260 (Abstr.).

9 FAO (1982): *Production Yearbook.* **36**, Rome: FAO.

10 Fahmy, A.H., Sirry, I.N. & Safwat, A. (1956): The size of fat globules and the creaming power of buffalo, sheep and goat milk. *Indian J. Dairy Sci.*, **9**, 80–83.

11 Goerner, G., Palo, V. & Bertan, M. (1968): Changes in the content of volatile substances during the ripening of yoghurt. *Milchwissenschaft*, **23**, 94.

12 Jenness, R. (1980): Composition and characteristics of goat milk: Review 1968–1979. *J. Dairy Sci.*, **63**, 1605–1630.

13 Lapido, J.K. (1973): Body composition of male goats and characterization of their fat depot. Ph.D. Thesis Cornell University, U.S.A.

14 Loewenstein, M., Speck, S.J., Barnhart, H.M. & Frank, J.F. (1980): Research on Goat Milk Products: A review. *J. Dairy Sci.*, **63**, 1631–1648.

15 Marshall, W.H., Smith, G.C., Dutson, T.R. & Carpenter, Z.L. (1977): Mechanically deboned goat, mutton and pork in frankfurters. *J. Fd Sci.*, **42**, 193–196.

16 N.R.C. (1981): *Nutrient requirements of goats.* Washington, DC: Nat. Acad. Sci. Press.

17 Owen, J.E., Norman, G.A., Fisher, I.L. & Frost, R.A. (1977): Studies on the meat production characteristics of Botswana goats and sheep. 2. General body composition, carcase measurements and joint composition. *Meat. Sci.*, **1**, 283–306.

18 Owen, J.E., Norman, G.A., Philbrooks, C.A. & Jones, N.D. (1978): Studies on the meat production characteristics of Botswana goat and sheep. 3. Carcase tissue composition and distribution. *Meat. Sci.*, **2**, 59–74.

19 Ueckermann, L. (1969): Produksies studies met Boer bokke. In utilisation of the Boer goat for intensive animal production. M.Sc. thesis. Trene, S. Africa: Anim. Dairy. Sci. Res. Inst.

20 WHO (1973): Energy and protein requirements. *Tech. Rep. Series No.* 252, Geneva.

Fish production for food in the tropics

E.A. HUISMAN and M.A.M. MACHIELS
Department of Fish culture and Fisheries, Wageningen Agriculture University, PO Box 338, Wageningen, The Netherlands.

Tropical fish culture is practised in a variety of husbandry and farming systems. In general five basic forms of husbandry systems are used in tropical fish farming: stagnant water bodies or ponds, ponds or waterbodies with water exchange, enclosures, cages and hatcheries.

This sequence represents a ranking order of increasing intensity of human control and production inputs, and at the same time a ranking order in decreasing popularity of the systems in the tropics. Hatcheries are used for reproduction and rearing of fry (fingerlings), while enclosures, cages and ponds with water exchange are used for fattening, whilst stagnant ponds serve both purposes.

Captural and cultural farming systems. In captural systems stocking takes place by fish (eggs, larvae, adults) entering 'the pond' through flooding, regulation of stocking being absent. This system is mainly found in rice fields and tidal ponds in Asia (several million hectares). Due to the adverse effects of intensification of rice culture this farming system is decreasing but some Asian countries still lay emphasis on it. Cultural systems exploit man-controlled stocking and use all five husbandry systems.

Subsistance and commercial systems. Both types are found in the tropics but commercial farming is poorly developed in Africa[2]. Subsistence farming is low-input farming, predominantly in stagnant ponds, and serves the objective of family nutrition, while commercial farming is practised in all 5 husbandry systems and focuses on local and foreign markets (food- and/or cash crops).

Integration of systems. *Monocultures* utilize the production potential by one species, or even by one sex (monosex culture of tilapias). All five husbandry systems are used. *Polycultures* consist of (balanced) mixtures of different fish species in the same production unit, which due to their species-specific food preferences do not compete with each other (phytophagous, herbivorous, piscivorous). It is mainly practised in stagnant ponds but also in enclosures and tidal ponds. *Integrated farming systems* consist of fish culture integrated into agriculture and/or animal husbandry. In such systems fish culture is used to add value to the waste products of the other component(s)[8]. It is almost exclusively practised in ponds with little or no water exchange.

Constraints to tropical food fish culture. Without underestimating cultural, technical, financial and/or political constraints, some present-day constraints in knowledge concern the following areas. *(1) Reproduction.* Of the ca 300 cultivated species only some tens can be reproduced in captivity and only a few of these throughout the year. To illustrate the extremes, the African catfish can be reproduced at any time throughout the year[5], but milkfish culture, covering ca 500 000 h in Asia completely depends on catch of fry from the wild, which is very variable. A major part of tropical fish farming concerns only fattening of fish caught in the wild. *(2) Nutrition.* Cultivated fish vary from herbivores to carnivores, however, present-day knowledge on nutritional requirements is limited to some ten, mainly carnivorous, and non-tropical, species. Lack of larval diets urges the fish farmer to cultivate micro-organisms to feed his fish. In pond fish culture more knowledge is required about the complexity of the food chains to direct the energy/material flow more efficiently to fish production. *(3) Health control* obviously is of extreme importance, but expertise in the tropics is scarce. The increased international trade in live fish (products) underlines the very need for fish health control to minimise risks of spreading disease. However, only five out of 139 selected fish culture research projects in the tropics are at present related to fish health control.

Table 1. *World fish culture production by region and by commodity group: estimate for 1985*, in metric tons (percentages in parentheses).

Region	Finfish	Molluscs	Crustaceans	Total
Asia & Oceania	2 912 150 (72.7)	4 466 150 (84.4)	133 550 (79.1)	7 511 850 (79.3)
Latin-America	21 500 (0.5)	38 500 (0.7)	17 900 (10.6)	77 900 (0.8)
Africa	11 550 (0.3)	250 (–)	– (–)	11 800 (0.1)
North America	154 950 (3.9)	144 800 (0.07)	17 450 (10.3)	317 200 (3.3)
Europe	908 150 (22.6)	643 900 (12.2)	100 (–)	1 552 150 (16.5)
Total	4 008 300 (42.3)	5 293 600 (55.9)	169 000 (1.8)	9 470 900 (100)

The role of fish culture in the tropics. Although reliable statistics are scarce, an estimate of current production is given in Table 1 based on recent FAO data. The role of fish culture based on a number of parameters is shown in Figs. 1–4 and the Appendix. All the data refer to 1980 except for income which refers to 1975. The data have been analysed by the BMDPIR regression programme[3].

As shown in Tables 2 and 3, Asia and Europe are the most advanced regions. Space precludes detailed discussion of these data here but it can be argued that: (a) fish consumption is income-dependent in general, fish availability playing a role in cases of extreme high or low availability; (b) also on a worldwide basis, the fish-to-meat consumption ratio is high for low-income countries and low for high-income countries (Fig. 3); (c) fish farming is correlated with fish consumption (which is income-dependent).

Although fish farming and fisheries essentially are competitors it seems that fisheries pave the way for fish farming (social acceptance, markets, marketing networks). In this respect it must be mentioned that for the majority of the Aquaculture Developed Countries (ADCs) the per caput fish catch far exceeds per caput fish consumption. Nevertheless it must be realized that fish farming is a husbandry activity and as such is promoted by favourable agriculture (animal husbandry) conditions[4]. This leads to an aquaculture expansion which can be characterized as a vicious circle with a momentum of 'autonomous growth' in itself. It is argued[4] that the threshold level to ensure such autonomous growth in finfish farming may be an annual production of 50–100 g/caput.

Why food fish culture in the tropics? As shown fish culture, already practised millenia BC, is unevenly distributed in the world, and it is difficult to enumerate sound scientific arguments for the fact that it has found its 'niche' in Asia and is struggling to find it in Africa, but there is high potential in tropical fish culture: First, fish, as poikilothermic animals have a low energy requirement for maintenance and as a consequence, efficient feed conversion; up to 80 per cent of the metabolizable energy can be retained. In addition, temperature has a double action on the production process: a rise — within species specific ranges — increases the food intake and improves the conversion of food into fish flesh. This — together with a growing 'season' of a whole year — contributes largely to the success of fish farming in the tropics and it explains the

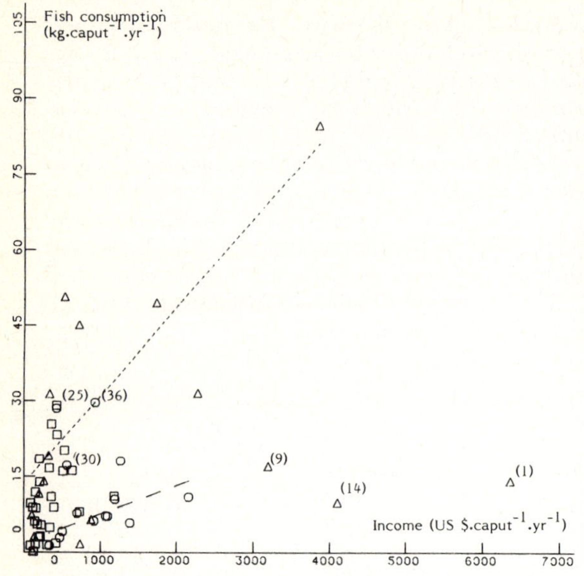

Fig. 1. *Fish consumption vs income (x). See text and Appendix.* △ Asia (r = 0.812; *P* < 0.01). ○ L. America (r = 0.631; *P* < 0.05). □ Africa.

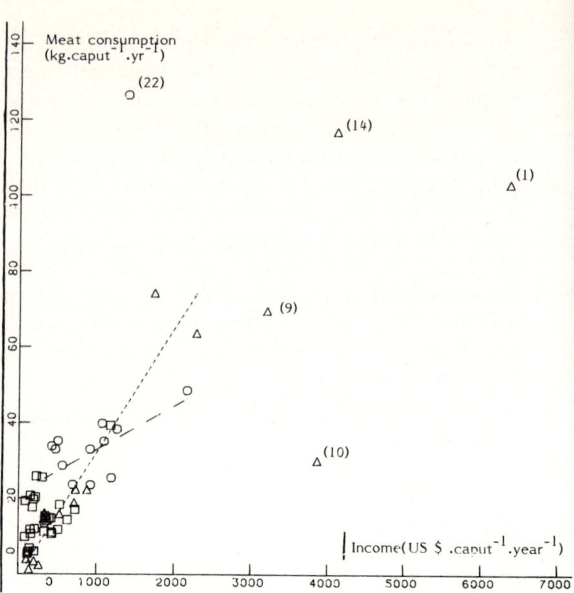

Fig. 2 *Meat consumption vs income (x) see text and Appendix.* △ Asia (r = 0.95; *P* < 0.01) ○ L. America (r = 0.645; *P* < 0.05) □ Africa.

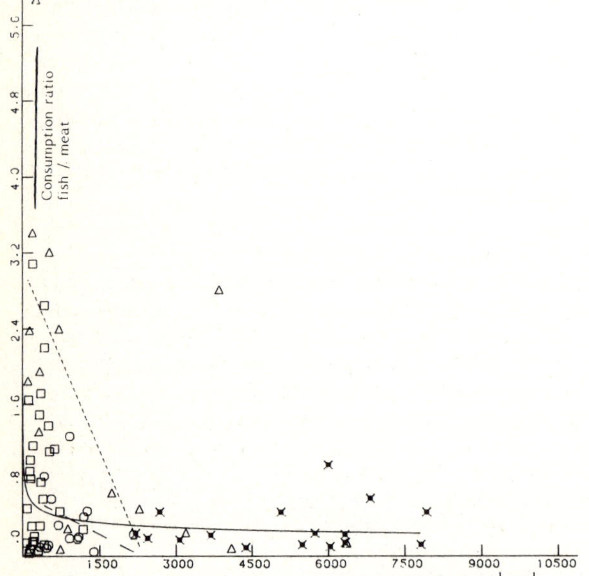

Fig. 3. *Fish/meat consumption ratio vs income.* △---Asia (r = 0.568; *P* < 0.1). ○--- L. America (r = 0.645; *P* < 0.05). □ Africa. × Europe/N. America. ——— all data (r = 0.250; *P* < 0.05).

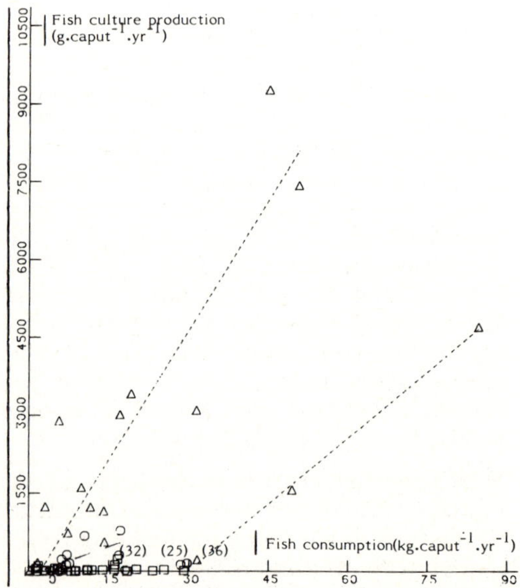

Fig. 4. *Fish culture production vs fish consumption (x) see text and appendix.* △ Asia (r = 0.999; *P* < 0.05, low income), (r = 0.942; *P* < 0.01, high income). ○ L. America (r = 0.690; *P* < 0.05). □ Africa.

Appendix. *Countries and their numbers as used in the Figures.*

1 Australia	24 Brazil	47 Lesotho	70 Bulgaria
2 Bangladesh	25 Chile	48 Liberia	71 Czechoslovakia
3 China[b]	26 Colombia	49 Madagascar	72 Denmark
4 Taiwan[a,b,d]	27 Costa Rica	50 Mali[c,d]	73 Finland
5 Cyprus[a,b]	28 Cuba[b]	51 Malawi	74 France
6 Hong Kong	29 Dom.Republic	52 Mauritius	75 Germany (Dem.)[b]
7 India	30 Equador	53 Niger[c,d]	76 Germany (Fed.)
8 Indonesia	31 El Salvador[a,b]	54 Nigeria	77 Greece
9 Israel	32 Honduras	55 Rwanda	78 Hungary
10 Japan	33 Jamaica	56 Senegal	79 Ireland
11 Rep.Korea	34 Mexico	57 Sierra Leone	80 Italy
12 Malaysia	35 Panama	58 S.Africa	81 Netherlands
13 Nepal	36 Peru	59 Sudan	82 Norway
14 New Zealand	37 Venezuela	60 Tanzania	83 Poland[b]
15 Papua New Guinea[a,b]	38 Benin	61 Tunisia	84 Romania
16 Philippines	39 Cameroun	62 Uganda	85 Spain
17 Singapore	40 Central African Republic	63 Upper Volta	86 Sweden
18 Sri Lanka	41 Congo	64 Zaire	87 Switzerland
19 Syria	42 Egypt	65 Zambia	88 United Kingdom
20 Thailand	43 Gabon[a]	66 Zimbabwe	89 USSR[b]
21 Turkey	44 Ghana	67 Canada	90 Yugoslavia[b]
22 Argentina	45 Ivory Coast	68 USA	
23 Bolivia	46 Kenya	69 Austria	

[a] = fish and meat consumption data unavailable; [b] = income data unavailable; [c] = fish culture production data unavailable, and [d] = fish catch data unavailable.

Table 2. *Fish consumption, fish culture production and the coverage-percentage*.*

Region	Fish consumption $(kg.caput^{-1}.yr^{-1})$ [A]	Fish production $(g.caput^{-1}.yr^{-1})$ [B]	%-Coverage $\left(\dfrac{B}{A} \times 100\%\right)$
Asia & Oceania	15.8	2 248	14.2
Latin-America	9.8	208	2.1
Africa	10.5	34	0.3
North America	16.6	749	4.5
Europe	18.0	1 566	8.6

*Production is a percentage of consumption.

popularity of warm water effluents for fish farming in the moderate zones[1].

Secondly, two groups of established and/or promising candidates for fish culture indigenous to the tropics but less represented in the temperate zones, must be mentioned. The first group is formed by fish with a short food chain (herbivores, detrivores, etc.), such as tilapias (Africa), characids (Latin-America), cyprinids (Asia) and others. The ability of herbivorous fish to control undesired aquatic weed growth — thus turning a problem (for instance in tropical irrigation systems) into protein — has largely contributed to their popularity[6]. The second group represents the so-called 'airbreathers', which due to an accessory organ can breath normal atmospheric air. These species can support very high densities since the production process is not limited to the few ppm's of dissolved oxygen in the water[7]. Annual yields of air-breathing catfish in Thailand amount to several tens of tonnes per hectare.

Conclusions. Based on the data and considerations as given, and on the fact that capture fishery is believed by many experts to have approached its maximum sustainable yield it is anticipated that fish culture can make a real and effective and increasingly important contribution to the food supply for human society. Bearing in mind the physiological nature of fish growth and the fish species available the implied potential for food fish farming in the tropical is obvious.

Table 3. *Aquaculture developed countries (ADCs) and relative ADCs: the top 15 in ranking of size.*

	ADCs		Relative ADCs*	
Country	Finfish production ($g.caput^{-1}.yr^{-1}$)		Country	%-Coverage†
Taiwan	7,181		Netherlands	74.9
Denmark	3,338		Hungary	68.8
Philippines	3,081		China	50.8
Israel	3,019		Bulgaria	46.8
Bulgaria	2,575		Yugoslavia	42.3
Hungary	2,472		India	40.0
Japan	2,136		Romania	30.6
Norway	1,953		Malaysia	20.6
Romania	1,861		Thailand	17.8
Hong Kong	1,524		Israel	17.7
Yugoslavia	1,303		Spain	16.5
USSR	1,280		New Zealand	16.3
India	1,213		France	15.3
Sri Lanka	1,158		Rep.Korea	14.7
Indonesia	1,071		Czechoslovakia	11.5

Total population:
1 378 965 000

Total population:
1 958 012 000

*Taiwan is excluded by lack of data.   †See footnote Table 2.

1 Backiel, T. (1981): Utilization of heated effluents for aquaculture in Europe. In *Aquaculture in heated effluents and recirculation systems, Vol. 2*, ed K. Tiews, pp. 357–371. Berlin: Heenemann.

2 CIFA (1983): Aquaculture development. *Committee for inland fisheries of Africa (CIFA)*, Report no. CIFA/83/5. Rome: FAO.

3 Dixon, W.J., Brown, M.B., Engelman, L., Franc, J.W., Hill, M.A., Jenrich, R.I. & Toporek, J.D. (1983): *BMDP statistical software*. Berkeley: University of California Press.

4 FAO (1984): A study of methodologics for forecasting aquaculture development. *FAO Fisheries technical paper*, No. 248, 1–47. Rome: FAO.

5 Hogendoorn, H. & Vismans, M.M. (1980): Controlled propagation of the African catfish. Clarias lazera (C&V), II. Artificial reproduction. *Aquaculture* **21**, 39–53.

6 Huisman, E.A. (1983): Grass carp (*Ctenopharyngodon idella* Val.) culture and weed control in irrigation systems —turning a problem into protein. In *Proc. 2nd int. fish farming conf.* pp. 131–144. Chislehurst: Janssen Services.

7 Huisman, E.A. (1985): The aquaculture potential of the African catfish (*Clarias gariepinus*, Burchell 1822). *Aquaculture Seminar*, 7–11 October 1985, Kisumu, Kenya. Stockholm: International Foundation for Science (In press).

8 Pullin, R.S.V. & Shehadeh, Z.H. (1980): *Integrated agriculture-aquaculture farming systems*, p. 238. Manila: International Center for Living Aquatic Resources Management (ICLARM).

Biological assessment of nutrient requirements and availability in fish: a workshop report

C.B. COWEY (Organizer)
Institute of Marine Biochemistry, St. Fittick's Road, Aberdeen AB1 3RA, UK.

Utilization of amino acids: speakers included T. Murai, Japan; S.J. Kaushik, France and B. Fauconneau, France. In general, fish do not appear to utilize dietary crystalline amino acids as well as certain other animals. Several studies have been conducted in order to explain this poor utilization and to develop improved amino acid test-diets for fish.

Improved growth rate and feed efficiency have been observed with increased frequency of feeding amino acid test-diets to young carp, a species that lacks a stomach and thus pepsin digestion. For example, feeding the fish to satiation four times daily improved the utilization of the test-diet as compared to feeding once, twice or three times per day. Plasma-free amino acids were analyzed in carp fed the above amino acid test-diets at various times after feedings. It was found that the levels of all essential amino acids reached their respective peaks in 2 to 3 hours after feeding and returned to fasting levels in about 4 hours. In an additional study, young carp fed a similar amino acid test diet were found to excrete substantial quantities of free amino acids through the gills and kidneys. In certain cases up to 40 per cent of the supplemental amino acids were excreted as the intact free amino acid.

Similar studies in another laboratory have also detected a very high level of nitrogen excretion from fish fed amino acid test-diets. These workers did not identify the compounds containing nitrogen that were being excreted. Feeding the fish a casein test-diet resulted in much less excretion of nitrogen. These results suggest one possible reason why fish do not utilize dietary free amino acids as effectively as some land animals.

Contribution of oxidation to the total amount of amino acid metabolism increases initially when external feeding by the fish first begins, decreasing as the fish grow. Protein synthesis and oxidation give only a small indication of the overall metabolism of amino acids taking into account the exchanges between tissues and recycling of amino acids in the different tissues (protein turnover and deamination). The adaptation of these processes and the yield of these steps of amino acid metabolism could give some information about changes in the requirement of amino acids.

The overall metabolism of amino acids in the whole animal is the sum of metabolic activities in different tissues. It has been demonstrated that there are great differences in protein turnover, in protein deposition efficiency, and in amino acid oxidation between 'active' tissues such as liver, gill or digestive tract on one hand, and the white muscle on the other. Thus, metabolic amino acid requirements can be analysed approximately as the sum of the requirements of these different tissues. The effects on amino acid metabolism in so-called 'active' tissues and in white muscle as they affect overall amino acid metabolism can be studied. In response to changes of nutritional state (diet composition, frequency of feeding) or changes of environmental conditions (temperature, salinity). An example was provided from sturgeon larvae fed natural food or an artificial diet. It appeared also that in response to environmental changes, there were alterations to the size of tissues or the size of cells in these tissues which compensated for the alteration in protein synthesis rate.

Utilization of energetic substrates: speakers included C.B. Cowey, UK; C.Y. Cho, Canada; J. Hilton, Canada; R.T. Lovell, USA; M. Furuichi, Japan; A. Kanazawa, Japan; and J. Atkinson, Canada. Several unique problems are associated with the study of energy utilization in fish. Since the animals are small, microtechniques have to be used to analyse faecal and urine samples or alternatively groups of fish must be used to obtain larger samples. The waste products are voided into water, and special techniques must be used to avoid leaching the dilution of the waste products. Care must be taken to avoid mixing of uneaten food with waste products. During the study, the fish should not be subjected to stress and they should be in positive nitrogen balance during the study.

Several methods have been developed to determine digestible energy and metabolizable energy values of fish foods and dietary ingredients. These methods include: (1) a metabolism chamber for the separate collection of faeces, urine and gill excretions, (2) use of suction to remove the faeces from the lower intestine, (3) a dissection techniques, (4) various other methods of removing the faecal material from the aquarium water. Each of these methods have advantages and disadvantages.

Several questions arise when evaluating the different methods used to determine the availability of gross energy in diet components for fish. These include: How accurately can digestible (DE) or metabolizable energy (ME) be measured? Do ME values vary with gross energy or with protein level in diet? How much additional information is provided by measuring ME rather than DE? Would net energy be a valuable measure of energy availability?

A method of determining ME based on carcass composition of the fish was described and compared to the use of the metabolism chamber. DE values should be determined for feed ingredients but ME values should be limited to the final diet. ME values for fish are not additive.

Digestible energy can be measured more accurately than ME and accounts for most of the variation in the availability of gross energy in feedstuffs fed to fish. Considering the increased accuracy and convenience in measuring DE over ME, and the small difference between DE and ME, DE should be the preferred measure of availability of energy for fish.

However, DE is not always a reliable measure of energy value of all feedstuffs for rainbow trout; DE tends to overestimate carbohydrates. Glucose is almost completely digested by trout but has relatively little protein-sparing value. Digestibility coefficients for proteins and lipids agree relatively well with the energy contribution from these nutrients.

The quantitative fate of absorbed glucose in rainbow trout cannot presently be adequately described. It does not seem to be efficiently oxidized to CO_2, converted to lipid stores, or used in protein (nonessential amino acid) synthesis. It is stored as glycogen and converted into glycoprotein but these processes are not quantitatively important. Also, urinary loss, gill losses, and metabolic dumping (heat production) do not seem to be important routes for glucose metabolism.

Digestible energy determinations in channel catfish for dehulled, solvent-extracted soybean meal, menhaden fishmeal, and a practical type diet formulation were not significantly different when fed voluntarily in a tank, when force-fed under anaesthesia and released, or when force-fed in a metabolism chamber. DE values determined indirectly, using chromic oxide, or directly, by total faecal collection in a metabolism chamber agreed closely. Faeces sampling by excision of the gut as compared to suction-stripping did not affect DE values, but collection of faeces anterior to the ileocecal valve in the lower gut reduced calculated DE coefficients and collection of faeces from the water gave increased values for the coefficients. Feeding the test feedstuff with 14 per cent cellulose fibre maximized DE coefficients, making them comparable to values determined by substituting the test feedstuff (30 per cent) in a standard diet.

Reducing water temperature from 30 to 22 °C reduced rate of movement of ingesta (practical-type diet) through the digestive tract of channel catfish by 58 per cent and reduced digestibility of starch by 17 per cent but did not reduce digestion of crude protein or fat. Extrusion processing (moist heating) of the practical-type diet increased digestibility of energy by 15 per cent of starch by 24 per cent and of protein by 6 per cent. Reducing particle size of the diet ingredients from 2 mm to 0.5 mm increased digestibility of energy by 4.8 per cent of starch by 8.4 per cent and of crude protein by 3 per cent.

Digestibility of dietary energy and protein was not significantly different among five genetic groups of channel catfish which varied greatly in growth rate (from 2.3 g/day to 4.8 g/day), indicating that digestion does not vary greatly among individual or genetic groups of channel catfish. Metabolizable energy (ME) values, determined with a metabolism chamber, were 4.6, 4.1 and 5.3 per cent lower than DE values for menhaden fish meal, soybean meal and the practical-type diet.

It had been suggested that the nutritive value of β-starch in carp is lower than that of α-starch, because of the lower digestibility of β-starch. However, investigations have shown that growth and feed efficiency of carp fed diets containing β-starch were higher than those of fish fed α-starch diets. Also, the groups fed β-starch exhibited a lower activity of hepatic pyruvate kinase and higher activities of hepatic phosphoenolpyruvate carboxykinase, aspartic amino-transferase, urocanase and citrate cleavage enzyme, although no such trend was evident in alanine aminotransferase activity. These results suggest that fish fed on diets containing β-starch will metabolize dietary protein more actively than those fed diets with α-starch. Accordingly, it may be questioned whether the nutritive values of diets containing large amounts of starch can be assessed on the basis of digestible energy content.

Measurements of energy utilization and metabolism are also difficult in Crustacea. The use of radioactively labelled lipids was demonstrated as a technique for determining the uptake, distribution and metabolism of lipids in the prawn, *Penaeus japonicus*. The technique was discussed.

XXIII: Nutrition education

NUTRITION EDUCATION FOR THE PUBLIC

Programmes to promote breast-feeding

E.F. Patrice JELLIFFE and D.B. JELLIFFE
School of Public Health, University of California, Los Angeles, CA 90024, USA.

Modern programmes to promote breast-feeding have become increasingly effective as it has been realized that success (or failure) depends on maternal reflexes, on *learned* knowledge concerned with practical 'management' and, to a lesser extent, on the health and nutrition of the mother. Until the recent resurgence of concern with breast-feeding in the early 1970s, the worst lactators were in the best nourished communities in the world, including North America and Western Europe. Conversely, poorly nourished women in many rural areas in less technically developed countries breast-feed surprisingly well, although often to their own detriment ('maternal depletion syndromes').

Community analysis. To develop a breast-feeding programme, some form of community analysis is required. Information needs to be sought not only on the prevalence of breast-feeding, but also on the main social forces influencing the lactation reflexes, maternal knowledge concerning practical management and the health of mothers. Experience suggests that this can most usefully be obtained from four sources — general information and attitudes, health services, women in the work force and the influence of the infant-food industry (Fig. 1).

From all four sources, information needs collecting on the occurrence of anxiety or confidence-inducing factors, the limitation or otherwise of opportunities for sucking, on the knowledge of the practical management of breast-feeding (modern or traditional methods) by mothers, and on maternal health and nutrition.

Similarly, situations which limit sucking and hence, prolactin secretion, such as separating the new-born and mother, or the use of complementary bottle-feeds, or the necessity for mothers to leave the baby at home while going out to work, need to be identified in such community analyses.

Fig. 1. *Community analysis and the development of a breast-feeding programme*

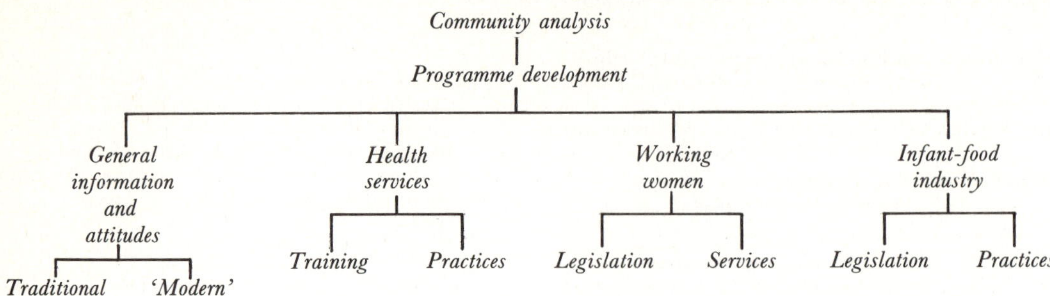

Especially in urban *doula*-less communities, the practical management of lactation needs to be investigated. Breast-feeding is *not* instinctive, but is partly reflex interaction and partly learned behaviour. Repeated studies have shown that minor-seeming modifications in management, such as mother neonate positioning, can increase both the supply and ejection of milk and avoid the two main avoidable anxiety-inducing problems — cracked nipples and engorgement. In addition, beneficial and potentially harmful traditional practices need to be known about, such as colostrum rejection.

The influence of these four areas on the general health and nutrition of mothers also needs to be investigated in relation to the possible impact on breast-feeding. Limitations in the dietary intake in pregnancy, in the puerperium and in lactation need to be known, and whether these are due to economic or cultural reasons, or to over-work. In particular, serious and substantial energy deficits are most likely to be relevant, especially in already malnourished mothers. Current evidence suggests a sliding scale of decreased milk production with increasing degrees of energy deficiency from adaptation (through known and unknown physiological mechanisms) to complete cessation of milk secretion, as in the severe energy deficiency of famine.

Groups needing conviction. There is a need to alter attitudes and to stimulate motivation in the general public, and especially to influence behaviour change in mothers (and fathers); there is also a need to convince and motivate other groups whose actions can support breast-feeding or make its accomplishment easier or more difficult. These include policy-makers and legislators, health workers of various types (including hospital administrators), research scientists, industrialists and the infant-food industry.

For the health professional, there are a number of procedures which need modification (notably 'rooming-in'), which facilitate the maternal reflexes, supply practical information and support, and make breast-feeding easier. Such changes also help reorient the training of medical and nursing staff *and* form an immediate part of direct health education of the public by visible example. For both the general health professional and especially for the research scientist, it is necessary to widen the perspective from over-attention to one, often very narrow, aspect (inevitably requiring ever more and more research) to a broad-spectrum view of the ranges of evidence available concerning the types of benefits obtained by breast-feeding (Fig. 2). The emphasis in this motivation will need to vary. In less technically developed countries, considerations of protection against enteral infection, over-all nutritional benefits, economics and child-spacing loom large. In more technically developed countries, the different psychophysiological interchange and detailed biochemical considerations (eg on requirements for taurine and carnitine) appear more relevant.

Details of programmes. *Small scale.* These can be (and have been) successfully undertaken on a relatively small scale, often in hospitals, by modification of maternity unit practices which have evolved with no rational scientific justification in the so-called Western world during the present century, and, unfortunately, have been exported to other cultures. Undoubtedly, the most significant 'package' of activities for the hospital is 'rooming-in'. The impact of changes in maternity unit procedures and follow-up home visits have been most dramatically demonstrated in the Puriscal region of rural Costa Rica[3], as regards decline in neonatal infection and increased duration of breast-feeding.

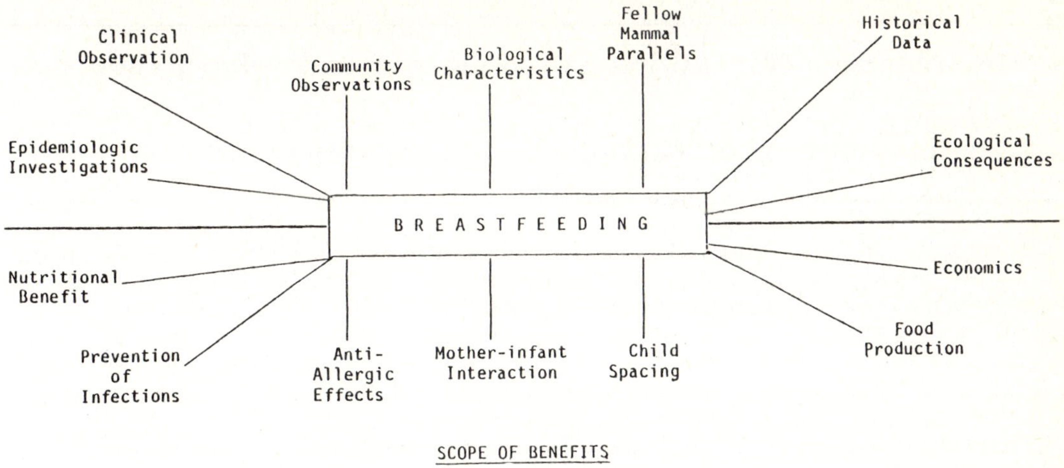

Fig. 2. *Ranges of evidence and scope of benefits from breast-feeding.*

National programmes. Various very different countries have shown a spontaneous increase in breast-feeding in the past 25 years. Most usually, this has been lead by mothers support groups, such as La Leche League in the USA, Nursing Mother's Association of Australia and *Ammehjelpen* in Norway. Their effectiveness is as *doula*-surrogates, making available psychological support and practical information.

During the past 10–15 years, national programmes of different degrees of complexity and coverage have been initiated in numerous countries, often with the backing of WHO, UNICEF and/or USAID. In all cases, such programmes have comprised consideration of the four aspects mentioned previously (Fig. 1) and have attempted to include motivation and action directed through one (or preferably all) of these channels. The blends of methods used have varied, but the results are striking in terms of coverage and of increase in breast-feeding in maternity units and some communities.

Briefly, breast-feeding programmes work when based on the 'tripod' approach — support of maternal reflexes, supply of practical information on management, and preservation of the health and nutrition of pregnant and lactating mothers[1]. Details of such programmes obviously will vary with different social, cultural, economic and geographical situations. Inclusion of legislation and services for working women seems usually (but *not* always) to represent a major activity, as does monitoring the activities of the infant-food industry's marketing practices[5]. The feasibility of breast-feeding mothers' support groups varies, but can be highly significant, as it usually involves the 'trend-setting' educated elite. However, probably the two most universal, initial components for such programmes are the modification of maternity health services (with accompanying reorientation of training of different categories of health professionals[4]) and information via the mass media, based on modern concepts of 'social marketing'[2]. However, above all else is the need for actively supportive legislators and for health professionals, including nutritionists, who are both well-informed and positive advocates.

1 Jelliffe, D.B. & Jelliffe, E.F.P. (1978): *Human milk in the modern world.* Oxford: Oxford University Press.
2 Manoff, R. (1985): *Social marketing.* New York: Praeger.
3 Mata, L., Carvajal, J.J. & Garcia, M.E. (1984): Promotion of breast-feeding, health and survival of infants through hospital and field interventions. In *Malnutrition determinants and consequences*, pp. 123–138. New York: Alan Liss.
4 Naylor, A. (1984): Learning the management of breast-feeding: experience of the San Diego Lactation Clinic. *Adv. Int. Mat. Child Hlth* **4**, 59–64.
5 World Health Organization (1981): *International code of marketing of breast-milk substitutes.* Geneva: WHO.

Nutrition education for children and adolescents in developed countries

M.A. CHURCH
Scottish Health Education Group, Woodburn House, Canaan Lane, Edinburgh EH10 4SG, UK.

The high fat and sugar levels in the diet of richer countries dramatically increase the energy density[2]. This results in children in richer countries being able to achieve adequate energy intakes much more easily than the children at risk of malnutrition in poorer countries. So, for example, a young British child on a typical diet with 8.4 kJ (2 kcal)/g only needs to eat half the weight of food that a typical child in Uganda does, with its low fat, high bulk staple diet, which only has 4.2 kJ (1 kcal)/g. Not surprisingly all British children easily achieve the energy intakes they need whereas Ugandan children often fail to.

The energy-rich diets of developed countries result in benefits such as: malnutrition (PEM) disappearing, children growing faster and reaching adult height earlier[5]; most vitamin and mineral deficiency diseases disappearing; with improved nutrition, a drop in childhood mortality from diseases such as measles and whooping cough[3].

These rich diets also cause new problems and challenges in nutrition and health education. Dental caries rapidly affects nearly everyone, from early childhood[8]. Obesity starts is early childhood, becomes more common in adolescence and then steadily rises with middle age[10]. Sexual maturity arrives much earlier. In Norway for instance, the age of menarche is now about 13 years whereas in the last century it was over 17. Most social and cultural institutions have not adequately acknowledged or adjusted to this change, for example its effect of precocious teenage sexual behaviour[12]. Lack of fibre in the diet causes digestive diseases, although the only serious one that is likely to affect children is appendicitis[1]. Arterial disease sets in prematurely, although it also is unlikely to cause symptoms in childhood[13].

The need for overall nutrition guide-lines. How best to acknowledge the benefits that have occurred and the new problems that have been caused by the diets that are typically high in fat and sugar but low in fibre? Some countries have produced proposed guide-lines for a more healthy diet, such as the one produced in Britain for the National Advisory Committee on Nutrition Education[7]. That report not only summarized the best current, authoritive data on nutrition and health but suggested realistic targets for change with the expected benefits to health. Previously, without such an overall view, nutrition education was fragmented as often conflicting, usually because of limited viewpoints. For instance dentists tend only to think about teeth and cardiologists about the heart!

An excellent recent book on the Scottish diet — *The Good Scots diet*[11] was the basis of a song by the Scottish singer/songwriter Adam McNaughtan, whose lyrics have beautifully summarized the situation:

> But the rot set in in the days o' Victoria;
> The 'Good Scots diet' tells the story o'
> How our alimentation has decayed.
> Oats disappeared frae the urban diet,
> Deficiency diseases ran riot,
> The pint-sized, rickety, bronchial Scot was made.
>
> So they tellt him meat and fish and eggs
> Would make short work o' his bowly legs,
> And his weans would grow up tall and strong and straight,
> So he ate these things plus cakes and candy,
> And Scotsmen now are seldom bandy;
> They're strong, they wear false teeth and they're overweight.
>
> Now being overweight can kill ya,
> So it's time that you become familiar
> With what the 'Good Scots Diet' has to say.

If you pay attention to what you hear,
You'll cut down fat and eat more cereal:
Eat for health the new, old-fashioned way.

Sweet snacks — a specific challenge. One of the most specific challenges is that of sweet snacks, which are largely responsible for the high rates of dental caries in children. But the attempts to change children's sweet-eating habits with nutrition education have never been very successful despite many years of effort. A clue to the reason for this and a useful new basis for planning better nutrition education is the 'Playpiece hypothesis'.

The 'Playpiece hypothesis'. In a study of the snack-eating habits of primary school children in Edinburgh, Rousseau[9] discovered a phenomenon called the 'playpiece' which was evidently very important to the children although quite strange to her as a visiting French Canadian. A playpiece is a child's food suitable for eating as a snack during playtime. When questioned, the children revealed strong views as to the acceptable features of a playpiece and those that were unacceptable. Significantly, most of the common health education suggestions for healthy snack alternatives to sweets failed the playpiece test badly!

Playpieces are integral to the young child's world of fantasy and fun. They are not really thought of as food, which is definitely in the adult world of meals, but as an essential part of play. A good playpiece will shock adults by its colour, taste or association. Jelly babies are a good example and children often relish biting the heads off. Another sweet called Dead man's finger is a more recent example. Playpieces must be small enough to share and swap and preferably come in a bag. They must be complete and tasty on their own, and must have exciting tastes, shapes, textures and colours. They must be dry enough to handle without getting messy fingers and must be able to be eaten without utensils such as knives, forks or spoons. Playpieces must be cheap and good value for money and easily available. Of course sweets fit the playpiece phenomenon well as their manufacturers have evidently understood. Crisps also are good playpieces and are favoured by dental health educators as healthy alternatives to sweets. Although there is some concern about the high fat content of crisps, there is probably little to worry about it they are eaten as snacks and the rest of the diet is healthy. Crisps have displaced sweets to an extent, probably mostly because of skilful marketing rather than health education. Crisps fit the playpieces criteria very well coming in more and more exotic flavours and shaped as creatures from outerspace or as monsters of fantasy.

Nutrition educators evidently need to get onto the child's wavelength — the playpiece phenomenon — if they hope to be more successful. The following commonly suggested healthy alternative snacks all badly fail the playpiece test: cream crackers or crispbreads, with cheese or meat paste; apples, grapes, bananas and pears, carrots and celery.

There is, however, real potential in a new range of snack products based on dried fruits and nuts. Tropical treat contains exotic dried fruit such a pawpaw and pineapple along with banana chips, coconut, raisins and nuts. There are also savoury snacks from India, such as Bengal mix, which is based on fried legumes such as chickpeas and extruded lentil flour.

The term playpiece seems to be specific to Scotland, but there is evidence of a very similar phenomenon in the north-east of England, where children refer to kets. A description of kets[4] shows them to have all the main features of playpieces. It would be very interesting to know if there are other examples of the playpiece phenomenon elsewhere.

Too fat or too thin: a specific challenge. After dental caries, obesity is the most common nutrition problem for children in developed countries. Taking obesity to be a weight-for-height more than 20 per cent above the expected level, some 2–3 per cent of young children in Britain are obese (about 10–15 per cent among teenagers). Nutrition education about obesity is difficult because so many factors are involved other than nutrition — genetics, metabolic rate and exercise. Energy requirements vary enormously and an average figure can only be misleading. Weight standards are similarly very wide and if they are made too narrow they can lead to problems of distorted body image, which is probably an important aspect of anorexia nervosa, present in about 1 per cent of adolescent girls.

Drama — a valuable way to explore complex issues with teenagers. The Scottish Health Education Group has used drama as a very effective way of engaging the attention and interest of teenagers in school. For several years now Theatre Workshop has been sponsored to produce and tour with a production, which last year was on nutrition — Foodstuff by Tony Mulholland[6]. Issues such as obesity, sugar and tooth decay, the effects of advertising and peergroup pressures were covered in a fast-moving production.

Integrated school nutrition policies — the most hopeful developments. Nutrition, if covered at all in schools tends to be highly fragmented and lacks any relationship to what children eat in their canteen or tuck shop. The most encouraging current developments in Scottish schools are where there has been a coordinated policy, supported by the head teacher, to place nutrition in the curriculum and to have a congruent policy for canteen and tuck shop. Pupils have a chance to cook and try out more healthy recipes in home economics classes.

Video is rapidly replacing film as a main visual aid and there is an abundance of useful educational material that can be recorded, such as the Channel 4 series last year Food for thought. The Open University has just produced a new course on Healthy eating. Computers are beginning to be used for nutrition teaching and probably one interesting development will be use of interactive programmes and video-discs.

1 Burkitt, D.P. (1975): In *Refined carbohydrate foods and disease*, ed D.P. Burkitt & H.C. Trowell, p. 87. London & New York: Academic Press.
2 Chirch, M.A. (1979): Dietary factors in malnutrition: quality and quantity of diet in relation to child development. *Proc. Nutr. Soc.* **38**, 41–49.
3 DHSS (1976): Childhood mortality from measles and whooping cough, 1871–1971. In *Prevention and health: everybody's business*, p. 23. London: HMSO.
4 James, A. (1979): Confections, concoctions and conceptions. *J. Anthropol. Soc.* **10**, 83–87.
5 Meredith, H.V. (1963): Change in the stature and body weight of North American boys during the last 80 years. *Adv. Child Dev. Behav.* **1**, 69–114.
6 Mulholland, T. (1985): Foodstuff — a play about food and nutrition produced by the Theatre Workshop for the Scottish Health Education Group, Edinburgh. (In press).
7 National Advisory Committee on Nutrition Education (1983): Proposals for nutritional guidelines for health education in Britain. ad hoc working party under the chairmanship of Professor W.P.T. James. London: Health Education Council.
8 Newburn, E. (1982): Sugar and dental caries: a review of human studies. *Science* **217**, 418–423.
9 Rousseau, N. (1983): Give us a playpiece, please; not lectures! *J. Roy. Soc. Hlth* **103**, 104–111.
10 Royal College of Physicians of London (1983): Obesity. *J. Roy. Coll. Physns* **17**, 3–58.
11 Steven, M. (1985): *The good Scots diet: what happened to it?* Aberdeen: Aberdeen University Press.
12 Udry, R.J. (1979): Age at menarche, at first intercourse, and at first pregnancy. *J. Biosoc. Sci.* **11**, 433–441.
13 WHO (1982): *Prevention of coronary heart disease*, p. 35. Tech. Rep. Ser. 678. Geneva: World Health Organization.

Nutrition education for children and adolescents in developing nations

Priyani SOYSA
Department of Paediatrics, University of Colmbo, Sri Lanka.

Nutrition education has long been considered a low-priority, low-cost programme. Indeed, some have doubted its value. This is partly due to the fact that conventional nutrition education has not been planned effectively for whatever population it has been addressed. It is often an additional component in a comprehensive intervention, as, for example, supplementary feeding. Nutrition education is a long-term type of intervention that politicians and policy makers do not favour as they look for quick results from the resources available to them and it does not seem to generate enough support for their policies.

Within the last decade, Sri Lanka has ventured on programmes that recognize the role and potential of nutrition education, encouraged by the success of the family planning programme, which demonstrated the importance of women's education in reducing family size and by the finding that, in the low income sector, the single most important variable in determining the nutritional status of the child is the level of the mother's education.

A major aim of the programme has been to reduce the problem of low birth weight. It is not enough to plan for supplementary feeding in pregnancy. The problem needs long-term intervention to improve the nutrition of young schoolgirls and adolescents.

Another aim was to encourage the consumption of home-grown produce since it was known that nutritional status was good in families who had home gardens.

For optimization of a programme, the *target group* must be selected well. It is believed that change of behaviour is best achieved among young people and a long-term programme of persuasion for schoolchildren and adolescents has therefore been launched. Change of behaviour can be achieved by knowledge but the type of knowledge imparted should overcome the inertia or disinterest of youth in a problem which may not be of immediate relevance to them, eg breast-feeding or weaning practices.

The point of educational entry was first focused on the primary-schoolchild where the curriculum is common to both girls and boys. Positive efforts were on a practical basis such as a visit to the local market to pick up nutritious foods. This was repeated using the school garden as the experimental field. Other activities were role-play on the theme of infection and nutrition and exhibitions organized by schools with a focus on nutrition. The accent has been on agricultural aspects, feeding practices, available foods and protective health interventions.Curricula for formal education have also been redesigned, a laborious task. Training workshops for primary-school-teachers have been organized by the Nutrition Society in collaboration with the Ministry of Education in successive years in order to increase their motivation.

The Association for the Advancement of Sciences, through its committee for popularisation of sciences, has helped to motivate schoolchildren to learn nutrition by organizing local 'science days'. A lecture programme is organized in a prestigious school in the district. Good science teachers participate in the programme together with nutrition experts and basic principles of nutrition, eg metabolism and biochemistry, are offered. Thus, examination-conscious schoolchildren are motivated to attend as the General Certificate Examination (GCE) advanced level syllabus is the basis for the programme and 700–1500 may be present at a session. This programme is followed by an exhibition organized by the schools.

School farms have been another focus. Funds were made available at district level through the local government administrators and the regional directors of schools. Produce is not only on sale to pupils, parents and teachers, but school meals are prepared from farm products. School attendance is improved with the preparation of a gruel or porridge made of rice, green leaves and coconut milk which is a traditional food in Sri Lanka. Recently efforts have been directed to improve the nutritional value of this meal by the use of soya milk rather than coconut milk. The motivation to learn nutrition is by satisfying the hunger of schoolchildren through a nutritious meal.

The criteria on which school farms are chosen are: availability of 10 perches of land; availability of water and a protective fence; ability to organize security for the farm and availability of an enthusiastic principal or teacher.

The main objectives of the farm project are to: disseminate the importance of nutrition among the community through schoolchildren; impart the scientific and technical knowledge and practical skills in relation to the cultivation of nutrition rich crops to students and the community; manage the farm as a model for the village, and train students in simple methods of preservation and storage of foods.

Knowledge of nutrition is also promoted by holding a 'nutrition week', with competitions in nutrition, essays, speeches and debates. Media-based nutrition education gives wide coverage through radio, television and newspapers. Radio and television quiz programmes for schoolchildren and crosswords in children's newspapers have been organized. Broader based programmes use nutrition jingles in English and the national languages, films and the nutrition magazine of the Food & Nutrition Policy Planning Division.

There has been no direct project focused on the evaluation of these projects. Although routine health education to adults is not evaluated in a special way, formal education in schools can be assessed by examinations and one must hope that education in this way leads to changes in behaviour. It is often stated that children take such knowledge back to their parents and this too could lead to a change of behaviour within and between families. However, it is not possible to relate this to an immediate change of nutritional status.

Radio programmes are often claimed to be effective when assessed in terms of the numbers listening in, regardless of whether or not the listener's attention has been gained. Very often, the radio is switched on from morning to night in rural homes and there are doubts about the effectiveness of such evaluation.

However, if competitions are organized on the account of a programme, success can be estimated on the recall of the message and its effectiveness can be assessed. Volumes of letters received by the radio station are also used as an index of effectiveness but this is no index of behaviour changes nor of a change in nutritional status. There is another aspect of broadcasting, especially when there is a commercial service with competing messages. The commercial advertisements of a processed food, put over in an attractive and fascinating style, may be more appealing to the audience than officially inspired nutrition messages. Newspaper messages are more lasting. They are pasted in a scrap book for reference and thus have longer effectiveness.

Television programmes are audiovisual and hence can be more effective than radio programmes, because the attention given is deeper as the visual image commands greater attention. However, the potential audience is less than for radio at present, notwithstanding the existence of community sets. Local teledrama is of a high standard, but in the long instalments of drama, the nutrition message may be lost. Also one has to avoid the notion that these programmes are 'government propaganda'.

Specific areas that need attention to make nutrition education effective are out-reach, the time of exposure to education, the content and quality of the nutrition message, the systematic method of communication, and the cost of evaluation, the cost of mass media programmes and incentives for those professionals who are either technical advisers or communicators designing programmes.

Dietary guide-lines for the general public in industrialized nations

Sushma PALMER

Food and Nutrition Board, National Academy of Sciences-National Research Council, 2101 Constitution Ave, NW, (Rm 341), Washington DC 20418, USA.

Emphasis on the role of nutrition in the aetiology and prevention of disease in industrialized nations has shifted from avoiding nutrient deficiency diseases in the first third of this century to refining knowledge of nutrient requirements in the second third. As the major causes of mortality shifted from infectious diseases to chronic degenerative diseases such as heart disease and cancer, attention turned to the role of dietary components in the maintenance of health and reduction of the risk of chronic diseases. However, as Fig. 1 shows, despite remarkable advances in research over the past century, the nutrition message remains essentially unchanged. Yet, the implications of today's message are vastly different for nutrition educators and the public. The average large supermarket in the USA now houses approximately 15 000 foods or 60 000 processed items compared to about 900 foods in 1928[14]. Food selection in the US market-place is influenced by multiple forces that compete for the public's attention: dietary guide-lines from national committees and government agencies coexist with commercial advertisements, popular literature and mass media coverage of nutrition, nutritional claims in health food stores, and pronouncements by self-proclaimed nutrition experts.

Taking developments in the United States as an example, what impact has nutrition advice on dietary practices in industrialized nations today?

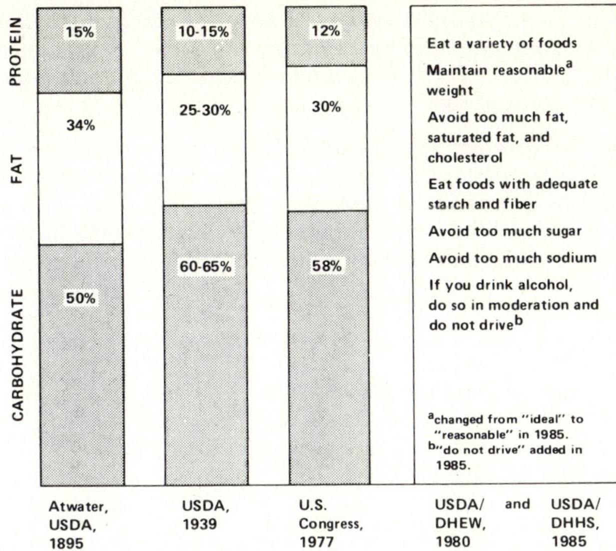

Figure 1. *U.S Dietary Goals, 1895 to 1985.*

Dietary guide-lines for health promotion and disease prevention in the United States and other industrialized countries. Overall, these guide-lines indicate that with two exceptions, all United States and overseas organizations have advised a reduction in total fat for the general population, usually to ~30 per cent of total energy. Although most groups favour a reduction in saturated fats, there is no unanimity about the intake of polyunsaturated fats and cholesterol. Most organizations have also advised increasing complex carbohydrate intake (or dietary fibre), with a concomitant decrease in simple sugars, and a reduction in sodium intake. Eating a variety of foods, maintenance of appropriate body weight, moderation in alcohol consumption, and exercise are universally advised.

Although these dietary recommendations are directed at different chronic diseases such as heart disease, cancer, diabetes, and hypertension or overall health promotion, there appears to be considerable agreement among many industrialized nations on these guide-lines. Nevertheless, dietary goals have generated enormous controversy, especially in the USA and the UK.

Implementation of dietary guide-lines. Despite lack of complete consensus on the guide-lines, innumerable steps have been taken by the public and the private sectors in the USA to implement *Dietary guide-lines for Americans* (the official and most widely accepted recommendations), as well as guide-lines for specific chronic diseases[10]. The role of the US government in this process is to lead, catalyse, and provide strategic support. This involves primarily the Department of Health and Human Services (DHHS) which focuses on nutrition, disease prevention and health promotion and coordinates its activities through a Nutrition Policy Board[12], and the Department of Agriculture (USDA) which has responsibility for research on 'normal' nutrition and which administers such food assistance programmes as the school lunch and the food stamp. The nutrition activities of the two departments are coordinated through several joint committees.

Other groups less directly involved in nutrition policy or its implementation include the Congress, nonprofit-independent organizations such as the Food and Nutrition Board, voluntary health organizations, such as the American Cancer Society, professional associations such as the American Dietetic Association, food and agriculture industries and consumer groups.

Since the 1960s, there has also been a series of government-sponsored dietary intervention trials and multi-level nutrition education programmes in the USA, designed to lower the risk of coronary heart disease[2,4]. More recently, several clinical trials involving dietary intervention have been initiated in an attempt to lower cancer risk.

Conclusions: Impact of dietary guide-lines. What is the impact of nutrition advice on dietary practices and the health of the US population? It is now apparent that the rates of mortality from coronary heart disease in the United States in the last 30 years have declined by approximately 30 per cent[7], and that some unknown proportion of the population has adopted a low-meat or essentially vegetarian lifestyle and adopted some form of regular exercise[3,6].

Table. *Trends in annual food use (per caput) in the United States: 1909–1913 and 1980 (adapted from[13])*

Item	1909–1913	1980	Item	1909–1913	1980
Food energy (kcal)	3480	3540	Vegetables (total)	92.3	95.0
(MJ)	14.6	14.8	dark green/yellow	6.4	10.9
Fats and oils (total)	18.6	27.7	total, fresh	84.5	65
butter	8.2	1.8	total, processed	7.7	35
Meat, poultry, and					
fish (total)	78.2	111.4	Grain products (total)	132	70[b]
beef	24.5	35.5[a]	Sugar and sweeteners		
poultry	8.2	28.2	(total)	41.4	65
fish	5.9	7.7			
Fruit (total)	80	89.5			
citrus	7.7	35			
total, fresh	76.4	48.6			
total, processed	3.6	40.5			

[a]18% decline between 1976–1980; [b]9% increase during 1972–1980.

Furthermore, as the Table shows, trends in food use in the United States have changed dramatically in this century. In particular, the use of saturated fats (eg butter and lard) has declined by about 80 per cent being largely replaced by vegetable fats and margarine and other edible fats and salad oils. Poultry consumption increased by over 200 per cent; dairy products generally increased with a quadrupling in the use of low-fat milk during the second half of the century and a 50 per cent reduction in the use of whole milk. Per capita citrus fruit intake has quadrupled. The use of sugars and other sweeteners, however, was at a record high in 1980 representating an increase of 50 per cent since 1903–1913[13].

Although there is evidence that the American public has changed its food habits, in many ways that are consistent with the various dietary recommendations, it is unclear to what extent these changes or the reduction in cardiovascular disease are due to nutrition education programmes aimed at producing such change. Furthermore, there is no concomitant decline in the prevalence of obesity, and dietary guide-lines for cancer are too recent for their impact to be assessed.

Recommendations: challenge for the future. Taking all these factors into account, what are the next steps? Clearly, better *implementation of existing knowledge* is warranted. There is a need to refine existing educational tools and to develop new ones; and government policies, strategic support, and agricultural incentives are needed to encourage more widespread adoption of guide-lines in commerce.

Furthermore, *additional research* is needed to permit evaluation of the outcome in relation to dietary change[5]. Research is needed to learn the 'natural history' of dietary patterns to determine factors which shape people's eating habits. In addition, to understand the obstacles to change, research is needed to analyze behaviours and motivations of persons who have already changed their diets in the desirable directions while simultaneously studying those who have not changed their diets.

1 Atwater, W.O. (1895): Food and diet. In *Yearbook of the United States Department of Agriculture, 1894*, p. 358. Washington DC: Government Printing Office.
2 Farquhar, J.W., Maccoby, N., Wood, P.D., Alexander, J.K., Breitrose, H., Brown, B.W. Jr., Haskell, W.L., McAlister, A.L., Meyer, A.J., Nash, J.D. & Stern, M.P. (1977): Community education for cardiovascular health. *Lancet* **1**, 1192–1195.
3 Marks Clements Research Inc. (1980): Highlights from a study of trends in nutrition. The benchmark survey, February 1980, conducted for Self Magazine (New York).
4 Multiple Risk Factor Intervention Trial Research Group (1982): Multiple risk factor intervention trials. Risk factor changes and mortality results. *J. Am. Med. Ass.* **248**, 1465–1477.
5 National Research Council, Committee on Diet, Nutrition, and Cancer (1983): *Diet, nutrition, and cancer: directions for research*. Washington DC: Commission on Life Sciences, National Academy of Sciences.
6 Rowland, M. & Roberts, J. (1982): Blood pressure levels and hypertension in persons ages 6–74: United States, 1976–80. *Advance Data from Vital and Health Statistics*, **84**, 1–11. Maryland: Public Health Service.
7 Stamler, J. (1985): Coronary heart disease: Doing the right things. *New Engl. J. Med.* **312**, 1053–1055.
8 US Congress, Senate Select Subcommittee on Nutrition and Human Needs (1977): *Dietary goals for the United States*, 2nd edn. Stock No. 052–070–94376–8. Washington DC: Governing Printing Office.
9 US Department of Agriculture (1939): *Food and life: Yearbook of agriculture, 1939*, pp. 7–8. Washington DC: Government Printing Office.
10 US Department of Agriculture and Department of Health and Human Services (1985): *Report of the Dietary Guidelines Advisory Committee on the dietary guidelines for Americans*. Washington DC: US Department of Agriculture and Department of Health and Human Services.
11 US Department of Agriculture and Department of Health, Education, and Welfare (1980): *Nutrition and your health-dietary guidelines for Americans*. Washington DC: US Department of Agriculture and Department of Health, Education, and Welfare.
12 US Department of Health and Human Services, Office of Disease Prevention and Health Promotion (1983): *Public health implementation plans for attaining the objectives of the nation*. Public Health Reports (Suppl. to Sept.–Oct. issues), PHS 83–50193A, pp. 132–154. Washington DC: Government Printing Office.
13 Welsh, S.O. & Marston, R.M. (1982): Review of trends in food use in the United States, 1909 to 1980. *J. Am. Diet. Ass.* **81**, 120–125.
14 Woteki, C. (1985): Improving estimates of food and nutrient intake: applications to individuals and groups. *J. Am. Diet. Ass.* **85**, 295–296.

Nutrition education for adults in developed nations: education of at-risk groups

Leena RÄSÄNEN
Department of Nutrition, SF-00710 Helsinki, Finland.

The content, emphasis and target-groups of nutrition education have been different in different times, due to changes in life-style and patterns of disease. The aim of this article is to consider the different ways of defining at-risk groups in nutrition education in developed nations today. The question of whether the content of nutrition education can be similar for groups which have been categorized as being 'at risk' by criteria of different types will also be discussed.

Criteria for defining at-risk groups in nutrition education. It is possible to distinguish three main principles used to categorize the groups believed to benefit most from the change in dietary habits to be achieved through nutrition education (Table).

The first way to define at-risk groups has been used in traditional nutrition education and in older textbooks of nutrition. It classifies individuals on the basis of their biological and physiological characteristics. The emphasis on nutrition education of the so-called vulnerable groups such as infants, adolescents, pregnant women or elderly people has been justified by the exceptionally great nutritional requirements for their supposed low intake of nutrients. Therefore, special educational efforts have been considered necessary to improve their diets. The results of most dietary surveys performed in industrialized countries show clearly, however,

Table. *Three different causes of nutritional risk in populations*

1. Risk of nutritional deficiency due to under-consumption
   (eg infants, adolescents, pregnant women, elderly people)
2. Health risk due to over-consumption
   (eg coronary heart disease, hypertension, dental caries, obesity)
3. Nutritional and health risk due to an imbalance in the composition of the diet and a simultaneous low energy consumption
   (eg refined diets)

that is not possible to use biological criteria to classify individuals so easily into groups inside which the diets are homogeneous but different from those of the other subgroups. Each of the so called vulnerable groups consists of individuals whose diet and nutritional situation may be completely different due to different social and economic background. It would be impractical, perhaps impossible, to give them identical nutrition education in the hope that each of them could easily apply the advice to his own situation.

The second way to define at-risk groups is to identify those individuals who are particularly susceptible to nutrition-related diseases because of either genetic or environmental factors. Examples of diseases common in all developed countries for which the possibilities of dietary prevention are considered good are cardiovascular diseases, certain types of cancer and dental caries as well as obesity, which increases the risk of many diseases. Common to all these conditions is that overconsumption of some dietary components, eg saturated fats, sodium, sugar or energy, are well-known risk factors for them.

When the prevalence and mortality rate of these diseases is high in a population, it also means that a considerable proportion of the so far healthy people will later fall ill. Neither morbidity nor mortality figures include the great number of people so far in the first asymptomatic phases of the diseases, at which time dietary changes can still play a decisive role in preventing the further development of the disease. In addition, there is no doubt of the usefulness of including in the target group of health and nutrition education not only the at-risk individuals themselves, but also the healthy members of their families and close relatives who also have a higher than average risk of getting the disease due to inherited characteristics and shared environment. This means that, using the increased susceptibility or early symptoms of diseases as criteria, the great majority of the population should be included in at-risk groups and thus into target groups of intensified nutrition education in most developed countries.

The third and newest way to examine nutritional at-risk groups is to classify individuals on the basis of the composition of their diets and their energy intakes. This approach can be argued by the following facts. The large share of refined, energy-yielding components such as fats, sugar and alcohol in the diet has become one of the most important nutritional problems in developed nations during the past few decades. In addition to the direct adverse effects these dietary components have on health, a high consumption of refined foods also means that the nutrient density or the concentration of vitamins, trace elements and fibre in the diet, and their total intake, tends to be low or inadequate. As a result of reduced habitual physical activity the energy consumption is now often so low in developed nations that it is impossible to satisfy the need of essential nutrients with the small amount of food eaten. The nutritional risk is aggravated when low energy intake is combined with a low nutrient density of diet (Fig.).

Thus in developed nations, at-risk groups nowadays consist more and more often of individuals whose diet has a low nutrient density and whose energy consumption is small. Such individuals have at the same time the risk of an inadequate intake of vitamins and minerals and the risk of a higher than recommended intake of such dietary components as saturated fats, sugar and alcohol, which play a role in the aetiology of several diseases.

The content of nutrition education directed to at-risk groups. It can be asked whether the three different types of risk groups presented above have any common characteristics or whether their special needs create problems or controversy when the content of nutrition education is planned. The recommendations presented in various connections for the different

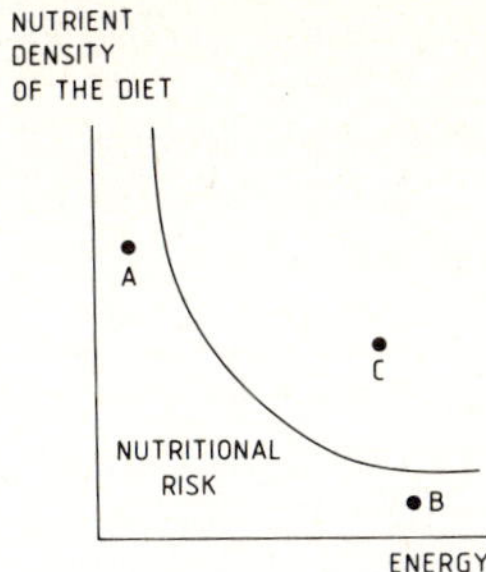

Fig. *Relationship between nutrient density of the diet and energy intake in causing nutritional risk.* A = low intake of vitamins and minerals due to small total intake of food; B = low intake of vitamins and minerals and high intake of fats, sugar and/or alcohol; C = adequate intake of vitamins and minerals and moderate intake of fats, sugar and/or alcohol.

types of at-risk groups have, however, a remarkably similar core content and lead, when applied in nutrition education, to very similar educational messages and practical advice.

The Finnish health authorities base the nutrition education of at-risk groups on the third principle presented above[1]. This approach is considered to cover also the at-risk groups defined by the other two criteria; that is, to take care of the special nutritional needs of the so-called vulnerable groups and to further the primary prevention of nutrition-related diseases. This strategy has been chosen because it is obvious that the risk factors and determinants of major diseases concern the majority of the population. Thus, the Finnish health authorities and nutrition educators have decided to recommend to the entire population such dietary changes which increase the nutrient density of the diet, decrease the risk of nutritional deficiencies and which at the same time are beneficial in the prevention of nutrition-relared diseases[2].

Concluding remarks. Nutrition education alone cannot realistically prevent or remedy the problems which orginate from individuals' behaviour, which is determined by environmental and social factors. It is not sufficient to try to persuade at-risk individuals to adopt a more healthy diet. To achieve this aim environmental modification is needed to remove barriers which hamper nutrition education.

Preventive nutrition involves not only nutrition education, but also other activities, ranging from regulating practices of the government — legislation, pricing policy — to general social policy aimed at changing the environment to support individuals' healthy food choices. The success of nutrition education is dependent on social policy, the feasibility of which is itself determined by the responsiveness created by education. Regulating practices or measures to change behaviour may prove to be unacceptable or inefficient if the population has not been prepared for them. The health-promoting alternative in nutrition has to be perceived as beneficial and sensible both for the individual and for the society.

1 Advisory Committee for Health Education (1983): General plan for the development of health education for 1984–88, p. 94. *Series Original Reports* 2/1983, Helsinki: The National Board of Health, Finland.
2 Finnish Nutrition Committee (1981): Summary of the report of the Finnish Nutrition Committee, p. 20. Helsinki: Ministry of Social Affairs and Health.

Nutrition education for adults in a developing country. Ten years of Philippine experience

F.S. SOLON
Nutrition Center of the Philippines, MCC PO Box 653, Makati, Metro Manila, Philippines.

As one of the developing countries seriously affected by malnutrition, the Philippines has long been engaged in nutrition education. The Philippine Nutrition Program (PNP) was set in motion soon after the establishment in 1974 of the National Nutrition Council (NNC) as the highest coordinating body on nutrition.

The problem of malnutrition then and now confronting the country took the form mainly of protein-energy deficiency, mostly affecting pre-school and schoolchildren. Other serious forms of the problem were iron deficiency, vitamin A deficiency and iodine deficiency.

Policy. Nutrition Information, Education, and Communication (NIEC) is one of the four major intervention schemes of the Philippine Nutrition Program. (The others are Food Assistance, Food Production, and Health Protection). The National Nutrition Council issued Policy Direction No. 4 (on Nutrition Education) which stated: 'Nutrition education, information and communication programmes shall be designed to stimulate demands for and encourage maximum utilization of indigenous foods which are nutritious'.

The NIEC goal is to improve the nutrition practices of the family, by increasing the knowledge of the family members of nutrition concepts and developing favourable attitudes particularly towards responsibility, self-reliance and cooperation in the family and the community.

Audience. The NIEC effort of the PNP is directed mainly at adult target audiences, especially those who wield a significant amount of influence in the shaping of opinion and policy, and who control the decision-making processes in the allocation and use of resources in the home, community, and country.

The major targets of nutrition education are at the household level, particularly depressed and malnourished families, who are the main beneficiaries of the programme. This audience category is generally rural and of low income, health, and educational status.

Approach. Because of socio-cultural conditions in the country, which require a flexible, personalized education approach especially in the rural areas, the use of face-to-face communications is predominant. Mass media are extensively used to reinforce this personal approach, but the educational effort relies heavily on the development of a nationwide task force which can provide a direct and credible link to the family at the grassroots level.

The personnel of more than 20 government and private agencies engaged in nutrition work participate in institutional and promotional work at various levels. The key educational link at the community level, however, is a local resident selected and trained to provide basic nutrition and health services to his own village. Called the barangay nutrition scholar (BNS), he/she serves as the final relay point for nutrition messages addressed to the household. There are now more than 10 000 BNS throughout the country.

Organization. At the national level is the National Nutrition Council consisting of the heads of the Ministries of Agriculture (chairman), Health, Education, Social Services and Development, Local Government, and National Science and Technology Authority, and of three private organizations: Philippine Medical Association, Nutrition Foundation of the Philippines, and the Nutrition Center of the Philippines. The NNC has its management committee and six technical committees. At sub-national levels are the regional, provincial, municipal, and barangay committees, each headed by the highest government official at that level (governor for the province, mayor for the municipality, barangay captain for the village). Under the barangay nutrition committee is the barangay network composed of all puroks (subdivisions) in the village. Each purok is headed by a teacher-coordinator and a purok leader and is, in turn, composed of several units, each made up of 20 households under a unit leader.

Activities. *(a) Initial drive.* Among the first thrusts of the PNP was a nutrition awareness campaign which focussed on the mass media. A concerted effort of government agencies and private organization, it combined the general public information approach with advertising techniques drawing the support of influential segments of the private sector. *(b) Nutrition 'School of the air'.* To provide continuing education to homemakers and sustain their awareness of and interest in the PNP classes on the air were organized in 1974 by the Food and Nutrition Research Center, Nutrition Foundation of the Philippines, and the Department (now Ministry) of Education. The course consisted of a series of 11 lessons divided into three sets based on priority information areas. It featured simple, but detailed, discussions on basic nutrition information, nutrition of vulnerable age groups, and related fields. *(c) Mass media nutrition education study.* The use of radio and modern marketing methods was the subject of an educational experiment conducted in the mid 1970s by Manoff International in a Philippine province (Iloilo)[1]. The project involved the use of commercial radio to broadcast recorded 60-second messages throughout the day for one year. Carefully designed and pretested, each radio spot sought to introduce new ways of infant care. The novella or soap opera (mini-drama) format was chosen to present these messages. The behavioural objectives were to increase the number of women beginning supplemental feeding to infants by the 6th month of age and who added chopped fish, green vegetables, and cooking oil to rice porridge by the 6th month. Results showed that a statistically significant number of mothers adopted the recommendations of the messages to enrich their rice porridge with cooking oil, fish and green vegetables. Consequent changes in behaviour as to child feeding habits were recorded in up to 25 per cent of the population. *(d) 'Nutri-bus' project.* A mobile comprehensive system called the 'nutri-bus' was organized in 1978 by the Nutrition Center of the Philippines to provide logistical, supervisory, and communication support to the barangay nutrition scholars (BNS). Using video tape to conduct community showings of educational modules, and well-trained nurse communicators to ensure successful audience reception of nutrition messages, the nutri-bus has proved to be cost-effective.

The nutri-bus offers: nutrition education of target populations through VTR showings and distribution of printed materials; promotion of the nutri-pak food supplement, and continuing education for the BNS. A nutri-bus unit reaches 90 villages (and their BNS) or an average population of 90 000 consisting of approximately 13 000 mothers, 360 teachers, 18 000 pre-schoolchildren and 12 000 schoolchildren.

As of June 1985, there were 23 nutri-bus units in operation in 13 provinces and eight cities in ten regions, assisting 1542 BNS. *(e) Radio campaign.* From July 1 to December 31, 1983, taped 60-second spots were aired thrice a day on radio to promote specific nutrition concepts, namely, breast-feeding, supplementary feeding weighing of pre-schoolchildren, BNS activities, and feeding the child with the family's food. *(f) Regional nutrition information group (RNIG).* This group was organized in the late 1970s, in order to make the nutrition information campaign fit the needs of identified regions. The 17 priority nutrition messages were translated into the local dialects and disseminated to target audiences through diverse media. *(g) Nutrition Institute for Distance Study (NIDS).* This further, multi-media, inter-agency effort was launched in 1976 to disseminate programmed information nationwide to specific professionals such as physicians, nurses and teachers, to mobilize their support for the nutrition effort. The NIST undertaking later evolved a unique system of extending nutrition education in schools to the household. Called the Teacher-child-parent (TCP) approach, the system involves a relay concept of transmitting nutrition messages to the home through the pupils in an interactive cycle. *(h) 'Strengthening community-based organizations for nutrition' (SCON).* This is a community-level educational effort which places emphasis on the training of local leaders and implementors in the planning and management of nutrition and related development programmes, bringing together NCP technical personnel and local nutrition committee workers. Approaches include the creation of awareness and sensitivity of target groups to nutrition concepts, organizational work and training, planning, and technical assistance to these groups in the development and implementation of programmes. *(i) 'People's adoption of total health self-sufficiency' (PATHS) training.* The Philippine Medical Association also undertook the training of barangay residents to provide basic health, family planning, and nutrition interventions in their localities. The project included training for gainful occupation and proper placement of the unemployed and underemployed barangay members, with built-in flexibility for integration into existing health programmes in the community.

NIEC Production. Much printed material has been placed in the mainstream of the PNP since its inception in 1974. Newsletters, leaflets, manuals, monographs, comic books, posters, flipcharts, brochures and calendars have been addressed to various target audiences. In addition use has been made of VTR modules and community video modules for the nutri-bus project, together with radio plugs, TV spots, and jingles on specific health and nutrition topics. Most of these materials have been translated into the major Philippines dialects for use in the overall NIEC campaign.

Evaluation. In 1978, an evaluation report[4] was prepared on the overall and strategic effectiveness of the PNP. General recipients scored high in awareness of nutrition concepts (functions and nutritive value of different food groups, food substitutability, food selection, and general sanitation) and in attitude (knowledge of the rationale behind specific food preparation techniques, the need to serve infant and young children prior to other family members, the need for proper feeding of sick children, and food sanitation). They also attained a high level of practice on the selected concepts (balanced diet, food preparation techniques, family food distribution, care for the sick child, food handling and sanitation, and general sanitation). Performance of pregnant/lactating mothers was similarly outstanding. These high levels of performance were indicative of the effectiveness of the NIE thrust, both through community activities and the mass media.

A subsequent evaluation was undertaken on the impact of the nutri-bus project in 1979 and 1981 to measure changes in knowledge, attitude, and nutritional status of the programme beneficiaries. 1979 results showed that mothers in villages exposed to more VTR showings were 55 per cent more likely to describe complete meals; 473 per cent more likely to name nutri-pak as a good snack; and 71 per cent more likely to give correct specific descriptions of nutri-pak than the BNS mothers. The 1981 study showed that the 1979 levels of knowledge had been well maintained. On nutritional status, a comparison of the results of the 1979 and 1981 studies indicated a 17 per cent decrease in second and third degree malnutrition and 12 per cent increase in normal and first degree malnutrition.

1 Cooke, T.M. (1977): *Radio, advertising techniques, and nutrition education: a summary of a field experiment in the Philippines and Nicaragua. A final report.* New York: Manoff International Inc.
2 Intengan, C. (1962): Forty-year review of nutrition progress in the Philippines. *Phil. J. Nutr.* **15**, 14–45.
3 Jose, A.M. (1982): Thirty-five years of food and nutrition work. *Phil. J. Nutr.* **35**, 158–170.
4 Philippines National Nutrition Council (1978): *Overall and strategic effectiveness of the Philippine Nutrition Program.* Manila: Sycip, Gorres, Velayo and Co.
5 Philippines National Nutrition Council (1981): *The Philippine nutrition program implementing guidelines.*
6 H.M. Sinclair & G.R. Howat, editors (1980): *World nutrition and nutrition education.* Oxford: Oxford University Press.
7 World Bank. Population, Health and Nutrition Dept. (1984): *Population, health and nutrition in the Philippines: a sector review.* Washington DC: World Bank.
References 2, 3, 5–7 are listed as further bibliography only.

★   ★   ★

PROMOTING AND COMMUNICATING NUTRITION

Indigenous food system: maintenance or replacement?
Prospects for nutrition education in broadening the food base with traditional food plants

A. MASCARENHAS
Institute of Resource Assessment, University of Dar es Salaam, Box 35097, Dar es Salaam, Tanzania.

Massive changes have been taking place in the food supply and dietary habits of various parts of sub-Saharan Africa. Only a few of the changes have been positive. Because most research on this question has lacked a multidisciplinary approach, the full implications of these changes have not been fully appreciated. Little attention, for example, has been paid to contributions by anthropologists and other social scientists. Yet if the nature of food and nutrition problems are better understood nutrition education may make a very significant impact.

Constraints to intervention. Professional agriculturalists working in Africa have traditionally been more interested in the promotion of export crops than in food crops required for local consumption. In the meantime the problems of food insecurity have become increasingly severe. As a consequence attention has even been diverted away from the longer-term priority of agricultural development[1].

The medical profession, on the other hand, has been so hard pressed just dealing with ever growing numbers of malnourished patients that useful non medical options have largely been over-looked. Nutrition intervention has concentrated on the symptoms of malnutrition. Thus, the planning and programming that was involved generally was centred around the role of the nutritionists themselves. This led to an impasse between economic and nutrition planning.

The scale of the crisis. It would not be an exaggeration to state that never in the history of the human race have so many people faced the spectre of malnutrition and starvation than in this decade. The food problem in Africa in less than 20 years has moved from local to national, then regional, and now to continental proportions. The rapidity of this deterioration has been complicated by the scale of the problem. In Ethiopia, the exact population is not known, but the 9 million or so presently affected require much more infrastructure than is nationally available.

Reasons for the distortion of the food base. The present calamity is mainly man-made and can be brought under control. What are the reasons for this distortion? Since changes in diets and food patterns take place within a specific physical and socio-economic context, Tanzania will be used as an example.

Many of the foods now common in most of Africa were introduced by movements of people. In Tanzania the crops such as cassava, cashew, pineapples, wheat and maize were largely introduced by the Portuguese in the 15th and 16th centuries. When changes are slow, over decades and centuries, there is time for people to adjust: the more recent trends have been much more sudden.

Uneven attention to the food and agricultural sector. In most sub-Saharan African countries, agriculture dominates the national economy. For a large number of them, as much as 30–60 per cent of their GNP is accounted for by the agricultural sector. In 29 out of 47 countries in sub-Saharan Africa, over 70 per cent of the labour force is in agriculture. Nevertheless investment has gone elsewhere, to such competing sectors as education or health.

Neglect of the subsistence sector. There has been another major flawed assumption — that the subsistence sector could fend for itself, despite changing social and economic conditions in the rural areas. Given the very poor technology was it realistic for peasants to be expected to produce the export crops, for the much-needed foreign exchange, as well as the food crops? Only under special conditions — such as in the coffee/banana agricultural system in the Kilimanjaro — was this a reasonable expectation. In Tanzania, as in most other parts of Africa, the emphasis was clearly on export crops; four specific research centres were established in the 1930s and 1940s to promote sisal, cotton, coffee and cotton.

Neglect of women as producers of food. Since most work by women in both rural and urban areas is generally related to food, any pressure on their time and well being negatively influences the food situation. At times even positive changes can be distorted. For instance, the introduction of hybrid maize has greatly increased yields in parts of Tanzania, but if village plots are several miles from women's homes, there is no way to carry back the harvest and time constraints are prohibitive. An important aspect of the change from subsistence to commercial agriculture is that such a shift undermines the production of crops for their nutrition — an aspect which is unlikely to change[2]. Related to this factor is that our knowledge of what women collected and cooked is so abysmal that any intervention has to be undertaken with great caution.

The urban bias. Perhaps no single factor in the distortion by decision-makers of the traditional food base is as significant as the urban bias. Although the percentage of the population living in urban areas is small, the pace of urbanization has been accelerating and the influence of urban dwellers is out of proportion to their numbers.

While all people in the urban areas have to eat, it does not follow that all have employment, nor that all can afford their preferred foods nor, were these foods conveniently available, in the right quality and amount. As the national agricultural sector began to decline because of neglect, it increasingly became necessary to import staples — maize, wheat and even rice — which were conveniently available from the developed countries. Because wages were low, imports were subsidized and the price of locally produced foods had to be artifically depressed.

The low price of food also has a pervasive influence provided they can be purchased in the rural areas. Economically, it makes more sense to purchase rather than produce the grains (provided they can be purchased at official prices!). During periods of stress — drought or floods — it was convenient for decision makers, living in capital cities, to make famine relief available from imported food items.

Narrow concept of food. Most national food strategies which have been drawn up recently have been strongly influenced by the crisis situation in Africa — specifically the droughts and related catastrophies and the problems of feeding the urban dwellers. As a result, the documents that have been hastily drawn focus on a few staples and are based on information which is relevant and available mainly to the urban areas. There is also an implicit assumption that manpower, research and infrastructure will be available.

The significance of supplementary staples has hardly been covered. It is generally assumed that wild plant foods are of a supplementary or emergency nature, implying that they are not eaten regularly. In many cases they are not at all peripheral to the diet[3]. Indeed, even in the urban areas supplement foods play a very important role.

The tradition that agricultural research and investment did not favour food crops continued long after independence. It has now become all too evident that although most developing countries have the prime objective of providing adequate levels of food, hunger has persisted and in some countries has reached calamitous levels. Weaknesses in policy design and failure to understand the complex linkages between production and consumption are responsible for this situation[4].

Food imports and negative aspects to development. Even with two-thirds of the country susceptible to drought from time to time due to inadequate rainfall, the resource base of Tanzania and the adjustment possibilities are adequate to produce enough food and even ensure a surplus. But hunger and malnutrition have persisted. The difference between good years and poor years is great. The ratio of food imports to total export revenue was of the order of 5.5 per cent per annum for the period 1967–76: in the 1974–75 crisis, the figure shot up to 22 per cent.

Prices for primary commodities are on the decline. In contrast, the prices of imported manufactured goods has spiralled upwards. Imported petroleum products contribute about 7 per cent of Tanzania's needs, yet absorb over 50 per cent of its earnings. This means that there is little purchasing power left over to import food. But like many poor countries Tanzania imports food. Concessional food aid for the three cereals — maize, rice, wheat — has literally doubled every year. In 1978–9 it was 12.8, in 1979–80 25, in 1980–1 42.8 and in 1981–2 88 million US dollars.

Most studies on food security in the third world have defined food solely as cereals. Yet the proportion of cereals varies from 85 per cent in Afghanistan to only 16 per cent in Zaire. In Africa and Latin America the role of non-cereals in consumption is very important and must be incorporated into any meaningful consumption equation[5].

Conclusion. The problems of food and nutrition touch almost every aspect of human development. The task ahead is very formidable. Still the central question remains — what are the prospects for nutrition education in broadening the food base with traditional food plants? There is no easy or single answer. There are many options and possibilities to take advantage of and to capitalize upon. The prospects depend to what extent we are prepared to be realistic. Only five areas will be touched upon.

If we accept that food and nutrition problems touch every aspect of development, then one thing should become very obvious — the problems are too large to be resolved by nutritionists alone. This means that there is need to redefine the role of nutrition educators and also to seek areas of collaboration with economists, agriculturalists, ecologists.

Secondly, the crisis in Africa indicates that there have been flaws in past development strategies. The blame must be accepted both by the developing countries as well as by developed countries and international institutions. The victims have been the producers of food. If the producers were to put their case first, it would probably result in the following; a greater reliance on foods that the producers know about rather than dependence on staples produced in distant places for quite different reasons.

Thirdly, the traditional food plants have to be promoted not by excluding viable 'modern' options but in the context of broadening the food base which was increasingly becoming narrow. The advantage of this strategy are tremendous — variety, improved security, a better and cheaper balance of diets.

Fourthly, the prospects for broadening the food base will be considerably enhanced if much more attention was paid to the central role of women in food and nutrition. Like all sensitive issues there are no major formulas — centuries of tradition cannot be changed overnight but neither should they be prolonged beyond what is reasonble. If the last decade was spent on being conscious of the other half of the human population (women), the next decade could well be spent on learning from them. This may well open new dimensions in the sciences — human and basic sciences.

Finally, food and nutrition issues have on the one hand to be looked at globally, but there is an equal need to look at the neglected end of the spectrum. At the household, village, district and national levels, the options which are possible are different. At the lower levels the dependence and security which the traditional foods offer are frequently greater than has been appreciated hitherto. This then is one of the biggest challenges we have.

1 Clay, E., Chambers, R., Singer, H. & Lipton, M. (1981): Food policy issues in low income countries. Staff Working Paper No. 473, Washington.
2 Dewey, K.G. (1979): Agricultural development, diet and nutrition. *Ecol. Food Nutr.* **8**, 265–273.
3 Fleuret, A. (1979): The role of wild foliage plants in the diet — a case study from Lushoto, Tanzania. *Ecol. Food Nutr.* **8**, 87–93.
4 Longhurst, R. (1983): Agricultural production and food consumption: some neglected linkages food and nutrition. *FAO* **9**, 2–5.
5 Valdes, A. & Konan Dreas, P. (1981): Food security in developing countries. In *Food security in developing countries*, ed A. Valdes. Boulder Co: Westview Press.

The newly industrializing countries — nutrition education in the face of rapid change. Experience in Bahrain

A.O. MUSAIGER
Nutrition Unit, Public Health Directorate, PO Box 42, Manama, Bahrain.

Bahrain, like other Gulf States, is small in size and population. The cultivated land is very limited as compared to the total land. The *per caput* income is relatively high (US $ 8000), when compared to other developing countries. The percentage of expatriates mainly from India, Pakistan and other middle-eastern countries is about 32 per cent of the total population.

Health and nutrition problems in Bahrain have changed as a result of an alteration in the socio-economic status. Infective and parasitic diseases were the major causes of deaths in the past. Nowadays, cardiovascular diseases are the leading cause of deaths. It is generally believed that the nutritional status of the people has improved. This is mainly due to the improvement in primary and secondary health care rather than the change in food habits. The decrease in illiteracy and the relative rise in health awareness are factors which have played an important role in improving health status.

However, despite the above advantages, undernutrition and overnutrition continue to exist. Malnutrition is still the most common nutritional disorder among infants and young children. Moderate and mild malnutrition are more frequent, while a severe case is very rare. Rickets and other vitamin deficiencies especially vitamin A and C are rarely reported by health practitioners. Iron deficiency anaemia, sickle-cell anaemia and thalassaemia are prevalent, particularly among young children[1].

Difficulties in teaching nutrition in Bahrain. *(1) The role of advertising in changing food habits.* Nutrition education faces a big challenge from advertising, particularly with the rapid growth of the mass media. In Bahrain, television and video occupy most of the leisure time of the public. This is due to a lack of other recreational facilities and the relatively high rate of illiteracy. Of households in Manama City (the capital of Bahrain) 98.7 per cent have one television set or more. The availability of television in almost all Bahraini households should facilitate the process of informal nutrition education. Unfortunately as reported by Al-Umran (unpublished) the health and nutrition programmes shown by Bahrain television are uninteresting and relatively ineffective. There is a lack of overall planning of programmes.

Where informal nutrition education is failing to capture the attention of the audiences, the advertising of food products is succeeding. Nutritionists always declare that food habits are difficult to change, but advertising induces many changes. A recent study[10] showed that 42.1 per cent and 47.1 per cent of Bahraini mothers 'believed' and 'moderately believed' food advertisement claims, respectively. It was reported that 48.5 per cent of mothers purchased food seen in the television advertisements and 39.5 per cent sometimes purchased[8].

Advertising is largely responsible for the growing consumption of sugar-products which increase the incidence of dental caries as well as obesity and its related problems[16]. Children are more vulnerable to advertisements for sugar foods such as chocolates and sweets. In Bahrain, it has been shown[7] that children enjoyed watching chocolates and sweets advertisements more than any other food advertisements. Of the children surveyed, 59 per cent always requested food advertised on television, whereas, 29.8 per cent and 11.2 per cent were sometimes and rarely requested, respectively. About 95 per cent of the mothers respond to their children's request, and almost 90 per cent stated that their children's requests affected the family expenditure.

(2) The conflict between advertising and nutrition education. Television food advertisements frequently contain little or no information on nutrition. Moreover, most of the foods advertised are of a poor nutritional value[2]. Advertising claims are highly accepted as fact by consumers, and this sharply affects the nutrition education message. For example if the advertisement claims that a certain food product will make your child grow strong and healthy, how can we nutrition educators convince the public that this claim is not true, especially when we lack the technique to compete with the advertising agencies?

A high percentage (55.7 per cent) of Bahraini mothers considered that television food advertisements helped to increase their nutrition knowledge. It was found that television advertisements were the main source of knowledge about food products[7]. The Table highlights how advertising influences the nutrition knowledge of Bahraini mothers.

The situation becomes more complicated when we realize that the majority of the younger generation have no understanding of what is meant for example by protein and starchy foods, vitamins and a balanced diet. Nutrition claims in food advertising can be misleading if

Table. *Responses of Bahraini mothers to questions on content of television food advertisements[7].*

Statements	*% Agreeing*
— Advertisements on TV keep me informed of good and healthy foods	74.4
— Food advertised on TV help children choose their food in a better way	62.8
— Foods advertised on TV are good and useful	62.8
— Baby foods advertised on TV encourage mother to use them and abandon breast-feeding	57.5
— Modern housewives are those who depend on food advertisements for purchasing food	46.8
— Food advertisements make one purchase unuseful foods	10.9

consumers misinterpret information because of a lack of knowledge about the meaning of nutrition words or concepts[17]. Girls are more knowledgeable on nutrition terms than boys and this difference may be due to the teaching of home economics to the girls as many educators still think that home economics is a subject only for girls. It seems that neither school nor nutrition education through the mass media can protect the public from the misleading food advertising claims, especially in the absence of advertising regulations.

(3) Illiteracy and ignorance. The percentage of illiteracy among Bahrainis is still high (31 per cent) as compared to inhabitants of other industrialized countries and is higher among females (41 per cent) than males (21 per cent). Booklets and leaflets are widely used as tools for nutrition and health education and the Ministry of Health in Bahrain spends thousands of dollars in printing these publications, which are hardly ever read. About one-third of visitors to the health centres in Bahrain read the booklets, while the majority did not read them, according to a pilot study[12]. Almost 19 per cent of the visitors could not read or write, and the percentage was higher among females (29 per cent) than males (8 per cent).

We do not know how much those who read the booklets benefited from them. It is well known that giving the people the facts about nutrition does not ensure that their food habits will change[15] and it is doubtful if this method of education is worthwhile continuing.

Ignorance about sound nutrition is the most important factor responsible for poor nutritional status in Bahrain. There is no scarcity of food. We currently have the most varied and nutritious foods to be found in the industrialized countries; the problem lies in the lack of a wise selection of these foods, as well as in food faddism. Many people accept false beliefs about food, despite having completed secondary or university education[3]. Surprisingly, we have found that all of the educated people attending health centres in Bahrain were practising many unsound food habits and believed in numerous food faddisms[13].

Even health practitioners are deficient in nutritional knowledge; there is inadequate knowledge about the nutritional value of various foods at all levels from physician to consumer[6]. Many nutritionists, food planners and health personnel, who are expected to be more knowledgeable about infant feeding, in fact often have little modern information and are ill-prepared to advise[5]. In Bahrain 69 per cent of the mothers thought that they were told to use bottle-feeding by health practitioners[9].

(4) The wrong selection of the target group. Mothers are always selected as the target group for communication messages either in Bahrain or in other developing countries. It has been shown that 90 per cent of the nutrition education programmes in the developing countries used mothers as the target group[4]. Several factors influence the selection of a particular group as the target. Among these factors, the socio-cultural and religious are the most important ones, particularly in Muslim countries. Nutrition educators often select their target group according to what is written in the text-books, without taking into consideration to socio-cultural customs which effect the nutritional status of the particular community. Most of these books were prepared for use in a different culture, eg African, Latin American, but not Arab communities. For example, in Bahrain, education of mothers would not help much in improving the nutritional status of the family because the father has a great influence on decision-making and food-purchasing. Even when the mother is well educated, the father is often the person who decides whether the mother should attend the nutrition education class or not. This is particularly true in low and middle socio-economic classes.

Groups which have the responsibility for making policy decisions which eventually influence nutritional status, such as government officials and health planners, should also be selected as a target group. Without convincing these people about the need of nutrition education programmes, it is difficult to get good support to run these programmes.

(5) The influence of foreign housemaids on food habits. Bahraini families have become more and more dependent on the services of housemaids. Most of these housemaids are poorly educated (60 per cent), and only 41 per cent of them can understand Arabic. They come from countries such as Sri Lanka, India, Pakistan and other Far-East countries. They are responsible for all levels of home management, in addition to feeding the infants and young children. Therefore, it is widely

accepted that these housemaids have a big influence on the food habits of the children in Bahrain[14].

Who, then, should be taught proper nutrition? Is it the mother or the father or the housemaid or may be all of them? The task of nutrition education has thus become more complicated, especially when the majority of housemaids do not understand Arabic. Therefore the medium of nutrition education should be in other languages in addition to Arabic in order to reach the expatriates engaged in domestic work.

(6) Television. The geographical location of Bahrain, allows its people to see as much as six to ten TV broadcasting channels from neighbouring countries. Thus, there is no guarantee that the nutrition message will reach the audience. I have shown that only 45 per cent of young people preferred to see Bahrain TV, the rest preferring to see other channels. This will create a difficult task for nutrition educators who aim to ensure that the nutrition message is being received by the target group. Coordination between the Arab Gulf countries in regard to nutrition education is highly recommended, in order to avoid contradiction in the information provided.

(7) Planning and staff. Planning is one of the most important prerequisites for establishing a programme. In Bahrain, Al-Umran (unpublished report) found that most of the health and nutrition education programmes were poorly planned and lacked coordination. Lack of technical staff, especially those responsible for production and script writing, has markedly affected the nutrition education programmes. The insufficient training of nutrition educators in the use of audio-visual techniques has also contributed to a deficiency of nutrition education programmes.

1 Autret, M. & Miladi, S. (1980): Assessment and analysis of services as related to the nutrition situation of children in the Gulf countries. In *Proceeding of first workshop on nutrition as related to child and mother in the Gulf countries*, ed O. Farrag, S. Miladi & E. Amine, pp. 13–24. Abu-Dhabi: UNICEF.

2 Council On Children, Media And Merchandising (1977): Edible TV: your child and food commercials. p. v. Washington DC: US Goverment Printing Office.

3 FAO (1971): *Food and nutrition education in the primary school*, pp. 6–11. Rome: FAO.

4 Gussow, J.D. & Contento, I. (1984): Nutrition education in a changing world. *Wld Rev. Nutr. Diet.* **44**, 1–56.

5 Jelliffe, D.B. & Jelliffe, E.F.P. (1971): An overview. *Am. J. Clin. Nutr.* **24**, 1013–1024.

6 Marriott, L. (1976): The mass media component of a food and nutrition policy. *Cajanus* **9**, 288–296.

7 Musaiger, A.O. (1980): The role of advertising in nutrition knowledge, attitudes and practices of Bahraini consumers. Doctoral thesis submitted to the High Institute of Public Health, University of Alexandria, Egypt.

8 Musaiger, A.O. (1982): Factors influencing food consumption in Bahrain. *Ecol. Fd Nutr.* **12**, 39–48.

9 Musaiger, A.O. (1983): The extent of bottle-feeding in Bahrain. *Food Nutr. Bull.* **5**, 20–22.

10 Musaiger, A.O. (1983): The impact of television food advertisements on dietary behaviour of Bahraini housewives. *Ecol. Fd Nutr.* **13**, 109–114.

11 Musaiger, A.O. (1985): *Nutritional knowledge and attitudes of the visitors to the health centers in Bahrain (a pilot study)*. Bahrain: Ministry of Health (in press, in Arabic).

12 Musaiger, A.O. (1985): *Youths and leisure in Bahrain*. Bahrain: Ministry of Health (in press, in Arabic).

13 Musaiger, A.O. & Abdulaziz, S.A. (1985): *Food beliefs in Bahrain*. Bahrain: Ministry of Health (in press, in Arabic).

14 Researches and Studies Department (1983): *The influence of housemaids on the characteristics of the family in Bahrain*. Bahrain: Ministry of Labour and Social Affairs (in Arabic).

15 Srinivasan, L. (1983): Nonformal approaches to nutrition education. In *Approaches to nonformal nutrition education*, pp 2–25. Paris: UNESCO.

16 Van Schaik, T.F.S.M. (1976): The role of carbohydrates and of sugar in particular in our diet. *J. Hum. Nutr.* **30**, 377–380.

17 Vermeersch, J.A. & Sweenerton, H. (1979): Consumer responses to nutrition claims in food advertisements. *J. Nutr. Educ.* **11**, 22–26.

Living at the top of the pyramid: does the confusion of abundance lead to an abundance of confusion?

Katherine L. CLANCY
Department of Human Nutriton, College for Human Development, Syracuse University, Syracuse, NY 13210, USA.

Several months ago, the following items made news in Washington DC within a day of each other.

Item 1. Americans eat 815 billion calories of food every day — roughly 200 billion more than they need to maintain a moderate level of activity, United Press International reports. That's enough extra calories to feed everyone in Mexico, a country of 80 million people[24].

Item 2. Henry Waxman opened hearings on the health consequences of hunger on children by saying, 'Hunger is something that isn't supposed to happen in America. Because we are the richest nation on earth, because we are the "breadbasket" of the world, we expect mothers and children to be adequately nourished. But they are not[25].'

Either of these facts is enough to illustrate the confusion, and even pathology, of food abundance in the USA. Although I write of the USA, much of what I am describing applies or will apply to many of the advanced industrialist countries as well. This abundance, which many citizens have claimed as a right and many more have never thought about, has of course come forth from and itself produced an affluent society which surpasses anything the world has known.

This society is marked by an exaggerated emphasis on the production of goods[8], because the functioning of the economic system is utterly dependent on steadily increasing consumption. Since, unlike other consumer goods, biology sets a limit to the amount of food that any one person can consume[11], it is not surprising that a good deal of confusion exists with regard to a number of food topics such as health, production, hunger, safety, even ethics.

Paradoxes abound in the US food system, but only the two most obvious ones will be examined here: (1) want in the midst of plenty and (2) disease as the result of affluence. The existence of hunger as grain bins overflow was experienced on a wide scale just 50 years ago[19] and this paradoxical situation still exists.

There have been recent widespread reports of hunger[18,23] amidst record expenditures for commodity storage. But the public outcry about the hunger reports has been muted. Perhaps this is because of a perception that the number of hungry are smaller than before (there are no data to support or refute this). Perhaps it is because the public has accepted the administration's Calvinistic view of the causes of poverty, even though children are the most impoverished group in America[17]. Or perhaps the public has finally come to realize that 'America's wealth has ceased to grow, that we can no longer raise the standard of living at one point without lowering it somewhere else'[20].

If that is true, we may perhaps look forward to a healthier population because of the second paradox: disease as the result of affluence. The pattern of increased mortality from the 'diseases of affluence' appears to be universal. The result of increasing income is not only an increase in energy intake but a reduction in the nutritional quality of the diet because of increased consumption of fat, sugar, and animal products. Therefore, as scientific knowledge about the relationship between dietary factors and disease accumulated in the last 50 years, at the same time that *per caput* incomes grew, there was a concomitant need to caution the public about their dietary habits. The paradoxes here are complicated. If affluence represents a higher state, why should it be accompanied by serious chronic disease caused by the very rewards of affluence? One is tempted to look for a religious answer in something like the seven cardinal sins, but whatever the cause, the prescription, as we all know, is moderation.

However, there *has* been a response from the public to the call for prevention of the chronic diseases, and it is the genius of the economic system to answer this need for moderation with a massive outpouring of new food products. In the last decade, there has been an incredible proliferation of 'healthy' products which comprised a $26 billion dollar market in 1982. Americans are being immoderate about diet and health[26]. Some are even cutting their energy intake so much that they are finding it difficult to procure adequate nutrients. This, in turn, has caused confusion about conflicting messages coming from different parts of the nutrition world regarding the need for, and benefits of, vitamin and mineral supplements in pill or food form.

The above might be what one would expect of a food system which is built on and filled with so much illusion and in some cases disillusion. The illusions are based in the consumption myth, the belief that the more we produce, the more we should consume[13] and are accompanied by partial myths about a number of other concepts like variety, new foods, cheap food, free enterprise, convenience, and self-sufficiency. These are all kept alive by that virtual fount of illusion, advertising.

It is probably true that the variety of foods in US markets surpasses that available in most other places and in some sense we must be grateful. However, the overwhelming number masks two major problems. The first is that a great deal (but of course, not all) of the 'variety' in the market and the 5 000 'new' products introduced every year are composed of products whose only difference is (a) size, (b) brand name, or (c) colour, flavour, shape, or any one of a number of different additives. In fact, after accounting for many of these spurious differences, it was shown (in 1981)[4] that the net increase of new products in any year is actually only about 5 per cent. The second problem relates to the wide array of out-of-season and out-of-country produce. This of course is made available through the wonders of the modern transport system and the use of enormous quantities of fossil fuel. While it could be argued that this cost in energy is worth it in the dead of winter in upstate New York, the practice: (1) uses up nonrenewable resources, (2) allows a marketing structure to exist such that consumers cannot find locally produced fruits and vegetables in season, which in turn (3) discourages the maintenance of local agricultural production, and (4) encourages the growth of sometimes inappropriate cash crops in developing countries.

Variety must also incorporate genetic diversity. There are about 20 000 species of plants, and the American diet is extraordinarily dependent on only four of them — corn, wheat, soybeans, and sugar beets[12]. Also, the number of varieties of any one fruit or vegetable is limited because high technology farming and the requirements of food processors have led to a narrowing of the genetic base[14]. We can see why nutrition educators (eg[16]) have encouraged the public to eat the most variable diet they possibly can. And what do we find when we measure the variety score in the US diet? The mean number of unique foods in the 3-day dietary records of a subsample of the National Food Consumption Survey is 26 and the mean number of total foods 42[21]. That number seems very low, considering what is available in the market-place.

Perhaps new and not yet developed foods will fill the holes. Ignoring one of their more candid colleague's honest assertions a few years ago that the public had no need of any new food product[1], manufacturers continue to churn out a dizzying array of them. The fact is that there has not been a truly new food product on the market since spun soybeans[22]. It has been too expensive for the companies to research them and bring them to market. But this may be about to change with the rush to embrace biotechnology both in the food-production and food-processing industries. The vision of the new genetic engineers is very wide and encompasses products from caffeine-free coffee beans and salt-tolerant plants to 'breads' with no nutritional value[15]. I suspect that the confusion about these new wonders may become pretty high among consumers, especially since it is not yet known how such foods are going to regulated. Are they to undergo only routine scrutiny because the product seems to be the same, even though the process by which it is synthesized is totally different, or are they to be regulated as new foods[6]? Whatever the decision, what is clear is that variety is being brought artificially into the food system under several guises: (1) high technology (which must not be hindered no matter what the consequences); (2) adequate food to solve the world's hunger problem (without questioning that we have enough food now but cannot distribute it equitably); and (3) the maintenance of a cheap food policy for Americans. This policy is a reality and illusion at the same time. It is true that most Americans spend a very small portion of their income on food (10–20 per cent). The fact that poor people in the US pay 30 to 40 or even 50 per cent of their income for food does not change the mean. But the cheap food policy belies several myths. The first is that farmers receive a good portion of the food dollar; they do not. The second is that we actually pay what food is worth, and the third is that the food-manufacturing sector provides food as efficiently and cheaply as possible.

While the farmer's dwindling share of the food dollar may not appear problematic, it is now of concern because the present crisis in American farming has direct effects on food quality. The debt burdens being carried by a large percentage of farmers have pressed them to produce way beyond the world's market capacity. This intense production has been at a high cost of soil loss, water depletion, and fertilizer, pesticide and herbicide, and fossil fuel use. Much of the water used in agriculture, particularly in the West, is subsidized and does not appear in the price of food, nor does the long-term cost of fossil fuel and soil depletion. And pesticides and herbicides, the residues of which are described as a serious hazard in the food supply by 73 per cent of consumers in a recent survey[7], account for what has been called 'one of the most serious calamities to befall modern industrial farming, that it turned food into a suspect, potentially dangerous commodity'[27]. A high price indeed to pay for cheap food.

Approximately 90 per cent of all foods sold in America are processed in some way, some minimally but others to a much greater extent. Also, the affluent society has allowed a large number of meals to be eaten outside the home, where not only do consumers have nothing to do except pay the bill, they have no way of knowing what they are eating. Because of this lack of control, and for other reasons, there is one place where citizens are showing interest in taking some responsibility for their own food and that is the huge number growing fruits and vegetables in their own back yards. The same urge has been felt in some states, particularly in the North East, which have found out that approximately 80-90 per cent of the food they consume comes from outside their boundaries. This does not bode well in the case of a water or energy emergency, and it has important long-term consequences for land use in the states. But it is unclear if any but the strongest-willed state governments and food systems can overcome the alleged competitive advantage of the mid-west and California. Of course, we produce so much food that it is something of a shock to discover that the US is also the world's largest food importer, $19 billion in 1984[5]. The rich get richer, as they say, and the poor do in fact get poorer as the result of our policies and appetites. This on top of using 30 per cent of the world's resources already for our 5 per cent of the world's population[3].

At this point the question can be asked, how do we manage to do all this? Why has logic not prevailed to make our wants decrease as our needs have been filled? The answer is that the economic system has done it — arranged it so that 'so long as the consumer adds new products — seeking variety rather than quantity — he may accumulate without diminishing the urgency of his wants'[8]. And the vehicle through which this legerdemain is wrought is advertising, to the tune of $7.5 billion in 1980[4]. Since we would probably all agree with Galbraith that 'a man who is hungry need never be told of his need for food', we are probably not amiss in claiming that food advertising is the pinnacle of the art of persuasion. Its usually manipulative techniques have led social scientists like Boorstin[2] to complain that 'we listen to commercials to discover functions, uses, needs, and perils of which we never dreamed and never would have known'. In this vein, the public's growing interest in the link between diet and health could not be more perfect for the admen who play on already present anxieties and turn, in many cases, a perfectly natural component of the diet into a magic potion.

Summary and conclusions. The paradoxes and confusion in the US food system have led to contradictions which range from vast to trivial. There is an ever-widening gap between the affluent population which is growing richer and somewhat healthier, and a fast-growing poverty population, composed mainly of women and children, which has inadequate resources to purchase adequate food (or health care, or housing). Many people are hungry right now while some commodity surpluses stand at record high levels. Production continues unabated, despite the fact that we know how much damage is being done to the environment by various agricultural practices. The consumption myth and conservation myth are clashing in the USA[13], and we are exporting the same destructive model around the world. A 'cheap' and short-term food policy is being pursued here even though it clearly is harmful to the environment, consumers, and the economic system itself, which has undervalued the worth of its natural resources.

I do not pretend to know how to resolve these contradictions, and I think we must ask whether nutrition educators can do much to improve the situation. But I am not totally pessimistic. I think that there are especially important roles for nutrition educators to play if they are willing to jump into the fray. The first thing nutritionists must do is widen the traditional definition of the discipline to incorporate topics like production and safety and economic development.

While we are defining things, I also think we should attempt to bring some useful meaning to the word 'moderation'. As Worster says, 'powerful elements in our society do not allow us to recognize that there is such a thing as too much productivity, too much chasing after wealth'[27]. Yet if we do not begin to define and recognize moderation and wait for dire economic conditions to accomplish this task, the affluent society will see itself becoming less so.

Related to this is a third admonition — that a much greater number of nutritionists must assume the role of advocates for the poor, both in the USA and in the third world. Domestically, support for food programmes must be increased, both for equity reasons and to ease the burden on the local level, where people have stepped in voluntarily to feed the hungry and been overwhelmed by the task. Nutritionists in the advanced industrial countries must support programmes in the third world which, as much as possible, encourage indigenous development projects and resist the myth that the model that I have described is an appropriate one for any country.

Fourth, nutrition educators must recognize the need for and become proponents of new policy, both at the federal and state levels. It may even be the time to take the bold step of developing policy which recognizes that there is a relationship between food production and consumption. The necessity of taking the long-term view with regard to regional food supplies is equally strong and appears, in fact, to have been recognized by some of the more enlightened states. Nutritionists have an important role to play in identifying adequate and appropriate regional dietary patterns and in responding to the scepticism usually shown toward the feasibility of such a concept.

Finally, I think that food and nutrition educators must accept greater responsibility for raising and addressing some of the ethical issues which underlie all of the concepts discussed here. They must give up some of their own illusions, eg that (a) scientists are value-free or neutral, (b) the diet is the way it is because it just evolved that way[10], or (c) the overwhelming food abundance in which Americans participate is their right by ownership. Just because economics, as Galbraith writes, 'has to be divorced from any judgment on the goods with which it is concerned'[8] does not mean that we must be also. There are very serious issues of inequity and injustice in the food system. I think that some of the confusion about food stems from a semi-conscious recognition on the part of the public that these are moral as well as economic and scientific issues. Perhaps food and nutrition educators can help their audiences identify some of these more profound issues and assist them in pursuing a more just and sustainable sustenance.

1 Albrecht, J. (1982): Technology's role in product development. *Fd Tech.* **35**, 73–76.
2 Boorstin, D. (1962): In Pollay, R., *The distorted mirror: reflections on the unintended consequences of advertising*, p. 14. Working Paper No. 1005, History of Advertising Archives. Vancouver: University of British Columbia.
3 Brown, L. (1981): *Building a sustainable society.* New York: Norton.
4 Connor, J. (1981): Food product proliferation: a market structure analysis. *Am. J. Agric. Econ.* **63**, 607–617.
5 *Farmline* (1985): Exports are weak, but imports ... they're booming. March, 13.
6 *Food Chemical News* (1985): Biotechnology use urged not to trigger food additive requirement. Washington: April 15, 6.
7 Food Marketing Institute (1985): *Trends: consumer attitudes and the supermarket.* Washington: FMI.
8 Galbraith, J.K. (1976): *The affluent society*, 3rd rev. edn. New York: Mentor.
9 General Accounting Office (1981): *Emerging issues from new product development in food manufacturing industries*, GAO-CED-81-138. Washington, August 19.
10 George, S. (1979): *Feeding the few: corporate control of food.* Washington DC: Institute for Policy Studies.
11 Gussow, J. (1980): What corporations have done to our food. *Business and Society Review* **35**, Fall, 19–25.
12 Hall, R.H. (1979): "A cell's eye view of the four food groups". Presented at *Third Conference on 'Nutrition and the American food system'.* Washington DC.
13 Keen, S. (1978): Eating our way to enlightenment. *Psychol. Today*, 62–87.

14 Merrill, R. (1976): Toward a self-sustaining agriculture. In *Radical Agriculture*, pp. 284–327. New York and London: Harper and Row.
15 Miller, S.A. (1984): Human health and safety in this biotechnical age. Presented at the *Food and Agriculture Forum* of the National Planning Association, Des Moines.
16 Morowitz, H. (1976): Food for thought. *Hops. Pract.* **11**, 179–180.
17 *Nutrition Week* (1985): Poverty in America singles out children. **15**(1), 3.
18 Physician Task Force on Hunger in America (1985): *Hunger in America, the growing epidemic.* Cambridge: Harvard University School of Public Health.
19 Poppendieck, J. (1985): *Breadlines knee deep in wheat: food assistance in the great depression.* New Brunswick, NJ: Rutgers University Press.
20 Potter, D. (1954): *People and plenty — economic abundance and the American character.* p. 121. Chicago and London: University of Chicago Press.
21 Smiciklas-Wright, H., Krebs-Smith, S. & Krebs-Smith, J. (1984): Variety in foods. Paper presented at *What is America eating?*, the annual symposium of the Food and Nutrition Board, Washington, December 10.
22 Solomon, G. (1983): New foods proliferate without high technology. *Nutrition Week* **13**(26), 4–5.
23 Texas Senate Interim Committee on Hunger and Nutrition (1984): *Faces of hunger in the shadow of plenty.* Austin: Senate Committee.
24 *Washington Post* (1985): On the pulse, May 22, health section, p. 5.
25 Waxman, H. (1985): Opening remarks at hearings on health consequences of hunger on children, US House of Representatives Subcommittee on Health and the Environment and House Select Committee on Hunger, Washington, May 23.
26 Williams, W. (1984): Cashing in on fitness foods. *New York Times* November 4, sect. 3, p. 1.
27 Worster, D. (1984): Good farming and the public good. In *Meeting the expectations of the land*, ed W. Jackson, W. Berry & B. Colman. San Francisco: North Point Press.

Women and food — who is in charge?

Barbara SMITH
Nutrition Education Coordinator, South Australian Health Development Unit, 1st Floor, Stoneham Chambers, Noarlunga Centre, South Australia 5168, Australia.

Women historically and in all cultures have been central in the preparation and provision of food. This role, whether mainly in the sphere of food production or as the managers of consumption, may appear to give women control over a vital area of human existence. A closer look at women's relationship to food however shows that it is almost always mediated by patriarchial culture or exploited by economic forces.

It is in the interests of both capitalism and patriarchy to keep women ill-informed, and mystified about food. Food is symbolic of the traditional female stereotypes which have contained women: stereotypes which have defined women only in relation to others as wives, mothers, housewives; stereotypes claimed to be variously ordained by God, evolution, biology, economics. Women are so intimately connected with food, that the process of confusing women about food, is to confuse women about themselves. This can contribute to the way in which women perceive themselves, how they define their role and therefore ultimately what they can choose to achieve.

The changing role of women in relation to food. In hunting and gathering societies of the Paleolithic era women played a major role in the provision of food. As Margaret Mead commented, 'Men had a delightful time chasing giraffes while women actually produced 80 per cent of the food'[12]. Men were the hunters, women the gatherers, although there is some evidence from foraging societies that these roles were not always hard and fast[4,8].

Settlement, approximately 10 000 years ago, saw the beginning of the agricultural production of food. Women's role in food production in traditional agricultural societies, particularly subsistence farming, has always been major, although there is usually a clear division of labour by gender[2,5,15,16]. The animals belonged to men and plants to women except, depending on the type of production, the smaller animals. 'If you are dairy farmers, chickens belong to women. There is a steady inverse relationship between the smaller animals, and vegetables and women'[12]. Women's work was more time consuming and generally of lower status. Nonetheless, there was a reciprocity within a family of a common endeavour — the production of food for survival. Women's tasks had real productive value. Women often played significant social and political roles and had considerable independence. Their economic contribution to the welfare of the family was usually recognized[16].

In the Western world, 19th century industrialization and the growth of capitalism needed constantly expanding markets. The beginning of the 20th century saw the creation of mass consumption and an urgent need for labour to manage it. Production, including food production, became male-dominated, public and paid: consumption primarily a female responsibility, domestic and unpaid. Women's relationship to food in industrialized countries is embedded in this role.

Women's domestic role. Women as the unpaid, domestic managers of consumption has been justified by the ideology that emphasises the primacy of women's domestic role[16]. One might expect that with industrialization the domestic role might become more specialized, less time-consuming and less emotionally involving. The reverse is true: the domestic role has become 'not just a job, but an expression of love and warmth performed by each women for her own little family'[9]. It is worth noting that in societies where paid servants perform the domestic tasks, food preparation, cleaning and so on are not seen as expression of love and femininity.

Not only has the domestic role become more emotionally involving, the time spent has not decreased. The introduction of household appliances and higher standards of hygiene, has resulted in increased frequencies for doing things such as washing daily instead of weekly. There is likely to be an increased number of daily contacts with food, different meals for each family member, frequent chauffeuring tasks and so on. Labour-saving devices tend to reduce men's contribution in the domestic sphere, 'When she is given a rubbish disposal unit and a dishwasher, he relinquishes any responsibility for washing up or putting the rubbish out'[1]. In addition domestic work has been deskilled and devalued. Production, preservation and much of the preparation of food are subsumed by the paid public sector. The monetisation of values has lead to only paid work being valued so that not only is domestic work deskilled it is devalued and trivialized. As this is the work culturally assigned to women they also become devalued. Further this work is most likely to be undertaken in suburban isolation — without kinship network support or reciprocity within the family.

The ideology that women's place is in the home has prevailed in spite of the fact that women have continuously been employed in the work-place[16]. What this does is create ambivalence among working mothers, justifies women's employment in unskilled, low wage industries and occupations and forces women, into the dual responsibilities of paid public work *and* unpaid domestic labour.

The same dynamics can be observed in developing countries. The ideology of women's place being in the home, has been introduced to many developing countries along with Western technology. Aid and education, apart from education for a domestic role, has been primarily directed at men. This has resulted in the displacement and marginalization of women in food production, denied them access to the cash economy and generally defined then as dependent or economically inactive. They too are being forced into the Western model of the unpaid managers of consumption.

Women as the managers of food consumption. Because of the emotionalization of the domestic role, feeding the family becomes one of the ways women are judged as 'good' or 'bad'. 'Good women feed their families 'properly' but does a 'good' woman feed her family take-aways or only home cooked food? Does a 'good' mother allow her children to eat sweets and soft drinks or is she a 'bad' mother if she succumbs to the pressures of her television indoctrinated children? Managing consumption is therefore a serious business for women, but knowing how to do it 'properly' can be difficult.

In modern food systems there is fierce competition for the available profits. Food manufacturers constantly develop new products to compete with similar products. Increasingly new products are of the more profitable, value-added kind — generally highly processed and of poor nutritional value. These foods are then vigorously promoted primarily to women as the main agents of consumption. In order to consume intelligently in such a competitive food environment, women need to be well informed. Frequently the main sources of information about food — the media, the food industry and nutrition educators — can contribute to women's confusion about food and their own role.

The media's role. Food advertising is a pervasive and influential aspect of the media, but it does not inform. In one study of television food advertising 56.9 per cent of all food advertisement provided no information, 30.6 per cent one piece of information, 11.8 per cent with two pieces and only 0.7 per cent with three pieces[14]. The main ways in which advertising sells food, is by the creation of images and illusions. The images sold to women are 'directed at her need to please ... husbands, boyfriends, children, even the dog and cat' (petfood)[9].

In most countries, perhaps particularly in third world countries, a hugh discrepancy exists between the media images of women and the reality of women's lives[13]. Although in the US women make up 51 per cent of the population and are well over 40 per cent of the work-force, relatively few working women are portrayed, for example, in the television media. When working women are portrayed they are frequently condemned, trivialized or in need of protection. Advertising distorts images of women so that they are predominantly young, slim, pretty, domestic in the sense of mostly appearing in bathrooms or kitchens, clean and dependent.

In the other sectors of the media food information is likely to be directed only to women. It is often guilt producing — 'how you can cheat by preparing a quick meal', 'the diets of children who have working mothers is poor' (don't their fathers work as well?), and patronizing. There is also the generalized problem of nutrition information being contradictory depending on which 'expert' is being reported or being out of context of overall dietary needs.

The food industry. As the first aim of the food industry is profit, not good nutrition, it would be naive to expect it to assume the role of nutrition educator when this obviously can represent a conflict of interests. One of the main sources of profit is the highly processed, value-added product, ie products which generally provide poor nutritional value for money. It is therefore unlikely that the food industry would want to make readily and easily available the information which might promote the sales of less profitable foods. Food labelling laws vary widely from country to country and can require the disclosure of information which can be very valuable to the food consumer. More often the information is not readily intelligible. In the United States, foods bear elaborate nutrition labels which predictably ordinary people are unable, not unwilling to understand[10].

Nutrition educators. The dual impact of technology and professionalism has lead to many different kinds of food experts working from very different assumptions about food and what is in the public interest. This fragmentation and mystification of knowledge makes it difficult for the consumer to get answers meaningful in *both* social and nutritional terms to questions such as 'What should I eat?' 'What is a good diet?' Home economics and nutritional science, serve as good examples of the ways in which experts can add to the confusion.

Home economics became a legitimized field of study for women on the grounds that it would help promote better wives and mothers. Home economics has reinforced women's domestic role and their role of feeding *others*. Frequently nutrition teaching was removed from home economics to male spheres of interest such as agricultural science, leaving home economics teaching food preparation and consumer skills without an adequate nutritional science base. In developing countries, home economics applied Western concepts of domesticity to third world women without attempting to understand their work in other than a domestic context. Home economics programmes tended to ignore nutritious, indigenous foods and promoted practices based on European food supplies. In this way traditional nutritional wisdom was eroded and devalued and women were made to feel they had been doing it 'wrong'.

Nutritional science. As nutritional science acquired the status of being scientific, men came to control nutrition knowledge in the sense that they are more likely to be the researchers and theorists. Women nutrition professionals tend to be the practitioners — dietitians and educators. When women do work in nutrition research they are more likely to research consumer issues[16]. Not only do men largely control nutrition knowledge, it is mostly men who control food policy at both national and international levels. Yet the day-to-day reality of nutrition remains the responsibility of women.

The result of this separation of theory and practice has been the mystification of nutrition knowledge. The value of food has largely been reduced by nutritional science to the value of nutrients. Nutrition educators have allowed themselves to be 'moved from foods to food groups, ... to the notion that we must teach not foods but nutrients'[10]. Nutritional science must take its share of responsibility for the process whereby food has become something which only the most sophisticated and literate can really understand and then only if it comes in a package with instructions on the label[10].

Women are increasingly trapped between social and nutritional values in their traditional roles; what the experts tell them they *should* feed their families, and what their families *want* to eat[7].

The consequences of women's nutritional health. Women are so intimately connected to food that this process of confusing women about food is to confuse women about themselves. Womens capacity to lactate is probably one of the reasons that they, to some extent, have been actually defined as food. The use of language describing women, demonstrates how deeply embedded the notion of an 'edible woman' is in our culture; 'sugar and spice', 'a luscious dish', 'chick' and 'peach'.

(1) Fat and thin responses to food. The extent of women's confusion over food and their own identity, is probably best evidenced in affluent societies by the fact that anorexia nervosa is almost exclusively confined to women and that overweight is more worrying for women than men. In countries with an abundance of food 'reed thinness' is valued in women: in countries with too little food 'soft plumpness' is likely to be the definition of feminine beauty. The common denominator is — 'passivity, lack of muscle, little strength — the enforcement of weakness in women'[17]. Men are usually considered attractive in a much greater range of sizes and shapes. In Western countries women constantly strive for this thin ideal, frequently consuming nutritionally inadequate diets and supporting a multi-million dollar 'slimming' industry.

(2) Malnutrition. In developing countries women and girls feel the scarcity of food earlier, more frequently and more severely than their husbands or brothers do. In a 1971 study in India, girls outnumbered boys four to three with kwashiorkor and more boys than girls were hospitalized[13].

A similar pattern of discrimination can be observed in many poor countries ... a woman is so dependent on her sons for immediate status and future security she is apt to nurse them longer and feed them better than her daughters. In Bangladesh the result is a mortality rate for girls that is 30 to 50 per cent higher than the rate for boys in the same age group[13].

For most nutritional deficiencies if there is sex difference in patterns of occurrence the higher occurrence occurs in females. The reasons for this are not all cultural, but undoubtedly the patriarchal notion that men are of greater value than women, and the fact that more women than men are likely to be poor, are major factors.

Conclusions. In all countries in the world women prepare, preserve and cook food. They are the main agents of food consumption and in the developing world 50–90 per cent of agricultural workers are women[3]. Yet this situation in no way reflects the control women have over food. Women cannot be regarded as in control of food when their role as food providers is used to contain or confine them; when they are defined as providing for others and not themselves; when their food budget is controlled by others; when they are manipulated in the market-place and blamed for their ignorance; when they have no power in food policy and production decisions; when their work in the home and work-place is devalued.

In order to begin to solve the problems of malnutrition there is a need for nutrition educators to confront the political issues surrounding food. The politics of women and food, along with the politics of maldistribution, and the proliferation of 'modern' highly processed food, is one such issue[6,11]. The extent to which nutrition educators fail to meet this challenge, is not only the extent to which they fail women, but the extent to which nutrition education itself may fail.

1 Bose, C. (1979): Technology and changes in the division of labour in the American home. *Women's Studies International Quarterly* **2–3**, 295–304.
2 Boserup, E. (1970): *Women's role in economic development*, pp. 160–173. New York: St. Martin's Press.
3 Cottingham, J. (1985): Women and health: an overview. In *Women in development*, p. 150. Geneva: ISIS International Womens Information and Communication Service.
4 Dahlberg, F.D. (ed) (1981): *Woman the gatherer*, pp. 10–15. New Haven and London: Yale University Press.
5 Davies, I. (1983): Women and subsistence agriculture. In *Women, aid and development*, ed L. Melville, pp. 39–44. Canberra: Women and Development Network of Australia.
6 Eide, W.B. (1978): Rethinking food and nutrition education under changing socio-economic conditions. *Paper from Tanzania Workshop. Education of the Public.* IUNS Committee 10/V.
7 Fine, P.A. (1971): Modern eating patterns; the structure of reality. *Paper for AMA Food Science Symposium*, New York.
8 Fisher, E. (1979): *Woman's creation; sexual evolution and the shaping of society*, p. 71. New York: Anchor Press/Doubleday.
9 Game. A. & Pringle, R. (1983): *Gender at work*, pp. 119–140. Sydney: George Allen & Unwin.
10 Gussow, J. (1981): Growth, prediction and responsibility. Food is the bottom line. 4th Annual Ellen S. Richards Lecture. pp. 9–11. University of North Carolina.
11 Gussow, J.D. & Contento, I. (1984): Nutrition education in a changing world. *Wld Rev. Nutr. Diet*, **44**, 1–56.
12 Mead, M. (1976): Comments on the division of labour in occupations concerned with food. *J. Am. Diet. Ass.* **68**, 321–325.
13 Newland, K. (1979): *The sisterhood of man, the impact of women's changing roles on social and economic life around the world*, pp. 45–68. New York and London: W.W. Norton & Co.
14 Resnik, A. & Stern, B.L. (1977): An analysis of information content in television advertising. *J. Marketing.* January: 50–53.
15 Rogers, B. (1980): *The domestication of women*, pp. 79–115. London and New York: Tavistock Publications.
16 Sachs, C.E. (1983): *The invisible farmers*, pp. 44–64. Totowa, New Jersey: Rowman and Allanheld.
17 Steinem, G. (1980): Politics of food. *Ms.* Feb. p. 91.

The challenge to the profession: how do we train for what we want to teach?

Joan Dye GUSSOW and Wenche Barth EIDE
Department of Nutrition Education, Teachers' College, Columbia University, New York, USA; Institute for Nutrition Research, University of Oslo, Norway.

People are much more influenced in their eating by their food environments than by their nutrition knowledge. In poor countries the eater's problem is often a lack of enough food of the right kind or not enough money to buy what there is. (Educators lack knowledge about what people actually *eat* or about resources they might potentially eat). In rapidly industrializing countries people living on traditional diets find themselves suddenly exposed to new, attractive and questionably nutritious foods that they do not know how to fit into their usual food patterns. And in rich, highly industrialized countries, consumers are faced with so many highly promoted foods of such baffling composition that wise decisions become difficult.

One school of thought in nutrition education says that the nature of the food supply is none of our business: our role is to teach people how to make use of it. One widely used definition of nutrition education is: 'any system of communication that teaches people to make better use of available food resources.' The difficulty with such a definition is that it does not tell the nutrition educator what to do if available food resources are inadequate, baffling or have an insecure future. We prefer to define the role of a nutrition educator as one who helps people of whatever social, economic, or political circumstance, to meet their need for nutritious food. This means helping them understand the real political, social, economic or other sources of their food problems and work to resolve those problems within the constraints imposed by a globe of finite resources. This means we must reconsider prevailing assumptions about the ignorance of ordinary eaters and pay more attention to the ignorance — or need for education — of the power-brokers and policy-makers whose decisions in a variety of settings affect the quality, distribution, comprehensibility, safety and sustainability of the food supply.

Obviously if they would undertake such a task, nutrition educators must know — or be willing to learn — about many things in addition to biochemistry and communication. A variety of fields could be mentioned as important to include in our curricula, but we are here concerned primarily with how students may be *educationally socialized* to become the kinds of nutrition educators who assume responsibility not only for what people eat with what effects, but also for whether they have anything to eat at all and if not, why not.

Major concerns that must underlie nutrition education. Let us first raise some major concerns that are — or will be — common to countries at all stages of development. First, there is the issue of women's responsibility for, and lack of control over, food; second, the largely reactive role of the nutrition educator in relation to the changing food supply; third, what most nutrition educators know versus what consumers want to know; and fourth, the nutrition educator's role in relation to the future availability of food.

Women and food. This first concern was, until recently, largely invisible to most decision-makers. Although women around the world are responsible for preparing, preserving and cooking food, and are, in many societies, also largely responsible for growing what their families eat, these heavy responsibilities in no way reflect any actual control over food. Women are traditionally the ultimate nutrition educators, the persons who want to provide well-chosen adequate food for their families. Yet powerful forces in both the developing and the developed worlds make it extremely difficult if not impossible for them to do so.

If nutrition educators (themselves very often women) do not begin to acknowledge and combat the powerlessness of the feeders, begin to organize women to assert their real power as producers and consumers — and as childbearers who wish to preserve the earth's capacity to provide for the next generation — then nutrition education will remain a marginal field, which those who have real power can exploit to justify their own irresponsibility.

Nutrition education: picking up the pieces? The traditional role of the nutrition educator has been to pick up the pieces — to try to talk people into eating well after a variety of factors visible in poor countries as well as rich ones — from colonialism to product promotion — have shattered what were once relatively rational eating patterns. This is not to suggest that traditional patterns were optimal, that all 'progress' in the food supply is wicked, or that there was once some pre-industrial paradise in which people lived to be centennarians with no nutritional deficiencies or excesses.

If nutritional science had developed without so many concurrent profit-driven changes in the available food supply, it might have had an opportunity to really improve people's diets. As it is, the drastic modification of agricultural systems, and the continual proliferation of food products, seem to create health dilemmas faster than nutrition scientists or educators can conceivably cope with them. In the USA, where product proliferation has reached a truly improbable level, those few nutrition educators who protest against the introduction of another children's breakfast cereal containing saturated fat or a new record level of sugar, are told that their job is to educate people to use the food supply, not to intervene in the free play of the market — and so the farce continues.

In effect, many nutrition educators in the USA, faced with the current food supply, find themselves unable to offer what they would consider really informed advice to ordinary people. Even experts do not fully understand either the composition or the long-term safety of a large percentage of the products on the shelves, nor do they know how to judge their actual nutritional value, or their potential for producing long-term health. Therefore, what sorts of rational advice can be given to ordinary people except that they should *avoid* much of what is in the market-place?

Consumers' versus educators' priorities. This brings up a third dilemma, faced now most often by nutrition educators in the most overdeveloped countries but certain to become increasingly troubling everywhere, namely that we often cannot answer the questions consumers want to know about food because we have been cut off, or cut ourselves off, from responsibility for knowing what happens to food before it gets to the market-place.

Therefore, however sophisticated our knowledge of how the biochemicals in food interact with the biochemicals in the body, that knowledge is entirely insufficient to enable us to give most people the answers they want about the foods they eat. In the USA these questions can include: which kind of cottage cheese should they buy from the dozens in the market; are they (whoever *they* are) still putting hormones in chickens and if so are those the same hormones thought to cause premature maturation in Puerto Rican children; are the tomatoes picked green in Florida and shipped to New York City as good for you as local tomatoes which have sat in the sun all day, and so on. Many nutrition educators greet such questions by deploring the public's ignorance about what a nutritionist is! Yet if our job is to teach people how to choose food wisely, is it up to us to decide which questions about food consumers are allowed to ask?

Conserve while consuming. The fourth concern is that of a sustainable food supply. Around the world the resources required to produce food are under stress. Soil and water, two obvious essentials for agriculture, are running short in many countries, including rich ones where the effects of continuing soil loss and water waste are more readily masked by what money can do. If we are to feed future generations, we must begin *now* to modify our demands on the biosystems, as we learn to create — or recreate — sustainable agriculture systems.

Thus an essential part of the nutrition educator's job should be to teach consumers about selecting food in relation to its environmental cost as well as its nutrient content. Such a linkage of nutrition education and agricultural sustainability should occur not only in rich, but, equally urgently, in poor countries since the latter have a smaller margin of safety. The rule in the third world, as was suggested at the August, 1985, Bangalore Conference on the environment, should be: Conserve while consuming, but it will be very difficult to conserve when eaters around the world depend increasingly on food grown far away. Many of the urban poor in the third world depend on the food exports of a few far-off countries even as their local croplands are used to produce luxuries for the affluent North. Leaving aside other arguments for greater local self-reliance, it can be argued on educational grounds alone that teaching people to worry about saving the resources necessary to produce food will be especially difficult when those resources are located a continent away.

A second generation of nutritionists? A fundamental issue facing us in the light of all these concerns is: How can we produce the second generation of nutritionists (generation here being used to mean type or kind) that we now see the need for? To ask that nutrition educators take on the role of being guardians of the food supply — present and future — is to give them an absurdly large task. Yet needed tasks cannot be neglected simply because they seem too large to be done. We would accept a much more modest role, even for nutrition educators trained to think about the whole thing as a *system for feeding people*, were it not for our acute awareness of how badly the other disciplines presumably concerned with food working from their own disciplinary boxes, have done in getting food to people. In asking how we can begin to train persons for this demanding role, we will concentrate on the formation of nutritionists at the university level, since we are persuaded that academic institutions will continue to function as generators of acceptable contemporary knowledge, providing the authority sought for by educators at lower educational levels.

We assume that most contemporary nutrition educators will recognize the need for graduates to know more than biochemistry and communication. But in trying to build a mosaic that will reflect the realities of people's existence, and, under varying circumstances, their access to food and its consumption as part of that existence, it will not help just to pull together different pieces carved out of totally different materials — ie, the different scholarly disciplines — since they might not fit together to form a real mosaic.

Unless carefully designed to apply to relevant *problems*, short introductions to different disciplines *as such* can be more confusing than helpful to students. This is especially so if students have already been socialized into thinking that the *real* nutritional knowledge is how nutrients are metabolized and function in the body, and how we must eat to maintain those functions. It is our experience that with such socialization all but a few already conscious students will continue to perceive wisdom from other disciplines as auxiliary and of less importance.

How can we make our students feel the need to acquire an understanding of when and how access to food and nutrients is, or is not, secured (and how they can go about studying such issues), even as we continue to ensure their appropriate grasp of nutrition at the level of the human organism? In other words, how can we make students see that what matters is the total system of resources and processes regarding food and nutrition, in the social as well as the biological world? Unless we can map the total territory before them, how can they select a direction, not only one that will most attract them personally, but one that will also be *useful* in the broader perspective?

It is sometimes said that there is no more need for generalist nutrition education but rather for focused training programmes that cater for specific sectors or problem areas. We believe there is today a greater need than even before, for an authentic generalist nutritionist, one who, able to understand linkages and to help establish interconnections, may *therefore* also be in a position to help direct the more specialist training programmes. What is now needed, in generalist nutrition education particularly, but also to varying degrees in more specialized nutrition training, is that we help students to acquire a birds' eye view of the food and nutrition system, from production and production relations, through nutrient metabolism and utilization. To make this possible, we may have to sacrifice some of the more subtle refinements that each of us loves to provide at some points in academic education (often *because* they are our specialities, rather than because they are needed) and instead introduce, as and when relevant, aspects from other disciplines' conceptual approaches, theories and methodologies, applied to issues identified as nutrition-relevant.

Students can thereby be made *aware* of the need for complementary approaches and methods that can tie in with theirs, and understand where to turn for interdisciplinary communication in trying to solve problems in real life. We have found that when students experience what they learn as having a much wider significance than they had originally imagined, they begin to see their own roles in a broader societal context.

Besides such a new approach to content, however, there is a need to rethink our educational methodology, or rather our basic educational philosophy. We propose that educators should consider themselves first as *resource persons* in the service of mature, searching individuals, individuals who should be assisted from the very first day to become inquiring, critical, and imaginative human beings, rather than passive recipients of whatever information we — who think we know — have decided should be passed on and stored in their brains.

Second, we should not abstain from exposing students to really controversial issues surrounding food, including who controls production, distribution, and marketing, who gains and who are the possible losers in the food game — internationally, nationally, at community level, and within households — as well as who the actors are behind actual policies affecting food supply and consumption, and what opportunities exist for influencing those we find do not serve the interests of different groups of people.

As resource persons, rather than teachers of dogmas, it is our duty to expose students to *problems*, and assist them in *finding out* their possible causes and solutions. This we can do by guiding students whenever an issue is controversial to a variety of sources and *opposing* views. Only then can students learn to think for themselves and to choose their future paths according to whatever their loyalties and ideologies may turn out to be — given the facts and their various interpretations.

One interesting aspect of the *problem-oriented* approach we advocate, is that students often want more information on issues they become turned on to, a contrast to the more common experience of teachers who meet resistance when they propose 'other readings' to enrich the learning process. This is only one sign that most students quickly demonstrate a remarkable openness, resourcefulness and imagination when they are allowed to take responsibility for their own learning, rather than being required to reproduce a certain amount of predetermined knowledge for exams. Such experiences give us hope that the second generation of nutritionists might on the whole be more aware, more concerned, and more relevant to society than the present one.

Having said that, however, we should not forget that there is still time for us in the first generation to change.

Upon this gifted age, in its dark hour
rains from the sky a meteoric shower
of facts … they lie unquestioned, uncombined.
Wisdom enough to leach us of our ill
is dark spun, but there exists no loom to weave it into fabric.
Edna St. Vincent-Millay (American Poet).

Advanced nutritional training: a workshop report*

S. BERGER (Organizer)
Human Nutrition Institute, Warsaw Agricultural University, Warsaw, Poland.

The scope of the workshop was to discuss existing gaps in nutrition training and moreover what actions for possible improvements could be taken. As far as gaps in subject-matter are concerned, several subjects were mentioned to be deficient in nutrition training, eg nutrition in agriculture, food science and technology (specifically food preservation and storage), management of nutritional planning, health education, methods in nutrition advising. However, since it is not possible to teach everything in all programmes, it was suggested that gaps could possibly be filled at a postgraduate level.

The urgent need for strengthening nutrition training in the developing world, specifically in Africa, was expressed because of the lack of qualified manpower in these countries. This could be reached by reinforcing existing institutions as well as by setting up new regional centres.

The distinction between training of professional nutritionists and nutrition training for non-professionals working in the field of health, agriculture, social sciences, education etc. and requiring an understanding of nutrition, was affirmed. Although the need for both types of training was agreed upon, the meeting stressed the importance of general public basic training, as nutrition training programmes for the non-professionals seems to be increasingly recognized, while there are only a limited number of general nutrition courses. Since a career structure in nutrition is badly needed for the improvement of the professional status of the nutritionist, top-level training, including PhD training, should be developed.

Other reasons put forward for the low professional status of the nutritionists were the existing lack of a professional profile and the confusion in curriculum development. Roles and responsibilities of nutritionists and other personnel in nutrition should be defined in order to get them official recognition as professionals with definite qualifications

The problem of the rather low status of nutrition — equating it with domestic science — seems to be getting better thanks to the development of women's studies, but there is still room for improvement as unfortunately this view still dominates.

As to the methodology of training it was stressed that this should be community-based and oriented in the direction of problem-solving. Unfortunately, training seems to be too often teacher- rather than learner-oriented. Internship should form part of the curriculum. Since there is a lack of visual aids, specifically of those dealing with the problems of rural development, assistance should be given to centres like TALC.

As it is not clear what is meant by advanced training, eg what is the cut-off point between basic and advanced training, it was recommended that IUNS should set up training standards based on a defined job-description for nutritionists. In addition, IUNS should take responsibility for the preparation of an inventory of advanced nutrition training giving basic information of the programmes listed. Because of its unique position, IUNS should coordinate all efforts and actions of UN and other organisations aiming at the improvement of nutrition training.

**This workshop incorporated a meeting of IUNS Committee V/8 on advanced degrees in nutrition science.*

The use of simulation techniques in training in nutrition, agriculture and health: a workshop report

Elizabeth DOWLER (Organizer)
Department of Human Nutrition, London School of Hygiene and Tropical Medicine, Gower St, London WC1E 7HT, UK.

Many participants in the Congress were involved in training programmes of one sort or another, whether in formal education courses or professional in-service training, or in communication, either with other professionals or with the general public. There is increasing interest in the use of simulation, games and role-play as a means of communication and education, and to widen the perspective of those being trained and taught. The Workshop was intended to offer an opportunity to share some of these experiences, discuss their implications and explore the potential for further use and development of ideas. About 30 Congress members took part in the workshop. To begin with, participants explained their interest and experience in simulation, and what they hoped to learn from the session. Two or three main issues were thus identified, and dealt with in turn by the group. There was also a strong if not universal interest in actually trying out a couple of short games; the constraints of time unfortunately prevented this wish being realized.

Participants came with a wide variety of professional backgrounds and interests. Some worked in nutrition/agriculture, some in the health sector, some in education (schools/colleges) and health education, and some, though laboratory-based, were simply curious. However, what was immediately clear was that they divided into two groups: those who had considerable experience of games and simulations and were keen to discuss problems; and those for whom the ideas were fairly new, and who wanted to discuss basic, elementary issues. As an agreed compromise therefore, the Organizer gave a brief, introductory presentation interrupted as appropriate by others in the group who wanted to contribute examples, to reinforce or disagree, or to introduce further ideas.

In defining terms at the outset, the speaker distinguished simulations between one individual and a computer (currently very popular in many countries) and between several people, whether with equipment, computers or not, and concentrated only on the latter. There is also a distinction to be made between formal education — where the teacher/trainer works to a specified syllabus with a set group — and non-formal education, such as that undertaken by health education or agricultural extension workers — where part of the job is to discover people's own perceptions of their needs and problems, or to enable them to discover and articulate them for themselves, and then provide information or solutions relevant to particular circumstances, and in a way that allows those people to make use of it/them, and not merely take in facts.

In most circumstances, simulations and games, broadly speaking, will nonetheless serve three main aims: to stimulate and engage the interest and participation of groups (which is why it would have been good to *play* some games, and not just theorise about them); to broaden the perspective and understanding of others' circumstances, or professional roles, or position, and why others might behave as they do; and to enable people to try out their knowledge and skills in circumstances where they can do no harm. The main problems that arise with using such techniques relate to understanding — and controlling — the knowledge they give: people can have the 'wrong messages' fixed by the experience (eg, because the strategy they adopted during the game had not worked very well, they conclude it would not work in 'real life' either, without analysing the difference between the two circumstances; simulations require considerable cooperation from the group to be successful, and can sometimes make unreasonable demands on a group — participation is enforced; and thirdly, it is difficult to evaluate such participation, both in terms of the knowledge and experience gained, and of individuals' performances.

Simulations demand a great deal of the trainer/communicator as well: physical control is more difficult than in traditional roles of 'teacher', who has all knowledge, at the front, and attendant 'pupils' who receive information sitting in rows; if a particular game confronts players with the contradictions in their knowledge/attitudes/positions, or exposes weakness, hostility either to other players, or to the leader, can result. Such arousal of strong feelings can of course be used constructively and may indeed be part of the purpose in playing on the leader's part, but it is obvious that considerable skill and sensitivity is needed in dealing with the immediate effects of conflict, and in drawing out positive insights and messages from the group as a whole.

In sharing experiences, good and bad, of these difficulties, many stressed how important discussion at the end was, both to enable all players to 'tell their own story', and to bring out a collective understanding of what went on and how these experiences relate to the real world. Some interesting examples were given of evaluation techniques, both by use of questionnaire and by panel observation and assessment; most of these had clearly been devised for particular circumstances. Several participants outlined difficulties they had encountered in obtaining or sustaining cooperation, and these problems were discussed by others in the group and several suggestions made.

One area which was touched on numerous times but not really addressed at length was peculiar to nutrition: that most people reasonably regard themselves as 'knowing how to eat', that food is in any case central to social exchange in most cultures and that decisions about what food to eat, how and when, are made in response to a variety of social, economic and cultural pressures, as well as those of knowledge and beliefs. People may look to the nutrition profession for advice and information, but make use of such in ways the profession may not approve of. There was continual lament over the difficulty of 'getting people to do what is good for them', discussion of the assumptions and responsibilities implied in such feelings, and agreement that whereas much formal training in nutrition deals with the 'scientific aspects' of metabolism and nutrients, the 'real world' of food and nutrition encompasses much more, with which many nutritionists are ill-equipped to deal. How to engage in dialogue with interested or disaffected members of the public, and how drama or role-play or games can be part of that process, was considered several times, though no general conclusions were drawn.

Finally, mention should be made of a brief discussion of the use of role-play or simulation by community workers in nutrition, agriculture or health to uncover the problems of a particular village or community, including how those problems might be viewed by different classes within the society concerned. Here, one is trying to use the techniques not so much to communicate information from outside, but to enable people to perceive and/or express information about themselves which they might otherwise find difficult to articulate.

Although no games were demonstrated or experienced in practice, it seemed that many useful ideas and contacts had emerged; a booklist and addresses of an International and British Society promoting the use of games and simulations were provided to those who requested them (further copies available from the organizer).

Nutrition in catering/food service: a workshop report

C. HUNT (Organizer)
Department of Catering Studies, Huddersfield Polytechnic, UK.

The aims of this workshop were: (1) to gain an overview of what is currently occurring in relation to nutrition education of the caterer/food service operator in the UK and other countries; (2) to provoke discussion and ideas for improving the nutrition training of caterers and facilitating caterers' efforts to implement dietary guide-lines. Topics were introduced by five speakers and the following is a summary of these topics and of the discussions that followed.

Nutrition education of the caterer working at craft level. (*Mary Duckworth*, William Angliss College, Melbourne, Australia). At the Melbourne College nutrition is taught to final (3rd) year apprentice cooks of whom there are about 200–300 a year.

About 85 per cent of them cook in restaurants and hotels, the rest work in hospitals, banks and other institutions. An important point to emerge is that cooks, chefs and caterers are notorious for their own poor eating habits brought about partly by overwork and anti-social hours. It was agreed that this is the case in Australia, Britain and some other countries and is undoubtedly a factor which can mitigate against them taking a keen interest in nutritionally well-devised menus for their customers. A feature, therefore, of the Melbourne course is to encourage 'personal' interest in their own eating habits. This is achieved partly by the students recording their own food and drink intakes, height and weight at the start, during and at the end of their nutrition course. Many felt that their habits did improve and certainly their awareness and interest in nutritional matters was considerably enhanced. Discussion in the workshop showed general agreement that this was a useful means of bringing nutritional points home to students.

Computerized food tables can obviously help considerably in this process but are not yet available in many colleges teaching at craft level. Collaboration with nearby institutions which do have this facility would therefore be worth pursuing.

It was felt that students should be given opportunities in college to actually devise, prepare and present meals for, eg, children, the elderly, businessmen, vegetarians, diabetics, overweight people, ethnic groups etc. The success of such menus from both the palatability and nutritional points of view can be monitored at a college without incurring excessive financial risk.

In Britain a major problem of teaching nutrition at craft level (mainly City and Guilds courses) is that the laid down syllabuses still specify preparation methods (eg sauces) which are at odds with recent dietary recommendations so that high fat, sugar and salt cookery practices are being perpetuated. Some of the cookery teachers themselves are resistant to change either through ignorance or apathy. However, City and Guilds syllabuses are currently being revised, hopefully for the better. Trends in customer demand and interest towards healthier eating are already apparent in various sectors so that caterers with no interest in this could find themselves 'left behind'.

Nutrition education of future catering managers. (*John Lawson*, Department of Catering Studies, Huddersfield Polytechnic, UK). *Lawson* dealt mainly with the teaching of nutrition on degree level catering courses in the UK. Hours of nutrition taught on each course range from none to 200 hours (the latter being in the BSc Hons Catering and Applied Nutrition course at Huddersfield Polytechnic). Course contents range from primarily administration and business-orientated to science-orientated, but even in the latter there appears to have been some pressure in recent years to reduce science (including nutrition) input. Some would feel this to be unfortunate and contrary to modern trends in catering.

Seventeen degree courses in catering are currently offered in the UK; four in universities, ten in polytechnics and three in colleges of higher education. Apart from the University courses the remainder are validated by the Council for National Academic Awards (CNAA). This body may therefore be influential in the future in encouraging the teaching of nutrition on the majority of degree courses in catering.

A quantitative assessment of the nutrition teaching on the above courses showed that three (18 per cent) contained more than 40 hours, nine (53 per cent) contained between 20 and 30 hours and five (29 per cent) had only a minimal content. A similar profile was observed in Catering degree courses awaiting validation by the CNAA in the next two years.

The teaching of nutrition was initially restricted to those courses involved with public sector catering since it was regarded as irrelevant to the commercial sector. However, recent developments in nutritional knowledge, an increasing awareness of nutrition amongst the population and an increasing tendency for nutrition to be used as a marketing ploy is causing the commercial sector to reappraise its position with regard to nutrition. To remain in tune with that demand, degree courses in catering will have to be similarly reappraised with regard to their nutrition input. The speaker recommended a minimum level of 40 hours for this purpose (ie, approximately 2.5 per cent of a degree course).

In-service education of caterers. (*Anneke Hekkens-Klaasen*, Bureau for Food and Nutrition Education, Netherlands). The Netherlands has a relatively privileged situation in having a government-funded Bureau which is specifically devoted to the nutrition education of both the general population and of special groups, including caterers. The Bureau has been established for many years and therefore has important experience of the most effective means of nutrition education of various groups. The point was made that whilst the training of higher-educated catering managers must not be neglected, the fact remained that the majority of customers were particularly dependent on the efforts of caterers with only craft training or no training at all. Hence schemes aimed at these people, including in-service courses, are important for the general nutritional improvement of menus. The Bureau has concentrated its efforts in the last 15 years on two target groups, ie the institutions and the factory canteens and it has become clear that whilst circulated literature, exhibitions etc appear to increase general nutritional awareness this is not readily translated by caterers into practice unless supported by detailed information and instructions, on how to incorporate better nutrition into the daily routine. Necessary information includes that on *buying* (eg buy low-sugar yoghurts, half-fat margarines, smaller individual packs of sugar), *preparing* (eg methods for low-fat sauces based on starch or yoghurt or vegetable purees; reduced use of fried food) and *portion weights*.

It appears to be more effective to consider and aim at the whole catering organization and staff in altering menus rather than attempting to teach pure nutrition principles to catering staff. Nutritional messages are best 'wrapped' within the whole context as a general package to improve 'food quality'. Also the publication of 'real-life' successful efforts at healthier menus in appropriate magazines seems to provide considerable impetus to their continuation and their adoption by other catering organizations. Another point that met with general agreement was that intermediaries between the food preparer and the customer have too long been neglected in terms of training, eg waiters in restaurants and food service assistants in institutions could be important informers of the customers if properly trained and motivated or conversely, if not, might contribute to a breakdown of any efforts towards healthier menus. Appropriate nutritional information on menus and displays can also help to reinforce such attempts and make the customer more aware of what the caterer is trying to achieve. Obviously, though, choice rather than 'imposition' must always by maintained in menus.

Implementation of dietary guide-lines by the caterer in Europe. (*Alison Dobson*, District Dietitian, Bloomsbury, London, UK). Attempts at implementation vary considerably from country to country in Europe. For example there appears to be relatively little of this nature occurring in Spain and Italy though it could be argued that there is less need, since Mediterranean diets tend to be more healthy than Northern European diets anyway. In the UK, approximately two-thirds of District Health Authorities are at various stages of planning or implementing their own food policies mainly in the hospital service. Lack of clear central government directions in this matter does not help and has led in some cases to confusing and conflicting advice being given to caterers. Also there is a danger of well meaning but misguided actions by caterers, eg over-zealous introduction of fibre; failure to differentiate between the very different nutritional needs of various categories of patients.

However, an encouraging move in the UK is the recent increase of in-service teaching of hospital staff which now includes a nutritional input. In hospitals, nurses are usually involved in serving food to patients so the current food and health campaign in the *Nursing Mirror* may prove helpful in reinforcing caterers attempts to implement dietary guidelines.

In schools there is still a worrying consumption by children of high-fat, -salt and -sugar, and low-fibre meals, but there are some that are trying to promote healthier eating. There are encouraging signs of more cooperation between teachers (home economists, biologists) and school caterers in this respect. Also one or two private caterers are launching healthier eating in some schools.

Nutrition education of caterers in developing countries. (Prepared by *Elisabeth Linusson* and delivered by *Dr Ronchi-Proja*, Food Policy and Nutrition Division, FAO, Rome, Italy). The training of caterers engaged in different institutional feeding programmes varies from country to country, eg the basic training in management and nutrition, in most countries in Latin America and Asia is well developed, whereas in African countries, with few exceptions, training in management without a nutrition component or no training at all is given. Therefore, there is a great need in such cases to provide caterers with basic knowledge of nutrition, hygiene and management skills. There is a trend in developing countries towards increased urbanization, more women working outside their homes, industrialization etc so that more people are eating away from home. This is increasing the need for mass catering for various categories of people. Therefore in recent years FAO has made an effort to collaborate with governments in the implementation of World Food Programme (WFP) assisted institutional feeding projects. Attention has been focused on the training of food supervisors or food managers and to a lesser extent of cooks in primary schools, boarding institutions, industrial canteens, hospitals, emergency or refugee feeding and supplementary feeding programmes for vulnerable groups. FAO has provided specialized staff to train them in different aspects of institutional management, including basic knowledge of nutrition, health and food safety both in theory and applied work. This experience has shown that nutrition education and training is most effective if given at local or regional level, when it can be made directly relevant to the staff and community needs. Teaching materials have been developed, adapted to local conditions and tested in several countries during workshop training. There is a considerable need to expand these activities and to introduce them to countries where they do not exist.

Conclusions. (1) The teaching of nutrition on full-time and in-service catering courses both at craft and higher levels should be maintained where its level is significant or introduced where absent. (2) This teaching should involve not just theory but practical exercises in implementing healthier menus. Students' interest can be enhanced by the study of their own eating habits. (3) Teaching of nutrition (and other aspects of food management) to caterers in developing countries should be increased. This instruction is most effective when performed at local or regional levels and when couched in clear practical terms that are directly relevant to the particular staff and communties involved.

XXIV: Nutrition and anthropology

Anthropology and nutrition: a discussion

Ellen MESSER
Department of Anthropology, Norton, MA 02766, USA and MIT International Food and Nutritional Planning Program

Anthropologists continually face two dilemmas: where do they fit into interdisciplinary teams and how can they best make an impact in socioeconomic and health projects in which anthropological information can improve the ultimate quality of life? These problems confront not only teams of anthropologists and nutritionists, but also teams that include other specialists, such as economists, public health professionals, and psychologists/child development experts. In each case, the team must decide what kinds of information (macro versus micro, quantitative versus qualitative) anthropologists should supply, and whether anthropological interpretations should be 'organic' or 'superorganic'. They must also determine how such information will be used, and the appropriate mix between research-oriented or applied (targeted) tasks.

In situations in which both quantitative nutritional data and qualitative sociocultural information is desired, anthropologists and nutritionists must also consider how to divide the work between them. This problem gives rise to questions concerning the education of nutritionists and anthropologists. Should nutritionists be trained in ethnographic research techniques in order to design and carry out the qualitative sociocultural components of studies, while anthropologists learn the quantitative research and analytical methods of nutritionists? That is, should schools of nutrition and departments of anthropology be producing a hybrid? Or, should the two disciplines continue separately, each informing and enriching joint studies?

Different types of anthropologists and nutritional anthropology. In elucidating the roles and directions anthropologists take in nutrition studies, it is important to keep in mind that there are different types of anthropologists. The discipline includes biological/physical as well as social/cultural anthropologists. At least in the United States, both subdisciplines are represented with 'nutritional anthropology' since both contribute anthropological studies to the food and nutrition field. Employing methods from biological and cultural anthropology, as well as methods from the nutrition sciences, nutritional anthropological studies approach topics such as the interaction of diet and human genetics (eg, the lactose-deficiency problem), relationships between food intake and energy expenditure (eg, energy balance in relation to time allocation and activity patterns), the congruence between local 'folk' and scientific analyses of nutritional problems and nutrient composition of foods, and cultural determinants of nutritional standards.

Nutritional anthropology in the USA is, thus, not so much a separate subdiscipline, as a network of anthropologists, all of whom are interested in food. They bring to discussions of particular topics in food and nutrition their own subdisciplinary perspectives in problem formation, methods of data collection, analysis and interpretation. They also try to use their specialists' skills in a broader, biocultural framework. To further communication about common research and project interests in 1974, biophysical and sociocultural anthropologists together formed the Council on Nutritional Anthropology (CNA) of the American Anthropological Association, a network for nutritionists and anthropologists, as well as for anthropologists of the various subdisciplines.

Overlap and division of labour between anthropologists and nutritionists. Overlap and division of labour between anthropologists and nutritionists is very much dependent on the type of problem being addressed and the kind of anthropologist involved. In some specialized areas, overlap in problem definition, research design, and methods is almost complete. Both physical anthropologists and nutritionists, monitoring growth in human populations, rely on survey methodologies and anthropometrics in their research design, data collection, and analysis. Both community nutrition and applied anthropological studies of food often employ the same research questions and methods. In these particular problem areas, anthropologists and nutritionists who have received comparable training may be interchangeable.

More generally, anthropologists and nutritionists often find themselve pursuing common research questions, but utilizing differing, complementary approaches. For example, both anthropologists and nutritionists study the nutritional consequences of particular cultural behaviours; the importance of nutrition in socioeconomic development; the significance of traditional foods; intra-household distribution of resources in order to explain differences in nutritional status; nutritional implications of famine and drought, often in the more general context of farming systems research. Moreover, both disciplines discuss critical issues of ethics in nutrition planning and nutrition programmes.

In such efforts, sociocultural anthropologists usually rely on nutritionists to design, carry out, and analyse the nutritional components, that is, the technical aspects of monitoring the nutritional consequences of particular behaviours. To provide anthropologists with clearer perspectives on nutritional research techniques and methodologies, the Council on Nutritional Anthropology, in conjunction with the Internation Commission on Anthropology and Food, the United Nations University, and the MIT International Nutrition Planning Program, has been providing a 'short course on nutritional methods for anthropologists' for the last 5 years. For one intensive week, nutritionists teach anthropologists methods of problem conceptualization, research design, data collection, analysis, and interpretation. Through lectures and laboratory exercises they learn anthropometrics, nutritional biochemical measures they can use in the field, how to record dietary intakes and analyse nutrient compositions of diets, and how to measure work capacity. By the end of the course they know how nutritionists address problems, the techniques they use, the advantages and difficulties of various methodologies in the field and their reliability or limitations for interpretation. They also have a better idea of whom to contact and what methods to trust in order to incorporate nutrition into their ethnographic research. But they hardly see themselves as substituting for nutritionists on research teams: each still has a specialty.

Complementarily, nutritionists ordinarily seek anthropologists' advice and skills in designing and carrying out the sociocultural or biocultural components of food and nutrition studies. They leave it to anthropologists to: (a) analyse the sociocultural determinants of food intake, folk classifications of food, cultural patterning and group-shared rules in diet; (b) identify appropriate social units of analysis; (c) characterize, label, and measure work and leisure activities; (d) decipher cultural concepts of nutrition and their relationship to disease, and (e) develop special topics, such as 'women and food' into meaningful food and nutrition policy objectives. In elucidating the sociocultural and biological implications of food selection, anthropologists are also called upon to frame and comment on broader questions of interrelationships of culture and biology.

Contributions of anthropological methods to nutrition studies. *Diet*. Anthropologists characterize local, regional, and national diets using a variety of distinctive approaches.

Archaeological, historical, and ethnographic data are used to define and to understand dietary patterns in the process of evolution. Using techniques from ethnobotany and ethnozoology, including participant observation, other types of observation, and interview, they identify distinctive foods and biological communities of plants and animals. By spending extended periods of time in communities they are able to describe principles of food classification: to delineate criteria for acceptance or rejection of food items and combinations and to define local concepts of hunger and satiety. They also examine local-regional-national-international food linkages according to general themes such as the effects of the Westernization and commercialization of the food supply. At the household level, cognitive and symbolic anthropologists characterize food patterns — meal formats, menus, and components — and decipher ethnic food classifications. Both ecological and cognitive anthropologists also specialize in ethnobotany and ethnozoology. They provide 'unusual' food identifications and investigate the effects of particular dietary patterns on the utilization of plants and animals and the consequent viability of the communities of plants and animals used as food. Archaeologists and ethnohistorians provide reconstructions of past diets and models of dietary evolution. Nutritionists are thus able to see geographical and historical patterns of food use and to evaluate the advantages and disadvantages of particular food combinations developed in indigenous and modernized areas. Biological anthropologists, in conjunction with sociocultural colleagues, trace genetic predispositions to, and interactions, with diet.

Social units of analysis. At a group level, anthropologists help nutritionists define the appropriate social group unit for a study, which may involve selection of communities, characterization of ethnic groups, regional groups, functional/regional groups, and tribal units. At the household level, anthropologists have refined the household concept for particular geographical areas and social groups, which aids in the study of intra- and inter-household distribution of resources. They may identify the appropriate units to follow (child? mother/child?) in investigating child nutrition and child-feeding rules, often by the method of 'child following' which anthropologists may have invented. Regarding other categories, anthropologists identify the appropriate age, sex, ethnic, class, and occupational categories for comparison in particular cases. In economics, they can help conceptualize the proper indicators of the material standard of living. Anthropologists also analyse the 'macro-micro' linkages in food systems, identifying appropriate socioeconomic units.

Characterizing, labelling, and measuring activities. In studies of energy flow, physical activities, diet, and nutrition in relation to dietary decision making and the time allocation of one principal household member (especially the mother), the observational methods of participant observation, timed observations, and spot observations are all anthropological techniques that can be used to advantage by an anthropologically-trained observer. In surveys, anthropologists can also provide the background information on cultural context, the appropriate social, occupational, and environmental context, and construct the appropriate questions and sampling techniques. They can also provide the culturally appropriate frameworks for eliciting respondent reports.

Nutrition issues. Anthropologists have developed the concept of 'ethno-nutrition,' a subject area that includes the study of local cultural concepts of what are nutritious foods; what are dangerous foods; what food combinations go together and produce health; and what quantities of foods are appropriate on a daily/annual schedule. They also investigate local ideas of the relationships between health and nutrition, including concepts of good growth and good appetite, as well as the relationships between appetite and health that affect local community, household, and individual food distribution and consumption. At the international, national, regional, local and household levels, anthropologists also trace the relationships between food production, food classification, social rules of food distribution, and good nutrition and health. Such information provides basic insights for predicting how people will respond to intervention programmes.

Food and nutrition policy issues. Anthropological studies can often help planners to anticipate the likely effects of food and nutrition programmes, given inter- and intra-household patterns of resource distribution, and to describe how various public health policies either succeed or fail. Participating in nutrition surveillance efforts, for example, they may note the uneven distribution of resources within and between communities, and over time, monitor the impact of national development policies. They investigate what people in local communities perceive as public health and socioeconomic problems, and how they respond to local project efforts. They discern between cultural and economic causes of malnutrition, document factors such as occupational stratification in socioeconomic status, diet, and nutritional levels, and compare 'cognitive' with 'behavioural' factors in diet, health, and nutrition outcomes. Studying the culture of both the 'consumers' and the 'planners', they offer explanations for why people underuse or fail to benefit fully from health and nutritional services by evaluating the expectations on both sides, along with data on implementation.

Anthropologists may be helpful to nutritionists in interpreting data on intra-community differences in nutritional outcomes by studying the influence of ecological differences on food habits, household decision making regarding the acquisition and distribution of food, food bias rules (such as discrimination against females) and also the socioeconomic levels and conditions in which food bias rules operate.

On specific questions, for example, why women in one community fail to participate in a particular mother-child health clinic programme and why they insist on giving supplementary foods to their infants at an early age, anthropological techniques can illuminate the time constraints that mothers face as well as the patterns of work and of surrogate mother-child care which encourage such feeding patterns. If they cannot solve the problem of work schedules and poverty, anthropologists can at least define the problem. They can also show how local responses are culturally patterned and perhaps cast such explanations in the larger framework of local concepts of adequate diet and its relationship to local concept of adequate child growth.

Implications for teamwork and anthropological studies for nutritionists. Although nutritionists might attempt to formulate and carry out these anthropological dimensions of nutrition research, most would probably rather leave such investigations to social scientists, especially anthropologists. In the interest of promoting teamwork, furthering nutritionists' understanding of anthropological concepts and methods, and attracting their anthropological colleagues to the study of food and nutrition, nutritional anthropologists have over the past 5 years produced three volumes of conceptual and methodological essays and several reviews of the field[1-6]. Jointly with nutritionists, anthropologists currently are addressing broad scientific, philosophical, and practical issues of data reliability in nutritional anthropological research. Through such efforts, nutritional anthropology may well become a new synthesis, a synthesis which stands to improve the quality of method and theory, our understandings of the relationships between culture and nutrition, and our abilities to solve food problems from the perspectives of both disciplines.

1 Jerome, N., Kandel, R. & Pelgo, G.H. (1980): *Nutritional anthropology*. NY: Redgrave.
2 Messer, E. (1984): Sociocultural aspects of nutrient intake and behavioral responses to diet. In *Nutrition and behavior: human nutrition*, ed J. Galler, **5**, 417–71. New York: Plenum Press.
3 Messer, E. (1984): Diet in cross-cultural perspective. *Ann. Rev. Anthropol.* **13**, 205–50.
4 Pelto, P.J. & Pelto, G.H. (1983): Culture, nutrition, and health. In *The anthropology of medicine from culture to method*, ed L. Romanucci-Ross, D.E. Moerman & L.R. Tancredi, pp. 221–30. NY: Praeger.
5 Pelto, G., Pelto, P. & Messer, E. (In prep): *Methods in nutritional anthropology*.
6 Quandt, S. & Ritenbaugh, C. (In prep): *Training manual in nutritional anthropology*

Anthropology of food, crossroads of biology and culture: its proper methodology from a case study in Zaïre

H. PAGEZY
C.N.R.S, ER 221, Université d'Aix-Marseille III, Pavillon de L'enfant, 346, route des Alpes, 13100-Aix en Provence, France.

Food anthropologists are often criticized for their methodology, in that they use a limited number of subjects, with whom they have privileged relationships, so that it is difficult to analyse the results statistically. On the other hand, human scientists are suspicious of the studies that draw conclusions from large amounts of somewhat crude data, crude mainly because of technical difficulties, and which are unlikely to reflect true reality.

The large-scale survey is essentially limited by the difficulty of increasing precision by increasing both the size of the sample and the accuracy of the observations and when collecting data, it is sometimes difficult to assess the correctness of what you are told. Furthemore, this type of survey is very costly and it becomes difficult to plan repeated visits, to identify any possible cyclical factor. For those reasons, we do not think that the anthropological method should be too hastily rejected by the epidemiologists. Firstly, it can be very useful in planning a large scale survey in choosing questions adapted to culture traits and food behaviour. Secondly, case studies can complete and reinforce the results of the large-scale survey. Finally, it can be very useful and indeed essential when establishing policies.

The subjects in their environment. Nzalekenga is a village located in the region of lake Tumba in Zaïre, called the 'basin'. Villages, 2 to 5 km apart, are separated by dams which are flooded during the rainy seasons, making movement difficult. They are inhabited by two genetically distinct populations, the tall Oto, descendants of agriculturalists and fishermen, and the pygmy Twa, descended from hunter-gatherers. Oto and Twa have developed a common culture and language, but do not intermarry, so they can be considered as two castes of a single ethnic group: the Ntomba. Traditionally, the Twa people are linked by specific trading relations to the Oto. They exchange game and gathered products for agricultural goods, essentials such as salt and tools, and nowadays, products such as cigarettes, alcohol and clothes. The Oto-Twa relationships have progressed and trading between the two castes is now based on the sale of labour, the Twa working for the Oto.

The anthropological approach of the Ntomba food system. A quantitative food consumption survey, carried out between 1980 and 1982 on 40 Oto and 40 Twa families, identified the similarities in the Oto and Twa diets, but showed that the two castes used very different methods of getting their food. Available throughout the year, cassava comes mainly from Oto plantations on which Twa are employed. Tubers, dug after 9 to 12 months, and steeped for 5–7 d in pools, are the staple food. Tubers are eaten with cassava leaves and animal foods prepared with palm kernal sauce or oil. Cassava leaves come from young leaves of 3-month-old plants. The sharing system permits everyone to get cassava leaves at any season.

Unlike cassava and palm nut, which are available throughout the year, animal foods are periodic. Dry and wet seasons alternate and food is abundant and diversified during the dry seasons. When the water level goes down, quantities of fish are caught by the Oto men setting traps in the currents, and shrimps are also caught. Although fish production seems to be sufficient for local consumption, conservation in the rainy forest is a major problem. Some 30 per cent of it can be destroyed by the adverse physical conditions combined with pests, mainly in the camp sites. Caterpillars are gathered in great amounts by the Twa and the Oto, just as the first rains start to fall and smoked fish appears in the diet with the rainy season, which should be a game season. The Ntomba do not catch much game nowadays, despite the number of traps set around the villages, although it still abounds 50 km away where less of the forest has been cleared for cash crops. The results of the survey have shown that the Ntomba are almost self-sufficient in food. Indeed, less than 2 per cent of the Oto and Twa diet comes from purchased products such as rice, sugar, flour, sardines, tomato sauce, sweet condensed milk and beer.

In 1979, we chose to study a village inhabited by some 850 people, 600 Oto and 250 Twa located on a secondary road, along which fewer than 5 vehicles per month passed. A precise census of the village was conducted every 3 months, using a system of cards on which were noted the name of the people sharing the same house and the number of each house as marked on a map. The village was divided into five blocks containing theoretically related families. The map also enabled the organization of consumption to be understood. There is a frequent exchanging of presents and various kinds of help are given within the family block.

The problem of identifying and isolating the consumers sharing the same dish is usually tricky, but is limited among the Ntomba by the fact that the staple, cassava, is eaten as a stick, or as roughly standardized portions. It is then easier to count the number of consumed units whenever they have escaped weighing. On the other hand, cassava leaves, fish and game are usually shared and eaten among a small group of people. Apart from the mother and her youngest child, who share the same food, we noticed that most of the undergroups were quite homogeneous in age and sex so that the results could be pooled. Nevertheless, the problem of sharing can be more acute in other regions. That is why C.M. Hladik has experimented with an electronic scale in Central Africa, which allows the precise measurement of each person's share among a small family group.

The census, besides demonstrating mobility, mainly among the Twa, showed the increase in size of the village during the rainy season and its spreading during the dry season, mainly towards the fishing camps. It showed how difficult it could be to determine the real number of residents at a given period, with subjects moving to and from their mothers' and fathers' villages, especially in the case of women at the end of their pregnancy and, escorted by the youngest of their children, during the first months of breast feeding. The primiparous woman goes back to her father's village after the first delivery, and stays there for 2 (Oto) to 4 (Twa) years apart from her husband, receiving special allocations of food, and not being allowed to perform any physical work[2]. Also, during school vacations, the teachers from surrounding villages go back home, whereas those originally from Nzalekenga return there. The results of the census led us to include the fishing camps in the study, although located some 10 km (4 to 8 hours journey) from the village; otherwise we would have left out some 30 per cent of the population.

Our methods enabled us to identify a few Oto and rather more Twa families that escaped the official census, which were, nutritionally speaking, most interesting: for instance, we discovered the only case of malnutrition among the Oto, a 3-year-old girl, who was kept hidden inside the hut, because of her parents' shame.

The detailed results of these surveys have been published[1,3] and underline the biological effects of the hungry season among certain categories.

Through the quantitative food consumption survey, we tried to answer the question 'what is the nutritional value of each group's diet for each season'? Living in the village made it easier for us to obtain random controls, thus increasing the precision of the investigation and the use of different sorts of scales and dynamometers allowed us to measure the individual consumption quickly. The use of the FAO food consumption tables allowed us were supplemented by measurements of the actual water content and by biochemical analyses of different preparations or different local species. Compared to the FAO tables, we noted a difference of 40 kcal (167 kJ)/100 g between different ways of cooking cassava, i.e. 20 per cent of its energy value. To identify local species, we collected plant and animal specimens, and made photographs. With regard to caterpillars, we showed that different species of caterpillars appeared in succession during a short period of time, and some years did not appear at all.

We also made some investigations with regard to the perception of the different categories of food by the population; for instance, the staple 'fills the stomach'; the lack of animal food-stuff is perceived as 'hunger'; food consumed as snacks (peanuts, fruit or even breadfruit or corn) is not 'real food'; some species normally consumed only by the Twa and rejected by the Oto e.g., certain caterpillars, wild leaves, ferns, seeds, could be consumed when food was short.

It can be important to note the way in which food is acquired, in order to form the basis of a food strategy. For instance, in the fishing camps, most of the fish eaten is caught directly or obtained from fishermen by exchange. On the other hand, cassava is brought regularly by the resident of the village, who go back with fish. Bachelors or fishermen whose wives have left temporarily, e.g. primiparous husbands, have to buy cassava every day. Cassava leaves are rare at the campsite, as they are brought from the villages as surplus and do not keep well. As they have no commercial value, they are constantly exchanged as gifts between and from the Oto.

The food system is also part of the economic system, so that investigations of who owns what and sells what can be instructive. It identifies the complementary strategies of the Oto and Twa, and the multiplicity of occupations and options of their economic life. We found a similar strategy in creating a succession of ties by marriage — the Ntomba frequently change spouses, which can be put to advantage, mainly in acquiring food. Fishermen are much sought after as husbands for these reasons.

We found that 50 per cent of mothers still breast-fed their children at 18 months of age for the Oto and 24 months for the Twa. Complementary food, not specially prepared for the child, is introduced before the age of 6 months and up to the age of 11–12 months, when they rely essentially on an adult diet. Complete weaning is more frequent at the end of the major rainy season (17 cases out of 69 in January), although it is a period biologically more constraining, and weaning never happens during the major dry season (one case out of 69 in July, none in August), despite the diversified and abundant food available. The mothers think that their child will 'not grow normally', will 'show behavioural troubles', will 'not endure the following hungry season', or will 'not accept the uniform foliage diet' after the dry season.

The anthropological outlook can be very important in nutritional studies because it allows one to link socioeconomic, cultural and environmental factors to biology. A good knowledge of the food system is interesting when faced with nutritional problems. Today, the Ntomba's diet, in accordance with their culture, is balanced and diversified. In the present local and economic conditions, we must encourage the preservation of the natural environment, which means the forest and its waterways by an appropriate type of action: otherwise the hungry season could be greatly extended.

Acknowledgements. I am grateful to the Medical and Scientific Center, University of Brussels (CEMUBAC) for material assistance.

1 Pagezy, H. (1982): Seasonal hunger, as experienced by the Oto and the Twa of a Ntomba village in the Equatorial forest (Lake Tumba, Zaïre). *Ecol. Fd Nutr.* **12**, 139–153.
2 Pagezy, H. (1983): The attitude of the Ntomba society towards the primiparous woman. *J. Biosoc. Sci.* **15**, 421–431.
3 Pagezy, H. (1984): Seasonal hunger as experineced by the Oto and the Twa women of a Ntomba village in the Equatorial forest (Lake Tumba, Zaïre). *Ecol. Fd Nutr.* **15**, 13–27.

Infant nutrition and growth in Madura, Indonesia

Jane A. KUSIN, Sri KARDJATI, C. de WITH and Wil M. van STEENBERGEN
Section of Nutrition and Food Technology, Royal Tropical Institute, Mauritskade 63, 1092 AD Amsterdam, The Netherlands; (S.K.) Department of Public Health, Faculty of Medicine, Airlangga University, Jl. Darmahusada 47, Surabaya, Indonesia.

In Indonesia, as in most developing countries, malnutrition is most prevalent at the age of 1–2 years[11]. However, the beginning of growth faltering is in early infancy, around the 3rd month[4,6]. To get a better insight into what happens in the process of infant growth, a longitudinal research programme is being undertaken from 1982–1985 in three villages in Madura, East Java — Gulbung, Apaan and Aengsareh.

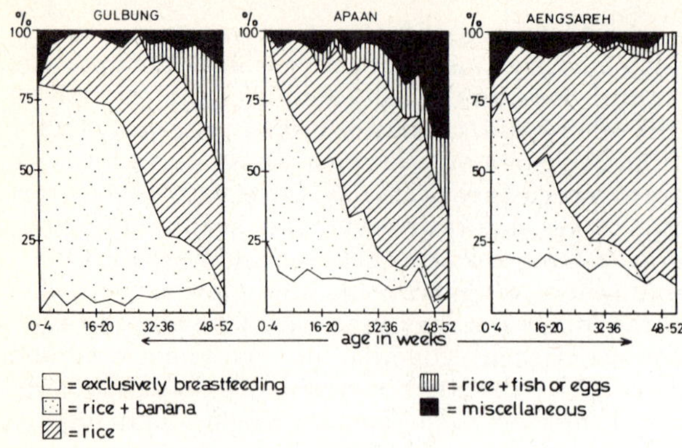

Fig. 1. *Changes with age in the feeding patterns of breast-fed infants in three villages.*

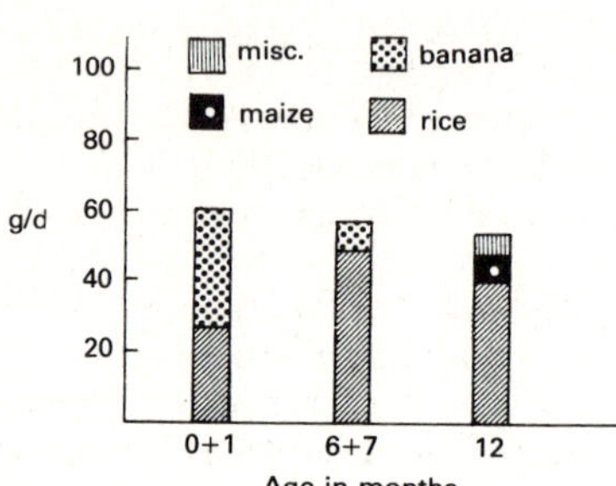

Fig. 2. *Consumption of supplementary foods by infants in Madura.*

Materials and methods. In August 1982 all infants were enrolled for the longitudinal study on postnatal growth, infant feeding, morbidity and mortality. New-borns were added to this sample in the subsequent months until 31 December 1984. Follow-up continues till the infant has reached the age of 12 months. This paper covers data of feeding pattern and growth of infants, examined in the period August 1982 through April 1983. Birth weight was measured with Salter scales within 24 h after birth by trained fieldworkers. New-borns were visited weekly to record information on feeding pattern and to measure weight and length. After the first month, the same information was collected at 4-weekly intervals. Breast-milk intake and amounts of additional foods consumed were measured in a subsample of 98 normal birth-weight infants. Fieldworkers stayed 48 h in a household and measured breast-milk intake by the test-weighing technique (Seca scales). Foods to be consumed by the infant were weighed before and after preparation and individual servings were measured. From these values the equivalent amount of raw ingredients was calculated and converted to amounts of energy and nutrients (Indonesian Food Composition Table).

Results. *Feeding pattern and food intake.* As observed in earlier studies[4], breast-feeding is the rule in these communities from the day of birth. However, new-borns are force-fed from the 1st week with mashed banana or a mixture of mashed banana and soft boiled rice. From the age of 7 months fish and eggs are given.

No difference in feeding pattern was observed between the sexes. On the other hand, differences between villages were noted. Exclusive breast-feeding was more common in Apaan and Aengsareh throughout infancy, while a larger percentage of infants received rice and fish or eggs at age 6–12 months in Gulbung and Apaan. (Fig. 1) Breast milk intake ranged from 650–775 ml per day in the 1st half year and from 600–650 ml in the 2nd half year. The additional food was about 35 g banana and 25 g rice in the first month. Rice replaced banana after the age of one month and by 9 months the infant received rice, maize and small amounts of side dishes. The amount of additional food did not increase with age. (Figure 2) The total energy

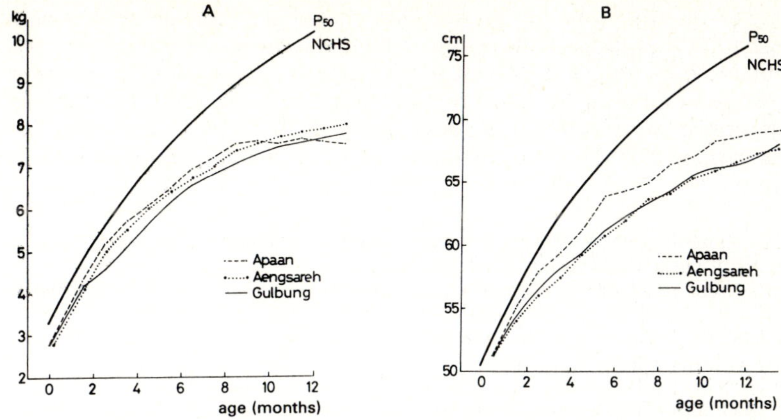

Fig. 3. *Growth in weight (A) and in length (B) of male infants in three villages in relation to National Centre for Health Statistics (NCHS) 50th centiles.*

intake per day ranged from 465–630 kcal (1.9–2.6 MJ). Mixed-fed infants had higher intakes than exclusively breast-fed infants. For reasons as yet unknown some infants were exclusively breast-fed after a period of mixed feeding.

Infant growth. Every 4-weeks, 71–128 infants of each sex were measured. Females were always lighter and smaller than males, but the pattern of growth did not differ. In Fig. 3 the growth curves for male infants are shown for the three villages separately. Weight started to falter at 12–16 weeks of age, length at 8–12 weeks. Growth curves deviated progressively from the standards, weight being more affected than length. At 12 months of age Madurese infants were not only much shorter (68 cm) and lighter (7.5 kg) than the reference, but also leaner. Growth in Apaan appeared the most favourable, while that in Gulbung was the most depressed.

Discussion. In children, failure to grow adequately is considered to be an indicator of poor health. It has been generally assumed that growth faltering before the sixth month of age is caused by low yields of breast-milk[2,13,14]. In our case, the average amount of breast-milk consumed was slightly lower than that of infants from well-nourished mothers. However, it is still within the range of 'normal' daily yields[1,3,5,10,15]. Lactation failure cannot therefore be the cause of growth faltering in our study population. Again, one would not expect a deviation from the reference growth curve during the first 6 months when total energy intake was about 600 kcal (2.5 MJ)/d. Mean birth weight of these infants was about 2800 g and energy requirement to maintain adequate growth at this age appears to be 85–90 kcal per kg B. wt. per day[1,15]. In these villages morbidity is certainly quite high but regular observations suggest that infants are generally healthy in the 1st half year of life. It may well be that the reference children grow abnormally fast and the Madurese infants grow 'normally' or 'physiologically', since at 6 months of age they have doubled their birth weight!

Undoubtedly, the growth curve after 6 months illustrates a discrepancy between intake and requirement. As far as feeding practices are concerned, two aspects need to be considered, ie the forced-feeding almost immediately after birth and the quantity of foods given in addition to breast-milk which did not increase with age. Questioning mothers about the reasons behind these practices will not provide the real background for their behaviour.

In general, the contribution of social sciences to a better understanding of what governs infant feeding practices, has been descriptive rather than analytical[8,9,12]. In our populations there are indications that an association exists between a mother's activities and the feeding and growth of her infant[7]. From what has been discussed, the interface between the medical-nutritional and the social-anthropological disciplines is crucial. The first can diagnose malnutrition but is ill-equipped to grasp the reasons why. Biomedical research has certainly elucidated some important causes of malnutrition, but has to be integrated in a more general assessment of what happens in households and the reasons people behave as they do. Until the underlying causes of malnutrition outside the biological framework are assessed, it is doubtful whether UNICEF's approach, i.e., Growth monitoring, Oral rehydration, Breast-feeding, Immunization — Food supplements, Family planning, Female education (GOBI-FFF) or the eight components of primary health care will make a contribution to solving the malnutrition problem in the forseeable future.

1 Dewey, K.G. & Lönnerdal (1983): Milk and nutrient intake of breastfed infants from 1–6 months: relation to growth and fatness. *J. Pediat. Gastro Enterol. Nutr.* **2**, 497–506.
2 Gopalan, C. (1985): Infant nutrition in West Bengal. Insights from recent studies. *Bull. Nutr. Foundation India*, **6** (2), 1–3.
3 Jelliffe, D.B. & Jelliffe, E.F.P. (1978): *Human milk in the modern world*, pp. 62–69. Oxford: OUP.
4 Kardjati, S., Kusin, J.A., de With, C. & Subidia, I.G.K. (1978): Feeding practices, nutritional status and mortality in preschool children in East Java, Indonesia: *Trop. Geogr. Med.* **30**, 359–371.
5 Kohler, L., Meeuwisse, G. & Mortensson, W. (1984): Food intake and growth of infants between six and twenty-six weeks of age on breastmilk, cow's milk formula and soy formula. *Acta Paed Scand.* **73**, 40–48.
6 Kusin, J.A., Sinaga, H.S.R.P., Khoma, J., Houtkoper, J.M. & Renqvist, V. (1978): The preschool child in Su a village, North Sumatra. II: Mixed longitudinal data of weight and height; *Paed. Indon.* **21**, 181–191.
7 Launer, L. (1985): The effects of maternal behaviour on growth velocity of infants in Madura, Indonesia: Poster C 20, XIII Intern. Congress of Nutrition, Brighton 18–23 August 1985.
8 Manderson, C. (1984): These are the modern times: infant feeding practices in peninsular Malaysia. *Soc. Sci. Med.* **18**, 47–57.
9 Pelto, G.H. (1981): Infant feeding practices in the Third World: beliefs and motivations. In *Infant and child feeding*, ed J.T. Boud *et al.* pp. 191–204, New York: Academic Press.
10 Picciano, M.F., Calkino, E.J., Garrick, J.R. & Deering, R.H. (1981): Milk and mineral intakes of breastfed infants. *Acta Paed. Scand.* **70**, 189–194.
11 Sajogyo, A.N.P. (1973): Evaluation study, 1973. Report of the Ministry of Health, Jakarta, Indonesia.
12 Sanjur, D., Cravioto, J. & van Veen, A.G. (1970): Infant nutrition and socio-cultural influences in a village in Mexico. *Trop. Geogr. Med.* **22**, 443–451.
13 Villar, J. & Belizan, J.M. (1981): Breastfeeding in developing countries. *Lancet* **2**, 621–623.
14 Waterlow, J.C. & Thomson, A.M. (1979): Observation on the adequacy of breast-feeding. *Lancet* **2**, 238–241.
15 Whitehad, R.G. & Paul, A.A. (1984): Infant growth and human milk requirements. *Lancet* **2**, 161–163.

Food practices in contrasting populations: an anthropological study of the Lepchas, Sherpas, Oraons and Mahishyas of West Bengal, India

Amitabha BASU, Susmita MUKHOPADHYAY, Partha P. MAJUMDER, Subrata K. ROY, Ba. MUKHOPADHYAY, Premananda BHARATI, and R. GUPTA
Biological Sciences Division and (PPM) Applied Statistics Division, Indian Statistical Institute, Calcutta 700035, India.

The objective of this paper is to illustrate the possible contribution of anthropology to nutrition, and the interface between the two disciplines with examples from our recent field studies on several contrasting ethnic groups and subgroups of West Bengal, India. Examples are cited on: (a) intake differences between and among subgroups of ethnic groups: (b) intake differences between and within ethnic groups inhabiting the same region and their health implications, and (c) intake differences among individuals within households, and the implications of these examples are discussed.

The study was undertaken as part of a broader multidisciplinary biomedical study programme, entitled 'Human adaptability Programme' initiated in the ISI in 1976. The general objective of the programme was to detect and measure the effects of physical, environmental, sociocultural and ethnic factors on health, as well as of health and activity patterns on the environment, and eventually to determine the limits to human adaptation, 'limits' defined in terms of a population's physical fitness and capacity for demographic survival (for a recent review, see[1]).

Materials and methods. Four populations and their subgroups were studied: *Lepchas*, indigenous to the medium altitudes of Sikkim-Darjeeling Himalaya; *Sherpas*, indigenous to high altitude Tibet and subsequently northeastern Nepal with a migrant section in the Sikkim-Darjeeling Himalaya; *Oraons*, indigenous to the Chotnagpur Plateau in Bihar with a migrant group in the tea gardens of Jalpaiguri district, West Bengal, in the eastern Himalayan foothills, and *Mahishyas*, an indigenous Hindu caste of deltaic West Bengal. Lepchas, Sherpas and Oraons are tribal groups.

The rural less-developed, rural developed and urban subgroups of the Buddhist Lepchas, agricultural and plantation labour subgroups of the Sherpas, two subgroups of tea labourers of the Oraons (ie, labourers of the adjacent Birpara and Dalgaon Tea Gardens) and high, medium and low economic subgroups of the Mahishyas were studied.

The types of data used are: (a) 1-day semi-quantitative dietary intake survey data by recall method using eight standard containers, on all four groups (container sizes in ml: No. 1, 3000; No. 2, 2000; No. 3, 1250; No. 4, 700; No. 5, 450; No. 6, 300; No. 7, 175; No. 8, 100); (b) 3-day weighed intake data on the Sherpas, Lepchas and Mahishyas; and (c) child growth data on body weight, also on Sherpas, Lepchas and Mahishyas. Semi-quantitative data were also collected on individual intakes.

The data on food consumption were converted to nutrient consumptions using Indian Council of Medical Research[2] conversion tables. Data on nutrient consumptions per capita and per consumption unit were calculated for four major nutrients: energy, animal protein, vegetable protein and fat. There are some limitations of the data which should be candidly admitted at this stage: sample sizes for all subgroups except the Oraons were fairly small; households were not randomly sampled — the samples were chosen depending on informant cooperation and time constraint; the data were subject to random fluctuations, being collected on a single day; and left-overs were not considered.

Results. The detailed results of this study will be published elsewhere and they can only be summarized here. Data for per caput and per Consumption Unit (CU) consumption of nutrients of the subgroups show that the Sherpas and Oraons are better-off than other populations in respect of intakes of most nutrients.

The results of multivariate analysis of variance indicate that, except for the Sherpas, the subgroups of every other group are significantly different in respect of nutrient intakes considered, for both per capita and per CU consumptions.

Stepwise discriminant analysis was also performed on the data. Where more than one significant discriminator existed they were arranged in order of importance. Of the four variables fat appeared to be a significant discriminator in most of the cases. Among the Oraeons, when per CU consumptions were considered, energy and vegetable protein were more important discriminators than fat. Among the Mahishyas, animal protein was the only, or relatively more important discriminator among the economic subgroups in respect of both per caput and per CU consumptions. Obviously, different sets of variables are involved in discriminating between subgroups of different groups.

The next question is 'how well can we predict the subgroup membership of a household by looking at its nutrient intakes'? To answer this question, the 'jackknifed classification' (a statistical technique) was performed.

The results of jackknifed classification showed that the probability of correct classification of a household into the subgroup to which it actually belonged was the highest in the case of the Mahishya low economic subgroup, followed by Lepcha rural developed subgroup, the other two Mahishya economic subgroups and Oraons of Birpara. In general then, with a few exceptions, households can be correctly classified into their actual subgroups with reasonably high probabilities, indicating that each subgroup has its own food intake specificity. Analysis based on weighed data from the Mahishyas also showed a high probability of correct classification. Results of this latter analysis as well as the methodology are discussed in detail elsewhere[3].

The data on energy and protein intakes of Lepchas, Sherpas and Mahishyas were then considered. It was found that the Mahishya high economic subgroup had higher intakes of all nutrients than the other two subgroups. Again, the Lepchas showed higher intakes than the Sherpas, except in the case of animal protein.

The child growth curves for body weight of the three economic subgroups of Mahishya showed that the high economic subgroup had the highest growth curve for both males and females.

The child growth curves for body weight of the Lepcha and Sherpa males, however, presented very different results. It was observed that the differences in nutrient intakes between these groups did not seem to affect their growth curves. In fact, the Lepcha curve lay within the range of one standard error unit from the data points of the Sherpa curve. This finding indicates the flexibility and the adaptability of human organisms to differential environmental (including nutritional) stresses. The body weight growth curves for Lepcha and Sherpa females showed similar results.

The data on ranking of individuals within the household in terms of the variable 'actual-recommended' showed that among the low and middle economic subgroups of the Mahishyas no inequity of food distribution occurred among members within a household. This suggests that each member receives food according to his or her need, where the need is defined in terms of sex and age-specific Recommended Dietary Allowances (RDA). However, among all subgroups of the Lepchas a consistent female bias was observed, irrespective of rural or urban and religious differences. Among the two Sherpa subgroups the pattern, however, was less clear; both husband and wife ranked among the four lower ranks. They perhaps sacrifice their shares in favour of others. Among the Oraons, no sex bias existed. Only the high economic subgroup of the Mahishyas showed a clear male bias, the highest rank being held by the male household head. These findings provide two major indications: the male bias may not be generally valid in case of tribal populations; and economic development does not automatically lead to equitable food distribution within the household.

Discussion. The above examples clearly show how the approach and method of anthropology can make a substantial contribution to the study of nutrition. For instance, recognition of micro-level differences in food intakes among and within ecological, regional and ethnic groups and subgroups should help in the formulation of practical nutritional and health programmes. Again, observation of the presence or absence in different situations of relationships of child growth with nutrient intakes may lead to further exploration of the human organism's intrinsic ability to cope with, and adapt to, nutritional stresses. Detection of the presence and absence of different kinds of biases in intra-household food distribution may emphasise the need for nutritional planning at the intra-household level, independent of general economic developments which may not necessarily raise intake levels equitably within the household.

While the contribution of anthropology to nutrition can thus be suggested from the above example, the converse is less easy to visualize. As a possible example, several studies have shown intake differentials among groups, subgroups, individuals. Studies on the extent to which physiological system can improve its own efficiency to be able to cope with nutritional stresses, and the mechanism thereof, by nutritionists can make important contribution to the anthropological problem of human adaptability.

1 Basu, A. (1985): Human biology in India: its possible role in a Third World society under rapid transformation. (Invited Lecture presented at the XI School of Biological Anthropology, Zagreb, 2–5 September 1985). *Collegium Antropologicum* (in press).

2 Indian Council of Medical Research (1981): *Nutritive value of Indian foods*. Hyderabad: National Institute of Nutrition.

3 Majumder, P.P., Bharati, P., Banerjee, D. & Basu, A. (1985): Dietary status of Mahishyas in Chakpota: Inter-and intra-economic group variations. *Ecol. Fd Nutr*. (In press).

Hunter-gatherer diet: an archaeological perspective and ethnographic method

Betty MEEHAN and R. JONES
Division of Anthropology, The Australian Museum, Sydney; Department of Prehistory, Research School of Pacific Studies, Australian National University, Canberra, Australia.

For all but the last 10–12 000 years of human history, before the emergence of tool making, a period of some two million years, human societies have lived entirely through hunting and foraging for meat and harvesting wild plants, with little modification of the environment except through the use of fire. We may posit that many of the fundamental biological parameters characteristic of the emergence of modern humans such as aspects of physiology, demography and perhaps biologically-based aspects of social behaviour were evolved under regimes analogous to those observed in contemporary and sub-contemporary hunter-gatherer cultures[24]. About 10 000 years ago in several parts of the world, such as the Middle-East, Middle America, China and New Guinea, subsistence modes of human societies became transformed with the development of agriculture and animal domestication, which led eventually to the formation of large-scale societies.

In analyses of hunter-gatherer societies, it is an interesting paradox that our weakest data base relates to the simplest and most fundamental parameters of the economy, what might be referred to as nutrition and subsistence. Indeed, this paucity of quantitative information has been a major limiting factor to the development of broadly-based theory concerning the evolution of hunting societies[10,16,20]. One of the main reasons for this was that, with the expansion of the European world in the 16th to 18th centuries into the Americas, Siberia, southern Africa and Australia, there was a massive phase of dislocation and eventual destruction of most indigenous hunter-gatherer societies at a period before the development of organized anthropological enquiry. Even in Australia, first occupied only 200 years ago by Europeans, the situation by the end of the 19th century was such that Aboriginal societies observed by the pioneer anthropologists Spencer, Haddon and Roth, were no longer carrying out their substantial traditional foraging activities. In the 1930s and 1940s it is probable that only in the remote desert areas of central Australia and on the coastal savannas of northern Australia in Arnhem Land and Cape York, were the Aborigines still operating with a largely foraging subsistence base. Even here, missions had had a profound influence in centralizing the residence of Aborigines away from their traditional lands so that most of the major anthropological treatises of that era omitted almost entirely any study of the subsistence base[19,23].

There were exceptions, e.g.[22] and studies in Arnhem Land[11–13]. The latter involved short-term (ie 1–2 weeks) quantitative analyses of the dietary intake of a small group of Aborigines living by hunting and gathering in the bush, together with the nutritional status of Aborigines living in government or mission settlements. While the main thrust of the analysis was to provide data for a Government programme for the improvement of health and nutritional status of Aborigines in northern Australia, implicit in it was also an appreciation of the broader relevance of the data to the understanding of hunter-gatherer economies in general (especially[13]).

It was generally believed in the 1950s and 1960s, that opportunity for any detailed observations of hunter-gatherer diet was over. However, with the initiation of systematic archaeological work in Australia in the 1960s, there was a pressing need for any sort of direct ethnographic information from which to build models of total economic systems which could be tested against the prehistoric data (eg[1,4,6]). Another factor was a political one, in that since 1967, when Aborigines became full citizens of Australia, they have enjoyed slowly increasing political and economic autonomy. Many Aborigines in northern Australia have moved away from government settlements and have re-established their religious and economic ties to the land, foraging again largely according to traditional methods, eg[15]. This has provided the opportunity for carrying out quantitative studies on subsistence economies such as those in Arnhem land[2,25], in Cape York[5,21], in Central Australia[17], and Devitt (pers. comm.), and in the Kimberley area of Western Australia[18].

The Gidjingali study 1972–73. The Gidjingali-speaking Aborigines, numbering some 400 people, occupy the flood plains of the Blyth River in central Arnhem Land in northern Australia at an average density of one person per 2 sq km[7]. In 1972–73, we spent 12 months living with some 35 members of the Anbarra community of this tribe, and during this time carried out systematic quantitative observations on their diet and subsistence ecology[9,14]. This community formed the core of a single camp, which itself was relocated several times during the year to take advantage of seasonal variation in food abundance. Being situated 12 degrees south of the equator within the tropical monsoon belt, there is marked seasonal variation in climate with most of the annual precipitation of 1200 mm falling in the wet season between December and March. Our field methods were to observe as comprehensively as possible all of the foods hunted and gathered by this small community during the annual cycle. Where possible direct measurements were made of the weight of each species collected. Samples of plants and animals were kept for scientific classification, and selected key foods were tested for their nutritional content. (Analyses done by P.M.A. Maggiore, Western Australian Institute of Technology Perth, and cf. Brand *et al.* 1983.) We also observed and quantified such factors as distances of foraging zones from base camps, time spent in various activities, gender-related division of labour, and the manufacture and maintenance of items of technology[14,15].

The total diet. Throughout the year, the people of the Anbarra community collected or hunted over 150 species, 29 species of shell fish, 45 fish, 10 reptiles, 20 birds, 10 mammals and 40 plant species: there was great seasonal variation in the relative proportions of foods obtained. In addition to animals hunted and vegetable foods gathered, they also had access to European flour and sugar, consumption of which we also monitored. To exemplify the nature of the data, the total dietary intake for 4 months, viz January in the full wet season; April in the late wet; May in the early dry; and September in the full dry are shown in the Table.

Per caput, the average daily energy inakes in each of these months were 1600, 2400, 2500 and 2100 kcals (6.7, 10.0, 10.5 and 8.9 MJ) respectively. Between 35 and 58 per cent of this came from European carbohydrates, indicating how the ready availability of these have replaced the carbohydrates previously obtained through hard labour in digging and preparing wild plant foods by the women. Nevertheless, important plant foods such as *Dioscorea* yams, *Tacca*, *Eleocharis* corms, de-toxified *Cycas* 'bread' and numerous tree fruits such as *Terminalia, Pandanus*, and *Syzygium* were still regularly gathered for their culinary properties. In the case of animal food, almost all was obtained by foraging with negligible contribution from European sources, and the average per capita daily protein intake was 140, 160, 190 and 170 g respectively for the four months indicated. People ate net weights of meat of all sorts at average rates of between 600 to 800 g per head per day, active male hunters taking the lion's share. Women made a sizeable contribution to the intake of animal protein especially through their collection of molluscs and reptiles, but it was primarily the work of men to get fish and exclusively theirs to hunt birds, turtles and mammal game such as wallabies and buffalo.

In terms of work, a woman could amass some 1200 kcal (5 MJ) energy per hour in most vegetable gathering and processing activities, and she could support herself in only about 2 hour's work. Men could, if they were to kill a wallaby, support their entire family on only an hour's work; however hunting was a low probability activity[9]. In general people worked about 2–3 h each day in foraging activities. They combined the lower productive and higher probability work of women with the higher productive and less predictable catch of men. This mix was done both casually on a day-by-day basis and also in the deeper organisation of work tasks for various members of the band.

Shell fish. To exemplify the complexity of the dietary patterns behind these average figures, we made a special study of the procuring and consumption of molluscs. During the study, a total of

Table. *Foods eaten by the Anbarra community during 4 months of the year 1972–73 expressed as percentages of total intake, data from Jones (1980); Meehan (1982)*

	Full wet season (January 1973)				Late wet/early dry (April 1973)				Early dry season (May 1973)				Late dry season (September 1972)			
	No. of species	Nett wt of edible food (%)	Protein (%)	Energy (%)	No. of species	Nett wt of edible food (%)	Protein (%)	Energy (%)	No. of species	Nett wt of edible food (%)	Protein (%)	Energy (%)	No. of species	Nett wt of edible food (%)	Protein (%)	Energy (%)
Flesh																
Shellfish	20	20	26	9	17	11	17	4.5	13	6.5	8	2.5	14	10.5	12	4
Crustacea	2	1	2	1	3	2	3	1	0	2	2	1	0	1.5	1	0.5
Fish	24	33	44	26	21	30	47	21.5	42	50	64	33.5	14	34	39	22
Reptiles	3	2	3	2	3	4	7	3.5	4	3.5	4.5	3	2	13	16	9.5
Birds	1+	1	1	2	p	0.5	0.5	0.5	p	0.5	0.5	1	3	4	4	6
Mammals	3	8	10	13	1	0.5	0.5	1	0	0	0	0	1	12	13.5	18
Vegetables																
Fruits and nuts	3	14	1	4.5	6	10.5	0.5	2	13	2	p	0.5	6	2	2	3
Roots/tubers	2	1	p	0.5	6	12	2	8	4	6	1	4	3	1	p	0.5
Honey	0				1	0.5	p	0.5	1	p	p	p	1	1.5	p	1
Foods bought																
Flour and sugar		20	13	42		29	23	58		30	20	55		20	12	35
Total	58				58				77				44			
No. of days observed	31				30				31				17			
Average no. of people	30				35				37				31			

29 species was collected in a total annual haul for the community of 7000 kg gross weight equivalent to 1500 kg flesh. This provided average intakes per head per day of the order of 100 g of flesh, 30 g protein and 105 k cal (440 kJ) energy. It was calculated the Anbarra ate shellfish at a rate five times that consumed by the Japanese and 200 times that eaten by the British. Sixty per-cent of this food came from only one species, the bivalve *Tapes hiantina*, and together with four other bivalves and one gastropod, the baler *Melo amphora*, they contributed 95 per cent of the total. During foraging expeditions people, usually women, concentrated on obtaining a marked preponderance of one species. Shell fish were most important in the wet season, which was the time of greatest nutritional stress. However they were also gathered at all other seasons. Their contribution to the total diet was relatively small, ranging from between 3 and 9 per cent of the total energy intake. However, shell fish gathering was the second most frequent foraging activity, occurring on 58 per cent of all days observed. The reasons for this were that it was the work of the women, it was a high probability activity that could be scheduled to fit in with other more risky foraging tasks, and it could be carried out by 'weak' members of society such as children, pregnant women and old women.

Conclusions. We do not suggest that the Anbarra system as observed in the 1970s represented all hunter-gatherer systems. We simply state that the detailed analysis of a single functioning system allows sophisticated models to be generated which can then be tested against the archaeological record. Such studies might give insights into the subsistence ecology that may have pertained under hunter-gatherer regimes over considerable periods of the human past. In terms of gross dietary intake, diversity of food categories eaten, the high meat intake and the relatively low work input, the Anbarra subsistence system is in stark contrast to the conditions which exist nowadays in most of the third world. While our perspective was primarily directed backwards in order to understand earlier societies, our data can also be used as a baseline from which to document changes in Aboriginal communities associated with assimilation into the broader Australian economy. As flour, sugar and alcohol become increasingly important in the diets of Aboriginal communities in northern Australia, associated health problems such as diabetes have become apparent[18]. Anthropology, archaeology and nutritional research are able in this instance to join forces in order to address the same problem.

1 Allen, H. (1974): The Bagundji of the Darling basin: cereal gatherers in an uncertain environment. *Wld Archael.* **5**, 309–22.

2 Altman, J.C. (1984): The dietary utilisation of flora and fauna by contemporary hunter-gatherers at Momega Outstation, north-central Arnhem Land. *Australian Aboriginal Studies* **1**, 35–46.

3 Brand, J.C., Rae, C., McDonnell, J., Lee, A., Cherikoff, V. and Truswell, A.S. (1983): The nutritional composition of Australian bush foods. *Fd Techn. Austr.* **35**, 293–8.

4 Gould, R. (1969): Subsistence behaviour among western desert Aborigines of Australia. *Oceania* **39**, 253–74.

5 Harris, D. (1978): Gardening and gathering. *Austr. Nat. Hist.* **19**, 206–9.

6 Hiatt, B. (see Meehan) (1967–68): The food quest and economy of the Tasmanian Aborigines. *Oceania* **38**, 99–133; 190–219.

7 Hiatt, L.R. (1965): *Kinship and conflict. A study of an aboriginal community in northern Arnhem Land.* The Australian National University, Canberra.

8 Jones, R. (1969): Fire stick farming. *Aust. Nat. Hist.* **16**, 224–228.

9 Jones, R. (1980): Hunters in the Australian savanna. In *Human ecology in savanna environments*, ed I.R. Harris pp. 107–146. London: Academic Press.

10 Lee, R. & I. DeVore, eds (1968) *Man the hunter.* Aldine-Atherton, Chicago.

11 McArthur, M. (1960): Food consumption and dietary levels of Aborigines living on naturally occurring foods. In *Records of the American-Australian scientific expedition to Arnhem Land*, Vol. 2, *Anthropology and nutrition* ed C. Mountford. pp. 14–26. Melbourne: Melbourne University Press.

12 McArthur, M. (1960): Food consumption and dietary levels of the Aborigines at the settlements. In *Records of the American-Australian scientific expedition to Arnhem Land*, Vol. 2, *Anthropology and nutrition* ed C. Mountford, pp. 90–135. Melbourne: Melbourne University Press.

13 McCarthy, F. & McArthur, M. (1960): The food quest and the time factor in Aboriginal economic life. In *Records of the American-Australian scientific expedition to Arnhem Land*, Vol. 2, *Anthropology and nutriton*, ed C. Mountford, pp. 145–94. Melbourne University Press.

14 Meehan, B. (1982): *Shell Bed to Shell Midden.* Australian Institute of Aboriginal Studies, Canberra.

15 Meehan, B. & Jones, R. (1980): The outstation movement and hints of a white backlash. In *Northern Australia. Options and implications*, ed R. Jones, pp. 131–57. Research School of Pacific Studies, Canberra.

16 Meggitt, M. (1964): Aboriginal food-gatherers of tropical Australia. In *Proceedings and Papers on the Ninth Technical Meeting of IUCN, Nairobi, Kenya*, pp. 30–37. Morges, Switzerland, International Union for the Conservation of Nature and Natural Resources.

17 O'Connell, J.F. & Hawkes, K. (1981): Alyawara plant use and optimal foraging theory. *Hunter-gatherer foraging strategies: ethnographic and archaeological analyses*, ed B. Winterhalder and E.A. Smith pp. 99–125. Chicago: University of Chicago Press.

18 O'Dea, K. (1982): The relationship between urbanisation and diabetes in Australian Aborigines. *Procs Nutr. Soc. Austr.* **7**, 30–36.

19 Radcliffe-Brown, A. (1930): Social organisation of Australian Aboriginal tribes, *Oceania* **1**, 34–63, 322–41, 426–56.

20 Sahlins, M.D. (1972): *Stone age economics*. Chicago: Aldine.

21 Taylor, J. (1977): Diet, health and economy: some consequences of planned social change on an Aboriginal community. In *Aborigines and change: Australia in the 70s*, ed R.M. Berndt. Australian Institute of Aboriginal Studies, Canberra.

22 Thompson, D. (1939): The seasonal factor in human culture. *Procs Prehistoric Soc.* **5**, 209–21.

23 Warner, W.L. (1937): *A black civilisation*. New York: Harper.

24 Weiner, J.S. (1980): Human biology of savanna peoples. In *Human ecology in savanna environments*, ed D.R. Harris, pp. 417–20 London: Academic Press.

25 White, N. (1978): A human ecology research project in the Arnhem Land region: an outline. *Australian Institute of Aboriginal Studies Newsletter* (n.s.) **9**, 39–52.

Tropical urban nutrition: a workshop report

R. GROSS and N.W. SOLOMONS (Organizers)
German Agency for Technical Cooperation at the Federal University of Rio de Janeiro, Institute of Nutrition, School of Health Sciences, Federal University of Rio de Janeiro, Brazil; Institute of Nutrition of Central America and Panama and Senior Scientist, Center for Studies of Sensory Impairment, Aging and Metabolism, Guatemala City, Guatemala, Central America.

The workshop's theme responded to the emerging realization that: (1) in the postwar years, most of the population and community-based studies in international human nutrition in developing countries have focused on *rural* populations: (2) that the population of the world is rapidly moving toward urbanization, with 80 per cent of the population of Latin America expected to live in urban or periurban areas by the year 2000, and (3) that little effort has been devoted to the study of the nutritional problems of the cities of third world nations.

The participants who attended the workshop represented a mix of professionals and students with widely differing and complementary experiences. Many lived and worked on the Indian Subcontinent representing the cities of Karachi, Dacca, Bombay, Delhi, Calcutta and Colombo. Others came from Jamaica. Still others work in urban communities of Latin America including Mexico City, Guatemala City, Lima, Rio de Janeiro and São Paulo. The workshop was constructed around invited presentations with ample time for discussion of points of interest between and among the participants assembled.

Solomons provided an introductory theme — 'Tropical urban nutrition: a new paradigm in international health', noting the small amount of research that had been devoted to urban populations, and speculating on the possible reasons for this neglect. Important among these is the fact that the poorest of the poor live in the countryside as rural peasants or in tribal groups and the fact that urban slum-dwellers are perceived as difficult to study by virtue of their reputation for aggressive behaviour (unlike the passive rural villagers) and have continuous movement within the cities, making longitudinal follow-up a major logistical concern. The demographic imperative, however, makes it *necessary* to study urban nutritional problems. It is doubtful if the lessons of the country-side can be extrapolated to the city.

Jay Schensul (Department of Anthropology, University of Connecticut) spoke on 'The central role of women in identifying and solving urban health problems' in which she built a model for the involvement of the mothers of the community in seeking and organizing the means for the protection of their own health and that of their children. Migration and the participation in the workplace were factors identified that conditioned the nature and success of these strategies. The focus of the presentation by *Maarten Immink*, an economist from INCAP Guatemala City, was complementary. He spoke of the role of the rural worker and its relation to energy expenditure and the need for dietary energy. He detailed the assumptions and the methodologies employed in the study of this phenomenon. He extrapolated from this rural experience to speculate on what differences and similarities would exist when a serious effort to approach the topic of worker productivity and energy output would be conducted in the city environment.

C. Monteiro, a nutritional epidemiologist from the University of São Paulo, expounded on the topic 'rural urban comparisons in the nutritional status of Brazilians' presenting data that demonstrated essentially no differences in the nutritional status of the population of São Paulo and that of the rural sectors of that huge South American country. Of note was the greater monetary cost of food and services paid by the slum-dwellers as compared to rural individuals or even by the well-to-do. Despite greater 'incomes' the consuming power of the urban poor of Brazil is no better than that of the rural poor. Again focusing on Brazil, *Roger Shrimpton* of the UNICEF office in São Luiz, Maranhão, Brazil, spoke on the theme 'UNICEF's experience in urban projects'. He cited examples of considerable current investment of that United Nations agency in urban areas and described the form of the UNICEF endeavour in the new campaign for improving infant survival in urban contexts in the developing world.

S. Schensul, Center for International Community Health Studies, University of Connecticut, spoke on approaches to establishing contact and rapport with urban sectors to be involved in research. His topic was 'Methods of public health research in urban poor communities in the developing and developed countries.' He emphasized a strategy that he had used in a Latin community in the USA and in Peruvian and Sri Lankan experience, that of participation *with* and advocacy *of* the community under study. Urban residents, wealthy or poor, are more sophisticated and more suspicious than their country cousins. A solid and viable relationship derives from a mutual commitment of community and academy to each other as well as to the issues under study. The importance of a two-way flow of communication was emphasized in this model.

Finally, the presentation by co-chairman Dr Gross was theoretical in its impact. He spoke on 'Urbanization and nutrition from a thermodynamic and cybernetic point of view'. His thesis represented the city as a thermodynamic and biological system, not simply as a chaotic deposit of inanimate streets and buildings and congregated people. As a system, it has a hierarchical organization of these elements, with periods of greater and lesser permeability, responding sooner or later to internal pressures and growing instability with reorganization and renewal. This is a continuous, but uneven, process, but at any point one sees the results of self-restructuring underway. This concept of cybernetic system sees the levels of regulation ordered from the level of the individual, through the family or household unit, to the neighbourhood, community and finally the metropolis itself. Thus, the usual reductionist approach of science in general, and nutrition in particular, may fail ultimately to understand nutrition in the city unless it takes into consideration the organic whole that is the metropolitan area.

Discussion throughout the morning was spirited, and led to a mutual appreciation of a deep interest in the field of nutrition in urban areas of tropical countries and to a flavour of diversity among different regions. There was also the sense that larger groups of interested individuals needed to be organized at future international meetings. The pursuit of new knowledge in nutrition in cities of the developing world cannot be achieved by the nutrition profession alone, but only with the assistance of other professionals including urban planners, and urban sociologists, with prior and ongoing experience in the study of cities and their populations. Mechanisms for continued communication among the participants and other interested parties were suggested and developed by a small working group which met with the organizers at the conclusion of the morning session. A small monograph of the proceedings of this Workshop is currently being prepared.

New and recent recommended dietary intakes and dietary guide-lines: a workshop report

A. Stewart TRUSWELL (Organizer)
Biochemistry Department, University of Sydney, NSW 2006, Australia.

These notes are informal. Written papers were not requested or given at this workshop. There has not been time for reported statements to be checked with individual speakers. Those speakers who are members of national or international committees were speaking unofficially and sharing their thoughts with scientists from other countries. These notes must be read as the personal impressions of the two rapporteurs — the organizer and *W. Becker*, (Swedish National Food Administration, Uppsala, Sweden). The workshop was organized on behalf of Committee 1/5 of IUNS (Recommended Dietary Allowances). The room was packed. Discussions were animated and friendly and people who attended said they found the workshop very interesting.

IUNS Committee 1/5 has published a *review* 'Recommended Dietary Intakes around the World'[8]. This shows the recommended intakes of nutrients for each of 41 countries or international agencies, together with comparative tables where for each nutrient the different countries' recommendations are shown all together. The introduction to the Committee's review suggests that there are *three levels of requirement* for any group of people: (1) the average requirement, the 50th percentile of individual physiological requirements for a nutrient, (2) the group requirement, the amount of the nutrient that meets the needs of nearly all healthy individuals and (3) recommended dietary intakes which usually exceed the group requirement because they add a margin of safety for reasons which differ for different nutrients and different committees.

Recommended intakes of nutrients are nowadays used for more purposes than was originally intended. Committee 1/5 therefore suggested that it would reduce confusion if national and international committees consider three levels of recommendations. (a) The primary recommendation is the traditional recommended dietary allowance (RDA). This is *a prescription — what everyone should aim to eat*. The figures are useful for a variety of professionals — home economists, caterers, economists, journalists and for the general public. (b) The traditional RDA cannot however be used to assess whether an individual's intake of a nutrient is adequate. It is too high for this diagnostic use. Nutritionists need a *lower diagnostic figure* for interpreting food intake data. New Zealand publishes such 'minimum safe intake' figures in its 1983 recommendations[4]. In current revisions of the Australian dietary recommendations lower diagnostic figures are proposed in the background papers, which are written for professional nutritionists, but not published for the general public[5,6]. (c) With megavitamin proponents believing that 'the sky's the limit' for vitamin intake it is becoming necessary to provide guidance for the public about what is the upper end of the safe intake for each nutrient, the *level above which toxic or adverse effects* may start to occur. For vitamin B_6, for example, the public needs to know that this figure is somewhere below 500 mg/d[1].

H. Kamin (chairman of the present US RDA Committee) described the philosophy adopted by his Committee. He thinks modern RDAs cover more than 95, 97 and probably even 99 per cent of people's individual requirements because deficiency features are rare in people who achieve the RDAs in their diet.

In the last 5 years there has been an enormous increase of awareness of nutrition among the public and media in the USA and the US Committee has been working under a huge spotlight. The present US Committee is making a complete reexamination of nutrient recommendations. They are aiming to protect people from the adverse effects on health of nutritional deficiencies. No one knows how to guarantee optimal health. For most nutrients there are inadequate data about the range and frequency distribution of individual physiological requirements. There is a useful amount of data for protein, but this is an exception. Balance studies, the US Committee concluded, should be used less for deriving RDAs than they have been. Balance study data can only be relied on for nutrients to which the body adapts rapidly, eg nitrogen.

They have paid much attention to breast-feeding. Recommendations for breast-fed infants have been based on a milk intake of 750 ml, which seems to be nearer what most infants get than the commonly used figure of 850 ml. They recognize that requirements for some nutrients may be different for formula-fed babies and breast-fed babies. (At the end of the IUNS Committee's report[8] it had been suggested that *different figures might be recommended for formula-fed and breast-fed infants*, as has been started in Bulgaria.) A difficulty in making recommendations for the 1st 6 months of life is the big range of energy intakes between the new-born and fast growing infant at 6 months.

Pregnancy is not a homogenous state: for some nutrients the requirements are different at each stage. The new US RDAs will be listed separately for each trimester.

The US Committee did not consider that the elderly should have different RDAs, provided adjustments are made where necessary for the smaller lean body mass of some old people.

The US RDA Committee did not reach the same conclusions about *calcium* requirements as the recent NIH Consensus development report on osteoporosis (raising the question whether this particular consensus was a real one).

Each section of the US RDA report will end with a discussion on toxicity and toxic intakes of the nutrient.

In discussion, the following were among the points made. (1) Chairmen of RDA Committees seem to have more humility about the numbers than most of the users. (2) It appeared to be agreed that shortage of basic information about nutrient absorption, losses, metabolism, etc. — and about the distribution of the variables within the population and how various factors influence requirements — makes it necessary to use informed guesswork in estimating RDAs. But 'there is a need for more research' is not the same thing as priority for research grants. (3) Because one does not have to eat the RDA for each nutrient every day one participant suggested that RDAs might be expressed as amount recommended per week. However, most people thought that this would make calculations more complicated. Nutrients per day is a rate, like miles per hour, and it is possible to explain the concept to the public.

Members of a British coronary prevention group were disappointed that the new US RDAs will not include a numerical recommendation for EFA (essential fatty acids). But it would be difficult to be precise about how much should be ω6 and how much ω3 in our present state of knowledge. Knowledge about dietary fibre needs is perhaps at a similar stage. The US RDA will not recommend precise numbers for fibre either.

There is an inertia in public viewpoints. Any change in the RDA is likely to be opposed by some group, no matter how carefully it has been worked out.

O. Levander reported major advances in information about *selenium* requirements. There is new information from: (a) animal experiments; (b) long-term human balances in the USA; (c) from China on intakes of people in Keshan Province with and without cardiovascular disease; (d) blood levels in the USA, New Zealand, China, etc. and (e) supplementation studies of the amount of Se needed in different communities to saturate plasma glutathione peroxidase.

It now appears that the physiological requirement is lower than the estimated safe and adequate daily dietary intake in the 9th edition of the US RDAs[3]. There is a possible benefit in preventing cancer with a higher intake, but selenium is one nutrient for which the safe range between requirement and toxicity is quite narrow.

A question was asked whether the US RDAs are applicable to the third world? The text of the report will be, but not the numbers because there are differences in body size, physical work, types of food, etc.

Zinc average intakes are often lower than the present US RDA. It has also been found that there is no correlation between intake and the degree of positivity of zinc balances. *Janet King* (California) reports that absorption adapts to a low intake of 5 mg/day, with faecal zinc diminishing with the adaptation. But absorption of zinc is better from some foods (eg, chicken) than from others (eg, vegetable foods) according to a Swedish report. It has lately been realized that seminal losses of zinc are considerable — 0.5 mg per ejaculate. This sexual loss of zinc in men corresponds in a way to sexual (menstrual) losses of iron in women.

V. Herbert described a new concept of four stages of depletion for folate and vitamin B_{12}, like the Bothwell-Finch concept[2] of decreasing body iron. *Folate-depletion* goes through these stages: (1) negative folate balance (serum folate $<$ 3 but red cell folate $>$ 200); (2) folate depletion (red cell folate $<$ 140); (3) folate-deficient erythropoiesis (hypersegmented polymorphs, liver folate now subnormal), and (4) folate-deficient anaemia. *Vitamin-B_{12}-depletion* similarly goes through these stages: (1) reduction of vitamin B_{12} on TCII (the main carrier protein), ie vitamin B_{12} absorption has ceased; (2) vitamin-B_{12}-depletion (low plasma vitamin B_{12}); (3) vitamin-B_{12}-deficient haemopoiesis (hypersegmented polymorphs), and (4) vitamin-B_{12}-deficient anaemia.

Transcobalamin II (TCII) is the predominant plasma protein carrier of vitamin B_{12}. Transcobalamins I and III reflect tissue stores. The normal degree of saturation of vitamin-dependent enzymes varies. It is only 10 per cent for vitamin B_{12} enzymes. We need an objective biochemical enzyme saturation test for all micronutrients.

In working out RDAs a valuable concept is the minimum amount that needs to be absorbed to meet requirements. Most interactions occur before this stage but not all, eg, vitamin E and polyunsaturated fat intake.

Efficiency of conversion of β-carotene to *vitamin A* varies. The 6 to 1 ratio used in previous US RDA reports will be used in the new report. This ratio is, of course, a rough average. Conversion of β-carotene is more efficient if it is in oil (eg, palm oil) rather than in vegetables and if it is in low concentration. Animals differ greatly in their ability to convert β-carotene to retinol and it is unreliable to extrapolate to man from experiments in any one animal species. *Brubacher* advised for these reasons that the carotenoid content of foods should be expressed as β-carotene equivalents in food tables so that nutritionists can allow for different efficiencies of conversion to vitamin A from individual foods and meals.

Only a little of the workshop's time was spent on *dietary goals and guide-lines*. An expert committee in Sweden reported to the National Food Administration on diet and health last year (an English translation is available). A report is being prepared in the Netherlands. The dietary guide-lines of the US Department of Agriculture have just been revised. New dietary guide-lines have been published in the German Federal Republic and in Japan. A list of dietary guide-lines up to 1982 has been compiled[7] and IUNS Committee 1/5 is hoping to prepare a summary of current guide-lines in different countries.

1 Berger, A. & Schaumburg, H.H. (1984): More on neuropathy from pyridoxine abuse. *New Engl. J.* **311**, 986–87.
2 Bothwell, T.H., Charlton, R.W., Cook, J.D. & Finch, C.A. (1979): *Iron metabolism in man*, p. 45. Oxford: Blackwell.
3 Committee on Dietary Allowances, Food & Nutrition Board (1980): Recommended dietary allowances, 9th rev. edn. Washington DC: National Academy of Sciences.
4 Nutrition Advisory Committee (1983): *Recommendations for selected nutrient intake levels of New Zealanders*. Wellington, NZ: New Zealand Department of Health.
5 Palmer, N., Rutishauser, I.H.E., Dreosti, I.E., English, R.M., Bullock, J. & Truswell, A.S. (1982): Background papers on new Australian dietary intakes for vitamin B-6, zinc, iodine, sodium and potassium. *J. Fd Nutr.* (Canberra), **39**, 157–93.

6 Palmer, N., Wood, B., Rutishauser, I.H.E., Dreosti, I.E., English, R. & Truswell, A.S. (1984): Background papers on new Australian recommended dietary intakes for thiamin, riboflavin, niacin, vitamin B-12 and folate. *J. Fd Nutr.* (Canberra), **41**, 109–54.
7 Truswell, A.S. (1983): The development of dietary guide-lines. *Fd Tech. Aust.* **35**, 498–502.
8 Truswell, A.S. *et al.* (1983): Recommended dietary intakes around the world. A report by Committee 1/5 of the International Union of Nutritional Sciences (1982). *Nutr. Abst. Rev.* **53**, 940–1015 and 1075–1119.

Analysis of international recommendations for energy and protein requirements: a workshop report*

B. TORUN (Organizer)
INCAP, Apartado Postal 1188, Guatemala, Guatemala.

In October 1981, FAO, WHO and UNU organized in Rome an Expert Consultation on Energy and Protein Requirements to revise the recommendations made 10 years earlier by a similar Expert Committee[1], as it was recognized that: (a) enough new knowledge had accumulated since 1971 to fill some of the gaps in the earlier committee's report, and (b) account had to be taken of man's capacity to adapt to different nutritional and environmental situations, thereby relating the requirements to the actual conditions of life. The Expert Consultation's report has not yet been published but is in the press[2]. Therefore, this workshop was organized to present and discuss the bases of the new recommendations, to identify the major differences with the 1973 Report and to make a critical analysis of the problem encountered in order to facilitate future revisions. The main issues discussed in the workshop were introduced by *B. Torun, V.R. Young, W.P.T. James, R.G. Whitehead* and *R. Vauy*, all of whom participated in the 1981 meeting in Rome.

The process of the 1981 Consultation and the subsequent events that led to modifications and delay in the publication of its report were summarized. A vast array of working papers were prepared by some Consultation members and other persons commissioned by the organizers. Discussions related to some assumptions that were necessary to estimate requirements, to problem of definition, to important concepts relating to the application of the recommendations, and to new analyses of the data evaluated in Rome and led to the preparation of five consecutive drafts. The first was prepared in December 1981 by the Consultation's rapporteur, H.N. Munro, and the subsequent drafts were prepared by the chairman, J.C. Waterlow, after discussions with the rapporteur and vice-chairpersons, D.H. Calloway and W.P.T. James. Some of those drafts or specific sections were circulated among all or selected members of the Consultation, who sent back their comments and provided additional information to the chairman and vice-chairpersons. The final draft and its revisions were sent to FAO and WHO in March 1985, and the latter was given the responsibility for printing the Report[2]. It is supposed to be a better document than that which came out from the initial deliberations in 1981, but it was felt that a delay of 4 years is difficult to justify and some of its considerations may be somewhat outdated.

Proteins and amino acids. Total nitrogen requirements for infants were based on human milk consumption data. Healthy babies who grow adequately while fed exclusively with their mother's milk consume an average of 750 ml/d. It was assumed that all its nitrogen, equivalent to 12 g crude protein/l (N × 6.25), was absorbed and utilized. This might overestimate requirements, since some proteins in human milk, such as SIgA, are not absorbed. Requirements for children 6–20 months' old and for adults were calculated from nitrogen

*This workshop incorporated a meeting of the IUNS Committee I/11 on Human Protein-Energy Requirements

balance data instead of the factorial approach and additional allowances were made from experimental data of sweat and miscellaneous losses. Based on the association observed between mean nitrogen requirements and basal metabolic rate, requirements for other age groups were interpolated between those of young children and adults. The values thus derived were in good agreement with the results of the nitrogen balance studies in older children that were available in 1981. Additional allowances for growth were estimated and added to the requirements of children.

The coefficient of variation (CV) from short- and longer-term nitrogen balance studies of different age groups was about 12.5 per cent. Therefore, the safe level of protein intake was calculated to be the mean requirement for an age group plus 25 per cent. Protein digestibility must be taken into account to calculate protein requirements using local diets in different parts of the world. The other component of protein quality, ie its essential amino acid composition, is important for children but not so much for adults, as it was considered that with almost all local diets, the satisfaction of total nitrogen needs for adults will fulfil their essential amino acid requirements. New experimental data on preschool children allowed a better definition of essential amino acid requirements for all age groups and the suggestion of modified amino acid scoring pattern for proteins that is lower in sulphur-containing amino acids, valine and isoleucine.

Energy. Requirements from birth to 10 years were estimated from energy intake data of healthy children who were growing normally plus 5 per cent to allow for a desirable level of physical activity. Energy requirements for adults and children over 10 years of age were assessed in terms of energy expenditure of people leading active lives consistent with physical and social health. Such expenditure was derived from the time spent in, and the energy cost of: (1) rest in bed; (2) occupational activities; (3) discretionary activities, and (4) residual time. Occupational activities include jobs and non-salaried chores, such as housework, looking after children or going to school. Discretionary activities include optional household tasks for men and women, socially desirable activities (such as interactions among family and community members, learning and exploration activities of children or participation in tasks for individual and social improvement), and exercise for physical fitness and cardiovascular health. The latter can be part of the energy-intensive occupational and other discretionary activities of many persons.

Energy costs were estimated as: (1) equivalent to BMR during sleep and rest in bed; (2) variable during occupational activities, which were assigned average factors related to BMR for high, medium and heavy activity of men and women; (3) 2 hours at $3 \times$ BMR for discretionary household tasks and social activities, and 20 min of vigorous exercise at $6 \times$ BMR; and, (4) $1.4 \times$ BMR during residual time to include BMR, metabolic response to food, minor physical movements and maintenance of muscle tone. Additional allowances were made for pregnancy, lactation and growth. It was recognized that more information is needed on the time allocated to different activities in different societies and on the energy cost of habitual activities, particularly of children and adolescents, as well as on BMR of different age groups in populations with different life-styles and ethnic backgrounds.

These recommendations are for population groups based on age, sex and average pattern of life, and not for individuals. For the latter, specific occupational and life-style demands must be considered. The variability of energy expenditure is high and a CV in BMR of ± 15 per cent can account for a difference of 500 kcal (2.1 MJ)/d between two men of the same age and size whose BMR's are within ± 1 S.D. Variability of energy intake is even greater. Estimates of CV within individuals are about ± 12–15 per cent in pregnant women and can be as high as ± 20 per cent.

To calculate dietary food intake for energy requirements, the FAO/WHO/UNU Consultation suggested adjustments for digestible energy so that in diets with low, moderate and high fibre contents the Atwater factors should be applied, respectively, without modifications or multiplied by 0.975 or 0.95.

Comparisons with 1973 report. The main differences between the new and the 1973 recommendations were partly because of the availability of more experimental data in 1981 but mainly because the principles and the assumptions adopted by the two Expert Groups were different in various respects.

Requirements for infants were based on data on breast-fed children who grew satisfactorily. Since their intakes fell more rapidly after 3 months than formerly acknowledged, the new energy recommendations are about 15 per cent lower for infants between 3 and 9 months of age, and about 4 per cent lower at ages 0–3 and 9–12 months. Energy requirements for preschool children were similar in both reports; for school-aged and adolescent children they are now approximately 10 per cent lower and more so (about 15 per cent) during puberty. Energy requirements calculated for *moderately active* adults between 18 and 30 years were similar to those of 1973, but they increased by around 5 per cent at ages 30–60 and about 12 per cent beyond 60 years. The differences with ageing decrease in persons with greater activity, indicating the care that must be given to apply the new report for groups of people with different levels of physical activity.

The safe level of protein intake for adults is increased by about 35 per cent. This had a marked effect on most safe levels estimated for children at different ages, since their maintenance needs were calculated by interpolation between infancy and adulthood. Additional allowances for growth were based on experimental and theoretical considerations about the interindividual variability and the efficiency of nitrogen utilization for growth. Consequently, protein recommendations were similar to those of 1973 for childen under 5 years of age and they increased gradually thereafter, from 12 per cent at 7 years to 43 per cent at 15. Energy and protein requirements for lactation remained similar in both reports. Total additional needs for pregnancy were also similar, but the 1981 Consultation divided the increment evenly in the three trimesters.

Although some of the protein recommendations may be too high, it was considered judicious to err on the side of safety until there is absolute certainty in making recommendations, especially for such vulnerable groups as young children and pregnant women.

Food intakes should be calculated correcting for protein digestibility and, in children, for the amino acid composition of the diet. Consequently, recommended food intakes may be large with many local diets of relatively poor quality. This may have important implications in food policy planning and indicates the need to test the recommendation in the field and to obtain more information in developing countries.

Problems faced by expert groups and application of their recommendations. Expert Groups usually include both scientists with previous experience in similar groups and newcomers. Most of the latter are actively engaged in research, whereas many of the former base their expertise on previous investigations and analysis of data from other scientists. The inputs from both types of experts are important but the difference in their approaches may be difficult to resolve. Universal representation and geographic balance may interfere with the inclusion of experts who can contribute signficantly, simply because their country is already represented by other scientists. This can be partly overcome by asking them to prepare background or position papers, but these should be prepared and sent to the Group members on time to allow careful analysis and to request clarifications before the Group convenes.

On the other hand, expert groups are faced with analysing solid, well-proven studies, as well as preliminary results supported by insufficient data and recent findings that have not undergone the critical test of peer review. This is compounded by the facts that many 'definitive' experiments may not be done for ethical reasons, and the complexity and high costs of controlled trials in humans and population studies do not always allow data to be obtained in quantities that will satisfy the statistically-oriented members of the committee. The group is then forced to make value judgements and estimates based on their knowledge and experience, which may be prone to error or must be stated as tentative.

These and other problems were faced by the 1981 Consultation and contributed to the multiple revisions and delays in preparing its report which, in its final stages, was in the hands of a limited number of participants. Although such revisions may have strengthened its conclusions and recommendations, new knowledge may indicate the need for additional revisions in the future.

The response of the users will be of utmost importance in evaluating the adequacy of current recommendations. An attempt to estimate the protein and energy needs for the population of

Chile identified a series of problems, especially in relation to energy requirements. This supports the need to provide specific orientation to the various categories of users, as a supplement to the report that deals with the application of the scientific principles and recommendations.

Additional discussion. In the ensuing discussions other important issues were raised. It is essential that an expert meeting be held as soon as the 1985 Report becomes available to deal with its applications and prepare a 'users' manual'. In addition to FAO, WHO and UNU, the appropriate IUNS Committees should be involved. More importance must be given to the protein and energy needs of persons over 60 years of age. The recommendations should be revised as more information about the elderly becomes available. The new report, as its predecessors, has dealt with healthy populations. More information is needed about the effects of frequent and chronic infections, which are quite common in developing countries, for the application of the recommendations. New, preliminary data on energy intake and expenditure of pregnant women suggest that the energy recommendations for pregnancy may be overestimated.

1 FAO/WHO (1973): *Energy and protein requirements. Report of a joint FAO/WHO Ad Hoc Expert Committee.* WHO Tech. Rep. Ser. No. 522. Geneva: WHO.
2 WHO (In Press): *Energy and protein requirements. Report of a joint FAO/WHO/UNU Expert Consultation.* Tech. Rep. Ser. No. 724. Geneva: WHO.

Implementation of dietary goals and the impact on the agricultural industries: a workshop report

V. WHEELOCK (Organizer)
School of Biomedial Sciences, University of Bradford, Bradford, Yorkshire BD7 1DP, UK.

It is now recognised that many of the major causes of death and disability such as obesity, coronary heart disease, certain cancers and diabetes are associated with diet. These conditions are responsible for well over 50 per cent of all deaths in the developed countries and are increasing in the developing countries, especially among the affluent. Although the precise role of diet in the aetiology of these disease cannot be defined at present, there is strong support for recommending changes in food consumption patterns. It is significant that when expert committees in many different countries have evaluated the scientific evidence, related to these diseases, virtually all have reached the same conclusions.

Very briefly, the recommendations are: (1) Reduce fat intake (from about 40 per cent of dietary energy), especially of saturated fat, (2) increase consumption of dietary fibre, (3) reduce sugar consumption, and (4) reduce salt intake.

In many countries the public are becoming increasingly aware of these recommendations, mainly because of a combination of government action and media exposure. The response of the food and agriculture industries can vary, but, in general, supermarket chains are positive about consumer requirements. Consequently, individuals are making changes in consumption. Very often this is achieved by substituting one product for another rather than by making major changes in the established pattern of eating. For example: (1) low fat milks are substituted for whole milk, (2) low fat spreads of 'diet margarines' are used instead of regular margarine or butter (3) lean meat instead of fatty meat — consumers may switch from beef and lamb to chicken and fish, (4) high-fibre breads consumed, instead of bread made from refined flour (5) low sugar alternatives used — or 'no added sugar', and (6) use of low salt alternatives.

Clearly, this means that the demand for some products is growing, while that for others must decline. This applies particularly to the developed countries where the scope for increasing total consumption of food is virtually nil. On the whole, the food manufacturing industries can cope with the changing market. Provided that a demand is identified, these industries respond by re-formulating existing products and developing new ones. This could mean that there would be a fall in the total demand for sugar and for saturated fat. Because the pricing and production of sugar is controlled to such a marked degree the Workshop considered it virtually impossible to predict what the effects on primary production would be. However, with saturated fat, this would mean a fall in its value, as a consequence of which there could be increased amounts of saturated fat incorporated into food products because of economic pressures. Concern was expressed that this would result in some people, especially those in the lower socio-economic groups, having an *increased* consumption of saturated fat.

It was suggested that the surplus fat could be exported to countries where there was a food shortage and that this would be one way of providing an increased supply of energy. This was strongly disputed by some of the participants who considered that such a strategy would undermine indigenous food production and eating patterns. There was general agreement that implementation of the dietary goals would mean a reduction in the demand for fat, especially saturated fat. Since most of this originates from meat and milk, it is evident that there would be a significant impact on these particular industries.

In many countries, agriculture, or at least certain sectors of it, is subject to very considerable state intervention. Yet there is little evidence that the nutritional dimension is taken into account in the formulation of agricultural policies. In some cases the policies may actually be in direct conflict with dietary goals: for example, farmers may be given financial incentives to produce saturated fat even though consumers are being recommended to reduce their intake. As a general rule, price support measures usually mean that farmers are insulated from the impact of changes in consumer demand.

There was general recognition that to facilitate the implementation of dietary goals it is essential to have close integration between nutrition policies and agricultural policies. Although many countries now realise the need for this kind of approach to be adopted, it was clear that progress was limited. Norway is one of the few countries to have tackled these issues and so the Workshop was fortunate to hear a short presentation from Anne Ditlefsen of the National Nutrition Council in Norway on what has been achieved there. In 1975–76, the Norwegian Parliament (the Storting) approved a report on Nutrition and Food Policy. In this report the Government took the view that 'measures of agricultural policy should be shaped in such a way that they also serve considerations based on nutrition and health grounds'. Having accepted this policy a number of steps have been taken. Consumers were encouraged to reduce consumption of milk fat by switching from whole milk to low fat milks. Hence, the demand for milk fat has fallen. In the past the price paid to producers for milk had been based on the fat content. On 1 Janury 1980, this was changed so that the prices paid to producers are determined by the milk protein content. Between 1959 and 1979, the fat content of milk dropped from 4.05 per cent to 3.86 per cent. From 1976–1979, the price of skimmed milk was the same as that for whole milk and since July 1980, the Agricultural Agreement has raised the price of skimmed milk less than that of whole milk. For meat, a price grading system has been introduced which pays considerably lower prices for fat carcases and has encouraged the production of leaner animals: the thickness of the dorsal fat layer in pigs for slaughter has been reduced by about half in the last 20 years.

The quality of wholegrain bread was improved by using strong American wheat instead of supplies from Sweden.

A system to improve the marketing of potatoes is to be introduced and there will be a subsidy to lower the price to consumers with the intention of increasing sales. In 1980–81, all subsidies on butter and margarine were withdrawn and a duty of N Kr 1.00 per kilo was to be placed on sugar. Special subsidies apply to the North of Norway, presumably because the high transport costs add to consumer prices. This was first introduced in 1970 for certain fruits, and in 1975 the subsidy levels were incrased by 20 per cent: in 1976 the range was extended so as to include virtually all fruit.

In Norway in 1980 N Kr 100 million was spent on 'commercial information' relating to food and beverages, which includes advertising. Of this about N Kr 30 million was devoted to snacks, soft drinks, sweets, chocolate bars, chocolates, and chewing gum. By contrast, only about N Kr 1 million is available for improving education on diet and nutrition. However, in addition, many official and voluntary organisations have conducted educational work on diet and nutrition on their own account. For example, a special co-ordinating committee has been appointed to facilitate communication between the Norwegian Medical Association and the Institute of Preventive Medicine at the University of Oslo to promote journalism concerning health and illness, social conditions, health and social policy.

Although this report on the developments in Norway is very limited, it does give an indication of what action can be taken when a government adopts a positive attitude. Although other countries have not yet achieved such a coherent food and nutrition policy, it is apparent that pressure is building up and that some progress is being made. In the United States the Dietary Goals were accepted during the Carter administration. At present, the USDA is actively considering the implications for the different agricultural sectors. In Australia, the States of Victoria and New South Wales already have food and nutrition policies and active steps are being taken by a number of bodies to promote the dietary guidelines. In the UK, a recent official Government report on 'Diet and Cardiovascular Disease' made specific recommendations on how the British diet should be changed and on how the guidelines could be implemented. This report has been adopted by the Government and steps are now being taken to put the recommendations into effect. Irrespective of Government action, the meat industry in the UK is making progress by reducing the amount of fat in carcases. This has been particularly successful with pigs so that there has been a progressive fall in the thickness of back fat in recent years.

It emerged very clearly from the discussions that initiatives to encourage 'healthy eating' are being taken in many countries. There may be some economic problems but the major difficulty is usually government support measures for agriculture which do not take nutrition into account. The Norwegian policy is extremely significant because it provides valuable lessons for other countries faced with similar issues.

The Workshop provided a forum for interaction between participants from many countries who have common interests. It was particularly valuable because it helped to establish a network of those working in this relatively new field. Hopefully, the topics raised will find a place in the formal agenda of future congresses.

Author index